Pediatric Orthopedic Imaging

Rebecca Stein-Wexler
Sandra L. Wootton-Gorges
M.B. Ozonoff
Editors

Pediatric Orthopedic Imaging

Springer

Editors
Rebecca Stein-Wexler
Department of Radiology
University of California Davis
Medical Center and UC Davis
Children's Hospital
Sacramento, CA
USA

M.B. Ozonoff
Department of Radiology
University of California Davis
Sacramento, CA
USA

Sandra L. Wootton-Gorges
Department of Radiology
University of California Davis
Medical Center and UC Davis
Children's Hospital
Sacramento, CA
USA

ISBN 978-3-642-45380-9 ISBN 978-3-642-45381-6 (eBook)
DOI 10.1007/978-3-642-45381-6
Springer Heidelberg New York Dordrecht London

Library of Congress Control Number: 2014956961

Printed on acid-free paper

Springer is part of Springer Science+Business Media (www.springer.com)

To all children and those who care for them
and
To our families for their love and support

Preface

In 1979, when the first edition of *Pediatric Orthopedic Radiology* was published, radiologic diagnosis relied almost entirely on radiography and occasional arthrography. Communication between radiologists and orthopedic surgeons was limited. The 1992 revision introduced ultrasound, computed tomography, and magnetic resonance imaging, but at the time these techniques were still relatively new, and their diagnostic potential not yet developed.

Medical imaging has changed a great deal since then. MRI has come to the forefront of musculoskeletal imaging, CT techniques are much more versatile and robust, many new applications for ultrasound are available, and PET-CT and molecular imaging offer a previously unimagined window into disease pathophysiology. At the same time, advances in medical research have greatly expanded our understanding of many disease processes. There is better communication between the orthopedic community and medical imagers, enabling imagers to make important contributions to patient care—not only by interpreting complex cases, but also by sharing their knowledge of radiation risks and appropriate choice of imaging modalities.

It is thus time for a new version of this text. The current volume has been retitled *Pediatric Orthopedic Imaging*, reflecting the impressive range of modalities that can be employed to answer complex orthopedic questions. Important parts of the previous version of this book have been preserved, but all the material has been updated, and much of it has been expanded. Parts of the text have been reorganized. We have endeavored to keep the book clinically relevant by soliciting input from orthopedic surgeons throughout the text.

The text begins with introductory material: Imaging Strategies addresses questions of when and how to image; the subsequent chapter provides a reference on basic *bone development and bone age assessment techniques*. The second part, Isolated Spine and Extremity Disorders: Congenital, Developmental, and Acquired, is organized according to *anatomical region*, with a pair of chapters for each area. Each extremity is divided into chapters that are centered on a joint. For example, the chapters on the upper extremity cover: (1) the shoulder, including the proximal humerus, (2) the elbow and adjacent humerus, radius, and ulna; and (3) the wrist and hand. The first chapter in each pair addresses congenital and developmental variants and abnormalities. The second addresses selected acquired pathology, focusing on entities that are unique to each region, emphasizing those that are exclusively or principally encountered in children. These chapters only briefly address more general pathological processes, such as infection, arthritis, and tumors, which are thoroughly covered in Part III.

The third part, Generalized and Systemic Diseases, is organized by *pathology type*. Two separate chapters address *trauma*, the first covering general considerations found in the growing skeleton, and the second covering non-accidental trauma. Chapters on *generalized disorders of orthopedic significance, neuromuscular disorders*, and *orthopedic procedures* have been updated, and the contents expanded. Due to increased contributions of cross-sectional imaging to diagnosis and treatment, several small sections from the previous version were greatly expanded, creating separate chapters on *infection, arthritis, bone tumors*, and *soft tissue masses*. Bone Marrow Imaging and Bone Densitometry are entirely new.

It was our goal in updating this text to provide practicing radiologists with a go-to reference, as well as to provide residents and fellows with a useful means for learning pediatric musculoskeletal imaging. Each chapter is therefore generously illustrated, and references include both classic papers and current works. We hope you find this book useful as you care for your young patients.

Sacramento, CA, USA Rebecca Stein-Wexler

Acknowledgement I

We would like to thank the pediatric radiology community at large for encouraging us. Tal Laor and Herman Kan provided important editorial and organizational advice, and contributed numerous excellent images. Many other pediatric radiologists graciously shared their images with us as well. Our orthopedic surgery colleagues (see page vii) have provided thoughtful criticism of almost every single chapter. Adult musculoskeletal imagers at the University of California, Davis—Jasjeet Bindra, Cyrus Batteni, Robert Boutin, Eva Escobedo, Adam Greenspan, and John Hunter—contributed images and advice. Raymond Dougherty, our department chair, helped make this project possible as well. Our pediatric radiology colleagues, Thomas Sanchez and Chirag Patel, generously and willingly helped in any way they could.

Sandra Baum, Mary Cardiff, Madison Dunitz, Galen Sanderlin, Michelle Stofa, and Hue To offered administrative assistance. Julie Ostoich contributed skillful and essential graphic art support, and Rachel Wexler provided excellent editorial assistance (and a few dinners). Flora Kim helped keep us on task. And many thanks to Ute Heilmann at Springer, whose enthusiasm and vision allowed this project to move forward.

Finally, words cannot begin to express the profound appreciation we feel toward our families for their patience and extraordinary support throughout the gestation of this book.

RSW, SWG, MBO

Acknowledgement II

Orthopedic consultation provided by orthopedic surgeons at Shriners Hospitals for Children Northern California and University of California Davis Children's Hospital:

Andrea Bauer, MD
Jennette Boakes, MD
Jon R. Davids, MD
Munish C. Gupta, MD
Brian M. Haus, MD
Michelle A. James, MD
Eric O. Klineberg, MD
Joel A. Lerman, MD
Debra Templeton Popejoy, MD
George T. Rab, MD

Contents

Contributors

Lauren W. Averill, MD Department of Medical Imaging, Nemours/AI duPont Hospital for Children, Wilmington, DE, USA

Paul Babyn, MDCM Department of Medical Imaging, University of Saskatchewan and Saskatoon Health Region, Saskatoon, SK, Canada

Kevin Coulter, MD Department of Pediatrics, University of California Davis Medical Center and UC Davis Children's Hospital, Sacramento, CA, USA

Steven Don, MD Mallinckrodt Institute of Radiology, Washington University School of Medicine, St. Louis, MO, USA

Vicente Gilsanz, MD, PhD Department of Radiology, Children's Hospital Los Angeles, Los Angeles, CA, USA

Angelo Don S. Grasparil II, MD Department of Radiology, Cardinal Santos Medical Center, San Juan, NCR, Philippines

Radiology Division Philippine Children's Medical Center, Quezon City, NCR, Philippines

Leslie E. Grissom, MD Department of Medical Imaging, Nemours/AI duPont Hospital for Children, Wilmington, DE, USA

Departments of Radiology and Pediatrics, Thomas Jefferson University, Philadelphia, PA, USA

Matthew R. Hammer, MD Department of Radiology, University of Texas Southwestern Medical Center and Children's Medical Center of Dallas, Dallas, TX, USA

Brian M. Haus, MD Department of Orthopaedic Surgery, UC Davis Children's Hospital and Shriners Hospitals for Children Northern California, Sacramento, CA, USA

J. Herman Kan, MD Department of Radiology, Texas Children's Hospital, Houston, TX, USA

Department of Radiology Baylor College of Medicine, Houston, TX, USA

Ingrid Kjellin, MD Radsource, Anaheim Hills, CA, USA

Elka Miller, MD Department of Diagnostic Imaging, Children's Hospital of Eastern Ontario, Ottawa, ON, Canada

Kamaldine Oudjhane, MD, MSc Diagnostic Imaging Department, The Hospital for Sick Children, University of Toronto, Toronto, ON, Canada

Deepa R. Pai, MD, MHSA Department of Radiology, C.S. Mott Children's Hospital, Ann Arbor, MI, USA

Debra Templeton Popejoy, MD Department of Orthopaedic Surgery, UC Davis Children's Hospital and Shriners Hospitals for Children Northern California, Sacramento, CA, USA

Jeffrey S. Prince, MD Department of Medical Imaging, Primary Children's Hospital, Salt Lake City, UT, USA

Marilyn Ranson, BSc, MD, FRCPC Radiology Department, The Hospital for Sick Children, University of Toronto, Toronto, ON, Canada

Glade E. Roper, MD Department of Musculoskeletal Imaging and Intervention, Kaweah Delta Medical Center, Visalia, CA, USA

Karen Rosendahl, MD, PhD Section of Paediatric Radiology, Department of Clinical Medicine, Faculty of Medicine and Dentistry, University of Bergen, Haukeland University Hospital, Bergen, Norway

Thomas Ray Sanchez, MD Department of Pediatric Radiology, University of California Davis Medical Center and UC Davis Children's Hospital, Sacramento, CA, USA

Department of Diagnostic Imaging, Shriners Hospitals for Children Northern California, Sacramento, CA, USA

Thomas L. Slovis, MD Department of Pediatric Imaging, Children's Hospital of Michigan, Wayne State University School of Medicine, Detroit, MI, USA

Ethan A. Smith, MD Section of Pediatric Radiology, Department of Radiology, C.S. Mott Children's Hospital, University of Michigan Health System, Ann Arbor, MI, USA

Rebecca Stein-Wexler, MD Department of Radiology, University of California Davis Medical Center and UC Davis Children's Hospital, Sacramento, CA, USA

Department of Diagnostic Imaging, Shriners Hospitals for Children Northern California, Sacramento, CA, USA

Jennifer Stimec, MD, FRCPC Department of Diagnostic Imaging, The Hospital for Sick Children, Toronto, ON, Canada

Peter J. Strouse, MD, FACR Section of Pediatric Radiology, Department of Radiology, C.S. Mott Children's Hospital, University of Michigan Health System, Ann Arbor, MI, USA

Benjamin H. Taragin, MD Division of Pediatric Radiology, Children's Hospital at Montefiore, Bronx, NY, USA

Mihir M. Thacker, MD Department of Orthopaedics, Nemours/AI duPont Hospital for Children, Wilmington, DE, USA

Department of Orthopedic Surgery, Sidney Kimmel Medical College of Thomas Jefferson University, Philadelphia, PA, USA

Mahesh M. Thapa, MD Department of Radiology, Seattle Children's Hospital, Seattle, WA, USA

Markus Uhl, MD, PhD Department of Radiology, RKK Klinikum, Freiburg, Germany

Nagwa Wilson, MS, MD, PhD Department of Medical Imaging, Montreal Children's Hospital, McGill University, Montreal, QC, Canada

Sandra L. Wootton-Gorges, MD Department of Radiology, University of California Davis Medical Center and UC Davis Children's Hospital, Sacramento, CA, USA

Department of Diagnostic Imaging, Shriners Hospitals for Children Northern California, Sacramento, CA, USA

Tishya A. L. Wren, PhD Children's Orthopaedic Center, Children's Hospital Los Angeles, Los Angeles, CA, USA

Abbreviations

2D	Two-dimensional
3D	Three-dimensional
3D-CT	Computed tomography with three-dimensional reconstruction
AAPM	American Association of Physicists in Medicine
ABC	Aneurysmal bone cyst
ABER	Abduction external rotation
aBMD	Areal bone mineral density
ACL	Anterior cruciate ligament
ACR	American College of Radiology
AD	Autosomal dominant
ADC	Apparent diffusion coefficient
AIGHL	Anterior inferior glenohumeral ligament
AIIS	Anterior inferior iliac spine
AIR	Abduction and internal rotation
AJCC	American Joint Commission on Cancer
AL	Annular ligament
ALARA	As Low As Reasonably Achievable
ALL	Acute lymphocytic leukemia/acute lymphoid leukemia
ALPSA	Anterior labroligamentous periosteal sleeve avulsion
AML	Acute myelogenous leukemia/acute myelocytic leukemia
ANA	Antinuclear antibody
AP	Anteroposterior
APL	Abductor pollicis longus
AR	Autosomal recessive
AVF	Arteriovenous fistula
AVM	Arteriovenous malformation
AVN	Avascular necrosis
BA	Bone area
BAGHL	Bony avulsion glenohumeral ligament
BEIR	Biological effects of ionizing radiation
BMC	Bone mineral content
BMD	Bone mineral density
BUA	Broadband ultrasound attenuation
CE	Contrast enhanced
CE	Center edge
CML	Classic metaphyseal lesion

CMT	Charcot-Marie-Tooth disease
CNS	Central nervous system
COMP	Cartilage oligomeric matrix protein
CP	Cerebral palsy
CPA	Cerebellopontine angle
CR	Computed radiography
CRMO	Chronic recurrent multifocal osteomyelitis
CRP	C reactive protein
CRPS-1	Complex regional pain syndrome – Type 1
CSF	Cerebrospinal fluid
CSVL	Central sacral vertebral line
CT	Computed tomography
CTA	Computed tomography arthrography
$CTDI_{vol}$	Volume CT dose index
DAP	Dose area product
DDH	Developmental dysplasia of the hip
DEMRI	Dynamic contrast-enhanced MRI
3D-DESS	3D dual echo steady state
DESS	Dual echo steady state
dGEMRIC	Delayed gadolinium-enhanced MRI of cartilage
DI	Deviation index
DIP	Distal interphalangeal
DLP	Dose length product
DMD	Duchenne muscular dystrophy
DR	Direct digital radiography
DRUJ	Distal radioulnar joint
DSA	Digital subtraction angiography
DWI	Diffusion-weighted imaging
DXA	Dual-energy x-ray absorptiometry
ECU	Extensor carpi ulnaris
EEC	Ectrodactyly-ectodermal dysplasia-cleft lip/palate syndrome
EES	Extraskeletal Ewing sarcoma
EI	Exposure index
EI_T	Target exposure index
EPB	Extensor pollicis brevis
ERA	Enthesis-related arthritis
ESR	Erythrocyte sedimentation rate
EWS gene	Ewing sarcoma gene
EXT	Exostosin
FAI	Femoral-acetabular impingement
FDG	Fluorodeoxyglucose
FDG-PET	Fluorodeoxyglucose photon emission tomography
FDG-PET	18 F-fluorodeoxyglucose positron emission tomography
FFE	Fast field echo
FGFR3	Fibroblast growth factor receptor type 3
FIESTA	Fast imaging employing steady state acquisition
FLI-1 gene	Friend leukemia virus integration 1 gene
FOPE	Focal periphyseal edema

FS	Fat suppressed
FSE	Fast spin echo
FSPR	Fast spoiled gradient recalled echo
FSS	Fast field echo
FT	Femoro-tibial
G-CSF	Granulocyte colony-stimulating factor
GBA	Glucocerebrosidae
GCT	Giant cell tumor
Gd-DTPA	Gadolinium-diethylene triamine pentaacetic acid
GE	Gadolinium enhanced
GE	Gradient echo
GI	Gastrointestinal
GIRD	Glenohumeral internal rotation deficit
GLAD	Glenolabral articular disruption
GMFCS	Gross motor function classification system
GRE	Gradient echo
Gy	Gray
HAGL	Humeral avulsion of the glenohumeral ligament
HIV	Human immunodeficiency virus
HLA	Human leukocyte antigen
HOX	Homeobox
HOXA11	Homeobox A11
HR-MRI	High-resolution magnetic resonance imaging
HR-pQCT	High-resolution peripheral quantitative computed tomography
HU	Hounsfield units
IFSSH	International Federation of Society for Surgery of the Hand
ILAR	International League of Associations for Rhematology
IR	Inversion recovery
ISCD	International Society for Clinical Densitometry
IV	Intravenous
JIA	Juvenile idiopathic arthritis
K-wires	Kirschner wires
LCH	Langerhans cell histiocytosis
LDF	Lateral distal femur
L	Lateral
LP	Legg-Perthes
LT	Lister tubercle
LUCL	Lateral ulnar collateral ligament
M	Medial
MATN3	Matrilin-3
MC	Metacarpals
MCE	Multiple cartilaginous osteochondromas
MCL	Medial collateral ligament
MCP	Metacarpophalangeal joint
MDP	Methylene diphosphonate
MED	Multiple epiphyseal dysplasia
MEDIC	Multi-echo data image combination
MFH	Malignant fibrous histiocytoma

mGy	Milligray
MHE	Multiple hereditary exostoses
MIBG	Metaiodobenzylguanidine
MIP	Maximum intensity projection
MPS	Mucopolysaccharidosis(es)
MPGR	Multiplanar gradient recalled echo
MPNST	Malignant peripheral nerve sheath tumor
MPZ	Myelin protein zero
MR	Magnetic resonance
MRA	Magnetic resonance arthrography/arthrogram
MRI	Magnetic resonance imaging
MRSA	Methicillin resistant *Staphylococcus aureus*
mSv	Millisievert
MTP	Metatarsophalangeal
NCRP	National Council on Radiation Protection
NEXUS	National Emergency X-Radiography Utilization Study
NF1	Neurofibromatosis type 1
NF2	Neurofibromatosis type 2
NIBIB	National Institute of Biomedical Imaging and Bioengineering
NIH	National Institutes of Health
NM	Nuclear medicine imaging
NOF	Nonossifying fibroma
NRDR	National Radiology Data Registry
NSAID	Non-steroidal anti-inflammatory drugs
OAR	Ottawa ankle rules
OCD	Osteochondritis dissecans
OI	Osteogenesis imperfecta
PA	Posteroanterior
PACS	Picture archiving computer system
PAO	Peri-acetabular osteotomy
PCL	Posterior cruciate ligament
PD	Proton density
PD-W	Proton density weighted
PET	Positron emission tomography
PET-MRI	Positron emission tomography-magnetic resonance imaging
PFFD	Proximal focal femoral deficiency
PIP	Proximal interphalangeal
PMR	Posteromedial release
pPNET	Peripheral primitive neuroectodermal tumor
pQCT	Peripheral quantitative computed tomography
PSFI	Posterior spinal fusion with instrumentation
PTEN	Phosphate and tensin homolog
PT/FT	Patello-tibial/femoro-tibial ratio
PTH	Parathyroid hormone
PV1	Polio virus 1
PVL	Panton-Valentin leukocidin
PVNB	Pigmented villonodular bursitis
PVNS	Pigmented villonodular synovitis

PVNTS	Pigmented villonodular tenosynovitis
QCSI	Quantitative chemical shift imaging
QCT	Quantitative computed tomography
QUI	Quantitative ultrasound index
QUS	Quantitative ultrasound
RCJ	Radiocarpal joint
RCL	Radial collateral ligament
RF	Rheumatoid factor
RVA	Rib-vertebral angle
RVAD	Rib-vertebral angle difference
SAPHO	Syndrome: synovitis, acne, pustulosis, hyperostosis, osteitis
SCD	Sickle cell disease
SCFE	Slipped capital femoral epiphysis
SCI	Spinal cord injury
SCT	Sacrococcygeal teratoma
SCIWORA	Spinal cord injury without radiologic abnormality
SE	Spin echo
SI	International system
SLAP	Superior labral anterior-posterior
SLC26A2	Sulphate transporter solute carrier family 26
SMA	Spinal muscular atrophy
SMA	Superior mesenteric artery
SMD	Spondylometaphyseal dysplasia
SMN	Survival motor neuron
SOS	Speed of sound
SPECT	Single-photon emission computed tomography
SPGR	Spoiled gradient recalled echo
SSDE	Size-specific dose estimate
SSFP	Steady state free procession
STIR	Short tau inversion recovery
T	Tesla
T1-W	T1-weighted
T2-W	T2-weighted
TAR	Thrombocytopenia absent radius
TBX5	T-box transcription factor gene
Tc-99m	MDP Technetium-99m methylene diphosphanate
TE	Echo time
TEF	Tracheo-esophageal fistula
TFCC	Triangular fibrocartilage complex
TL	Thoracolumbar
TLSO	Thoracolumbosacral orthosis
TMJ	Temporomandibular joint
TRPV4	Transient receptor potential cation channel subfamily V member 4
TT-TG	Tibial tuberosity to trochlear groove
UCL	Ulnar collateral ligament
US	Ultrasound
VATER	Vertebral-anorectal-TEF-radial

VACTERL	Vertebral, anorectal, cardiac, tracheoesophageal, renal, and limb anomalies
VCA	Vertical center anterior margin angle
VEPTR	Vertical expandable prosthetic titanium rib
WB-MRI	Whole body MRI
WBC	White blood cell
WHO	World Health Organization
WS-bSSFP	Water selective balanced steady state free precession
ZPC	Zone of provisional calcification

Part I

Introductory Material

Musculoskeletal Imaging Strategies and Controlling Radiation Exposure

1

Steven Don and Thomas L. Slovis

Contents

S. Don, M.D. (✉)
Mallinckrodt Institute of Radiology,
Washington University School of Medicine,
510 South Kingshighway, St. Louis, MO 63110, USA
e-mail: dons@mir.wustl.edu

T.L. Slovis, M.D.
Department of Pediatric Imaging,
Children's Hospital of Michigan,
Wayne State University School of Medicine,
3901 Beaubien Drive, Detroit, MI 48201, USA
e-mail: tslovis@med.wayne.edu

Abstract

The chapter begins by discussing the development of imaging techniques and then addresses the tremendous importance of clinical evaluation in selecting the "best" first imaging test. Issues of appropriateness based on indications and cost containment are reviewed. Imaging modalities are presented with their risks and benefits. Techniques for reducing radiation exposure and the risks of anesthesia in imaging are examined.

The discovery of x-rays by Wilhelm Conrad Roentgen on November 8, 1895, revolutionized the diagnosis and management of pediatric diseases. By May 1896 the first image of an infant, which took 14 min (Fig. 1.1), was published in the Archives of Skiagraphy [1]. Ever since, radiography has been the mainstay of orthopedic imaging. A second revolution in orthopedic imaging took place between the 1960s and 1980s, with the development of nuclear medicine (NM), computed tomography (CT), ultrasound (US), and magnetic resonance imaging (MRI). A wide variety of imaging choices are now available to diagnose and manage pediatric orthopedic problems.

Imaging, of course, is not without risk. In 1904, Clarence Dally, Thomas Edison's x-ray assistant, died from metastatic radiation-induced carcinoma after having radiation burns on his face, ulcers on his hands, and both arms amputated

R. Stein-Wexler et al. (eds.), *Pediatric Orthopedic Imaging*,
DOI 10.1007/978-3-642-45381-6_1, © Springer-Verlag Berlin Heidelberg 2015

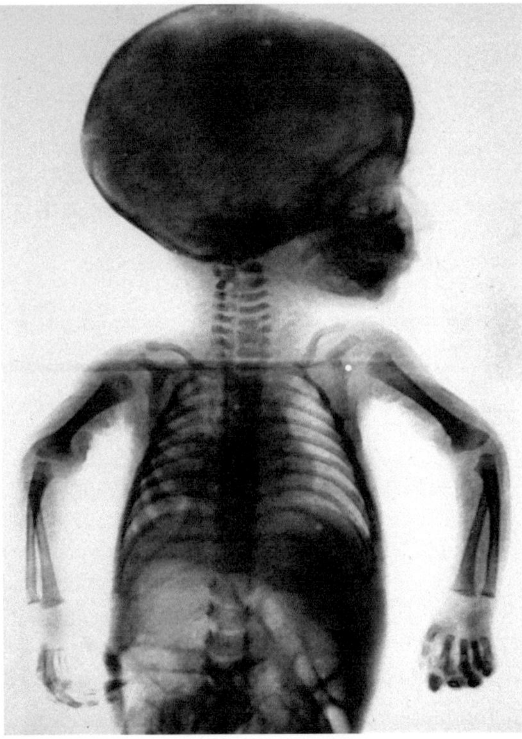

Fig. 1.1 The first recorded image of an infant, published in the Archives of Clinical Skiagraphy in May 1896. Note the apparent situs inversus (no markers to indicate side)

[2]. Although there is currently no increased incidence of cancer mortality among radiologists, the incidence was as high as 41 % for the earliest radiologists [3]. However, increasing evidence suggests that low-level radiation may cause fatal cancer [4, 5]. In 2005, the National Institute of Environmental Health Sciences formally added x-rays and gamma rays to the list of known carcinogens.

The overriding goal of imaging is to provide a timely and accurate diagnosis while limiting risks and controlling costs. Strategizing the appropriate imaging choice should utilize evidence-based medicine, usually starting with radiographs before moving to complex studies. This chapter discusses how clinical assessment affects imaging choices and introduces appropriateness criteria that can help determine the "best" imaging study. It reviews the strengths and weaknesses as well as costs, benefits, and risks of different imaging techniques. It also presents a brief review of technical factors that affect image quality and radiation exposure.

1 Assessing the Patient

1.1 Clinical Evaluation

Clinical evaluation, including history, physical examination, and laboratory investigation, is paramount to any imaging strategy. The history, beginning with the patient's age, assesses the character of symptoms, their chronicity, and whether there has been trauma (although, especially in children, lack of trauma history does not necessarily exclude trauma). Physical examination may indicate point tenderness or the presence of regional or generalized pathology; there may be signs of inflammation or complex findings of congenital abnormalities. Laboratory investigation can help differentiate infectious/inflammatory conditions, malignancy, and systemic disease.

The radiographic evaluation of a limping infant or child, a common reason for imaging, illustrates how clinical information affects the imaging evaluation [6, 7]. The history may indicate an acute condition, such as a fracture, or a chronic condition, such as developmental dysplasia of the hip (DDH). The specific gait abnormality and the point of maximum tenderness can help focus the radiographic workup. For instance, if a toddler acutely stops walking and there are no signs of infection, then a toddler's fracture is likely and radiographs of the tibia and fibula are indicated [8]. If this study is negative, imaging the pelvis and remainder of the affected limb may be appropriate. Limited motion, fever, and elevated inflammatory markers (white blood cell count, C-reactive protein, and erythrocyte sediment rate) suggest infection or inflammation that may require further workup to evaluate for septic joint or osteomyelitis.

1.2 Importance of the Point of Maximum Tenderness

Knowledge of the point of maximum tenderness is essential. This both allows the clinician to order the appropriate imaging study and helps the radiologist deliver a correct interpretation. In a large series of diagnostic errors from a United Kingdom emergency department, 5.4 % of fractures and

32 % of dislocations were missed because the wrong radiographs had been ordered [9].

Knowledge of the point of maximum tenderness helps the clinician order the appropriate imaging study in the setting of acute trauma. A strict imaging protocol can eliminate 12 % of upper extremity and 19 % of lower extremity radiographs, missing only 1 fracture out of 287, with significant savings in costs [10]. If the Ottawa ankle rules (OAR) are applied on children older than 5 years of age, a meta-analysis of 12 studies found a fracture detection sensitivity of 98.5 % (missing 10 out of 671 fractures), while 24.8 % of the radiographs could have been eliminated [11]. A smaller multicenter study validating the Ottawa knee rules in children reduced knee radiographs by 31.2 % without missing a single fracture [12]. Applying clinical evaluation criteria to trauma patients can eliminate unnecessary radiation and save costs. Though it takes time to assess patients for these protocols, it is better for the patient and for healthcare.

Understandably, knowing the location of maximum tenderness allows for more focused and intense evaluation of the site of injury. Radiologists improved their fracture detection rate by 6 % when they learned the location of pain [13]. Orthopedic surgeons' fracture detection improved by 11 % [14] (Fig. 1.2).

A small percentage of acute fractures will be radiographically occult. Therefore, if a fracture is strongly suspected yet radiographs are normal, the patient's injury should be immobilized and imaged again 2 weeks later, by which time radiographs should show evidence of a healing fracture, such as resorption along the fracture line and development of periosteal reaction [15].

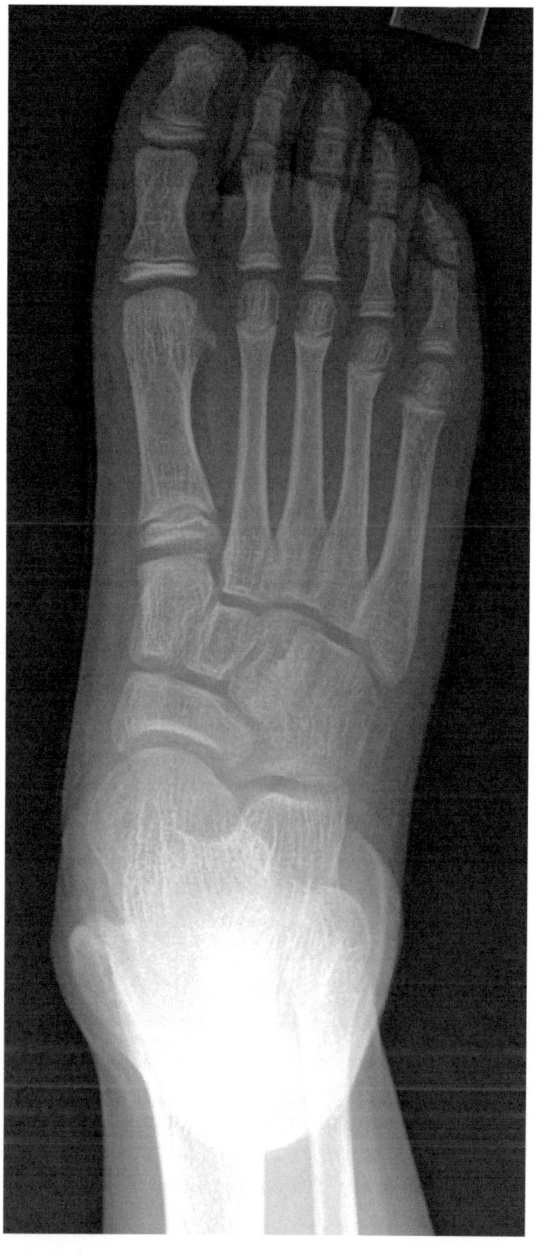

Fig. 1.2 Importance of knowledge of the point of maximal tenderness. There are subtle metaphyseal buckle fractures of the distal third and fourth metacarpals in a 12-year-old boy. However, the history did not identify the point of maximal tenderness, and the fractures were not recognized at the outside institution. One week later, the child was referred to our orthopedic clinic, where the same image was reviewed, this time with knowledge of the location of maximal tenderness. The fractures were now correctly identified

1.3 Imaging Acute Trauma in the Emergency Room Setting

Of all emergency imaging requests, those for skeletal trauma are probably the most common. It is estimated that over 50 % of emergency department visits are for minor injuries, many of which require radiographs. Radiographs help triage patients and sometimes direct further workup. It has been found that triage nurses can expedite visits and improve patient satisfaction by ordering radiographs before a physician sees the patient. Furthermore, radiographs ordered by appropriately trained triage nurses demonstrate fractures at a significantly higher rate than those ordered by senior house officers [16].

Imaging in the setting of acute blunt trauma is controversial but is frequently driven by hospital-based protocols. Protocols and literature-based evidence sometimes disagree, leading to over (or under) utilization of imaging. Many centers routinely obtain radiographs of the cervical spine, chest, and pelvis regardless of the clinical situation. However, the National Emergency X-Radiography Utilization Study (NEXUS) evaluated pediatric cervical spine injury to identify candidates for imaging studies [17]; they suggest that in the absence of midline cervical tenderness, intoxication, altered level of alertness, focal neurologic deficit, or distracting painful injury, there were no cervical spine injuries; 20 % of imaging studies would be eliminated if these criteria were applied. The Canadian cervical spine rules simplify the algorithm for determining the need for imaging the cervical spine. This system is based on assessing high-risk factors (age, dangerous mechanism, or paresthesia), low-risk factors that allow for safe assessment of range of motion, and the patient's ability to rotate the neck 45° to the right and left. Almost half of the radiographs in a study population could have been eliminated by following these rules [18]. There is, however, much debate about applying NEXUS or Canadian cervical spine rules, especially for those under 10 years of age [19].

Similarly, pelvic radiographs may be ordered more often than necessary in the setting of blunt trauma. A study evaluating clinical correlates with pelvic fracture found no pelvic fractures if a child had not injured the lower extremity, had a normal physical examination of the pelvis, and had no indication for an abdomen/pelvic CT [20]. In another study of pelvic trauma, if there was no high-risk mechanism of injury, high-risk clinical findings, or pelvic tenderness, and if the Glasgow Coma Scale was ≥14, fracture could be excluded in 152/504 trauma patients, and pelvic radiographs could have been eliminated in 30 % of patients [21]. Multicenter prospective trials are needed to optimize blunt trauma imaging protocols in children.

2 Choices of Imaging Technique

2.1 Radiography

Imaging of the pediatric patient usually starts with radiographs, which are readily available, inexpensive, deliver minimal radiation, and often answer the clinical question [8, 22–28]. Even for soft tissue masses, radiography can help identify calcification, bony erosion or disruption, and foreign bodies [28].

Radiography is often sufficient in the acute setting of trauma [15]. The point of maximum tenderness should be imaged in at least two orthogonal planes, with three views for such complex areas as the foot/ankle and hand/wrist.

Routine contralateral imaging is generally unnecessary [29, 30], but in select cases, imaging the opposite side for comparison can help diagnose occult fractures, including subtle plastic bending fractures, hairline fractures, impaction fractures, Salter–Harris fractures, and buckle fractures [31]. Opposite side imaging is usually performed in pelvic radiography to assess femoral head ossification and acetabular development [29]. In unique cases, comparison views may avoid more expensive imaging tests such as CT and MRI (Fig. 1.3).

2.2 Ultrasound

Limited research suggests that US can detect radiographically occult fractures with high sensitivity and specificity (Fig. 1.4), but it is uncertain to what extent detection of these occult fractures alters management [32].

In some situations, radiographs are not appropriate for initial imaging. For example, US is recommended to evaluate for DDH in infants less than 6 months old. US stratifies patients best, reduces the number of patients in Pavlik harness, does not increase the incidence of "missed" DDH at age 2 years, and does not increase costs [33].

US is also the appropriate second imaging test (after radiographs) for most soft tissue and joint issues, as it is relatively inexpensive and does not involve ionizing radiation or sedation [28]. US readily detects radiolucent foreign bodies,

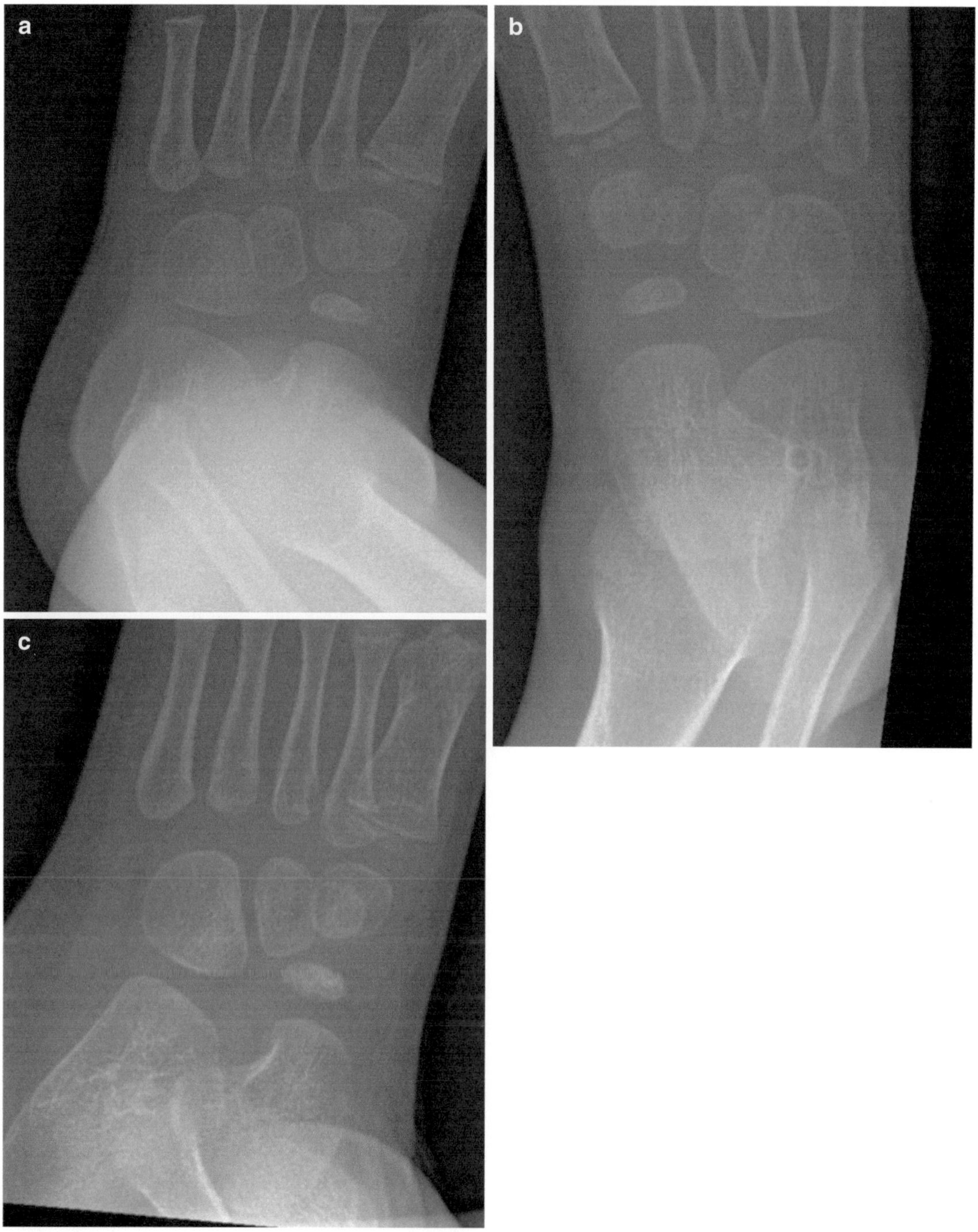

Fig. 1.3 Use of selected comparison view. Kohler disease in a 3-year-old girl with pain at the left mid-foot. The patient had been limping for 4 weeks and had no history of trauma or signs of infection. (**a**) Initial radiograph of the left foot shows subtle flattening of the tarsal navicular bone, more obvious when compared with (**b**), a radiograph of the right foot obtained at the same time. (**c**) Three weeks after supportive treatment in an orthopedic shoe, oblique view of the left foot shows patchy sclerosis, denoting early healing. In this case, initial correlation with the normal contralateral side confirmed that the tarsal navicular on the left was indeed abnormal and also allowed confident diagnosis. While not routinely performed, selective opposite extremity views can help establish the diagnosis and eliminate the need for complex imaging such as MRI (expensive, with attendant sedation risks in a 3-year-old) or nuclear medicine bone scan (radiation risk and costs)

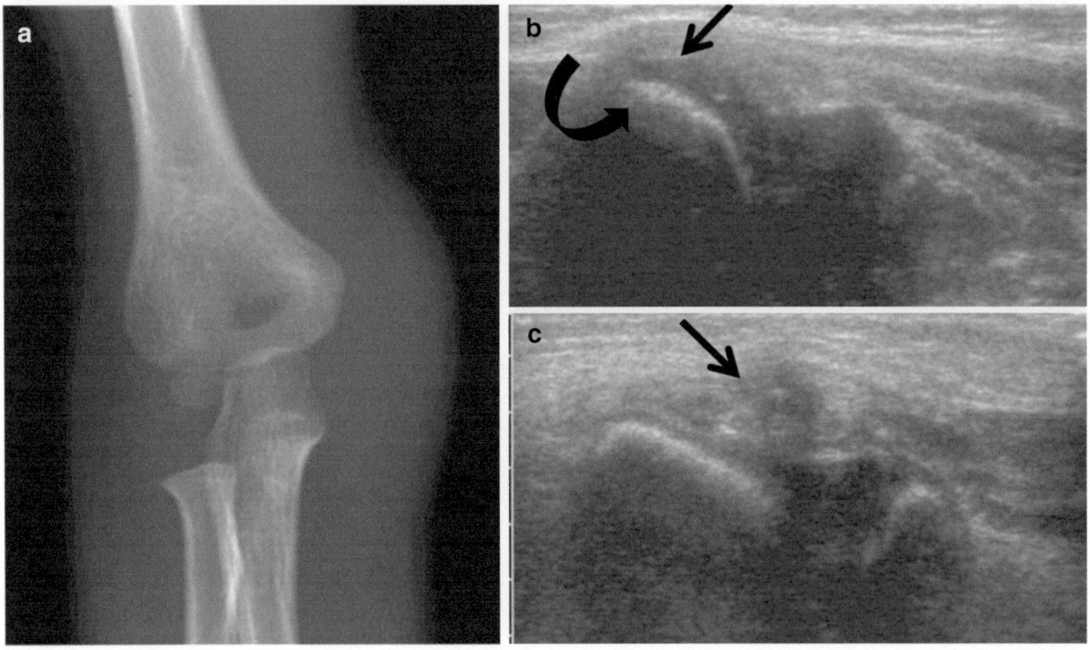

Fig. 1.4 Use of US to identify cartilaginous fracture in a 4-year-old who landed on the right elbow after jumping off a couch. (**a**) Frontal elbow radiograph shows soft tissue swelling over the non-ossified medial epicondyle. (**b**) Longitudinal US of the normal left medial epicondyle (for comparison) shows the normal relationship of the hypoechoic medial epicondyle (*arrow*) to the echogenic medial condylar cortex (*curved arrow*). (**c**) Comparable US of right medial epicondyle demonstrates fractured cartilage (*arrow*)

classifies soft tissue masses as cystic or solid, and characterizes vascular flow. The main limitations to US include limited operator and interpreter expertise, long learning curve, and resistance on the part of referring physicians (as US images are difficult to understand without experience). Furthermore, although US can evaluate bone cortex for abnormalities such as fractures, it is otherwise limited in its ability to assess bones. It is employed in adults to assess tendon/ligament pathology and rheumatologic diseases of the shoulder, elbow, and wrist. Although its use is less widespread in children, increased concern about radiation exposure has led investigators to study US to evaluate congenital and developmental anomalies, ligament injury, and arthropathies.

2.3 Computed Tomography

CT is in general readily available and rapidly performed; multiplanar isotropic voxel imaging allows reconstruction in any plane at submillimeter thickness. It is superb for evaluation of cortical bone, periosteal reaction, and soft tissue calcification. CT provides excellent anatomic detail in evaluation of acute trauma, especially for complex pelvic fractures or Salter–Harris injuries of the knee or ankle. Contrast CT angiography is as effective as angiography for assessing vascular extremity injury in acute trauma [34]. CT accurately assesses biological response of osteosarcoma to chemotherapy [35], but in general MRI surpasses CT in evaluating soft tissues and bone marrow in patients with suspected infection and tumor. High radiation exposure and cost are CT's main drawbacks.

2.4 Magnetic Resonance Imaging

MRI has revolutionized musculoskeletal imaging. Multiplanar imaging is routinely performed without ionizing radiation. MRI excels at evaluating muscle, soft tissue, and bone marrow pathology because of its exquisite detail and tissue contrast. Sequences that accentuate differences in T1 and T2 relaxation times between normal and pathological tissues help characterize lesions. Contrast is rarely needed in post-traumatic evaluation of muscle, tendon, cartilage, and bone. MRI arthrography (MRA) may help evaluate labral injuries of the hip and shoulder. Gadolinium-based intravenous contrast agents help assess tumors as well as infection/inflammation and abscesses. Whole-body MRI techniques that evaluate bone marrow are becoming more common [36]. While MRI has superior sensitivity to bone scintigraphy in the detection of skeletal metastases, it has significantly decreased sensitivity to small extraskeletal metastases, especially in the lung and liver [37].

However, MRI is expensive and may require sedation or general anesthesia. Nephrogenic systemic fibrosis develops after gadolinium administration in some patients with renal insufficiency, and, although there are few reports of this in children [38], this has led to more cautious application of contrast material in all age groups. Metallic implants may cause localized artifact. Furthermore, both known and unknown metallic material within the patient can move, with potentially disastrous results (MRI safety of different devices can be reviewed at http://www.mrisafety.com/default.asp or by contacting the device manufacturer).

2.5 Nuclear Medicine Imaging

Nuclear medicine imaging (NM) contributes to evaluation of many orthopedic disorders, including tumors, occult trauma, child abuse, and osteomyelitis/inflammation. Bone scans are sensitive at detecting lesions in the child with subacute or chronic nonlocalizable musculoskeletal pain. Positron emission tomography (PET) and PET/CT are important for oncologic imaging [39]. Recent research suggests that sodium fluoride (18F-NaF) has higher spatial resolution and performs better than technetium-99m methylene diphosphonate (Tc-MDP) bone scan at a comparable dose, such as in the setting of child abuse [40], but currently it is not widely used. Bone scintigraphy, like CT, involves relatively high radiation exposure [39].

3 Cost and Optimizing Imaging Selection

Decisions about which study to perform should be based on the most cost-effective test that answers the clinical question. Two-thirds of referring physicians rely on advice from radiologists when selecting imaging tests [41]. The American College of Radiology (ACR) has developed evidence-based guidelines to help determine the best imaging test [8, 22–28]. However, only 30 % of radiologists use the musculoskeletal appropriateness criteria in their practice [42], and few referring physicians are aware of or employ these criteria. When general practitioners employ appropriateness criteria in ordering MRI's, the studies are more likely to be approved at insurance review [43].

In a survey of high-litigation risk specialists (emergency medicine, general surgery, orthopedic surgery, neurosurgery, and obstetrics/gynecology), over 50 % practice defensive medicine by ordering more tests than are medically indicated [44]. Seventy-six percent of emergency medicine physicians order imaging tests that are not medically indicated because of malpractice concerns. These tests, of course, increase costs as well as radiation exposure.

Medicare musculoskeletal imaging costs in the USA in 2010 were estimated to be $969 million for MRI and $851 million for radiographs. By 2020, these costs are projected to increase to $2,046 million for MRI and $1,266 million for radiographs. By 2020, $736 million per year could be saved by substituting US for MRI when appropriate [45]. The 2005 Deficit Reduction Act was enacted to reduce imaging payments to control Medicare costs. This Act attempted to decelerate the growth of imaging examinations, but the number of tests continues to increase, particularly MRIs performed by non-radiologists in the office setting [46]. Cost containment can be achieved when ordering imaging studies in pediatric patients by using objective evidence-based imaging strategy (such as the OAR) along with appropriateness criteria.

4 Radiation Exposure

Between 1987 and 2006, the average yearly total radiation a person living in the USA received nearly doubled, from 3.6 millisievert (mSv) to 6.2 mSv [47]. This increase was due to medical imaging. In 1987, medical radiation accounted for 15 % of the annual radiation (0.53 mSv); in 2006 it accounted for 48 % (3.0 mSv) (Fig. 1.5). CT currently accounts for nearly 25 % of annual background radiation exposure (Fig. 1.6).

The International System (SI) terms describe radiation exposure: the two most important metrics are gray (Gy) and sievert (Sv). Gray is the energy imparted to a tissue in joules/kilogram. One Gy is equal to 100 rads. The Gy is frequently used to indicate the absorbed organ dose. Sievert is the equivalent or effective dose. The Sv is typically used to equate an imaging test that covers a limited area, such as a chest CT, to uniform, whole-body irradiation. One Sv equals 100 rem. Because some organs are more susceptible to radiation, the Sv is calculated by multiplying the organ dose in Gy by a tissue weighting factor [49]. The breast, lung, red bone marrow, stomach, and colon are the most radiosensitive organs, each with a tissue weighting factor of 0.12 (Table 1.1).

4.1 Biological Effects of Ionizing Radiation

Diagnostic radiation has two biological effects: deterministic (tissue-effect) and stochastic. Deterministic effects have a definite exposure threshold below which there is no effect; once the threshold is exceeded, the severity of the effect correlates to the dose. Classic examples are skin

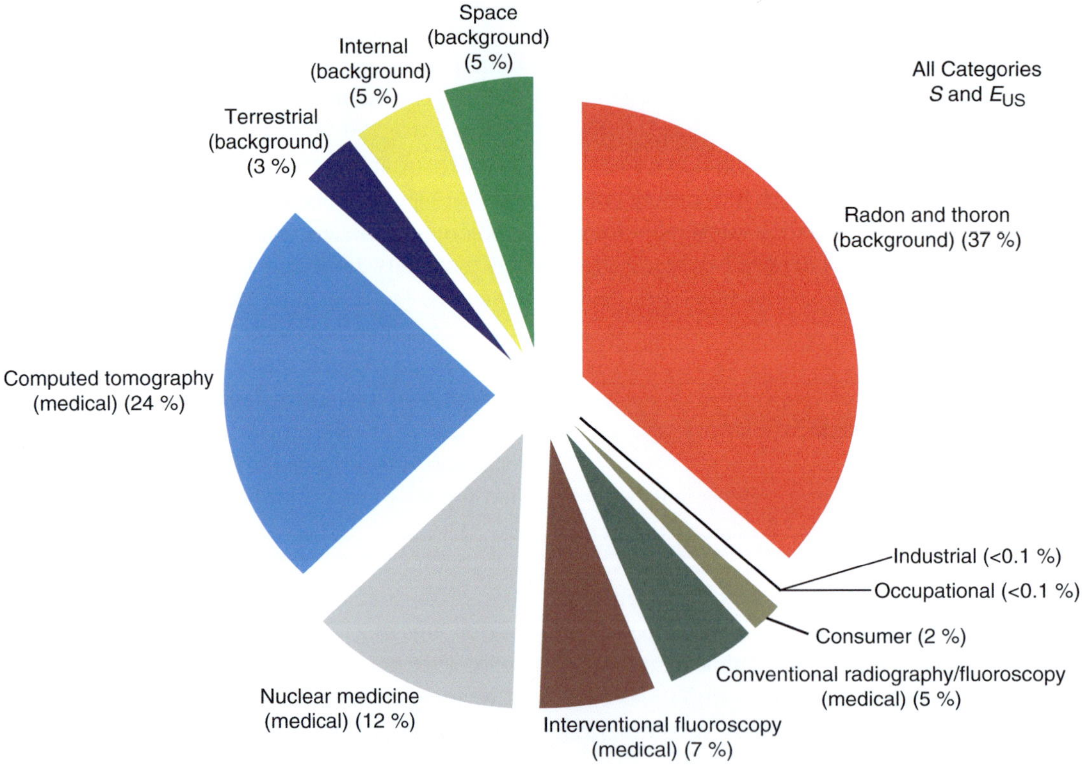

Fig. 1.5 Contribution of different forms of background radiation and different forms of medical radiation to overall radiation exposure in 2006. The total effective dose per individual was 6.2 mSv (whereas it was 3.6 mSv in the early 1980s). In 2006, medical radiation accounted for 48 % of the effective dose, whereas in the early 1980s it accounted for only 15 %. (Percent values have been rounded to the nearest 1 %, except for those less than 1 %.) (Reprinted from Ref. [48], with permission of the National Council on Radiation Protection and Measurements, http://NCRPpublications.org)

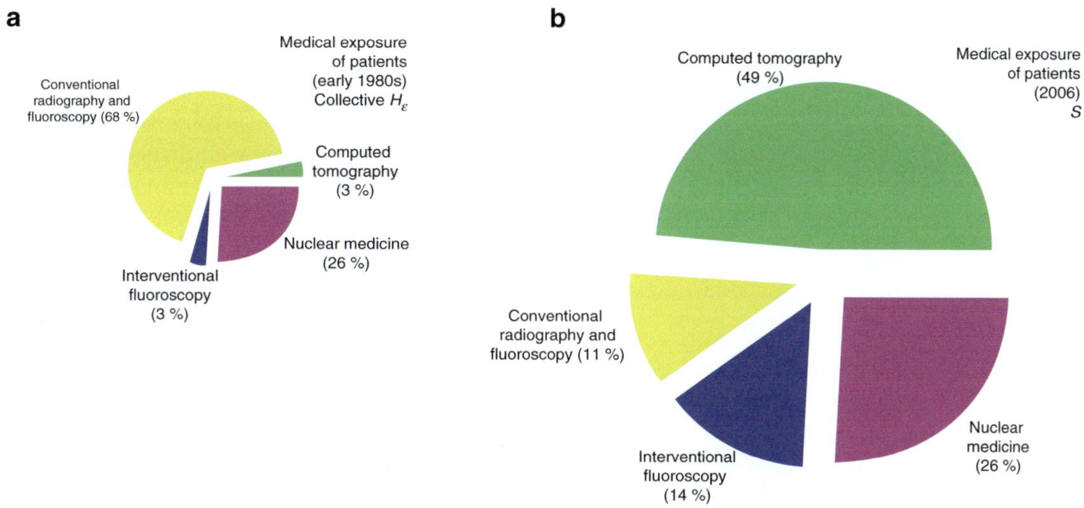

Fig. 1.6 Comparison of collective doses for computed tomography, conventional radiography and fluoroscopy, interventional fluoroscopy, and nuclear medicine (as percent of total collective dose) as reported for the early 1980s (**a**) and for 2006 (**b**). The percentage of effective dose from conventional radiograph and fluoroscopy decreased from 68 % to 11 %, while CT increased from 3 % to 49 % and interventional fluoroscopy increased from 3 % to 14 %. Note the disproportionate size of the pie charts reflecting the nearly 6-fold increase in medical radiation in the intervening years (Data from National Council on Radiation Protection Report 160. Reprinted from Ref. [48], with permission of the National Council on Radiation Protection and Measurements, http://NCRPpublications.org)

Table 1.1 Tissue weighting factors (W_T) ICRP 103

Organ	(W_T)
Breast	0.12
Red bone marrow	0.12
Lung	0.12
Colon	0.12
Stomach	0.12
Gonads	0.08
Thyroid	0.04
Esophagus	0.04
Liver	0.04
Bladder	0.04
Bone surface	0.01
Brain	0.01
Salivary glands	0.01
Skin	0.01
Remainder[a]	0.12

Adapted from Ref. [49]

[a]Remainder includes adipose tissue, adrenal glands, connective tissue, extrathoracic airways, gallbladder heart wall, kidneys, lymph nodes, muscle, pancreas, prostate, small intestine, spleen, thymus, and uterus/cervix

reddening and hair loss, which occur if 2 Gy are delivered to a localized area and which have been reported after excessive radiation during CT brain perfusion studies [50]. Skin reddening and hair loss can also occur after high-dose interventional fluoroscopic procedures [51].

Stochastic effects are random events that have no threshold dose. The probability of their effect increases with higher radiation dose. Radiation-induced cancer data best fits with a linear, no-threshold model, with potential risk of cancer induced by even the smallest dose [52]. It is estimated that for a single exposure of 100 mSv of radiation, one additional cancer per 100 people will develop (as a baseline, 42 people out of 100 will develop cancer) [52].

Ionizing radiation delivered in the course of orthopedic imaging may, therefore, eventually cause malignancy, either as an indirect x-ray interaction of hydroxyl radicals with DNA or as a direct x-ray interaction with DNA. The indirect method is more common, but both interactions can cause a double-stranded DNA break [53]. Children are up to ten times more likely to develop cancer than are middle-age adults (Fig. 1.7) [55]. Furthermore, patients with some inherited diseases have increased sensitivity to radiation (Table 1.2) [56].

Radiation doses over 100 mSv are clearly associated with fatal malignancy, and some argue that doses as low as 10–50 mSv can cause malignancy [57]. The Life Span Study has

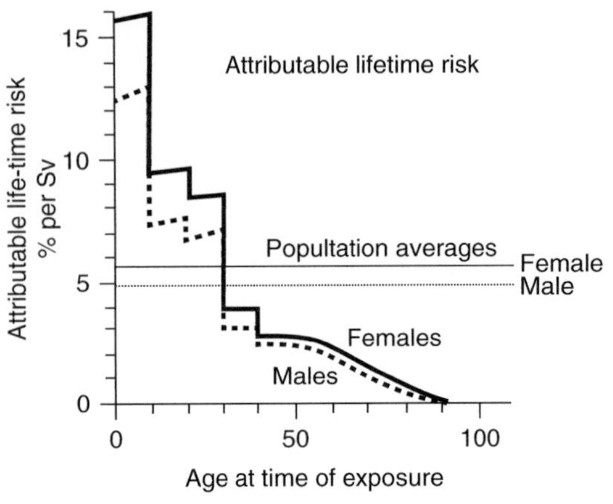

Fig. 1.7 Lifetime risk of excess cancer per sievert as a function of age at the time of exposure (based on data from A-bomb survivors). While the average risk for a population is about 5 % per sievert, the risk varies considerably with age. Children are much more sensitive than adults (Reprinted from Ref. [54], with kind permission from Springer Science+Business Media)

Table 1.2 Selected inherited syndromes associated with increased sensitivity to radiation. This list contains syndromes associated with mutations in DNA repair that increase the risk of developing cancer after ionizing radiation causes DNA damage. There are many other syndromes that are associated with increased risk of cancer including syndromes related to cancer predisposition genes [56]

Ataxia–telangiectasia
Ataxia–telangiectasia-like disorder
Seckel syndrome
Nijmegen breakage syndrome
Fanconi anemia
Homologues of RecQ–Bloom syndrome, Werner syndrome, and Rothmund–Thomson syndrome

Adapted from Ref. [56]

followed atomic bomb survivors over 60 years; this provides the best stochastic risk data [4, 5]. Studies have also implicated diagnostic imaging. As far back as 1958 [58], in utero exposure was associated with a 6 % increase in absolute risk of cancer per Gy; 10 milligray (mGy) in utero exposure was associated with increased childhood cancer deaths [59]. A study that followed women with scoliosis for 50 years found a 1.69-fold increased incidence of breast cancer deaths (the mean breast dose from scoliosis radiographs was 108 mGy). As the number of radiographs increased, so did the risk of breast cancer death [60]. PA rather than AP frontal views reduce the breast cancer risk by three- to fourfold [61]. Furthermore, recent retrospective pediatric studies have linked CT scans with a small increased incidence of leukemia and brain tumors (one extra case of either per 10,000 head CTs) in one UK study [62] and small increased incidence of multiple types of cancers in an Australian study [63]. More pediatric CT cohort studies examining the radiation risk will be reported in the next few years [64]. These studies are based on actual patient exposure data.

Many high-profile journal articles have used theoretical, population-based risk estimates from low-dose radiation, based on such sources as the Biological Effects of Ionizing Radiation (BEIR) VII report and atomic bomb survivors. For example, Berrington de González and Darby estimated a cumulative cancer risk from diagnostic imaging at 0.6 % in the UK, from 0.6 % to 1.8 % in 13 other developed countries, and at greater than 3 % in Japan [65]. Brenner and Hall estimate that 1–2 % of all future cancers will be caused by CT [66].

Physicists have developed position statements in response to theoretical studies on population-based risk estimates from low-dose radiation. For example, the American Association of Physicists in Medicine (AAPM) cautions that "Predictions of hypothetical cancer incidence and deaths in patient populations exposed to such low doses [less than 100 mSv] are highly speculative and should be discouraged. These predictions are harmful because they lead to sensationalistic articles in the public media that cause some patients and parents to refuse medical imaging procedures, placing them at substantial risk by not receiving the clinical benefits of the prescribed procedures" [67]. Similarly, the Health Physics Society, in "accordance with current knowledge of radiation health risks… recommends against quantitative estimation of health risks below an individual dose of 5 rem [50 mSv] in one year or a lifetime dose of 10 rem [100 mSv] above that received from natural sources" [68].

The International Atomic Energy Agency is attempting to change the focus from collective

Table 1.3 Relative radiation exposure from different imaging studies. Actual patient doses in these procedures vary according to body habitus, the region exposed to ionizing radiation, the number of images, and technique factors. The range of doses is based on the ACR Appropriateness Criteria® Radiation Dose Assessment Introduction [70] and the corresponding ACR Appropriateness Criteria as referenced except for the dose range specified for scoliosis series [71] and PET/CT [72, 73]

Relative radiation level [70]	Adult effective dose estimate range (mSv)	Pediatric effective dose estimate range (mSv)	Example examinations
O	0	0	Ultrasound; MRI
☢	<0.1	<0.03	Chest radiographs; hand radiographs
☢☢	0.1–1	0.03–0.3	Pelvis radiographs, cervical spine trauma series [74]
☢☢	0.1–1	0.03–0.3	CT foot or CT knee without contrast [22, 26]
☢☢☢	1–10	0.3–3	Scoliosis series (2 views) [71]
☢☢☢	1–10	0.3–3	Tc-99m bone scan
☢☢☢	1–10	0.3–3	Abdomen CT
☢☢☢☢	10–30	3–10	Whole body PET
☢☢☢☢☢	30–100	10–30	Whole body PET with diagnostic CT [72, 73]

dose to the population to individual dose protection by launching a Smart Card/SmartRadTrack project that tracks patient examinations and cumulative dose [69]. If technique is known, organ dose and effective dose can be estimated, though precise estimation of the risk from a specific study requires calculations performed by a qualified medical physicist. A simpler approach is comparing the relative risk of radiographs, CTs, fluoroscopy, and NM in order to put the radiation risk from common orthopedic imaging tests in context. The American College of Radiology (ACR) has a relative radiation level scale that provides reasonable estimates of dose (Table 1.3) [70].

Although we do not have precise risk estimates for low-dose radiation, it is prudent to treat ionizing radiation as increasing the risk of developing cancer. If there is no benefit to a study, it should not be performed. If there is a benefit to performing the study, the risks should be mitigated. The "as low as reasonably achievable" (ALARA) principle aims to minimize the risk of cancer and was initially developed to protect medical and dental personnel. ALARA has been adapted for patients. It states that the small risk of developing cancer must be weighed against the benefits of performing an examination that employs ionizing radiation and, when feasible, MRI or US should be performed. The Image Gently® campaign (Alliance for Radiation Safety in Pediatric Imaging, Cincinnati, Ohio) recommends adjusting dose for patient size.

4.2 Radiography

Radiography accounts for the greatest number of all ionizing radiation imaging examinations in children (84.7 %); CT, fluoroscopy, and NM—in descending order of frequency—account for the remainder [75]. Digital radiography has replaced screen-film radiography in many imaging centers. There are two types of digital radiography: computed radiography (CR) and direct digital radiography (DR).

CR uses a photostimulable storage-phosphor imaging plate to create a latent image on a cassette. The cassette is then placed in a laser reader, and a digital image is produced in 30–40 s. Powder phosphor imaging plates are the most common type of CR. More recently, needle phosphors have been developed [76], reducing patient exposure [77].

DR eliminates the need for a separate scanning step because the x-ray detector is bonded directly onto integrated thin-film transistors, allowing the readout to appear in less than 10 s. DR can use either direct detection that converts x-rays into electronic charge or indirect detection that converts x-rays first into light and then into electronic charge.

Digital radiography has many advantages over screen-film radiography. Image storage and distribution permit simultaneous viewing in the radiology suite and in clinical areas. Digital radiography has a latitude of exposure approximately 100 times greater than screen-film radiography [78], reducing the number of repeat examinations due to under- or overexposure. Image manipulation (processing) can enhance subtle characteristics in an image. Although digital images have lower spatial resolution than screen-film radiographs, their improved contrast and image processing can result in superior studies [76].

Controlling patient exposure with digital radiography is more complex than with screen-film radiography because of the latitude of digital radiography. Unlike screen-film radiography, where film darkening is directly related to exposure, there is a disconnect between the final image and the actual dose used with digital radiography. Image processing can adjust the gray scale to produce the correct brightness despite under- or overexposure, making it difficult to determine whether the study was actually under- or overexposed. While digital radiography can reduce dose by eliminating repeat exposures, overexposure is common. In one report, 43 % of pediatric CR images were overexposed [79]. This may in part be due to "exposure creep": since overexposed images have less quantum mottle, or noise, than underexposed images and can be processed so they do not appear dark, the overexposed image looks like an excellent radiograph that radiologists prefer. Over time technologists may gradually increase technical parameters to obtain images with little noise [80].

Confusing proprietary exposure terminology that differs among manufacturers contributes to exposure creep. Some manufacturer exposure values are directly related to exposure, whereas others are inversely related to exposure; some use logarithmic scales. Standard terminology to report exposure factor adequacy has recently been adopted, replacing confusing proprietary terminology. Three terms describe exposure: target exposure index (EI_T), exposure index (EI), and deviation index (DI) [81]. The EI_T represents the ideal exposure to the imaging receptor and is set by the manufacturer or imaging facility based on the body part and detector. Target values have not been established. The EI is the nonproprietary exposure indicator term that measures radiation exposure at the image receptor. At a fixed kVp, it has a direct, linear relationship with mAs (doubling the mAs doubles the EI). The lower the EI, the greater the quantum mottle or noise. A thicker patient requires more exposure than a thinner patient. With appropriate technique adjustment for patient thickness, the EI should be relatively constant for a given body part. The DI, the base 10 logarithm of EI/EI_T, is a measure of how much the target exposure varies from the ideal exposure. The DI indicates the adequacy of the exposure and provides an immediate feedback indicator to the technologist and radiologist.

The EI is not a patient dose metric. Many factors must be considered in order to estimate dose: technique (kVp, total filtration), grid, source-to-patient distance, positioning, entrance skin exposure, age, target organ, and area exposed [82]. If the radiography unit records these technique factors, patient dose can be calculated. Alternatively, the dose-area product (DAP) meter can serve as a surrogate for patient dose [83]. DAP meters are required in many European countries, but not in the USA. The technique factors, exposure indicators, and DAP results can be displayed directly on the image, allowing the viewer to assess whether imaging technique is appropriate. To prevent exposure creep, the radiologist and the technical staff need to review these values for each image. Errors in technique or protocols can be recognized and corrected to avoid exposure creep.

In US children's hospitals, digital radiography technique varies considerably [84]. A 1992 study of screen-film radiography in 89 European centers found the measured entrance skin dose for neonatal examinations ranged over a factor of 50 [85]. In 2010, this large variation showed little to no change despite extensive publicity about the risk of ionizing radiation [86].

We may repeat radiographs because of concern that noise will obscure disease processes.

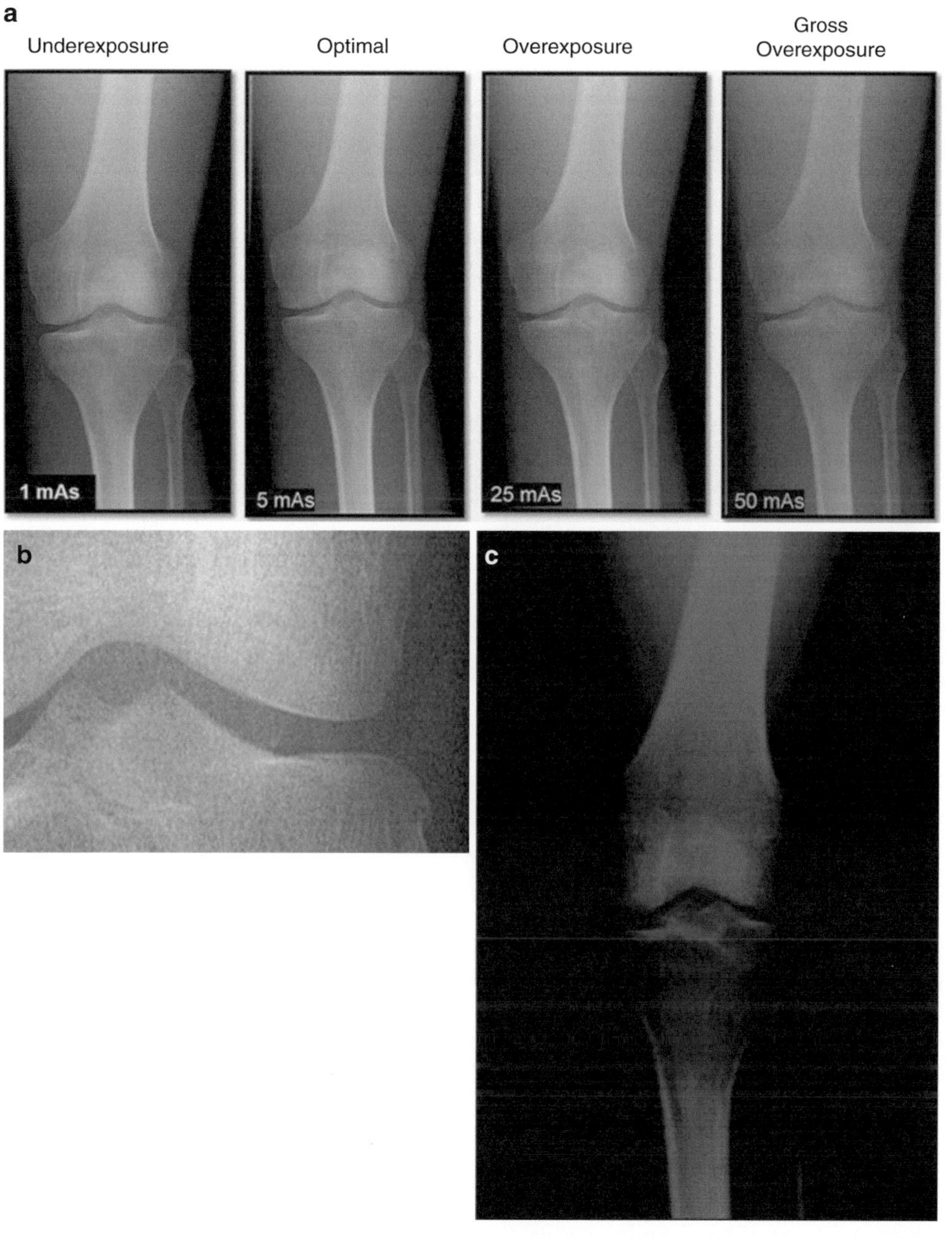

Fig. 1.8 Effect of different exposures on appearance of an adult knee phantom. (**a**) A series of exposures at a 75 kVp and increasing mAs shows little difference in appearance despite a 50-fold increase in exposure. (**b**) Magnification view at 1 mAs exposure shows a relatively noisy appearance (high quantum mottle). (**c**) Radiograph at 160 mAs shows loss of soft tissue and bone detail (image saturation) (Reprinted from Ref. [87], with permission from the Alliance for Radiation Safety in Pediatric Radiology)

To control patient exposure, radiologists must understand the relationship between exposure and noise and develop a noise tolerance level. Since noise has relatively little effect on visualization of high-resolution structures, such as bone detail (Fig. 1.8) [79], lower-dose studies tailored to answer a specific question (such as fracture follow-up) should be considered.

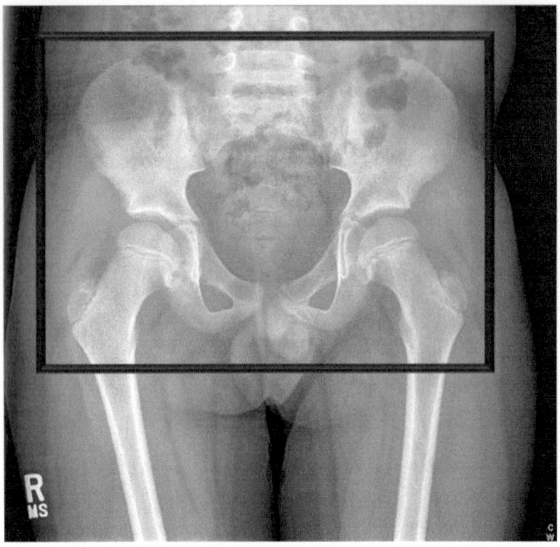

Fig. 1.9 Cropping of a digital image after exposure. The collimators were wide open when this pelvis was radiographed. Before being sent to the radiologist's workstation, the image was cropped to exclude the lower femurs and mid-abdomen. Lack of collimation results in unnecessary radiation to extraneous body parts as well as increased scatter (and decreased detail) (Reprinted from Ref. [87], with permission from the Alliance for Radiation Safety in Pediatric Radiology)

Other factors also help control exposure. Grids can be eliminated for most extremity imaging [88]. Technologists report they often do not collimate before exposure but instead crop the processed images before submitting them for interpretation (Fig. 1.9) [89]. Pre-exposure collimation both reduces patient dose by minimizing the exposed area and improves image quality by reducing scatter.

4.3 Computed Tomography

Since its invention in 1971, CT has become essential to diagnose disease as well as to plan and evaluate treatment. CT represents 11.9 % of all ionizing radiation imaging examinations in children [75]. The average child in the USA will have one CT before age 18. In the USA, the use of pediatric CT in US emergency departments increased by a factor of 5 between 1995 and 2008 [90]. However, at least at children's hospitals, CT use has decreased since 2003, likely due to concern about radiation and increased reliance on MRI [91].

A CT delivers more ionizing radiation than any other study routinely performed in children. As with digital radiography, CT exposure involves a trade-off between radiation dose and diagnostic performance—image noise correlates inversely with radiation dose. The National Council on Radiation Protection (NCRP) concluded that "The dose received by some patients, particularly children, is higher than desired and must and can be reduced without a significant loss of diagnostic information" [92]. The NCRP further suggested performing only medically justified examinations and using the minimum necessary exposure.

CT exposure simulation facilitates evaluation of the relationship between noise and diagnostic performance. Simulation has been shown to accurately produce qualitatively realistic images and has been used to assess the effect of lower radiation dose on tissue contrast and lesion conspicuity in the chest and abdomen (Fig. 1.10) [93, 94], although similar studies have not been performed on pediatric orthopedic CT. However, since orthopedic imaging involves high-contrast structures, relatively large dose reduction should be possible.

Many manufacturers now install pediatric CT protocols. The Image Gently® web site also has a worksheet to help adjust CT techniques [95]. The Image Gently® 10 Steps article suggests methods for reducing exposure [96]. In brief, it recommends scanning only the indicated area and scanning only once, centering the patient in the gantry, reducing technique for the scout image, reducing kVp, and using tube current modulation/automatic exposure control. Iterative image reconstruction algorithms, just being introduced by the manufacturers, should also decrease dose [97].

Bismuth shields for the eye, thyroid, and breast are sometimes used to reduce dose during CT [98–101]. However, their efficacy is controversial as they may affect automatic exposure control/tube current modulation, degrade image quality and accuracy, and waste radiation exposure [102]. The AAPM instead recommends reducing the tube current by the same percentage as the shield would reduce dose and refraining from shielding.

The standard dose metrics in CT—the volume CT dose index ($CTDI_{vol}$) and dose-length product

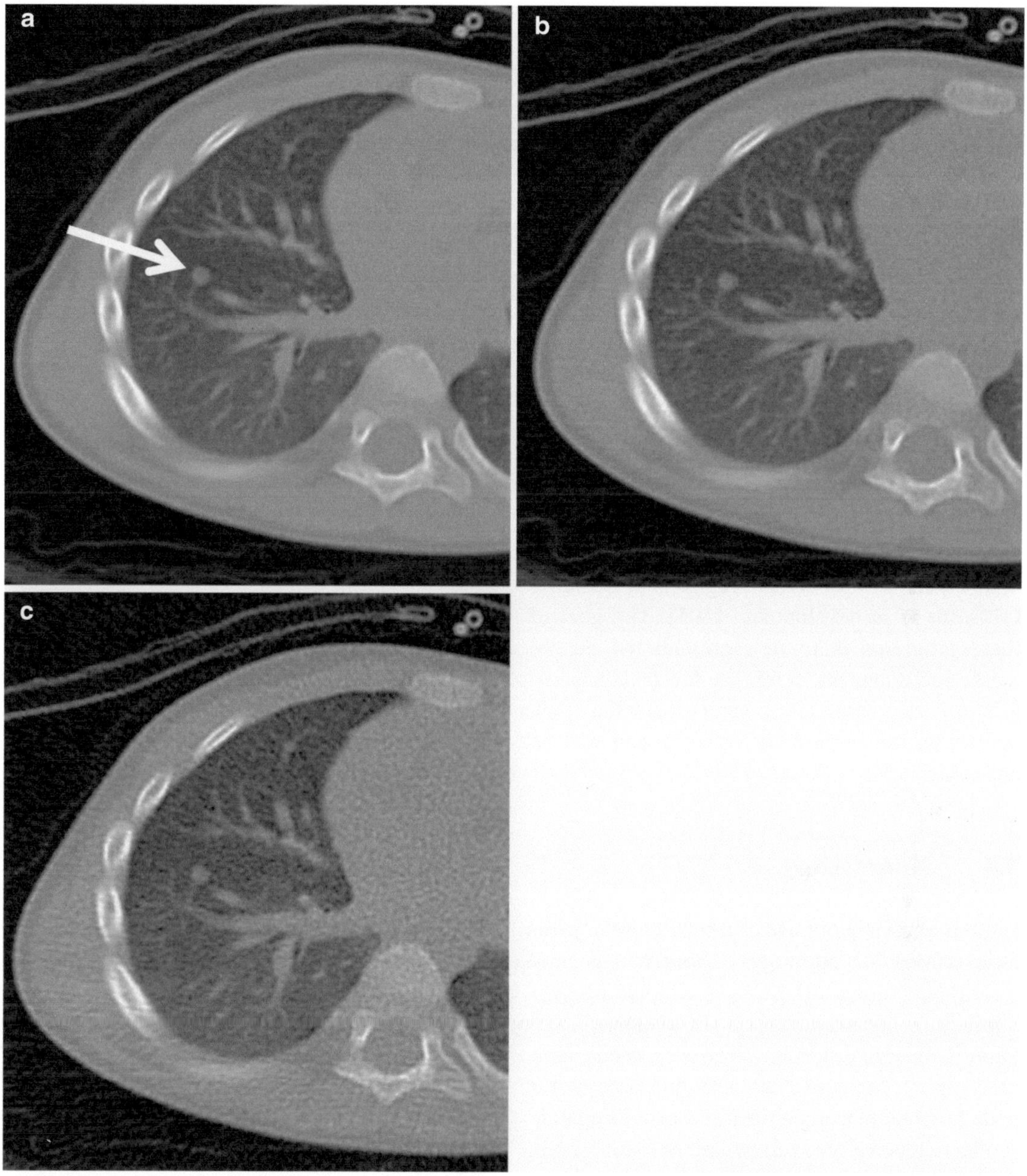

Fig. 1.10 Effect of dose reduction on conspicuity of pulmonary nodule and on bone detail in a 3-year-old with metastatic disease. (**a**) Full-dose CT. (**b**) Simulated 50 % dose reduction. (**c**) Simulated 90 % dose reduction. The pulmonary nodule (*white arrow* in **a**) adjacent to the major fissure is easily seen on all three images. However, bone detail is decreased on (**c**), best recognized at the cortex of the vertebral body and sternum. Bone detail is similar on the full-dose image (**a**) and on that obtained with 50 % dose reduction (**b**)

(DLP)—use phantoms to compare radiation output between different scanners. However, when these measures are employed to estimate pediatric CT dose, they can be off by a factor of 2–3. Several other approaches have been suggested for use in children. The size-specific dose estimate (SSDE), which corrects the $CTDI_{vol}$ for body habitus, is probably the simplest [103]. Unfortunately, it has been developed only for body, not extremity, protocols.

Due to extensive media coverage of the potential health consequences of CT radiation exposure as well as concern in the medical community, the National Institute of Biomedical Imaging and Bioengineering (NIBIB) cosponsored a meeting in 2011 to determine the feasibility of achieving sub-mSv scans, essentially lowering conventional dose by an order of magnitude. Numerous technical innovations were identified that could potentially transform CT examination practices to achieve this goal [104].

In 2012, the Centers for Medicare & Medicaid Services in the USA began to require accreditation for the technical component of advanced diagnostic imaging procedures, including CT, MRI, NM, and PET. The ACR, an accreditation organization, has launched a National Radiology Data Registry (NRDR) Dose Index Registry for CT. A quality improvement registry for pediatric CT scans is in development [105]. The goal of these programs is to develop national benchmarks and diagnostic reference levels. If a facility's reported dose is greater than the 75th percentile, review and corrective action will be necessary.

4.4 Fluoroscopy

Little is known about use of fluoroscopy in pediatric orthopedic radiology, although in general fluoroscopy represents 2.5 % of all ionizing radiation imaging examinations in children [75]. Dose to operative staff has, however, been evaluated. Spine surgeons who use fluoroscopy for pedicle screw placement in adolescent idiopathic scoliosis receive an average annual whole-body radiation dose of 13.49 mSv [106]. A study of radiation exposure to the orthopedic surgery team found that the operating surgeon, estimated to be 12 in. from the beam, received 0.02 mSv/min of fluoroscopy of whole-body exposure, while the scrub nurse, estimated to be 36 in. from the field, received none [107].

Many techniques can reduce radiation dose [108, 109]. These include reducing the mAs [109], using pulsed fluoroscopy at a low rate rather than continuous fluoroscopy [110], employing last image hold, removing the grid [110], avoiding magnification, collimating, limiting duration of radiation administration, blocking patient exposure with lead shielding, and using knowledge of patient anatomy—rather than fluoroscopy—to appropriately position the fluoroscope.

4.5 Nuclear Medicine Imaging

Nuclear medicine represents only 0.9 % of all ionizing radiation imaging examinations in children [75]. A quarter of the increase in annual background radiation is due to NM studies [48]; however, this is primarily from adult myocardial perfusion imaging. Approximately 180,000 pediatric NM examinations are performed annually in the USA [111]. Bone and joint studies represent almost half of pediatric nuclear imaging. NM studies are more commonly used during the teenage years.

Before 2008, there were no universal standards for pediatric radionuclide administration despite established adult-dose adjustments based on body mass or body surface area. That year, a dosimetry survey of 16 pediatric NM examinations at 13 North American pediatric institutions was reported [112]. Most centers reported dose per unit of body mass, not body surfacc arca; minimum dosage, typically given to neonates and infants, varied by up to a factor of 20, while the maximum activity and the activity per kilogram varied by a factor of only 2 (perhaps because the latter were based on adult dosages). Modern equipment, such as multidetector single positron emission computed tomography (SPECT) cameras and iterative reconstruction algorithms, may render historical standards for minimum-dose calculations obsolete.

The Pediatric Nuclear Medicine Dose Reduction Workgroup created pediatric radiopharmaceutical dose guidelines for North America [113], and these were approved in 2010 by the Society of Nuclear Medicine and the Society for Pediatric Radiology. These guidelines address three issues: (1) which method should be used to calculate pediatric administered activities, (2) how should positron-emitting radiopharmaceuticals be adjusted, and (3) what should be the minimum and maximum dose for each of 11 radiopharmaceuticals. These doses are mostly based on weight, with the exceptions of NM cystograms and gastric-emptying studies.

The European Association of Nuclear Medicine also developed pediatric dosage guidelines, based on baseline dosage (equated to a 3 kg child) multiplied by a factor [114–116]. As a general rule, the North American standards recommend lower doses than do the European standards.

The Society of Nuclear Medicine suggests how to minimize and communicate radiation risk in pediatric NM [111]. It recommends comparing the radiation dose a child and parent receive for a particular study to the amount of background radiation the child receives in 1 year and the amount the parent receives in a transcontinental flight. Alternatively, the relative risk of death from everyday activities can be compared to the risk of death from cancer induced by NM studies.

PET/CT presents a special case in patient exposure management [72]. PET/CT is mainly used in pediatric oncologic imaging, including assessment of bone and soft tissue tumors, but with the addition of newer radiopharmaceuticals, potential applications include other forms of bone pathology as well [117]. The dosage of radiopharmaceutical, as well as the accompanying CT scan, must be considered. The CT scan often includes a larger portion of the body than routine diagnostic CTs, extending from the head through the mid-thigh. Furthermore, the dose varies depending on whether the scan is performed only for attenuation correction (lowest dose), anatomic localization, or complete diagnosis (highest dose) [72]. A study of 78 pediatric oncology patients found that the mean effective dose per subject was 20.3 mSv from CT and only 4.6 mSv from PET [73], perhaps because a large number of fully diagnostic CTs were performed. SPECT/CT and PET/CT face similar issues related to dose management; again, both the radiopharmaceutical dose and the CT scan must be considered [118].

5 Risks of Non-radiation-Based Imaging Techniques

When appropriate, ultrasound and MRI offer excellent alternatives to imaging with ionizing radiation. Ultrasound is essentially risk-free, with its use limited both by technical limitations and by the skill of the ultrasonographer. Although MRI lacks radiation risk, other inherent problems limit its use. As discussed earlier in this chapter, in patients with renal insufficiency, there is the risk of nephrogenic systemic fibrosis, and metal within the patient can move—with disastrous results. In addition, general anesthesia is often required in young patients (especially those under 6 years). One medical center reported three general anesthetic deaths in MRI over a 10-year period. The patients weighed less than 7 kg and were considered high anesthetic risk. Their risk of death of 1 in 3,900 was nearly double the risk of intraoperative anesthesia—1 in 7,138 [119]. Furthermore, some studies in rodents and primates suggest behavioral and learning disorders after administration of anesthesia, but this does not necessarily apply to humans. Currently no anesthetic practice changes are indicated [120, 121]. Communication among the ordering physician, radiologist, and anesthesiologist to determine the best option for high-anesthetic-risk patients is recommended. Children who are high anesthetic risks may benefit from CT performed without anesthesia, despite the radiation dose.

References

1. Roberts RE. Our heritage. Br J Radiol. 1938;11(121):38–45.
2. Brown P. American martyrs to radiology. Clarence Madison Dally (1865–1904). 1936. Am J Roentgenol. 1995;164(1):237–9.
3. Berrington A, Darby SC, Weiss HA, Doll R. 100 years of observation on British radiologists: mortality from cancer and other causes 1897–1997. Br J Radiol. 2001;74(882):507–19.
4. Pierce DA, Preston DL. Radiation-related cancer risks at low doses among atomic bomb survivors. Radiat Res. 2000;154(2):178–86.
5. Preston DL, Ron E, Tokuoka S, Funamoto S, Nishi N, Soda M, et al. Solid cancer incidence in atomic bomb

survivors: 1958–1998. Radiat Res. 2007;168(1):1–64. PubMed PMID: 17722996. Epub 2007/08/29. eng.

6. Barkin RM, Barkin SZ, Barkin AZ. The limping child. J Emerg Med. 2000;18(3):331–9. PubMed PMID: 10729672. Epub 2000/03/24. eng.
7. Flynn JM, Widmann RF. The limping child: evaluation and diagnosis. J Am Acad Orthop Surg. 2001;9(2):89–98. PubMed PMID: 11281633. Epub 2001/04/03. eng.
8. ACR Appropriateness Criteria® limping child: ages 0–5 years. [Internet]. American College of Radiology; 2012 [cited 27 Aug 2012]. Available from: http://www.acr.org/~/media/ACR/Documents/AppCriteria/Diagnostic/LimpingChildAges0To5Years.pdf.
9. Guly HR. Diagnostic errors in an accident and emergency department. Emerg Med J. 2001;18(4):263–9.
10. Brand DA, Frazier WH, Kohlhepp WC, Shea KM, Hoefer AM, Ecker MD, et al. A protocol for selecting patients with injured extremities who need X-rays. N Engl J Med. 1982;306(6):333–9.
11. Dowling S, Spooner CH, Liang Y, Dryden DM, Friesen C, Klassen TP, et al. Accuracy of Ottawa Ankle Rules to exclude fractures of the ankle and midfoot in children: a meta-analysis. Acad Emerg Med. 2009;16(4):277–87. PubMed PMID: 19187397. Epub 2009/02/04. eng.
12. Bulloch B, Neto G, Plint A, Lim R, Lidman P, Reed M, et al. Validation of the Ottawa Knee Rule in children: a multicenter study. Ann Emerg Med. 2003;42(1):48–55. PubMed PMID: 12827123. Epub 2003/06/27. eng.
13. Berbaum KS, el-Khoury GY, Franken EA, Kathol M, Montgomery WJ, Hesson W. Impact of clinical history on fracture detection with radiography. Radiology. 1988;168(2):507–11.
14. Berbaum K, Franken E, el-Khoury G. Impact of clinical history on radiographic detection of fractures: a comparison of radiologists and orthopedists. Am J Roentgenol. 1989;153(6):1221–4.
15. Coris EE, Zwygart K, Fletcher M, Pescasio M. Imaging in sports medicine: an overview. Sports Med Arthrosc Rev. 2009;17(1):2–12. PubMed PMID: 19204546. Epub 2009/02/11. eng.
16. Lindley-Jones M, Finlayson BJ. Triage nurse requested x rays—are they worthwhile? J Accid Emerg Med. 2000;17(2):103–7.
17. Viccellio P, Simon H, Pressman BD, Shah MN, Mower WR, Hoffman JR, et al. A prospective multicenter study of cervical spine injury in children. Pediatrics. 2001;108(2):e20.
18. Stiell IG, Wells GA, Vandemheen KL, Clement CM, Lesiuk H, De Maio VJ, et al. The Canadian C-spine rule for radiography in alert and stable trauma patients. JAMA. 2001;286(15):1841–8.
19. Booth TN. Cervical spine evaluation in pediatric trauma. Am J Roentgenol. 2012;198(5):W417–25.
20. Wong AT, Brady KB, Caldwell AM, Graber NM, Rubin DH, Listman DA. Low-risk criteria for pelvic radiography in pediatric blunt trauma patients. Pediatr Emerg Care. 2011;27(2):92–6.
21. Lagisetty J, Slovis T, Thomas R, Knazik S, Stankovic C. Are routine pelvic radiographs in major pediatric blunt trauma necessary? Pediatr Radiol. 2012;42(7):853–8.
22. ACR Appropriateness Criteria® chronic foot pain [Internet]. American College of Radiology; 2008 [cited 27 Aug 2012]. Available from: http://www.acr.org/~/media/ACR/Documents/AppCriteria/Diagnostic/ChronicFootPain.pdf.
23. ACR Appropriateness Criteria® nontraumatic knee pain [Internet]. American College of Radiology; 2008 [cited 27 Aug 2012]. Available from: http://www.acr.org/~/media/ACR/Documents/AppCriteria/Diagnostic/NontraumaticKneePain.pdf.
24. ACR Appropriateness Criteria® acute hand and wrist trauma [Internet]. American College of Radiology; 2008 [cited 27 Aug 2012]. Available from: http://www.acr.org/~/media/ACR/Documents/AppCriteria/Diagnostic/AcuteHandAndWristTrauma.pdf.
25. ACR Appropriateness Criteria® developmental dysplasia of the hip—child [Internet]. American College of Radiology; 2010 [cited 27 Aug 2012]. Available from: http://www.acr.org/~/media/ACR/Documents/AppCriteria/Diagnostic/DevelopmentalDysplasiaOfHipChild.pdf.
26. ACR Appropriateness Criteria® acute trauma to the knee [Internet]. American College of Radiology; 2011 [cited 27 Aug 2012]. Available from: http://www.acr.org/~/media/ACR/Documents/AppCriteria/Diagnostic/AcuteTraumaKnee.pdf.
27. ACR Appropriateness Criteria® suspected physical abuse—child [Internet]. American College of Radiology; 2012 [cited 27 Aug 2012]. Available from: http://www.acr.org/~/media/ACR/Documents/AppCriteria/Diagnostic/SuspectedPhysicalAbuseChild.pdf.
28. ACR Appropriateness Criteria® soft-tissue masses [Internet]. American College of Radiology; 2009 [cited 27 Aug 2012]. Available from: http://www.acr.org/~/media/ACR/Documents/AppCriteria/Diagnostic/SoftTissueMasses.pdf.
29. McCauley RGK, Schwartz AM, Leonidas JC, Darling DB, Bankoff MS, Swan CS. Comparison views in extremity injury in children: an efficacy study. Radiology. 1979;131(1):95–7.
30. Merten DF. Comparison radiographs in extremity injuries of childhood: current application in radiological practice. Radiology. 1978;126(1):209–10.
31. Swischuk LE, Hernandez JA. Frequently missed fractures in children (value of comparative views). Emerg Radiol. 2004;11(1):22–8. PubMed PMID: 15278701. Epub 2004/07/28. eng.
32. Cho KH, Lee SM, Lee YH, Suh KJ. Ultrasound diagnosis of either an occult or missed fracture of an extremity in pediatric-aged children. Korean J Radiol. 2010;11(1):84–94. PubMed PMID: 20046499. Pubmed Central PMCID: 2799655. Epub 2010/01/05. eng.
33. Elbourne D, Dezateux C, Arthur R, Clarke NM, Gray A, King A, et al. Ultrasonography in the diagnosis and

management of developmental hip dysplasia (UK hip trial): clinical and economic results of a multicentre randomised controlled trial. Lancet. 2002;360(9350):2009–17. PubMed PMID: 12504396. Epub 2002/12/31. eng.
34. Peng PD, Spain DA, Tataria M, Hellinger JC, Rubin GD, Brundage SI. CT angiography effectively evaluates extremity vascular trauma. Am Surg. 2008;74(2):103–7. PubMed PMID: 18306857. Epub 2008/03/01. eng.
35. Mail J, Cohen M, Mirkin L, Provisor A. Response of osteosarcoma to preoperative intravenous high-dose methotrexate chemotherapy: CT evaluation. Am J Roentgenol. 1985;144(1):89–93.
36. Darge K, Jaramillo D, Siegel MJ. Whole-body MRI in children: current status and future applications. Eur J Radiol. 2008;68(2):289–98.
37. Siegel MJ, Acharyya S, Hoffer FA, Wyly JB, Friedmann AM, Snyder BS, et al. Whole-body MR imaging for staging of malignant tumors in pediatric patients: results of the American College of Radiology Imaging Network 6660 Trial. Radiology. 2013;266(2):599–609. Epub 2013/2/1.
38. Karcaaltincaba M, Oguz B, Haliloglu M. Current status of contrast-induced nephropathy and nephrogenic systemic fibrosis in children. Pediatr Radiol. 2009;39 Suppl 3:S382–4.
39. Treves ST, Baker A, Fahey FH, Cao X, Davis RT, Drubach LA, et al. Nuclear medicine in the first year of life. J Nucl Med. 2011;52(6):905–25.
40. Drubach LA, Johnston PR, Newton AW, Perez-Rossello JM, Grant FD, Kleinman PK. Skeletal trauma in child abuse: detection with 18F-NaF PET1. Radiology. 2010;255(1):173–81.
41. Bautista AB, Burgos A, Nickel BJ, Yoon JJ, Tilara AA, Amorosa JK. Do clinicians use the American College of Radiology Appropriateness Criteria in the management of their patients? Am J Roentgenol. 2009;192(6):1581–5.
42. Tigges S, Sutherland D, Manaster BJ. Do radiologists use the American College of Radiology Musculoskeletal Appropriateness Criteria? Am J Roentgenol. 2000;175(2):545–7.
43. Levy G, Blachar A, Goldstein L, Paz I, Olsha S, Atar E, et al. Nonradiologist utilization of American College of Radiology Appropriateness Criteria in a preauthorization center for MRI requests: applicability and effects. Am J Roentgenol. 2006;187(4):855–8.
44. Studdert D, Mello MM, Sage WM, et al. Defensive medicine among high-risk specialist physicians in a volatile malpractice environment. JAMA. 2005;293(21):2609–17.
45. Parker L, Nazarian LN, Carrino JA, Morrison WB, Grimaldi G, Frangos AJ, et al. Musculoskeletal imaging: Medicare use, costs, and potential for cost substitution. J Am Coll Radiol. 2008;5(3):182–8.
46. Kennedy S, Forman HP. Deficit reduction act: effects on utilization of noninvasive musculoskeletal imaging. Radiology. 2012;264(1):146–53.
47. Schauer DA, Linton OW. National Council on Radiation Protection and Measurements report shows substantial medical exposure increase. Radiology. 2009;253(2):293–6.
48. National Council on Radiation Protection and Measurements. Report no. 160 – Ionizing radiation exposure of the population of the United States. Bethesda; 2009.
49. The 2007 Recommendations of the International Commission on Radiological Protection. ICRP publication 103. Ann ICRP. 2007;37(2–4):1–332.
50. Zarembo A. Hospital error leads to radiation overdoses after Cedars-Sinai reset a CT scan machine in February 2008, more than 200 brain scans on potential stroke patients were performed at eight times the normal dose of radiation, the hospital says. Los Angeles Times. 2009; 13 Oct 2009.
51. Ukisu R, Kushihashi T, Soh I. Skin injuries caused by fluoroscopically guided interventional procedures: case-based review and self-assessment module. Am J Roentgenol. 2009;193(6 Supplement):S59–69.
52. National Research Council Committee to assess health risks from exposure to low levels of ionizing radiation: BEIR VII Phase 2. Washington, DC: The National Academies Press; 2006.
53. Hall EJ, Giaccia A. The physics and chemistry of radiation absorption. Radiobiology for the radiologist. 7th ed. Philadelphia: Lippincott Williams and Wilkins; 2012. p. 3–11.
54. Hall EJ, Session I. Helical CT and cancer risk. Introduction to session I. Pediatr Radiol. 2002;32:225–7.
55. Beir V. Health effects of exposure to low levels of ionizing radiation. Washington, DC: The National Academies Press; 1990.
56. Hall E, Giaccia A. Cancer biology. Radiobiology for the radiologist. 7th ed. Philadelphia: Lippincott Williams & Wilkins; 2012. p. 273–302.
57. Brenner DJ, Doll R, Goodhead DT, Hall EJ, Land CE, Little JB, et al. Cancer risks attributable to low doses of ionizing radiation: assessing what we really know. Proc Natl Acad Sci. 2003;100(24):13761–6.
58. Stewart A, Webb J, Hewitt D. A survey of childhood malignancies. Br Med J. 1958;1(5086):1495–508.
59. Doll R, Wakeford R. Risk of childhood cancer from fetal irradiation. Br J Radiol. 1997;70(830):130–9.
60. Doody MM, Lonstein JE, Stovall M, Hacker DG, Luckyanov N, Land CE. Breast cancer mortality after diagnostic radiography: findings from the U.S. Scoliosis Cohort Study. Spine. 2000;25(16):2052–63.
61. Levy ARM, Goldberg MSP, Mayo NEP, Hanley JAP, Poitras BMDF. Reducing the lifetime risk of cancer from spinal radiographs among people with adolescent idiopathic scoliosis. Spine. 1996;21(13):1540–7.
62. Pearce MS, Salotti JA, Little MP, McHugh K, Lee C, Kim KP, et al. Radiation exposure from CT scans in childhood and subsequent risk of leukaemia and brain tumours: a retrospective cohort study. Lancet. 2012;380(9840):499–505. PubMed PMID: 22681860. Pubmed Central PMCID: 3418594. Epub 2012/06/12. eng.
63. Mathews JD, Forsythe AV, Brady Z, Butler MW, Goergen SK, Byrnes GB, et al. Cancer risk in 680,000

people exposed to computed tomography scans in childhood or adolescence: data linkage study of 11 million Australians. Br Med J. 2013;346:f2360. Pubmed Central PMCID: 3660619. Epub 2013/05/23. eng.
64. Einstein AJ. Beyond the bombs: cancer risks of low-dose medical radiation. Lancet. 2012;380(9840):455–7. PubMed PMID: 22681861. Epub 2012/06/12. eng.
65. Gonzalez A, Darby S. Risk of cancer from diagnostic X-rays: estimates for the UK and 14 other countries. Lancet. 2004;363(9406):345–51. PubMed PMID: 15070562. Epub 2004/04/09. eng.
66. Brenner DJ, Hall EJ. Computed tomography–an increasing source of radiation exposure. N Engl J Med. 2007;357(22):2277–84. PubMed PMID: 18046031. Epub 2007/11/30. eng.
67. AAPM position statement on radiation risks from medical imaging procedures. American Association of Physicists in Medicine; 2011 [cited 12 May 2012]. Available from: http://www.aapm.org/org/policies/details.asp?id=318&type=PP&current=true.
68. Position statement of the Health Physics Society. Radiation risk in perspective. Health Physics Society; 2010 [cited 1 Aug 2012]. Available from: http://hps.org/documents/risk_ps010-2.pdf.
69. Rehani MM, Frush DP. Patient exposure tracking: the IAEA smart card project. Radiat Prot Dosimetry. 2011;147(1–2):314–6. PubMed PMID: 21778155. Epub 2011/07/23. eng.
70. ACR Appropriateness Criteria® radiation dose assessment introduction [Internet]. American College of Radiology; 2007 [cited 27 Aug 2012]. Available from: http://www.acr.org/~/media/ACR/Documents/AppCriteria/RRLInformation.pdf.
71. Mogaadi M, Ben Omrane L, Hammou A. Effective dose for scoliosis patients undergoing full spine radiography. Radiat Prot Dosimetry. 2011;7:2011.
72. Fahey FH. Dosimetry of pediatric PET/CT. J Nucl Med. 2009;50(9):1483–91.
73. Chawla S, Federman N, Nagata K, Zhang D, Nuthakki S, Angel E, et al. Estimated cumulative radiation dose from PET/CT in pediatric patients with malignancies: a 5-year retrospective review. Pediatr Radiol. 2008;38 Suppl 2:s338.
74. ACR Appropriateness Criteria® suspected spine trauma. Reston: American College of Radiology; 2012 [cited 27 Aug 2012]. Available from: http://www.acr.org/~/media/ACR/Documents/AppCriteria/Diagnostic/SuspectedSpineTrauma.pdf.
75. Dorfman AL, Fazel R, Einstein AJ, Applegate KE, Krumholz HM, Wang Y, et al. Use of medical imaging procedures with ionizing radiation in children: a population-based study. Arch Pediatr Adolesc Med. 2011;165(5):458–64. PubMed PMID: 21199972. Epub 2011/01/05. eng.
76. Korner M, Weber CH, Wirth S, Pfeifer KJ, Reiser MF, Treitl M. Advances in digital radiography: physical principles and system overview. Radiographics. 2007;27(3):675–86. PubMed PMID: 17495286. Epub 2007/05/15. eng.
77. Cohen M, Corea D, Wanner M, Karmazyn B, Gunderman R, Applegate K, et al. Evaluation of a new phosphor plate technology for neonatal portable chest radiographs. Acad Radiol. 2011;18(2):197–8. PubMed PMID: 21232684. Epub 2011/01/15. eng.
78. Willis C. Computed radiography: a higher dose? Pediatr Radiol. 2002;32(10):745–50.
79. Don S. Radiosensitivity of children: potential for overexposure in CR and DR and magnitude of doses in ordinary radiographic examinations. Pediatr Radiol. 2004;34 Suppl 3:S167–72. discussion S234–41. PubMed PMID: 15558258. Epub 2004/11/24. eng.
80. Willis CE. The ALARA concept in pediatric CR and DR: dose reduction in pediatric radiographic exams. Pediatr Radiol. 2004;34 Suppl 3:S159–247. PubMed PMID: 15558256. Epub 2004/11/24. eng.
81. Don S, Whiting BR, Rutz LJ, Apgar B. New exposure indicators for digital radiography simplified for radiologists and technologists. Am J Roentgenol. 2012;199(6):1337–41. PubMed PMID:23169727 Epub 2012/5/1.eng.
82. McCollough CH, Schueler BA. Calculation of effective dose. Med Phys. 2000;27(5):828–37.
83. Le Heron JC. Estimation of effective dose to the patient during medical x-ray examinations from measurements of the dose-area product. Phys Med Biol. 1992;37(11):2117–26. PubMed PMID: 1438564. Epub 1992/11/01. eng.
84. Don S, Goske M, Uzenoff R, Rodriguez G, Mills T, Spelic D. Image gently: a survey of technique factors for CR-DR users. Pediatr Radiol. 2012;42 Suppl 2:s284.
85. Schneider K, Fendel H, Bakawski C, Stein E, Kohn M, Kellner M, et al. Results of a dosimetry study in the European community on frequent X ray examination in infants. Radiat Prot Dosimetry. 1992;43(1–4):31–6.
86. Billinger J, Nowotny R, Homolka P. Diagnostic reference levels in pediatric radiology in Austria. Eur Radiol. 2010;20(7):1572–9.
87. Back-to-basics Image Gently® campaign. The Alliance for Radiation Safety in Pediatric Imaging. Available from: http://www.pedrad.org/associations/5364/ig/?page=824.
88. Cartlon RR, Adler AM. The grid. Principles of radiographic imaging: an art and a science. 4th ed. Clifton Park: Delmar Cengage Learning; 2013.
89. Morrison G, John SD, Goske MJ, Charkot E, Herrmann T, Smith SN, et al. Pediatric digital radiography education for radiologic technologists: current state. Pediatr Radiol. 2011;41(5):602–10. PubMed PMID: 21491200. Epub 2011/04/15. eng.
90. Larson DB, Johnson LW, Schnell BM, Goske MJ, Salisbury SR, Forman HP. Rising use of CT in child visits to the emergency department in the United States, 1995–2008. Radiology. 2011;259(3):793–801.
91. Townsend BA, Callahan MJ, Zurakowski D, Taylor GA. Has pediatric CT at children's hospitals reached its peak? Am J Roentgenol. 2010;194(5):1194–6.

92. Linton OW, Mettler Jr FA. National conference on dose reduction in CT, with an emphasis on pediatric patients. Am J Roentgenol. 2003;181(2):321–9.
93. Frush DP, Slack CC, Hollingsworth CL, Bisset GS, Donnelly LF, Hsieh J, et al. Computer-simulated radiation dose reduction for abdominal multidetector CT of pediatric patients. Am J Roentgenol. 2002;179(5):1107–13.
94. Li X, Samei E, DeLong DM, Jones RP, Gaca AM, Hollingsworth CL, et al. Pediatric MDCT: towards assessing the diagnostic influence of dose reduction on the detection of small lung nodules. Acad Radiol. 2009;16(7):872–80.
95. Image Gently®. Worksheet. The alliance for radiation safety in pediatric imaging. Available from: http://pedrad.org/associations/5364/ig/index.cfm?page=368.
96. Strauss KJ, Goske MJ, Kaste SC, Bulas D, Frush DP, Butler P, et al. Image gently: ten steps you can take to optimize image quality and lower CT dose for pediatric patients. Am J Roentgenol. 2010;194(4):868–73. PubMed PMID: 20308484. Epub 2010/03/24. eng.
97. Singh S, Kalra MK, Shenoy-Bhangle AS, Saini A, Gervais DA, Westra SJ, et al. Radiation dose reduction with hybrid iterative reconstruction for pediatric CT. Radiology. 2012;263(2):537–46.
98. Hohl C, Wildberger JE, Suss C, Thomas C, Muhlenbruch G, Schmidt T, et al. Radiation dose reduction to breast and thyroid during MDCT: effectiveness of an in-plane bismuth shield. Acta Radiol. 2006;47(6):562–7. PubMed PMID: 16875333. Epub 2006/08/01. eng.
99. Hopper KD, Neuman JD, King SH, Kunselman AR. Radioprotection to the eye during CT scanning. Am J Neuroradiol. 2001;22(6):1194–8. PubMed PMID: 11415918. Epub 2001/06/21. eng.
100. Leswick DA, Hunt MM, Webster ST, Fladeland DA. Thyroid shields versus z-axis automatic tube current modulation for dose reduction at neck CT. Radiology. 2008;249(2):572–80. PubMed PMID: 18780826. Epub 2008/09/11. eng.
101. Mukundan Jr S, Wang PI, Frush DP, Yoshizumi T, Marcus J, Kloeblen E, et al. MOSFET dosimetry for radiation dose assessment of bismuth shielding of the eye in children. Am J Roentgenol. 2007;188(6):1648–50. PubMed PMID: 17515389. Epub 2007/05/23. eng.
102. AAPM Position Statement on the use of bismuth shielding for the purpose of dose reduction in CT scanning. American Association of Physicists in Medicine; 2012 [cited 12 May 2012]. Available from: http://www.aapm.org/org/policies/details.asp?id=319&type=PP&current=true.
103. Boone J, Strauss K, Cody D, McCollogh C, McNitt-Gray M, Toth T. Size-Specific Dose Estimates (SSDE) in pediatric and adult body CT examinations. AAPM report no. 204; 2011.
104. McCollough CH, Chen GH, Kalender W, Leng S, Samei E, Taguchi K, et al. Achieving routine submillisievert CT scanning: report from the summit on management of radiation dose in CT. Radiology. 2012;264(2):567–80.
105. Goske MJ, Strauss KJ, Coombs LP, Mandel KE, Towbin AJ, Larson DB, et al. Diagnostic reference ranges for pediatric abdominal CT. Radiology. 2013;268(1):208–18. PubMed PMID:23513245. Epub 2013/03/21. Eng.
106. Ul Haque M, Shufflebarger HL, O'Brien M, Macagno A. Radiation exposure during pedicle screw placement in adolescent idiopathic scoliosis: is fluoroscopy safe? Spine. 2006;31(21):2516–20.
107. Mehlman CT, DiPasquale TG. Radiation exposure to the orthopaedic surgical team during fluoroscopy: "how far away is far enough?". J Orthop Trauma. 1997;11(6):392–8.
108. Hernanz-Schulman M, Goske MJ, Bercha IH, Strauss KJ. Pause and pulse: ten steps that help manage radiation dose during pediatric fluoroscopy. Am J Roentgenol. 2011;197(2):475–81. PubMed PMID: 21785097. Epub 2011/07/26. eng.
109. Strauss K. Pediatric interventional radiography equipment: safety considerations. Pediatr Radiol. 2006;36 Suppl 2:126–35.
110. Brown PH, Thomas RD, Silberberg PJ, Johnson LM. Optimization of a fluoroscope to reduce radiation exposure in pediatric imaging. Pediatr Radiol. 2000;30(4):229–35.
111. Fahey FH, Treves ST, Adelstein SJ. Minimizing and communicating radiation risk in pediatric nuclear medicine. J Nucl Med. 2011;52(8):1240–51. PubMed PMID: 21764783. Epub 2011/07/19. eng.
112. Treves ST, Davis RT, Fahey FH. Administered radiopharmaceutical doses in children: a survey of 13 pediatric hospitals in North America. J Nucl Med. 2008;49(6):1024–7. PubMed PMID: 18483096. Epub 2008/05/17. eng.
113. Gelfand MJ, Parisi MT, Treves ST. Pediatric radiopharmaceutical administered doses: 2010 North American consensus guidelines. J Nucl Med. 2011;52(2):318–22.
114. Lassmann M, Biassoni L, Monsieurs M, Franzius C, Dosimetry E, Paediatrics C. The new EANM paediatric dosage card: additional notes with respect to F-18. Eur J Nucl Med Mol Imaging. 2008;35(9):1666–8. PubMed PMID: 18574583. Epub 2008/06/25. eng.
115. Lassmann M, Biassoni L, Monsieurs M, Franzius C, Dosimetry E, Paediatrics C. The new EANM paediatric dosage card: additional notes with respect to F-18. Eur J Nucl Med Mol Imaging. 2008;35(11):2141.
116. Lassmann M, Biassoni L, Monsieurs M, Franzius C, Jacobs F, Dosimetry E, et al. The new EANM paediatric dosage card. Eur J Nucl Med Mol Imaging. 2007;34(5):796–8. PubMed PMID: 17406866. Epub 2007/04/05. eng.
117. Williams J, Treves ST. PET/CT imaging in children: current techniques and indications. Appl Radiol. 2012;June:8–13.

118. Gelfand MJ, Lemen LC. PET/CT and SPECT/CT dosimetry in children: the challenge to the pediatric imager. Semin Nucl Med. 2007;37(5):391–8.
119. Girshin M, Shapiro V, Rhee A, Ginsberg S, Inchiosa Jr MA. Increased risk of general anesthesia for high-risk patients undergoing magnetic resonance imaging. J Comput Assist Tomogr. 2009;33(2):312–5. PubMed PMID: 19346867. Epub 2009/04/07. eng.
120. Cauldwell C. Anesthesia risks associated with pediatric imaging. Pediatr Radiol. 2011;41(8):949–50.
121. Greenberg S. Rebalancing the risks of computed tomography and magnetic resonance imaging. Pediatr Radiol. 2011;41(8):951–2.

Normal Development

2

Kamaldine Oudjhane

Contents

Abstract

The development of the musculoskeletal system encompasses the embryonic period, fetal development, and the lengthy postnatal period of growth and maturation. This chapter emphasizes the growth of the infant, child, and adolescent but briefly reviews key points of prenatal development. Understanding cartilage maturation is key to understanding bone development, as well as imaging of normal development and pathology. After reviewing the process of physeal bone deposition, the chapter presents MRI appearance of cartilage, focusing on the primary and secondary physes. It discusses normal developmental physiologic periostitis of infancy. The chapter concludes by discussing several different systems for establishing skeletal maturity and reviewing for which ages each is most applicable.

The development of the musculoskeletal system encompasses the embryonic period, fetal development, and the lengthy postnatal period of growth and maturation. This chapter emphasizes the development of the infant, child, and adolescent but briefly reviews key points of the prenatal period. Understanding cartilage maturation is key to understanding bone development, as well as imaging of normal development and pathology. After reviewing the process of physeal bone deposition, the chapter reviews the magnetic

K. Oudjhane, MD, MSc
Diagnostic Imaging Department,
The Hospital for Sick Children, University of Toronto,
555 University Avenue, Toronto, ON M5G 1X8, Canada
e-mail: kamaldine.oudjhane@sickkids.ca

R. Stein-Wexler et al. (eds.), *Pediatric Orthopedic Imaging*,
DOI 10.1007/978-3-642-45381-6_2, © Springer-Verlag Berlin Heidelberg 2015

resonance imaging (MRI) appearance of cartilage, focusing on the primary and secondary physes. It discusses normal developmental physiologic periostitis of infancy. The chapter concludes by discussing several different systems for establishing skeletal maturity and reviewing for which ages each is most applicable. Bone marrow maturation is presented in Chap. 25, which addresses both normal and pathologic bone marrow.

1 General Cartilage and Bone Development

1.1 Embryonic and Fetal Development

Musculoskeletal development starts during the embryonic period, or the first 8 weeks after conception. Following formation of the trilaminar embryonic disk during the first 2 weeks, induction starts the process of tissue specialization and subsequent organogenesis [1]. Primordial organogenesis occurs during the first 4 weeks, and major defects in limb development can occur at this time. Key landmarks of skeletal development in the embryo and fetus are summarized below.

Embryonic Development:

- Week 3: The embryonic disk develops, with individualization of somites and the neural tube.
- Week 4: The somites differentiate into three segments—dermatome (skin), myotome (muscle), and sclerotome (cartilage and bone). The embryo is very sensitive to major defects in limb development during this period. During week 4, the limb buds originate as elevations of the fetal unsegmented mesenchyme. The upper limb buds appear shortly before those of the lower limb, and the upper extremity continues to develop more quickly than the lower until about age 2 years.
- Week 5: Mesenchyme condenses in the limbs, and the hand plate is formed.
- Week 6: Mesenchyme chondrifies. Digits individualize.
- Week 7: Notching occurs between the digits, and the upper and lower limbs rotate in opposite directions.
- Week 8: The embryo is recognizably human.

Fetal Development:

The fetal stage is characterized by rapid changes in body proportions, with the following highlights:

- Week 12: Bone development spreads beyond the clavicle, the first bone to ossify. The relatively short lower limbs grow rapidly.
- Week 14: Clefting of mesenchyme results in the formation of synovial joints. This is followed by chondrification and cavitation.
- Week 16: The development of the neuromuscular system allows for spontaneous limb activity. Hematopoiesis, which had started in the yolk sac and then liver, begins in bone as the marrow space develops [2].
- Week 20: Growth and remodeling of body proportions continue, and the fetus develops an infant-like form.

Much of the skeleton forms by endochondral ossification. Mesenchyme condensation occurs first, forming cartilage, which is then transformed to bone [3]. This occurs at the skull base, long and tubular bones, clavicles, and vertebral column. Primary ossification centers develop within the diaphyses of the long bones, in the vertebrae, in a few epiphyses, and in some of the smaller bones before birth. Their formation requires changes in the perichondrium: degeneration of hypertrophic cells and increased vascularity form an ossified core at the cartilage-bone interface. Most of the epiphyses and small bones ossify after birth. The flat bones—such as the pelvis, scapula, skull, and facial bones—form by intramembranous ossification, which occurs without a cartilaginous precursor.

1.2 Infancy and Childhood

Fetal woven bone is flexible and has a high collagen content; it is replaced by lamellar bone during infancy. Most of the smaller bones develop primary ossification centers during infancy.

During childhood, the long bones undergo further growth, with tremendous increase in length as well as thickness. Secondary ossification centers develop at the ends of the long bones. Longitudinal growth of long bones depends principally on the primary physis, adjacent to the metaphysis. The secondary physis, which surrounds the epiphysis, results in the more spherical configuration at the ends of the long bones. Transverse growth at the diaphysis occurs by intramembranous bone formation at the periosteum, which consists of an outer fibrous layer and an inner layer composed of osteoprogenitor cells.

Physis

The physeal cartilage includes three well-defined histologic zones: resting, proliferative, and hypertrophic. Its composition is the same whether at the primary physis (abutting the metaphyses) or at the secondary physis (surrounding the secondary ossification centers), but the secondary physis is thinner. The resting zone is closest to the metaphysis or secondary ossification center and contains an abundant, disorganized matrix of chondrocytes. These are the germinator stem cells of the physis. The proliferative zone has longitudinal columns of rapidly dividing chondrocytes responsible for increased bone length. It is rich in glycogen; rapid extracellular matrix turnover takes place here. Chondrocyte proliferation and differentiation are highly regulated by secreted growth factors that activate chondrocyte-specific transcription factors [4]. The hypertrophic zone abuts the cartilage and includes a segment where chondrocytes mature, a segment of degeneration (with disintegration of mucopolysaccharides and declining blood supply), and a zone of provisional calcification. The zone of provisional calcification is closest to the metaphysis and marks the transition from bone to cartilage; this is the weakest part of the growth plate.

The periphery of the metaphysis, adjacent to the physis, is a very vascular site of active bone formation and remodeling. The perichondrial ring of LaCroix and the groove of Ranvier constitute the periphysis, a fibro-chondro-osseous structure that encircles the growth plate and the most recently developed portion of the metaphysis [5]. The periphysis and bone formed by the gradual transverse growth of the physis make up the metaphyseal collar in the young child; this may protrude from the metaphyseal contour and must be differentiated from a corner metaphyseal fracture (see Chap. 18).

The vascular system plays a major role in growth plate physiology [6]. Three major pathways supply the physis: the epiphyseal arteries of the secondary ossification center reach the proliferative segment, the diaphysial nutrient arteries provide a capillary network to the metaphyseal-physeal junction, and the perichondrial arteries supply the periphysis. Bone remodeling occurs by funnelization, with bone resorption and deposition; longitudinal growth and shaping at the epiphysis, metaphysis, and diaphysis result. The acrophyses, including the epiphyses, apophyses, carpals, tarsals, and growth plates at nonphyseal ends of the small tubular bones, make up the growth plates of the secondary ossification centers [7].

Cartilage

The ends of the long bones are composed of hyaline cartilage. Although all hyaline cartilage consists of chondrocytes and water within a matrix of collagen and glycosaminoglycans, the architecture and the exact composition vary. Epiphyseal cartilage, physeal cartilage (whether at the primary physis or at the secondary physis that surrounds the epiphyseal ossification center), and articular cartilage therefore appear different on some MRI sequences.

Articular cartilage is hypocellular and avascular; it consists predominantly of a collagen and proteoglycan matrix. Physeal cartilage is very cellular, especially the hypertrophic zone; it is vascular until age 18 months and then becomes avascular. Epiphyseal cartilage is very vascular while the ossification center is developing [8, 9]. The articular cartilage functions to transmit and buffer force, whereas the epiphyseal and physeal cartilage contribute to growth. With maturation, the appearance of epiphyseal and physeal cartilage changes.

2 Cartilage Imaging

MRI differentiates between joint fluid and articular cartilage; it can also differentiate between epiphyseal, physeal, and articular cartilage because of their different compositions [10]. At histological examination, hyaline cartilage of the epiphysis demonstrates chondrocytes within a matrix rich in water, collagen, glycoproteins, and glycosaminoglycans. The water is bound to collagen fibers, and only a small fraction is free. The orientation of the collagen fibers is uniform in the physeal and epiphyseal cartilage. However, in the articular cartilage—where it is less tightly bound to water—its pattern varies depending on location. The superficial collagen fibers parallel the articular surface, whereas those in the deep zone are perpendicular to the surface; those in the intermediate zone have a more random arrangement [11]. Some MRI sequences demonstrate subtle differences in signal intensity, corresponding to these different zones.

A variety of sequences have been developed to image cartilage, and others allow molecular and functional imaging. As a general rule, cartilage imaging requires at least a 1.5 tesla (T) magnet. Cartilage is, in general, isointense to muscle on T1-weighted (T1-W) imaging (Fig. 2.1) and relatively hypointense on fluid-sensitive sequences [12]. T1-W and intermediate-weighted proton density (PD) sequences are superb for showing morphology of ligaments and menisci. However, these sequences offer little information about architecture of the hyaline cartilage of the epiphysis, as its signal intensity is uniform on these sequences [13] (Fig. 2.2). Hyaline cartilage also shows uniform signal intensity (high to intermediate) on gradient echo (GRE) sequences. Decreasing the flip angle (to 15–20°) on these sequences increases T2 weighting and thus helps differentiate hypointense cartilage from more hyperintense joint fluid [8].

Fluid-sensitive sequences, such as short tau inversion recovery (STIR) and T2-weighted (T2-W) (especially fat-suppressed (FS) sequences), characterize cartilage architecture better than T1-W sequences (Fig. 2.3). On these fluid-sensitive sequences, signal intensity of physeal and articular cartilage is higher than that of epiphyseal cartilage, probably due to increased cellularity and free water in the growth plate cartilage compared with epiphyseal cartilage. Because the physeal cartilage has longer T2 values, increasing the echo time (TE) enhances the contrast between epiphyseal and physeal cartilage. 3D dual-echo steady-state imaging (3D-DESS) is also useful for imaging cartilage, improving the accuracy of cartilage thickness assessment (Fig. 2.4). Regardless of the sequence employed, adequate spatial resolution is essential for satisfactory imaging of cartilage.

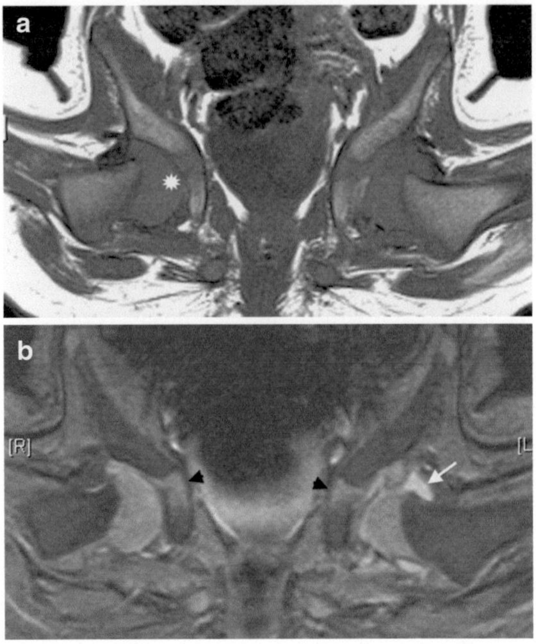

Fig. 2.1 Homogeneous appearance of femoral head cartilage in a 6-month-old. (**a**) Coronal T1-weighted (T1-W) image shows the epiphysis (*asterisk*) is of homogeneous intermediate signal intensity. (**b**) Coronal gradient echo (*GRE*), fast field echo (*FFE*) image shows moderately hyperintense cartilage signal, along with a small amount of very hyperintense joint fluid (*white arrow*) on the left. Note cartilaginous triradiate cartilage (*black arrowheads*), which has similar signal intensity to the femoral head

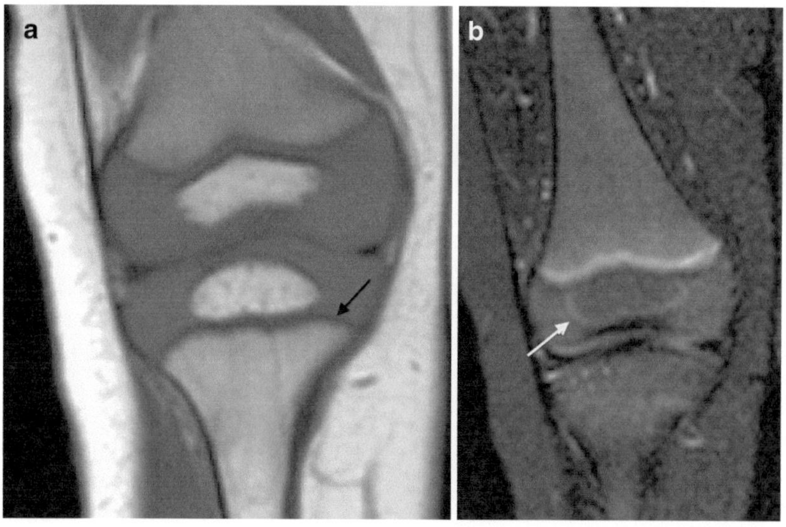

Fig. 2.2 Normal infant knee. (**a**) Coronal T1-W image shows the growth plate and epiphyseal cartilage have homogeneous intermediate signal. The zone of provisional calcification (*ZPC*) is hypointense (*arrow*) adjacent to the hyperintense metaphysis. (**b**) Coronal STIR image shows the primary physis is hyperintense, compared to the intermediate signal epiphyseal cartilage. The secondary physis, surrounding the epiphyseal ossification center, is also hyperintense (*arrow*) but much thinner than the primary physis (Courtesy of Marilyn Ranson)

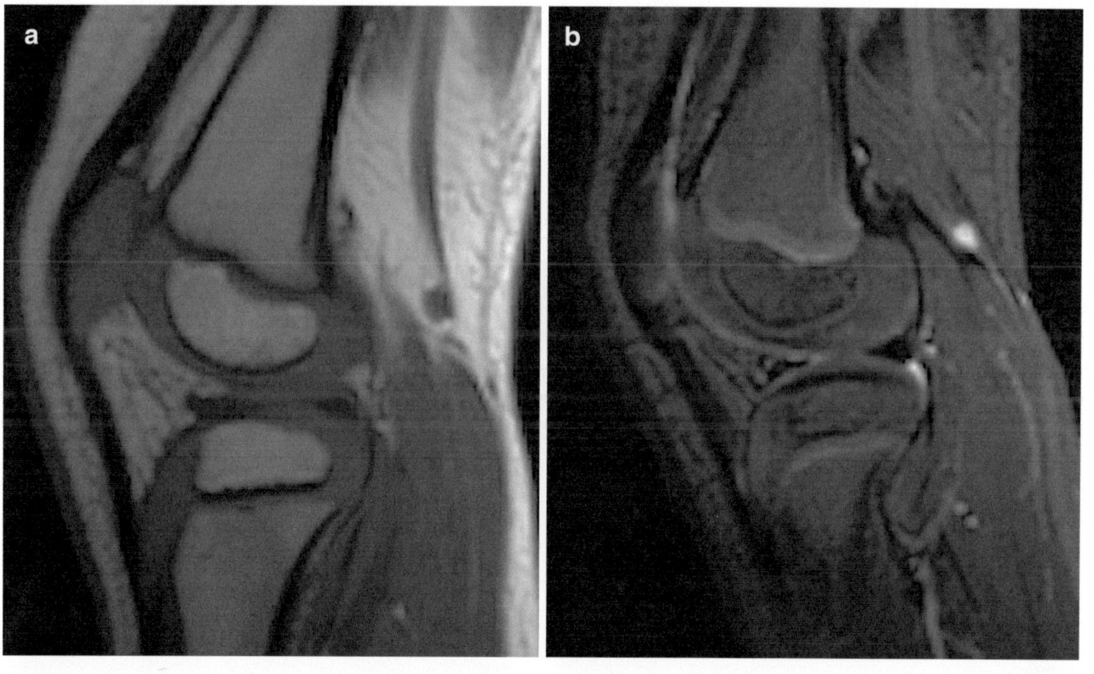

Fig. 2.3 Epiphyseal cartilage in a 4-year-old boy. (**a**) Sagittal T1-W image shows uniformly isointense cartilage (compared to muscle). (**b**) Sagittal inversion recovery (*IR*) image shows isointense signal intensity (compared to muscle) in the cartilage surrounding the ossified epiphysis and hyperintense physeal cartilage (Courtesy of Rebecca Stein-Wexler)

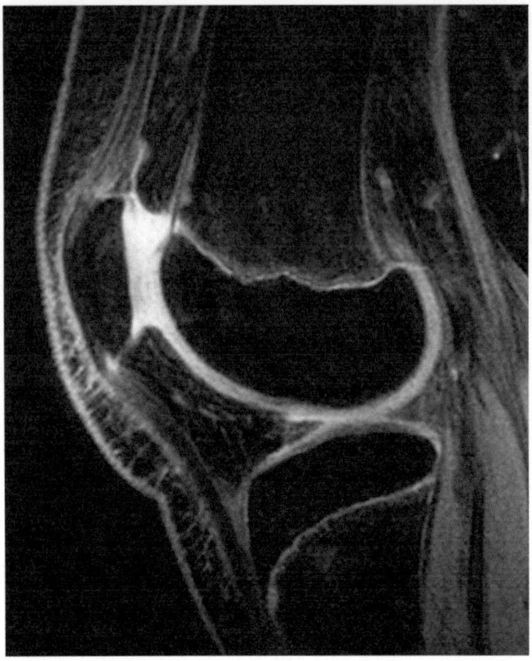

Fig. 2.4 Epiphyseal cartilage contrasted against joint fluid on sagittal 3D double-echo steady-state (*3D-DESS*) image of the knee in a 13-year-old boy. The epiphyseal and articular hyaline cartilage is slightly less bright than the joint fluid

With development, the cartilage changes in several ways. Epiphyseal cartilage evolves from its infantile appearance of uniform intermediate signal on T1-W images and moderate hyperintensity on fluid-sensitive sequences [12]. As ossification begins, fluid-sensitive sequences demonstrate patchy, heterogeneous (more hyperintense) areas, likely due to increased free water. These are most evident at the posterior distal femoral condyle and the trochlea of the distal humerus, but are also seen elsewhere [14] (Fig. 2.5). Cartilage at weight-bearing areas (e.g., the acetabulum and the distal and proximal femur) develops decreased T2 signal as the child begins walking, probably as water is displaced from cartilage [15] (Fig. 2.6).

The physeal cartilage at both the primary physis and at the peri-epiphyseal secondary physis has specific architecture that yields a trilaminar appearance on MRI (Figs. 2.7 and 2.8). The portion that abuts the metaphysis, the zone of provisional calcification, is densely mineralized and thus markedly hypointense on all sequences. The remainder of the physeal cartilage, like the articular cartilage, resembles unossified epiphyseal cartilage on T1-W images and is predominantly hypointense. However, on fluid-sensitive sequences, this portion of the physis (the germinal and proliferative zones as well as part of the hypertrophic zone) is brighter than epiphyseal cartilage, yielding the second identifiable layer [13]. The

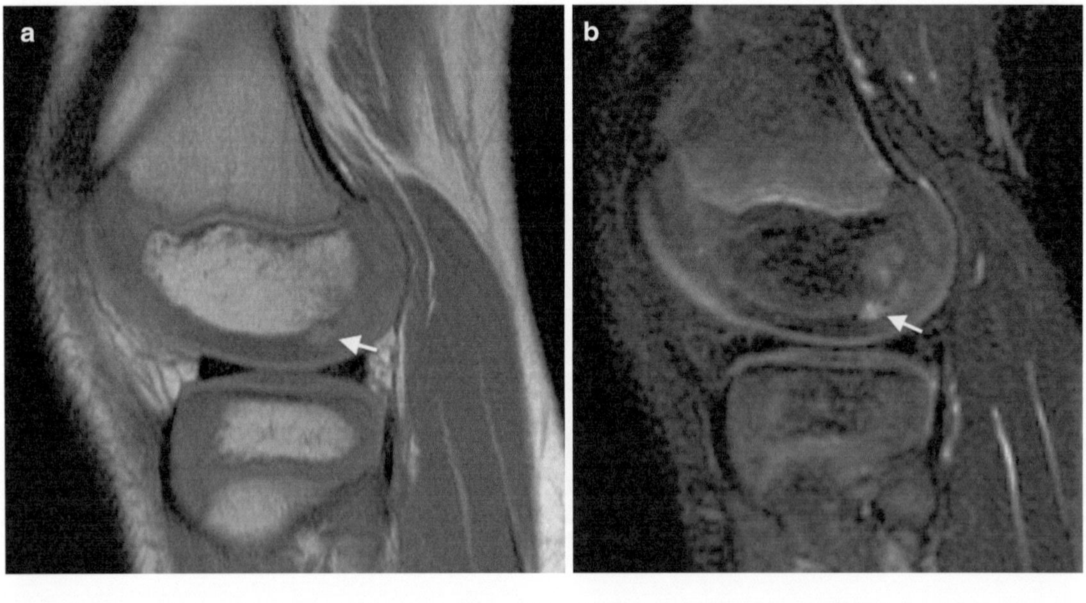

Fig. 2.5 Normal hyperintense pre-ossification centers within epiphyseal cartilage. Sagittal PD (**a**) and fast spin echo (*FSE*) T2-W FS (**b**) show pre-ossification (*arrows*) (Courtesy of Marilyn Ranson)

Fig. 2.6 *Morphological* changes in cartilage with maturation in a 6-year-old boy. Sagittal T2-weighted (*T2-W*) image with fat-suppressed (*FS*) knee image shows the weight-bearing epiphyseal cartilage of the femoral condyle has a relatively low signal, likely related to displacement of water from cartilage (*arrow*). A focus of increased signal in the posterior epiphyseal cartilage of femoral cartilage (*curved arrow*) likely represents the hyperintense fluid condensation that can be seen prior to the onset of ossification. In addition, the hyperintense articular cartilage (*arrowhead*) contrasts against the more intermediate signal of the epiphyseal cartilage

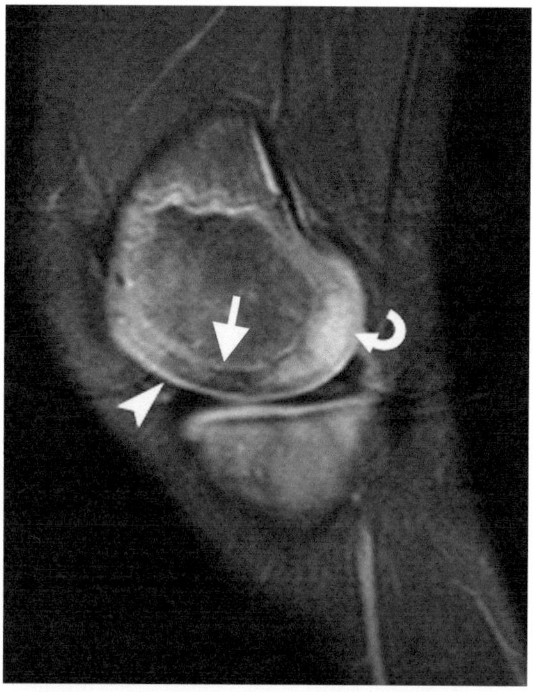

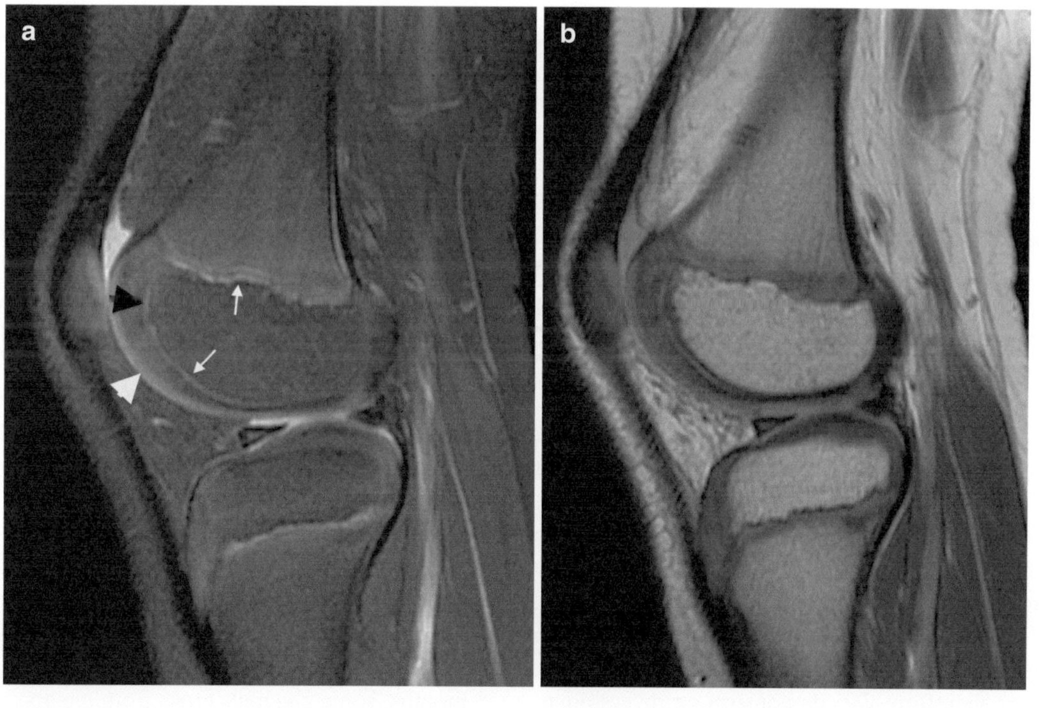

Fig. 2.7 Normal appearance of physeal, epiphyseal, and articular cartilage in a 7-year-old boy. (**a**) Sagittal PD FS image shows hypointense ZPC (*white arrows*), moderately hyperintense physeal cartilage (*black arrowhead*), and moderately hyperintense articular cartilage (*white arrowhead*). The ossified portion of the epiphysis is hypointense, and the remainder of the epiphyseal cartilage is heterogeneously hyperintense. (**b**) Sagittal PD image also demonstrates the various cartilage regions (Courtesy of Rebecca Stein-Wexler)

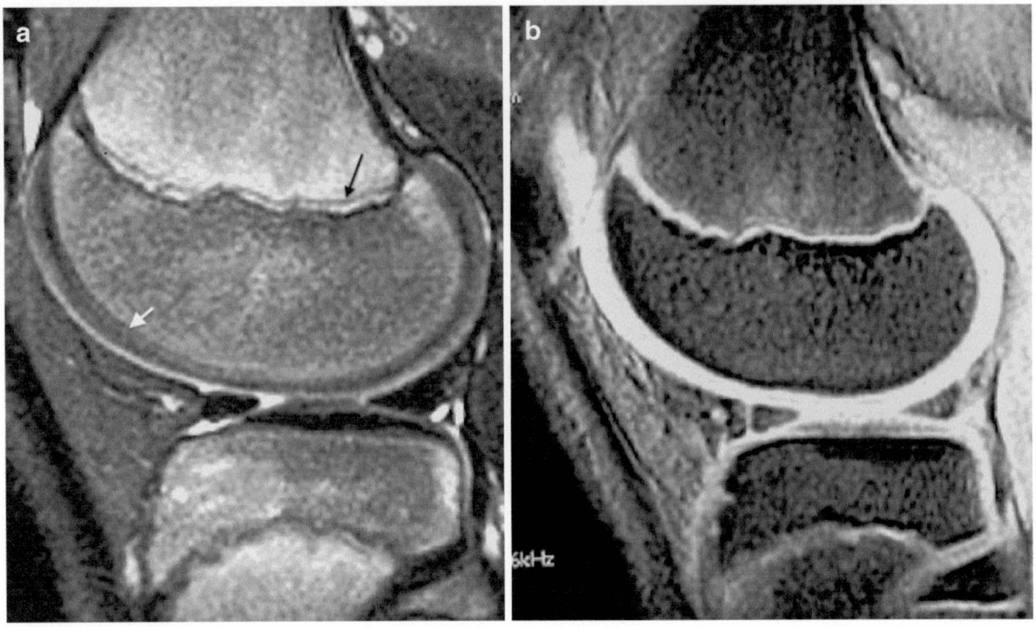

Fig. 2.8 Normal appearance of cartilage in an adolescent knee. (**a**) Sagittal FSE T2-W FS image shows trilaminar appearance with hyperintense metaphyseal spongiosa, hypointense ZPC (*black arrow*), and hyperintense physis. The epiphyseal cartilage (*white arrow*) has lower signal than articular cartilage. (**b**) Sagittal multiplanar T1-W GRE image shows uniformly bright cartilage signal (Courtesy of Marilyn Ranson)

physis that surrounds the ossification center in the epiphysis, the secondary physis, has similar architecture and signal intensity but is thinner.

Epiphyseal ossification begins in a single ossification center (as at the distal femur), in two centers (as at the proximal humerus), or in several centers (as at the trochlea of the distal humerus). The contour may be irregular. Normal signal intensity at MRI helps differentiate multiple ossification centers from fragmentation of a single center. If there is a single focus of ossification, ossification begins in the center of the epiphysis. Initially spherical, as endochondral bone forms, the shape changes to hemispheric, with the flat portion adjacent to the primary physis [16]. Although epiphyseal marrow is initially, like the adjacent metaphysis, hematopoietic, within a few months it becomes uniformly fatty (see Chap. 25).

Development of carpal bones, tarsal bones, and apophyses is similar to that of epiphyses. They therefore also demonstrate conversion to fatty marrow much sooner than do the metaphyses of long bones.

In very young children, the primary physis is flat and smooth, but with growth its contour begins to undulate [8]. It should still have uniform thickness, unless it has been damaged (e.g., after fracture or as a result of chronic stress in athletes). The physis thins with maturation and eventually fuses and disappears, sometimes leaving a very thin hypointense linear scar. Physeal fusion usually begins in the center of the physis and spreads to the periphery. The exception to this is at the distal tibia, where the anteromedial physis fuses first (at Kump's bump) and fusion progresses posterolaterally.

Epiphyseal cartilage is initially perfused by vessels within cartilage canals; these gradually become smaller and less numerous. Vascularization is most readily appreciated after administration of intravenous gadolinium, on fat-suppressed T1-W images. The vascular channels of the cartilaginous epiphysis exhibit linear and punctate areas of high signal intensity (the punctate areas are vascular channels viewed on end). Before the age of 18 months, some channels cross from metaphysis to epiphysis, and vascular canals are arrayed parallel to each other and to the long axis of the bone. As the secondary ossification center develops, the orientation of the vascular channels changes, so

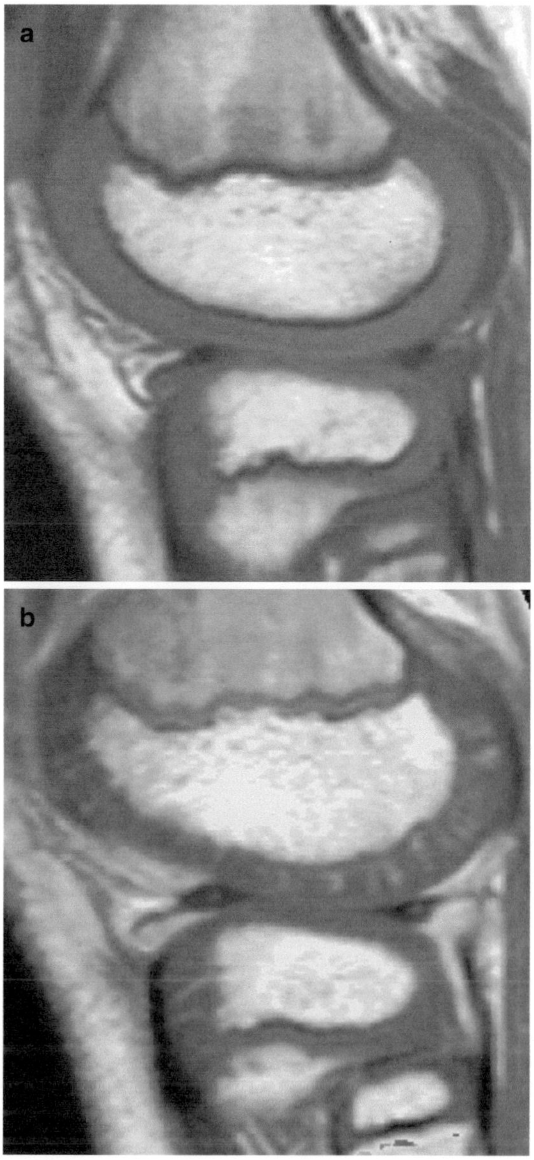

Fig. 2.9 Radiating array of epiphyseal vessels in a young child. (**a**) Sagittal T1-W MRI shows homogeneous intermediate signal of the epiphyseal and articular cartilage. (**b**) With GRE, radiating vascular channels are evident. The physes also enhance (Courtesy of Marilyn Ranson)

that they are arrayed in a spoke-like fashion around the ossifying epiphysis [9] (Fig. 2.9). During most of childhood, metaphyseal and epiphyseal blood flow are separate, with important consequences for trauma as well as spread of infection and tumor.

Gadolinium-enhanced sequences allow definition of the fibrovascular cuff and the primary

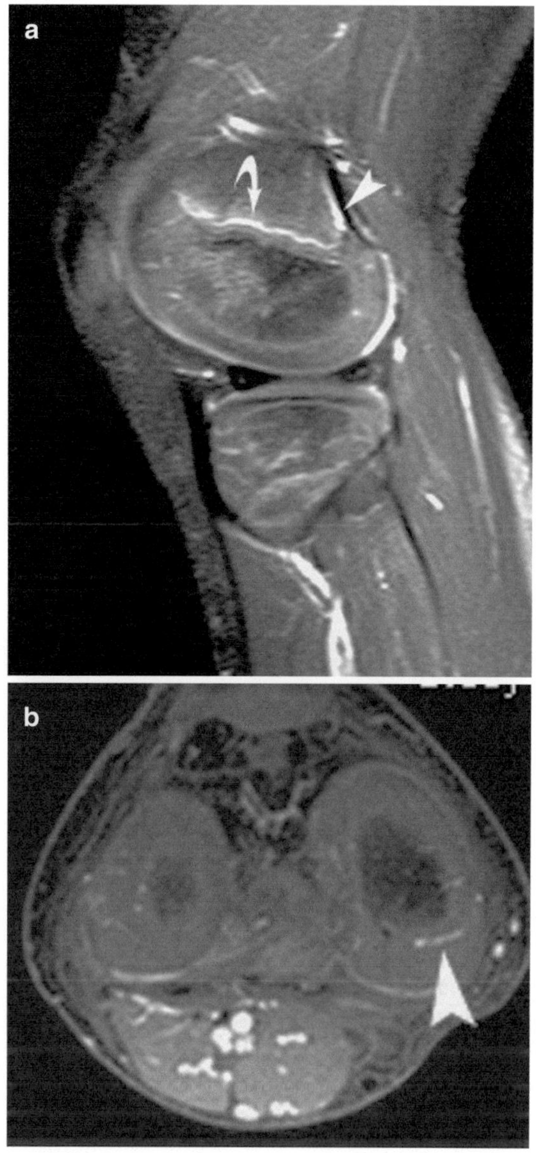

Fig. 2.10 Normal appearance of epiphyseal vasculature in a 6-year-old. Gadolinium-enhanced T1-W fast field echo (*FFE*) fat-suppressed (*FS*) MRI shows, on sagittal view (**a**), enhancement of the primary spongiosa of new metaphyseal bone (*curved arrow*). There is also enhancement of the subperiosteal fibrovascular tissue that forms the posterior metaphyseal stripe (*arrowhead*). (**b**) Axial image shows typical spoke-wheel pattern of vascular channels in the epiphyseal cartilage (*arrowhead*)

spongiosa of new bone formation; it also delineates the posterior metaphyseal stripe, which is a subperiosteal band of fibrovascular tissue that contributes to growth (Fig. 2.10). In older patients, specialized MRI techniques such as delayed gadolinium-enhanced MRI (dGEMRIC) and T2 mapping allow visualization of the four unique zones of articular cartilage: superficial or tangential, middle or transitional, deep or radial, and calcified [11]. In higher field-strength magnets, 3D isotropic techniques can be applied to cartilage imaging [17].

3 Physiologic Periostitis of Infancy (Box 2.1)

> **Box 2.1: Physiologic Periostitis of Infancy**
>
> 1–4 months old (residual findings occasionally seen to 6 months old)
>
> Bilateral in 40–70 %
>
> Frequency: tibia > femur > humerus > ulna > radius
>
> <2 mm thick
>
> Diaphysis

Physiologic periostitis of infancy is a normal physiologic process wherein new bone forms rapidly by intramembranous ossification along the periosteum of the diaphysis of long bones. This can be identified in one third to one half of infants between 1 and 4 months of age. The residual finding of subperiosteal bone blending into cortex can be seen occasionally as late as 6 months of age [18]. Periosteal new bone results from the rapid growth that is characteristic of early infancy, combined with the fact that in children the periosteum is relatively thick and loosely attached. It generally involves both the upper and lower extremities [19] and is bilateral in 40–75 % (especially at the femur) [18]. The tibia is affected most often, followed by the femur, humerus, ulna, and radius.

The periosteal new bone initially appears as a faint amorphous line paralleling the diaphysis of the long bone, separated from the cortex by a thin lucent line. Not necessarily concentric, it may be seen on only one projection (Fig. 2.11). As the child grows, the layer of new bone thickens and becomes denser, briefly resembling a double cortex. It is gradually absorbed into the cortex, where it contributes to bone width.

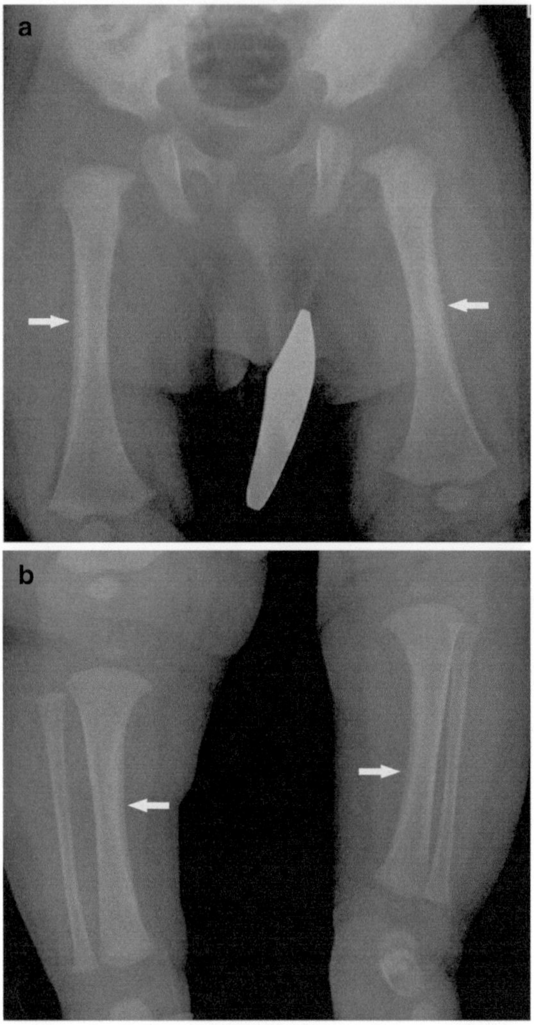

Fig. 2.11 Physiologic periostitis of infancy in a 2-month-old boy. Frontal views show bilateral lamellar bone formation (*arrows*) along the lateral diaphyseal cortex of both femurs (**a**) and along the medial diaphyseal cortex of both tibias (**b**)

Physiologic periostitis is differentiated from pathologic periostitis by its thinness (less than 2 mm), by the fact that it spares the metaphysis, and by the typical age at presentation, 1–4 months [18]. It should not be confused with osteomyelitis, infantile cortical hyperostosis, trauma, vitamin A intoxication, leukemia, or metastatic neuroblastoma.

4 Skeletal Maturation

Assessment of skeletal maturity is important in several clinical scenarios: in the setting of a suspected hormonal abnormality (e.g., precocious puberty), to help predict adult height (especially important in children with short stature), and to determine appropriate timing of surgery for scoliosis or for leg-length discrepancy. Radiologic assessment of skeletal maturity relies on evaluation of mineralization, maturation, and morphology of the ossification centers and comparison of these observations to standards.

Many methods of bone age assessment have been developed, but they are plagued by questions about accuracy, statistical validity, and interobserver variability [20, 21]. Furthermore, there are marked sexual, racial, familial, and environmental influences on bone development. For example, the sequence of ossification in the hand and wrist varies such that the triquetrum may ossify in any order ranging from the 3rd to the 24th of the 28 centers [22]. Some standards are based on a specific population group and do not necessarily apply to others [21, 23]. Girls differ from boys, not only in their advanced maturity but also in the order of ossification, and black infants are more skeletally mature than white infants. Therefore it is important to consider the standards as approximations and to always include a range of two standard deviations in estimating bone age. Computer-assisted measurement appears to increase statistical power [24].

Skeletal maturity in different parts of the body can be discordant, and this affects timing of surgical intervention. Discrepancy may be striking in the hand and wrist, where carpal maturation may lag behind or precede phalangeal maturation by several years. This can be syndromic or associated with disease but is more often inconsequential. However, up to 40 % of patients demonstrate a 1-year difference in physeal fusion between the distal forearm and the leg, and physeal closure in the hand may precede or follow physeal closure in the tibia by up to 2 years. This has important implications for timing of surgery. More important than the precise stage of skeletal maturity of the hand, elbow, or iliac crest is the state of maturation in the bone (or bones) being considered for potential intervention.

Skeletal maturity may be assessed by several methods, depending on patient age. In premature infants and during the prenatal period, the presence of specific ossification centers correlates with patient age. During the first year of life, the method of Sontag can be used (see below) [25]. During much of childhood, skeletal age determination is based on a PA view of the left hand, according to the methods of Greulich and Pyle, Tanner, Gilsanz and Ratib, and others [26–28]. However, during the pubertal growth spurt, these methods become less accurate, and skeletal age can be determined by the configuration of the olecranon apophysis [29] and then, later, by the status of the iliac crest apophysis [30].

Before birth and in premature infants, age can be assessed by determining whether ossification has begun in key centers. A few important prenatal ossification standards follow:

- Dental buds at 20–21 weeks, +/− 2 weeks
- Calcaneus at 24 weeks
- Talus at 28 weeks
- Distal femur epiphysis at 36 weeks
- Proximal tibial epiphysis at 38 weeks
- Proximal humeral epiphysis at 40–41 weeks

In addition, throughout childhood, multiple ossification centers provide rough landmarks for skeletal maturity [20] (see Table 2.1).

In infants less than 1 year old, skeletal maturation can be determined by the Sontag method [25]. This method counts secondary ossification centers in half of the skeleton, based on a radiograph of the entire left upper extremity (including the shoulder to the distal epiphyses of the fingers) and a second radiograph of most of the left lower extremity (from the mid-femur to the distal epiphyses). All secondary ossification centers except the talus and calcaneus are counted, including the coracoid and other centers at the shoulder. The total number of ossification centers in the hemiskeleton is compared with normal values for children up to age 1.5 years (see Table 2.2).

From age 1 year through adolescence, evaluation of the hand is generally performed, though interpretation is plagued by questions of statistical accuracy. Specificity is lower and standard deviations greater during the adolescent growth spurt, and other bones may be evaluated at this age, as discussed below. The Greulich and Pyle

Table 2.1 Selected ossification centers, 50th percentile age at appearance

	50th percentile age at appearance	
	Boys	Girls
1. Infancy		
Capitate	3 m	2 m
Hamate	4 m	2 m
Capitellum of humerus	4 m	3 m
Capital femoral epiphysis	4 m	4 m
Cuneiform 3	6 m	3 m
Humerus greater tuberosity	10 m	6 m
2. Early childhood		
Cuneiform 1	2 y, 2 m	1 y, 5 m
Cuneiform 2	2 y, 8 m	1 y, 10 m
Navicular of the foot	3 y	1 y, 11 m
Fibula proximal epiphysis	3 y, 6 m	2 y, 7 m
Patella	4 y	2 y, 6 m
3. Childhood		
Radius head	5 y, 3 m	3 y, 10 m
Medial epicondyle of humerus	6 y, 3 m	3 y, 5 m
Calcaneal apophysis	7 y, 7 m	5 y, 4 m
Olecranon of ulna	9 y, 8 m	8 y
Lateral epicondyle of humerus	11 y, 3 m	9 y, 3 m
4. Adolescence		
Tibial tubercle	11 y, 10 m	10 y, 3 m
Adductor sesamoid of thumb	12 y, 9 m	10 y, 9 m
Acromion	13 y, 9 m	11 y, 11 m
Iliac crest	14 y	12 y, 9 m
Coracoid apophysis	14 y, 4 m	12 y, 3 m
Ischial tuberosity	15 y, 3 m	13 y, 11 m

Adapted from Ref. [20]
y year, *m* month

Table 2.2 Age based on presence of hemi-skeleton ossification centers in the infant

	Number of centers in boys		Number of centers in girls	
Age (months)	Mean	1 S.D.	Mean	1 S.D.
1	4.1	1.4	4.6	1.8
3	6.6	1.9	7.8	2.2
6	9.6	1.9	11.4	2.5
9	11.9	2.6	15.4	4.9
12	14	4.0	22.4	6.9
18	19.3	6.6	34.1	8.4

Adapted from Ref. [25]

method compares the appearance, growth, modeling, and fusion of the metacarpal and phalangeal epiphyses as well as the carpal centers to standard hand radiographs [26]. Table 2.3 is based on the atlas of Greulich and Pyle and summarizes changes during the early adolescent period after ossification of the adductor sesamoid. Tanner's method assigns a score to the carpal bones (except the pisiform) and to the epiphyses of the distal ulna, distal radius, and metacarpals and phalanges of the first, third, and fifth rays. These are summed to establish an individual's skeletal maturity scale and do not directly refer to patient age [27]. A digitally formatted atlas of the hand, developed by Gilsanz and Ratib, includes a large range of sample populations and is statistically more accurate [28].

Assessment of skeletal maturity around puberty is very important, because the success of some surgical interventions depends on the precise timing of when they are performed. Puberty can be divided into two phases: acceleration and deceleration [31]. The pubertal growth spurt (on average, age 11–13 for girls and 13–15 for boys) is considered accelerational. Growth is rapid—and the rate of growth increases—during this time. The subsequent 3 years (on average, age 13–16 for girls and 15–18 for boys) are considered decelerational, as growth gradually ceases. Different methods of bone age assessment have varying utility during these periods.

The Sauvegrain method, which evaluates the ossification centers of the elbow, assesses maturation during growth acceleration but is static during deceleration, when all physes have fused. The Risser method, in contrast, which evaluates the iliac crest apophysis, is static during acceleration but useful during deceleration. The method of Greulich and Pyle is fairly accurate before the pubertal growth spurt but relatively imprecise during both the accelerational and decelerational growth phases.

During the acceleration phase of skeletal maturation, the ossification centers of the elbow change dramatically, from being predominantly cartilaginous to being fully fused. Indeed, they change enough in the course of 6 months to allow determination of skeletal maturity on a semiannual basis, which helps fine-tune surgical planning. The Sauvegrain method analyzes the size and shape of the lateral condyle and epicondyle, trochlea, olecranon, and radial head apophyses on

Table 2.3 Estimation of skeletal age in adolescence

	Skeletal age in boys		Skeletal age in girls	
Bone	Age (years)	1 S.D. (months)	Age (years)	1 S.D. (months)
Small adductor sesamoid	13	10.4	11	11.9
Large adductor sesamoid	13.5–14	10.7	12	10.2
DP 1, fusion almost complete DP 2–5, partial fusion in male	15	11.3	13	10.6
DP, all fused PP, partial fusion	15.5	–	13.5	–
DP, all fused MP, partial fusion PP, fusion almost complete	16	12.9	14	11.3
DP, MP, PP, all fused	17	13	15	9.2
Radius, partial fusion	18	–	16	7.3

Adapted from Ref. [26]
DP distal phalanx epiphysis, *MP* middle phalanx epiphysis, *PP* proximal phalanx epiphysis

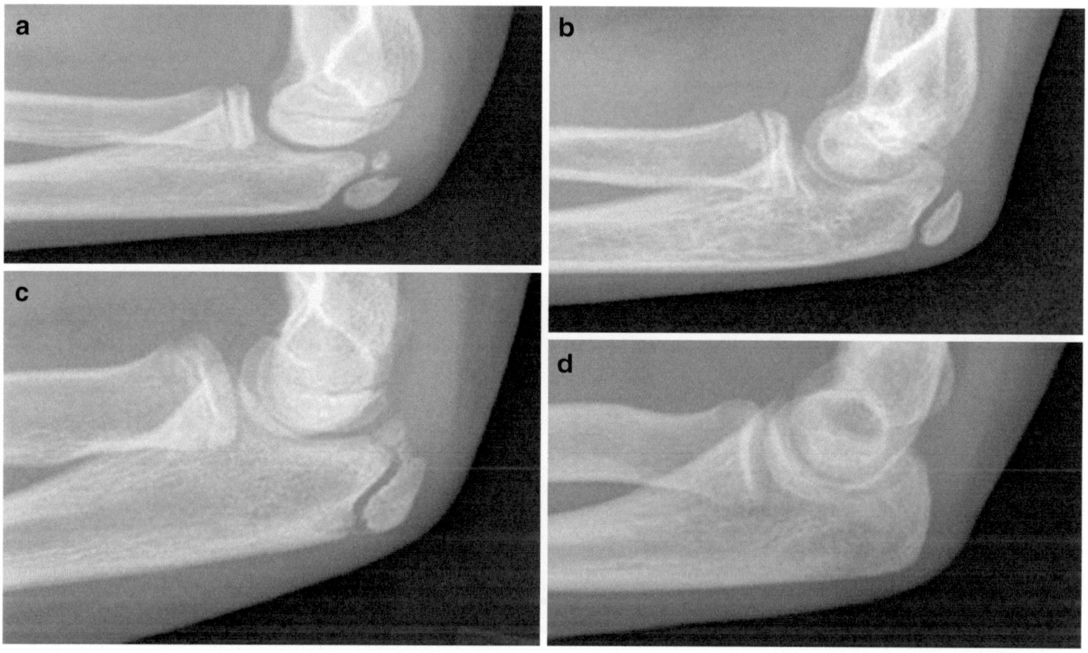

Fig. 2.12 Maturation of the olecranon. According to the simplified Sauvegrain method, the configuration of the olecranon ossification changes from (**a**) two ossific centers, to (**b**) a single half-moon-shaped center, to (**c**) a rectangular center, to (**d**) a center that has completely fused to the ulna

frontal and lateral views to provide a relatively accurate means of assessing skeletal maturity [29]. It is also possible to employ a simplified Sauvegrain method, which focuses on the appearance of the olecranon apophysis viewed on a lateral radiograph [31]. The olecranon changes from having two ossification centers initially (at age 11 in girls, 13 in boys) to resembling a half-moon 6 months later and to appearing more rectangular after another 6 months. It then begins fusion (age 12.5 in girls, 14.5 in boys) and 6 months later is fully fused to the ulna [31] (Fig. 2.12) (Table 2.4).

The configuration of the iliac crest apophysis begins to change 6 months after the elbow physes close, so Risser staging is applied to the decelerational growth phase. The apophysis at the iliac crest ossifies in a predictable manner—initially lateral, with progressive ossification of the more

Table 2.4 Skeletal maturation indices in the second decade

Girls	Boys	Risser scale	Olecranon	Fusion of epiphyses
11 y	13 y	0	2 centers	
11.5 y	13.5 y		Half-moon	
12 y	14 y		Rectangle	
12.5 y	14.5 y		Begins fusion	
13 y	15 y		Fusion complete	
13 y, 8 m	14 y, 7 m	1		Distal phalanx epiphyses [2–5]
14 y, 6 m	15 y, 7 m	2		Proximal phalanx epiphyses
				Greater trochanter apophysis
15 y, 2 m	16 y, 2 m	3		Distal phalanx epiphyses [1, 2]
16 y, 2 m	17 y	4		Distal ulnar epiphysis
18 y, 1 m	18 y, 6 m	5		Distal radial epiphysis

Adapted from Refs. [26, 30–32]
y year, *m* month

central portions as the more peripheral portions undergo fusion. At Risser 0, the apophysis has not yet ossified, and at Risser 5 it is fully formed and fused. The intermediate stages divide the iliac crest into quartiles (see Chap. 3 for additional discussion of the Risser method).

Maturation of the hand, elbow, and iliac crest should correlate (Table 2.4). The olecranon matures during early puberty (11–13 years in girls, 13–15 years in boys), when the iliac crest registers as Risser 0 (non-ossified apophysis). Risser 1 occurs at the same time as fusion of the distal phalanges in the hand. At Risser 2, the greater trochanter fuses to the femur, and the metacarpal epiphyses fuse. Risser 3 occurs at the same time as closure of the epiphyses of the middle phalanges. At Risser 4, the distal ulna fuses. Finally, Risser 5 is a lengthy period during which the distal radius epiphysis gradually fuses to the radius.

Skeletal maturity can also be used to estimate adult stature. The Bayley and Pinneau tables [33] are easy to use, but a more accurate system devised by Roche and colleagues integrates variables such as present height, weight, skeletal age, and parental stature [34].

References

1. Hall BK. The embryonic development of bone. Am Sci. 1988;76(2):174–81.
2. Babyn PS, Ranson M, McCarville ME. Normal bone marrow: signal characteristics and fatty conversion. Magn Reson Imaging Clin N Am. 1998;6(3):473–95. PubMed PMID: 9654581.
3. Dietz FR, Morcuende JA. Embryology and development of the musculoskeletal system. In: Morrissy RT, Weinstein SL, editors. Lovell and Winter's pediatric orthopedics: sixth edition. 6th ed. Philadelphia: Lippincott Williams & Wilkins; 2005. p. 1–33.
4. Wuelling M, Vortkamp A. Chondrocyte proliferation and differentiation. Endocr Dev. 2011;21:1–11. PubMed PMID: 21865749.
5. Oestreich AE, Ahmad BS. The periphysis and its effect on the metaphysis: I. Definition and normal radiographic pattern. Skeletal Radiol. 1992;21(5):283–6. PubMed PMID: 1502578.
6. Gray H, Standring S, Ellis H, Berkovitz BKB. Gray's anatomy: the anatomical basis of clinical practice. 39th ed. Edinburgh/New York: Elsevier Churchill Livingstone; 2005. xx, 1627 pp.
7. Oestreich AE. The acrophysis: a unifying concept for enchondral bone growth and its disorders. I. Normal growth. Skeletal Radiol. 2003;32(3):121–7. PubMed PMID: 12605274.
8. Jaramillo D, Laor T. Pediatric musculoskeletal MRI: basic principles to optimize success. Pediatr Radiol. 2008;38(4):379–91. PubMed PMID: 18046547.
9. Barnewolt CE, Shapiro F, Jaramillo D. Normal gadolinium-enhanced MR images of the developing appendicular skeleton: Part I. Cartilaginous epiphysis and physis. AJR Am J Roentgenol. 1997;169(1):183–9. PubMed PMID: 9207522.
10. Khanna PC, Thapa MM. The growing skeleton: MR imaging appearances of developing cartilage. Magn Reson Imaging Clin N Am. 2009;17(3):411–21, v. PubMed PMID: 19524193.
11. Potter HG, Foo LF. Magnetic resonance imaging of articular cartilage: trauma, degeneration, and repair. Am J Sports Med. 2006;34(4):661–77. PubMed PMID: 16365371.
12. Laor T, Jaramillo D. MR imaging insights into skeletal maturation: what is normal? Radiology. 2009;250(1):28–38. PubMed PMID: 19092089.
13. Jaramillo D, Connolly SA, Mulkern RV, Shapiro F. Developing epiphysis: MR imaging characteristics and histologic correlation in the newborn lamb.

Radiology. 1998;207(3):637–45. PubMed PMID: 9609885.
14. Chapman VM, Nimkin K, Jaramillo D. The preossification center: normal CT and MRI findings in the trochlea. Skeletal Radiol. 2004;33(12):725–7. PubMed PMID: 15322770.
15. Varich LJ, Laor T, Jaramillo D. Normal maturation of the distal femoral epiphyseal cartilage: age-related changes at MR imaging. Radiology. 2000;214(3):705–9. PubMed PMID: 10715034.
16. Rivas R, Shapiro F. Structural stages in the development of the long bones and epiphyses: a study in the New Zealand white rabbit. J Bone Joint Surg Am. 2002;84-A(1):85–100. PubMed PMID: 11792784.
17. Naraghi A, White LM. Three-dimensional MRI of the musculoskeletal system. AJR Am J Roentgenol. 2012;199(3):W283–93. PubMed PMID: 22915419.
18. Kwon DS, Spevak MR, Fletcher K, Kleinman PK. Physiologic subperiosteal new bone formation: prevalence, distribution, and thickness in neonates and infants. AJR Am J Roentgenol. 2002;179(4):985–8. PubMed PMID: 12239052.
19. Shopfner CE. Periosteal bone growth in normal infants. A preliminary report. Am J Roentgenol Radium Ther Nucl Med. 1966;97(1):154–63. PubMed PMID: 5938033.
20. Graham CB. Assessment of bone maturation–methods and pitfalls. Radiol Clin North Am. 1972;10(2):185–202. PubMed PMID: 4339776.
21. Ontell FK, Ivanovic M, Ablin DS, Barlow TW. Bone age in children of diverse ethnicity. AJR Am J Roentgenol. 1996;167(6):1395–8. PubMed PMID: 8956565.
22. Garn SM, Rohmann CG, Silverman FN. Radiographic standards for postnatal ossification and tooth calcification. Med Radiogr Photogr. 1967;43(2):45–66. PubMed PMID: 6056078.
23. Gilsanz V, Skaggs DL, Kovanlikaya A, Sayre J, Loro ML, Kaufman F, et al. Differential effect of race on the axial and appendicular skeletons of children. J Clin Endocrinol Metab. 1998;83(5):1420–7. PubMed PMID: 9589632.
24. Gross GW, Boone JM, Bishop DM. Pediatric skeletal age: determination with neural networks. Radiology. 1995;195(3):689–95. PubMed PMID: 7753995.
25. Sontag LWS D, Anderson M. Rate of appearance of ossification centers from birth to the age of five years. Am J Dis Child. 1939;58:949–56.
26. Greulich WW, Pyle SI. Radiographic atlas of skeletal development of the hand and wrist. 2nd ed. Stanford: Stanford University Press; 1959. xvi, 256 pp.
27. Tanner JM. Assessment of skeletal maturity and prediction of adult height (TW2 method). London/New York: Academic; 1975. vii, 99 pp.
28. Gilsanz V, Ratib O. Hand bone age: a digital atlas of skeletal maturity. 2nd ed. New York: Springer; 2012.
29. Sauvegrain J, Nahum H, Bronstein H. Study of bone maturation of the elbow. Ann Radiol. 1962;5:542–50. PubMed PMID: 13986863.
30. Risser JC. The Iliac apophysis; an invaluable sign in the management of scoliosis. Clin Orthop. 1958;11:111–9. PubMed PMID: 13561591.
31. Dimeglio A, Charles YP, Daures JP, de Rosa V, Kabore B. Accuracy of the Sauvegrain method in determining skeletal age during puberty. J Bone Joint Surg Am. 2005;87(8):1689–96. PubMed PMID: 16085606.
32. Scoles PV, Salvagno R, Villalba K, Riew D. Relationship of iliac crest maturation to skeletal and chronologic age. J Pediatr Orthop. 1988;8(6):639–44. PubMed PMID: 3192691.
33. Bayley N, Pinneau SR. Tables for predicting adult height from skeletal age: revised for use with the Greulich-Pyle hand standards. J Pediatr. 1952; 40(4):423–41. PubMed PMID: 14918032.
34. Roche AF, Wainer H, Thissen D. Predicting adult stature for individuals. Monogr Paediatr. 1975;3:1–114. PubMed PMID: 1109427.

Part II

Isolated Spine and Extremity Disorders: Congenital, Developmental, and Acquired

The Spine: Congenital and Developmental Conditions

3

Benjamin H. Taragin and Sandra L. Wootton-Gorges

Contents

B.H. Taragin, MD
Division of Pediatric Radiology,
Children's Hospital at Montefiore,
111 E. 210 St., Bronx, NY 10467, USA
e-mail: btaragin@montefiore.org

S.L. Wootton-Gorges, MD (✉)
Department of Radiology,
University of California Davis Medical
Center and UC Davis Children's Hospital,
4860 Y Street, Suite 3100, Sacramento, CA 95817, USA

Department of Diagnostic Imaging,
Shriners Hospitals for Children Northern
California, Sacramento, CA, USA
e-mail: sandra.gorges@ucdmc.ucdavis.edu

Abstract

The chapter initially discusses normal spinal development and variants. Pathology is addressed first in terms of general structural vertebral anomalies. These are then applied to congenital scoliosis, kyphosis, and lordosis, as well as anomalies involving the craniovertebral junction. Discussion of spinal dysraphism follows, including tethered filum terminale, hydrosyringomyelia, and diastematomyelia. Congenital intraspinal tumors are briefly reviewed. Klippel-Feil syndrome and caudal regression are presented, as well as spine manifestations of neurofibromatosis and several other syndromes. Idiopathic scoliosis is discussed in detail, including curve measurement, imaging techniques, and treatment options. Neuromuscular scoliosis is briefly reviewed. The chapter concludes with juvenile kyphosis.

R. Stein-Wexler et al. (eds.), *Pediatric Orthopedic Imaging*,
DOI 10.1007/978-3-642-45381-6_3, © Springer-Verlag Berlin Heidelberg 2015

Congenital abnormalities of the spine are relatively common and occur as an isolated finding or as part of a syndrome or association. Anomalies can be severe and lead to debilitating physical deformities with significant neurological consequences. Others have relatively mild clinical manifestations and may even be initially overlooked. Correct categorization depends in part on an adequate understanding of vertebral development, as well as the ability to recognize variant anatomy. Congenital scoliosis may result from segmentation abnormalities, including hemivertebrae and vertebral fusion. In addition, depending on severity, spinal dysraphism may be associated with extensive anomalous development of the spine.

1 Normal Development and Variant Ossification

1.1 Normal Development

Vertebral body development begins during embryogenesis and continues until the third decade [1]. Development occurs in four overlapping stages: the mesenchymal stage, chondrification, primary ossification, and secondary ossification. During the mesenchymal stage, the notochord forms; cells migrate from the bilaminar embryonic disc toward the primitive knot where the notochord forms. This occurs between the endodermal yolk sac and the ectodermal neural plate; the latter then folds, forming the neural tube. The notochord then induces differentiation of the ectoderm and mesoderm. By day 20 of embryonic life, the paraxial mesoderm is ready to separate into lateral plates, from which the genitourinary system later forms (thus explaining the close relationship between vertebral and renal anomalies), and medial columns, from which the myotomes and sclerotomes develop. By the end of the fifth gestational week, the paraxial mesoderm has divided into between 42 and 44 somites (Fig. 3.1). Each consists of three cell groups: the sclerotome, or future vertebra; the myotome, or future skeletal muscle; and the dermatome, or future dermis [2].

The sclerotome grows to surround the notochord and neural tube and then forms the annulus fibrosus. The enveloped notochord goes on to form the infantile and childhood nucleus pulposus. Once adjacent to the notochord and neural tube, the sclerotome divides, allowing the spinal nerves to emerge from the neural tube. When division of the sclerotome is complete, the caudal half of the sclerotome above merges with the cranial half of the sclerotome below to form the vertebra precursor. Fibrocartilagenous cells gradually replace the original notochord cells of the nucleus pulposus.

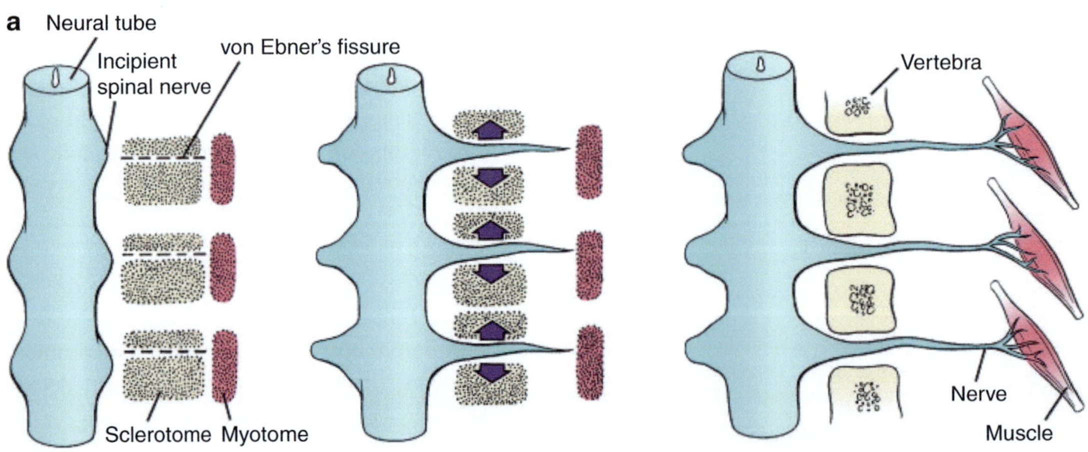

Fig. 3.1 Sclerotome division and reconvergence. Sclerotome division allows the spinal nerves to emerge from the neural tube and extend to the periphery (**a**). The sclerotome then reconverges to form the final vertebrae (**b**) (Reprinted with permission from Schoenwolf et al. [127])

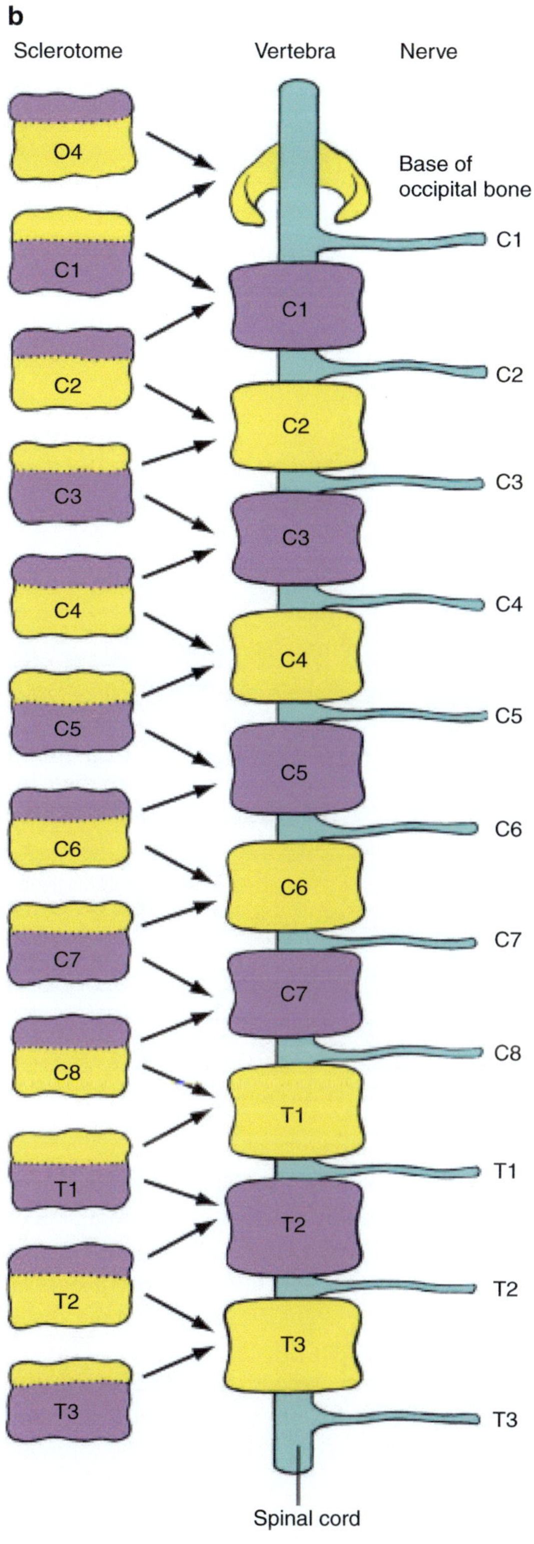

Fig. 3.1 (continued)

Chondrification of the membranous vertebrae occurs between fetal weeks 4 and 7. Two cartilaginous centers form in the centrum (either dorsal-ventral or side-by-side). Every neural arch and every costal/transverse process develop one center as well. Ossification begins in the neural arches at fetal weeks 8–9, starting at the upper cervical region. Ossification of the vertebral bodies starts in the lower thoracic and upper lumbar region and moves caudally and cranially; this process is complete by about week 20. All vertebrae below C2 and above the level of the sacrum have three ossification sites: one for the vertebral body and for each neural arch (Fig. 3.2). The single vertebral body ossification center results from coalescence of the

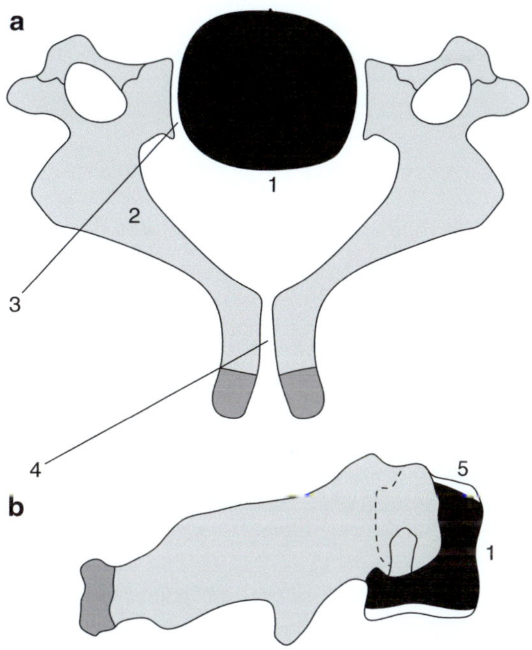

Fig. 3.2 Formation of a lower cervical vertebra. Axial (**a**) and sagittal (**b**) views. The body (*1*) appears by the fifth fetal month. Neural arches (*2*) appear by the seventh to ninth fetal week and are separated from the body by the neurocentral synchondroses (*3*), which close between 3 and 7 years of age. The posterior synchondrosis (*4*) between the spinous processes usually closes by age 2–4 years. Superior and inferior epiphyseal rings (*5*) appear at puberty, contribute to the vertical growth of the vertebral body, and unite with it at about age 25 years (Reprinted from Ghanem et al. [4] with kind permission from Springer Science and Business Media)

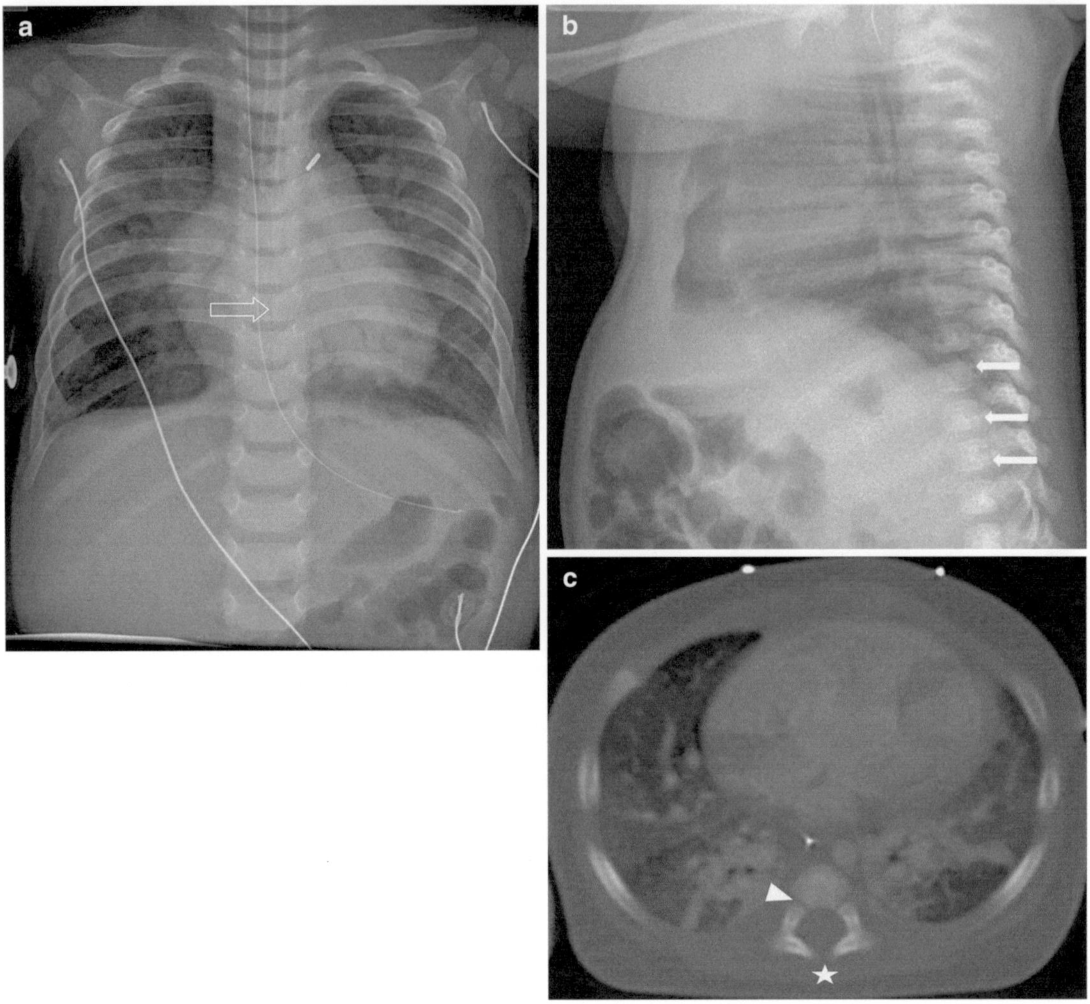

Fig. 3.3 Normal spine synchondroses. (**a**) Frontal view shows unfused neural arches (*arrow*) in a 3-month-old infant. (**b**) Normal neurocentral synchondrosis (*arrow*) in a neonate, shown on a lateral radiograph. (**c**) Computed tomography (*CT*) shows normal unfused neural arch (*asterisk*) and bilateral unfused neurocentral synchondroses (*arrowhead*)

two chondral centers that are transiently present (dorsal-ventral or side-by-side), which helps explain the occurrence of posterior and lateral hemivertebrae.

The strip of cartilage that separates the two neural arch centers from the single vertebral centrum, the neurocentral synchondrosis, is slightly anterior to the base of the pedicles (Fig. 3.3). The age at closure of the neurocentral synchondroses varies by position—cervical (3–7 years), lumbar (4–10 years), and thoracic (5 to >10 years) [3, 4]. The ossified portions of each neural arch fuse with each other dorsally by 2–4 years of age; the radiolucent lines seen on the frontal projection of the spine before this age should therefore be recognized as normal (Fig. 3.3). Between 3 and 6 years of age, this synchondrosis disappears as bone bridges the segment, although more distal levels may fuse later [5].

Around puberty, secondary ossification centers appear at the tips of the spinous, transverse, and mammillary processes, as well as in the cartilaginous ring apophysis surrounding the vertebral end plate (note that this ossification can appear as early as 2–6 years of age) [6]. Complete rings are rarely visible—on lateral radiographs, they appear as small ossification centers in notches adjacent to the anterior and posterior borders of the vertebral end plates. These secondary ossification centers fuse with the vertebral body in the third decade, usually by age 25.

Ossification of the atlas and axis is somewhat different. Most of the cranial half of the first cervical sclerotome normally merges with the occipital condyles, with a small portion forming the tip of the dens. The caudal half of the first cervical sclerotome forms the anterior, lateral, and posterior masses as well as the posterior arch of the atlas (C1). In the atlas, three separate ossification centers are present in the lateral masses and anterior arch (Fig. 3.4). The anterior arch's center is ossified at birth in only 20 % of infants and may not be radiographically evident until 2 years of age [7]. Incomplete incorporation or failure of segmentation of the first cervical sclerotome can cause a broad spectrum of fusion anomalies involving the craniocervical junction and accessory structures.

The usual pattern of ossification occurs in the centrum and neural arches of the axis. However, two additional centers form in the base of the dens and fuse into a single odontoid center, either by birth or a few months later (Fig. 3.5) [8, 9]. The ossification centers of the body and dens are separated by a well-demarcated synchondrosis, the homologue of the disc between C1 and C2

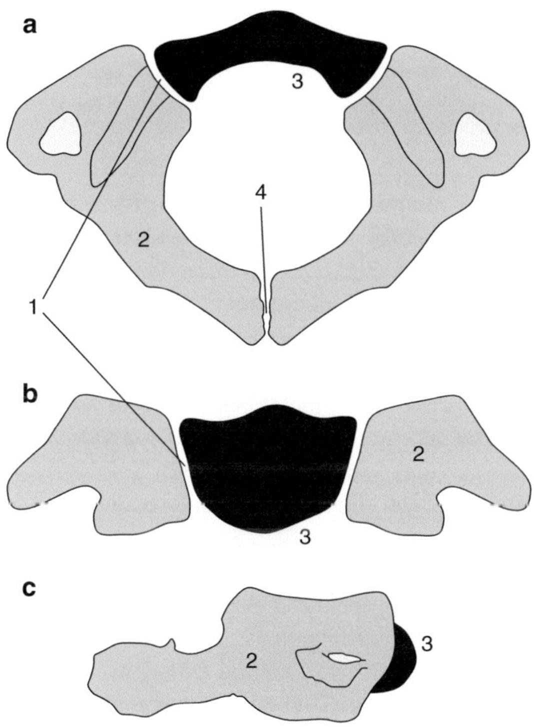

Fig. 3.4 Development of the atlas (C1). Axial (**a**), coronal (**b**), and sagittal (**c**) views. The neurocentral synchondrosis (*1*) unites the neural arch (*2*) to the anterior arch (*3*) of the atlas. The ossification center of the anterior arch (*3*) appears between age 6 months and 2 years. The posterior synchondrosis at the spinous process (*4*) unites by 4–6 years of age, followed by the neurocentral synchondrosis (*1*), which fuses by about age 7 (Reprinted from Ghanem et al. [4] with kind permission from Springer Science and Business Media)

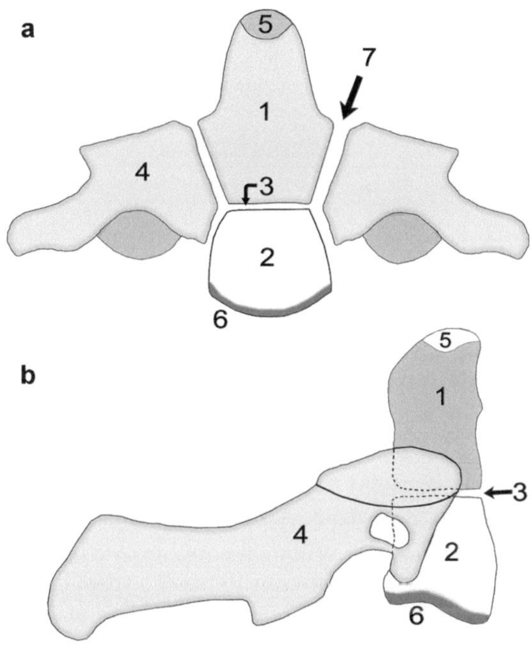

Fig. 3.5 Development of the axis (C2). Coronal (**a**) and sagittal (**b**) views. The dens (odontoid process) (*1*) develops from two primary ossification centers that usually coalesce within the first 3 months of life. The C2 centrum (*2*) appears by the fifth fetal month and is separated from the dens (*1*) by the dentocentral synchondrosis (*3*). The dentocentral synchondrosis fuses between ages 3 and 11, though it usually closes by age 6–7 years. The bilateral neural arches (*4*) appear by the seventh fetal month and fuse posteriorly by age 3 years. The neurocentral synchondroses (*7*), located on each side between the dens/vertebral body and neural arch, close between 3 and 7 years. The ossiculum terminale (*5*) at the tip of the dens appears between 3 and 10 years of age and fuses to the dens between ages 10 and 12. The inferior epiphyseal ring (*6*) appears at puberty and fuses at about age 25

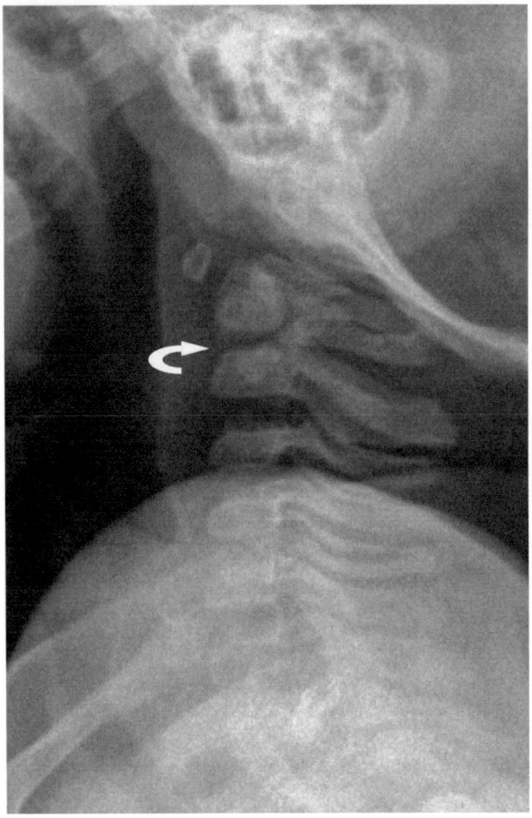

Fig. 3.6 Dentocentral synchondrosis at the base of the odontoid (*curved arrow*) in a 3-year-old boy

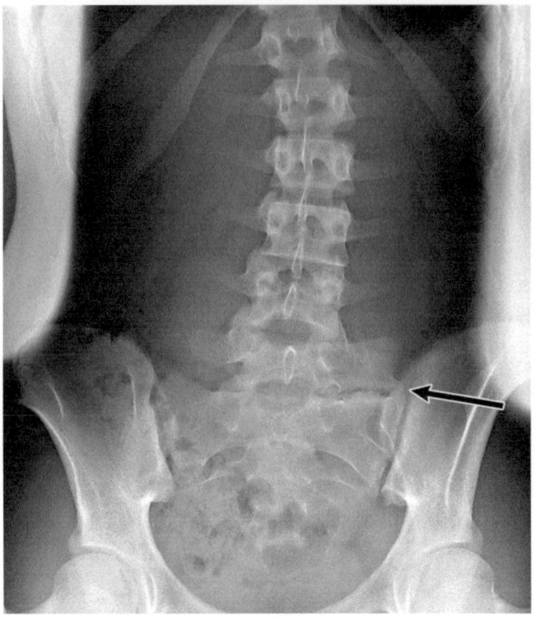

Fig. 3.7 Transitional S1 vertebra in a 14-year-old girl with scoliosis. Note pseudoarticulation of S1 and S2 on the left (*arrow*) (Courtesy of Thomas Ray Sanchez)

(Fig. 3.6). This synchondrosis closes between 3 and 11 years [5] and the neurocentral synchondroses by 3–7 years. A small ossification center appears at the tip of the odontoid between 3 and 10 years; it fuses between 10 and 12 years [5].

At the sacrum, in addition to the usual three centers for the body and neural arches of each segment, there are two epiphyseal plates that provide secondary ossification centers to form the superior and inferior portions of the sacral ala of the first through third segments.

Most people have 33 vertebrae: 7 cervical, 12 thoracic, 5 lumbar, 5 sacral, and 4 coccygeal. About 5 % have variant distribution (e.g., 6 lumbar and 11 thoracic vertebrae) but still have a total of 33 vertebral bodies. Three percent have one or two extra vertebrae, and 2 % have only 32 vertebrae [10, 11].

The lumbosacral junction is unstable during embryogenesis, and variations in formation and ossification are common in this area. Transitional vertebrae occur in approximately 20 % and often involve the sacrococcygeal and lumbosacral junctions. These vertebrae retain some features of the adjacent segments and often do not alter the overall number of vertebrae. Common variants include "sacralized" L5 and "lumbarized" S1 vertebrae (Fig. 3.7). Hemi-sacralization or lumbarization can be seen in up to 6.5 % and can cause back pain due to nonuniform articulation. Symptomatic abnormal articulation, known as Bertolotti syndrome, may be characterized on magnetic resonance imaging (MRI) by adjacent edema (Fig. 3.8). Confusion is common when it comes to labeling levels of transitional vertebrae—complete evaluation of the spinal axis before surgical intervention will allow correct assignment of vertebral levels.

The individual vertebral bodies enlarge circumferentially by the process of periosteal apposition and grow vertically by endochondral

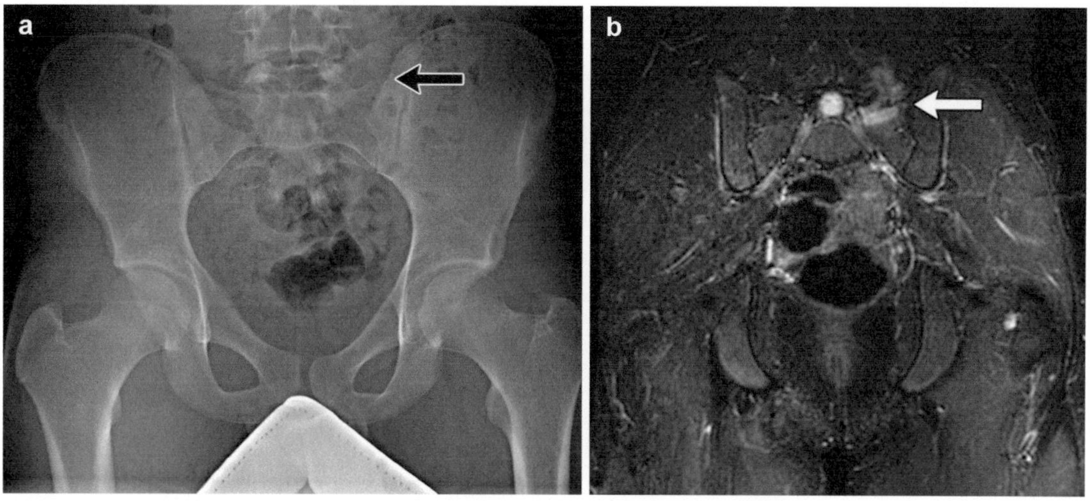

Fig. 3.8 Bertolloti syndrome in a 15-year-old girl with back pain. (**a**) Transitional vertebral segment with pseudoarticulation on the left (*black arrow*). (**b**) Coronal inversion recovery (IR) image shows hyperintensity due to marrow edema on both sides of the pseudoarticulation (*white arrow*) (Courtesy of Chirag V. Patel)

ossification; the cartilage of the vertebral end plates functions like other growth plates. The ring apophyses do not contribute to vertical growth. Following a relatively rapid length increase during the first 2 years of life, the spine grows linearly until age 16 [12]. Normal weight bearing helps balance vertical and horizontal growth and maintains an acceptable ratio between axial diameter and vertebral height. Without normal upright or walking postures, as in children with spinal muscular atrophy or cerebral palsy, vertebral bodies grow disproportionately tall and thin, developing biconvex end plates and decreased disc space height (Fig. 3.9).

1.2 Variant Ossification

Common developmental features as well as unusual normal variants can be easily mistaken for pathologic processes. The variants described below are common but not exhaustive. Ultimately, consultation with atlases of normal variants when bony defects are uniform, disproportionate to physical exam findings, or asymptomatic should prevent mischaracterization of congenital variants as disease.

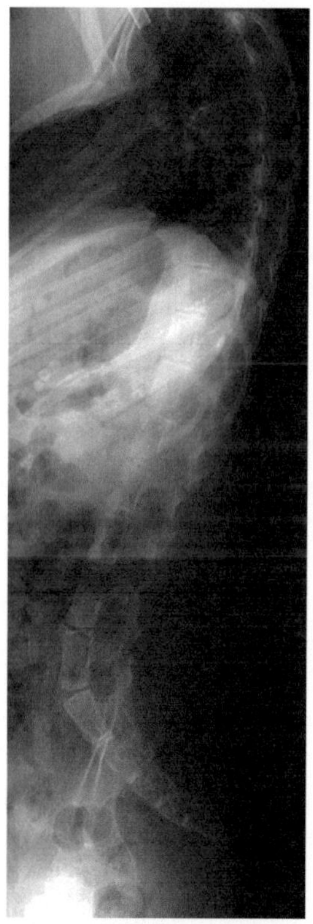

Fig. 3.9 Increased height of vertebral bodies (caninization) in an 11-year-old boy with congenital myopathy

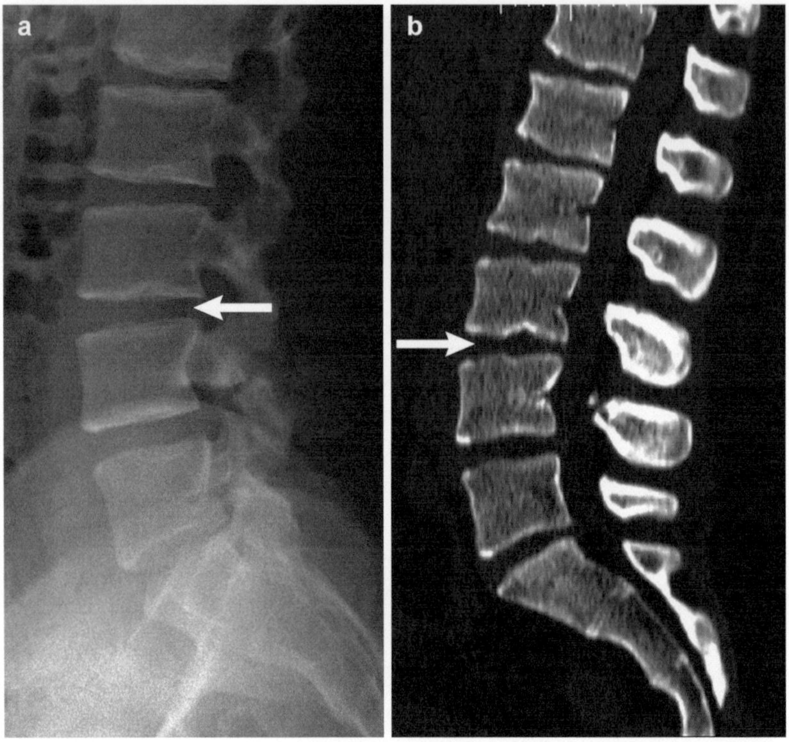

Fig. 3.10 Multiple Schmorl nodes in a 17-year-old male. *Arrows* delineate L3–4 on radiograph (**a**) and sagitally reformatted CT (**b**) (Courtesy of John Hunter)

The multiple primary and secondary ossification centers and their intervening synchondroses are often mistaken for fractures or avulsion fragments. Ossification in the superior and inferior ring apophysis may begin in children as young as 6 years of age and may persist well into adolescence.

During adolescence, the nucleus pulposus may herniate through the vertebral end plate, resulting in Schmorl nodes (Fig. 3.10). Additionally, notochord remnants may appear as impressions on consecutive inferior end plates, mimicking erosive or lytic lesions. Similarly, anterior intraosseous herniation of the intervertebral disc, also referred to as a limbus vertebra (Fig. 3.11), may be mistaken for a teardrop fracture. These normal variants may be differentiated from fractures by examining the edge of the lesion: physeal plates should be smooth and regular, with subchondral sclerotic lines, whereas acute fractures are irregular and non-sclerotic; fractures can occur at any location.

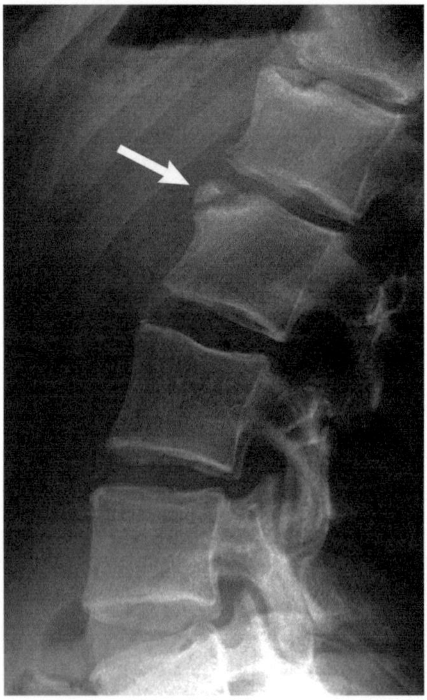

Fig. 3.11 Limbus vertebra at L2 (*arrow*) in a 16-year-old girl

During the first two decades, the appearance and physiology of the cervical spine varies tremendously. Until age 15, a normal atlantoaxial

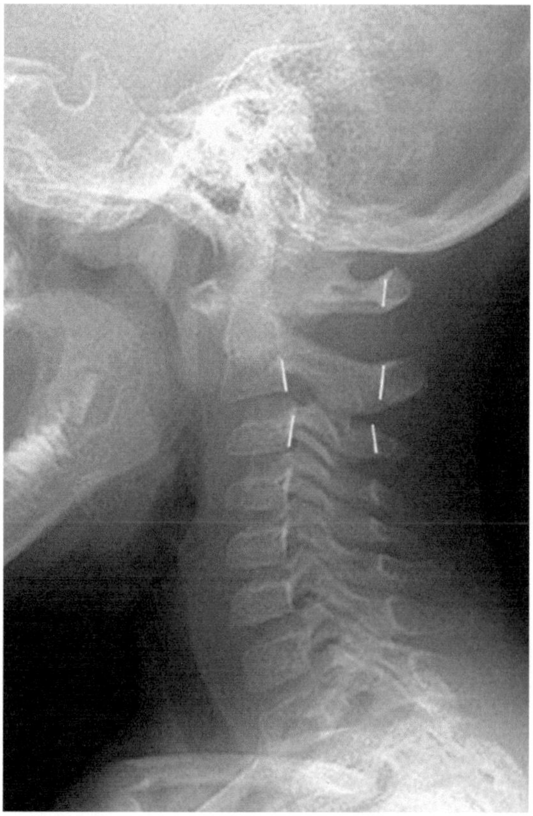

Fig. 3.12 Normal pseudosubluxation of C2 on C3. A discontinuous line connects the posterior C2 and C3 vertebral bodies, but the posterior cervical line along C1–3 is continuous and normal (Reprinted from Cakmakci [14] with kind permission from Springer Science and Business Media)

interval can be as large as 5 mm and occasionally even 6 mm. More accurate assessment evaluates for change in distance between passive flexion and extension, which should not exceed 2 mm.

Physiologic displacement of C2 anteriorly on C3 is common in normal children due to ligamentous laxity (Box 3.1). Known as pseudosubluxation, this occurs because until age 10, flexion and extension are centered at the C2–3 level (Figs. 3.12 and 3.13). (In adolescence and throughout adulthood, maximum mobility is at C4–6.) In order to determine whether subluxation results from this normal variant or from a C2 arch fracture and pathologic subluxation, one can draw a curved "posterior cervical" line, connecting the anterior cortices of the C1 and C3 spinous processes (Fig. 3.12). With physiologic subluxation, this line either passes through the C2 posterior arch or passes less than 2 mm anterior to it.

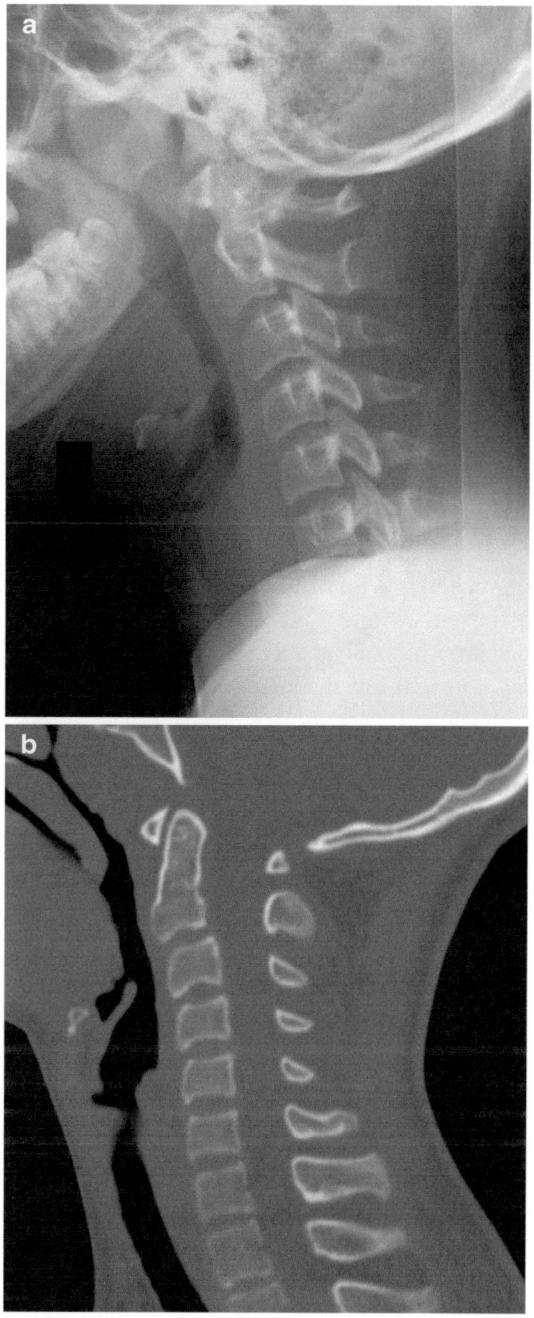

Fig. 3.13 Normal pseudosubluxation of C2 on C3. Radiograph (**a**) and sagitally reformatted CT (**b**) show forward displacement of C2 on C3. However, the posterior cervical line is normal

In the presence of an arch fracture, the distance will be greater, since the atlas and the C2 centrum slip forward at the fracture site while the spinous process remains posterior [13, 14].

Box 3.1: Pseudosubluxation of C2–3

Before about age 10 years

Due to normal ligamentous laxity

Posterior cervical line connects the anterior cortex of spinous processes of C1 and C3

- Passes through the posterior arch of C2 or <2 mm anterior to it

Developmental pseudospread of the atlas is a normal phenomenon that occurs because the growth of the atlas is linked to the relatively rapid growth of the skull base, whereas the growth of the axis is influenced by the slower growth of the spine. With pseudospread, the lateral margins of C1 lie symmetrically lateral to the margins of C2, mimicking the bilateral lateral displacement of a Jefferson fracture of the arch of the atlas. This disparity generally resolves after age 2. The overlap is usually less than 2 mm, whereas in the case of fracture, it generally exceeds 3 mm [15].

In up to 5 % of newborns, a coronal cleft is apparent on a lateral radiograph of the thoracic or lumbar spine. This appears as a vertical lucency at the junction of the anterior two thirds and posterior third of the vertebral body [16]. The cleft is filled with hyaline cartilage, possibly a remnant of the division between dorsal and ventral ossification centers. The coronal cleft ossifies during infancy and does not persist or lead to other anomalies.

A horizontal cleft in the midportion of the vertebral body, also referred to as a Hahn cleft, may also be visible on a lateral view. It marks both the boundary of fusion between sclerotomes and the nutrient foramen (Fig. 3.14) and may persist as a sclerotic line throughout adolescence.

Bone-in-bone is another common finding during infancy (Fig. 3.15). This results from rapid growth during the first postnatal months, before remodeling of the fetal spine begins [14]. The outline of a smaller replica of the vertebral body is seen within the centrum.

Incomplete bony fusion at the neural arch of L5 or S1 is very common in children, but the incidence decreases during childhood. Cartilage usually fills this apparent gap, so it is

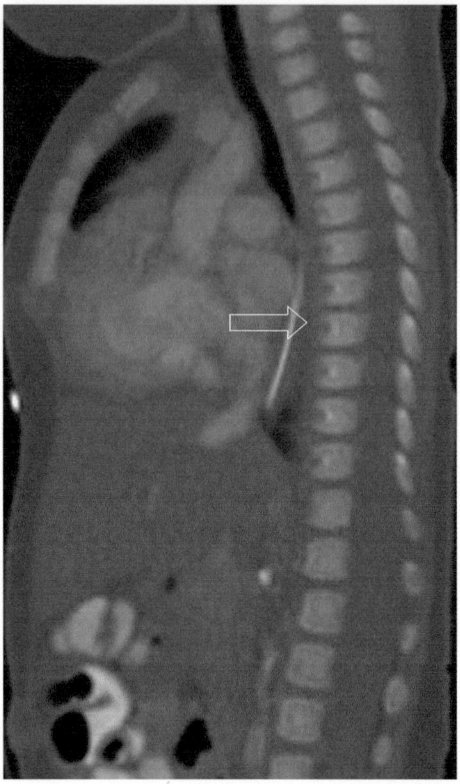

Fig. 3.14 Hahn clefts (*arrow*), the boundary of fusion of the reformed sclerotomes and also the level of arterial entry into the vertebral bodies (sagittally reformatted CT)

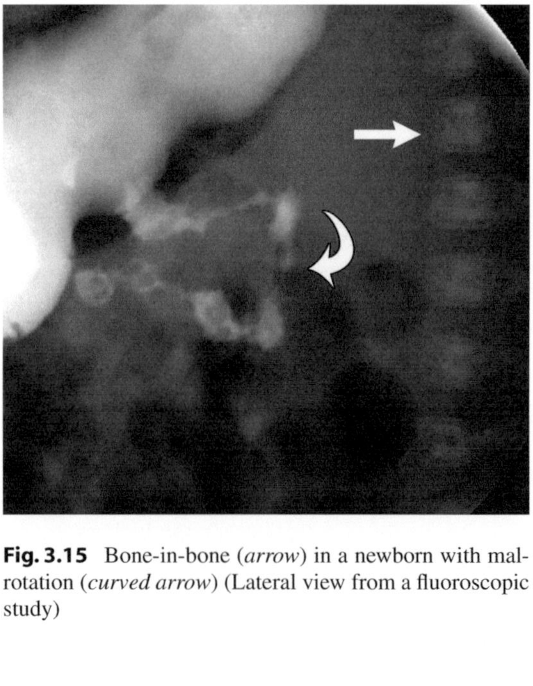

Fig. 3.15 Bone-in-bone (*arrow*) in a newborn with malrotation (*curved arrow*) (Lateral view from a fluoroscopic study)

not functionally open [17]. The S1 neural arch is incompletely fused in up to 58 % at age 8, 48 % at age 12, and 10–26 % of adults. A separation of 3 mm or less is normal and will often ossify during childhood. Occasionally, a similar narrow cleft may be encountered as an isolated finding at the T11 or T12 level. The term spina bifida occulta has been applied to this appearance (at any isolated level), but this term may be misleading as it implies pathology. Misreporting of this finding may result in confusion and unnecessary imaging.

At the T12 and L1 vertebrae, localized moderate to marked pedicle thinning occurs in 7 % of normal children and adults. The developmentally aberrant pedicle may be differentiated from a pedicle that is being deformed by mass effect because the lateral border of the aberrant pedicle is flat or concave, rather than rounded.

2 Structural Vertebral Abnormalities

Spinal defects may be restricted to the vertebrae or may involve neural and non-neural structures [18]. Sixty-one percent of those with congenital spinal defects have other abnormalities as well. For example, a prenatal neural crest and sensory nerve injury may lead to a field defect that causes the constellation of upper limb, vertebral, and rib anomalies. The mnemonic *VACTERL* describes the clinical confluence of *v*ertebral, *a*norectal, *c*ardiac, *t*racheo*e*sophageal, *r*enal, and *l*imb anomalies [19]. It is important to recognize that VACTERL is an association *not* a syndrome. Less common associated abnormalities are found in the ear, choanae, lips, palate, intestinal tract, abdominal wall (hernias), and genital system.

Scoliosis may develop if vertebrae fail to form, as with wedge vertebrae (unilateral hypoplasia) or hemivertebrae (unilateral aplasia). Less often, a hemivertebra may be supernumerary, resulting from partial duplication. Failure of segmentation may be unilateral or bilateral, resulting in an osseous bar (or bars) connecting the posterior elements, vertebral bodies, or both (Fig. 3.16). If anomalies are multiple and balanced, alignment may be normal.

2.1 Vertebral Anomalies

Wedge vertebrae (Fig. 3.16) form asymmetrically such that one side is hypoplastic and the other develops normally. Both pedicles are present, but one is larger than the other. A single wedge vertebra results in scoliosis, with the apex at the abnormal vertebra. However, bilateral wedge vertebrae may balance each other and result in a straight spine [20].

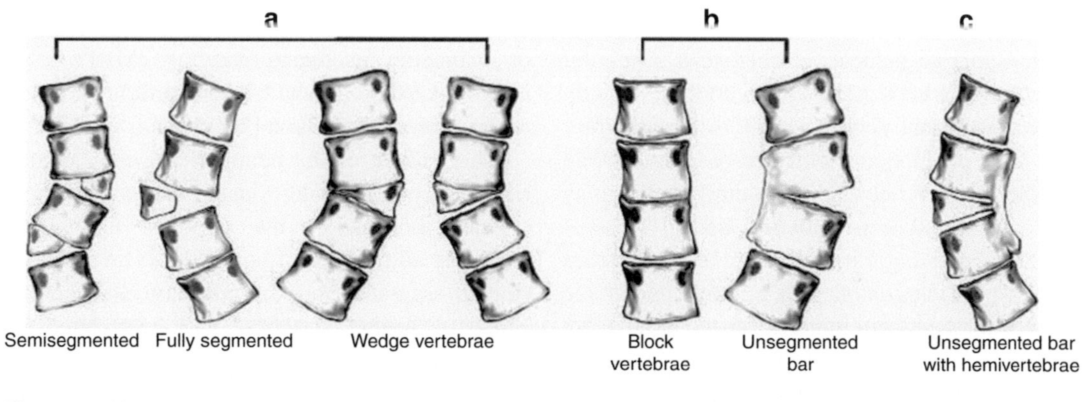

Fig. 3.16 Diagrammatic representation of the classification system of congenital scoliosis. (**a**) Failures of formation: various types of hemivertebrae (semisegmented, fully segmented, wedge vertebra). (**b**) Failures of segmentation: block vertebra, unsegmented bar. (**c**) Mixed: combination of hemivertebra and unsegmented bar (Reprinted with permission from Erol et al. [128])

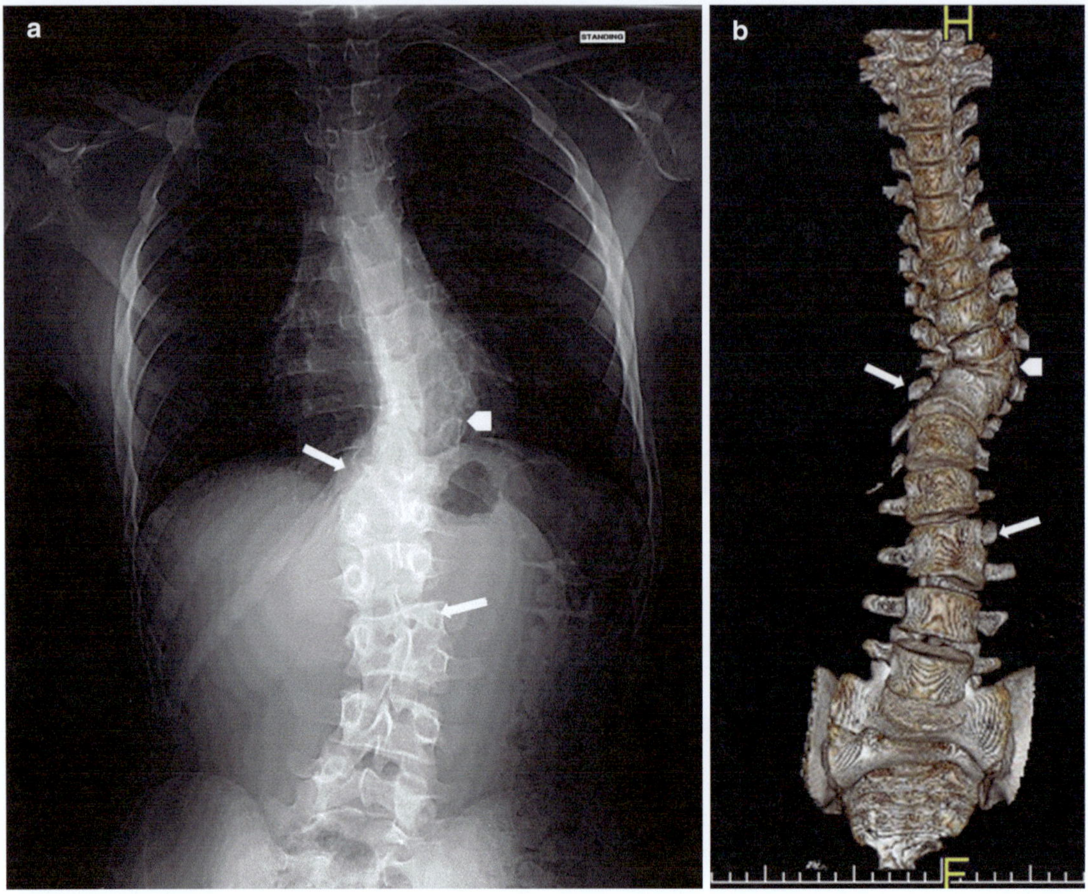

Fig. 3.17 Congenital scoliosis. Radiograph (**a**) and 3-dimensional (3D)-CT reconstruction (**b**) show three hemivertebrae on the left. The most cephalad (*arrowhead*) is fully segmented, whereas the more caudad are semisegmented (*arrows*), fused to the vertebra below

Hemivertebrae (Figs. 3.16, 3.17, and 3.18) are completely aplastic on one side, resulting in a single unpaired pedicle attached to a triangular vertebral half-body [21]. Hemivertebrae usually replace a normal vertebra but if supernumerary tend to be positioned slightly more laterally than are the other vertebrae. The hemivertebra may fuse with an adjacent vertebral body ("nonsegmented"), creating a tripediculate block vertebra with two pedicles on one side but only one on the other. If the hemivertebra is not fused to adjacent vertebrae ("fully segmented"), it is more likely to cause continued asymmetrical growth [21], since it has two functioning—and tilted—growth plates. However, curve progression is less likely with a tripediculate block vertebra. The hemivertebra may also be semisegmented, in which case one growth plate is fused to the adjacent vertebra and the other is not. Computed tomography (CT) or magnetic resonance imaging (MRI) helps assess the extent to which a hemivertebra is fused to the adjacent vertebrae [22].

The pedicle of the hemivertebra may induce rib development. Additionally, ribs at the most concave portion of the scoliosis may fuse. Counting all the ribs on both sides is an essential step in assessing the configuration and significance of wedge vertebrae and hemivertebrae. Since hemivertebrae may be supernumerary, accurate assessment of vertebral level requires evaluation of the entire spine, from C1 through the coccyx.

Butterfly vertebrae (Fig. 3.19) have a partial sagittal cleft resulting in two approximately sym-

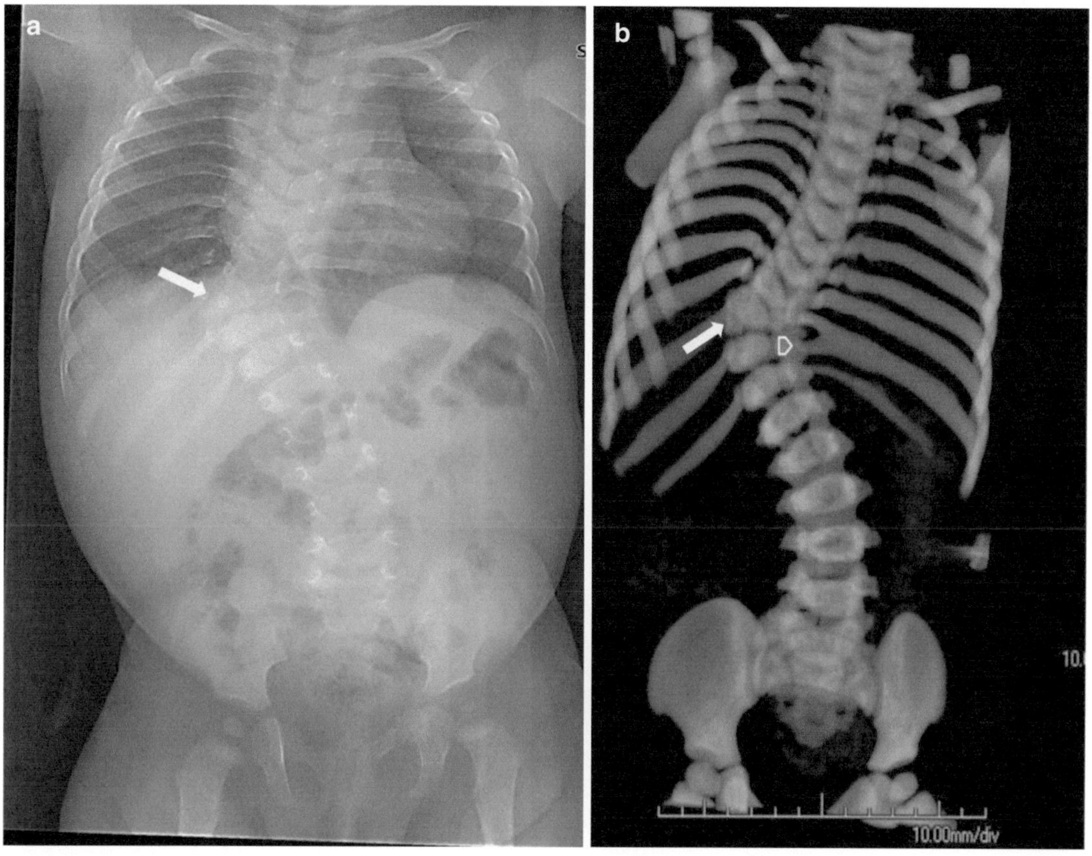

Fig. 3.18 Congenital rotatory scoliosis. Radiograph (**a**) and 3-dimensional (3D)-CT reconstruction (**b**) demonstrate a right-sided hemivertebra at T9–T10 interspace (*arrow*). Even though the ribs end at same level, the right side has 12 ribs and the left has 11, because of the extra rib induced by the right hemivertebra. Also note fusion of the left 9th and 10th ribs (*arrowhead*)

metric segments that can be otherwise normal or appear as bilateral wedge vertebrae or—if completely divided—hemivertebrae. If balanced, butterfly vertebrae do not cause significant scoliosis, but they may suggest the presence of a syndrome or other anomalies.

Isolated absence of the pedicle (Fig. 3.20) is most common in the cervical and lumbar region and is uncommon in the thoracic spine. It is important to distinguish this congenital anomaly from pathologic destruction of the pedicle. With congenital absence of the pedicle, the pedicle outline is completely absent, and the associated intervertebral foramen is enlarged. In older children, the opposite pedicle and lamina may be hypertrophied.

Congenital vertebral bars (Fig. 3.21) develop when the laminae or pediculate bases of adjacent vertebrae fuse. Fusion that is limited to the laminae and facets dorsal to the intervertebral foramina leads to lordo-scoliosis. If the vertebral bodies at the base of the pedicles are also fused, the intervertebral foramina will be small. If there are no ribs in this region, a large conglomerate foramen develops, through which multiple nerve roots pass. If these anomalies are bilateral and symmetric, growth will be restricted but alignment may be normal. If unilateral, more problematic angular deformity occurs.

If cleavage of somites fails, normal segmentation does not occur, and *block vertebrae* form.

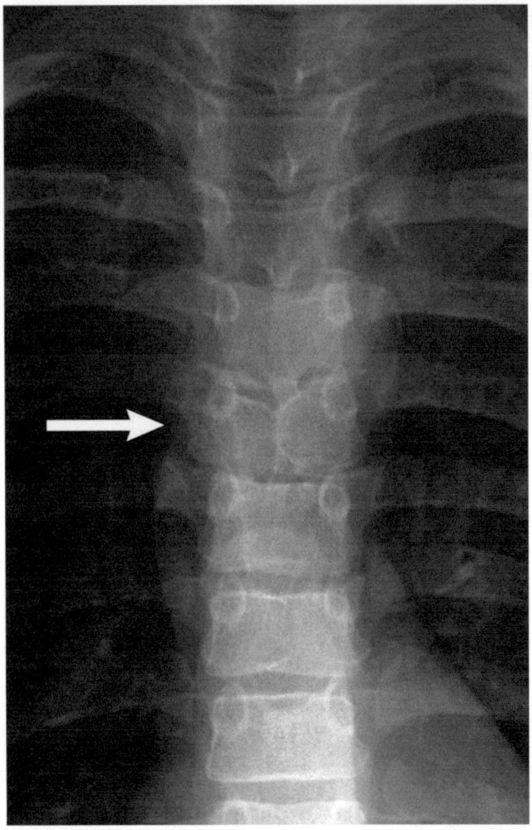

Fig. 3.19 Butterfly vertebra (*arrow*) in an 11-year-old boy with Alagille syndrome

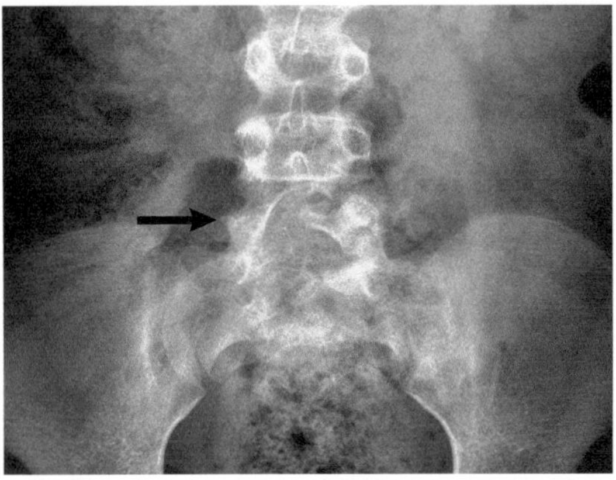

Fig. 3.20 Transitional lumbosacral vertebra in a 6-year-old girl. The pedicle on the right (*arrow*) is absent

Vertebral bodies do not separate, and there is no (or very little) intervening disc space. The vertebral block appears constricted at the level of the disc, and the height of the structure is slightly less

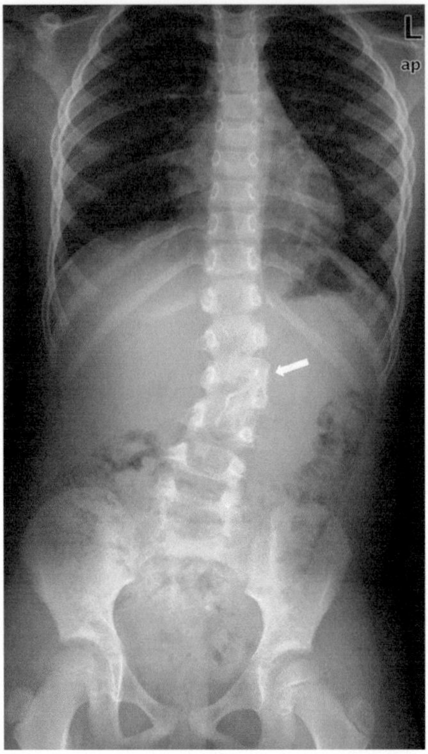

Fig. 3.21 Laminopediculate bar. The lamina of the hemivertebra has fused to the lamina of the pedicle above (*arrow*)

than that of two normal vertebral bodies (excluding the height of a disc). A thin sclerotic linear density may replace the disc, or a rudimentary disc may be present.

Fusion in young children is often cartilaginous and thus may be radiographically occult. In older children, a frontal radiograph demonstrates a laminopediculate bar as a discrete sclerotic curved line connecting pedicles at two or more levels (see Fig. 3.21). The ipsilateral vertebral body and disc space are often hypoplastic, and the vertebral bodies may be fused as well. If the fusion is coronal rather than sagittal, the anterior aspect of the vertebral body is almost invariably wedge shaped or entirely absent, resulting in kyphosis or lordosis (further discussed below). In young children, radiographs may fail to demonstrate fusion, but MRI readily depicts block vertebra formation by demonstrating absence of intervertebral disc signal (Fig. 3.22).

CT is valuable in showing associated spinous process obliquity, transverse process hypoplasia,

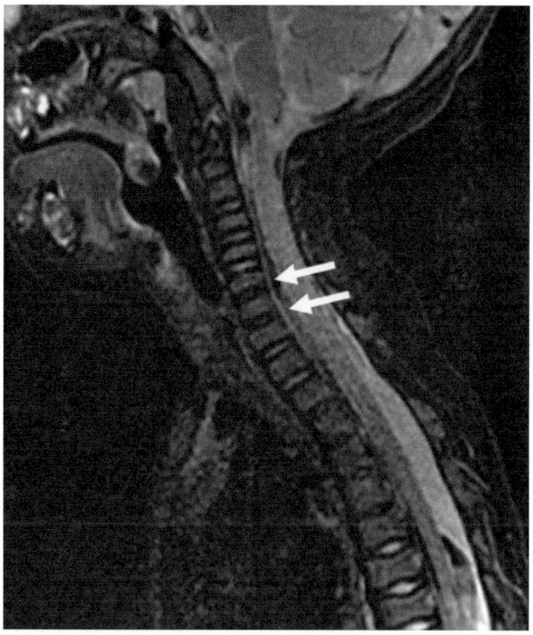

Fig. 3.22 Lack of normal hyperintense intervertebral disc signal in the upper thoracic and lower cervical region (*arrows*) denotes areas that will develop into block vertebrae when ossification is complete (sagittal T2-weighted (T2-W) fat-suppressed (FS) magnetic resonance image (MRI)) (Incidental flow artifact dorsal to the spinal cord)

abnormally shaped spinal canal, anomalous facet and rib articulations, and hypoplasia of pedicles at adjacent levels. It also delineates hypoplastic or malpositioned pedicles that are not apparent on routine radiography. MRI best images nerve root compression, myelomalacia, and contralateral laminar stress fracture, all of which can cause back pain.

2.2 Congenital Scoliosis (Table 3.1)

Spinal curvature in the coronal plane is caused by unbalanced anatomy and growth potential of the two sides of the spine. Unlike idiopathic scoliosis, congenital scoliosis progresses in up to 75 % of patients and most often affects the thoracic spine (thoracolumbar scoliosis is the second most common). Once curvature starts to increase, it will continue to do so, often accelerating during the preadolescent growth spurt. Since ribs and vertebrae form from the same mesenchymal

Table 3.1 Anomalies that cause congenital scoliosis (Fig. 3.7)

I. Failure of formation
A. Unilateral hypoplasia (wedge vertebra)
B. Unilateral aplasia (hemivertebra)
II. Partial duplication (supernumerary hemivertebra)
III. Failure of segmentation
A. Unilateral nonsegmentation (unilateral bar)
1. Posterior elements only
2. Vertebral body only
3. Vertebral body and posterior elements
IV. Combined lesions

Adapted from Refs. [23, 125]

somites, associated developmental and fusion anomalies are common. However, it is difficult to predict exactly what effect a single anomaly will have.

Multiple lesions are sometimes balanced, canceling each other out and causing little overall effect on spinal alignment. Ribs that fuse centrally near the spine may contribute to scoliosis, but peripheral rib fusion generally does not affect spinal curvature [23].

Hemivertebrae function both as the apex of the curve and as an unbalanced growth center that contributes to increased curvature. Congenital bars have the opposite effect of hemivertebrae, restricting growth on one side of the spine while the other side continues to grow. Congenital bars are present in 40 % of patients with multiple hemivertebrae. A hemivertebra at the same level as a contralateral bar has the worst prognosis, especially if thoracolumbar. However, in young children it can be difficult to predict exactly where and how a segment will fuse to adjacent bodies.

Imaging

Radiographic evaluation includes frontal and lateral radiographs. Curves can be measured according to a variety of techniques; the Cobb technique is commonly employed and is presented later in this chapter. Cross-sectional imaging is indicated for exact delineation of anomalies [24]. CT and MRI may demonstrate occult hemivertebrae as well as vertebral fusion. Additionally, MRI of the entire spine is typically performed before surgery in order to assess asymptomatic associated anomalies such as tethered cord, syringomyelia, and diastematomyelia, which are cumulatively described in up to 40 % of patients with congenital scoliosis [25].

Up to 18 % of patients with congenital scoliosis have associated genitourinary tract abnormalities, with renal agenesis being the most common [26]. Urologic evaluation is therefore indicated in all patients with congenital anomalies of the spine. Screening ultrasound (US) to assure the normal site and structure of both kidneys usually suffices, although occasionally additional imaging is necessary. Patients may also have congenital heart disease (7 % incidence), undescended scapula (6 %), thumb anomalies (4 %), and other malformations.

2.3 Congenital Kyphosis and Lordosis

Congenital kyphosis is another manifestation of unbalanced longitudinal development of vertebrae, with the curvature occurring along the sagittal axis. As with coronal scoliosis, these developmental anomalies generally manifest as failure of formation, failure of segmentation, or both.

Kyphosis in the thoracic spine is defined as curvature greater than the 40° [27–29]. It can be caused by posterior overgrowth, restricted anterior growth, or anomalies of segmentation [30]. The most common form of congenital kyphosis is caused by a dorsal hemivertebra (although infrequently the entire vertebral body is absent but the neural arch elements are formed) (Fig. 3.23). Both the anterior and the lateral portions of the vertebra may be deficient, causing a combination of scoliosis and kyphosis [31]. If kyphosis is severe, an anterior pseudoarticulation may develop above or below the defect. Anterior block vertebra formation rarely causes kyphosis, usually without scoliosis, since such fusion tends to be symmetric [32].

Congenital nonsegmentation and fusion must be distinguished from progressive anterior vertebral body fusion, in which erosion of the anterior end plates is followed by anterior fusion and later

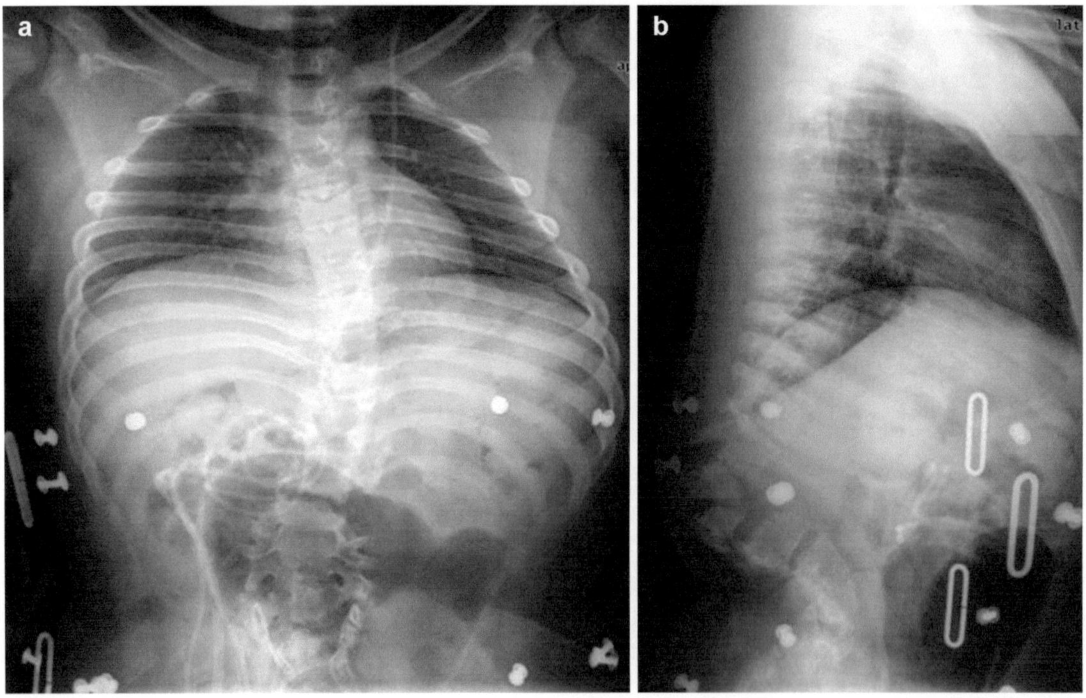

Fig. 3.23 Congenital thoracolumbar kyphosis and posterior spinal dysraphism. (**a-frontal**, **b-lateral**) Multiple anterior vertebral body segments are hypoplastic, and posterior elements have not fused. The patient is in a brace, and there is a ventriculoperitoneal shunt catheter

disc fusion. Muscle imbalance in severe myelomeningocele may also cause kyphosis.

Congenital lordosis, a lumbar angle over 40°, is usually severe but fortunately uncommon. In this condition, posterior elements fuse while the anterior vertebral bodies continue to grow. Extreme thoracolumbar lordosis may also result from intrauterine positioning. Posterior rib synostosis contributes to growth inhibition.

Kyphosis and lordosis are usually assessed with standing radiographs, with flexibility determined by placing the patient on a bolster. As with congenital scoliosis, CT clearly delineates osseous causes of kyphosis or lordosis. MRI best evaluates for spinal cord compression and other cord abnormalities. A complete investigation includes cardiac and urologic screening due to the high associated incidence of these anomalies.

2.4 Craniovertebral Junction

Like the lumbosacral area, the craniovertebral junction is developmentally unstable. Congenital anomalies and developmental variants in this region are therefore common. Anomalous development here often results in multiple abnormalities, and therefore recognition of a single variant should trigger evaluation for additional problems. Many patients with abnormal development at the craniocervical junction can further be classified as syndromic [33]. While many abnormalities at the craniocervical junction are minor and asymptomatic, clinically significant spinal cord compression can result from somatic growth or recurrent motion.

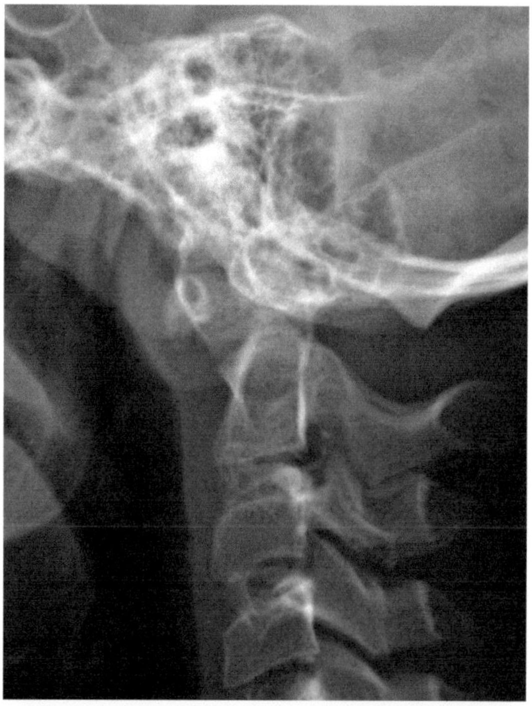

Fig. 3.24 Occipitalization of atlas. There is continuity of the cortex between the skull base and C1 (Same patient as Fig. 3.27)

Occipitalization of the Atlas

Occipitalization of the atlas (Fig. 3.24) occurs in up to 0.75 % of the population and ranges from complete osseous fusion between the atlas and occiput to more focal osseous bridging. Most commonly, the anterior arch of the atlas fuses to the skull base. However, fusion may involve the posterior arch or the lateral masses, and multiple sites of fusion are not uncommon [33]. Atlantoaxial instability is common in those with occipitalization of the atlas, as is encroachment on the spinal cord, sometimes resulting in myelopathy. Since development of the neural elements is closely intertwined with that of bony elements, basilar invagination, Chiari 1 malformation, and tonsillar ectopia may be present as well. Fifty-seven percent of patients with occipitalization of the atlas also have a syndrome [33].

Occipitalization of the atlas must be distinguished from an unusually high atlas, which can occur as a normal variant due to relatively flat occipital condyles. In some cases, occipitalization is associated with a short clivus, the latter due to primary growth failure (as in achondroplasia) or premature fusion of the spheno-occipital synchondrosis [4].

The posterior arch at C1 may be open in some patients with craniocervical fusion [33], but this finding can be seen until age 4 years in normal children and indeed persists as a normal variant in up to 4 % of adults. Complete absence of the posterior arch of the atlas is rare (Fig. 3.25). Defects in the anterior arch of C1 are less

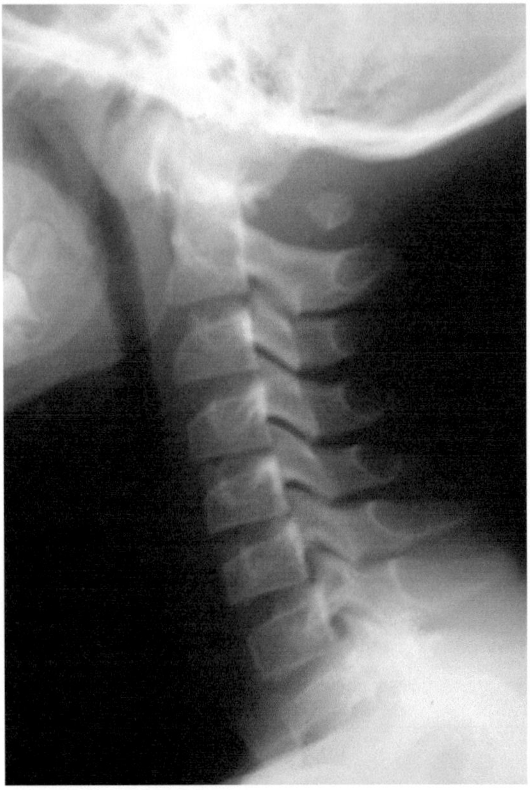

Fig. 3.25 Near complete absence of the posterior arch of C1 in a 12-year-old girl

common than defects in the posterior arch. The anterior arch of the atlas rarely fuses to the dens. The occipital condyles may be asymmetrical, and similar asymmetry may be seen at the atlantal and axial articulations. One third of patients have associated fusion of C2–3 vertebrae.

Patients with craniocervical junction abnormalities may complain of neck pain and stiffness, with neurological signs and symptoms usually beginning insidiously in the third decade and progressing slowly. However, earlier onset is being reported with increasing frequency. Sometimes symptoms occur acutely, and sudden death may result from relatively mild trauma at the craniocervical junction.

Imaging

Fusion may be apparent on a lateral radiograph, showing a fused block of bone or continuous cortex. Lack of mobility on flexion and extension radiographs can indicate fusion as well. This finding is especially valuable in skeletally immature children. However, if there is reasonable suspicion for fusion, CT with sagittal and coronal reformats as well as three-dimensional (3D) reconstructions is most useful to delineate bony anatomy, and MRI may be useful to evaluate cord impingement or myelopathy.

C2 Developmental Anomalies

Multiple anomalies can affect the dens. Some have significant clinical implications, whereas others may contribute to diagnostic uncertainty in the setting of trauma. The dens may be hypoplastic or hypertrophied, or it may be composed of ossicles that fail to fuse to each other or to C2.

The normal odontoid terminates just below the foramen magnum, with a normal basion to (top of) dens measurement of 8.3–10 mm [34]. If the odontoid extends above or below this level, neurologic symptoms may result, especially if there is also transverse ligament laxity [35]. In odontoid hypoplasia, also known as stubby dens, the odontoid process is underdeveloped and does not reach its normal height at the superior surface of the atlas. In the severe form, odontoid aplasia, the dens does not extend above the body of C2. These congenital anomalies of formation may be isolated or associated with syndromes such as mucopolysaccharidoses, spondyloepiphyseal dysplasia, and metatropic dwarfism.

Anomalous development of the odontoid can take several forms. Os odontoideum describes a small fragment of bone that does not fuse with the subjacent portion of the odontoid. The ossific fragment usually lies directly behind the anterior arch of the atlas, but it is sometimes displaced (Fig. 3.26). Occasionally, there is a transverse cleft between the odontoid and the adjacent C2 vertebral body. A history of neck trauma is common in patients with this finding, and the phenomenon may sometimes result from an incomplete or partially healed fracture rather than aberrant development. The unfused ossicle usually moves with the atlas and occasionally fuses to the anterior lip of the foramen magnum.

Differentiating os odontoideum from acute fracture can be difficult [36]. Features that suggest a chronic process such as os odontoideum include a relatively thick anterior arch of C1 with a convex posterior border. MRI can also help differentiate by demonstrating normal signal intensity in the bone and surrounding soft tissues.

Atlantoaxial Subluxation

In atlantoaxial subluxation, the transverse, alar, and other ligaments binding the odontoid to the atlas are lax or absent whereas bones are normal. Laxity of the transverse and other stabilizing ligaments allows the anterior arch of the atlas to subluxate anteriorly [37] (Box 3.2). Atlantoaxial subluxation may be associated with structural abnormalities. Alternatively, it may be a component of various syndromes, such as Ehlers-Danlos syndrome and other connective tissue disorders or trisomy 21. The condition can also follow trauma or be associated with local osteomyelitis, pharyngitis and cervical adenitis, and juvenile idiopathic arthritis. Rotational and atlanto-occipital instability as well as skeletal anomalies may be present, and scoliosis occurs in up to 50 % of cases.

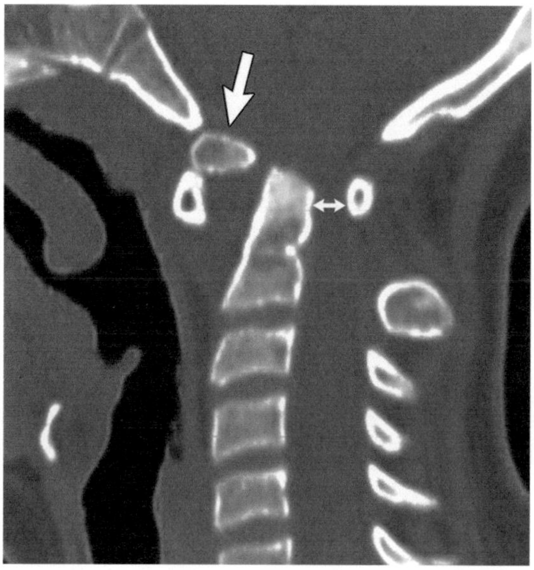

Fig. 3.26 Os odontoideum in an 11-year-old girl with Down syndrome. Sagittally reformatted CT shows the os (*arrow*) is displaced, positioned just behind and superior to the anterior arch of C1, with the remainder of the dens posterior to the os. There is marked narrowing of the spinal canal (*double arrow*)

Imaging

In normal older children and adults, the gap between the posterior surface of the anterior arch of the atlas and the anterior surface of the odontoid is 2–3 mm, whereas in younger children the presence of cartilage may cause this distance to be as large as 5 mm or occasionally even 6 or 7 mm. Although slight laxity and instability can be present in normal children, the atlanto-dens interval usually does not change with flexion or extension. In atlantoaxial subluxation, the distance is usually normal on standard neutral lateral radiographs but increases 2 mm or more with flexion (Fig. 3.27). However, in some patients with trisomy 21, the atlanto-dens interval is abnormal on neutral images yet normal with flexion [37].

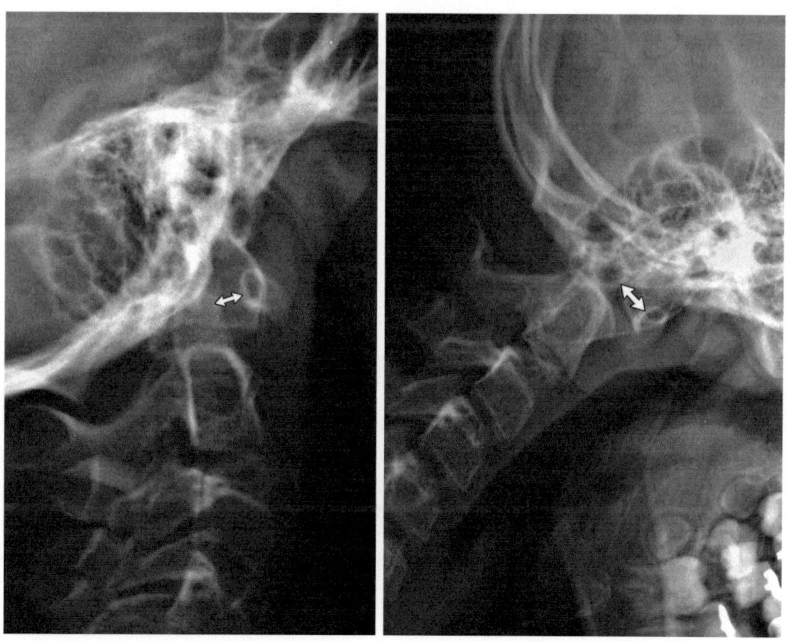

Fig. 3.27 Abnormal motion between the anterior arch of C1 and the dens (*double arrows*) in patient with occipitalization of the atlas (Same patient as Fig. 3.24)

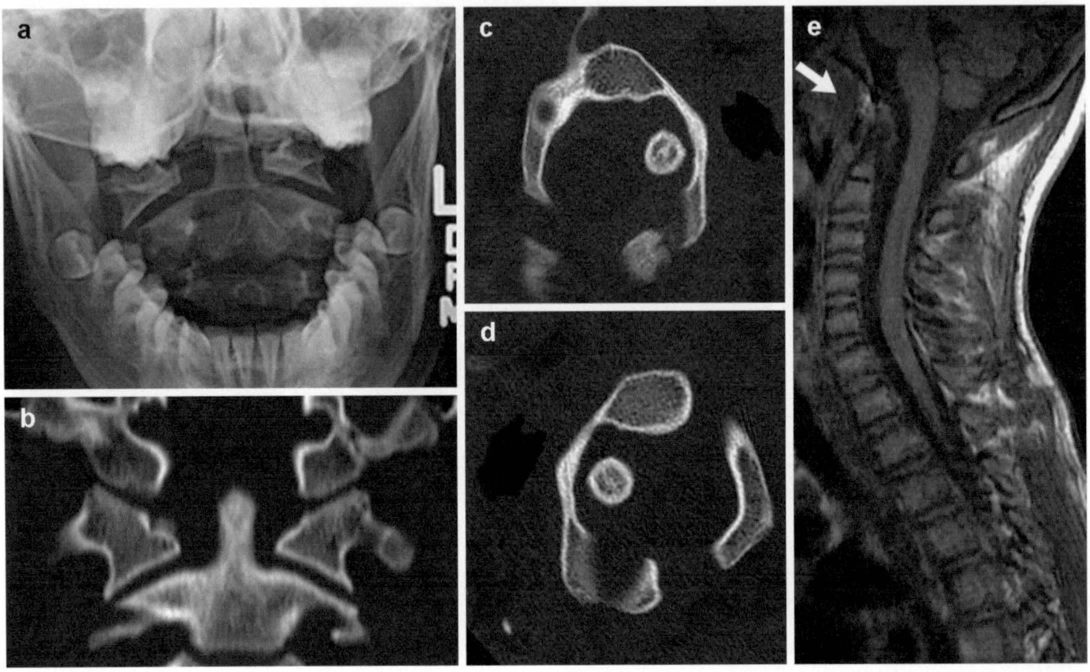

Fig. 3.28 Atlantoaxial rotary fixation in a preteen. (**a**) Frontal radiograph shows asymmetry between the lateral masses of C1 and the dens, with the head tilted to the right. (**b**) Coronally reformatted CT in neutral confirms this finding. Axial CT images with the head turned to the right (**c**) and left (**d**) show asymmetrical widening on the right persists. (**e**) Sagittal T1-weighted (T1-W) MRI shows subacute hemorrhage at the alar ligament (*arrow*)

Box 3.2: True Atlantoaxial Subluxation

Associated with structural abnormalities, trisomy 21 and other syndromes, arthritis, trauma, and pharyngitis

Increased distance between the anterior arch of C1 and dens

- Normal <5 mm in young children
- Normal <2–3 mm in older children

Increases with flexion

Atlantoaxial Rotary Subluxation

Atlantoaxial rotary subluxation may follow trauma or occur with Grisel syndrome (local inflammation in the pharynx) [38]. In the latter condition, inflammation around the dens and pharyngo-vertebral venous plexus causes the ligaments to weaken [39]. Relatively minor trauma to this area that would not affect an adult may lead to rotary subluxation in children, perhaps due to more steeply angled facets.

Imaging

The atlantoaxial facets and occiput-C1-C2 articulation are best investigated with CT as the patient passively rotates their head. Sagittal and coronal reformatted images or 3D-CT reconstructions demonstrate the abnormal relationships well (Fig. 3.28). On fluid-sensitive MRI sequences, abnormal signal in the transverse and alar ligaments is sometimes evident; this may be reactive or causative.

3 Spinal Dysraphism Complexes

Dysraphism describes the failure of midline vertebral structures to fuse. The term encompasses not only structural vertebral defects but also associated anomalies of neurologic, gastrointestinal, genitourinary, and other systems. The sequence of neural tube-notochord-yolk sac differentiation is disrupted, and thus structures that develop from the primordial layers may be affected. There may be abnormal induction of structures that develop later as well. Dysraphism is categorized as open (uncovered) or closed (covered) and the later further subdivided according to configuration (Fig. 3.29) [40]. Most open defects (meningocele (Fig. 3.30), meningomyelocele (Fig. 3.31), and myelocele) are clinically obvious, but dermal sinuses may be difficult to detect. Closed defects are completely covered with skin, which may be dysplastic and have an associated nevus, hairy

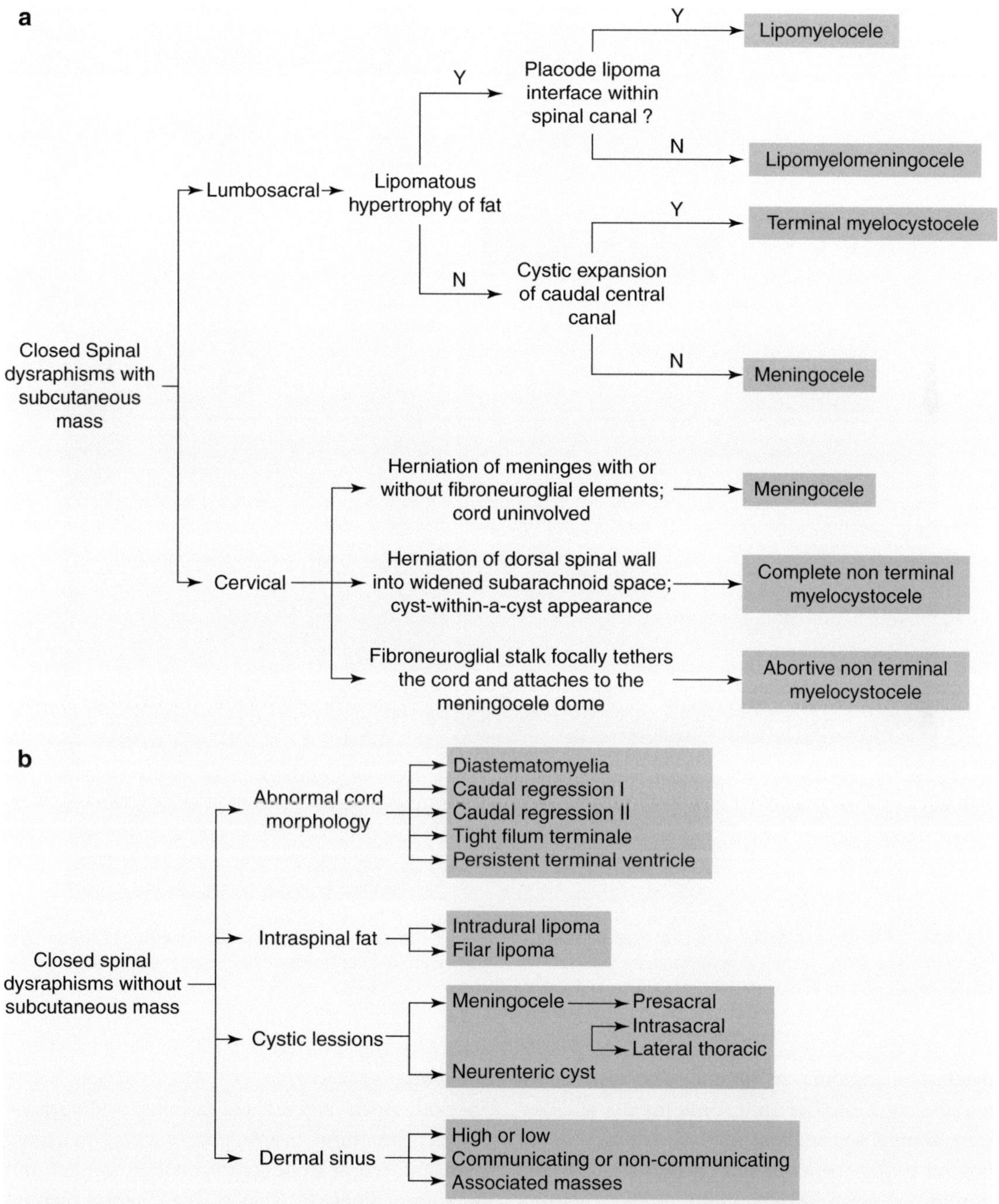

Fig. 3.29 Diagnostic algorithm of closed spinal dysraphism presenting with (**a**) and without (**b**) a subcutaneous mass (Reprinted from Badve et al. [129] with kind permission from Springer Science and Business Media)

Fig. 3.30 Anterior pelvic meningocele. Sagittally reformatted (**a**) and axial CT (**b**) images show an anterior pelvic meningocele at the mid-sacral level. Dorsal elements are dysmorphic, and there is lower lumbar and sacral dysraphism with partial sacral agenesis

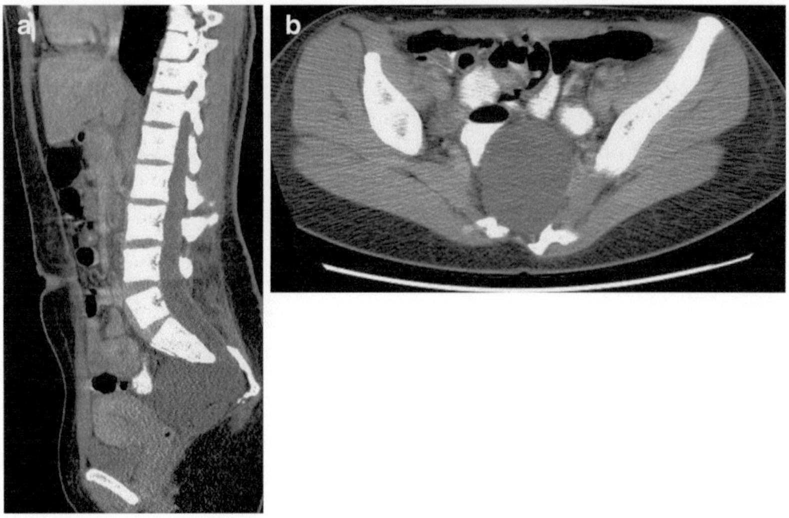

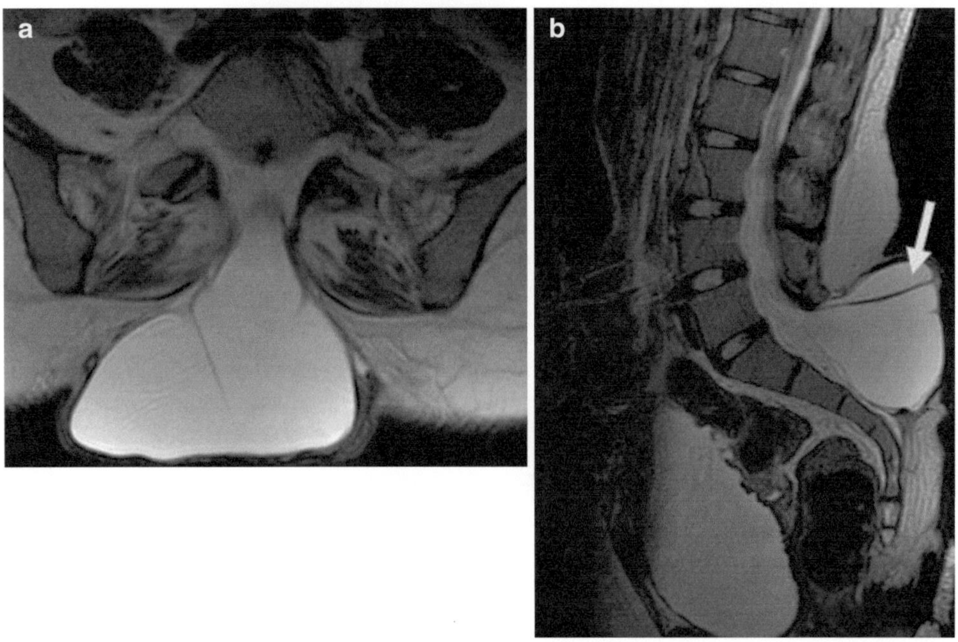

Fig. 3.31 Meningomyelocele. Axial (**a**) and sagittal (**b**) T2-W images demonstrate a myelomeningocele at the L5–S1 level with posterior spinal dysraphism and extension of the neural placode into the dorsal aspect of the cyst (*arrow*). Note the trabeculated neurogenic bladder

patch, hemangioma, or lipoma. The spinal cord may be duplicated or split (diplomyelia and diastematomyelia), or there may be overgrowth of normal tissues (lipoma and dermoid) or herniation of one germ layer through another (neurenteric cyst).

Imaging

In both open and closed lesions, radiographs reveal structural vertebral defects in most patients. Neural arches appear widely spread, and laminar/pediculate fusion or intersegmental fusion is common, often affecting more than one level. The spinal canal may appear diffusely enlarged. Vertebral bodies are often hypoplastic, deformed, or scalloped, and there may be hemivertebrae (see Fig. 3.23). These findings may be present at the level of the neurologic defect or elsewhere in the spine. Associated mediastinal or pelvic masses may result from ectopic neurenteric rests.

Cross-sectional imaging provides essential information for skin-covered lesions. If cutaneous stigmata are present, US can help evaluate for tethered cord until about age 3 months (Figs. 3.32 and 3.33), with subsequent MRI if needed. CT is rarely performed to better delineate the bony abnormalities, while MRI exquisitely depicts the extent of neural and soft tissue abnormalities (see Figs. 3.30 and 3.31). MRI may occasionally be performed before surgery for open lesions, as it allows more precise diagnosis and surgical planning.

3.1 Tethered Filum Terminale

Low conus or tethered cord generally occurs because either the terminal cord fails to involute or the filum terminale fails to lengthen. Low conus (Fig. 3.33) is characterized by abnormal termination of the cord, whereas abnormal thickening of the filum, fibrolipoma, and/or a filar cyst characterize an abnormal filum terminale (Fig. 3.34). If the conus is abnormally low, nerve roots emerge more horizontally than usual, and stretching of the vascular supply may

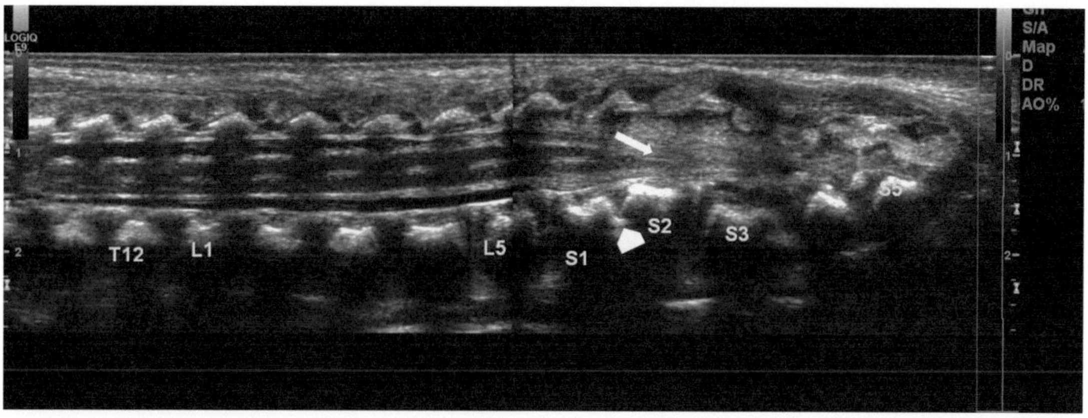

Fig. 3.32 Tethered cord in a newborn. Longitudinal ultrasound (US) shows the spinal cord extends to the sacral-level dysraphism (*arrow*). Additionally there is a lipoma of the filum. Note the fused vertebrae compatible with VACTERL association (*arrowhead*)

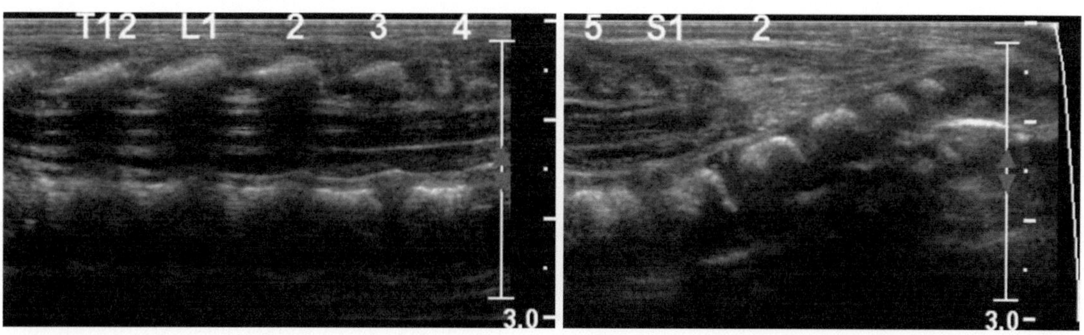

Fig. 3.33 Tethered cord. Longitudinal US shows conus at the S1 level, with increased fibro-fatty tissue in the canal below this level

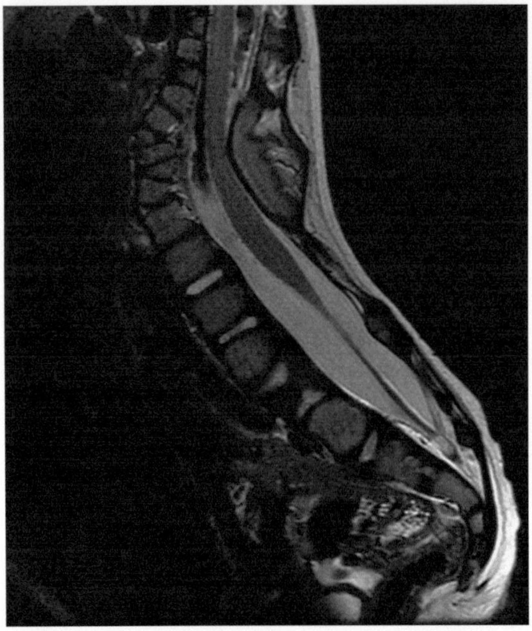

Fig. 3.34 Tethered cord and multiple segmentation anomalies in a 3-year-old. Sagittal T2-W image shows the distal cord is dorsally positioned and kinked over dysmorphic posterior elements at the thoracolumbar junction. Multiple dorsal and ventral hemivertebrae

lead to myelopathy. Tethering occasionally presents late with such symptoms as lower extremity spasticity, bladder incontinence, and toe walking. Hairy tufts, midline vascular malformations, and other cutaneous findings should prompt evaluation.

A conus terminating at the superior half of the L3 vertebral body can be considered normal in newborns, provided that normal ascent follows [41]. The inferior tip of the conus should lie at the adult level, T12 to L2/3, by 2 months of age. Absence of normal motion with cerebrospinal fluid (CSF) pulsation is another feature of tethered cord [42]. Even if surgery reveals that the conus is not tethered, symptoms sometimes occur. Tethering can also occur or recur after surgical repair of myelomeningocele, diastematomyelia, and other lesions.

Imaging

Ultrasound (US), performed between birth and 3 months of age, readily evaluates the level of the conus. Additionally, evaluation of cerebrospinal fluid pulsations can identify abnormal cord motility. If US identifies tethered cord, MRI of the entire neural axis should be performed to evaluate for occult concomitant issues. The filum is abnormally thick if it measures more than 2 mm in diameter at L5–S1 or if it is infiltrated by fibrous or fatty tissue. In addition, the filum may adhere to other structures, which limits its normal compliance and may lead to signs of traction, even if the conus terminates at a normal level. Very thin sagittal T2-weighted (T2-W) or balanced steady-state free precession images may be necessary to image the filum.

3.2 Syringohydromyelia

Hydromyelia and syringomyelia are both characterized by the presence of fluid within the central cord. Hydromyelia involves the central canal, whereas syringomyelia does not. However, the pathogenesis of these abnormalities is similar, and they are clinically indistinguishable and frequently lumped together as "syrinx", or syringohydromyelia. A congenital syrinx may develop from an obstructed fourth ventricle in the fetus [43], but a syrinx can also develop from posttraumatic/ischemic myelomalacia or obstruction due to adhesions, compression, or tumor. Syrinxes occur in 63 % of patients with myelomeningocele and scoliosis, and therefore, preoperative MRI is recommended prior to scoliosis instrumentation [44]. A syrinx often accompanies cord tethering, congenital hydrocephalus, and other congenital abnormalities. Hydrosyringomyelia is a common component of Chiari I malformations, probably due to obstruction. Occasionally, isolated primary hydromyelia becomes evident only in late childhood [45].

Imaging

If the syrinx is large, radiographs rarely may reveal fusiform enlargement of the spinal canal, with widening of the interpediculate distance and of the sagittal diameter of the canal. This may be limited to a portion of the spine (often cervical) but in severe cases extends inferiorly into the thoracic and even lumbar spine. MRI is necessary to evaluate the spinal cord, allowing differentiation of syrinx from, for example, a long-standing neoplasm. It can also demonstrate tonsillar herniation, indicating Chiari malformation.

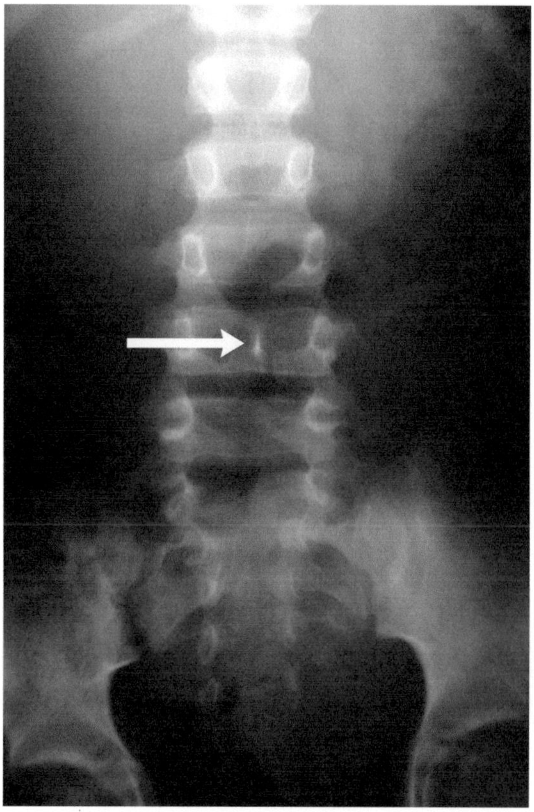

Fig. 3.35 Diastematomyelia with bony septum (*arrow*)

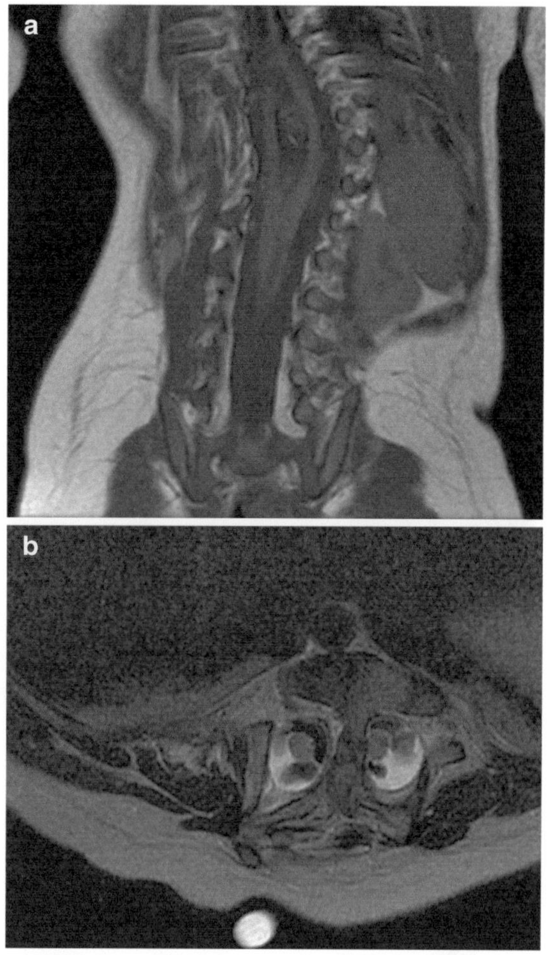

Fig. 3.36 Diastematomyelia. (**a**) Coronal T1-W image shows the two hemicords unite below a bony spur. (**b**) Axial fluid-sensitive sequence shows two hemicords

3.3 Diastomatomyelia

This refers to a longitudinal split in the spinal cord that develops when the notochord divides during cell migration [11]. The two parts are usually asymmetric in size and are separated by a bony (Fig. 3.35), cartilaginous, or fibrous septum; the cord usually unites distally [46]. Diastematomyelia is most common in the upper lumbar region (Fig. 3.36) but can occur anywhere from the lower thoracic spine to the sacrum. Cervical and basicranial diastematomyelia are rare and usually associated with Klippel-Feil (see Fig. 3.40 below) and Chiari malformations [47].

The conus is almost always low, and neurologic signs are likely related to tethering or stretching of the spinal cord. In up to 70 % of cases, each hemicord is encased in its own dural sheath. Skin changes are present in up to 80 % of patients and are similar to those found in other occult spinal dysraphisms. The location of the skin abnormality does not necessarily correlate with the septum level. Diastematomyelia should be distinguished from cord duplication or diplomyelia.

Because the notochord gives rise to vertebral bodies, diastematomyelia can be accompanied by neurenteric cysts, dorsal enteric fistulas, and abnormal vertebral bodies such as hemi- and/or butterfly vertebrae.

Imaging

Radiographs may demonstrate associated increased interpediculate distance and narrow intervertebral discs with possible vertebral body fusion. A subtle linear density may be apparent at the midline if the septum is osseous (see Fig. 3.35). CT depicts a bony septum but will identify the hemicords and a fibrous or

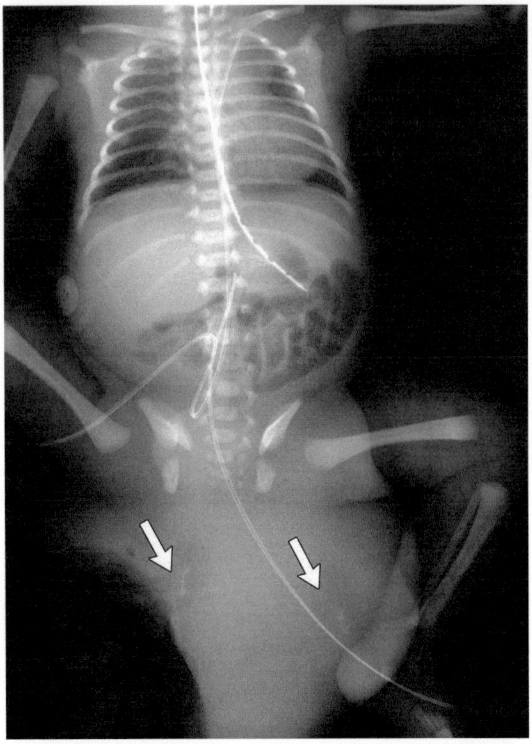

Fig. 3.37 Huge exophytic type I sacrococcygeal teratoma in a newborn boy. There are ill-defined calcifications within the mass (*arrows*) (Umbilical catheters are malpositioned)

cartilaginous septum only if CT myelography is performed. MRI depicts the cord anomaly as well as the dural sac(s) and demonstrates a fibrous, cartilaginous, or bony septum (see Fig. 3.36). The septum often extends anteriorly from the neural arch and thus may not be visibly fused to the vertebral body.

3.4 Congenital Intraspinal Tumors

Lipomas represent 1 % of all spinal cord tumors and may be intramedullary, extradural, or mixed; these lesions are often associated with meningocele, in which case they are termed lipomeningocele. Extravertebral lipomas may enter the spinal canal and cord or remain totally subcutaneous; associated anomalous bony structures may be present. Intraspinal lipomas are strongly associated with large sacral sacs, a low conus, and vertebral abnormalities. Occasionally, neural elements may enter these extraspinal tumors.

Sacrococcygeal teratomas (SCT) (Figs. 3.37 and 3.38) are the most common tumor of the

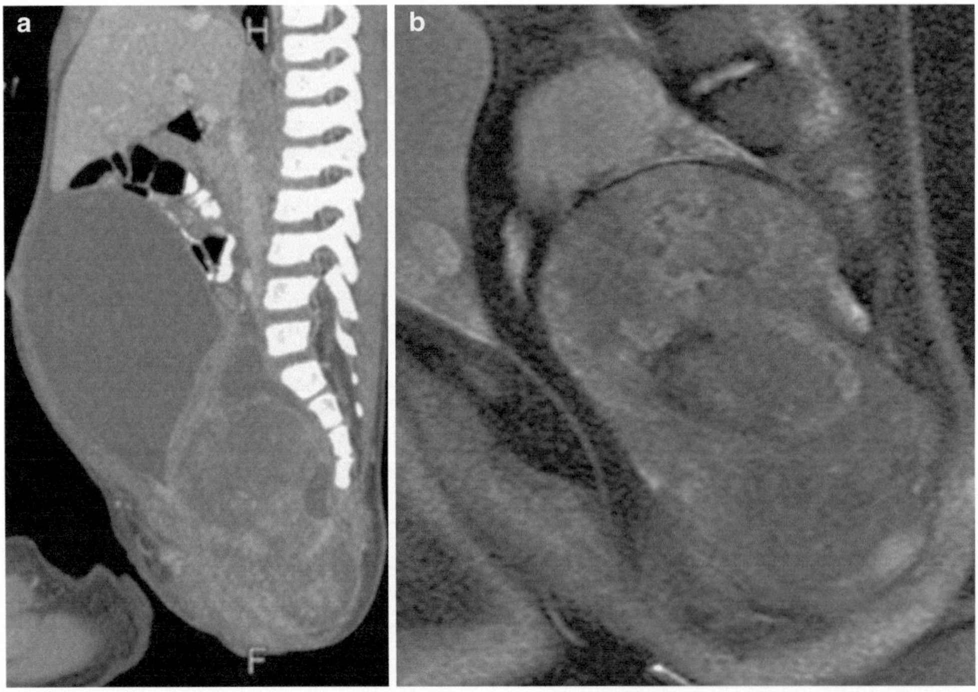

Fig. 3.38 Type IV sacrococcygeal teratoma. Sagittally reformatted contrast-enhanced CT (**a**) and sagittal T2-W MRI (**b**) show a large, inhomogeneous, predominantly solid presacral mass, which elevates and obstructs the bladder

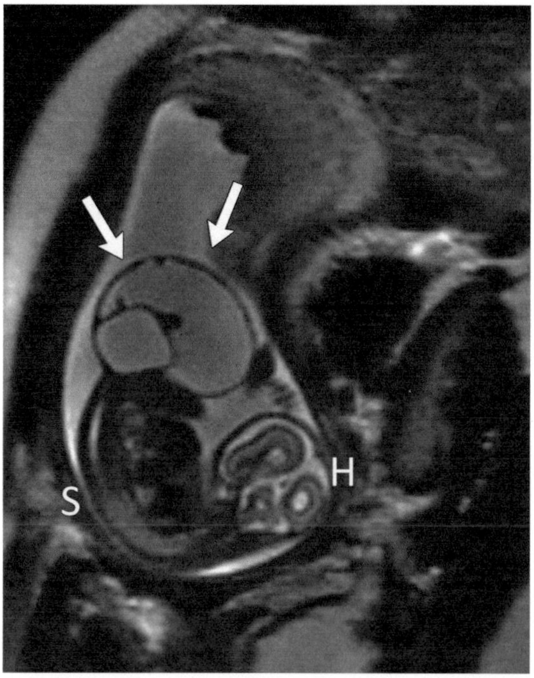

Fig. 3.39 Large exophytic predominantly cystic sacrococcygeal teratoma in a 30-week fetus (single-shot fast-spin echo MRI). *Arrows* delineate teratoma. *H* fetal head, *S* fetal spine

fetus and newborn and are more common in girls [48]. They are closely associated with the coccyx and may involve the spinal canal. By definition they contain three germ cell layers (ectoderm, mesoderm, and endoderm). SCT may be mature or immature and may develop malignant transformation especially if internal (see staging below), in males, or if diagnosed after 2 months of age (Box 3.3). Fetal SCT may present with maternal increased fundal height and polyhydramnios, prompting imaging evaluation and diagnosis of the mass by US and subsequently MRI (Fig. 3.39) [48]. Prenatal hydrops due to a highly vascular tumor portends a poor outcome.

Newborns usually present with a mass. Associated genitourinary anomalies include hydronephrosis and renal dysplasia. Rectal atresia/stenosis or Currarino triad (presacral mass, scimitar sacrum, and anal malformation) may be present. Treatment is complete surgical resection, including resection of the coccyx.

Box 3.3: Sacrococcygeal Teratoma (SCT)

Most common tumor of fetus/newborn
Contains all three germ cell layers
May be malignant, especially if detected after 2 m of age, in male, or completely internal
Associated genitourinary abnormalities
Heterogeneous mixed solid/cystic mass

Sacrococcygeal teratomas may be classified [49] as type I, external (these account for half of the cases [50]) (see Fig. 3.37); type II, predominantly external with presacral internal extension; type III, external and internal with extension into the abdominal cavity; and type IV, entirely internal (see Fig. 3.38).

Imaging
Radiographs may show segmentation abnormalities in the case of lipomas and lipomyelomeningoceles or show a presacral or external SCT mass (see Fig. 3.37). Pre or postnatal US may identify presacral masses and characterize SCT as solid, cystic, or—most often—heterogeneous (15 % are purely cystic) [48]. The vascular/shunting nature of the solid portion of the tumor may be ascertained by Doppler interrogation. MRI provides greater anatomic detail for lipomas, lipomyelomeningoceles, and associated spinal cord abnormalities and may better delineate the extent and characteristics of internal SCT (see Fig. 3.38).

4 Syndromes with Spinal Dysplasia

4.1 Klippel-Feil Syndrome

In Klippel-Feil syndrome, the cervical and upper thoracic spine fuses partially or completely, forming a bony mass (Box 3.4). In its most extreme form, the neck is essentially absent [51]. However, the term can describe any degree of congenital cervical spine fusion if the clinical triad of short neck, low posterior hairline, and limited range of motion at the neck is evident. External and middle ear atresia and malformation may be present as well. Many patients have brain stem or high vertebral anomalies, making them vulnerable to cord impingement if manipulated.

Box 3.4: Klippel-Feil Syndrome

Clinical triad of short neck, low posterior hairline, and limited range of motion at neck
Cervical and upper thoracic spine fusion and/or segmentation anomalies
  C2–3 and C5–6, the most commonly affected
May also have rib fusion anomalies
Sprengel anomaly in up to 50 %
Renal anomalies in about 50 %

Neurologic dysfunction is associated with increased mobility at unfused levels and may progress slowly or decompensate acutely after trauma. Spinal cord compression occurs either anteriorly in flexion or posteriorly due to an hypertrophied ligamentum flavum. Additionally, excess motion above or below fused levels may result in vertebral artery occlusion [52].

Twenty-five percent of patients with congenital scoliosis or kyphosis demonstrate structural malformations of the cervical spine, and 60 % of children with Klippel-Feil have scoliosis that exceeds 15° [53]. Undescended scapula, or Sprengel anomaly (see Chap. 5), occurs in up to 42 % of patients with Klippel-Feil syndrome. In up to half of children with Sprengel deformity, there is an omovertebral bone which extends from the medial border of the scapula to the posterior elements of C5–C7 [54].

Primitive renal tissue is closely linked with the developing cervicothoracic junction, and therefore renal anomalies accompany Klippel-Feil syndrome in more than 50 % of patients. Unilateral renal agenesis is most common, but ectopia and horseshoe kidney may be seen. US should therefore be performed on all patients with congenital cervical spine abnormalities.

Imaging

Radiographs demonstrate total or partial fusion of cervical spinous processes, laminae, pedicles, and vertebral bodies (Fig. 3.40). C2–3 and C5–6

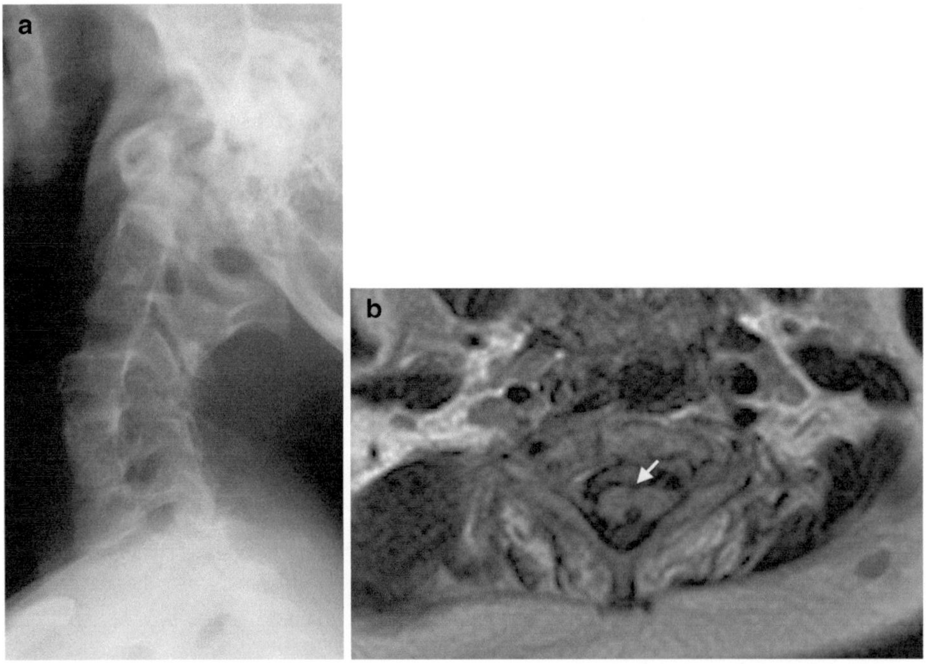

Fig. 3.40 Klippel-Feil syndrome with associated diastematomyelia in a teen. (**a**) Multilevel fusion of vertebral bodies and posterior elements. (**b**) Axial T1-W MRI shows split cord (*arrow*). Also note asymmetric musculature (Courtesy of Rebecca Stein-Wexler)

are most often affected. Upper thoracic segmentation anomalies, scoliosis, rib fusion abnormalities, and Sprengel deformity may also be seen. Progressive fusion incorporating additional vertebral bodies has been observed as these patients mature. The complex anatomy in this area lends itself to CT evaluation, and sagittal or coronal reformatted images as well as 3D reconstructions are often helpful. MRI may delineate associated pathology, such as diastematomyelia (Fig. 3.40).

4.2 Lumbosacral Agenesis (Caudal Regression)

As with many abnormalities of the spine, caudal regression varies from mild to severe. At least one sacral segment is usually present, but the entire sacrum and lumbar spine can be absent, and in especially severe cases, even the distal thoracic spine may fail to form. Unilateral sacral maldevelopment/agenesis results in a sickle-shaped sacrum and sometimes a protruding anterior meningocele. The constellation of scimitar sacrum, presacral mass, and anorectal malformation is termed Currarino triad. Currarino syndrome is the familial autosomal dominant form of the triad related to mutations of a homeobox gene, HLXB9, on chromosome 7 [55].

The spinal cord segments distal to the aplastic vertebrae are usually absent, and bowel/bladder dysfunction is common (indeed, the astute radiologist may diagnose partial sacral agenesis when performing fluoroscopy to assess vesicoureteral reflux, neurogenic bladder, or constipation). Flexion contractures may be seen at the hips and knees. Hip dysplasia occurs in 20 % of cases (Fig. 3.41) and foot deformities in up to 50 %. More than 50 % of patients have scoliosis [56]. Up to 20 % of patients with this abnormality are children of diabetic mothers.

Imaging

The radiographic appearance varies with the level of agenesis. If the sacrum is completely absent, the iliac bones may fuse at the midline or articulate with each other below the lowest intact vertebral segment—lumbar or thoracic. If any portion of the sacrum is present, its position is normal, between the iliac wings.

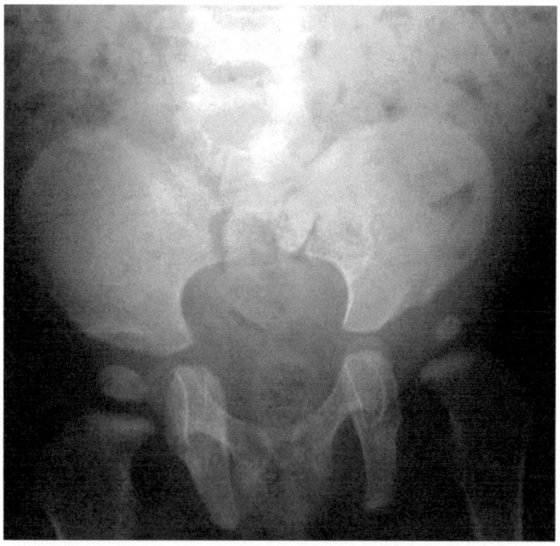

Fig. 3.41 Sacral agenesis and left hip dysplasia in a 1-year-old girl. The iliac wings articulate with each other. The left hip is dislocated superolaterally, and the left acetabulum is dysplastic and shallow (Image copyright Shriners Hospital for Children Northern California)

US evaluation of the urinary tract is essential, since all patients with more than one absent sacral segment have neurogenic bladder and many also have abnormalities of the upper urinary tract. Lower tract disorders such as megalourethra and congenital urethral valves as well as strictures and duplications are common [57]. Gastrointestinal anomalies may be encountered as well.

MRI of the abdomen and spine should be performed early. Spine MRI (Fig. 3.42) may demonstrate dural sac stenosis, intradural adhesions, and cord tethering, whereas abdomen MRI may demonstrate visceral and musculoskeletal abnormalities important for staged surgical repair.

4.3 Neurofibromatosis Type 1

Neurofibromatosis type 1 (NF1) is inherited as an autosomal dominant trait that involves chromosome 17. Mesodermal dysplasia results in a wide variety of skeletal and soft tissue findings (see Chap. 23 for more extensive discussion of NF1).

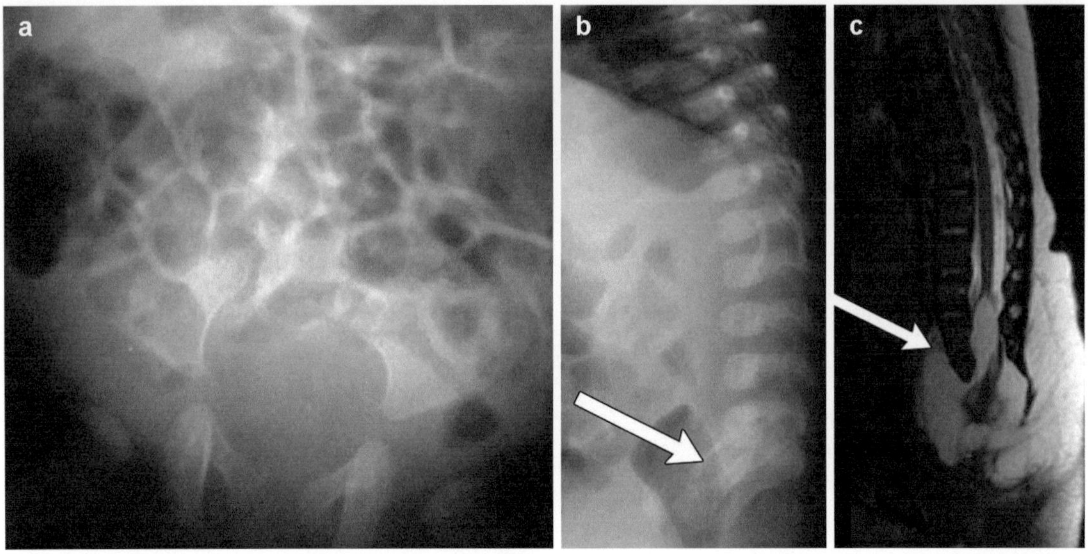

Fig. 3.42 Sacral agenesis in a 6-month-old. (**a**) The iliac wings are positioned too closely together, and most of the sacrum is absent. (**b**) There are no vertebral segments below S1 (*arrow*). (**c**) Sagittal T2-W image shows no vertebral segments below S1 (*arrow*), along with tethering of the spinal cord into a large lipoma that involves the canal, retrorectal space, and subcutaneous tissues

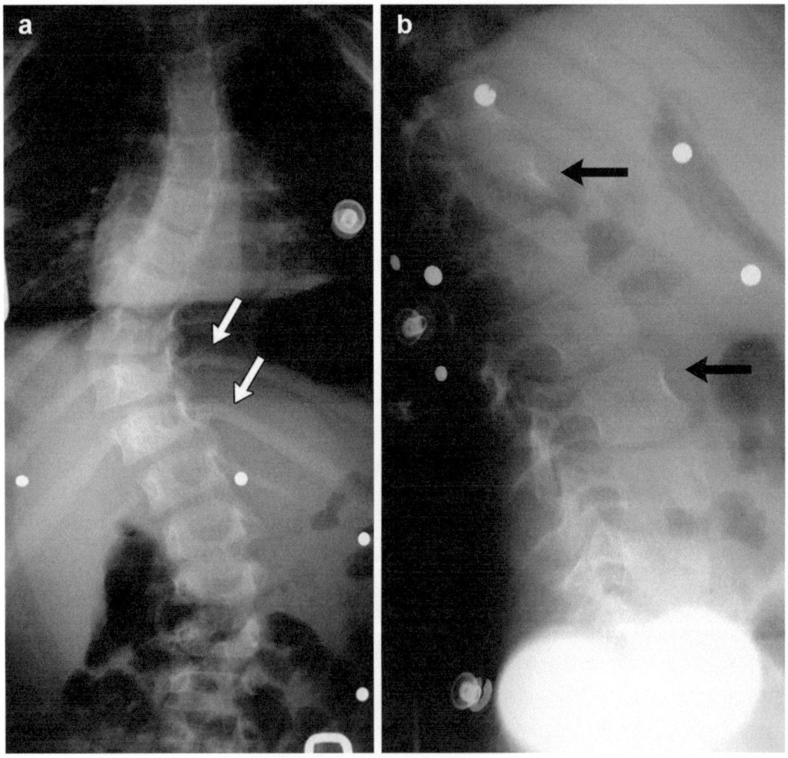

Fig. 3.43 Neurofibromatosis. (**a**-frontal, **b**-lateral) Radiographs in brace show a sharp-angle lower thoracic dystrophic scoliosis and anterior vertebral scalloping (*black arrows*). There is also penciling of the posterior left tenth and 11th ribs (*white arrows*) (Images copyright Shriners Hospital for Children Northern California)

More than 50 % of patients have skeletal abnormalities, including scoliosis and kyphosis. Mesodermal dysplasia may result in vertebral wedging, concave scalloping of the anterior and lateral borders of vertebrae, and irregularities of the vertebral margins (Fig. 3.43). Posterior vertebral scalloping may result from lack of a strong, intact dura (dural ectasia) or from intraspinal

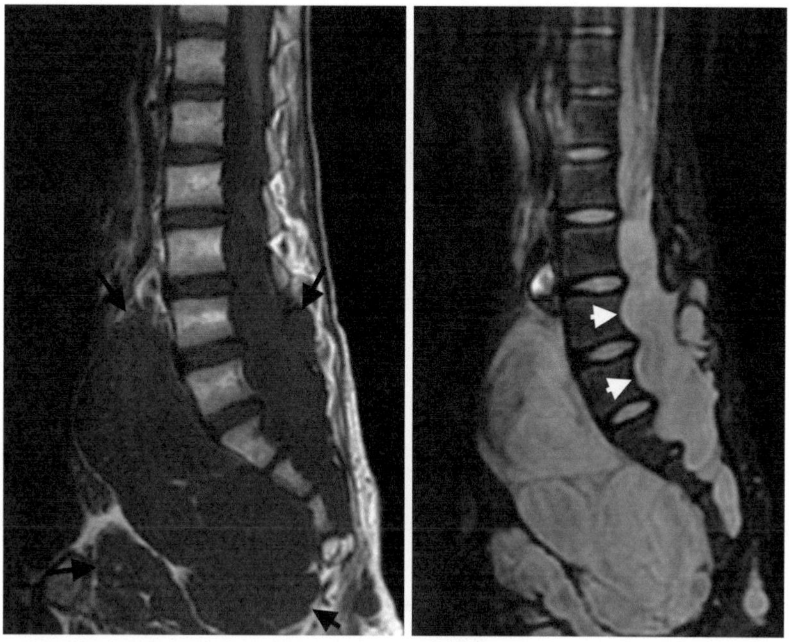

Fig. 3.44 Neurofibromatosis. There are massive plexiform neurofibromas (*arrows*) as well as posterior vertebral scalloping (*arrowheads*)

neurofibromas (Fig. 3.44). This may also be seen with other mesenchymal abnormalities and collagen vascular diseases, such as Marfan, Ehlers-Danlos, and Déjerine-Sottas syndromes [58].

Spinal deformity—most often kyphoscoliosis—is seen in 10–69 % of patients with NF1 and is most common in the thoracic region [59]. Curves may be dystrophic or nondystrophic. Nondystrophic scoliosis is more common and resembles the idiopathic form, although it can modulate to the dystrophic form. As many as 80 % of curves in children younger than 7 years of age will indeed eventually become dystrophic [60].

Dystrophic scoliosis is characterized by a sharply angulated, short-segment curve of four to six vertebral levels (see Fig. 3.43). Neurofibromas may be present, and vertebral bodies at the apex are dysplastic and may appear wedged, scalloped, and rotated. Foramina may be enlarged (usually due to meningeal ectasia and CSF pulsations), and transverse processes can be quite narrow; this configuration contributes to spine instability. The ribs may appear thin ("penciled"), twisted, and irregular. If very thin, they may penetrate the spinal canal at the apex of the curve and cause neural compression [59]. Dystrophic kyphoscoliosis progresses rapidly and requires aggressive treatment.

Severe kyphosis of the cervical spine can suggest the diagnosis of NF1. Cervical spine abnormalities resemble those elsewhere in the spine and occur in as many as 40 % of those with scoliosis [61]. Instability, including atlantoaxial instability, and neurologic deficits may be present in addition to kyphosis [62].

Imaging

Radiographs depict the bony findings described above. Preoperative MRI is essential for patients with NF1, and many advocate routine spine MRI. This allows characterization of dural ectasia, anterior and lateral meningoceles, myelopathy, thecal volume (often increased), and potential intraoperative cord compression. Neurofibromas are readily identified because of their markedly increased T2 signal, characteristic dumbbell or plexiform appearance, and avid enhancement.

4.4 Additional Syndromes

Abnormal formation and growth of the spine are common in many bone dysplasias and heritable syndromes. Kyphosis occurs in 70 % of some dysplasias, especially achondroplasia (Fig. 3.45), mucopolysaccharidoses, spondyloepiphyseal

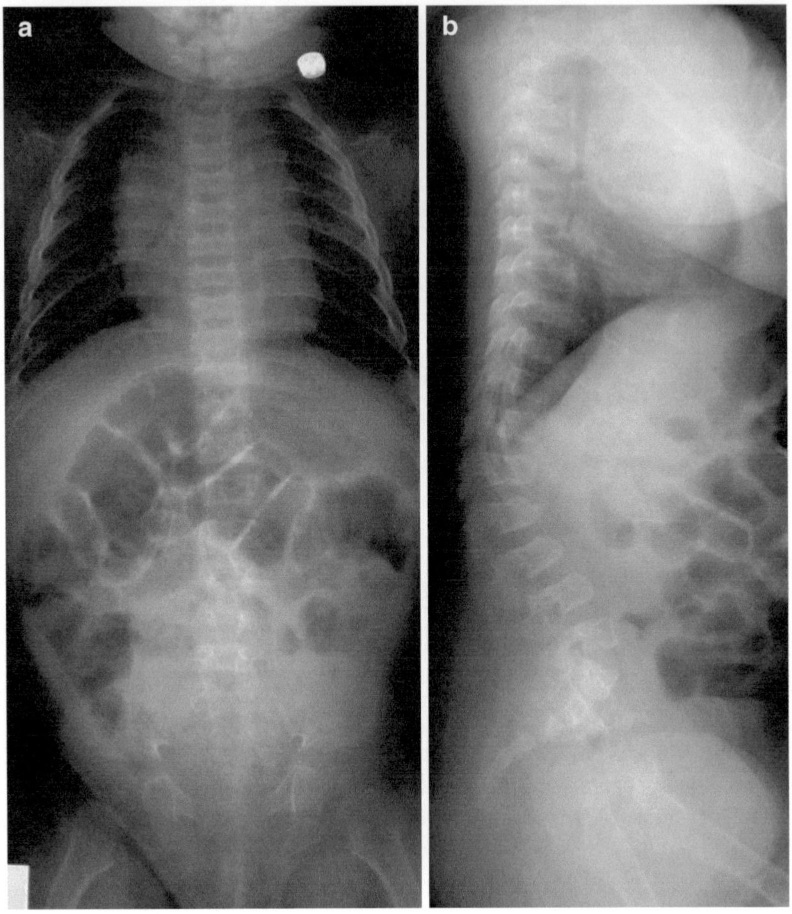

Fig. 3.45 Achondroplasia. (**a**) There is progressive decrease in the interpediculate distance in the lumbar spine. The pelvis also shows typical features of achondroplasia. (**b**) The pedicles are short, and there is focal thoracolumbar kyphosis. The discs are nearly as tall as the vertebral bodies (Images copyright Shriners Hospital for Children Northern California)

dysplasia congenita, diastrophic dysplasia, and metatropic dwarfism. Scoliosis occurs in about one fourth of patients with spondyloepiphyseal dysplasia (Fig. 3.46), diastrophic dysplasia, and metatropic dwarfism. Clinical and skeletal factors can assist with diagnosis, but genetic mapping is necessary in order to differentiate between similar syndromes.

Some of the more common syndromes and dysplasias are discussed in Chap. 23 (such as achondroplasia, osteogenesis imperfecta, and trisomy 21). A few unusual syndromes are discussed briefly below, but thorough presentation is beyond the scope of this text. Texts on skeletal dysplasias offer a more complete review [63].

Spondylocostal dysostosis (Jarcho-Levin syndrome) is an autosomal recessive disorder, characterized by congenital abnormalities of the spine and associated dysplasia of the ribs, leading to severe lordosis and variable thoracic insufficiency (Fig. 3.47). Spondylothoracic dysostosis (Lavy-Moseley syndrome) has less severe lumbar and rib anomalies, but there is a crab-like thoracic deformity due to posterior element fusion, and the clinical prognosis is worse (Fig. 3.48). It is seen predominantly in children of Puerto Rican descent [64].

Marfan syndrome is characterized by reduced amounts of stable collagen and such abnormalities as ectopia lentis, thoracic kyphoscoliosis, dural ectasia, arachnodactyly, pectus excavatum deformity, and cardiovascular lesions. Any of these traits may be partially expressed. Scoliosis is present in 40–60 % of patients. Vertebral scalloping and intrasacral meningoceles may also occur. With autosomal dominant inheritance, Marfan syndrome should be considered in tall, myopic children with pectus excavatum deformity and a family history of scoliosis.

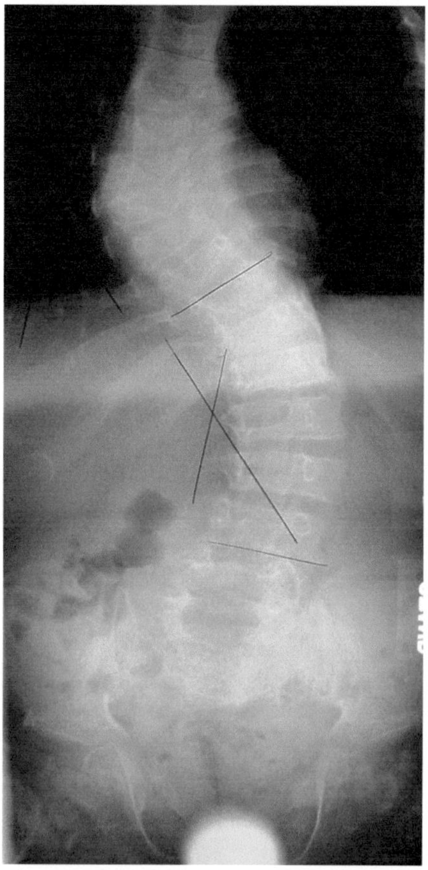

Fig. 3.46 Spondyloepiphyseal dysplasia. There is diffuse platyspondyly and biphasic scoliosis. Fragmentation of the femoral heads

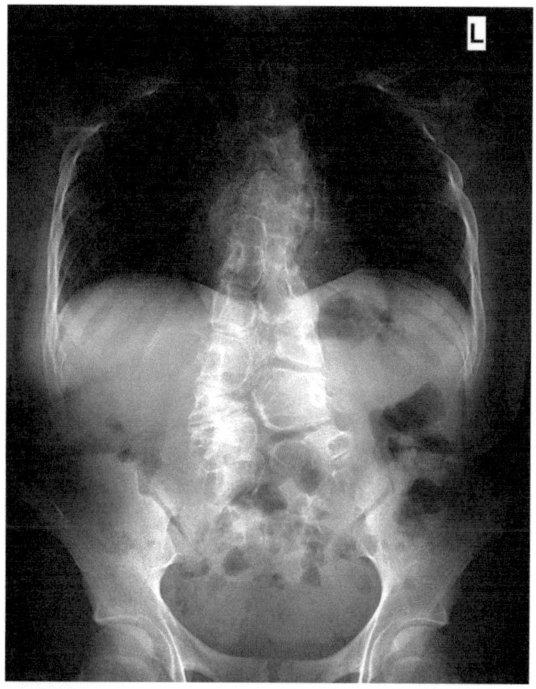

Fig. 3.47 Spondylocostal dysostosis with multiple hemivertebrae and butterfly vertebrae

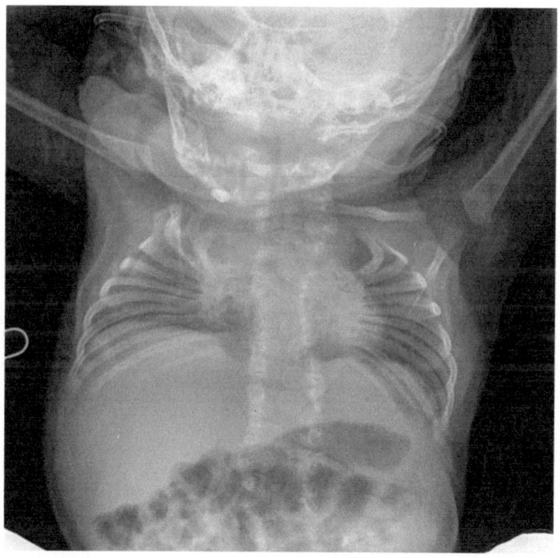

Fig. 3.48 Spondylothoracic dysostosis with crab-like deformity of the thorax due to posterior rib fusion

The most important feature of trisomy 21 is the malformation, aplasia, or laxity of the transverse ligament that holds the odontoid to the axis, resulting in C1–2 subluxation in 20 % of patients (discussed in the section above on atlantoaxial subluxation). In addition, cervicothoracic kyphosis may develop in young adults. It resembles juvenile kyphosis radiographically, with decreased disc space height and with end plate irregularities.

Significant abnormalities of the spine occur in many other dysplasias. For example, kyphoscoliosis is a prominent feature of diastrophic dwarfism, and extreme platyspondyly is seen with metatropic dwarfism. Patients with osteogenesis imperfecta (Fig. 3.49) may have severe scoliosis, or their spine may be normal. Butterfly vertebrae may be seen in patients with Alagille syndrome (see Fig. 3.19), also known as arteriohepatic dysplasia [65]; these patients also have a paucity of bile ducts (resulting in chronic cholestasis) and congenital heart abnormalities such as tetralogy of Fallot and pulmonary artery stenosis.

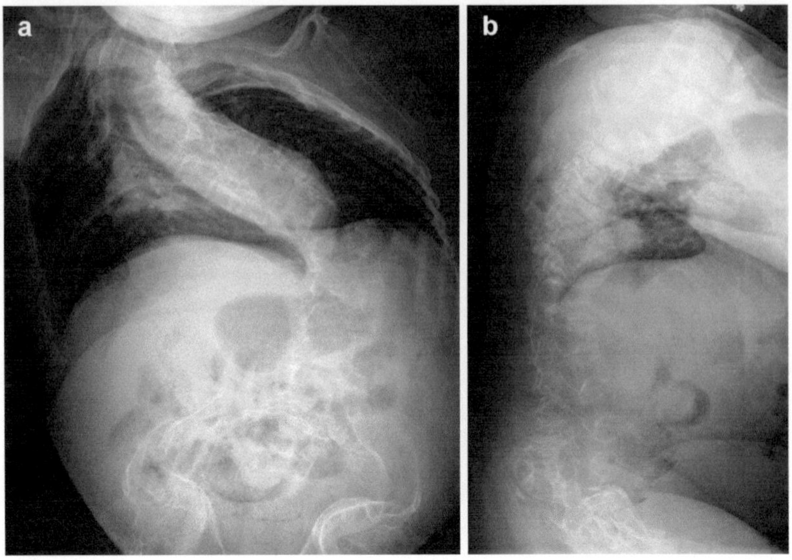

Fig. 3.49 Osteogenesis imperfecta, characterized by severe scoliosis, biconcave vertebral bodies, osteoporosis, and acetabular protrusion (**a**-frontal, **b**-lateral)

Table 3.2 Etiologies of scoliosis

Category	Subtype	Example
Idiopathic	Infantile	
	Juvenile	
	Adolescent	
Congenital	Osteogenic	Segmentation anomalies
	Neurogenic	Spinal dysraphism
		Chiari malformations
Developmental dysplasia/dysostosis	Bony dysplasia	Achondroplasia
	Mesenchymal dysplasia	Neurofibromatosis
Neuromuscular	Neurogenic	Cerebral palsy
	Myopathic	Duchenne muscular dystrophy
Tumor	Osseous	Osteoid osteoma
	Intracanalicular, extramedullary	Neurofibroma
	Intracanalicular, intramedullary	Astrocytoma
	Paraspinous	Ganglioneuroma
Trauma		
Infection	Tuberculous	
Rheumatoid	Juvenile idiopathic rheumatoid arthritis	

Adapted from Refs. [66, 86, 104]

5 Idiopathic Scoliosis

The word scoliosis, derived from the Greek word for curvature or crookedness, refers to curvature of the spine in the coronal plane. About 80 % of cases of scoliosis [66] are of seemingly spontaneous origin and thus termed idiopathic. Non-idiopathic causes of scoliosis include congenital spinal anomalies, neuromuscular disease, and irritative, traumatic, metabolic, or extraspinal lesions (Table 3.2). Non-idiopathic scoliosis may also be associated with neuroectodermal or mesodermal diseases or syndromic dysplasias.

Many theories have been advanced to explain idiopathic scoliosis, etiology, including connective tissue abnormalities, unusual growth patterns, neuromuscular and central nervous system (CNS) aberrations, and hormonal variations, but none seems to explain all the features that may be encountered [67]. There is evidence for multifactorial inheritance [67–69], as the rate of scoliosis occurring in first-degree (10–11 %) or first- through third-degree (26 %) relatives is up to 20 times that expected in the normal population. Geographic variation in the incidence of scoliosis is also well recognized. Estimates of the prevalence of adolescent idiopathic scoliosis in the normal population (in patients 10–16 years old) varies from 2 % to 4 %, depending on how scoliosis is defined [68].

It is important to remember that spinal curvature is three dimensional [66]. Biomechanical initiation of scoliosis appears to begin with axial rotation of the involved thoracic vertebral bodies, resulting in increased pressure on the more ventrally placed vertebrae and decreased pressure on the more dorsally placed vertebrae [70]. In the immature skeleton, bone growth is inhibited by growth plate compression and accelerated by growth plate tension; this results in the more ventral part of the spine becoming the concave side of the curve and the dorsally located vertebrae the convex side. Mechanical imbalance accelerates during skeletal growth, with resultant progression of scoliosis. Supporting this, the pedicles and laminae are short and thick on the concave side of the curve, and the cartilage of the ipsilateral end plates demonstrates degeneration and decreased chondrogenesis along with osteogenesis, consistent with growth inhibition.

Scoliosis may progress during growth but ceases with skeletal maturity unless the curve is severe (more than 30°) [66].

5.1 Clinical Variants

Idiopathic scoliosis has been divided into three temporal classes, defined by age of onset/recognition/main period of progression: infantile (0–3 years), juvenile (4–10 years), and adolescent (11–18 years) (Box 3.5). It can alternatively be grouped into early onset (<5 years of age) and late onset (>5 years of age), based upon the risk of developing cardiopulmonary complications; progressive early-onset scoliosis can lead to cardiopulmonary compromise in later life, whereas late onset does not [71]. The following discussion employs the classic division into three different age groups.

Box 3.5: Idiopathic Scoliosis

Infantile

Onset <3 years old, 75 % resolve by age 2 years

0.5–4 % of cases of scoliosis

Usually thoracic levoconvex

More likely to progress if	Onset after age 1 year
	Double major curve
	>35°
	Altered articulation between ribs and vertebrae

Juvenile

Onset 4–10 years old, almost all will progress

12 % of cases of scoliosis

Usually dextroconvex

Adolescent

Onset 11 years old to skeletal maturity

Most common

Usually thoracic dextroconvex, compensatory lumbar levoconvex

Curve increases most quickly during growth spurt (Risser 0–1)

Infantile scoliosis is diagnosed before the age of 3 years and accounts for 0.5–4 % of all idiopathic scoliosis. The clinical picture is typical: it is more common in boys than girls, is usually not present at birth but develops during the first 6 months of life, and is associated with hip dysplasia in 25 % [72]. Plagiocephaly is also commonly associated [73]. Almost all (85–90 %) curves are thoracic and convex to the left (levoconvex) (Fig. 3.50). The curves resolve without treatment during the first 2 years of life in three quarters of these patients. Factors that suggest a curve will progress include: (1) double major curves, (2) curvature of more than 35°, (3) onset after the age of 1 year, and (4) changes in the normal relation of the rib articulation with the vertebra [74, 75]. The rib-vertebral angle difference (RVAD) also predicts progression (see discussion on measurement, below).

Juvenile idiopathic scoliosis is first diagnosed between the ages of 4 and 10 years and represents about 12 % of all idiopathic scoliosis. There is a male predominance in younger patients (4–6 years), but after that age, the curve is more common in girls. Most curves in patients in the United States are convex to the right (dextroconvex). Scoliosis

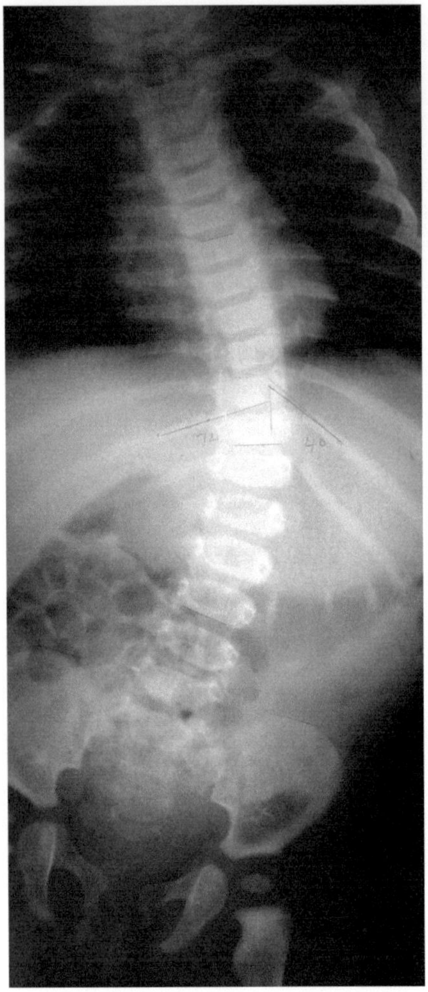

Fig. 3.50 Infantile scoliosis. There is levoconvex thoracolumbar scoliosis, but no segmentation anomalies. The RVAs are 74° and 30°, and the RVAD is 74°–30° = 34°, indicating increased risk of curve progression (see Fig. 3.58 and text) (Image copyright Shriners Hospital for Children Northern California)

first recognized at this age almost invariably progresses.

Adolescent scoliosis is the most common type of idiopathic scoliosis and is diagnosed in patients after age 11 years and before skeletal maturity has been attained. On average, girls present at 13 years of age and boys at 14. There is a female predominance of 4:1–8:1. The majority of these curvatures are dextroconvex in the thoracic region with a levoconvex lumbar compensatory curve (Fig. 3.51), but other patterns are common. Curvature increases most rapidly during the normal growth spurt, coincident with development of pubic hair and breast buds; by the time of menarche and male axillary hair development, about 18 months of growth (and potential curvature increase) remain. Curves are thus most likely to progress in patients between age 9 and 13 years, in those with progression skeletal maturity between 9 and 14 years, if the Risser stage is 0 or 1 (see following discussion), or if annual vertical growth exceeds 2 cm [66]. The younger the patient and the greater the curve, the faster the curve will progress [76].

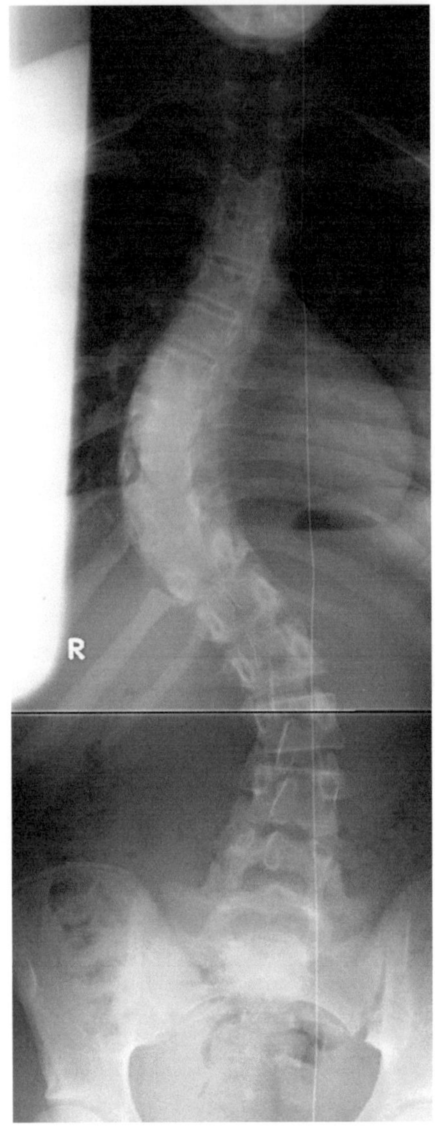

Fig. 3.51 Adolescent idiopathic scoliosis in a 15-year-old girl. Primary dextroconvex thoracic and secondary levoconvex curves. Incidental ununited spinous process at T12 (Same patient as Fig. 3.69) (Image copyright Shriners Hospital for Children Northern California)

5.2 Curve Patterns and Terminology

The Scoliosis Research Society has attempted to standardize terminology [77]. The curve is identified by the level of the apical and end vertebrae, as well as the side of convexity. There are five possible patterns: (1) cervicothoracic, (2) thoracic (most common), (3) thoracolumbar, (4) lumbar, and (5) double structural (double thoracic, combined thoracic and lumbar, combined thoracic and thoracolumbar) [77]. Although the length and severity of the curve may change during growth, the pattern usually does not.

The direction of curvature is labeled according to its convexity. Thus, a curve whose convex side faces the left is termed "levoconvex," whereas a curve whose convex side faces the right is termed "dextroconvex."

All curves can be identified as structural (also called major) or nonstructural (minor). Nonstructural curves are flexible with lateral bending to both sides, straightening when the patient bends toward the convexity (Fig. 3.52). Structural curves are less flexible and retain some deformity with lateral bending. With severe or long-standing curves, vertebral bodies become wedged and thoracic kyphosis is reduced, leading to straightening of the thoracic spine. A compensatory curve that returns spinal alignment to the midline is usually present above or below a structural curve of any significant magnitude. This compensatory scoliosis is initially flexible but may become structural with time. The most characteristic idiopathic pattern is a structural dextroconvex thoracic curve with a compensatory levoconvex lumbar curve.

Finally, the severity of the curvature can be graded into the following groups: I, less than 20°; II, 20 to 30°; III, 31 to 50°; IV, 51 to 75°; V, 76 to 100°; VI, 101 to 125°; and VII, more than 125°.

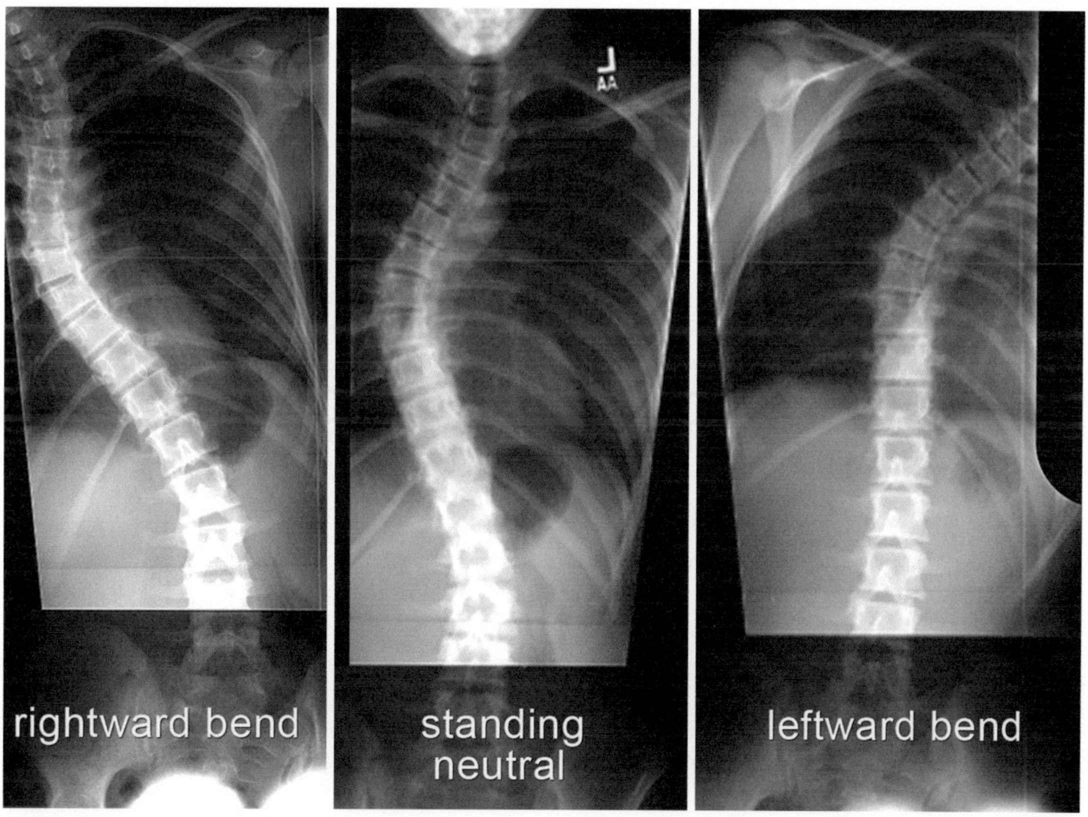

Fig. 3.52 Scoliosis with lateral bending views. Neutral view shows primary dextroconvex thoracic and secondary levoconvex lumbar scoliosis. With rightward bending, the rightward thoracic curve does not significantly change. With leftward bending, there is complete correction of the leftward compensatory curve (Images copyright Shriners Hospital for Children Northern California)

5.3 Imaging Techniques

Radiology plays an essential role in identifying and following any type of scoliosis. To analyze alignment from C5 to the level of the hips, a frontal (coronal) standing projection of the spine is obtained (without shoes), from the lower edge of the mandible to the level of the top of the greater trochanters. Although some centers obtain the initial frontal image in the anteroposterior projection in order to achieve greater bone detail at the spine, the posteroanterior projection is generally preferred, since it delivers a lower radiation dose to the breasts and thyroid. If the patient is unable to stand, a sitting or supine view may be performed.

Structures outside the field of view are excluded by collimation and using a gonadal shield. To reduce breast and thyroid exposure, a combination of posteroanterior positioning, breast shields, high tube voltage, contoured beam filtration, high-speed films and screens, replacement of anti-scatter grids with air gap techniques, and segmented field radiography with beam collimation can be employed [78, 79]. Using computed radiography or digital imaging systems also reduces dosage. For example, the EOS 2D/3D low-dose digital imaging device (EOS Imaging SA, Paris, France) simultaneously captures frontal and lateral standing images that can then undergo 3D reconstruction to create 3D surface images (Fig. 3.53). These

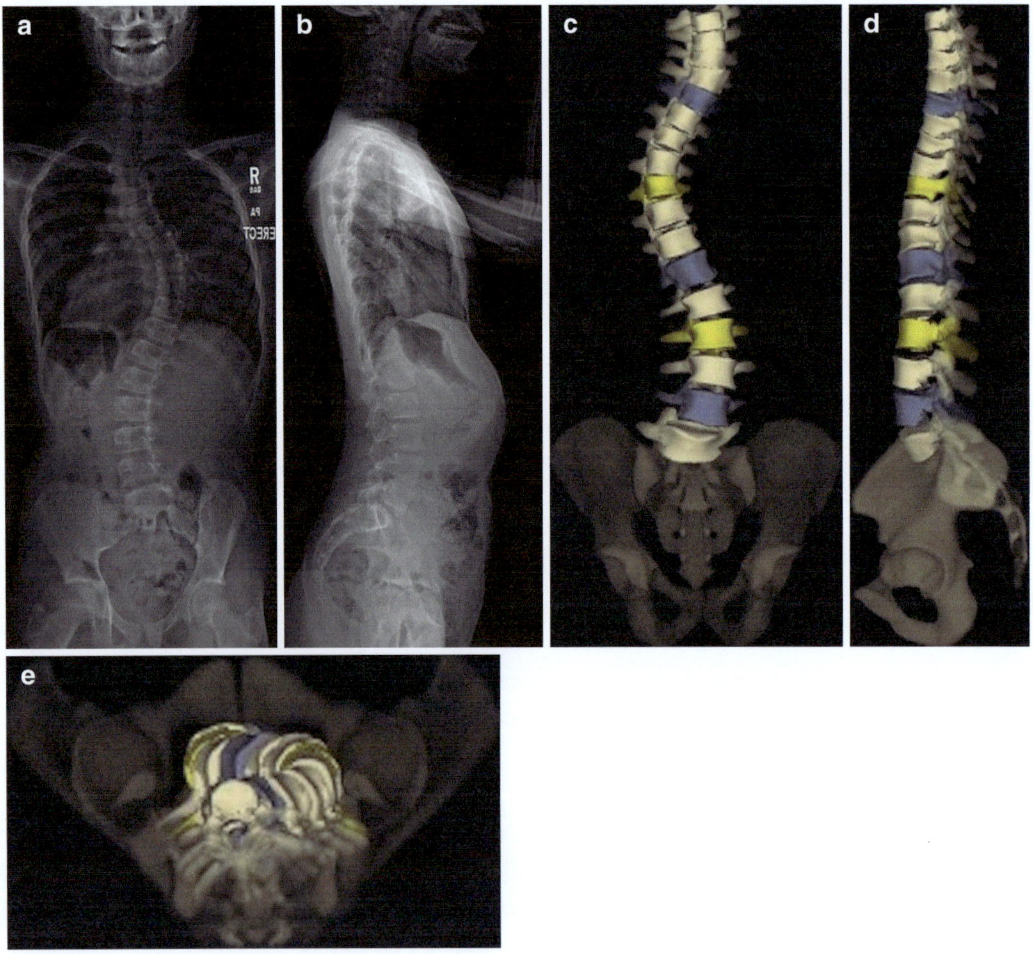

Fig. 3.53 Spine image obtained with low-dose digital EOS 2D/3D device. Frontal (**a**) and lateral (**b**) images of the spine can be processed into a variety of 3D images, including coronal (**c**), sagittal (**d**), and axial (**e**). In this case, the apical and end vertebrae have been highlighted with *yellow* and *blue*. The axial 3D image shows the degree of rotation and displacement (Courtesy of Leslie E. Grissom)

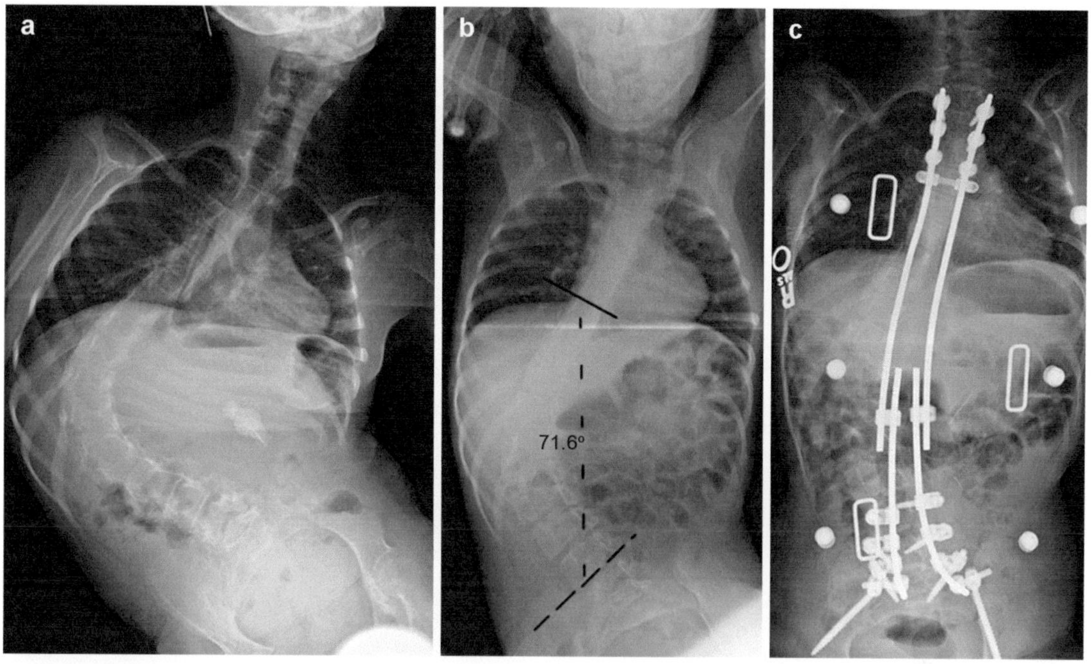

Fig. 3.54 Neurogenic scoliosis in a 7-year-old girl. (**a**) Standing view shows severe dextroconvex thoracolumbar C-shaped scoliosis. Note pelvic tilt, gastrostomy button, and gracile long bones. (**b**) Stretch supine view shows improvement in the rightward scoliosis. (**c**) Sitting view in brace after posterior instrumentation and fusion shows significantly improved curvature (compared to preoperative study) (Images copyright Shriners Hospital for Children Northern California)

can be manipulated further to allow detailed analysis of curve structure [80]. All of these measures should be employed in any facility performing a significant number of spine examinations, as radiographic monitoring of scoliosis has been shown to increase the risk of breast cancer, thyroid cancer, and infertility [76, 81–84].

Since scoliosis is a three-dimensional process and the sagittal component of the thoracic curve must also be assessed, initial evaluation includes a lateral projection of the spine. Further lateral projections are usually only performed if there is evidence of abnormal kyphosis or lordosis. The sagittal image is obtained with the same field limits, shielding, and technique described above. To remove the effect of upper extremity positioning on forward or backward lean, the arms should be extended parallel to the floor with the wrists resting on a support (usually an intravenous [IV] pole) so they do not bear weight.

Other imaging techniques may be necessary for surgical planning or to determine the need for bracing. In these situations, the degree of flexibility and correctability of curvatures is evaluated with supine maximal bending images. If the patient cannot cooperate with bending studies, a stretch or traction supine view may be obtained (Fig. 3.54). Since dose-reduction techniques do not provide optimal visualization of osseous anatomy, detailed anteroposterior (AP) images are indicated to further evaluate suspicious areas. In addition, complex osseous abnormalities may be assessed on noncontrast CT with three-dimensional (3D) reformation. All of these examinations should be ordered judiciously to minimize radiation exposure.

Additional imaging may be helpful. For example, skeletal maturity can affect treatment decisions; the hand, elbow, and iliac crest apophyses provide information about skeletal maturity at different ages (see Chap. 2). If leg length discrepancy (Fig. 3.55) is suggested by clinical evaluation or significantly unequal iliac crest height, leg length measurement may be performed

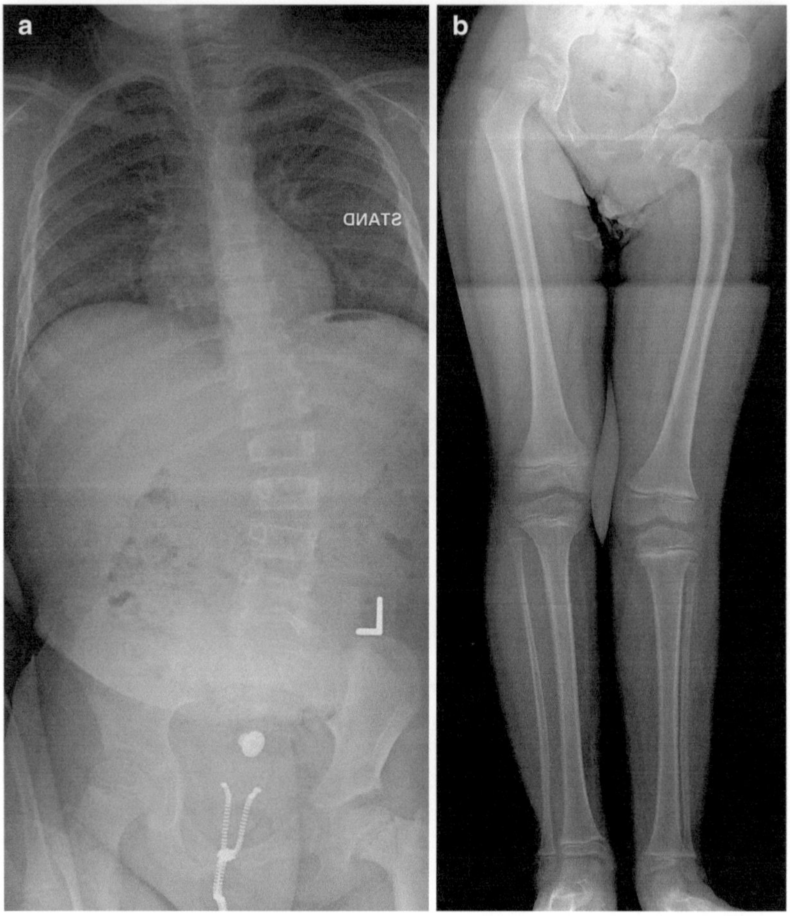

Fig. 3.55 Scoliosis resulting from leg length inequality in an 8-year-old boy. (**a**) The right hemi-pelvis is higher than the left, and there is levoconvex thoracolumbar scoliosis. (**b**) Left femoral (and to a lesser degree tibial and fibular) hypoplasia (Images copyright Shriners Hospital for Children Northern California)

by a variety of techniques (see Chap. 13). In order to eliminate the effect of leg length disparity on spinal curvature, erect spine radiographs can be obtained with the patient sitting (Fig. 3.56), or a standing view can be obtained with blocks elevating the short extremity. Nuclear scintigraphy is reserved for demonstrating whether an irritative focus (e.g., osteoid osteoma) is causing scoliosis and for evaluating postoperative pseudarthrosis.

In cases of congenital scoliosis, the urologic system should be evaluated by screening US, whereas the presence of symptoms dictates the need for renal US in cases of idiopathic scoliosis. MRI is useful in assessing underlying or occult spinal pathology in scoliosis. MRI should be performed when intraspinal tumors are suspected based on clinical or radiologic examination; indeed, 27 % of patients with intraspinal tumors also have scoliosis [85] (Fig. 3.57). Other clinical indications for spine MRI include spinal dysraphism, early age of onset of scoliosis, painful scoliosis, abnormal neurologic exam, rapidly progressive curve (more than 1° per month),

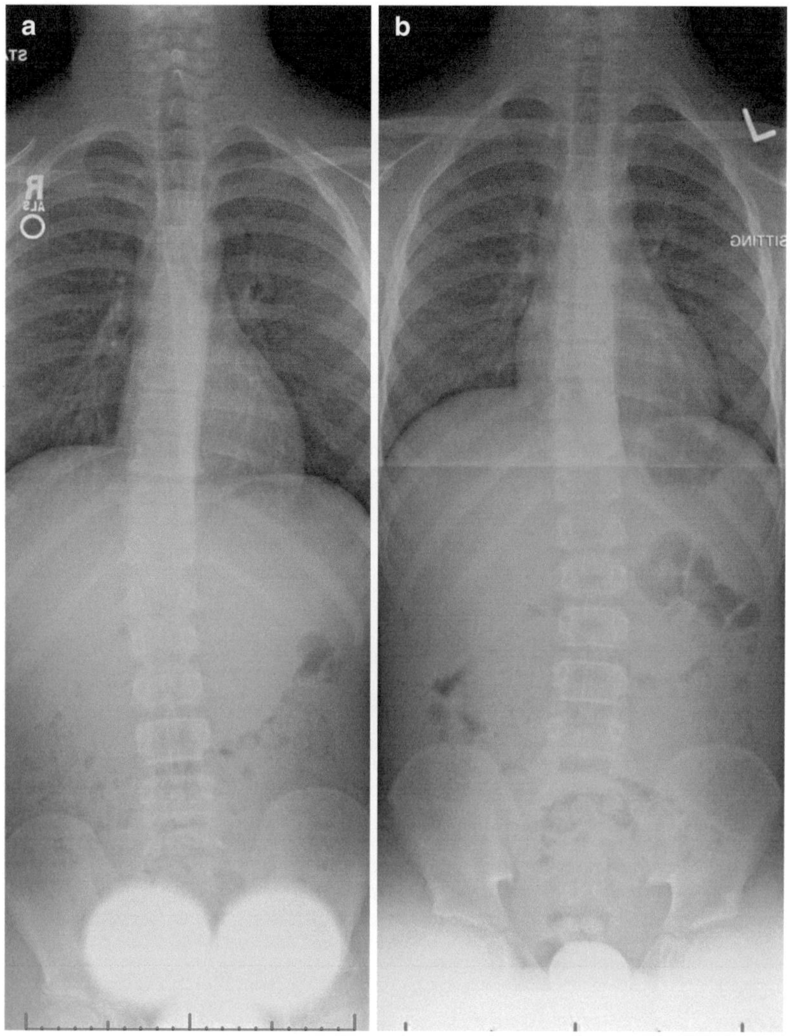

Fig. 3.56 Flexible positional spinal curvature due to leg length inequality. (**a**) Standing view shows dextroconvex spinal curvature with pelvic tilt (*left side* higher due to short right lower extremity). (**b**) Curvature flips when the patient sits (Images copyright Shriners Hospital for Children Northern California)

atypical curve (such as levoconvex thoracic), developmental abnormalities such as neurofibromatosis or Klippel-Feil syndrome, and for surgical clearing or to assess for postoperative complications [79, 86].

Two to four percent of neurologically normal patients with idiopathic adolescent scoliosis have CNS abnormalities [87–89], the most common being Arnold-Chiari I malformation, subtle syrinx, tethered cord, and filar lipoma [86]. In the absence of a neurologic deficit, the first two would usually not be treated [90]. However, treating a CNS lesion may prevent neurological deterioration and progression of scoliosis, and the presence of an untreated lesion may compromise successful surgical correction [91].

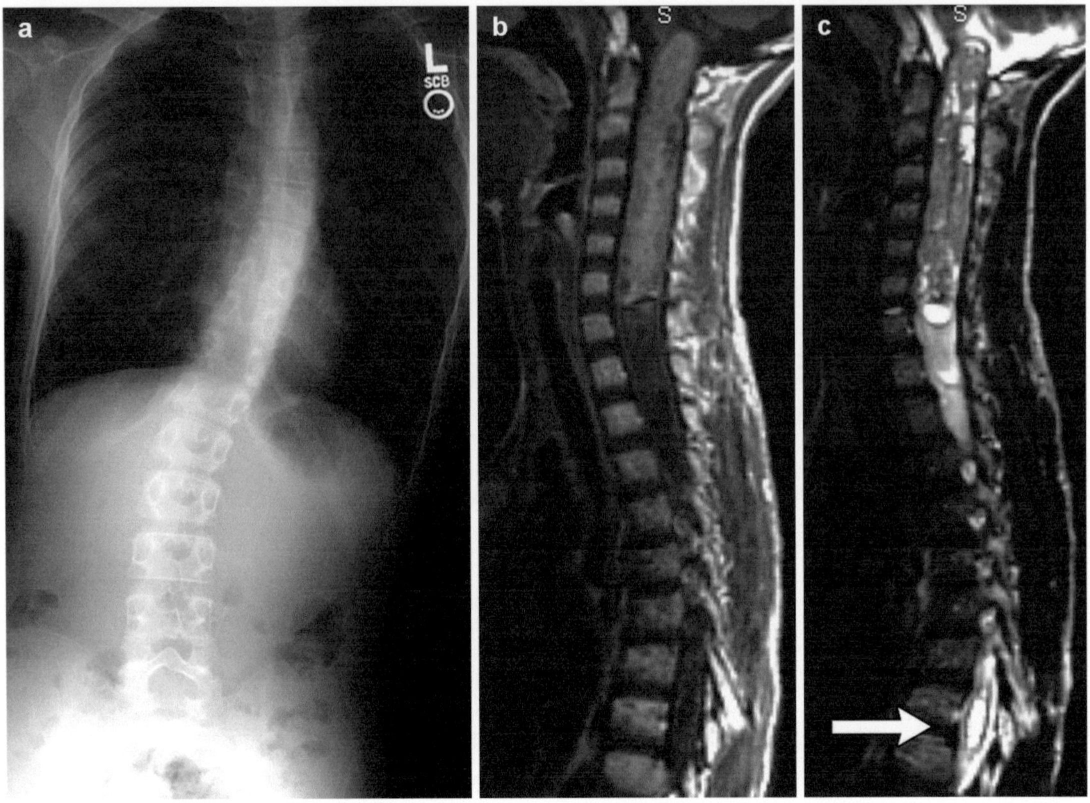

Fig. 3.57 Scoliosis in a 13-year-old boy with hyperactive reflexes and and positive Babinski test. (**a**) Levoconvex thoracic and dextroconvex lumbar spinal curve. Sagittal T1-W gadolinium-enhanced (**b**) and T2-W (**c**) images show an enhancing, partially cystic ependymoma in the cervical and upper thoracic cord, bulging upward into the posterior fossa. There is also a thoracic syrinx (*arrow*)

5.4 Radiologic Analysis and Imaging Techniques (Boxes 3.6, 3.7)

Box 3.6: Techniques for Measuring Scoliosis

Cobb: assesses angle of curvature in coronal or sagittal plane

- Angle between lines parallel to end plates or pedicles of upper and lower vertebrae
- Difference of 6° indicates progression

Rib-vertebral angle difference (*RVAD*): indicates likelihood of progression

- Evaluate apical vertebra on frontal projection
- Based on comparing bilateral rib-vertebral angles (RVA)
  - RVA: angle between line connecting/extending from the head and neck of each rib (where neck widens into shaft)
  - Vertical line perpendicular to vertebral end plate
- RVAD = concave side RVA minus convex side RVA
- RVAD >20° indicates progression is likely

Box 3.7: Nash and Moe Technique to Assess Vertebral Body Rotation

Evaluates position of pedicle on convex side of curve on frontal projection

Divides convex side of vertebral body into thirds

- 1+ Pedicle in lateral third
- 2+ Pedicle in middle third
- 3+ Pedicle in medial third or at midline
- 4+ Pedicle projects over other side of the vertebral body

Several key components of every curve must be assessed, including identifying the apical and transitional vertebrae. The apical vertebra is the one that is most rotated and most laterally displaced; its end plates are the least tilted (Fig. 3.58). Rotation and lateral displacement of the vertebrae above and below this apical vertebra will diminish until either no curve remains or an opposite curve begins. The vertebrae at the termination of the curvature are called either "end" or "transitional," respectively. These vertebrae may be identified by their lack of rotation and by the fact that lines drawn along their superior and inferior end plates point maximally toward the concavity of the curve. Additionally, at the transitional or end vertebrae, the intervertebral disc space will be maximally wedged, with the greatest width on the convex side of the curve.

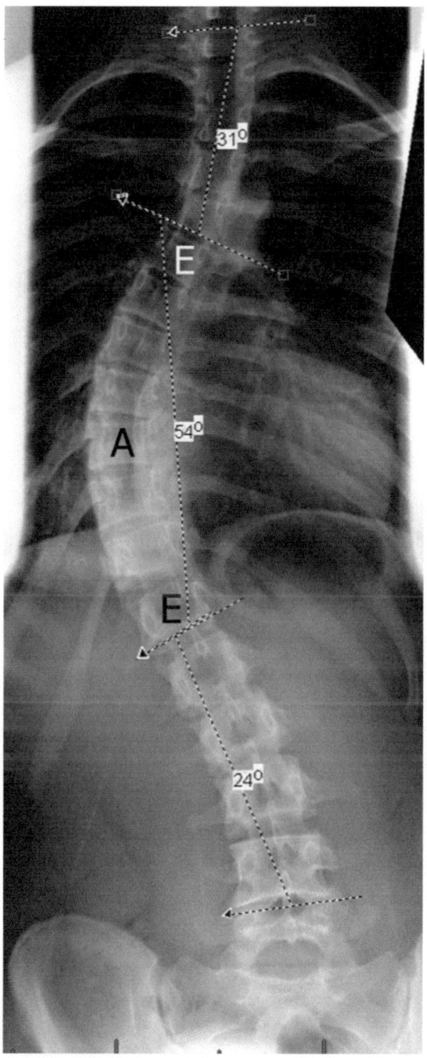

Fig. 3.58 Triphasic idiopathic scoliosis in a 16-year-old girl. The primary dextroconvex thoracic curve Cobb angle measures 54° (*A* apical and *E* end vertebrae of this curve). There are compensatory levoconvex lumbar and upper thoracic curves. The thorax is centered to the right of the pelvis

Once the curve extent has been determined, all subsequent measurements should use the same vertebral end points, unless the curve becomes longer or shorter. In that case, the new examination should be compared with the most recent, assessing the alteration in curve extent.

The Scoliosis Research Society recommends the standardized Cobb method of calculation. A line is drawn along the superior end plate of the upper end (or transitional) vertebra, and another is drawn along the inferior end plate of the lower end (or transitional) vertebra (Fig. 3.58). If the end plates are indistinct, the tops or bottoms of the pedicles may be used. The angle between these two lines (or between lines drawn perpendicular to them, if the angle is not sufficiently acute to allow measurement) is the degree of curvature. Severe vertebral wedging may exaggerate the true curve measurement.

When two oppositely convex curves are present but contiguous, the lower end vertebra of the upper curve represents the upper end vertebra of the lower curvature and is therefore included in both measurements. This technique has an interobserver error of 7–9° [92, 93]. The 95 % confidence level for any observed change between serial measurements is 3.3–10° for scoliosis and 11° for kyphosis [93–95]. The variation is less with computer-generated measurements [79]. Generally, a difference of 6° between serial radiographs indicates curve progression [79].

The rib-vertebral angle difference (RVAD) predicts curves that are more likely to progress. The rib-vertebral angle (RVA), which is determined on a frontal radiograph at the apical vertebra and its corresponding ribs, is formed by the intersection between a line drawn along the midpoint of the head and neck of each rib and a vertical line drawn perpendicular to the superior or

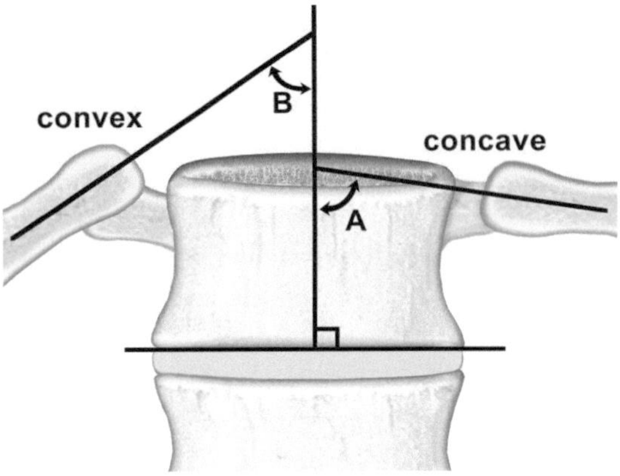

Fig. 3.59 Rib-vertebral angle (RVA) and rib-vertebral angle difference (RVAD) calculation. The RVA is the angle formed between a perpendicular line drawn to either the upper or lower end plate of the apical vertebra with a second line drawn from the midpoint in the rib head to the midpoint in the rib neck just medial to the region where the neck widens into the shaft of the rib (angle *A* for concave side, *B* for convex side). The RVAD is the difference between the RVA on the concave and convex sides of the curve (*A-B*)

inferior end plate of the vertebra (Fig. 3.59). The RVA is usually smaller on the convex side of the curve. The RVAD is obtained by subtracting the RVA on the convex side from the RVA on the concave side. If the RVAD is greater than 20° and if the head of the rib projects over the vertebra, the curve will likely progress. In addition, when both the RVA is less on the concave side than the convex side of the curve and the eleventh and twelfth ribs are very oblique to the spine, a double structural progressive curve is likely.

The Cobb method is also used to determine the degree of lordosis or kyphosis on the lateral projection (Fig. 3.60). Thoracic kyphosis is usually measured between the superior end plate of T3 and the lower end plate of T12; lumbar lordosis is measured between the top of Ll and the lower edge of L5. Normal thoracic kyphosis ranges from 21 to 42°, and normal lumbar lordosis ranges from 31 to 50° [27]. These values do not change with patient age, sex, height, or weight [96]. Severe scoliosis is often associated with thoracic lordosis and straightening of normal lumbar lordosis.

Rotation is maximal in the apical vertebra of the structural curve. One or more of the vertebrae above or below the maximally tilted end vertebra may also be rotated. Generally, the vertebral body rotates anteriorly toward the convexity, although CT studies have shown both opposite rotation with scoliosis and the presence of some rotation in patients without scoliosis [97].

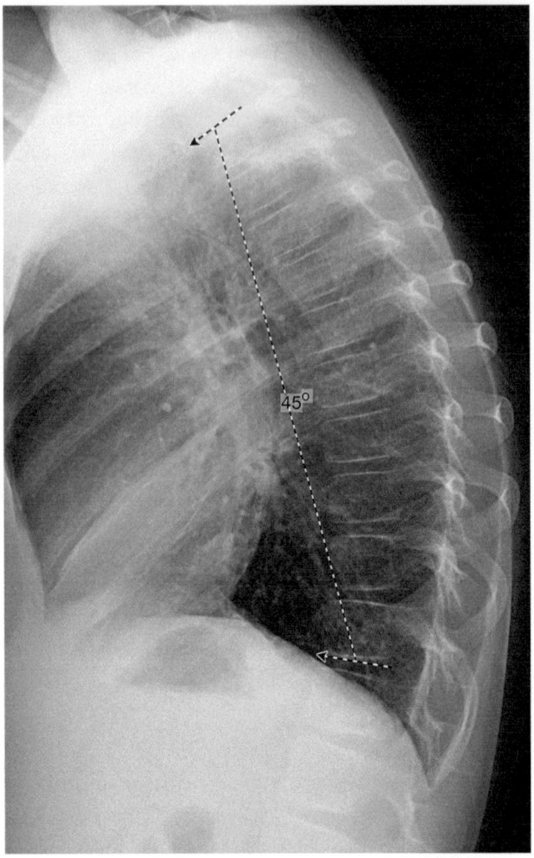

Fig. 3.60 Mildly increased thoracic kyphosis in an 8-year-old girl. Cobb measurement technique delineates 45° of kyphosis

Rotation is common but not obligatory; occasionally, fairly severe curves have no rotation. Nash and Moe describe a method for estimating rotation, mild to severe, and this should be sufficient for clinical purposes [66, 98] (Fig. 3.61). The pedicles of a non-rotated vertebra are symmetrically positioned, tangent to the edges of the vertebral body. With rotation, the body usually turns toward the convex side of the curve, and the pedicle on this side appears to move away from the edge of the vertebral body and toward the

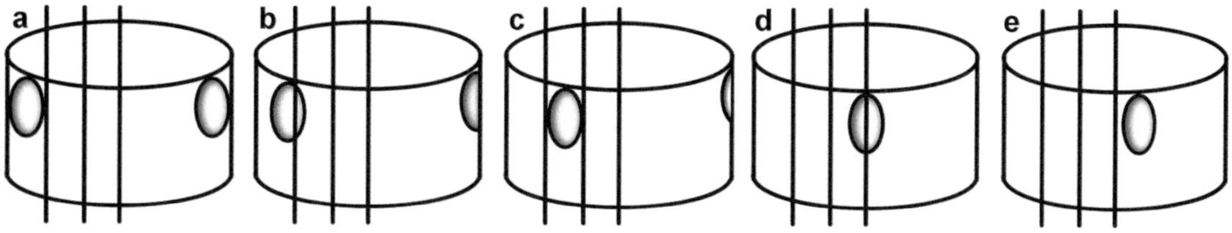

Fig. 3.61 Grading of vertebral rotation by the Nash-Moe method. (**a**) No rotation. (**b**) Grade 1. (**c**) Grade 2. (**d**) Grade 3. (**e**) Grade 4. On a frontal spine radiograph, each involved vertebra is bisected by an imaginary line, and the half vertebra on the convex side is then divided into outer, middle, and inner thirds. Rotation is quantified on the basis of the location of the convex-side pedicle in one of these segments and the visibility of the concave-side pedicle, which gradually disappears as rotation progresses. The pedicles are shown as vertically oriented ovals (Reprinted with permission from Kim et al. [66])

midline. The pedicle on the concave side becomes progressively less apparent.

Rotation can be estimated by assessing the pedicle position relative to the vertebral body (evaluating the pedicle on the convex side of the curve). The distance between the vertebral edge and its midline is divided into thirds. If the pedicle lies in the lateral one third, rotation is termed 1+; in the middle one third, 2+; and in the medial one third or in the midline, 3+. Rotation greater than this is denoted 4+. Roughly speaking, the percentage of migration of the pedicle equals the degree of rotation of the body; for example, 50 % pedicle displacement (pedicle in midline, or 3+) equals 50° rotation. CT may be employed if this determination affects critical surgical decisions.

How a curve changes with bending determines whether or not it is structural (see Fig. 3.52). While a nonstructural curve corrects scoliosis and vertebral rotation (returning to normal, straight alignment), morphologic changes prevent structural curves from correcting. Nonstructural curves are usually either compensatory to structural scoliosis or secondary to irritative or extraspinal causes, most often leg length discrepancy. With leg length discrepancy, the convexity of the curve is ipsilateral to the short limb (see Fig. 3.55). A nonstructural curve usually does not progress; however, it may become structural due to growth retardation on the concave side of the curve and subsequent ligament shortening [66]. Additionally, wedging of the vertebral body indicates a permanent structural change. The degree of wedging can be graded from 1+ to 4+ [99].

Coronal and sagittal balance is measured using a plumb line from the center of the C7 vertebral body (Fig. 3.62). On the frontal view, this line is compared with the central sacral vertebral line (CSVL). The CSVL bisects the sacrum and is drawn perpendicular to a tangent connecting the iliac crests [66]. The normal CSVL is within 2 cm of the plumb line. On the lateral view, the plumb line should be within 2 cm of the sacral promontory (defined as the most cephalad part of the ventral sacrum) [100].

On the lateral view, the gravity line and pelvic incidence assess gravitational alignment between the trunk and feet. The center of balance, or gravity line, should be located anterior to the spine on the lateral view [101]. Since anteroposterior translation and/or rotation of the pelvis attempts to maintain sagittal balance, evaluating pelvic alignment is essential in patients with scoliosis [101]. Pelvic incidence, which is the sum of pelvic tilt and sacral slope, is utilized to describe pelvic alignment and guide corrective surgery (Fig. 3.63).

Evaluation of maturity is crucial when following idiopathic scoliosis, as curvature may increase until the spine is mature. Radiologic observation of the iliac apophyses can gauge maturity [102]. The Risser stages of maturity, which correlate with standard bone age determinations, progress as follows: the iliac apophysis first ossifies laterally (stage 1), and the maturation process extends medially until there is complete capping of the crest (stage 4); complete fusion of the apophysis (stage 5) occurs some years later, often after age 20 (Table 3.3) (Fig. 3.64). However, average age

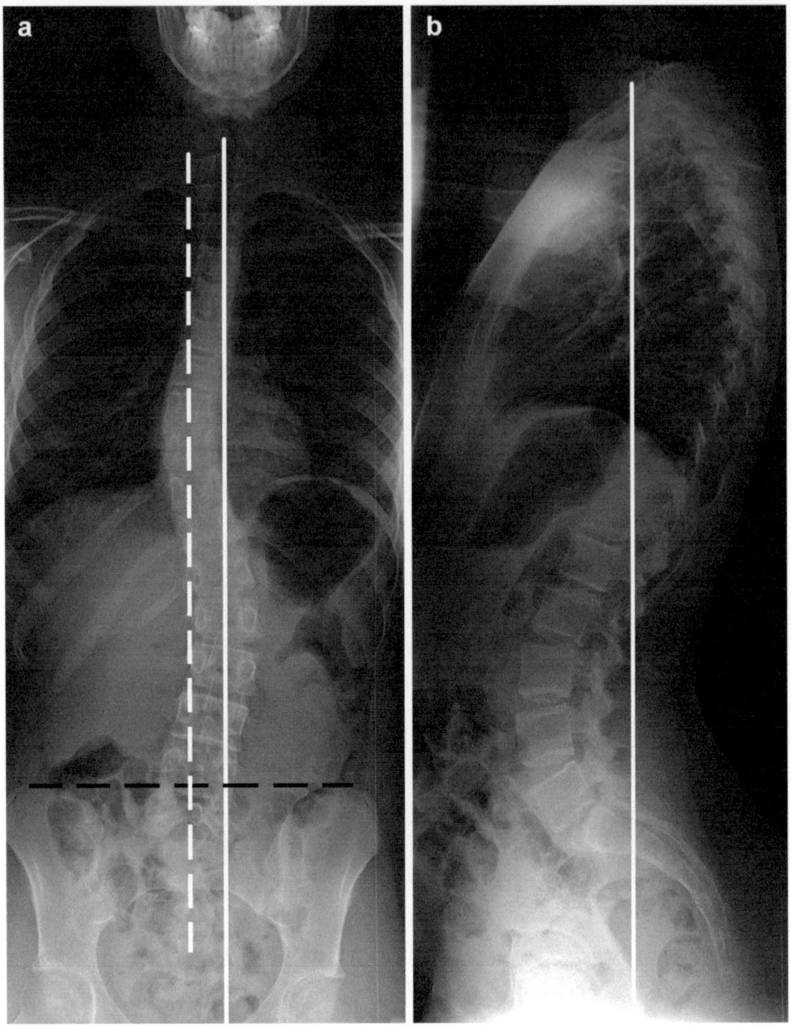

Fig. 3.62 Idiopathic scoliosis in a 14-year-old girl. (**a**-frontal, **b**-lateral) The C7 plumb line is the solid white line on the frontal and lateral views dropped from the center of the C7 vertebral body. The central sacral vertebral line (CSVL) (*dashed white line*), which bisects the sacrum, is drawn perpendicular to a line connecting the tops of the iliac crests (*dashed black line*)

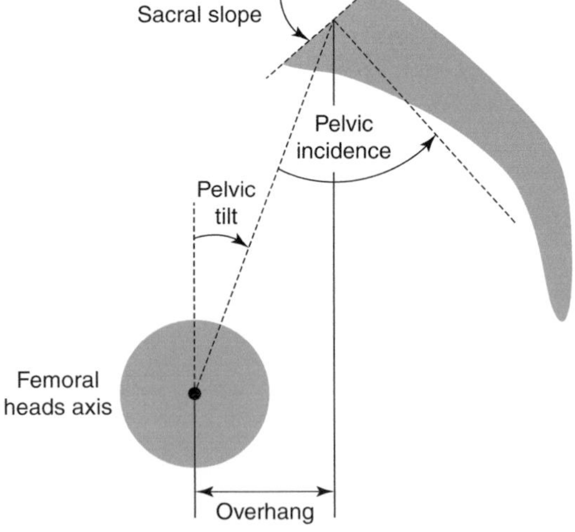

Fig. 3.63 Determining pelvic incidence. The sacral slope is the angle between the horizontal and the sacral plate. Pelvic tilt is the angle between the vertical and a line drawn between the midpoint of the femoral head and the midpoint of the sacral plate. Pelvic incidence is the sum of these two angles (Reprinted with permission from Schwab et al. [101])

Table 3.3 Correlation of Risser stage with mean bone age

	Mean bone age (years, months)	
Risser stage	Girls	Boys
1	13, 8	14, 7
2	14, 6	15, 7
3	15, 2	16, 2
4	16, 2	17, 0
5	18, 1	18, 6

Adapted from Ref. [126]

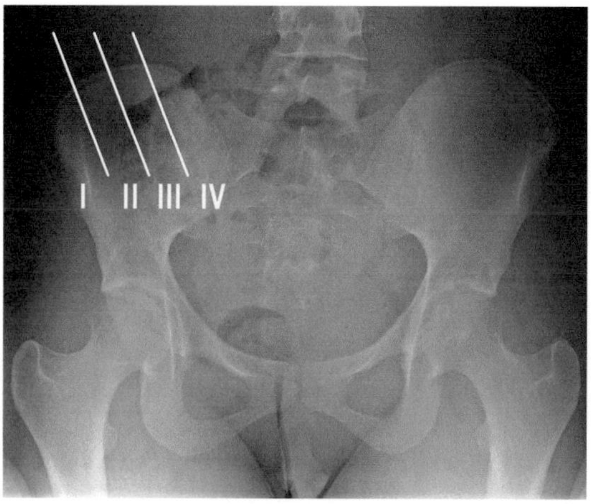

Fig. 3.64 Risser staging. The iliac crest apophysis ossifies from anterior and lateral to posterior and medial. At stage 0, the apophysis has not ossified. For stages I to IV, divide the iliac crest into four equal parts and assign the Risser stage according to the most advanced point of ossification of the apophysis (this patient is Risser stage IV). At stage V, the apophysis has fused (Image copyright Shriners Hospital for Children Northern California)

of menarche and thus maximal spinal growth occurs 8 months before stage 1. During the period of accelerational growth, before ossification of the iliac crest apophysis, skeletal maturation may be assessed by evaluating the olecranon apophysis (Sauvegrain method) or the configuration of the hand (Greulich and Pyle, among others) (see Chap. 2 for additional discussion of techniques for assessing skeletal maturation). The vertebral ring apophyses tend to fuse at the same time as the iliac crest apophyses. Thus the spine may continue to grow and scoliosis to progress, until Risser stage 5 and after extremity growth plate fusion [103].

Sequential monitoring is performed at intervals of 4–12 months, depending on the nature of the curve and age of the child [71]. At each visit, the same end vertebrae should be measured and compared to several previous examinations. After growth stops, curves greater than 30° should be monitored for progression about every 5 years [66].

5.5 Treatment

Treatment depends on the etiology and severity of the scoliosis, associated symptoms, and the patient's perception of the deformity. Options include observation, bracing, and surgery.

Orthotic Management

Nonoperative treatment of scoliosis generally involves orthotic (brace) control of curvature and is usually indicated when curvature approaches the 25–30° range and when children have significant growth remaining (Fig. 3.65); it is also indicated at lesser degrees of scoliosis in younger children with rapid progression. For most curvatures, however, a plastic, molded, underarm thoracolumbosacral orthosis (TLSO) is adequate. The brace can be expected to somewhat decrease the curvature (e.g., from 30 to 20°) and maintain the curvature at this value. In general, the Cobb angle should decrease about 30 % when the brace is in place [104]. After bracing therapy concludes, the curvature may remain improved or gradually return to its original value by the time spinal growth is complete. In that case, the orthosis has served to halt progression.

Surgical Management

Spinal fusion is indicated when scoliosis approaches or exceeds 50°. The primary goal is to prevent curve progression by fusing the involved segments; secondary goals include restoration of truncal balance, improvement in spinal curvature, and improved cosmesis (such as diminishing a rib hump) [71]. Occasionally, surgery corrects cardiopulmonary impairment caused by thoracic deformity. As each case is different, the decision for surgical treatment varies, based on likely outcomes with or without surgery [71]. Fusion is most commonly performed

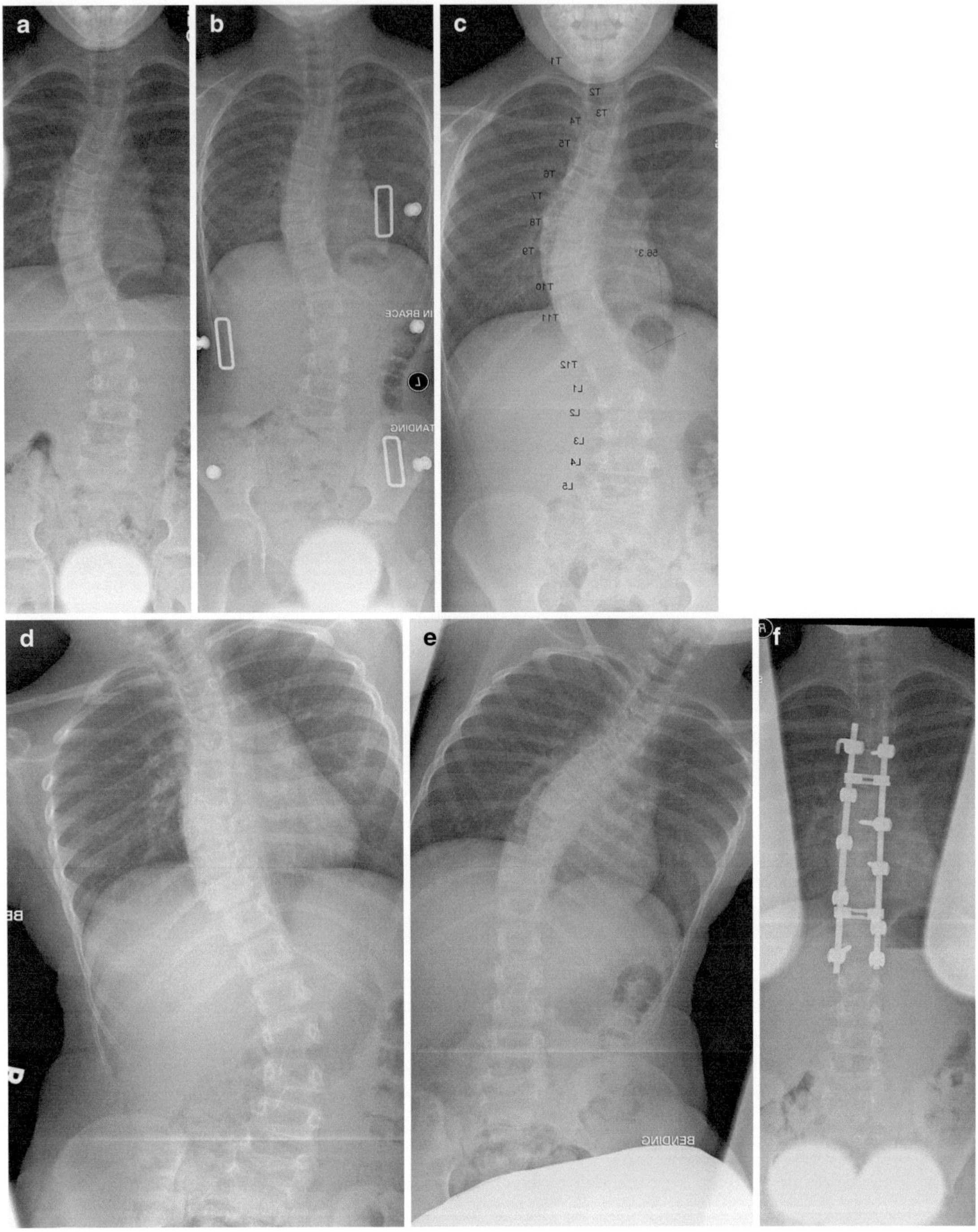

Fig. 3.65 Idiopathic scoliosis. At age 11 years, this girl had a 43° dextroconvex scoliosis (**a**) that decreased to 33° after bracing (**b**). At age 12, after completion of brace therapy, her thoracic curve had worsened to 56° (**c**). Bending views show that the dextroconvex thoracic curve decreases to 28° with rightward bending (**d**) and the 25° levoconvex secondary curve completely corrects with leftward bending (**e**). After posterior spinal fusion (**f**), the thoracic curve measures 7°, and the secondary levoconvex lumbar curve has resolved (Images copyright Shriners Hospital for Children Northern California)

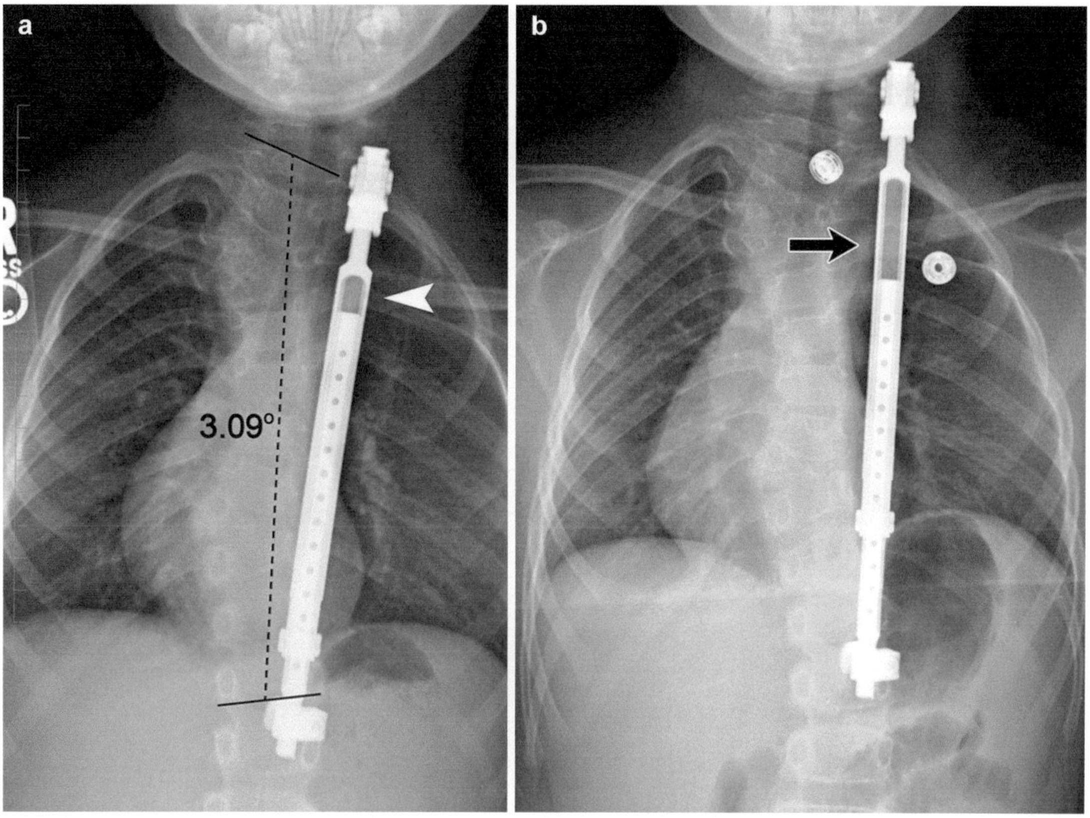

Fig. 3.66 VEPTR instrumentation in an 8-year-old boy. Radiographs before (**a**) and after (**b**) lengthening show distraction (*arrow* vs. *arrowhead*) at the tandem connector (Image copyright Shriners Hospital for Children Northern California)

posterior to the laminae; fusion of the anterior vertebral column is generally combined with posterior fusion and performed for cases of severe neuromuscular, congenital, and dysplastic scoliosis. Hardware, technique, and nomenclature are continually being modified. While detailed explanation is beyond the scope of this text, some typical procedures are illustrated in Chap. 27.

Posterior Spinal Fusion (see Fig. 3.65)
Permanent growth arrest and halt in curve progression are obtained by bone grafting and facet obliteration, with instrumentation holding the spine in place during the period of graft maturation. The original stabilization apparatus was the Harrington rod, but many methods of segmental fusion offering greater correction and stability have since been developed. These include custom rods, pedicle screws, laminar hooks, sublaminar wires, and crossbars (see Fig. 3.65). Growing implants may be employed in young patients with severe early-onset congenital scoliosis, syndromic scoliosis, or scoliosis due to cerebral palsy, spinal muscular atrophy, or chromosomal abnormalities. When growing rods are used, the spine is not fused; this allows for continued spinal growth while stabilizing or improving curvature (Fig. 3.66).

Anterior Spinal Fusion
This may be performed alone or in combination with posterior fusion; the latter is useful when severe neuromuscular forces would defeat isolated posterior fusion or when bone is dystrophic or the configuration of posterior elements is suboptimal (e.g., with spinal dysraphism). In this procedure, the intervertebral discs are excised and the gap is filled with bone. Instrumentation is applied to the vertebral bodies along the convex

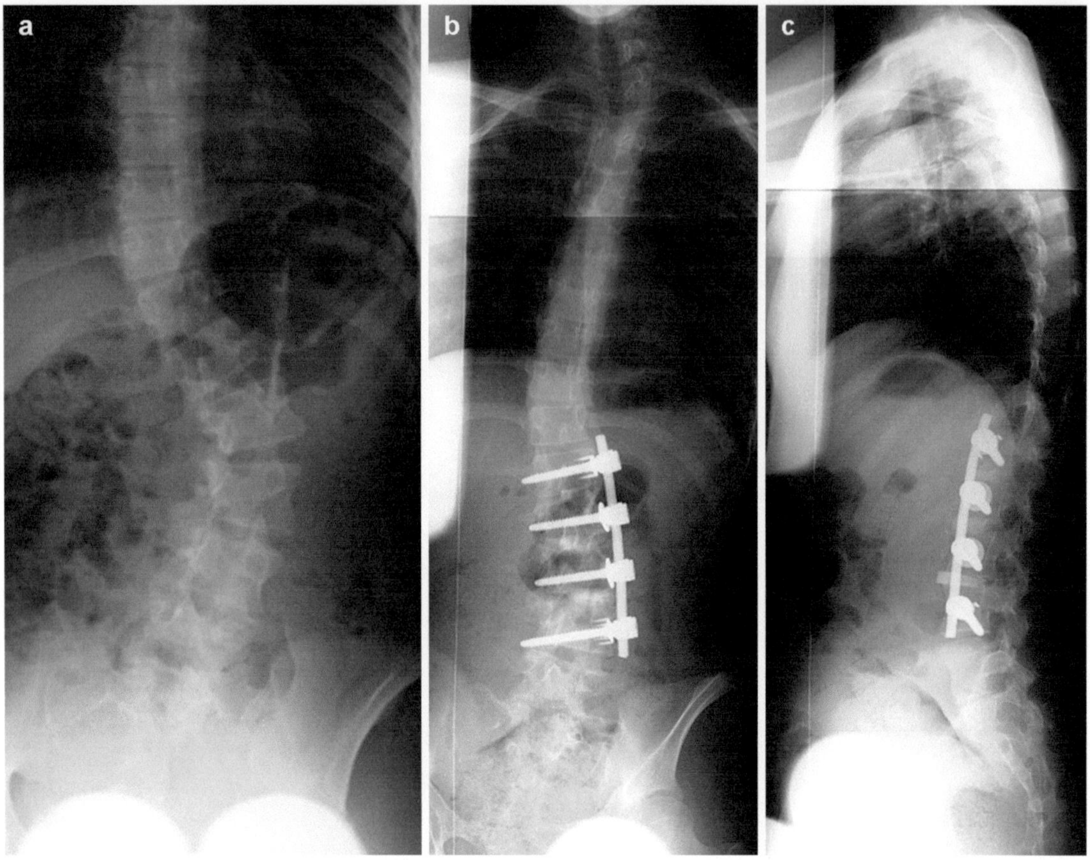

Fig. 3.67 Focal lumbar rotoscoliosis in a teenage girl. (**a**) Asymmetric pedicles indicate rotation. (**b**, **c**) Postoperative images show scoliosis has improved after anterior spinal instrumentation

side of the structural curve, compressing the vertebrae and correcting the curve (Fig. 3.67). If needed, bone struts are applied to the anterior aspect of the vertebral bodies. With anterior fusion, fewer levels may need to be fused.

5.6 Postoperative Evaluation

In the immediate postoperative period, a chest radiograph is often obtained to evaluate lung expansion and possible pneumothorax (especially if a transthoracic approach was used for anterior fusion). Very rarely, acute neurological postoperative symptoms may necessitate CT to evaluate for hardware malplacement/displacement or MRI to evaluate for cord or nerve injury. Postoperative infection or abscess is best defined by contrast-enhanced CT. Before hospital discharge, it is necessary to confirm that instrumentation is intact and has not displaced.

Occasionally, gastroduodenal obstruction develops during treatment, attributed to compression of the third part of the duodenum by the superior mesenteric artery (SMA). Although the exact mechanism is uncertain, the duodenum may become trapped in the angle formed by the SMA and the aorta due to elongation of the spine and stretching of the mesentery. Weight loss may contribute to compression of the duodenum between the SMA and the aorta. Abdominal radiographs show gastric dilatation, and the diagnosis can be confirmed by administration of a small amount of barium after gastric decompression. Extrinsic compression of the SMA is characteristic, appearing as a sharp, oblique termination of the barium column in the transverse duodenum (Fig. 3.68). This obstruction may partially correct after the patient is placed in the left lateral decubitus or prone position. Surgical intervention is rarely necessary; instead, nasojejunal feeding with continued gastric drainage usually suffice until symptoms resolve.

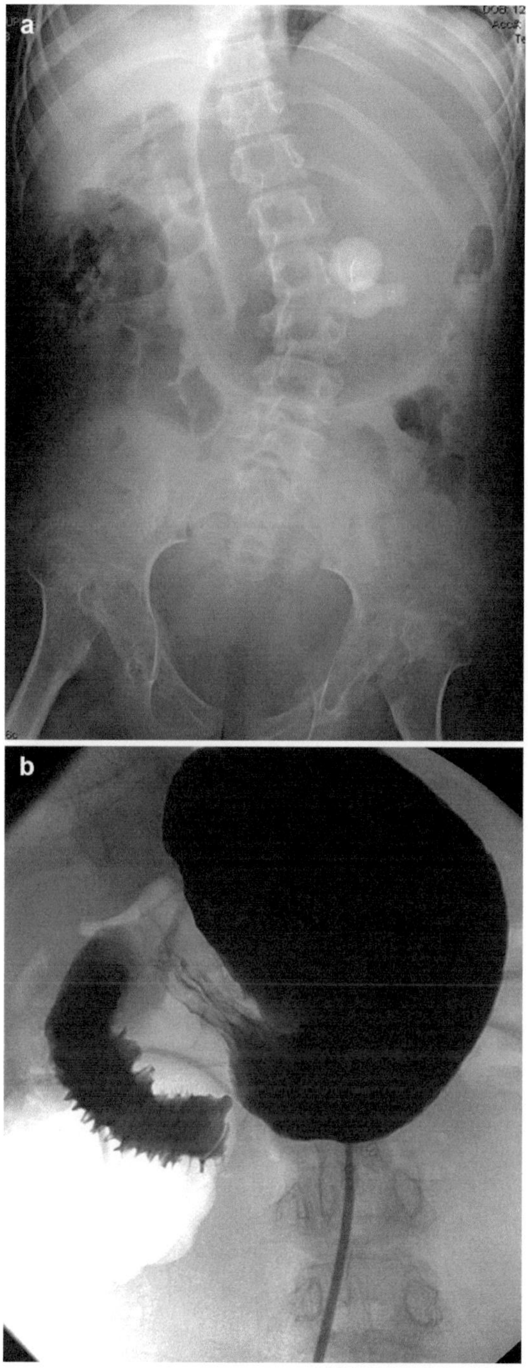

Fig. 3.68 Superior mesenteric artery (SMA) syndrome in a patient with cerebral palsy and scoliosis. (**a**) Abdomen radiograph shows lumbar levoscoliosis and gaseous distension of the stomach, along with bilateral dislocated hips. (**b**) Image from the upper gastrointestinal tract shows a dilated proximal duodenum with abrupt vertical cutoff at the level where the SMA crosses the transverse duodenum (Images copyright Shriners Hospital for Children Northern California)

After spinal instrumentation, the patient must be monitored at least for skeletal maturity to ensure security of fixation, confirm integrity of hardware, exclude pseudarthrosis development, and evaluate for recurrent or new deformity [71]. Successful surgical spinal fusion prevents further increase in the length of the fused segment, although some anterior growth may occur and result in narrowing of the anterior disc space. This may then lead to lateral bulging of intervertebral discs [71, 105].

The fusion mass is best seen along the concavity of the curvature. Oblique radiographs may be necessary to evaluate all portions. Eventually, the facets and intervertebral discs are obliterated by bone ingrowth. Surgical complications may include rod and wire breakage (Fig. 3.69), hook slippage, spondylolysis at levels of increased stress below the fusion, and dislocation of facets above the site of fusion after severe trauma.

At each postoperative evaluation, the density and maturity of bone fusion should be evaluated. Pseudarthroses are recognized as clearly

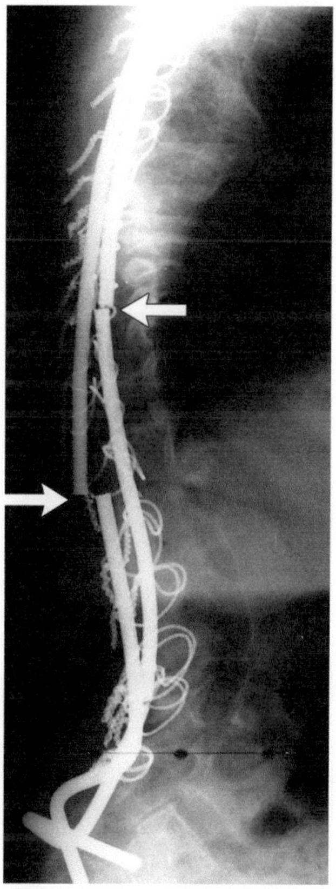

Fig. 3.69 Fractured spinal instrumentation rods (*arrows*)

demarcated gaps in the continuity of bone fusion, with sclerosis at the edges of the discontinuity; motion shown on bending films proves true functional pseudarthrosis is present. However, only 68 % of surgically proven pseudarthroses are visible on radiographs [106]. Furthermore, areas of decreased bone density on radiographs as well as irregular uptake on nuclear scintigraphy, without sharp edges or sclerosis, are very common during the healing process and do not indicate nonunion unless they persist unchanged for longer than 6 months. Although oblique images can be obtained, CT is the standard to confirm pseudarthrosis (Fig. 3.70) [107]. Hardware failure late after fusion suggests but is not always associated with pseudarthrosis.

Gallstones have been reported in almost 20 % of patients on average of 4.5 years postoperatively, attributed to blood loss and hemolysis [108].

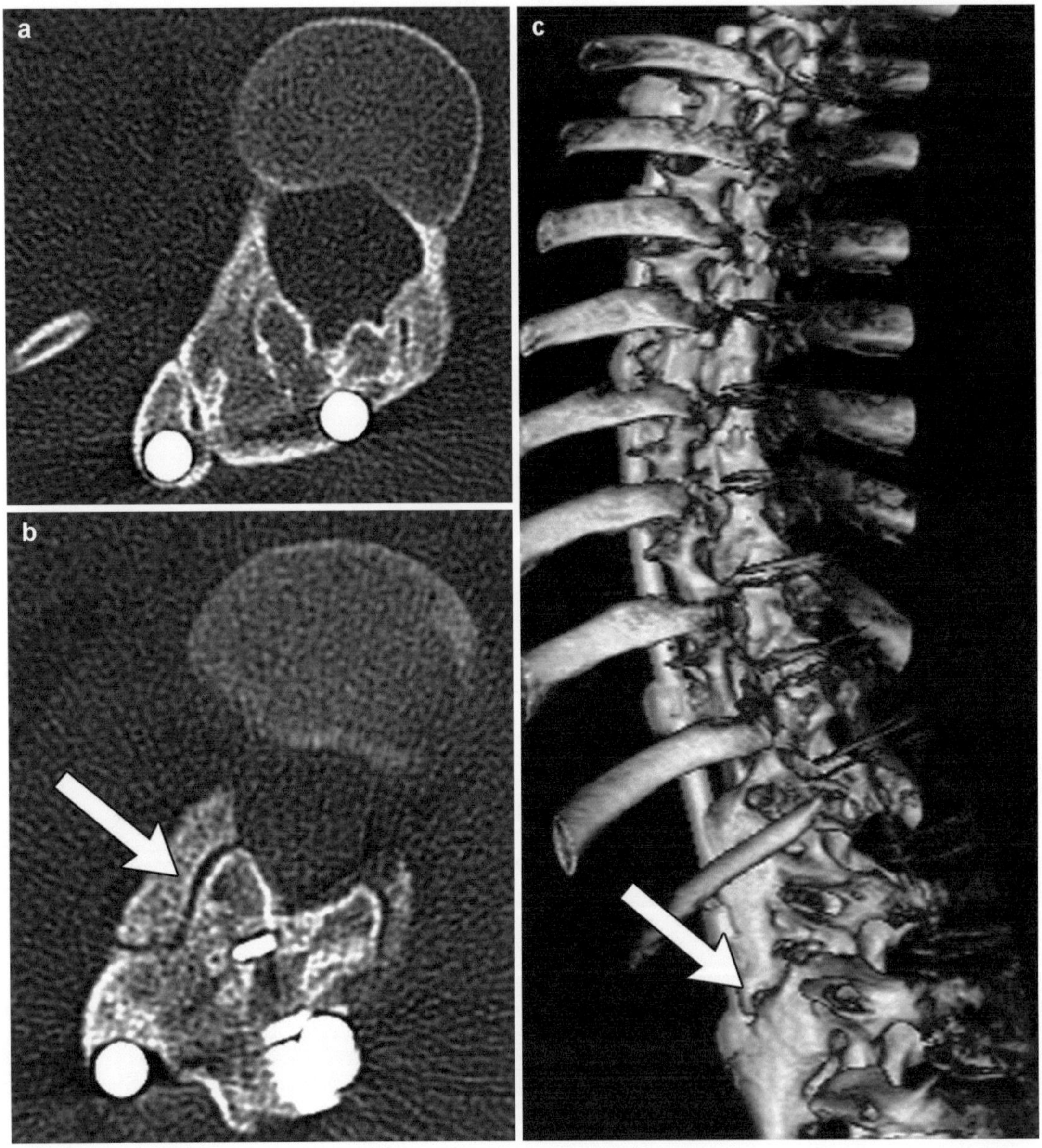

Fig. 3.70 Pseudarthrosis after posterior spinal fusion. Axial CT images at the (**a**) T12–L1 and (**b**) L1–2 levels show a pseudarthrosis on the right (*arrow*) at L1–2 while the fusion mass at T12–L1 is intact. Pseudarthrosis (*arrow*) is also seen on the 3D-CT reformatted image (**c**) (Same patient as Fig. 3.51)

5.7 Differential Diagnosis (Box 3.8)

Box 3.8: Clues to Non-idiopathic Scoliosis

Findings	Diagnosis
Dysmorphic vertebrae	*Congenital scoliosis*
Levoconvex thoracic curve	Syrinx or spinal cord tumor
Short segment severe dystrophic curve with kyphosis	*Neurofibromatosis*
Rib dysplasia, vertebral deformities	
Lumbar curve convex to short leg	Compensatory (leg length discrepancy)
Flexible, corrects with lateral bending	
Long, C-shaped, without compensatory curves	*Neuromuscular*
Marked pelvic obliquity	
Hip may be dislocated on concave side	
Levoconvex or double thoracic curve	Congenital cardiac disease
Early onset, fails bracing	
Pedicle or lamina at curve apex is sclerotic or overgrown	*Vertebral osteoid osteoma*
Tumor, fracture, infection, spondylolysis/spondylolisthesis	Pain

Although the usual pattern of idiopathic scoliosis is a dextroconvex thoracic structural curve with levoconvex nonstructural curve(s) above and/or below, almost any pattern can be seen. There are, however, some intrinsic or associated features that may suggest the scoliosis is not completely idiopathic.

Intraspinal pathology. Levoconvex thoracic curves are reported to be more often associated with hydrosyringomyelia and spinal cord tumors (see Fig. 3.57). If clinical findings suggest this, MRI is indicated.

Congenital scoliosis (see Figs. 3.17, 3.18, 3.21, and 3.23). Any congenital vertebral anomaly, when not sufficiently severe to cause the patient's scoliosis, should prompt a search for an occult bar or fusion.

Neurofibromatosis (see Figs. 3.43 and 3.44). Dystrophic curves associated with neurofibromatosis are frequently short, severe, and accompanied with kyphosis. The presence of rib dysplasia and vertebral deformities, along with other findings of neurofibromatosis, may confirm this etiology (see Chap. 23).

Compensatory scoliosis due to underlying leg length discrepancy (see Figs. 3.55 and 3.56). Lumbar curvature is convex on the side of the short leg; it is flexible and corrects with lateral bending. There should be significant disparity in iliac crest level on standing radiographs. Scoliosis improves with a lift under the short leg.

Neuromuscular scoliosis (see Fig. 3.54 and further discussion below). These curves are frequently long and C shaped, without compensatory curves above or below. Pelvic obliquity is usually marked, often with hip dislocation on the concave side of the curve. The femoral necks have valgus deformity. The combination of scoliosis and pelvic obliquity is almost pathognomonic for a neuromuscular imbalance.

Vertebral osteoid osteoma. The pedicle or lamina at the curve apex is sclerotic or overgrown. Back pain is the presenting complaint (see Chap. 4).

Painful scoliosis. Idiopathic scoliosis is not painful. If spine pain is significant, consideration should be given to the presence of osteoid osteoma or other vertebral tumor, fracture, infection, spondylolisthesis, or intraspinal tumor.

Scoliosis in association with other diseases. The incidence of scoliosis is increased in patients with a great variety of disorders, often without an underlying structural osseous anomaly. Scoliosis occurs in 5–16 % of patients with congenital heart disease [109]. These patients show an increased incidence of levoconvex and double thoracic curves, and early onset and brace failure are characteristic [110]. As many as 48 % of patients with ulnar longitudinal deficiency, radial longitudinal deficiency, or phocomelia have scoliosis, and up to 50 % of those with unilateral and 100 % of those with bilateral amelia have scoliosis [111]. Scoliosis has been reported in 13–23 % of those with spondylolysis and in 25–48 % of those with spondylolisthesis (see Chap. 4). About 20 % of patients with pectus excavatum have scoliosis [112]. Scoliosis is common in diseases characterized by abnormal collagen and osteopenia, such as osteogenesis imperfecta (see Fig. 3.49) and idiopathic juvenile osteoporosis. Patients with posterior rib resection and prior thoracotomy may develop scoliosis whose curve is concave to the abnormal side, whereas those with a fractured transverse process may develop a curve that is convex to the injured side.

6 Neuromuscular Scoliosis

Scoliosis is a common and frequently disabling concomitant of neuromuscular disease (see Chap. 24). Its incidence varies with the type of disease and patient age; progression of scoliosis correlates with the severity and symmetry of muscle involvement. Gravity and growth affect the unstable spinal column and significantly influence otherwise nonprogressive conditions, such as myelomeningocele and poliomyelitis.

A discussion of all of the types of neuromuscular disease associated with scoliosis is beyond the scope of this chapter. A few of the more common are presented below.

Scoliosis is common in patients with cerebral palsy and tends to be worse in those who are more severely neurodevelopmentally impaired (Fig. 3.71). Most of these patients eventually develop associated pelvic obliquity, and this is thus an important radiologic sign. Furthermore, severe pelvic tilt causes the pelvis to move away from the femoral head on the concave side of the spinal curvature, contributing to hip dysplasia/dislocation.

Muscular dystrophies are characterized by a variety of spinal curvatures. In Duchenne muscular dystrophy, early muscular changes are usually symmetric, so scoliosis typically does not progress until the child is wheelchair bound (Fig. 3.72) (see Chap. 24). At that point, pelvic obliquity, combined with gravitational and growth effects, induces progressive and frequently severe scoliosis. Chest radiography is important during adolescence, since the cardiomyopathy associated with this disease will eventually cause cardiac failure and death. Chest radiographs characteristically show soft tissue wasting, humeral shaft thinning, and obliquity of the clavicles and ribs due to weak intercostal muscles. The different subtypes of spinal muscular atrophy (Fig. 3.73) manifest scoliosis at different ages. Scoliosis occurs in 60–70 % of patients with spinal muscular atrophy, and the average age at onset is between 7 and 8 years.

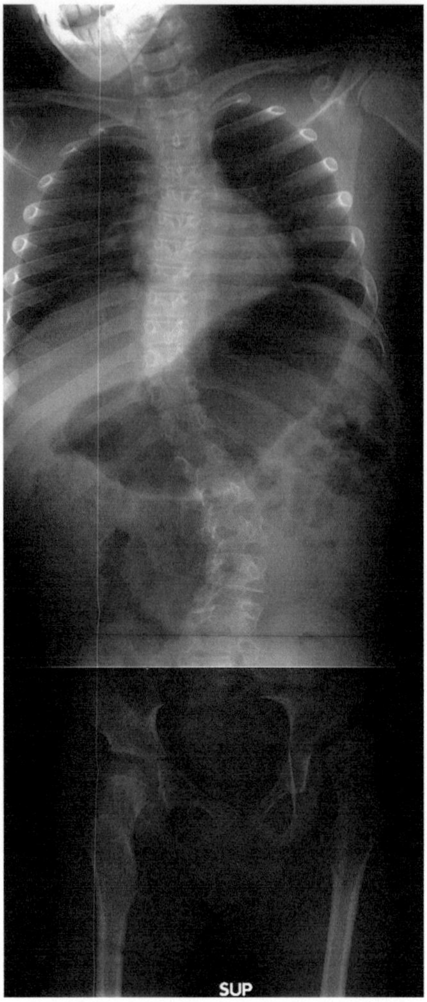

Fig. 3.71 Biphasic scoliosis in a 13-year-old boy with severe cerebral palsy. There is also a small pelvis compared to the size of the chest, bilateral coxa valga, and superolateral subluxation of the left femoral head (supine view)

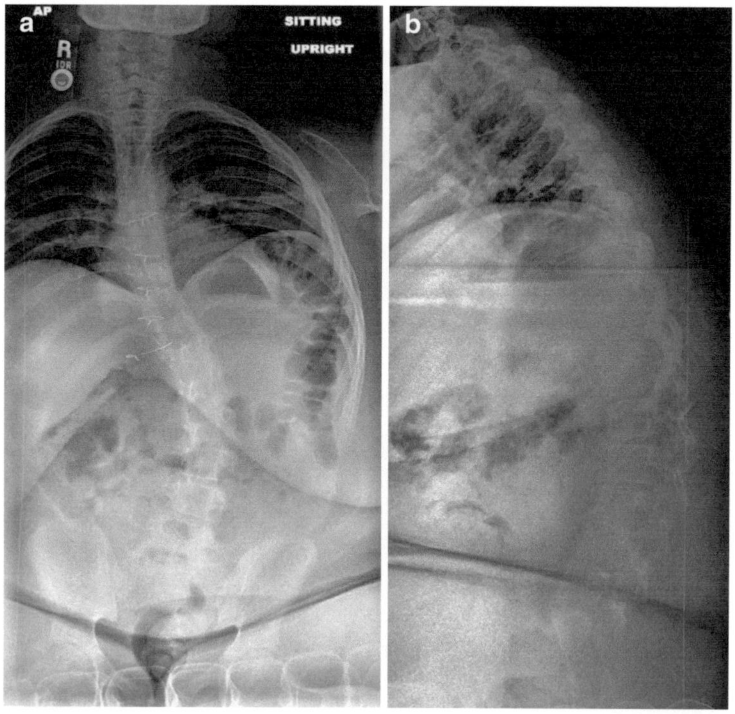

Fig. 3.72 Duchenne muscular dystrophy. Sitting radiographs show neurogenic (**a**) levoconvex C-shaped thoracolumbar curve and (**b**) accentuated thoracic kyphosis and straightening of lumbar lordosis (Images copyright Shriners Hospital for Children Northern California)

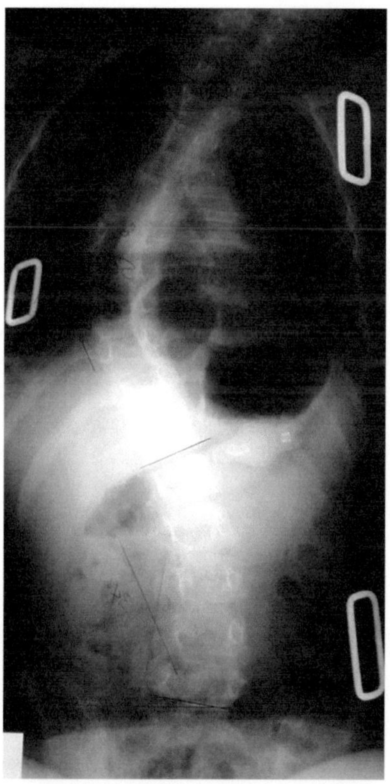

Fig. 3.73 Neuromuscular scoliosis in an 8-year-old girl with spinal muscular atrophy. 53° long C-shaped scoliosis (sitting, braced). Incidental hiatal hernia (Image copyright Shriners Hospital for Children Northern California)

Imaging

The typical neuromuscular curve is single, C shaped, dextroconvex, and long thoracolumbar. Radiographs may show the patient is sitting (often supported) or supine. Traction radiographs assess flexibility of the curvature, as these patients cannot participate in bending exams. Other imaging clues can include decreased bone density, caninization of vertebral bodies (see Fig. 3.9), coxa valga with or without hip dislocation, prominent fecal burden, and/or indwelling gastrostomy button.

7 Juvenile Kyphosis

Thoracic kyphosis and lumbar lordosis develop as the child adopts an erect posture. Interference with this normal process results in persistence of the infantile continuous smooth upper thoracic-to-lower-lumbar kyphotic curve. Recognizing persistence of the infantile pattern allows diagnosis of developmental delay or generalized muscle weakness.

Norms for thoracic kyphosis depend on patient age, measurement limits, and placement of the subject's arms. To standardize radiologic evaluation, the patient should stand with arms extended forward and parallel to the floor, supported to reduce any tendency to lean forward. Measurements are made from T3, or the highest visible superior end plate below this, to the inferior end plate of T12. In children aged 2–9, kyphosis averages 21–24°, with a maximum of 40° [28]. In those aged 10–19, kyphosis averages 25–34°, with a maximum of 45° [28, 29]. In general, the normal upper limit in adolescents is 40°. For repeated measurements, the 95 % confidence limit is 11° [94].

Abnormal kyphosis either results from a primary structural cause or is associated with another condition. Structural causes include congenital anomalies, fracture, neoplasm, dysplasias, syndromes, and post-laminectomy and postradiation states. Conditions that are associated with kyphosis include neuromuscular disorders, myelomeningocele, vertebral and spinal cord inflammation, and collagen, metabolic, and skeletal diseases. There is of course some overlap among these categories. The two main types of idiopathic juvenile kyphosis are postural kyphosis and Scheuermann kyphosis (or disease). Postural kyphosis exceeds 40° and lacks additional abnormalities including those described below.

Scheuermann disease (Box 3.9) is characterized by gradual development of abnormal kyphosis during adolescence (Fig. 3.74) [113].

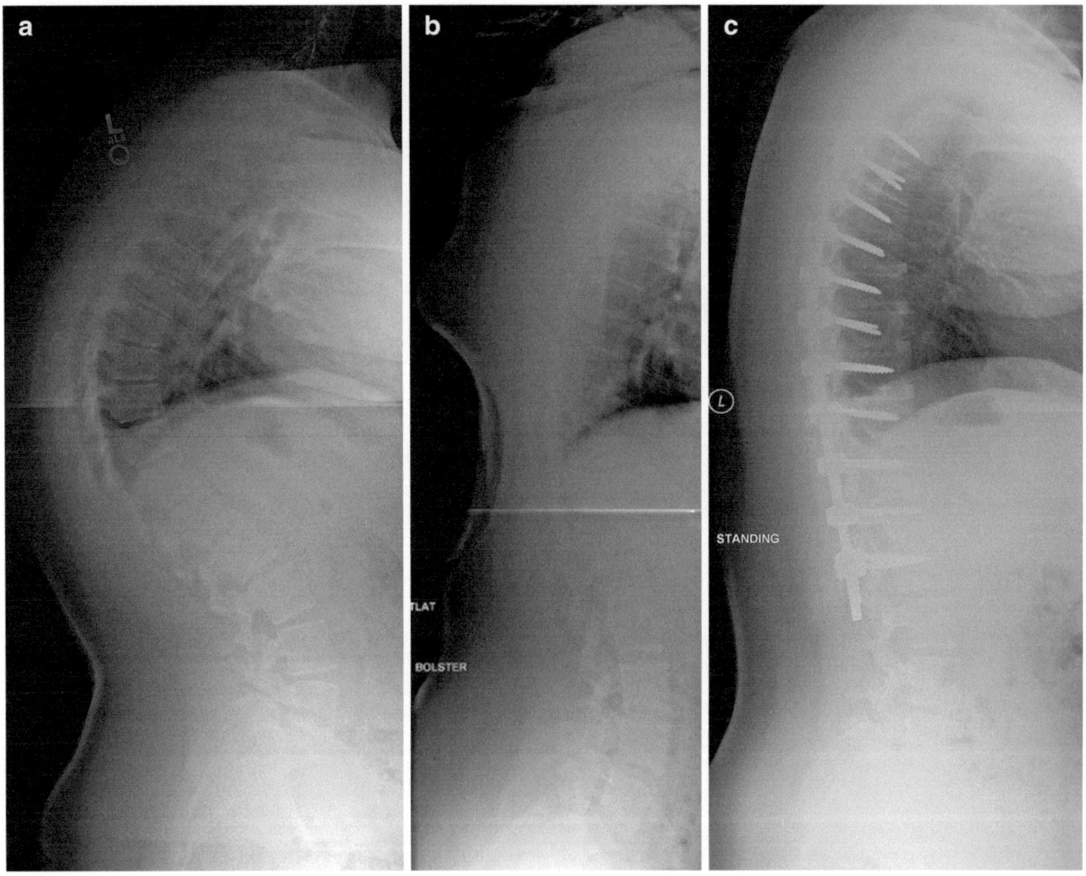

Fig. 3.74 Scheuermann disease in a 15-year-old girl. (**a**) Standing radiograph shows disc space narrowing and anterior vertebral wedging at T8–10, with 82° of kyphosis. (**b**) Lateral radiograph with patient lying on a bolster placed at the apex of the kyphosis shows marked improvement. (**c**) Standing radiograph after anterior and posterior fusion shows correction of abnormal kyphosis

Kyphosis exceeds 40°, and at least three adjacent vertebrae are wedged 5 or more degrees [114]. Clinical vertebral deformity and back pain are present in slightly more than half of these patients. Males and females are affected equally, and symptoms are rarely described in those younger than 11 years of age. Statistics obtained from young male military recruits indicate that 5–6 % of the population may be affected, although most have no symptoms [115]. Scheuermann kyphosis appears to be inherited, with probable autosomal dominant transmission and variable penetrance and expression [113, 116]. There is an increased incidence of spondylolyses and spondylolisthesis in patients with Scheuermann disease; this may cause low back pain.

Box 3.9: Scheuermann Kyphosis

Etiology unknown
5–6 % of population, M = F
Asymptomatic deformity or back pain
Thoracic kyphosis >42° with anterior wedging of at least three adjacent vertebrae
- Decreased disc space height (worse anteriorly), Schmorl nodes
- Increased vertebral anterior-posterior length
- Irregular ossification of ring apophyses
- Hyperlordosis of lumbar spine

Many cases are incorrectly attributed to poor posture, delaying correct diagnosis and treatment. Clinically, Scheuermann disease is differentiated from postural kyphosis by the Adam test, in which the patient is observed from the side while forward bending. Those with Scheuermann disease have acute angular deformity, while those with postural kyphosis have uniform rounding of the spine [114].

Scheuermann disease is considered benign, as it causes negligible deformity and limited symptomatology after skeletal maturity [113]. Treatment depends on patient age, the severity and position of the deformity, and the degree of pain; surgery is infrequently performed [114]. If the thoracic kyphosis is between 55 and 80°, the patient should participate in an exercise regimen to increase flexibility and also wear a brace. Brace treatment of Scheuermann kyphosis may not only halt progression but also decrease the severity of kyphosis. If the thoracic kyphosis is more than 80°, posterior instrumentation and fusion with posterior column shortening may be performed [113]. Severe or rigid kyphotic curves may require additional anterior release. It is important to consider preoperative MRI to evaluate for cord compression from thoracic disc herniation or from accompanying spinal epidural lipomatosis [114, 117, 118].

The etiology of this condition is incompletely understood; extensive pathologic investigation has shown no evidence of inflammation, osteochondritis, or avascular necrosis. Histopathological evaluation shows disorganized enchondral ossification similar to Blount disease, thinning or absence of vertebral end plates and ring apophyses, as well as a decrease in collagen fibrilism, altered proteoglycan content, and increased muccopolysaccharides in the end plates [113]. However, it is unclear whether these changes are primary or secondary. Biomechanical abnormalities have been suggested, including lack of anterior pelvic tilt with forward bending resulting from hamstring tightness commonly found in these patients [113]. Since Scheuermann disease has been reported in chimpanzees and gorillas, upright posture may not be essential in the development of this deformity [119]. Trabecular bone structure is normal [120].

Classic work by Schmorl has found fissures in the cartilaginous end plate adjacent to the nucleus pulposus, with nuclear material herniating through these areas [121]. It is uncertain why these fissures develop, however—perhaps because cartilage in this area is relatively thin or because unrecognized variability in cartilage structure or cartilage-osseous boundary predisposes to fissuring. In any case, once trauma or the usual stresses of childhood open these fissures, herniation of disc material occurs, followed by fibrosis and reactive sclerosis. The so-called Schmorl nodes are formed by sclerosis outlining the cystic areas where nucleus pulposus has herniated through fissures (see Fig. 3.10). However, Schmorl nodes alone do not indicate the presence of Scheurmann disease, since isolated central end plate disc herniation without vertebral wedging is seen in almost the same proportion of normal teenagers.

Loss of disc material causes decreased disc space height, most notable anteriorly, since the posterior height of the intervertebral space is maintained by facet articulations. The loss of elasticity and increased pressure anteriorly retard growth in this area, eventually resulting in wedging of the vertebral body. It is important to recognize that the wedging is an anterior growth dysfunction and not analogous to the compressive wedging seen with osteoporosis. Abnormal pressure dynamics presumably cause irregular ossification of the ring apophysis.

Imaging

Radiologic examination should include erect frontal and lateral projections of the thoracic and lumbar spine. The vertebral bodies are anteriorly wedged, slightly flattened, and often elongated from front to back. The cortical outlines may be irregularly marginated or indistinct. Only one or two vertebrae may be affected, but in most cases three or more are abnormal; half of the patients have five or more wedged vertebrae. Vertebrae between T3 and T12 are characteristically involved, with T7 most frequently abnormal. Occasionally, the upper lumbar vertebrae are affected—many of these cases are associated with severe stress, such as weightlifting. Persistent vascular channels in the anterior face have been reported in 24 % of patients [115]. Ring apophyses may ossify irregularly. Instead of the usual homogeneous continuous pattern, a fragmented pattern of irregular thickness is noted, and the steplike corners into which the ossification centers fit may be enlarged. In 10 % of cases, at least one ring will remain unfused into adulthood. There is usually hyperlordosis of the lumbar spine [114].

Scoliosis is present in one third of patients but is rarely severe, usually around 15°. In about two thirds of patients, the scoliotic curve is above or (more often) below the level of the kyphosis, in the region of compensatory lordosis. In one third of patients, the level of scoliosis is the same as the level of kyphosis [122]. Secondary hypertrophic changes are common later in life. Spastic paraparesis may develop, associated with a posteriorly herniated thoracic disc.

The angle of kyphosis should be measured according to the Cobb technique, with lines drawn along the superior and inferior vertebral end plates at each end of the curvature (Fig. 3.74). The degree of flexibility is estimated by comparing the curvature when the patient lies supine on the radiographic table versus supine over a bolster placed at the apex of the kyphosis (Fig. 3.74).

Radiographic findings are consistent with pathologic findings. The intervertebral disc spaces are decreased in height, with greater narrowing anteriorly. Herniation of nuclear material into the anterior or central portions of the vertebral body may appear as typical Schmorl nodes in up to 75 % of patients, visible on frontal or lateral projections as well as reformatted CT images.

Nuclear scintigraphy is normal [123]. MRI demonstrates the bony and disc findings described above as well as abnormal disc signal (decreased signal of the nucleus pulposus on T2-W images). Discs with the most decreased height demonstrate the most striking signal abnormalities (Fig. 3.75) [124]. MRI may also define disc herniation, usually at the apex of the kyphosis (often affecting T7–T9). Spinal epidural lipomatosis and extradural cysts have been reported [116, 118].

Differential diagnosis of juvenile kyphosis is occasionally problematic. Simple postural round back has none of the disc changes or vertebral wedging described above and will be fairly supple in hyperextension. Tumor and infection rarely affect a series of vertebrae so uniformly, without extensive deformity or destructive changes. Isolated severe trauma may cause anterior disc herniation and vertebral wedging.

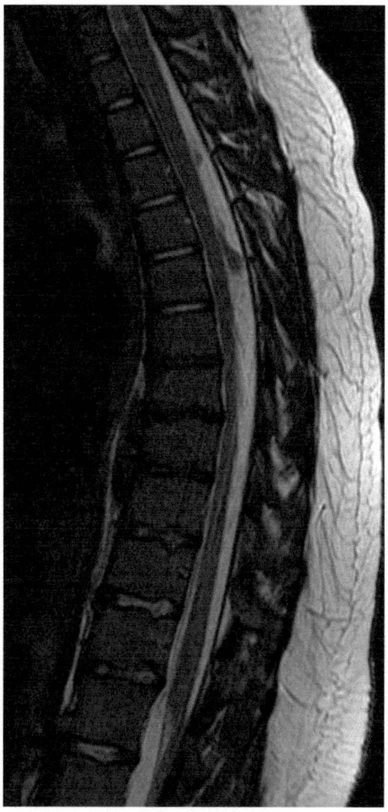

Fig. 3.75 Scheuermann disease in a 15-year-old boy. Sagittal T2-W image shows mild anterior wedging of T7–9, with disc space narrowing and irregularity as well as decreased signal of the nucleus pulposus at T7–8, T8–9, and T9–10. Schmorl nodes at T10–11, T11–12, and T12–L1 (For reference, the conus medullaris is at L1)

References

1. Bess S, Varma V. Embryology and anatomy: spine/spinal cord. In: Akbarnia B, Yazici M, Thompson G, editors. The growing spine. Berlin/Heidelberg: Springer; 2010. p. 3–12.
2. Diel J, Ortiz O, Losada RA, Price DB, Hayt MW, Katz DS. The sacrum: pathologic spectrum, multimodality imaging, and subspecialty approach. Radiographics. 2001;21(1):83–104.
3. Zhang H, Sucato DJ, Nurenberg P, McClung A. Morphometric analysis of neurocentral synchondrosis using magnetic resonance imaging in the normal skeletally immature spine. Spine. 2010;35(1):76–82. Epub 2010/01/01.
4. Ghanem I, El Hage S, Rachkidi R, Kharrat K, Dagher F, Kreichati G. Pediatric cervical spine instability. J Child Orthop. 2008;2(2):71–84.
5. Lustrin ES, Karakas SP, Ortiz AO, Cinnamon J, Castillo M, Vaheesan K, et al. Pediatric cervical spine: normal anatomy, variants, and trauma. Radiogr Rev Publ Radiol Soc N Am Inc. 2003;23(3):539–60. Epub 2003/05/13.
6. Hindman BW, Poole CA. Early appearance of the secondary vertebral ossification centers. Radiology. 1970;95(2):359–61. Epub 1970/05/01.
7. Ogden JA. Radiology of postnatal skeletal development. XI. The first cervical vertebra. Skeletal Radiol. 1984;12(1):12–20. Epub 1984/01/01.
8. Ogden JA. Radiology of postnatal skeletal development. XII. The second cervical vertebra. Skeletal Radiol. 1984;12(3):169–77. Epub 1984/01/01.
9. Ogden JA, Murphy MJ, Southwick WO, Ogden DA. Radiology of postnatal skeletal development. XIII. C1-C2 interrelationships. Skeletal Radiol. 1986;15(6):433–8.
10. Moore K. The developing human: clinically oriented embryology. 5th ed. Philadelphia: Saunders; 1997.
11. Barkovich AJ. Pediatric neuroimaging. 4th ed. Philadelphia: Lippincott Williams & Wilkins; 2005.
12. Currarino G, Williams B, Reisch JS. Linear growth of the thoracic spine in chest roentgenograms from birth to 16 years. Skeletal Radiol. 1986;15(8):628–30. Epub 1986/01/01.
13. Swischuk L. Normal variations. Imaging of the cervical spine in children. New York: Springer; 2002. p. 13–38.
14. Cakmakci H. Essentials of trauma: head and spine. Pediatr Radiol. 2009;39(3):391–405.
15. de Beer JD, Hoffman EB, Kieck CF. Traumatic atlantoaxial subluxation in children. J Pediatr Orthop. 1990;10(3):397–400.
16. Wollin DG, Elliott GB. Coronal cleft vertebrae and persistent notochordal derivatives of infancy. J Can Assoc Radiol. 1961;12:78–81. Epub 1961/09/01.
17. Boone D, Parsons D, Lachmann SM, Sherwood T. Spina bifida occulta: lesion or anomaly? Clin Radiol. 1985;36(2):159–61. Epub 1985/03/01.
18. Osborne J, Masel J, McCredie J. A spectrum of skeletal anomalies associated with pulmonary agenesis: possible neural crest injuries. Pediatr Radiol. 1989;19(6–7):425–32.
19. Beals RK, Rolfe B. VATER association. A unifying concept of multiple anomalies. J Bone Joint Surg Am. 1989;71(6):948–50. Epub 1989/07/01.
20. Hensinger RNMD. Congenital scoliosis: etiology and associations. Spine. 2009;34(17):1745–50.
21. McMaster MJ, David CV. Hemivertebra as a cause of scoliosis. A study of 104 patients. J Bone Jt Surg Br. 1986;68(4):588–95.
22. Kawakami NMD, Tsuji TMD, Imagama SMD, Lenke LGMD, Puno RMMD, Kuklo TRMD, et al. Classification of congenital scoliosis and kyphosis: a new approach to the three-dimensional classification for progressive vertebral anomalies requiring operative treatment. Spine. 2009;34(17):1756–65.
23. Marks DSFF, Qaimkhani SAF. The natural history of congenital scoliosis and kyphosis. Spine. 2009;34(17):1751–5.

24. Chan GMD, Dormans JPMD. Update on congenital spinal deformities: preoperative evaluation. Spine. 2009;34(17):1766–74.
25. McMaster MJ. Occult intraspinal anomalies and congenital scoliosis. J Bone Joint Surg Am. 1984;66(4):588–601. Epub 1984/04/01.
26. MacEwen GD, Winter RB, Hardy JH. Evaluation of kidney anomalies in congenital scoliosis. J Bone Joint Surg Am. 1972;54(7):1451–4. Epub 1972/10/01.
27. Lee CS, Noh H, Lee DH, Hwang CJ, Kim H, Cho SK. Analysis of sagittal spinal alignment in 181 asymptomatic children. J Spinal Disord Tech. 2012;25(8):E259–63. Epub 2012/06/13.
28. Fon GT, Pitt MJ, Thies Jr AC. Thoracic kyphosis: range in normal subjects. AJR Am J Roentgenol. 1980;134(5):979–83. Epub 1980/05/01.
29. Singer KP, Jones TJ, Breidahl PD. A comparison of radiographic and computer-assisted measurements of thoracic and thoracolumbar sagittal curvature. Skeletal Radiol. 1990;19(1):21–6. Epub 1990/01/01.
30. Mayfield JK, Winter RB, Bradford DS, Moe JH. Congenital kyphosis due to defects of anterior segmentation. J Bone Joint Surg Am. 1980;62(8):1291–301. Epub 1980/12/01.
31. Tsou PM. Embryology of congenital kyphosis. Clin Orthop Relat Res. 1977;128:18–25. Epub 1977/10/01.
32. Winter RB. Congenital kyphosis. Clin Orthop Relat Res. 1977;128:26–32.
33. Gholve PA, Hosalkar HS, Ricchetti ET, Pollock AN, Dormans JP, Drummond DS. Occipitalization of the atlas in children morphologic classification, associations, and clinical relevance. J Bone Jt Surg. 2007;89(3):571–8.
34. Bulas DI, Fitz CR, Johnson DL. Traumatic atlanto-occipital dislocation in children. Radiology. 1993;188(1):155–8. Epub 1993/07/01.
35. Hosalkar HS, Sankar WN, Wills BPD, Goebel J, Dormans JP, Drummond DS. Congenital osseous anomalies of the upper cervical spine. J Bone Jt Surg. 2008;90(2):337–48.
36. Schuler TC, Kurz L, Thompson DE, Zemenick G, Hensinger RN, Herkowitz HN. Natural history of os odontoideum. J Pediatr Orthop. 1991;11(2):222–5. Epub 1991/03/01.
37. Pueschel SM, Scola FH. Atlantoaxial instability in individuals with Down syndrome: epidemiologic, radiographic, and clinical studies. Pediatrics. 1987;80(4):555–60. Epub 1987/10/01.
38. Kawabe N, Hirotani H, Tanaka O. Pathomechanism of atlantoaxial rotatory fixation in children. J Pediatr Orthop. 1989;9(5):569–74.
39. Parke WW, Rothman RH, Brown MD. The pharyngovertebral veins: an anatomical rationale for Grisel's syndrome. J Bone Joint Surg Am. 1984;66(4):568–74. Epub 1984/04/01.
40. Tortori-Donati P, Rossi A, Cama A. Spinal dysraphism: a review of neuroradiological features with embryological correlations and proposal for a new classification. Neuroradiology. 2000;42(7):471–91. Epub 2000/08/22.
41. Thakur N, Lowe L. Borderline low conus medullaris on infant lumbar sonography: what is the clinical outcome and the role of neuroimaging follow-up? Pediatr Radiol. 2011;41(4):483–7.
42. Unsinn KM, Geley T, Freund MC, Gassner I. US of the spinal cord in newborns: spectrum of normal findings, variants, congenital anomalies, and acquired diseases. Radiographics. 2000;20(4):923–38.
43. Porensky P, Muro K, Ganju A. Nontraumatic cervicothoracic syrinx as a cause of progressive neurologic dysfunction. J Spinal Cord Med. 2007;30(3):276–81. Epub 2007/08/10.
44. Ozerdemoglu RA, Denis F, Transfeldt EE. Scoliosis associated with syringomyelia: clinical and radiologic correlation. Spine (Phila Pa 1976). 2003;28(13):1410–7. Epub 2003/07/03.
45. Nakamura M, Ishii K, Watanabe K, Tsuji T, Matsumoto M, Toyama Y, et al. Clinical significance and prognosis of idiopathic syringomyelia. J Spinal Disord Tech. 2009;22(5):372–5. Epub 2009/06/16.
46. Rufener SL, Ibrahim M, Raybaud CA, Parmar HA. Congenital spine and spinal cord malformations–self-assessment module. AJR Am J Roentgenol. 2010;194(3 Suppl):S38–40. Epub 2010/03/05.
47. Huisman TAGM, Rossi A, Tortori-Donati P. MR imaging of neonatal spinal dysraphia: what to consider? Magn Reson Imaging Clin N Am. 2012;20(1):45–61.
48. Woodward PJ, Sohaey R, Kennedy A, Koeller KK. From the archives of the AFIP: a comprehensive review of fetal tumors with pathologic correlation. Radiogr Rev Publ Radiol Soc N Am Inc. 2005;25(1):215–42. Epub 2005/01/18.
49. Altman RP, Randolph JG, Lilly JR. Sacrococcygeal teratoma: American Academy of Pediatrics Surgical Section Survey-1973. J Pediatr Surg. 1974;9(3):389–98. Epub 1974/06/01.
50. Kocaoglu M, Frush DP. Pediatric presacral masses. Radiogr Rev Publ Radiol Soc N Am Inc. 2006;26(3):833–57. Epub 2006/05/17.
51. Hensinger RN, Lang JE, MacEwen GD. Klippel-Feil syndrome; a constellation of associated anomalies. J Bone Joint Surg Am. 1974;56(6):1246–53. Epub 1974/09/01.
52. Winter RB, Moe JH, Lonstein JE. The incidence of Klippel-Feil syndrome in patients with congenital scoliosis and kyphosis. Spine (Phila Pa 1976). 1984;9(4):363–6. Epub 1984/05/01.
53. Theiss SM, Smith MD, Winter RB. The long-term follow-up of patients with Klippel-Feil syndrome and congenital scoliosis. Spine (Phila Pa 1976). 1997;22(11):1219–22.
54. Azouz EM. CT demonstration of omovertebral bone. Pediatr Radiol. 2007;37(4):404. Epub 2007/02/03.
55. Lynch SA, Wang Y, Strachan T, Burn J, Lindsay S. Autosomal dominant sacral agenesis: Currarino syndrome. J Med Genet. 2000;37(8):561–6. Epub 2000/08/03.
56. Pang D. Sacral agenesis and caudal spinal cord malformations. Neurosurgery. 1993;32(5):755–78. Discussion 78–9; Epub 1993/05/01.

57. Torre M, Buffa P, Jasonni V, Cama A. Long-term urologic outcome in patients with caudal regression syndrome, compared with meningomyelocele and spinal cord lipoma. J Pediatr Surg. 2008;43(3):530–3. Epub 2008/03/25.
58. Mitchell GE, Lourie H, Berne AS. The various causes of scalloped vertebrae with notes on their pathogenesis. Radiology. 1967;89(1):67–74. Epub 1967/07/01.
59. Ton J, Stein-Wexler R, Yen P, Gupta M. Rib head protrusion into the central canal in type 1 neurofibromatosis. Pediatr Radiol. 2010;40(12):1902–9.
60. Tsirikos AI, Saifuddin A, Noordeen MH. Spinal deformity in neurofibromatosis type-1: diagnosis and treatment. Eur Spine J Off Publ Eur Spine Soc Eur Spinal Deformity Soc Eur Sect Cervical Spine Res Soc. 2005;14(5):427–39.
61. Calvert PT, Edgar MA, Webb PJ. Scoliosis in neurofibromatosis. The natural history with and without operation. J Bone Jt Surg Br. 1989;71(2):246–51. Epub 1989/03/01.
62. Vitale MG, Guha A, Skaggs DL. Orthopaedic manifestations of neurofibromatosis in children: an update. Clin Orthop Relat Res. 2002;401:107–18. Epub 2002/08/02.
63. Taybi HLR. Radiology of syndromes, metabolic disorders, and skeletal dysplasias. 5th ed. Chicago: Year Book Medical Publishers; 2006.
64. Berdon W, Lampl B, Cornier A, Ramirez N, Turnpenny P, Vitale M, et al. Clinical and radiological distinction between spondylothoracic dysostosis (Lavy-Moseley syndrome) and spondylocostal dysostosis (Jarcho-Levin syndrome). Pediatr Radiol. 2011;41(3):384–8.
65. Turnpenny PD, Ellard S. Alagille syndrome: pathogenesis, diagnosis and management. Eur J Hum Genet Eur J Hum Genet. 2012;20(3):251–7. Epub 2011/09/22.
66. Kim H, Kim HS, Moon ES, Yoon CS, Chung TS, Song HT, et al. Scoliosis imaging: what radiologists should know. Radiogr Rev Publ Radiol Soc N Am Inc. 2010;30(7):1823–42. Epub 2010/11/09.
67. Miller NH. Cause and natural history of adolescent idiopathic scoliosis. Orthop Clin North Am. 1999;30(3):343–52, vii. Epub 1999/07/07.
68. Roach JW. Adolescent idiopathic scoliosis. Orthop Clin North Am. 1999;30(3):353–65, vii–viii. Epub 1999/07/07.
69. Yang T, Jia Q, Guo H, Xu J, Bai Y, Yang K, et al. Epidemiological survey of idiopathic scoliosis and sequence alignment analysis of multiple candidate genes. Int Orthop. 2012;36(6):1307–14. Epub 2011/12/21.
70. Stokes IA. Mechanical effects on skeletal growth. J Musculoskelet Neuronal Interact. 2002;2(3):277–80. Epub 2005/03/11.
71. Cassar-Pullicino VN, Eisenstein SM. Imaging in scoliosis: what, why and how? Clin Radiol. 2002;57(7):543–62. Epub 2002/07/05.
72. Ceballos T, Ferrer-Torrelles M, Castillo F, Fernandez-Paredes E. Prognosis in infantile idiopathic scoliosis. J Bone Joint Surg Am. 1980;62(6):863–75. Epub 1980/09/01.
73. Wynne-Davies R. Infantile idiopathic scoliosis. Causative factors, particularly in the first six months of life. J Bone Joint Surg. 1975;57(2):138–41. Epub 1975/05/01.
74. James JI. The management of infants with scoliosis. J Bone Joint Surg. 1975;57(4):422–9. Epub 1975/11/01.
75. Thompson SK, Bentley G. Prognosis in infantile idiopathic scoliosis. J Bone Joint Surg. 1980;62-B(2):151–4. Epub 1980/05/01.
76. Jaramillo D, Poussaint TY, Grottkau BE. Scoliosis: evidence-based diagnostic evaluation. Neuroimaging Clin N Am. 2003;13(2):335–41, xii. Epub 2003/09/19.
77. Goldstein LA, Waugh TR. Classification and terminology of scoliosis. Clin Orthop Relat Res. 1973;93:10–22. Epub 1973/06/01.
78. Fearon T, Vucich J, Butler P, McSweeney WJ, Taylor GA, Markle BM, et al. Scoliosis examinations: organ dose and image quality with rare-earth screen-film systems. AJR Am J Roentgenol. 1988;150(2):359–62. Epub 1988/02/01.
79. Khanna G. Role of imaging in scoliosis. Pediatr Radiol. 2009;39 Suppl 2:S247–51. Epub 2009/05/19.
80. Wybier M, Bossard P. Musculoskeletal imaging in progress: the EOS imaging system. Jt Bone Spine revue du rhumatisme. 2013;80(3):238–43.
81. Levy AR, Goldberg MS, Hanley JA, Mayo NE, Poitras B. Projecting the lifetime risk of cancer from exposure to diagnostic ionizing radiation for adolescent idiopathic scoliosis. Health Phys. 1994;66(6):621–33. Epub 1994/06/01.
82. Levy AR, Goldberg MS, Mayo NE, Hanley JA, Poitras B. Reducing the lifetime risk of cancer from spinal radiographs among people with adolescent idiopathic scoliosis. Spine (Phila Pa 1976). 1996;21(13):1540–7. Discussion 8. Epub 1996/07/01.
83. Doody MM, Lonstein JE, Stovall M, Hacker DG, Luckyanov N, Land CE. Breast cancer mortality after diagnostic radiography: findings from the U.S. Scoliosis Cohort Study. Spine. 2000;25(16):2052–63.
84. Goldberg C, Thompson F, Dowling F, Regan BF, Blake NS. Pilot study for a scoliosis screening project in South Dublin. Ir Med J. 1980;73(7):265–8. Epub 1980/07/01.
85. Tachdjian MO, Matson DD. Orthopaedic aspects of intraspinal tumors in infants and children. J Bone Joint Surg Am. 1965;47:223–48. Epub 1965/03/01.
86. Musson RE, Warren DJ, Bickle I, Connolly DJ, Griffiths PD. Imaging in childhood scoliosis: a pictorial review. Postgrad Med J. 2010;86(1017):419–27. Epub 2010/07/17.
87. Do T, Fras C, Burke S, Widmann RF, Rawlins B, Boachie-Adjei O. Clinical value of routine preoperative magnetic resonance imaging in adolescent idiopathic scoliosis. A prospective study of three hundred and twenty-seven patients. J Bone Joint Surg Am. 2001;83-A(4):577–9. Epub 2001/04/24.
88. Maiocco B, Deeney VF, Coulon R, Parks Jr PF. Adolescent idiopathic scoliosis and the presence of spinal cord abnormalities. Preoperative magnetic resonance imaging analysis. Spine. 1997;22(21):2537–41. Epub 1997/12/31 23:39.

89. Davids JR, Chamberlin E, Blackhurst DW. Indications for magnetic resonance imaging in presumed adolescent idiopathic scoliosis. J Bone Joint Surg Am. 2004;86-A(10):2187–95. Epub 2004/10/07.
90. Malfair D, Flemming AK, Dvorak MF, Munk PL, Vertinsky AT, Heran MK, et al. Radiographic evaluation of scoliosis: review. AJR Am J Roentgenol. 2010;194(3 Suppl):S8–22. Epub 2010/03/05.
91. Inoue M, Minami S, Nakata Y, Otsuka Y, Takaso M, Kitahara H, et al. Preoperative MRI analysis of patients with idiopathic scoliosis: a prospective study. Spine. 2005;30(1):108–14. Epub 2005/01/01.
92. Oda M, Rauh S, Gregory PB, Silverman FN, Bleck EE. The significance of roentgenographic measurement in scoliosis. J Pediatr Orthop. 1982;2(4):378–82. Epub 1982/10/01.
93. Morrissy RT, Goldsmith GS, Hall EC, Kehl D, Cowie GH. Measurement of the Cobb angle on radiographs of patients who have scoliosis. Evaluation of intrinsic error. J Bone Joint Surg Am. 1990;72(3):320–7. Epub 1990/03/01.
94. Carman DL, Browne RH, Birch JG. Measurement of scoliosis and kyphosis radiographs. Intraobserver and interobserver variation. J Bone Joint Surg Am. 1990;72(3):328–33. Epub 1990/03/01.
95. Shea KG, Stevens PM, Nelson M, Smith JT, Masters KS, Yandow S. A comparison of manual versus computer-assisted radiographic measurement. Intraobserver measurement variability for Cobb angles. Spine. 1998;23(5):551–5. Epub 1998/04/08.
96. Propst-Proctor SL, Bleck EE. Radiographic determination of lordosis and kyphosis in normal and scoliotic children. J Pediatr Orthop. 1983;3(3):344–6. Epub 1983/07/01.
97. Armstrong GW, Livermore 3rd NB, Suzuki N, Armstrong JG. Nonstandard vertebral rotation in scoliosis screening patients. Its prevalence and relation to the clinical deformity. Spine. 1982;7(1):50–4. Epub 1982/01/01.
98. Nash Jr CL, Moe JH. A study of vertebral rotation. J Bone Joint Surg Am. 1969;51(2):223–9. Epub 1969/03/01.
99. McAlister WH, Shackelford GD. Measurement of spinal curvatures. Radiol Clin North Am. 1975;13(1):113–21. Epub 1975/04/01.
100. Van Goethem J, Van Campenhout A, van den Hauwe L, Parizel PM. Scoliosis. Neuroimaging Clin N Am. 2007;17(1):105–15. Epub 2007/05/12.
101. Schwab F, Lafage V, Boyce R, Skalli W, Farcy JP. Gravity line analysis in adult volunteers: age-related correlation with spinal parameters, pelvic parameters, and foot position. Spine. 2006;31(25):E959–67. Epub 2006/12/02.
102. Risser JC. The iliac apophysis; an invaluable sign in the management of scoliosis. Clin Orthop. 1958;11:111–9. Epub 1958/01/01.
103. Dickson RA, Deacon P. Spinal growth. J Bone Joint Surg. 1987;69(5):690–2. Epub 1987/11/01.
104. Thomsen M, Abel R. Imaging in scoliosis from the orthopaedic surgeon's point of view. Eur J Radiol. 2006;58(1):41–7. Epub 2006/01/28.
105. Hefti FL, McMaster MJ. The effect of the adolescent growth spurt on early posterior spinal fusion in infantile and juvenile idiopathic scoliosis. J Bone Joint Surg. 1983;65(3):247–54. Epub 1983/05/01.
106. Lauerman WC, Bradford DS, Transfeldt EE, Ogilvie JW. Management of pseudarthrosis after arthrodesis of the spine for idiopathic scoliosis. J Bone Joint Surg Am. 1991;73(2):222–36. Epub 1991/02/01.
107. Selby MD, Clark SR, Hall DJ, Freeman BJ. Radiologic assessment of spinal fusion. J Am Acad Orthop Surg. 2012;20(11):694–703. Epub 2012/11/03.
108. Teele RL, Nussbaum AR, Wyly JB, Allred EN, Emans J. Cholelithiasis after spinal fusion for scoliosis in children. J Pediatr. 1987;111(6 Pt 1):857–60. Epub 1987/12/01.
109. Roth A, Rosenthal A, Hall JE, Mizel M. Scoliosis and congenital heart disease. Clin Orthop Relat Res. 1973;93:95–102. Epub 1973/06/01.
110. Farley FA, Phillips WA, Herzenberg JE, Rosenthal A, Hensinger RN. Natural history of scoliosis in congenital heart disease. J Pediatr Orthop. 1991;11(1):42–7. Epub 1991/01/01.
111. Powers TA, Haher TR, Devlin VJ, Spencer D, Millar EA. Abnormalities of the spine in relation to congenital upper limb deficiencies. J Pediatr Orthop. 1983;3(4):471–4. Epub 1983/09/01.
112. Hong JY, Suh SW, Park HJ, Kim YH, Park JH, Park SY. Correlations of adolescent idiopathic scoliosis and pectus excavatum. J Pediatr Orthop. 2011;31(8):870–4. Epub 2011/11/22.
113. Tsirikos AI. Scheuermann's kyphosis: an update. J Surg Orthop Adv. 2009;18(3):122–8. Epub 2009/10/22.
114. Lowe TG. Scheuermann's kyphosis. Neurosurg Clin N Am. 2007;18(2):305–15. Epub 2007/06/09.
115. Williams HJ, Pugh DG. Vertebral epiphysitis: a comparison of the clinical and roentgenologic findings. Am J Roentgenol Radium Ther Nucl Med. 1963;90:1236–47. Epub 1963/12/01.
116. Graat HC, van Rhijn LW, Schrander-Stumpel CT, van Ooij A. Classical Scheuermann disease in male monozygotic twins: further support for the genetic etiology hypothesis. Spine. 2002;27(22):E485–7. Epub 2002/11/19.
117. Kapetanos GA, Hantzidis PT, Anagnostidis KS, Kirkos JM. Thoracic cord compression caused by disk herniation in Scheuermann's disease: a case report and review of the literature. Eur Spine J Off Publ Eur Spine Soc Eur Spinal Deformity Soc Eur Cervical Spine Res Soc. 2006;15 Suppl 5:553–8. Epub 2006/01/20.
118. Abul-Kasim K, Schlenzka D, Selariu E, Ohlin A. Spinal epidural lipomatosis: a common imaging feature in Scheuermann disease. J Spinal Disord Tech. 2012;25(7):356–61. Epub 2011/06/28.

119. Farrell BM, Kuo CC, Tang JA, Phan S, Buckley JM, Kondrashov DG. Scheuermann kyphosis in nonhuman primates. Spine. 2012;37(23):E1432–7. Epub 2012/08/28.
120. Gilsanz V, Gibbens DT, Carlson M, King J. Vertebral bone density in Scheuermann disease. J Bone Joint Surg Am. 1989;71(6):894–7. Epub 1989/07/01.
121. Schmorl G. Uber Knorpelknotchen an der Wirbelbandscheiben. Fortschr Roentgenstr. 1928;38:265–79.
122. Deacon P, Berkin CR, Dickson RA. Combined idiopathic kyphosis and scoliosis. An analysis of the lateral spinal curvatures associated with Scheuermann's disease. J Bone Joint Surg. 1985;67(2):189–92. Epub 1985/03/01.
123. Winter WA, Veraart BE, Verdegaal WP. Bone scintigraphy in patients with juvenile kyphosis (M. Scheuermann). Diagn Imaging. 1981;50(4):186–90.
124. Swischuk LE, John SD, Allbery S. Disk degenerative disease in childhood: Scheuermann's disease, Schmorl's nodes, and the limbus vertebra: MRI findings in 12 patients. Pediatr Radiol. 1998;28(5):334–8. Epub 1998/05/07.
125. Winter RB. Congenital scoliosis. Clin Orthop Relat Res. 1973;93:75–94. Epub 1973/06/01.
126. Scoles PV, Salvagno R, Villalba K, Riew D. Relationship of iliac crest maturation to skeletal and chronologic age. J Pediatr Orthop. 1988;8(6):639–44. Epub 1988/11/01.
127. Schoenwolf GC, Bleyl SB, Brauer PR, Francis-West PH. Development of the musculoskeletal system. In: Schoenwolf GC, Bleyl SB, Brauer PR, Francis-West PH, editors. Larsen's human embryology. 4th ed. New York: Churchill Livingstone; 2009.
128. Erol B, Kusumi K, Lou J, et al. Etiology of congenital scoliosis. Univ Pennsylvania Orthop J. 2002;15:37–42.
129. Badve CA, Khanna PC, Phillips GS, Thapa MM, Ishak GE. MRI of closed spinal dysraphisms. Pediatr Radiol. 2011;41(10):1308–20.

The Spine: Acquired Disorders

4

Sandra L. Wootton-Gorges

Contents

Abstract

The chapter begins with the discussion of spondylolysis and spondylolisthesis, including a section describing various methods for imaging these conditions. Intervertebral disc disease follows, with discussion of intervertebral calcification and disc prolapse. Spinal trauma is addressed, along with inflammatory and neoplastic destructive vertebral lesions. The last section of the chapter covers salient features of tumors that occur in the spine, including osteoid osteoma, osteoblastoma, aneurysmal bone cyst, Langerhans cell histiocytosis, and osteochondroma.

The pediatric spine is affected by a variety of processes that are unique to children or that manifest in children in unusual ways. Spondylolysis represents a response to chronic stress injury and may lead to spondylolisthesis, wherein one vertebra slips forward on the subjacent vertebra. Spine fractures in young children differ greatly from those in adults and are especially common in the upper cervical spine. Discitis, an uncommon idiopathic inflammatory process, is essentially limited to children, whereas disc herniation and spine infection in children resemble these processes in adults. Several bone tumors, such as osteoid osteoma/osteoblastoma, Langerhans cell histiocytosis, and osteochondroma have unique appearances in the spine. (Inflammatory,

S.L. Wootton-Gorges, MD
Department of Radiology,
University of California Davis Medical Center and UC Davis Children's Hospital,
4860 Y Street, Suite 3100, Sacramento, CA 95817, USA

Department of Diagnostic Imaging,
Shriners Hospitals for Children Northern California, Sacramento, CA, USA
e-mail: sandra.gorges@ucdmc.ucdavis.edu

R. Stein-Wexler et al. (eds.), *Pediatric Orthopedic Imaging*,
DOI 10.1007/978-3-642-45381-6_4,

infectious, and neoplastic processes are discussed in greater depth in Chaps. 19, 20, 21, and 22.)

1 Spondylolysis

Spondylolysis is a cleft or fissure in the pars interarticularis of the neural arch. If the two fragments of bone separate, the portion of the vertebra anterior to this defect may slip forward. Spondylolysis is most common in the lumbar spine. In this location it is considered to be an acquired lesion that cannot be explained by embryologic processes and has never been seen in a fetus or newborn. The L-4 to S-1 region is subject to severe stress, and in some people the facets are oriented such that when subject to stress they act like pincers, compressing the lamina between them. However, only about 6 % of the population develop a corresponding fatigue fracture in the lamina [1].

Histologic examination has not revealed any primary abnormality of the bone in this area. It is possible that an as yet unrecognized abnormality may predispose certain people to fatigue fractures. Some people may have an impaired ability to repair minor microfractures or an inherited predisposition to spondylolysis due to decreased bone density or increased angulation of laminae. These factors may combine with such developmental features as posture, body habitus, and athletic activities to predispose certain individuals to fatigue fracture of the lamina and resultant isthmic spondylolysis. In fact, up to 47 % of young athletes complaining of low back pain have spondylolysis [2].

The fracture fissure may persist in a quiescent state (usually filled with fibrocartilage), heal completely, or allow the vertebral body above to slip forward (spondylolisthesis). The lamina may heal in the slipped position, resulting in an elongated, sclerotic, or thinned lamina that has no visible fracture.

The youngest patient reported with spondylolysis was 4 months old. By 7 years of age, 5 % of a normal population will develop spondylolysis. By age 18, less than one additional percent will have developed the defect. Thus, while this condition may only become symptomatic in adulthood, it is a disease of children. Fifteen to 35 % of close relatives of those with spondylolisthesis have isthmic defects. Heritable predisposition is recognized in certain genetic groups: spondylolysis is three times more common in Caucasians than in those of African descent [3], and prevalence reaches up to 28 % in certain Inuit populations.

The lowermost lumbar neural arch is typically involved; 95 % of isthmic spondylolysis is reported at L5 and most of the remaining at L4. A non-united spinous process is fairly common at these levels and may lead to additional stress at the pars interarticularis. In the absence of severe trauma, repeated stress (e.g., back spasm in cerebral palsy), or distal structural dysplasia, defects in the upper lumbar spine are unusual [4]. Lumbar spondylolysis is bilateral in more than 75 % of cases [1].

Spondylolysis occurs in 6 % of the total population regardless of the presence of idiopathic scoliosis. However, between 13 % and 23 % of those with spondylolysis have scoliosis, and in those with spondylolisthesis, the incidence of scoliosis is even higher—25–48 %. The incidence of lumbar pars defects in Scheuermann deformity is definitely increased: up to 50 % of those with Scheuermann kyphosis and lumbar hyperlordosis also have spondylolysis [5]. Spondylolysis and spondylolisthesis cause symptoms about half the time, often developing with the adolescent growth spurt even though the defect occurs earlier. Neurologic symptoms may result from foraminal stenosis with nerve root compression or disc herniation, although the latter usually occurs above the defect.

Certain rare entities may mimic pars interarticularis defects of isthmic spondylolysis. Pediculate clefts occur anterior to the isthmus and at T12 or below; these, however, are rare in children, often associated with pediculate dysplasia and sometimes indicative of stress fractures. Retroisthmic congenital defects lie more posteriorly, near the spinous process. On the frontal projection, the facets, which run caudally and medially, should not be mistaken for pars interarticularis defects.

Unlike the more common lumbar defect, spondylolysis in the cervical spine is generally congenital. Associated congenital anomalies in the cervical spine include interbody fusion, pediculate hypoplasia, laminar dysplasia, hyperplasia of adjacent facets, and non-fused neural arches [6]. Spondylolysis appears as well-corticated defects in the articular pillars and is most commonly noted at C6. It may be either unilateral or bilateral. Familial occurrence has been reported. On a lateral radiograph, defects at C2 may mimic hangman fracture.

Imaging (Box 4.1)

In general, the work-up for spondylolysis begins with radiographs. Frontal, coned lateral, and oblique views demonstrate most pars defects. A coned lateral projection of the lumbosacral area demonstrates the greatest number of defects (84 %) (Fig. 4.1). Thirty-degree cranial angulation on anteroposterior and oblique projections may help define the pars defects that routine radiographs fail to detect. Indeed, if oblique views are not performed, up to 19 % of spondylolysis cases will be missed. However, oblique views do carry a heavy radiation burden.

Box 4.1: Spondylolysis

Frontal	30° cranial angulation helps visualization
Oblique/lateral	Lucency crossing neck of "Scottie dog"
Unilateral	Spinous process tilts toward lytic side
	Contralateral lamina sclerotic, hypertrophied

On the oblique or lateral view, the typical isthmic spondylolysis appears as lucency below the eyelike intervertebral foramen and crossing the pars interarticularis at the neck of the "Scottie dog" (Fig. 4.2). The margins of the defect may be ragged and square or smooth and tapered. The size of the gap varies, and there may be fragmentation in the fracture interval. After the fracture heals, the gap may close and the isthmus may appear normal, elongated, or sclerotic (reflecting repair).

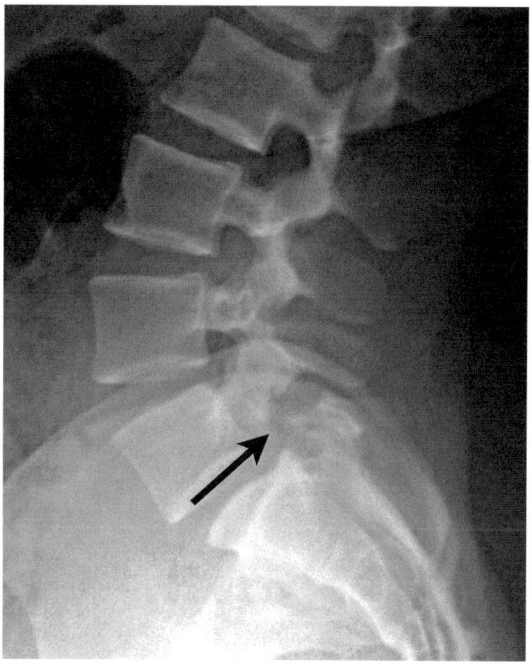

Fig. 4.1 Spondylolysis at L5. The *arrow* points to the bony defect in the pars interarticularis (Image copyright Shriners Hospital for Children Northern California)

When only one lamina is involved, the facet on the unstable side will advance, causing the spinous process of that vertebra to tilt toward the defective side. Additionally, increased stress on the normal side causes sclerosis and hypertrophy of this lamina and pedicle [7]. In the typical isthmic or superior facet defect, this change occurs at the level of the abnormal lamina; in uncommon inferior laminar defects, the hypertrophied pedicle is below the lesion [8]. In a child with back pain, the affected pedicle may be mistaken for osteoid osteoma, since it is sclerotic and also shows increased uptake on nuclear scintigraphy.

Nuclear Medicine Imaging

Bone scan with single-photon emission computed tomography (SPECT) is very useful for diagnosing spondylolysis (Fig. 4.3). SPECT may show increased uptake at the pars interarticularis when radiographs are normal. In addition, it can help distinguish between symptomatic spondylolysis (increased activity) and silent spondylolysis (normal activity) [9].

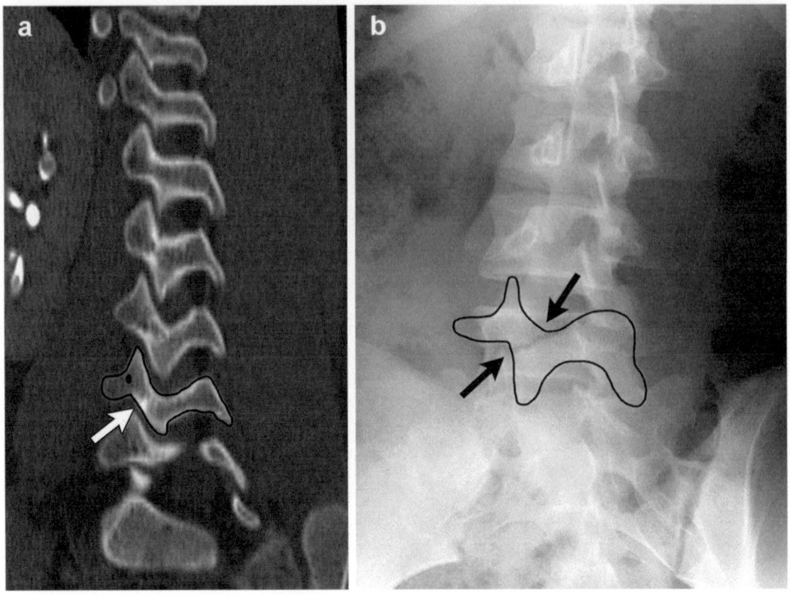

Fig. 4.2 Spondylolysis of L5 in a teen. (**a**) For comparison, normal pedicle, pars interarticularis (*white arrow*), and articulating facets of the L4 vertebra on an oblique sagittal reformatted computed tomography (CT) image. (**b**) "Scottie dog" formed by the "neck" of the Scottie dog is broken (*black arrows*)

Computed Tomography (CT) (Box 4.2)

CT is a valuable tool for diagnosing spondylolysis, as it provides excellent bony detail and can be reformatted in multiple planes (Fig. 4.4). On the axial projection, it may be challenging to distinguish between a spondylolytic defect and a normal facet joint, and all the contiguous slices in the series must be studied in sequence. The facet is smoothly marginated, slightly curved, and level with the disc, whereas the pars defect is usually irregularly marginated, fragmented, or sclerotic and both more superior (at the level of the pedicle) and anterior to the normal facet joint [10]. Sagittal and coronal reformatted images show pars defects well. The anteroposterior diameter of the canal is often increased, and disc herniation is occasionally associated, usually at the level above the laminar defect. Spondylolisthesis may cause a false impression of herniation.

Box 4.2: Spondylolytic Lucency Vs Normal Facet Joint CT

Spondylolysis	Facet
Superior to disc, anterior to facet joint	Level with disc
Irregular margins	Smooth margins
Fragmented and sclerotic	Slightly curved

Magnetic Resonance Imaging (MRI)

MRI is as accurate as CT in the diagnosis of lower lumbar spondylolysis [11]. It is characterized by interruption of marrow signal in the lamina and increased T2 signal in the defect. A sclerotic but continuous pars interarticularis may result in a false positive. On all pulse sequences, the cleft is best shown in the sagittal plane as a zone of intermediate signal that is perpendicular to the facets; signal varies with the amount of fibrous tissue, cartilage, and fluid in the defect (Fig. 4.4). Surrounding marrow edema appears hyperintense on T2-weighted (T2-W) images. If spondylolisthesis is present, the disc may appear prolapsed and may be split into two parts [12].

2 Spondylolisthesis

Spondylolysis may lead to spondylolisthesis, as the fracture allows one vertebral body to slip forward over the one below. This lesion is almost exclusively limited to the lower lumbar spine, usually with L5 slipping forward over S1 (Fig. 4.5). The most common cause of spondylolisthesis is an isthmic (pars interarticularis) defect in which the posterior neural arch remains stationary while the anterior body slides forward. In

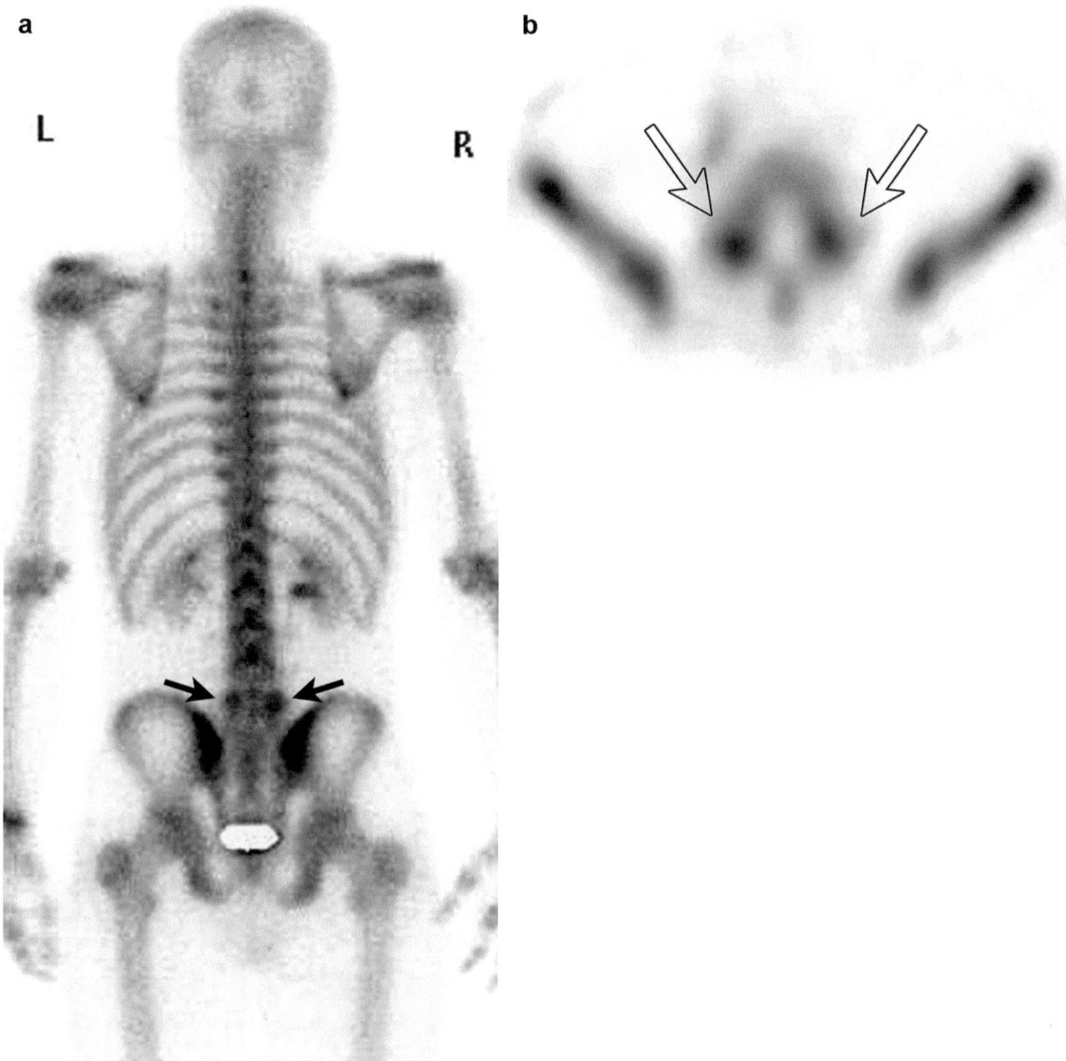

Fig. 4.3 Bilateral spondylolysis at L5 in a 16-year-old athlete. (**a**) Note the increased uptake on the posterior view planar bone scan (*black arrows*). (**b**) Increased uptake at the pars interarticularis at L5 on axial single-photon emission computed tomography (SPECT) (*white arrows*) (Courtesy of Cameron Foster)

rare cases, neural arch dysplasia allows slippage, when facet and laminar defects insufficiently restrain forward movement. This can occur with myelomeningocele and neurofibromatosis. Degenerative and traumatic causes are rare in children. Spondylolisthesis is very unusual in the cervical spine.

Spondylolisthesis develops in less than half of those with spondylolysis. This slipping process rarely starts before age 7 and often begins or accelerates between the ages of 9 and 12, rarely increasing after age 20. While no prognostic radiographic or clinical factors can predict the progression of mild slips [13], in most cases ultimate vertebral displacement is less than 25 or 30 %.

Dysplastic spondylolisthesis is more common in girls, whereas the isthmic form is more common in boys. Most patients with spondylolysis alone are asymptomatic. When spondylolisthesis develops, low back pain and hamstring spasm are often noted.

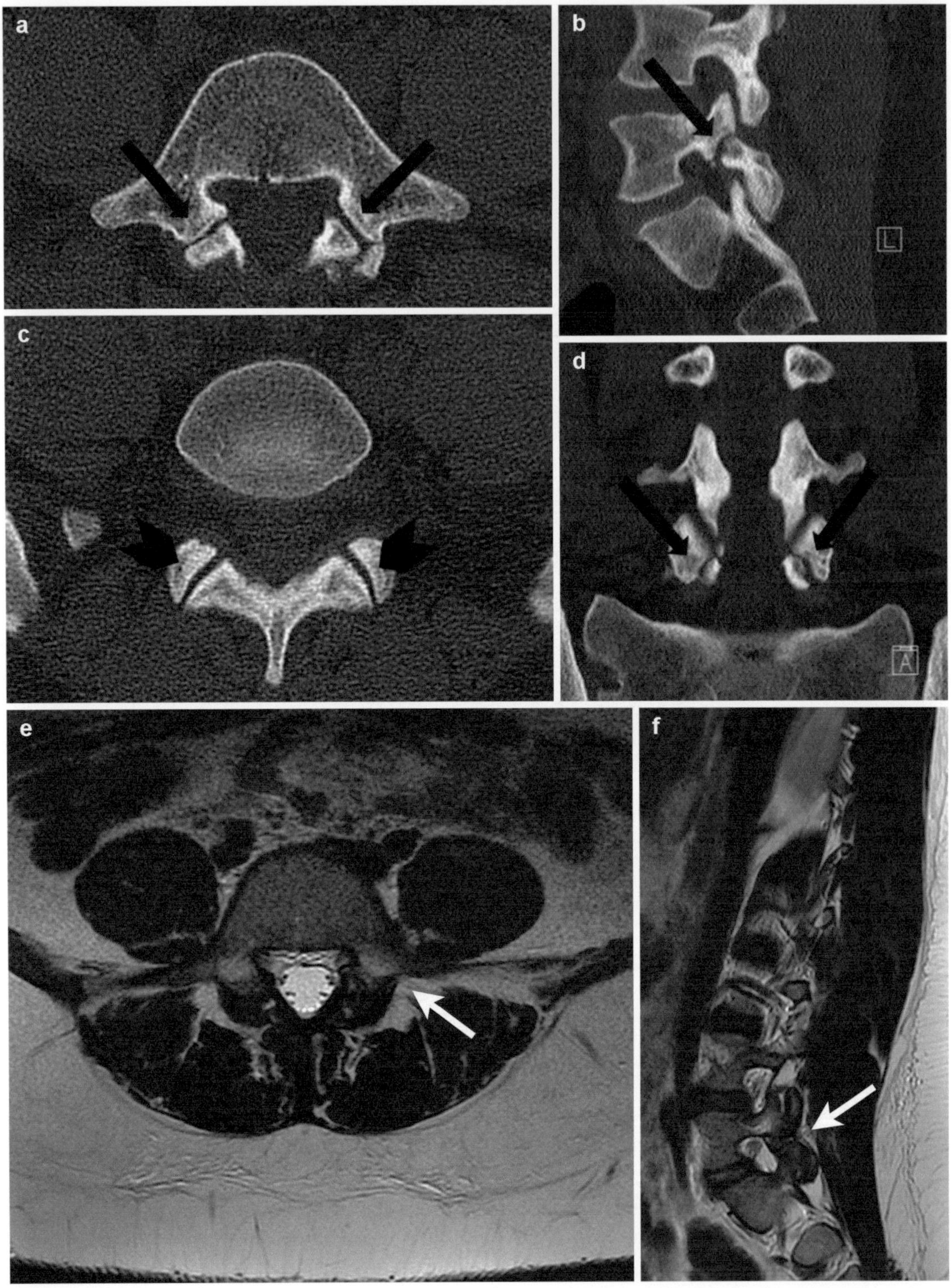

Fig. 4.4 Bilateral spondylolysis in an 11-year-old. (**a**, **b**) Axial CTs show that the irregular pars interarticularis defects (*arrows*) are located at the level of the pedicles. These must be differentiated from the normal facet joints (*arrowheads*) that are located at the level of the disc. Sagittal (**c**) and coronal (**d**) reformatted CTs show the spondylolysis defects. Axial (**e**) and sagittal (**f**) T2-W images show hyperintense edema anterior to the hypointense pars defects (*arrows*)

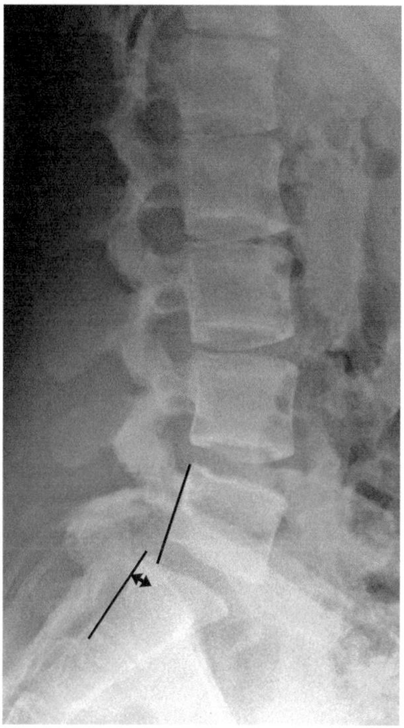

Fig. 4.5 Bilateral spondylolysis and grade 1 spondylolisthesis in an 11-year-old girl. Forward slip of L5 on S1 is less than one fourth the width of the S1 vertebra (Image copyright Shriners Hospital for Children Northern California)

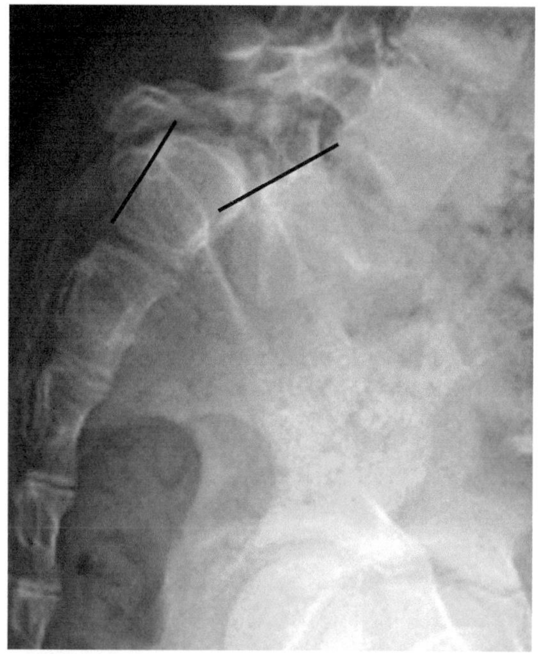

Fig. 4.6 Grade IV spondylolisthesis in a 12-year-old girl with spondylolysis and about 90 % anterior slip of L5 on S1 (Image copyright Shriners Hospital for Children Northern California)

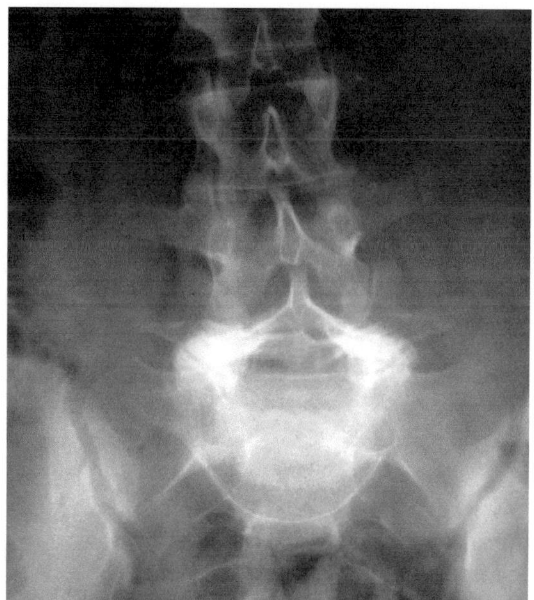

Fig. 4.7 Grade IV spondylolisthesis. The inverted cocked hat, or tricorn hat, creates a double density on frontal projection (Image copyright Shriners Hospital for Children Northern California)

Imaging

The vertebra above slips forward on the one below, usually L5 on S1 (Fig. 4.6). On a frontal view, if L5 is slipped significantly forward on S1, a double density results, resembling an inverted cocked hat (Fig. 4.7). A reliable method for recognizing (but not quantifying) spondylolisthesis on the oblique projection is noting that each successive facet is located anterior to the one just above. If this progression is reversed, corresponding slip must have occurred.

Erect lateral radiographs may show more extensive slip than recumbent cross-table lateral examinations. Hypoplasia or scoliotic rotation of L5 can result in a false impression of spondylolisthesis. Using the lateral view, magnitude is grading from I to V: the superior surface of the sacrum is divided into four zones and the location of the slipped vertebra's posteroinferior corner is determined (Fig. 4.8). An alternate, more reproducible assessment determines the percentage of

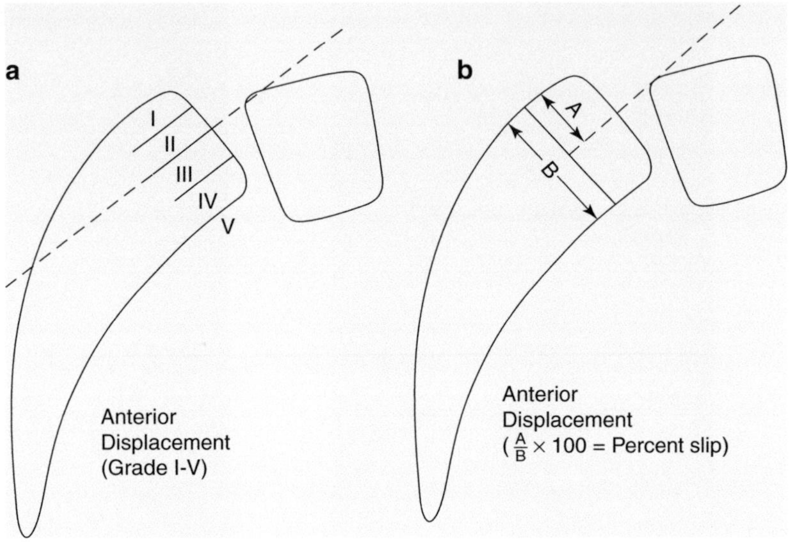

Fig. 4.8 Methods for assessing severity of spondylolisthesis. (**a**) shows technique for grading spondylolisthesis, and (**b**) shows technique for calculating the percentage of slip. Grade I is forward slip of the posterior corner of the affected vertebra (usually L5) by less than one fourth (0–25 %) of the width of the vertebra it slips on (usually S1). Grade II is 1/4–1/2 (26–50 %) of the width. Grade III is 1/2–3/4 (51–75 %). Grade IV 3/4–1 (76–100 %). Grade V is more than 100 % slip; the displaced vertebral body falls forward and is angled caudally

slip by dividing the distance slipped by the width of the body below.

In long-standing spondylolisthesis, the slipped vertebral body becomes trapezoidal and its anterior face longer than the posterior due to underdevelopment of the posteroinferior corner. The superior surface of the sacrum becomes rounded because of abnormal pressure and impaired growth.

3 Spinal Trauma

Stability of the vertebral column depends on the vertebrae; the posterior muscular, ligamentous, and capsular structures; the intervertebral disc; and the anterior and posterior longitudinal ligaments. The mechanisms that cause traumatic stress include flexion, rotation, extension, compression, and shearing. The anatomic peculiarities of various segments determine the type of lesion: horizontal facets of the cervical region promote dislocation and disc tear without fracture, whereas the more vertical lumbar facets predispose to facet fracture and slice-type fracture of the vertebral body. Dissolution of bone, for example, in the odontoid, may follow trauma.

The cervical spine is fractured in 37–80 % of pediatric spine injuries, and there is a higher incidence of neurologic injuries in younger children (less than 8 years of age) than in older children or adults [14]. Fractures in younger children are more likely to affect the upper cervical spine—from the occiput to C3. This is in part because movement occurs at a higher fulcrum, about C2–3 in young children versus C5–6 in adults and older children. It is also a consequence of their relatively large head and small body as well as increased mobility due to lax ligaments and underdeveloped neck muscles. In young children the geometry of the cervical vertebrae differs from that in adults, further predisposing them to upper cervical spine injury [15]. Elasticity of the ligaments also increases the likelihood of cord injury without osseous injury. Common upper cervical injuries include occiput-C1 injury, with possible rupture of ligaments and craniocervical separation; Jefferson fractures of the atlas; atlantoaxial separation or rotation; odontoid fractures; and hangman fracture of C2.

Older children are subject to similar fractures as adults. Most fractures involve the thoracic and lumbar spine, though the mid and lower cervical spine may be affected. Vertebral body compression fractures are most common. It is important to evaluate for additional fractures if one fracture is identified, as the presence of injury at multiple noncontiguous levels in children is associated with an increased probability of neurologic injury [16].

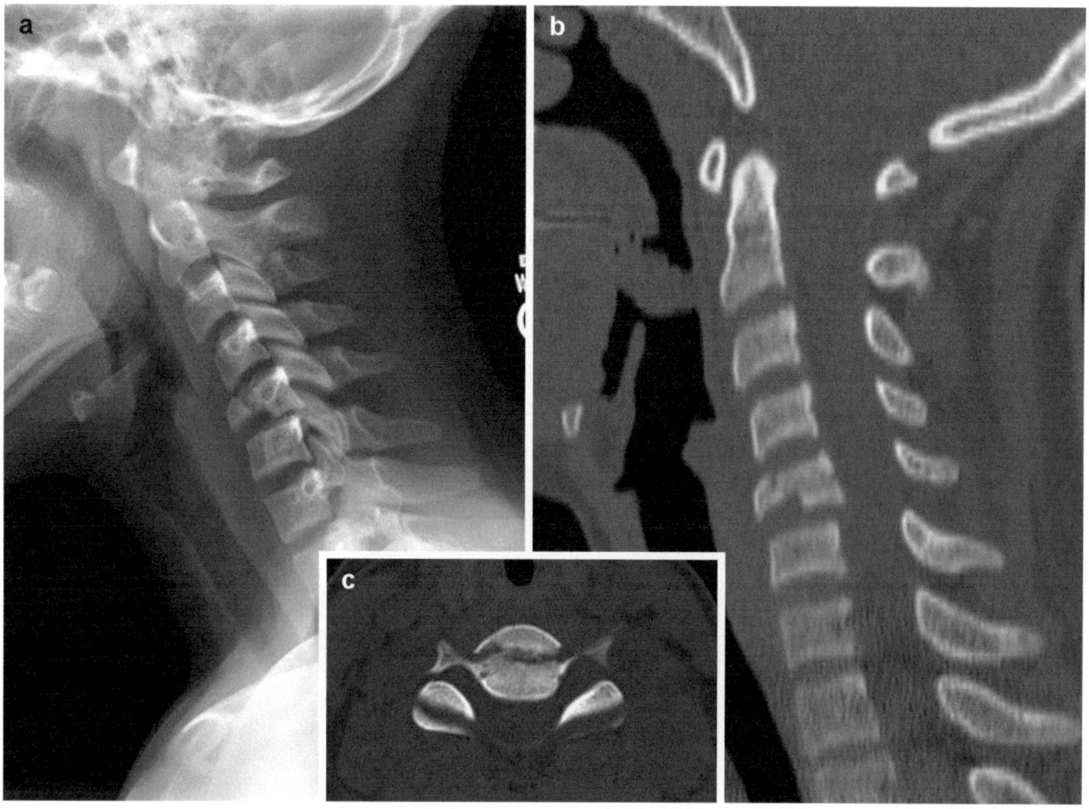

Fig. 4.9 Flexion-distraction fracture at C5–6 in a 12-year-old boy. (**a**) The C5–6 injury shows the C6 vertebral body is fractured, and there is increased distance between the spinous processes of C5 and C6, suggesting ligamentous injury. Loss of normal cervical lordosis. (**b**) Sagittal reformatted CT confirms these findings. (**c**) Axial CT shows the fracture bisects the vertebral body

Imaging

Radiographs provide initial evaluation of spine injury (Fig. 4.9). Flexion and extension radiographs can help identify unstable ligamentous injury and clarify questionable abnormalities but are fraught with problems and can be unsafe to perform [14]. Patients with radiographic abnormalities and those with high-risk mechanism of injury require CT examination with coronal and sagittal reformatting. CT is superior to all other modalities in detecting and delineating spinal fractures, while MRI best defines muscular, ligamentous, and spinal cord injury (Fig. 4.10) [17]. MRI can delineate significant craniocervical junction injury in young children with normal CTs and may be considered if there is a high likelihood of injury [18].

Flexion injury results in tears and sprains of posterior spinal muscles and ligaments, as well as vertebral body compression fractures. Rotational forces may contribute to subluxation. The cervical spine is prone to hyperextension injury caused by blows to the head, collisions, and whiplash. The thoracic and lumbar spine can suffer posterior element avulsion fractures [17].

Burst fractures, secondary to axial compressive loading, show up clearly by CT (Fig. 4.11). A retropulsed fragment may be rotated and displaced craniad or caudad. Callus extending into the spinal canal may cause late neurologic deterioration. MRI may investigate spinal cord injury. Acute intraspinal hemorrhage or cord laceration along with late myelopathy, syrinx formation, and atrophy may be evident, as well as neural injury remote from the region of skeletal injury.

The Chance fracture of the spine (Fig. 4.12) is an unstable flexion-distraction transverse disruption through the posterior elements and into the vertebral body [19]. It typically occurs at the T12–L2 level. Chance fractures are frequently associated with the lap belt injury complex: acute flexion of the abdomen over a lap belt during rapid deceleration. The abdominal viscera are compressed, possibly resulting in hollow viscus injury, as the spine flexes over the fulcrum of the belt. Sagittal reformatted CT images best show Chance fractures. Fortunately, associated spinal cord injury is rare.

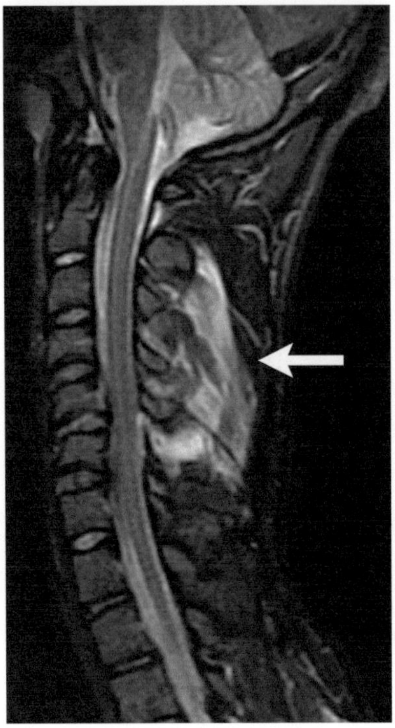

Fig. 4.10 C5–6 flexion-distraction injury. Sagittal short tau inversion recovery (STIR) MRI shows C5 and C6 are fractured, and C6 is deformed with mild retropulsion of the posterior aspects of the vertebrae and resultant cord compression. Extensive soft tissue edema and ligamentous injury (*arrow*)

Hyperflexion compression fractures may occur in children under age 2 who are subject to nonaccidental trauma [20]. These fractures may be clinically silent or associated with neurologic injury (Fig. 4.13). Subluxation and kyphosis may result. Extreme vertebral compression may suggest the dysostosis multiplex picture of mucopolysaccharidoses, and loss of disc space from traumatic intravertebral herniation may mimic pyogenic infection.

4 Intervertebral Disc Disorders

4.1 Discitis

Discitis is a relatively rare disorder of the pediatric spine, possibly inflammatory or due to low-grade bacterial infection (see Chap. 19 for additional discussion). Clinical findings may include back pain and stiffness, limp, fever, and increased sedimentation rate. Interestingly, children under 28 months of age tend not to complain of back pain, while older children do [21]. In most cases, blood cultures are sterile; occasionally, biopsy material from the involved disc shows bacterial growth—usually *Staphylococcus*

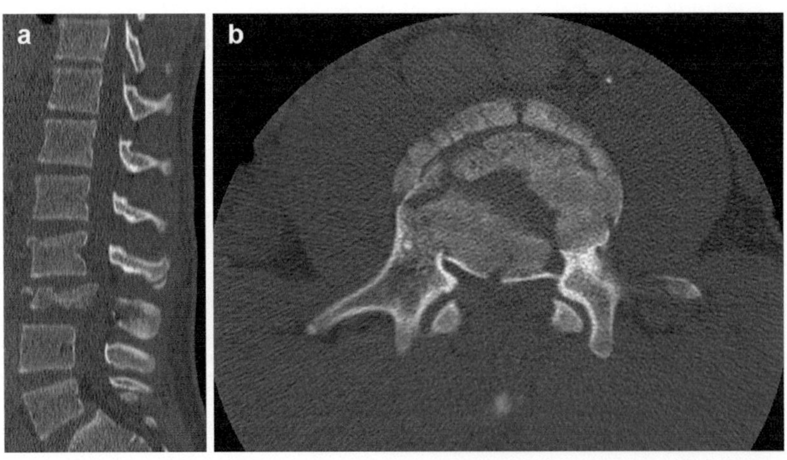

Fig. 4.11 Burst fracture in a teen. Sagittal reformatted (**a**) and axial (**b**) CT images show a burst fracture of L3. Retropulsion of posterior fragments significantly narrows the spinal canal

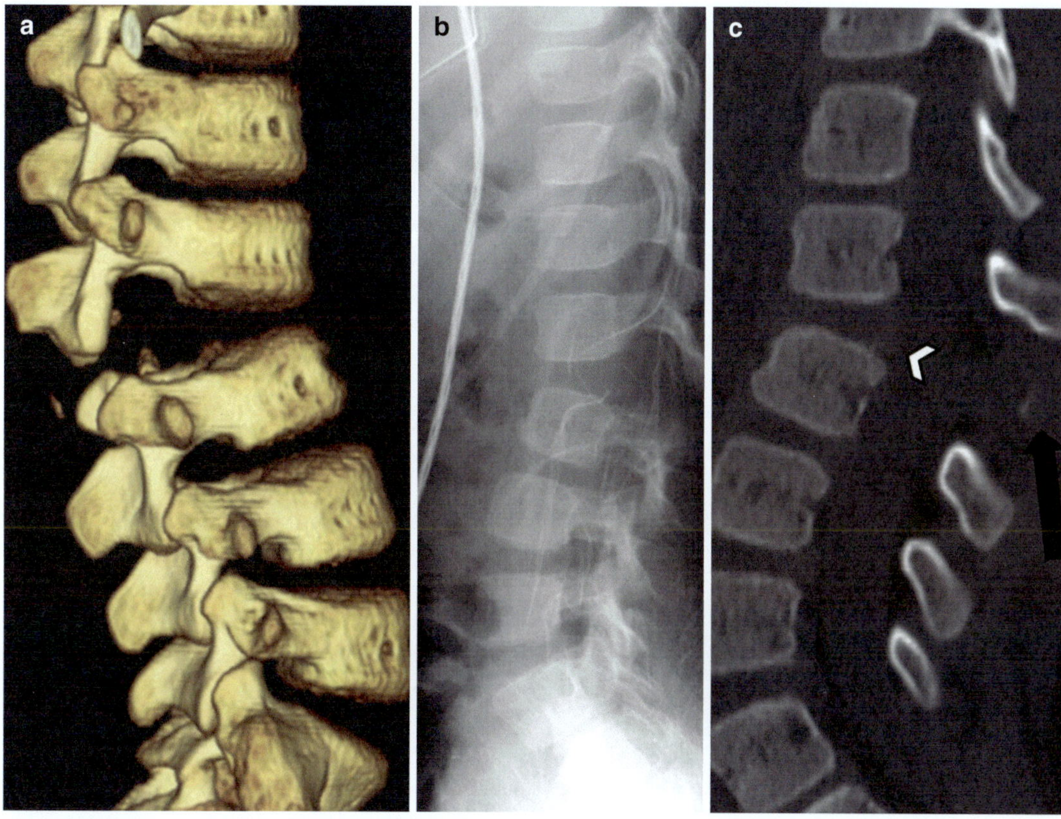

Fig. 4.12 Chance fracture in an 8-year-old girl who was a restrained backseat passenger in a motor vehicle accident and presented with a lap-belt bruise across her lower abdomen. Three-dimensional (3D) CT (**a**), radiograph (**b**), and sagittal reformatted CT (**c**) all show the fracture with distraction of the spinous processes at L2–3. A fragment avulsed from the L2 spinous process is displaced into the gap (*black arrow*). Vague lifting of bony density at the posterosuperior L3 vertebral body likely results from fracture through the ring apophysis (*arrowhead*). Widening of the disc space indicates disc fracture

aureus. Typically, biopsy or aspiration is unnecessary unless antibiotic treatment fails. Prognosis for full recovery is good. The lumbar spine is involved in three fourths of patients, whereas the cervical spine is rarely affected. Occasionally, lesions are present at more than one level.

At early stages of the disease, radiographs are normal. Vertebral end plate irregularities and narrowing of the intervertebral disc are seen after a few weeks (Fig. 4.14). Narrowing may in part be due to destruction of the disc itself and in part due to disc herniation through an eroded vertebral end plate. MRI best evaluates discitis, showing inflammation at the disc and reactive signal change in the adjacent vertebral body end plates (Fig. 4.14). MRI can also depict significant complications, including epidural abscess or cord compression. As healing progresses, end plate irregularity, cavitation of the adjacent vertebral cortex, and reactive sclerosis become radiographically apparent. With healing, the disc may increase in height and the vertebral body may increase in anteroposterior dimension. Fusion of adjacent vertebrae across the affected disc space is uncommon. The posterior elements are unaffected.

4.2 Intervertebral Disc Calcification (Box 4.3)

This condition is uncommon in childhood, and its cause is unknown. It occurs more often in boys, and the peak age at diagnosis is 7–8 years but ranges from 1 day to 20 years. Children

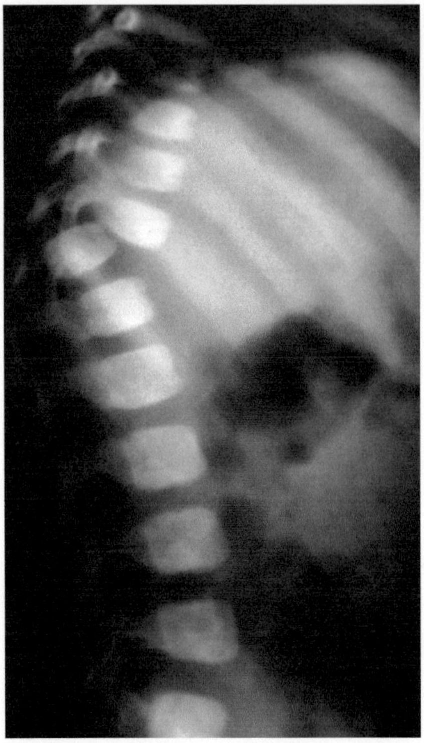

Fig. 4.13 T11–12 hyperflexion dislocation in an abused infant who was slammed buttocks first onto a table

Box 4.3: Intervertebral Disc Calcification

Cervical spine in 75 % (C6–7)
Often affects more than one level
Calcifications round, oval, fragmented, and flat
Adjacent vertebrae deformed
Eventual resorption and loss of disc height

may be asymptomatic or may present with pain, spasm, limitation of motion, leukocytosis, and increased inflammatory markers. Less common symptoms include torticollis, neurologic symptoms including focal weakness and sensory loss, and compressive myelopathy resulting from herniation of the calcifications through the annulus fibrosus. Anterior herniation rarely causes dysphagia.

Symptoms usually improve within 1 month. Conservative treatment including immobilization and analgesic therapy is usually successful even if neurologic signs are present. Significant and persistent sensorimotor deficits caused by root or spinal cord compression are managed surgically [22].

The cervical spine is affected in nearly 75 % of cases, especially between C6 and C7 (Fig. 4.15). In up to half of patients, two discs are involved, and three or more are calcified in almost 20 % of patients. The calcifications are located in the nucleus pulposus and may be round, oval, flat, bilobed, or fragmented. Adjacent vertebral bodies may be deformed. At MRI, the affected disc is hypointense on both T1-weighted (T1-W) and T2-W images. MRI is excellent in defining disc herniation and determining cord or nerve root involvement [22].

During the early stages of resorption (which may last months to years), calcified material becomes fragmented. Eventually there is loss of disc height, with increased height of the adjacent vertebra and osteophyte formation in some cases.

Differential Diagnosis

Idiopathic disc calcification must be distinguished from that associated with spinal fusion, which may result from degenerative change following decreased normal mechanical stress. This may occur with Klippel-Feil syndrome, myositis ossificans progressiva congenita, juvenile rheumatoid arthritis, and ankylosing spondylitis, as well as after surgical spinal fusion [23].

4.3 Intervertebral Disc Herniation

This is an infrequent but not rare cause of back pain in adolescents—about 3 % of disc herniations occur in this age group. In teens, herniated discs are usually posttraumatic rather than degenerative [24] and may result from hyperextension or excessive loading. Adolescent disc herniation is five times more common in those with a positive family history [25]. Two thirds of teens with disc herniation complain of back pain, while only one third have sciatica. Associated avulsion fracture of the ring apophysis may occur [17]. An apophyseal fracture may destabilize the annulus fibrosis, allowing for herniation of the nucleus pulposus.

Slightly more than one half of the lesions occur at the L5–S1 level (Fig. 4.16) and the rest

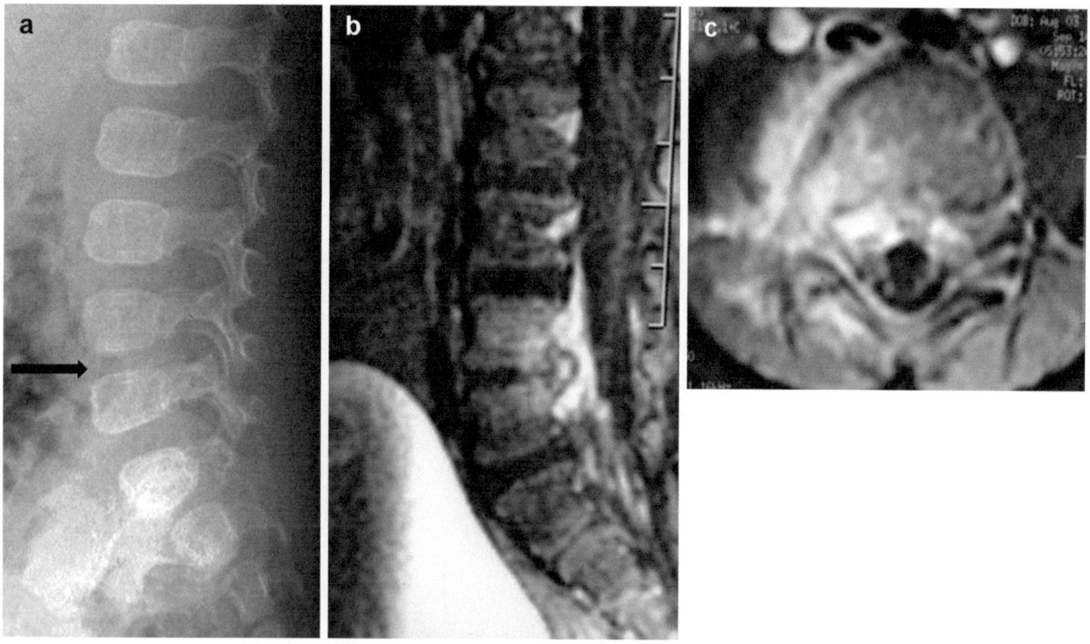

Fig. 4.14 Discitis in a 13-month-old who presented with a limp. (**a**) Subtle disc space narrowing at L3–4 (*arrow*). (**b**) Sagittal T2-W MRI shows hyperintensity at the posterior disc and adjacent vertebral body end plates. (**c**) A gadolinium-enhanced T1-W fat-suppressed (FS) axial image shows enhancement at the disc and right paraspinous soft tissues

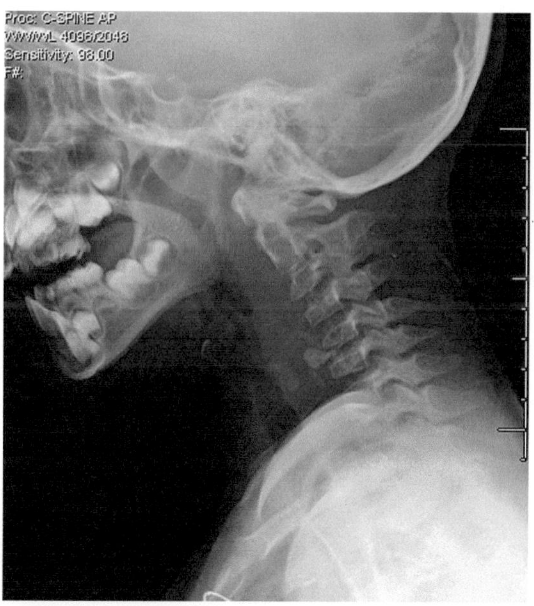

Fig. 4.15 Calcified discitis in a 6-year-old who presented after a motor vehicle accident. There is calcified, extruded disc material anteriorly at C5–6. No acute cervical spinal injury was detected. Incidental partial fusion of C2–3

at the interspace above. Radiographs are rarely helpful, although decreased disc space height may be seen in about 20 %. MRI is the study of choice to diagnose both disc bulge and herniation. Interestingly, in 75 % of adolescents (ages 14–19) with clinical findings of disc prolapse, MRI shows abnormal T2 signal in discs at other lumbar levels as well. Adolescent disc herniations tend to be larger than those in adults.

5 Infectious Destructive Disorders

Visible destruction of one or several vertebrae is an important finding in patients with back pain or systemic symptoms. At times it is difficult to separate inflammatory from neoplastic lesions, for, although a specific finding or constellation of findings may occasionally suggest one lesion or agent in preference to another, there are few pathognomonic signs. The more common considerations include bacterial infection,

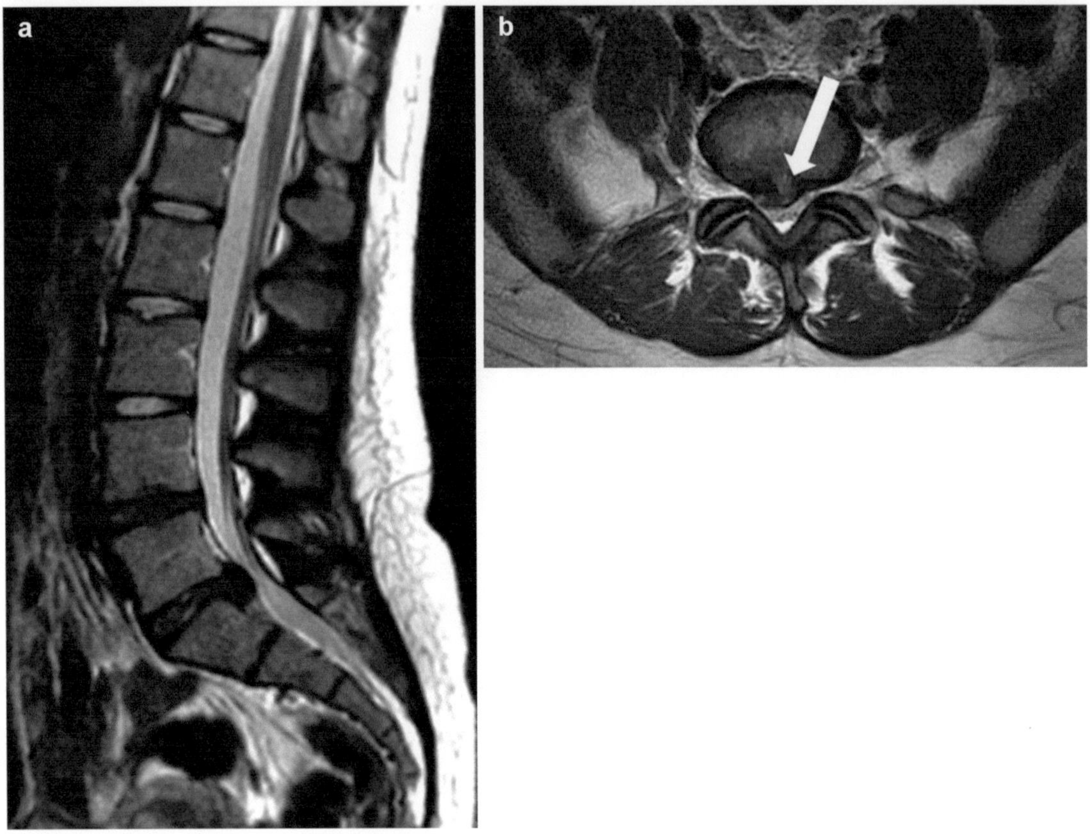

Fig. 4.16 Disc herniation in a 15-year-old girl who presented with back pain. (**a**) Sagittal T2-W image shows disc herniation at L5–S1. (**b**) Axial T2-W image shows the slightly eccentric herniation (*arrow*) narrowing the spinal canal and right S1 neural foramen

spinal tuberculosis, Langerhans cell histiocytosis (LCH), and metastatic diseases including leukemia/lymphoma and neuroblastoma. (See Chap. 19 for additional discussion of infectious processes and Chap. 21 for discussion of bone tumors (as well as Sect. 4.6, below).)

5.1 Bacterial Infections

Agents commonly responsible for pyogenic infection of the spine are *Staphylococcus aureus* and *Streptococci*. Local paravertebral soft tissue swelling is the earliest finding, followed by disc space diminution and vertebral destruction (Fig. 4.17). Later, reactive sclerosis with lytic changes and vertebral collapse may supervene. In infantile-onset disease, vertebral bodies can fuse; this may be indistinguishable from congenital kyphosis, which is caused by an anterior bar or posterior hemivertebra [26]. Based solely on radiography, discitis (discussed above and in Chap. 19) is almost impossible to distinguish from pyogenic osteomyelitis. The differential features characterizing nonpyogenic disc space inflammation are absence of sepsis, negative bacteriologic findings, relatively benign clinical course, and the uncommon occurrence of late vertebral body fusion (although the latter can only be assessed at follow-up).

5.2 Tuberculosis

Worldwide, tuberculosis is the most common pediatric spinal infection (Fig. 4.18). Extensive destruction and large abscesses characterize spine disease in children younger than 10 years

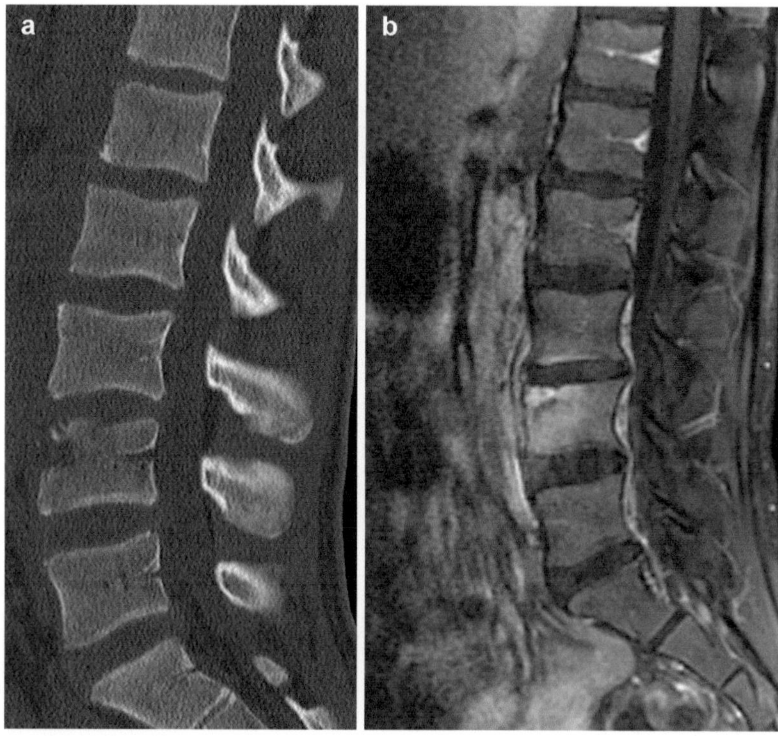

Fig. 4.17 *Staphylococcus aureus* osteomyelitis of L4. (**a**) Sagittal reformatted CT shows irregularity and partial destruction of the superior portion of the L4 vertebral body. (**b**) Sagittal T1-W FS gadolinium-enhanced MRI shows vertebral body enhancement, most marked at the anterosuperior corner of the L4 vertebra

of age, but paraplegia is more common in older children [27]. Lesions generally occur between T8 and L3, and T9 is involved most often. In almost 90 % of patients, at least two vertebrae are affected, and some patients may have two or three separate levels of involvement. As with pyogenic infection, there may be paravertebral masses, bone destruction, and loss of disc space. There is good evidence that much of what seems to be disc destruction is really a sequel of herniation of the disc material through the destroyed vertebral end plate.

Tuberculosis lacks diagnostic pathognomonic changes. Typical findings of anterior vertebral destruction, disc narrowing, and paraspinal mass are common to most inflammatory lesions. However, a few features that may suggest tuberculosis include visible sequestra, anterior scalloping of the vertebral bodies (due to prevertebral cold abscess formation), and increased density or calcification of the psoas regions indicating psoas abscess. CT is valuable in evaluating these findings.

Posterior elements are rarely involved. Scoliosis may follow asymmetric vertebral body collapse, and kyphosis is frequent and most common in the thoracic region. Spontaneous fusion of contiguous vertebral centers may occur. Sarcoidosis can exhibit similar findings, such as disc space narrowing, vertebral lysis, and paravertebral masses. A malignant lesion may also cause extensive bony destruction, but usually only one vertebra is involved and disc spaces are intact.

6 Vertebral Tumors

Several tumors occur relatively often in the vertebrae and have a unique appearance in this region. Osteoid osteoma, osteoblastoma, and aneurysmal bone cyst (ABC) tend to cause focal lysis without involving the adjacent vertebrae or the intervertebral disc. Osteoid osteoma is usually confined to the posterior elements, but osteoblastoma and ABC may extend into the vertebral body. Langerhans cell histiocytosis (LCH) may result in near complete destruction of the vertebral body and resultant vertebra plana. Osteochondromas are exophytic and may protrude into the spinal canal. (See Chap. 21 for a more complete discussion of bone tumors in children.)

6.1 Osteoid Osteoma (Box 4.4)

Box 4.4: Osteoid Osteoma and Osteoblastoma

Characteristic	Osteoid osteoma	Osteoblastoma
Vertebral body involvement	Rare	>30 %
Reactive sclerosis	Common	50 %
Size	</=2 cm	>2 cm
Central ossification	Sometimes	>75 %
MRI enhancement	In lesion and marrow	Intense perilesional

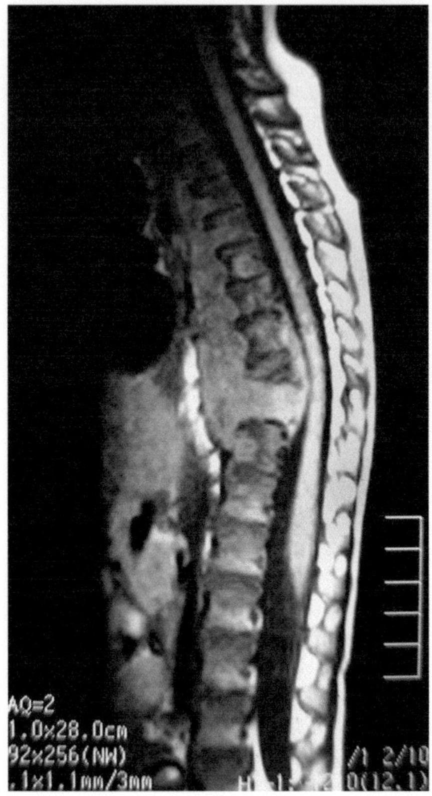

Fig. 4.18 Spinal tuberculosis in an infant. Sagittal T1-W MRI shows focal kyphosis with extensive underlying vertebral destruction. Inflammatory tissue tracks under the anterior spinous ligament as well as in the anterior epidural space, resulting in cord compression

Ten to twenty percent of osteoid osteomas are located in the spine, with the lumbar spine most often affected. The histology of this tumor is indistinguishable from osteoblastoma, but osteoblastomas are larger. Most patients are male and younger than age 16. Back pain, spasm, vertebral tenderness, and scoliosis are common. Scoliosis is generally concave toward the lesion, and the apex is normally at the level of the lesion. However, osteoid osteomas in the spinous processes or sacrum may not be associated with scoliosis. If the lesion has been symptomatic for a short time (9–15 months), scoliosis usually regresses after surgery, but if symptoms have been present for a longer time, the curve may become structural.

Osteoid osteoma usually occurs in the posterior elements, with less than 10 % of cases affecting the vertebral body. Common findings include reactive sclerosis as well as overgrowth of one lamina, pedicle, or transverse process (Fig. 4.19); rarely does an adjacent vertebral body show reactive sclerosis. While it may not be visible as a lytic area on routine studies, noncontrast CT usually shows the tumor nidus. CT frequently detects central nidus calcification as well. On MRI, the nidus has T1 intermediate and T2 hypointense signal. On T2-W images, surrounding marrow edema is hyperintense, and intralesional calcification results in signal voids. After gadolinium administration, the nidus/peri-nidal marrow may enhance [28]. Osteoid osteomas are usually smaller than 2 cm.

Nuclear scintigraphy can assist with diagnosis. Osteoid osteoma and osteoblastoma typically exhibit diffuse regional increased uptake with a central hyperintense focus. SPECT imaging localizes the lesion precisely within the vertebra.

6.2 Osteoblastoma

Osteoblastoma also occurs during adolescence and like osteoid osteoma affects males more often than females. Back pain, muscle spasm, and scoliosis are common.

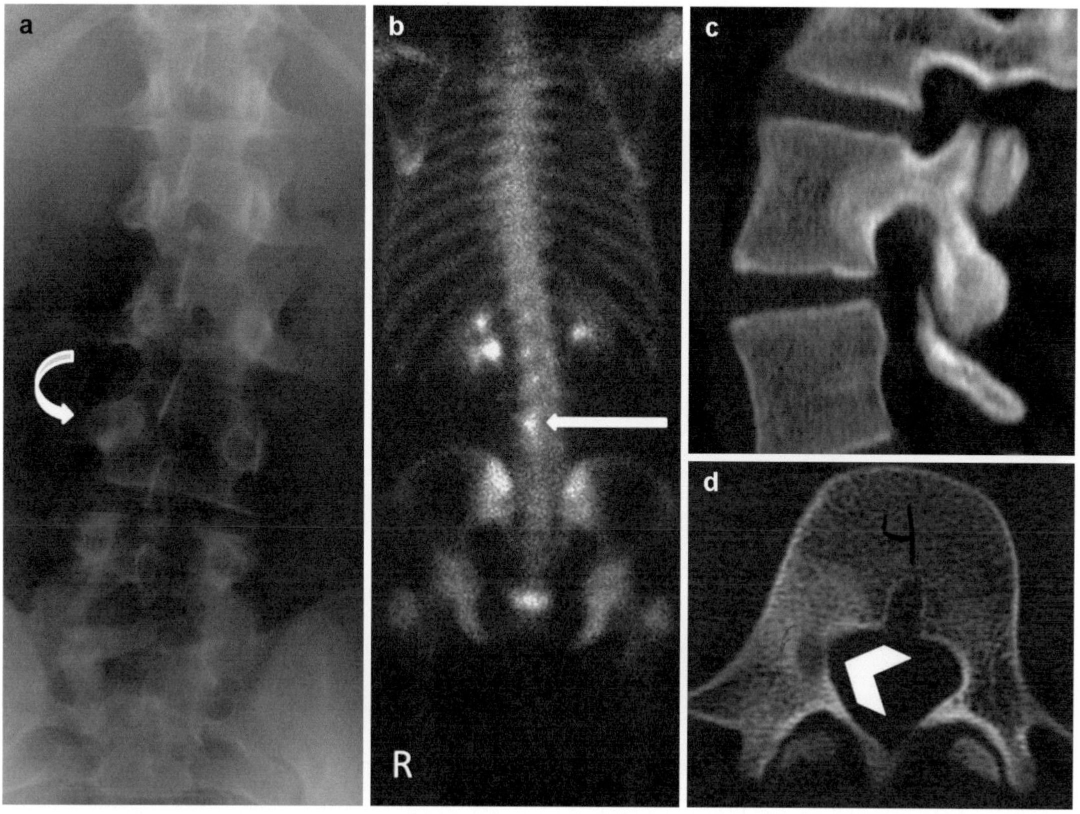

Fig. 4.19 Osteoid osteoma in a boy with back pain. (**a**) The right L4 pedicle is sclerotic (*curved arrow*), and there is spinal curvature concave to the right. (**b**) Bone scan shows increased uptake at this location (*arrow*). (**c**) Sagittal reformatted CT shows sclerosis in the affected pedicle. (**d**) Axial CT shows the radiolucent nidus (*arrowhead*) with surrounding sclerosis causing widening of the pedicle (Images copyright Shriners Hospital for Children Northern California)

Osteoblastoma is an expansile osteolytic lesion of the lamina, transverse or spinous processes, or adjacent rib, often with a thin shell of periosteal reaction at the periphery. In 75 % of cases, ossification is seen within the lucency, and a soft tissue mass may be associated.

Clinically, histologically, and radiographically, it may be difficult to distinguish this lesion from osteoid osteoma, although osteoblastoma is larger (larger than 2 cm) and more often centrally ossified (Fig. 4.20). While with osteoid osteoma surrounding sclerosis is almost the rule and involvement of the vertebral body quite uncommon, only half of osteoblastomas result in significant reactive sclerosis, and over one third extend to a portion of the vertebral body. On MRI, intense inflammatory response and enhancement surrounding the tumor may lead to overestimation of tumor size [29]. Since treatment is generally based on lesion size, the necessity for preoperative differentiation between these two entities is generally academic.

6.3 Aneurysmal Bone Cyst (Box 4.5)

Box 4.5: Aneurysmal Bone Cyst

- Often lumbar
- Affects lamina, may spread to vertebral body
- Pathological fracture
- Expansile, lytic
- Internal septations (unlike osteoblastoma)
- Fluid-fluid levels (hematocrit equivalent)
- Large soft tissue mass may span vertebral segments

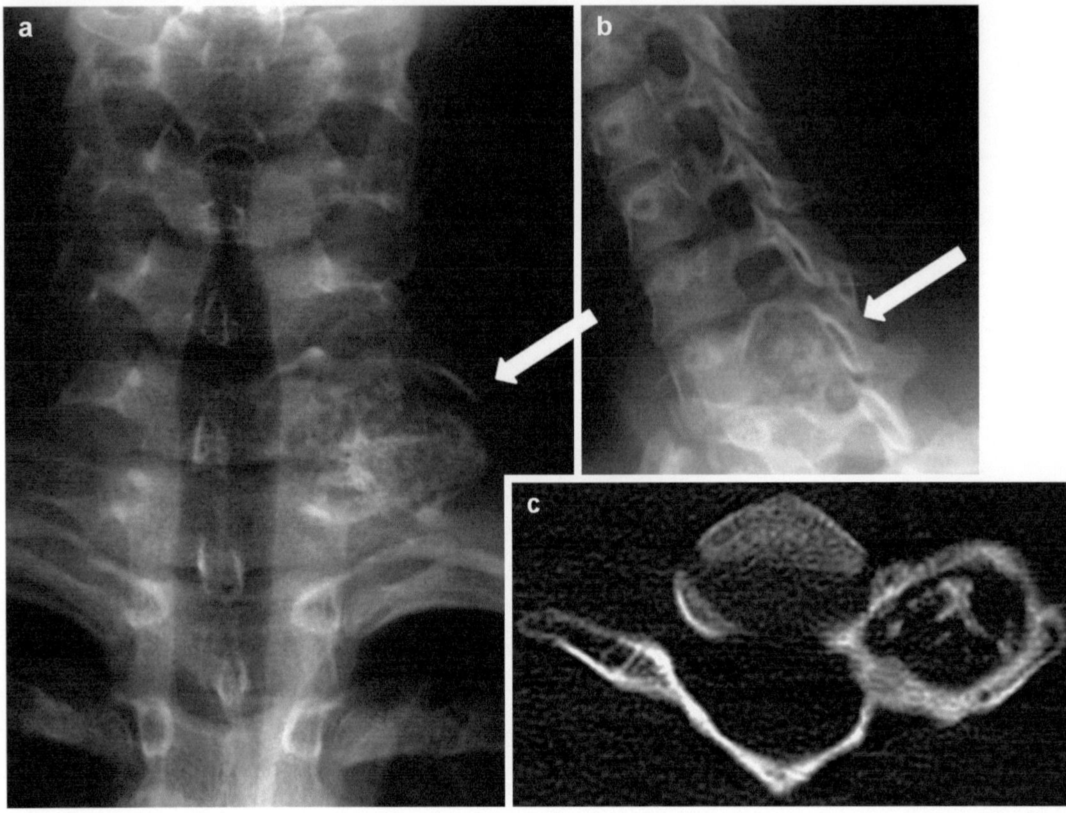

Fig. 4.20 Osteoblastoma in a 15-year-old boy with neck pain. (**a**) There is an expansile mass (*arrow*) of the left posterior elements of C7. (**b**) Irregular calcification within the expansile mass (*arrow*). (**c**) Axial CT shows expansion of the pedicle with osteoid matrix within the lytic lesion

Primary aneurysmal bone cysts (ABC) of the spine are locally aggressive but benign tumors that may recur locally after resection. Although ABCs are relatively rare, half of spinal cases occur in children [30], most often in the lumbar spine [31]. Pain, weakness, and radiculopathy are typical manifestations. The lamina alone is most often involved (Fig. 4.21), although the vertebral body may be invaded and later collapse. This highly vascular lesion can also cause pathological fracture and spinal instability.

The presence of internal septations helps distinguish primary ABC of the spine from osteoblastoma. On radiographs, the lesion appears expansile and lytic, with a thin cortical shell. CT can be useful in defining the bony extent of the ABC and in visualizing pathological fracture. On MRI, the expansile, lobulated, septated mass is hypointense on T1-W images and hyperintense on T2-W images. Septations typically enhance after gadolinium administration [29]. Fluid-fluid levels are common and result from serum and blood separating in the cavernous spaces [32]. There may be a large soft tissue mass extending along more than one vertebral segment.

6.4 Langerhans Cell Histiocytosis

About 17 % of children with Langerhans cell histiocytosis (LCH) have spinal involvement, most commonly presenting with dull back or neck pain [31]. LCH can cause the vertebral body to collapse into a wafer-like sclerotic plate (vertebra plana)

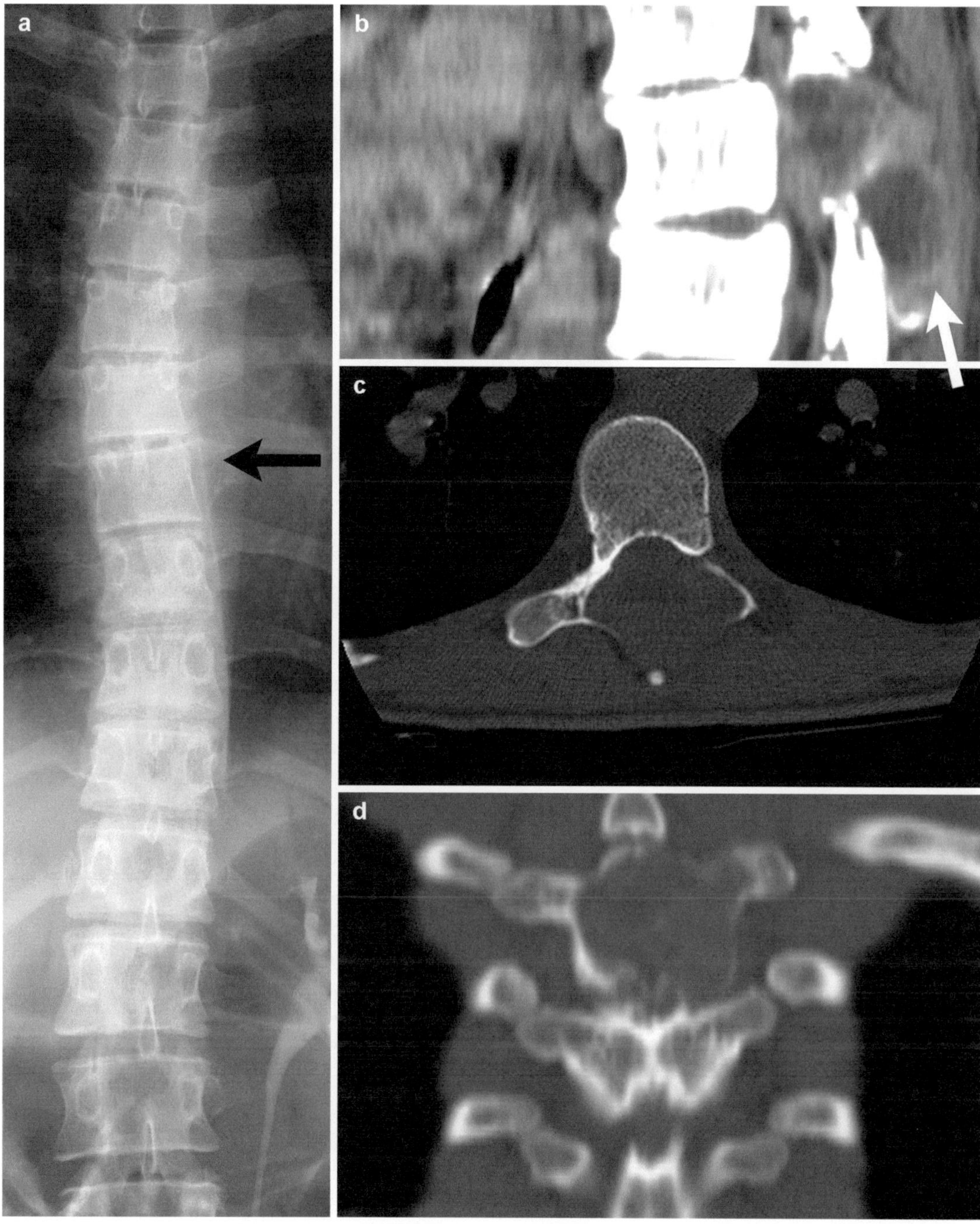

Fig. 4.21 Aneurysmal bone cyst in a 16-year-old girl. (**a**) Absent left pedicle at T8 (*black arrow*). (**b**) Sagittal reformatted CT imaging in soft tissue window shows lucent mass replacing pedicle as well as intraspinal extension. Suggestion of a fluid-fluid level (*arrow*). Axial (**c**) and coronal reformatted (**d**) CTs show expansile lytic mass with cortical thinning and destruction (Courtesy of Arthur Dublin)

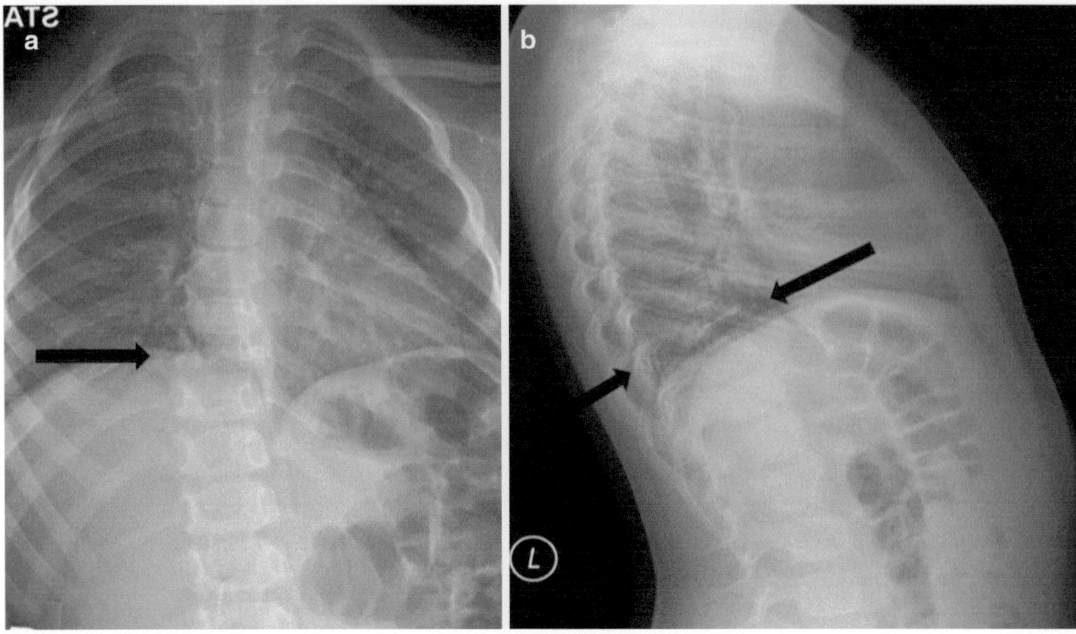

Fig. 4.22 Vertebra plana of T9 (*black arrows*) in a 3-year-old with Langerhans cell histiocytosis (**a**, **b**)

(Fig. 4.22). This is common in the thoracic spine and may be accompanied with epidural extension or a fusiform soft tissue mass. Posterior elements are spared and adjacent disc spaces preserved [33]. Intervertebral disc space height is normal or even slightly increased. During recovery, the vertebra may remarkably return to normal height.

Vertebra plana is not pathognomonic for LCH but can also result from spinal tuberculosis along with a variety of malignant tumors, including lymphoma [31].

6.5 Osteochondroma

Osteocartilaginous exostoses are benign lesions that are frequently found in the metaphyses of long bones and rarely in the spine. However, spinal lesions may acutely compress the spinal cord (Fig. 4.23), resulting in sudden neurological decompensation. To prevent neurological compromise, patients with multiple hereditary exostoses should have systematic neurological screening as well as spinal imaging [34, 35].

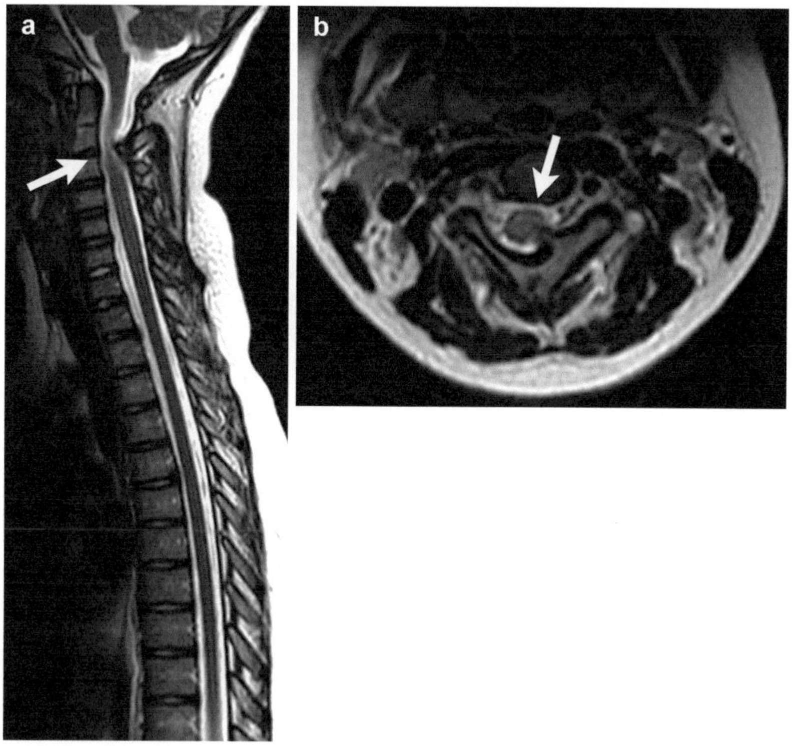

Fig. 4.23 Osteochondroma in an 11-year-old girl with multiple hereditary exostoses and new long tract signs. Sagittal (**a**) and axial (**b**) T2-W images show an intraspinal osteochondroma (*white arrows*) at C2 that compresses the cord

References

1. Belfi LM, Ortiz AO, Katz DS. Computed tomography evaluation of spondylolysis and spondylolisthesis in asymptomatic patients. Spine. 2006;31(24):E907–10. Epub 2006/11/17.
2. Micheli LJ, Wood R. Back pain in young athletes. Significant differences from adults in causes and patterns. Arch Pediatr Adolesc Med. 1995;149(1):15–8. Epub 1995/01/01.
3. Afshani E, Kuhn JP. Common causes of low back pain in children. Radiographics. 1991;11(2):269–91. Epub 1991/03/01.
4. Lowe J, Libson E, Ziv I, Nyska M, Floman Y, Bloom RA, et al. Spondylolysis in the upper lumbar spine. A study of 32 patients. J Bone Joint Surg. 1987;69(4):582–6. Epub 1987/08/01.
5. Hensinger RN. Spondylolysis and spondylolisthesis in children and adolescents. J Bone Joint Surg Am. 1989;71(7):1098–107. Epub 1989/08/01.
6. Forsberg DA, Martinez S, Vogler 3rd JB, Wiener MD. Cervical spondylolysis: imaging findings in 12 patients. AJR Am J Roentgenol. 1990;154(4):751–5. Epub 1990/04/01.
7. Yochum TR, Sellers LT, Oppenheimer DA, Peterson CK, Kirton CW, Dal Mas EC, et al. The sclerotic pedicle–how many causes are there? Skeletal Radiol. 1990;19(6):411–7.
8. Maldague BE, Malghem JJ. Unilateral arch hypertrophy with spinous process tilt: a sign of arch deficiency. Radiology. 1976;121(3 Pt. 1):567–74.
9. McCleary MD, Congeni JA. Current concepts in the diagnosis and treatment of spondylolysis in young athletes. Curr Sports Med Rep. 2007;6(1):62–6. Epub 2007/01/11.
10. Grogan JP, Hemminghytt S, Williams AL, Carrera GF, Haughton VM. Spondylolysis studied with computed tomography. Radiology. 1982;145(3):737–42. Epub 1982/12/01.
11. Ganiyusufoglu AK, Onat L, Karatoprak O, Enercan M, Hamzaoglu A. Diagnostic accuracy of magnetic resonance imaging versus computed tomography in stress fractures of the lumbar spine. Clin Radiol. 2010;65(11):902–7. Epub 2010/10/12.
12. Birch JG, Herring JA, Maravilla KR. Splitting of the intervertebral disc in spondylolisthesis: a magnetic resonance imaging finding in two cases. J Pediatr Orthop. 1986;6(5):609–11.
13. Frennered AK, Danielson BI, Nachemson AL. Natural history of symptomatic isthmic low-grade spondylolisthesis in children and adolescents: a seven-year follow-up study. J Pediatr Orthop. 1991;11(2):209–13. Epub 1991/03/01.

14. Egloff AM, Kadom N, Vezina G, Bulas D. Pediatric cervical spine trauma imaging: a practical approach. Pediatr Radiol. 2009;39(5):447–56.
15. Cakmakci H. Essentials of trauma: head and spine. Pediatr Radiol. 2009;39 Suppl 3:391–405.
16. Firth GB, Kingwell SP, Moroz PJ. Pediatric noncontiguous spinal injuries: the 15-year experience at a level 1 trauma center. Spine. 2012;37(10):E599–608.
17. Maxfield BA. Sports-related injury of the pediatric spine. Radiol Clin North Am. 2010;48(6):1237–48. Epub 2010/11/26.
18. Junewick JJ, Meesa IR, Luttenton CR, Hinman JM. Occult injury of the pediatric craniocervical junction. Emerg Radiol. 2009;16(6):483–8.
19. Bernstein MP, Mirvis SE, Shanmuganathan K. Chance-type fractures of the thoracolumbar spine: imaging analysis in 53 patients. AJR Am J Roentgenol. 2006;187(4):859–68. Epub 2006/09/21.
20. Cullen JC. Spinal lesions in battered babies. J Bone Joint Surg. 1975;57(3):364–6. Epub 1975/08/01.
21. Spencer SJ, Wilson NI. Childhood discitis in a regional children's hospital. J Pediatr Orthop B. 2012;21(3):264–8. Epub 2011/10/22.
22. Lernout C, Haas H, Rubio A, Griffet J. Pediatric intervertebral disk calcification in childhood: three case reports and review of literature. Childs Nerv Syst ChNS. 2009;25(8):1019–23. Epub 2009/05/09.
23. Renshaw TS, Solga PM, Drennan JC, Donskoy E. Studies of an L-rod sublaminar wire spinal fusion. J Pediatr Orthop. 1991;11(2):226–9. Epub 1991/03/01.
24. Khoury NJ, Hourani MH, Arabi MM, Abi-Fakher F, Haddad MC. Imaging of back pain in children and adolescents. Curr Probl Diagn Radiol. 2006;35(6):224–44. Epub 2006/11/07.
25. Varlotta GP, Brown MD, Kelsey JL, Golden AL. Familial predisposition for herniation of a lumbar disc in patients who are less than twenty-one years old. J Bone Joint Surg Am. 1991;73(1):124–8. Epub 1991/01/01.
26. Eismont FJ, Bohlman HH, Soni PL, Goldberg VM, Freehafer AA. Vertebral osteomyelitis in infants. J Bone Joint Surg. 1982;64(1):32–5.
27. Hsu LC, Leong JC. Tuberculosis of the lower cervical spine (C2 to C7). A report on 40 cases. J Bone Joint Surg. 1984;66(1):1–5.
28. Ropper AE, Cahill KS, Hanna JW, McCarthy EF, Gokaslan ZL, Chi JH. Primary vertebral tumors: a review of epidemiologic, histological and imaging findings, part II: locally aggressive and malignant tumors. Neurosurgery. 2012;70(1):211–9; discussion 9; Epub 2011/07/20.
29. Woertler K. Benign bone tumors and tumor-like lesions: value of cross-sectional imaging. Eur Radiol. 2003;13(8):1820–35. Epub 2003/04/18.
30. Novais EN, Rose PS, Yaszemski MJ, Sim FH. Aneurysmal bone cyst of the cervical spine in children. J Bone Joint Surg Am. 2011;93(16):1534–43. Epub 2011/12/29.
31. Ropper AE, Cahill KS, Hanna JW, McCarthy EF, Gokaslan ZL, Chi JH. Primary vertebral tumors: a review of epidemiologic, histological, and imaging findings, part I: benign tumors. Neurosurgery. 2011;69(6):1171–80. Epub 2011/07/05.
32. Alyas F, James SL, Davies AM, Saifuddin A. The role of MR imaging in the diagnostic characterisation of appendicular bone tumours and tumour-like conditions. Eur Radiol. 2007;17(10):2675–86. Epub 2007/03/08.
33. De Schepper AM, Ramon F, Van Marck E. MR imaging of eosinophilic granuloma: report of 11 cases. Skeletal Radiol. 1993;22(3):163–6. Epub 1993/01/01.
34. Lotfinia I, Vahedi P, Tubbs RS, Ghavame M, Meshkini A. Neurological manifestations, imaging characteristics, and surgical outcome of intraspinal osteochondroma. J Neurosurg Spine. 2010;12(5):474–89. Epub 2010/05/04.
35. Aldea S, Bonneville F, Poirier J, Chiras J, George B, Carpentier A. Acute spinal cord compression in hereditary multiple exostoses. Acta Neurochir. 2006;148(2):195–8; discussion 8; Epub 2005/11/29.

The Shoulder: Congenital and Developmental Conditions

5

Rebecca Stein-Wexler

Contents

Abstract

Three important congenital or developmental disorders affect the shoulder. Congenital pseudarthrosis of the clavicle is discussed at length, followed by congenital undescended scapula, or Sprengel deformity. A similar section focusing on glenohumeral dysplasia follows. The typical presentation, etiology, pathology, treatment, and imaging are discussed.

Three important congenital or developmental disorders affect the shoulder. Congenital pseudarthrosis of the clavicle is uncommon and generally important for cosmetic reasons. Undescended scapula (Sprengel deformity) is often accompanied by significant spine abnormalities. Glenohumeral dysplasia (brachial plexus birth palsy) is an unusual complication of birth trauma, and although many patients recover fully, a few experience persistent shoulder instability and upper extremity weakness. All these entities have a unique imaging appearance and can be readily identified. However, knowledge of normal development as well as a few variants is helpful.

R. Stein-Wexler, MD
Department of Radiology,
University of California Davis Medical
Center and UC Davis Children's Hospital,
4860 Y Street, Suite 3100, Sacramento, CA 95817, USA

Department of Diagnostic Imaging,
Shriners Hospitals for Children Northern California,
Sacramento, CA 95817, USA
e-mail: rebecca.steinwexler@ucdmc.ucdavis.edu

R. Stein-Wexler et al. (eds.), *Pediatric Orthopedic Imaging*,
DOI 10.1007/978-3-642-45381-6_5, © Springer-Verlag Berlin Heidelberg 2015

1 Normal Development of the Upper Extremity

The upper limb buds appear in the fourth fetal week as elevations of fetal unsegmented mesenchyme. They develop before those of the lower limb, and until age 2 the upper extremities dominate in terms of both size and degree of maturation. The cartilaginous models of the humerus, radius, and ulna form in the seventh week. Primary ossification centers can be seen in the humerus and ulna by eight fetal weeks, and in the radius by 12. The metacarpals begin to ossify by four fetal months, and the phalanges by six.

The secondary ossification centers in the upper extremity appear during childhood and adolescence. The humeral head ossifies first, between 37 fetal and 16 postnatal weeks, whereas the medial epiphysis of the clavicle ossifies last, appearing at approximately 17 years and fusing by age 25. (Additional information about secondary ossification centers of the shoulder is presented in Chap. 6.) Secondary ossification centers of the elbow occasionally cause concern in the diagnosis of traumatic lesions, and it is therefore important to understand both their timing of ossification and their normal appearance (see Chap. 8).

Most growth in the arm occurs at the wrist and shoulder. For each bone, the relative percentage contributions of the upper and lower epiphyses, respectively, are humerus, 80/20; radius, 25/75; and ulna, 20/80 [1]. Because the wrist (and knee) grow most rapidly and therefore have greater metabolic turnover, radiographs of these areas are useful for detecting metabolic bone disease such as rickets.

2 Variant Ossification of the Shoulder

Several normal features and projectional lucencies must be recognized in evaluating radiographs of the pediatric shoulder. One edge of the proximal humeral growth plate may project below the other, forming a linear lucency that may mimic a fracture line. The greater tuberosity may normally appear as a well-demarcated lucency. Older children may have normal bony ridges along the bicipital groove of the proximal humerus that should not be mistaken for periosteal reaction [2]. Infants between 1 and 6 months of age may demonstrate smooth periosteal thickening, a benign and generally symmetric condition known as periostitis of infancy (discussed in greater depth in Chap. 2).

3 Congenital Pseudarthrosis of the Clavicle (Box 5.1)

Box 5.1: Congenital Pseudarthrosis of the Clavicle

- Middle third of clavicle, usually right
- Sternal segment usually larger, tapered, points anterosuperiorly
- Acromial segment smaller, bulbous, points superomedially
- Differential: birth trauma, nonunion of old fracture, cleidocranial dysostosis

Congenital pseudarthrosis of the clavicle presents as a painless, palpable, and often visible prominence in the middle one third of the clavicle, usually on the right. The lump may increase during growth, and hypermobility may result in an unattractive forward drooping of the shoulder. Parasthesias are uncommon, but thoracic outlet syndrome may develop in adulthood. Most patients present during the first 2 years of life. More than 200 cases have been reported in the literature [3]. Most are isolated abnormalities, but some result from autosomal recessive inheritance; bilateral lesions are extremely rare and may result from autosomal dominant inheritance.

The embryological development of the clavicle helps explain congenital pseudarthrosis. The clavicle, which is the first bone to ossify, develops from two ossification centers. Subsequent failure of these centers to coalesce results in congenital pseudarthrosis [4, 5]. Both vascular pulsations and bony impingement have been implicated in this lack of fusion. The almost-exclusive right-sided occurrence may result from the fact that the right subclavian artery is normally higher than the left. It must therefore pass through a narrow gap between the first rib and midclavicle, where it can apply pressure on the developing bone [6]. Most reported cases of congenital pseudarthrosis on the left occur in patients with dextrocardia, supporting the theory that vascular pulsations contribute to the lesion. Furthermore, cervical ribs or superior extension of the thorax and first rib are often present, exacerbating impingement. Bilateral lesions are rare, with only nine reported cases [7]. They are associated with bilateral high subclavian arteries, cervical ribs, and/or high, vertically oriented upper ribs [8].

Histological studies of resected specimens have shown that both ends of bone are covered with hyaline cartilage caps composed of columnar chondrocytes, resembling normal growth cartilage. Fibrocartilage connects these hyaline caps [4, 5].

Treatment is generally surgical, although there is a high rate of failure and complications [4, 7, 9]. Surgery usually consists of resection, bone graft placement, and internal fixation [3, 7, 10].

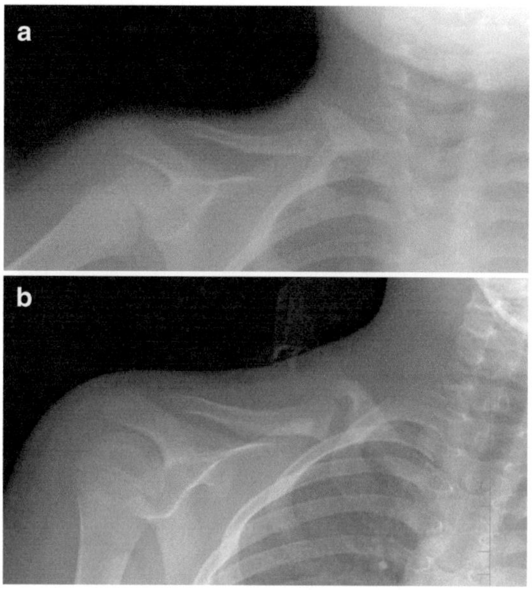

Fig. 5.1 Congenital pseudarthrosis of the clavicle in a 3-year-old who presented with a palpable mass. (**a**) At presentation, there are typical smooth, tapered contours without evident callus formation. (**b**) 5 years later, nonunion persists, although the medial fragment abuts the lateral fragment (Images copyright Shriners Hospital for Children Northern California)

Imaging

On radiographs, absence of bone in the midportion of the clavicle is obvious in young children, but the configuration varies [10]. The classic appearance consists of a large sternal portion that protrudes anteriorly and superiorly and a smaller more caudally positioned acromial segment that points superiorly and medially (Fig. 5.1). Typically the lateral end of the sternal segment is tapered, and the medial end of the acromial fragment is expanded or bulbous [11]. However, both the configuration of and the relationship between the ends of the two clavicular fragments may vary (Fig. 5.2) [10]. There is no callus or periosteal reaction. Radiographs are almost always diagnostic, but very rarely—if the pseudarthrosis is hidden behind the apex of the deformity and if the history is atypical—additional imaging such as computed tomography with three-dimensional reconstruction (3D-CT) may be necessary to exclude such lesions as Ewing sarcoma [12].

Differential Diagnosis

If a radiograph is obtained in the newborn, the typical configuration often allows differentiation from birth fracture; lack of subsequent callus formation helps in equivocal cases. A postnatal fracture is usually differentiated by typical history and development of callus [10]. If there is nonunion of an old fracture, both ends are usually attenuated [8]. Differentiation from cleidocranial dysostosis is more difficult, since the appearance can be identical—in 40 cases of cleidocranial dysostosis, 17 of the clavicular lesions were unilateral and affected only the right side [13]. A careful search for cranial sutural and fontanelle defects, pubic symphysis diastasis, and the other characteristic spine and hand abnormalities should be made, especially if there is a family history of similar abnormalities in this autosomal dominant dysplasia.

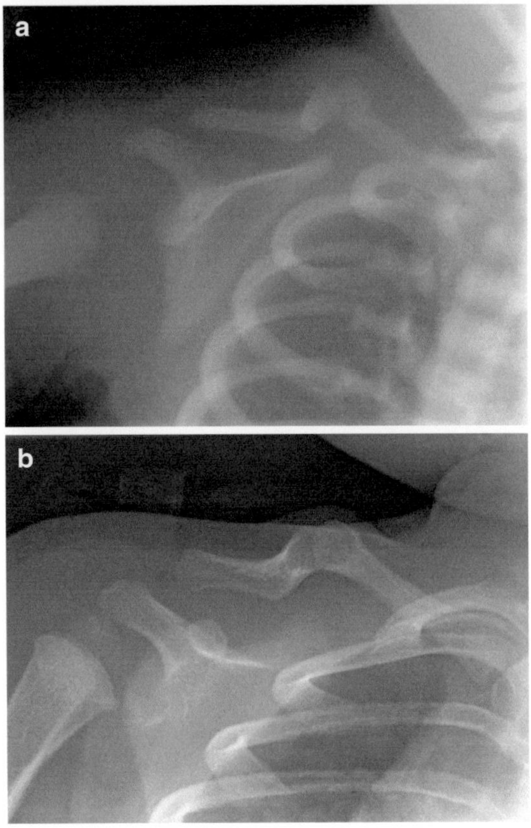

Fig. 5.2 Congenital pseudarthrosis of the clavicle in a newborn, discovered incidentally during evaluation for respiratory distress. (**a**) Right clavicular defect with ends that are smoothly contoured, tapered, and sclerotic. The medial fragment is elevated by pull of the sternocleido-mastoid muscle. (**b**) One year later, the ends are more closely apposed and remain smooth (Images copyright Shriners Hospital for Children Northern California)

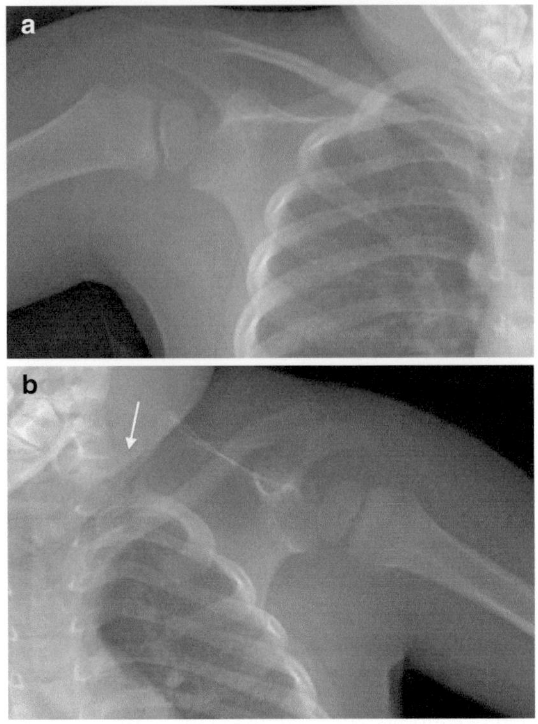

Fig. 5.3 Sprengel deformity on the left. (**a**) The right shoulder is normal. (**b**) The left scapula is elevated, rotated, and medially displaced. The omovertebral bone is difficult to see (*arrow*), extending laterally from the lower cervical spine (Images copyright Shriners Hospital for Children Northern California)

4 Congenital Undescended Scapula (Sprengel Deformity) (Box 5.2)

> **Box 5.2: Sprengel Deformity (Congenital Undescended Scapula)**
>
> Klippel-Feil associated in 20 %
> Omovertebral bone in 50 %
> Scapula tilted, lifted, medially displaced
> Acromion elongated

Patients with Sprengel deformity typically present with fullness at the base of the neck and loss of shoulder motion; average age at diagnosis is 3 years [14]. Three times more common in girls, it is usually on the left but occasionally bilateral or on the right. Almost all patients have accompanying anomalies. Scoliosis occurs in 39 %, usually convex on the same side as the scapular elevation. Accessory, absent, fused, or bifid ribs are seen in 25 %. Twenty percent have developmental anomalies of the cervical spine, such as hemivertebrae and vertebral fusion (constituting the Klippel-Feil anomaly) (Fig. 5.3). Meningocele or dysraphism occur in 7 %, and genitourinary abnormalities are common [15]. The adjacent musculature is typically hypoplastic and fibrotic [16].

Sprengel deformity occurs when the scapular anlage fails to descend from the C4–C5 level to its normal position below T3. A physical connection between the medial angle or edge of the scapula and the lamina, spinous, or transverse process of the spine from C4–T1 is common [17], but it is uncertain whether this tethering causes or results from

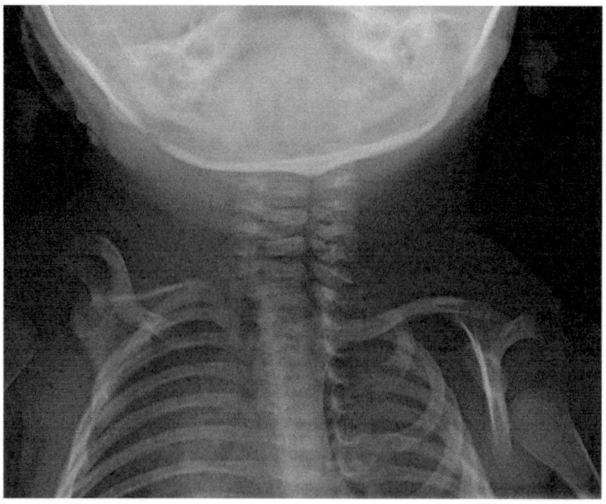

Fig. 5.4 Sprengel deformity on the right in a 3-week-old girl. The scapula is elevated, angulated, and medially displaced

the anomaly. The site of insertion appears to affect scapular shape [18]. A bony connection between the scapula and occiput has rarely been described [19].

A fibrous or cartilaginous connection to the spine is common. Osseous condensation occurs in up to 50 % of patients and is termed the omovertebral bone [15, 19]. This bone may represent a rudimentary cervical rib or the homologue of the suprascapular bone seen in some lower vertebrates [20].

Children with mild deformity can be treated with physical therapy to maintain range of motion and are generally followed until skeletal maturity. For more severe deformities, various surgical procedures have been developed, including repositioning and osteotomy of the scapula and resection of the omovertebral bone [1]. These procedures are thought to be most successful before 6 years of age [14].

Imaging

On radiographs, the extent of scapular elevation and medial displacement varies; often the scapula is tilted with the medial angle high but the glenoid and shoulder at near-normal level. The scapula appears small but is actually larger than normal [18]. Its shape is infantile, with an increased horizontal and decreased vertical length—the latter may be partly due to projectional foreshortening, since the scapula is often angulated forward (Fig. 5.4). The acromion may be elongated and carried downward, and there is generally a rotational component to the deformity as well. Minor changes in projection can dramatically alter the apparent position of the scapula [14], and overlapping structures limit visualization. 3D-CT provides more accurate information and can assist with surgical planning (Fig. 5.5) [18]. Either computed tomography (CT) or magnetic resonance imaging (MRI) allows improved identification of the omovertebral bone [21].

5 Glenohumeral Dysplasia (Box 5.3)

Box 5.3: Glenohumeral Dysplasia

US up to 12 months	Delineates cartilage, quantifies subluxation
Radiography	Humeral head—small, flat, and deformed
	Scapula—elevated and rotated out with small glenoid
	Acromion process—elongated and hooked
MRI	Glenoid fossa—normal, flat, or biconcave

The brachial plexus is injured during obstetric delivery in 2.3–3.3 per 1,000 live births [22]. Several identifiable syndromes result from these nerve injuries. In 80 % of patients, C5 and C6 branches are affected and a classic upper arm (Erb's) palsy results—paralysis of the external rotators and tightness of the internal rotators result in loss of both active and passive external rotation. The arm hangs in internal rotation, the forearm is pronated, and the wrist flexed—the "waiters tip" deformity. The upper arm may appear foreshortened if there is posterior dislocation at the glenohumeral joint, which causes telescoping of the soft tissues and extra skinfolds. There may be fullness of the posterior aspect of the shoulder. Persistent muscle imbalance results in progressive posterior shoulder dislocation; this has usually been diagnosed after the age of 1 year, but studies have shown that it can develop as early as 4 months in 7–8 % of patients with

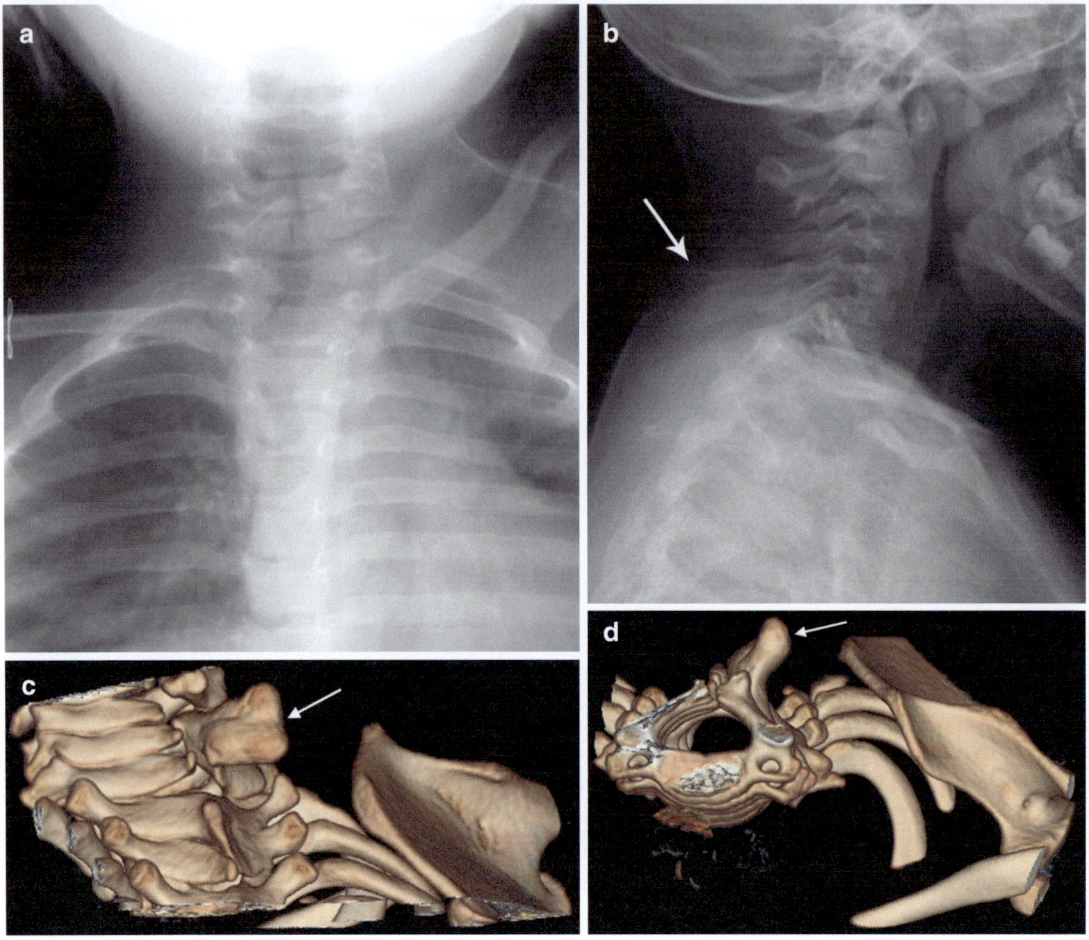

Fig. 5.5 Sprengel deformity in a 15-month-old girl. (**a**) The left scapula is elevated, rotated, and medially displaced. (**b**) Note bulbous fusion of spinous processes of the lower cervical spine. (**c**, **d**) 3D-reconstructed CT images suggest omovertebral bone (*arrows*) extending toward the superomedial scapula, probably with an intervening fibrous segment

brachial plexus birth injury [22, 23]. The phrenic nerve, predominantly C4 but with contributions from C5, may also be involved.

When the whole arm is involved (C5–Tl lesions of Duchenne-Erb-Klumpke), flaccidity is obvious and there may be an associated Horner's syndrome. However, muscle damage tends to be more balanced, resulting in less glenohumeral dysplasia [24, 25].

The brachial plexus is usually injured in the course of breech deliveries. Birth weight over 4,000 g increases the risk of brachial plexus injury by a factor of 2.5 [26]. Other risk factors include multiparous pregnancies, shoulder dystocia in vertex deliveries, and vacuum-assisted deliveries [27]. Reversible hemorrhage and edema may result from nerve plexus traction, and thus gradual near-complete recovery occurs in 93–95 % [22, 26]. When partial or total nerve transection occurs, full recovery is unlikely; injury is irreversible if the nerve root is torn from the spinal canal injury [27]. With progressive neuromuscular imbalance, the cartilage of the glenoid and humerus becomes increasingly dysplastic, as with developmental dysplasia of the hip. Eventually, there is bony remodeling.

Treatment is intended to restore range of motion and establish a stable glenohumeral relationship in order to maximize the functional potential of the affected arm. There is some evidence that glenoid remodeling is facilitated by rebalancing musculature, although it is unclear how much glenohumeral dysplasia can be reversed and at what age [28, 29]. Botulinum toxin injection, splinting, and stretching are useful initial treatment for children under 1 year of age, and physical therapy is often continued throughout childhood. In those less than 6–9 months of age, microsurgery may be employed to reconstruct the brachial plexus. Tendon transfers and capsular releases (either open or arthroscopic) are useful in children over 1 year of age who develop glenohumeral dysplasia and/or persistent limited external rotation. Humeral derotational osteotomy may be performed in older children with advanced dysplasia [30]. Other surgical procedures including tendon transfers and osteotomies are used throughout the upper extremity to address dysfunction of the elbow, wrist, and hand as needed.

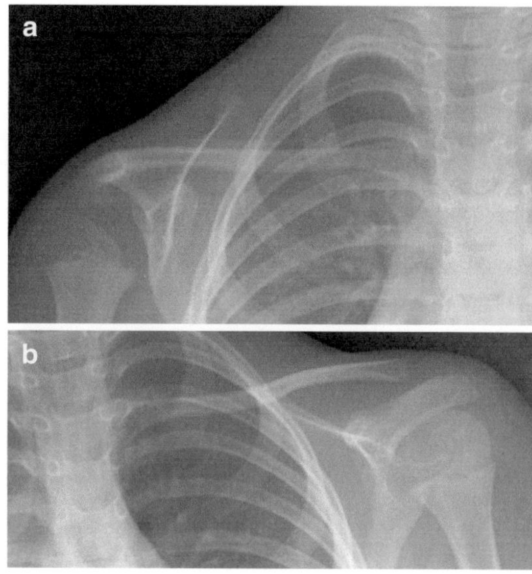

Fig. 5.6 Brachial plexus birth palsy. (**a**) The right scapula is small, elevated, and rotated outwardly with a prominent acromion. The humeral head is small and flattened, positioned inferior to its normal location. (**b**) The left shoulder is normal (Images copyright Shriners Hospital for Children Northern California)

Imaging

Radiographic evaluation should be performed as soon as the diagnosis is entertained to rule out associated clavicular and humeral epiphyseal trauma; ultrasound (US) diagnosis of the latter in the newborn is possible [31]. Although MRI can assess nerve root avulsion or pseudomeningocele [32], MRI of the plexus is rarely helpful in determining prognosis. The appearance of the ossification centers for the humeral head and greater tuberosity (usually radiographically apparent by the first and ninth month, respectively) may be delayed, limiting utility of radiographs in infants. However, dislocation of the humeral head has been identified by US as early as 3 months of age [23].

Frontal and lateral shoulder radiographs in infants are usually nondiagnostic, and axillary views are often improperly positioned. However, as the bones mature and there is increased ossification, the humeral head may appear laterally displaced from the glenoid and internally rotated. The scapula is elevated and rotated outward (Fig. 5.6). With phrenic nerve injury, the diaphragm may be paralyzed and elevated. In later childhood, decrease in soft tissue muscle mass becomes obvious. The humeral head is small, flattened, and often deformed. If the growth plate of the upper humerus was injured initially, premature union or impaired growth may take place, with resultant shortening of the humerus (since this growth plate contributes 80 % of the total length). Relative overgrowth of the greater tuberosity may occur. The acromion process often elongates and hooks downward, and the coracoid may be prominent. The clavicle may also be short and the lateral aspect hooked inferiorly. Humeral head dislocation is not uncommon and usually occurs in the first 6 months, before contractures develop [33].

The bones of the arm, forearm, and hand may be smaller and shortened, and overall the limb is on average 95 % of the length and girth of the normal side [34]. Up to one fourth of patients develop posterior dislocation of the radial head or medial subluxation of the ulna [35].

US readily evaluates the degree of posterior subluxation of the humeral head and is easily performed up to age 12 months [36, 37]. Early US screening of patients with brachial plexus birth injury allows earlier diagnosis of displacement of the humeral head, and this in turn allows earlier and potentially more successful intervention. Posterior dislocation has been diagnosed in 11 % of at-risk infants [23].

The shoulder is scanned from a posterior oblique/axial approach, and the degree of

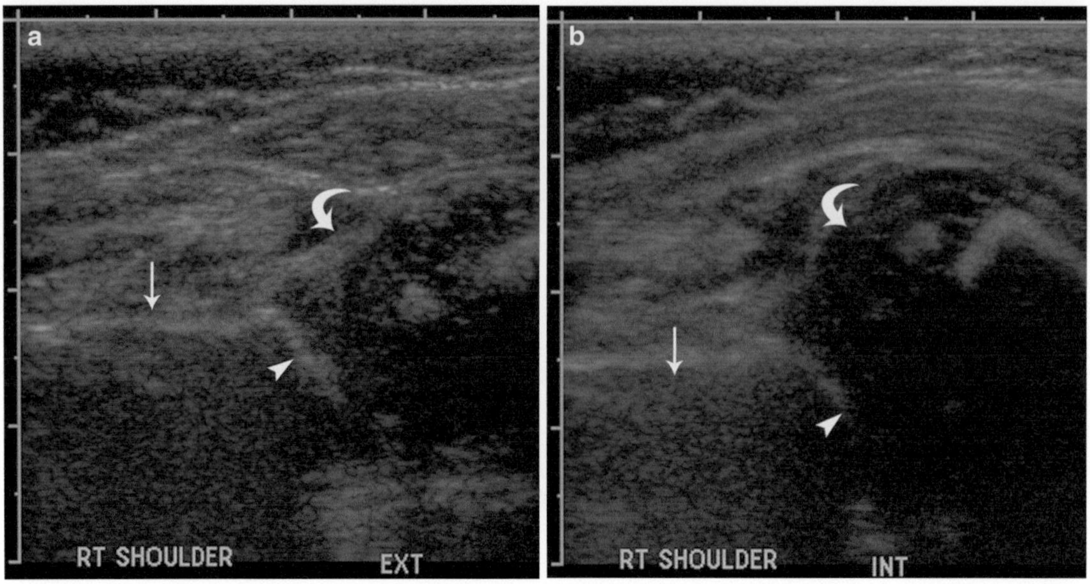

Fig. 5.7 US of brachial plexus birth palsy, posterior oblique axial approach. The *straight arrows* indicate the posterior margin of the scapula, the *curved arrows* the posterior aspect of the humeral head, and the *arrowheads* the glenoid fossa. (**a**) With external rotation, the humeral head is normally seated in the glenoid. (**b**) With internal rotation, the humeral head subluxates posteriorly (Images copyright Shriners Hospital for Children Northern California)

posterior subluxation is assessed during internal and external rotation of the arm (Fig. 5.7). Subluxation can be quantified by determining the angle between a line tangential to the posterior margin of the scapula and a line drawn tangentially to the humeral head and the posterior edge of the glenoid (alpha angle) [38, 39]. In normal patients, the humeral head ossification center is positioned anterior to the posterior margin of the scapula, and the alpha angle is less than 30°. Decreased size of the humeral head and a smaller ossified humeral head nucleus are evident in those with glenohumeral dysplasia [38]. Ultrasound screening at 3 and 6 months of age can be employed in patients with history of shoulder dystocia, as it may identify clinically occult subluxation [38].

CT provides excellent evaluation of the glenohumeral relationship but only limited assessment of non-osseous structures (Fig. 5.8). It is most useful in older children.

MRI provides exquisite delineation of cartilage, muscles, and tendons and is especially useful up to age 5, when the humeral head and glenoid are predominantly composed of unossified cartilage. In suspected brachial plexus birth injury, both shoulders should be imaged to permit comparison. Axial and oblique coronal gradient echo sequences are the most useful; the hyaline cartilage of the glenoid fossa, glenoid labrum, and humeral epiphysis appears bright [30]. Features demonstrated at MRI include (1) shape, size, ossification, and position of the humeral head; (2) shape and degree of retroversion of the glenoid fossa; (3) configuration of the glenoid labrum; (4) position and configuration of the coracoid process; and (5) degree of muscular atrophy (Fig. 5.9).

With MRI, the humeral head appears round, oval, or flattened. The degree of subluxation is assessed in the transverse plane by determining the percentage of the humeral head that is positioned anterior to a line transecting the scapular spine and the midportion of the glenoid fossa [40]. Ossification of the nucleus for the greater tuberosity of the humerus is delayed [41]. The glenoid fossa is described as concentric (normal), flat, or biconcave; a "pseudoglenoid fossa" (wherein the humeral head articulates with a retroverted, posterior articular surface) is analogous to the pseudoacetabulum of developmental dysplasia of the hip [42, 43]. Glenoid fossa retroversion is

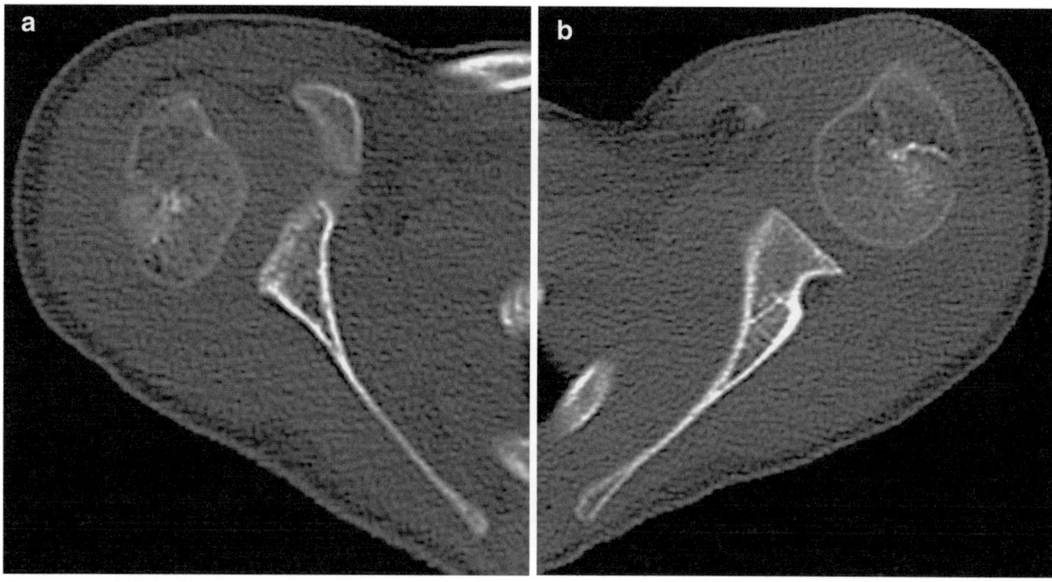

Fig. 5.8 CT of brachial plexus birth palsy. (**a**) The right glenoid is convex and irregular, and the humeral head is flattened. (**b**) The left shoulder is normal

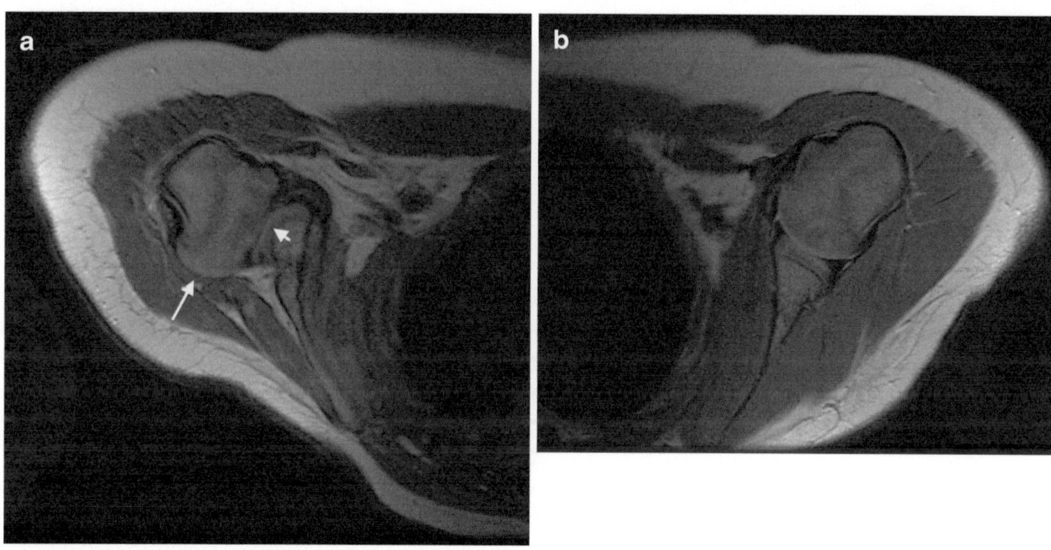

Fig. 5.9 Brachial plexus birth palsy on the right. Axial T1-weighted (T1-W) MRI shows (**a**) the right glenoid is biconvex (*short arrow*), and the posterior labrum is thinned. An irregular, flattened humeral head (*long arrow*) is posteriorly subluxated. Muscle bulk is severely diminished. (**b**) The left shoulder is normal

normally within 5° of that on the opposite side [40]. Glenohumeral deformity may progress from normal (I), to posterior glenoid deformity (II), to humeral head subluxation and further glenoid dysplasia (III), to the development of a false glenoid (IV), to flattening of both the glenoid and the humeral head (V) [27]. The posterior corner of the glenoid labrum may be blunted, and the posterior articular cartilage thin [26]. The coracoid process may appear retroverted [44]. Denervation atrophy is most common in the subscapularis muscle, but—depending on which nerves are damaged—additional muscles may be involved [25].

Differential diagnosis

The differential diagnosis of glenohumeral dysplasia is limited. Infants with birth-trauma-related fractures of the clavicle or humerus present with pseudoparalysis that resolves rapidly as the fracture heals. Occasionally, a child with mild hemiplegic or monoplegic cerebral palsy can have similar findings on physical exam, but the birth history is much different and the infant usually small or premature. Infants with tumors involving the brachial plexus may present with clinical findings mimicking brachial plexus injury. Glenoid and scapular neck hypoplasia with acromial and coracoid overgrowth are seen in glenoid dysplasia, which is usually an isolated, sporadic abnormality, with occasional familial occurrence [45]. Sometimes, an undescended scapula (Sprengel lesion) may be difficult to differentiate radiographically, as elongation and downward hooking of the acromion may be present in both conditions. However, the presence of an omovertebral bone or extensive cervical spine anomalies—along with the absence of changes in the glenoid and proximal humeral epiphysis—may help confirm the diagnosis of congenital scapular elevation. Nontraumatic glenohumeral dysplasia rarely results from local edema secondary to infantile cortical hyperostosis (Caffey disease) of the scapula.

References

1. Blount WP. Fractures of the forearm in children. Pediatr Clin North Am. 1955:1097–119. PubMed PMID: 13266453.
2. Keats TE, Anderson MW, editors. Atlas of normal roentgen variants that may simulate disease. 8th ed. Philadelphia: Mosby; 2006.
3. Beslikas TA, Dadoukis DJ, Gigis IP, Nenopoulos SP, Christoforides JE. Congenital pseudarthrosis of the clavicle: a case report. J Orthop Surg (Hong Kong). 2007;15(1):87–90. PubMed PMID: 17429126. Epub 2007/04/13. eng.
4. Hirata S, Miya H, Mizuno K. Congenital pseudarthrosis of the clavicle. Histologic examination for the etiology of the disease. Clin Orthop Relat Res. 1995;315:242–5. PubMed PMID: 7634675. Epub 1995/06/01. eng.
5. Gomez-Brouchet A, Sales De Gauzy J, Accadbled F, Abid A, Delisle MB, Cahuzac JP. Congenital pseudarthrosis of the clavicle: a histopathological study in five patients. J Pediatr Orthop B. 2004;13(6):399–401. PubMed PMID: 15599233. Epub 2004/12/16. eng.
6. Lloyd-Roberts GC, Apley AG, Owen R. Reflections upon the aetiology of congenital pseudarthrosis of the clavicle. With a note on cranio-cleido dysostosis. J Bone Joint Surg (Br). 1975;57(1):24–9. PubMed PMID: 1117020. Epub 1975/02/01. eng.
7. Lorente Molto FJ, Bonete Lluch DJ, Garrido IM. Congenital pseudarthrosis of the clavicle: a proposal for early surgical treatment. J Pediatr Orthop. 2001;21(5):689–93. PubMed PMID: 11521043. Epub 2001/08/25. eng.
8. Herring JA. Tachdjian's pediatric orthopaedics. 4th ed. Philadelphia: Saunders; 2007.
9. Padua R, Romanini E, Conti C, Padua L, Serra F. Bilateral congenital pseudarthrosis of the clavicle report of a case with clinical, radiological and neurophysiological evaluation. Acta Orthop Belg. 1999;65(3):372–5. PubMed PMID: 10546362. Epub 1999/11/05. eng.
10. Currarino G, Herring JA. Congenital pseudarthrosis of the clavicle. Pediatr Radiol. 2009;39(12):1343–9. PubMed PMID: 19763557. Epub 2009/09/19. eng.
11. Owen R. Congenital pseudarthrosis of the clavicle. J Bone Joint Surg (Br). 1970;52(4):644–52. PubMed PMID: 5487564. Epub 1970/11/01. eng.
12. Sloan A, Paton R. Congenital pseudarthrosis of the clavicle: the role of CT-scanning. Acta Orthop Belg. 2006;72(3):356–8. PubMed PMID: 16889151. Epub 2006/08/08. eng.
13. Jarvis JL, Keats TE. Cleidocranial dysostosis. A review of 40 new cases. Am J Roentgenol Radium Ther Nucl Med. 1974;121(1):5–16.
14. Leibovic SJ, Ehrlich MG, Zaleske DJ. Sprengel deformity. J Bone Joint Surg Am. 1990;72(2):192–7. PubMed PMID: 2303505. Epub 1990/02/01. eng.
15. Cavendish ME. Congenital elevation of the scapula. J Bone Joint Surg (Br). 1972;54(3):395–408. PubMed PMID: 4559837. Epub 1972/08/01. eng.
16. Carson WG, Lovell WW, Whitesides Jr TE. Congenital elevation of the scapula. Surgical correction by the Woodward procedure. J Bone Joint Surg Am. 1981;63(8):1199–207. PubMed PMID: 7026567. Epub 1981/10/01. eng.
17. Ogden JA, Conlogue GJ, Phillips MS, Bronson ML. Sprengel's deformity. Radiology of the pathologic deformation. Skeletal Radiol. 1979;4(4):204–11. PubMed PMID: 394335. Epub 1979/01/01. eng.
18. Cho TJ, Choi IH, Chung CY, Hwang JK. The Sprengel deformity. Morphometric analysis using 3D-CT and its clinical relevance. J Bone Joint Surg (Br). 2000;82(5):711–8.
19. Mooney 3rd JF, White DR, Glazier S. Previously unreported structure associated with Sprengel deformity. J Pediatr Orthop. 2009;29(1):26–8. PubMed PMID: 19098640. Epub 2008/12/23. eng.
20. McClure JG, Raney RB. Anomalies of the scapula. Clin Orthop Relat Res. 1975 Jul–Aug(110):22–31. PubMed PMID: 808367. Epub 1975/07/01. eng.
21. Azouz EM, Oudjhane K. Disorders of the upper extremity in children. Magn Reson Imaging Clin N Am. 1998;6(3):677–95. PubMed PMID: 9654591. Epub 1998/07/09. eng.

22. Dahlin LB, Erichs K, Andersson C, Thornqvist C, Backman C, Duppe H, et al. Incidence of early posterior shoulder dislocation in brachial plexus birth palsy. J Brachial Plex Peripher Nerve Inj. 2007;2:24. PubMed PMID: 18081937. Pubmed Central PMCID: 2225400. Epub 2007/12/18. eng.
23. Moukoko D, Ezaki M, Wilkes D, Carter P. Posterior shoulder dislocation in infants with neonatal brachial plexus palsy. J Bone Joint Surg Am. 2004;86-A(4):787–93. PubMed PMID: 15069145. Epub 2004/04/08. eng.
24. Bahm J, Wein B, Alhares G, Dogan C, Radermacher K, Schuind F. Assessment and treatment of glenohumeral joint deformities in children suffering from upper obstetric brachial plexus palsy. J Pediatr Orthop B. 2007;16(4):243–51. PubMed PMID: 17527100. Epub 2007/05/29. eng.
25. Hogendoorn S, van Overvest KL, Watt I, Duijsens AH, Nelissen RG. Structural changes in muscle and glenohumeral joint deformity in neonatal brachial plexus palsy. J Bone Joint Surg Am. 2010;92(4):935–42. PubMed PMID: 20360518. Epub 2010/04/03. eng.
26. Gudinchet F, Maeder P, Oberson JC, Schnyder P. Magnetic resonance imaging of the shoulder in children with brachial pLexus birth palsy. Pediatr Radiol. 1995;25 Suppl 1:S125–8. PubMed PMID: 8577503. Epub 1995/11/01. eng.
27. Waters PM. Update on management of pediatric brachial plexus palsy. J Pediatr Orthop. 2005;25(1):116–26. PubMed PMID: 15614072. Epub 2004/12/23. eng.
28. Waters PM, Bae DS. Effect of tendon transfers and extra-articular soft-tissue balancing on glenohumeral development in brachial plexus birth palsy. J Bone Joint Surg Am. 2005;87(2):320–5. PubMed PMID: 15687154. Epub 2005/02/03. eng.
29. Van Heest A, Glisson C, Ma H. Glenohumeral dysplasia changes after tendon transfer surgery in children with birth brachial plexus injuries. J Pediatr Orthop. 2010;30(4):371–8. PubMed PMID: 20502238. Epub 2010/05/27. eng.
30. Chauvin NA, Jaimes C, Laor T, Jaramillo D. Magnetic resonance imaging of the pediatric shoulder. Magn Reson Imaging Clin N Am. 2012;20(2):327–47, xi. PubMed PMID: 22469407. Epub 2012/04/04. eng.
31. Broker FH, Burbach T. Ultrasonic diagnosis of separation of the proximal humeral epiphysis in the newborn. J Bone Joint Surg Am. 1990;72(2):187–91. PubMed PMID: 2406274. Epub 1990/02/01. eng.
32. Martinoli C, Gandolfo N, Perez MM, Klauser A, Palmieri F, Padua L, et al. Brachial plexus and nerves about the shoulder. Semin Musculoskelet Radiol. 2010;14(5):523–46. PubMed PMID: 21072730. Epub 2010/11/13. eng.
33. Babbitt DP, Cassidy RH. Obstetrical paralysis and dislocation of the shoulder in infancy. J Bone Joint Surg Am. 1968;50(7):1447–52. PubMed PMID: 5677299. Epub 1968/10/01. eng.
34. Bae DS, Ferretti M, Waters PM. Upper extremity size differences in brachial plexus birth palsy. Hand (N Y). 2008;3(4):297–303. PMID: 18780022. Pubmed Central PMCID: 2584210. Epub 2008/09/10. eng.
35. Adler JB, Patterson Jr RL. Erb's palsy. Long-term results of treatment in eighty-eight cases. J Bone Joint Surg Am. 1967;49(6):1052–64. PubMed PMID: 6038856. Epub 1967/09/01. eng.
36. Grissom LE, Harcke HT. Infant shoulder sonography: technique, anatomy, and pathology. Pediatr Radiol. 2001;31(12):863–8. PubMed PMID: 11727022. Epub 2001/12/01. eng.
37. Hunter JD, Franklin K, Hughes PM. The ultrasound diagnosis of posterior shoulder dislocation associated with Erb's palsy. Pediatr Radiol. 1998;28(7):510–1. PubMed PMID: 9662568. Epub 1998/07/15. eng.
38. Poyhia TH, Lamminen AE, Peltonen JI, Kirjavainen MO, Willamo PJ, Nietosvaara Y. Brachial plexus birth injury: US screening for glenohumeral joint instability. Radiology. 2010;254(1):253–60. PubMed PMID: 20032156. Epub 2009/12/25. eng.
39. Vathana T, Rust S, Mills J, Wilkes D, Browne R, Carter PR, et al. Intraobserver and interobserver reliability of two ultrasound measures of humeral head position in infants with neonatal brachial plexus palsy. J Bone Joint Surg Am. 2007;89(8):1710–5. PubMed PMID: 17671008. Epub 2007/08/03. eng.
40. Waters PM, Smith GR, Jaramillo D. Glenohumeral deformity secondary to brachial plexus birth palsy. J Bone Joint Surg Am. 1998;80(5):668–77. PubMed PMID: 9611027. Epub 1998/06/04. eng.
41. Clarke SE, Chafetz RS, Kozin SH. Ossification of the proximal humerus in children with residual brachial plexus birth palsy: a magnetic resonance imaging study. J Pediatr Orthop. 2010;30(1):60–6. PubMed PMID: 20032744. Epub 2009/12/25. eng.
42. Pearl ML, Edgerton BW. Glenoid deformity secondary to brachial plexus birth palsy. J Bone Joint Surg Am. 1998;80(5):659–67. PubMed PMID: 9611026. Epub 1998/06/04. eng.
43. Pearl ML, Edgerton BW, Kon DS, Darakjian AB, Kosco AE, Kazimiroff PB, et al. Comparison of arthroscopic findings with magnetic resonance imaging and arthrography in children with glenohumeral deformities secondary to brachial plexus birth palsy. J Bone Joint Surg Am. 2003;85-A(5):890–8. PubMed PMID: 12728041. Epub 2003/05/03. eng.
44. Soldado F, Kozin SH. The relationship between the coracoid and glenoid after brachial plexus birth palsy. J Pediatr Orthop. 2005;25(5):666–70. PubMed PMID: 16199952. Epub 2005/10/04. eng.
45. Borenstein ZC, Mink J, Oppenheim W, Rimoin DL, Lachman RS. Case report 655: congenital glenoid dysplasia (congenital hypoplasia of the glenoid neck and fossa of the scapula, with accompanied deformity of humeral head, coracoid process, and acromion). Skelet Radiol. 1991;20(2):134–6. PubMed PMID: 2020862. Epub 1991/01/01. eng.

The Shoulder: Acquired Disorders 6

J. Herman Kan

Contents

Abstract

The chapter begins with an in-depth discussion of glenohumeral instability and dislocation. Proximal humeral fractures and Little Leaguer's shoulder are described, followed by a concise discussion of glenohumeral internal rotation deficit (GIRD). Fractures of the clavicle and the scapula are then discussed in depth. A section on chondral injuries of the glenohumeral joint follows, and the chapter concludes with a short description of soft tissue injuries around the shoulder.

The shoulder is composed of three bones: the humerus, scapula, and clavicle. The pediatric shoulder is biomechanically balanced by a very mobile but unstable ball and socket glenohumeral joint and a gliding acromioclavicular joint, with both supported by multiple active (shoulder girdle muscles) and passive (ligaments and labrum) soft tissue stabilizers. It is prone to extra-articular fractures due to its open physis and apophysis, the weakest components of the musculoskeletal unit of the skeletally immature patient [1]. The physis and apophysis tend to fail before soft tissues (ligaments and muscles). Injuries to the pediatric shoulder are frequent and increasing due to the popularity of organized youth sports.

J.H. Kan, MD (✉)
Department of Radiology, Texas Children's Hospital, 6701 Fannin Street, Suite 470, Houston, TX 77005, USA

Department of Radiology, Baylor College of Medicine, Houston, TX, USA
e-mail: jhkan@texaschildrens.org

R. Stein-Wexler et al. (eds.), *Pediatric Orthopedic Imaging*,
DOI 10.1007/978-3-642-45381-6_6, © Springer-Verlag Berlin Heidelberg 2015

1 Glenohumeral Instability and Dislocation (Box 6.1)

> **Box 6.1: Anterior Shoulder Dislocation**
>
> Hill-Sachs fracture: subchondral fracture along the posterolateral humeral head
>
> Bankart fracture: anteroinferior glenoid fracture

Glenohumeral dislocations usually result from direct injury during contact sports. In children, these injuries are most common in the second decade [2]. Forty percent of patients present before age 22 [3]. The younger the child is at the time of dislocation, the higher the likelihood of recurrent dislocation and glenohumeral shoulder instability. Approximately 65–90 % of teenagers who suffer one shoulder dislocation will have additional dislocations [4]. Children with collagen disorders such as Ehlers-Danlos or Ulrich collagen VI deficiency have increased incidence of shoulder dislocation.

Most dislocations are anterior, and the child presents with the arm abducted and externally rotated [5]. Less commonly, glenohumeral dislocations may be posterior, inferior (luxatio erecta), or superior. Seizures may cause posterior dislocation. An additional consideration—particularly for atraumatic recurrent posterior dislocations—is underlying primary glenoid dysplasia with excessive retroversion, which can predispose to posterior dislocation.

The glenohumeral joint is a ball and socket joint invested by glenohumeral ligaments, capsule, and shoulder girdle muscles. The static stabilizers include the capsule, labrum, and glenohumeral ligaments. The active stabilizers include the rotator cuff and biceps tendon [6]. The glenoid cavity is concave and slightly retroverted (approximately 2–4°) with respect to the body of the scapula (i.e., the articular surface is directed posteriorly with respect to the scapula). The glenoid cavity itself is shallow, and its perimeter is reinforced by the fibrocartilaginous labrum to increase contact and depth of apposition with the humeral head. Although the glenohumeral joint is technically a ball and socket joint, the relatively small glenoid fossa (compared with a relatively large humeral head) allows for greater mobility at the cost of relative instability. The glenohumeral joint is more predisposed to dislocation than are hinge-type joints.

Atraumatic glenohumeral instability is usually multidirectional and may be bilateral [6]. In addition to underlying glenohumeral dysplasia, risk factors include hypermobility syndromes encountered in mixed connective tissue disease such as Marfan disease and Ehlers-Danlos syndrome [7] or activities that lead to repetitive overstretching such as swimming and gymnastics [8]. Traumatic glenohumeral dislocation tends to be unilateral and unidirectional.

Patients may respond well to rehabilitation after one traumatic dislocation, but primary repair is recommended after two or more, due to the high incidence of recurrent dislocation [9]. In one study, the incidence of recurrent dislocation was 19 % in patients treated operatively, compared with 60 % for a similar group treated nonoperatively [10]. Arthroscopic Bankart repair may be performed if the bone of the glenoid is relatively preserved. If greater than 25 % of the inferior glenoid is deficient as a result of a Bankart fracture, a Latarjet procedure may be indicated [11, 12]. In this procedure, a portion of the coracoid is transferred to the area of bone loss along the anteroinferior glenoid, improving glenoid and humeral head congruency. However, the Latarjet procedure has a relatively high incidence of complications, and, if bone loss is very severe, grafting with iliac crest bone graft may be necessary.

Traumatic multidirectional instability is treated with physical rehabilitation. If physical rehabilitation is unsuccessful, anterior capsular shift is recommended [13]. This procedure tightens the anterior and inferior capsule.

Imaging

Suspected glenohumeral dislocation is evaluated with an axillary view along with frontal radiographs in internal and external rotation. The normal glenohumeral joint has a smooth, round scapulohumeral arch, which is formed by the axillary border of the scapula, the inferior portion of the humeral neck, and the proximal humeral shaft (Fig. 6.1). In both anterior and

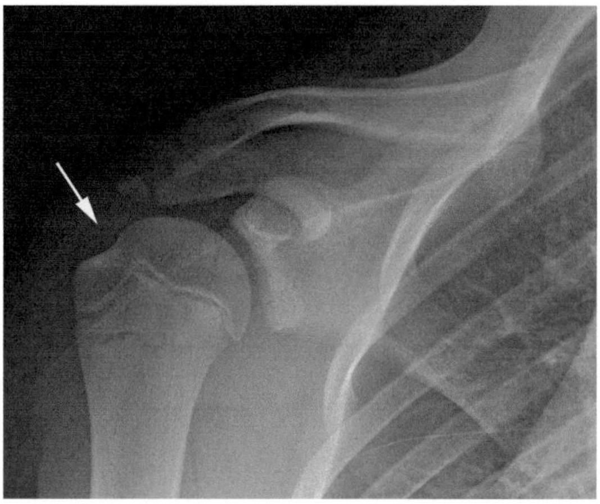

Fig. 6.1 Normal shoulder radiograph with humerus in external rotation in a 13-year-old boy. Note normal smooth scapulohumeral arch. Do not confuse the normal concavity at the interface of the greater tuberosity and humeral head (*arrow*) on this view (or on a poorly obtained frontal internal rotation radiograph) for a Hill-Sachs fracture

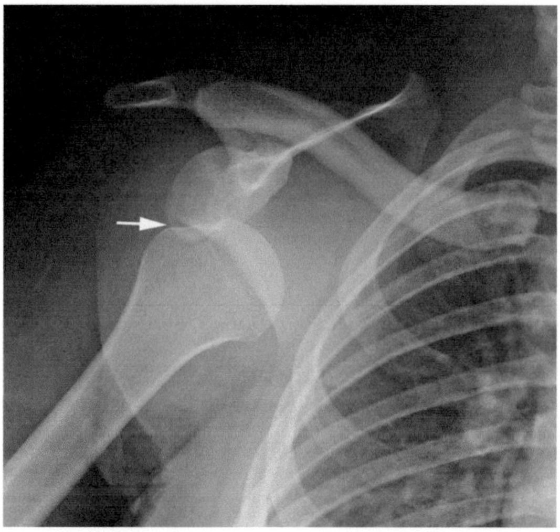

Fig. 6.2 Anterior shoulder dislocation in a 17-year-old girl. The humeral head is displaced inferomedially. Hill-Sachs fracture of the humeral head and bony Bankart fracture of the anteroinferior glenoid rim are also present (*arrow*)

posterior shoulder dislocations, the humeral head moves medially, and the arch is no longer aligned (Fig. 6.2). The extent of medial displacement is subtler with posterior dislocations than anterior dislocations. Axillary, Velpeau, and "Y" views help distinguish posterior from anterior glenohumeral dislocation (Fig. 6.3). The axillary view also evaluates for a glenoid fracture (bony Bankart) and determines if a Hill-Sachs fracture is either engaging (Hill-Sachs fracture depression is locked in place along the inferior glenoid rim) or non-engaging. The Velpeau view provides similar information and is useful for patients who cannot tolerate a traditional axillary view. The "Y" view principally helps determine the anteroposterior relationship but also supplements the frontal views for evaluation of the glenoid (Fig. 6.4). Hill-Sachs and Bankart fractures are presented in greater detail below.

Secondary signs of anterior shoulder dislocation include a Hill-Sachs fracture and osseous Bankart fracture (Figs. 6.5 and 6.6). These fractures result as the posterolateral humeral head and anteroinferior glenoid collide as the humeral head anteriorly dislocates. These fractures are less common in children than in adults and—like shoulder dislocation in general—are more likely in the second decade. The Hill-Sachs fracture occurs along the posterolateral humeral head and is optimally seen on a frontal internal rotation view (Fig. 6.7). The normal concavity at the interface between the humeral head and the greater tuberosity may mimic a Hill-Sachs fracture on a poorly obtained internal rotation AP view. Furthermore, normal glenoid fragmentary ossification may mimic an osseous Bankart fracture. Whereas the former is usually distributed evenly throughout the glenoid rim, the Bankart fracture is more focal, at the anteroinferior glenoid.

Less common glenohumeral dislocations include luxatio erecta (inferior dislocation) and posterior dislocation. Luxatio erecta occurs when the humeral head displaces inferiorly; as a result, the arm is fully abducted and held upward. Secondary signs of posterior shoulder dislocation include a reverse Hill-Sachs fracture and reverse osseous Bankart fracture. A reverse Hill-Sachs fracture occurs along the anteromedial humeral head.

Computed tomography (CT) helps determine the type of surgical stabilization necessary to repair the glenohumeral joint. Sagittal and coronal reformatted images along with three-dimensional (3D) maximum intensity projections (MIPs) are especially helpful for determining the amount of bone loss at the anteroinferior glenoid. The normal glenoid is pear-shaped. It

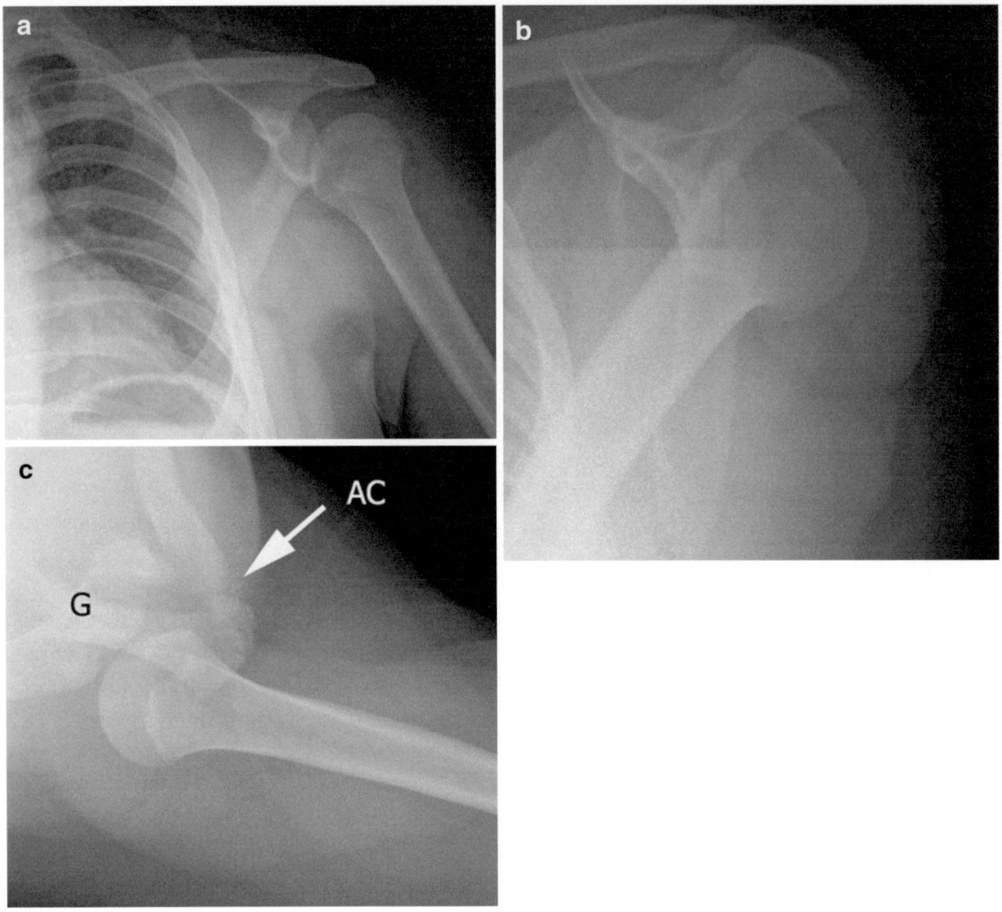

Fig. 6.3 Posterior shoulder dislocation in a 15-year-old girl. (**a**) There is subtle disruption of the scapulohumeral arch with medial humeral head displacement. The "Y" (**b**) and axillary (**c**) views confirm posterior shoulder dislocation. *AC* acromioclavicular joint. *G* glenoid

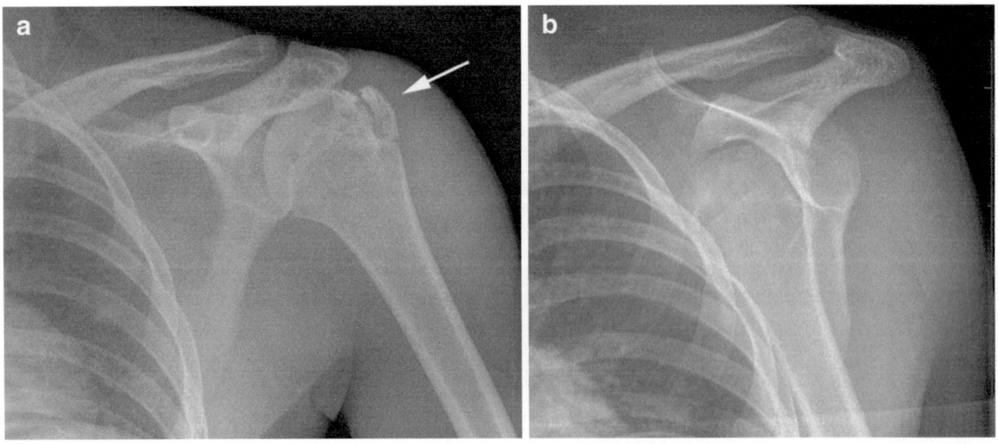

Fig. 6.4 Greater tuberosity fracture in an 11-year-old boy. (**a**) On the frontal view, the fracture fragment (*arrow*) is slightly separated, and glenohumeral alignment appears normal. (**b**) The "Y" view shows the humeral head is actually dislocated

may become an "inverted pear" (large end up) if a Bankart fracture causes bone loss along the anteroinferior quadrant (Fig. 6.8). If more than 25 % of the glenoid is deficient, surgical fixation with a Latarjet procedure or iliac crest grafting may be indicated [11, 12].

Magnetic resonance arthrography (MRA) delineates the status of the static stabilizers of the glenohumeral joint and the various soft tissue Bankart injuries [14]. Although CT arthrography (CTA) and MRA may have comparable accuracy for the evaluation of Bankart injuries [15], MRA avoids radiation and can also evaluate marrow and soft tissue edema, as well as delineate subtypes of Bankart injuries. In the acute setting, posttraumatic glenohumeral joint fluid may have an arthrographic effect, making intra-articular gadolinium injection unnecessary.

Anteroinferior glenoid and labroligamentous injuries are classified into two subtypes: osseous Bankart and soft tissue Bankart lesions. The true soft tissue Bankart lesion is an anteroinferior labral tear with a torn scapular periosteum (Fig. 6.9), but there are many subtypes for soft tissue injuries (Fig. 6.10). It is more important

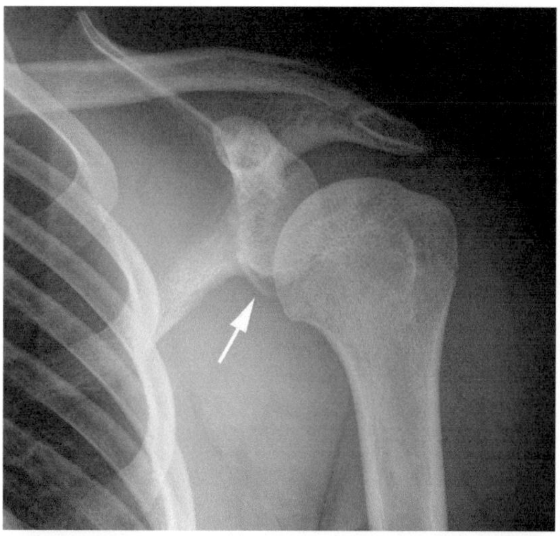

Fig. 6.5 Anterior shoulder dislocation in a 17-year-old boy. There is a bony Bankart fracture (*arrow*)

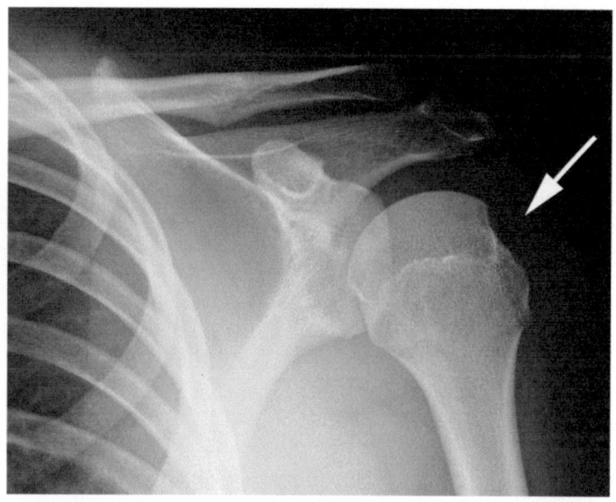

Fig. 6.7 Sequela of anterior shoulder dislocation in a 15-year-old boy. There is a large Hill-Sachs fracture (*arrow*) on this frontal view with internal rotation

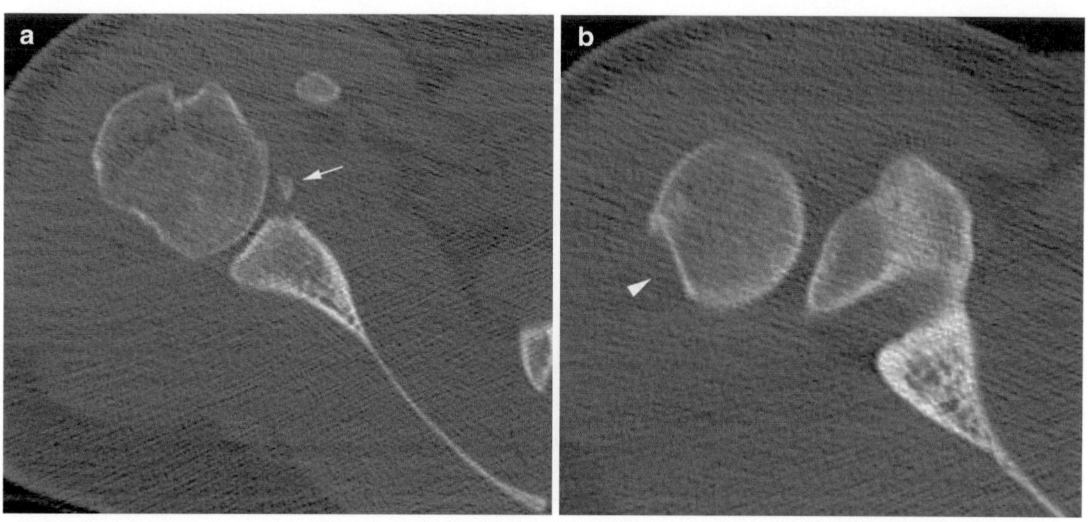

Fig. 6.6 Fractures in a 16-year-old girl with prior anterior shoulder dislocation. Axial CT images show (**a**) mildly displaced bony Bankart (*arrow*) and (**b**) depressed Hill-Sachs (*arrowhead*) fractures

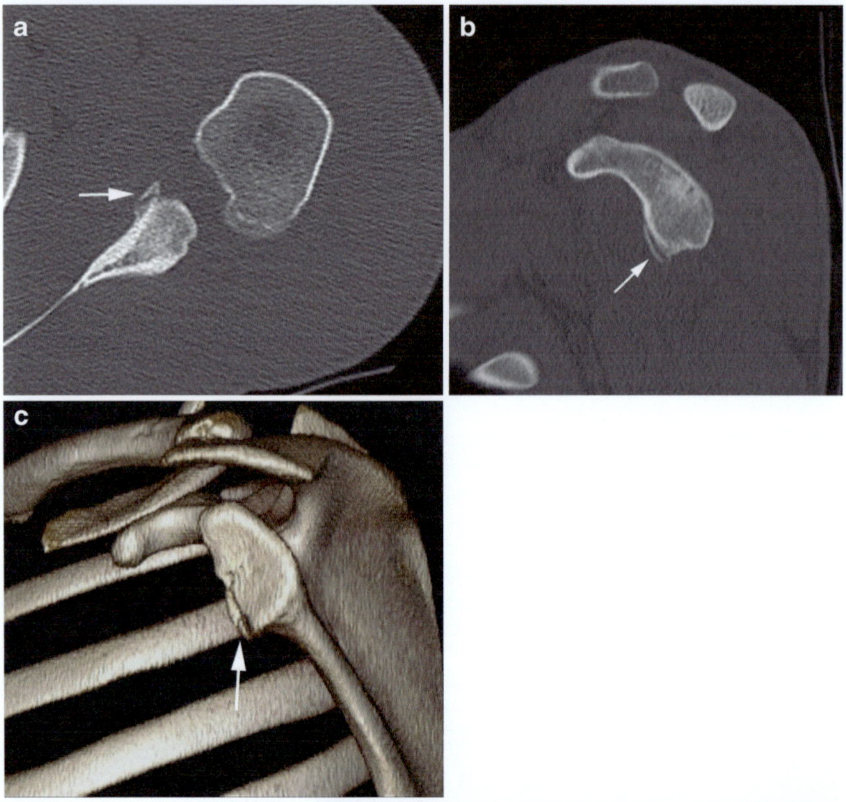

Fig. 6.8 A 16-year-old girl with osseous Bankart (*arrows*) demonstrated on axial (**a**), sagittal (**b**), and 3D (**c**) reconstructions. 3D-CT best delineates the inverted pear appearance of the glenoid due to anteroinferior deficiency after Bankart fracture (Courtesy of Tal Laor, Cincinnati Children's Hospital)

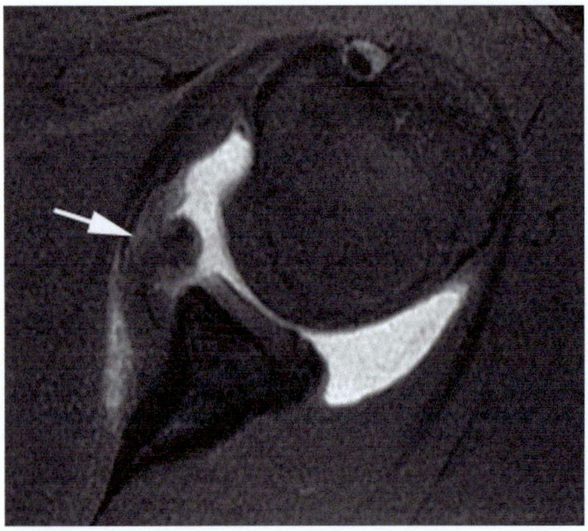

Fig. 6.9 Soft tissue Bankart lesion in a 16-year-old boy. Axial T1-weighted (*T1-W*) fat-suppressed (*FS*) image from MR arthrography (*MRA*) shows intra-articular contrast material insinuating between the glenoid and the displaced, torn, mass-like labral tissue (*arrow*)

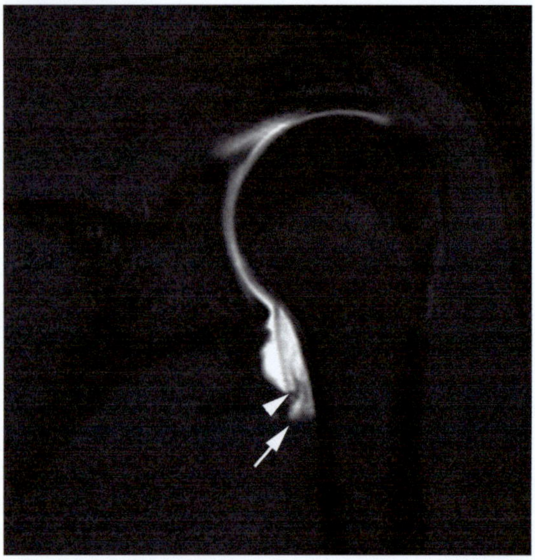

Fig. 6.10 Humeral avulsion of the glenohumeral ligament injury (*HAGL*) in a 16-year-old girl. Coronal T1-W FS MRA shows extra-articular contrast extension (*arrow*) and retracted inferior glenohumeral ligament (*arrowhead*)

Table 6.1 Soft tissue Bankart variations

Soft tissue Bankart variations	Description
Bankart lesion (Fig. 6.9)	Anteroinferior labral tear with a torn scapular periosteum
Perthes	Non-displaced Bankart with intact scapular periosteum
Anterior labroligamentous periosteal sleeve avulsion (ALPSA)	Bankart lesion with medial displacement with intact scapular periosteum
Glenolabral articular disruption (GLAD) (Fig. 6.11)	Bankart with associated glenoid chondral defect
Humeral avulsion glenohumeral ligament (HAGL) (Fig. 6.10)	Avulsion of the anterior inferior glenohumeral ligament at its humeral insertion
Bony avulsion glenohumeral ligament (BAGHL)	HAGL but with a humeral bone avulsion injury
Floating anterior inferior glenohumeral ligament (AIGHL)	Combined Bankart and HAGL lesion

Adapted from Ref. [16]

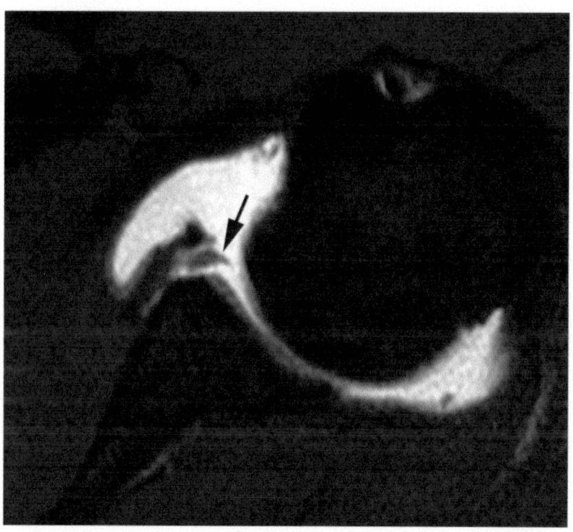

Fig. 6.11 Glenolabral articular disruption (*GLAD*) subtype of soft tissue Bankart lesion in a 17-year-old boy. Axial T1-W FS MRA shows a component of cartilage has been stripped (*arrow*)

to accurately describe findings than to label the exact subtype (Table 6.1). The status of the glenoid cartilage (Fig. 6.11), inferior glenohumeral ligament, labrum, and glenoid bone must all be closely evaluated.

Superior labral anterior-posterior (SLAP) injuries are sometimes associated with glenohumeral instability and at least in adults occur in approximately 20 % of patients with glenohumeral instability [17]. However, treatment is not always necessary.

There are no specific imaging findings for atraumatic multidirectional shoulder instability other than a patulous glenohumeral capsule, which is best seen along the axillary recess after distention during arthrography. Therefore, the diagnosis is generally made on gestalt interpretation in conjunction with clinical findings [8]. Associated findings include articular and labral injuries resulting from recurrent dislocations.

2 Proximal Humeral Fractures

Proximal humeral fractures comprise 0.5 % of all fractures in children and between 4 and 7 % of all epiphyseal fractures [18]. The mechanism and force of injury resemble those for shoulder dislocations, but the force decompresses along the proximal humerus. The unbalanced biomechanical pull of muscle insertions proximal and distal to the site of fracture leads to angular and displacement deformities.

An understanding of the timing and appearance of the ossification centers of the proximal humerus helps in interpreting radiographs in the setting of trauma and elbow ossification centers also helps determine the clinical significance of different fracture patterns. There are three ossification centers at the proximal humerus. The humeral head epiphysis begins to ossify at or shortly after birth, and the greater tuberosity apophysis begins to ossify at age 3 years. The lesser tuberosity begins to ossify at age 5 years, and the humeral head, greater tuberosity, and lesser tuberosity fuse at age 6 [19]. The proximal humeral physis remains open until age 14–17 in girls and 16–18 in boys [20]. Damage to this physis can result in significant growth disturbance, as it is responsible for 80 % of the longitudinal growth of the humerus. However, as a general rule, proximal humeral fractures are more likely to remodel in younger children than in older children due to the open physis.

Non-displaced or minimally displaced proximal humeral fractures are treated nonoperatively. Severely angulated or displaced fractures may require operative fixation in children older than 10–13 years of age [18, 21]. In children under 11 years of age, most if not all fractures will remodel without long-term sequelae and can be treated nonoperatively [19]. Surgical reduction is indicated in open proximal humeral fractures or if there is evidence of neurovascular compromise.

Imaging

Three-view shoulder (frontal internal and external rotation along with axillary) or two-view humerus radiographs adequately assess most proximal humeral fractures. It is important to determine the amount of displacement, as this predicts prognosis and determines appropriate treatment. The Neer classification offers a convenient way to categorize proximal humeral fractures (Table 6.2), although it is not generally used with children [19]. Angulation should also be addressed (Fig. 6.12), although the need to report the precise degree of fracture angulation varies with institution and orthopedic surgeon preference [18]. In older children, fractures are frequently complete (Fig. 6.12), while in younger children, buckle fractures are common (Fig. 6.13). The fracture line orientation, physeal involvement (humeral head, greater tuberosity, lesser tuberosity) (Fig. 6.14), and presence of

Table 6.2 Neer classification of proximal humeral fractures

Grade	Displacement
I	<5 mm
II	<1/3 shaft width
III	2/3 shaft width
IV	>2/3 shaft width

Adapted from Ref. [19]

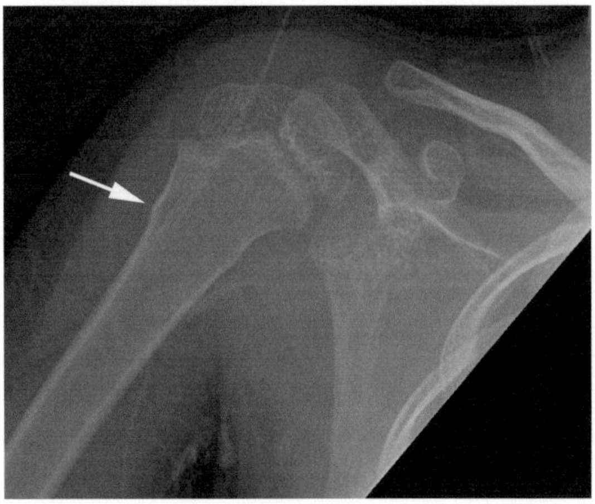

Fig. 6.13 Non-displaced buckle fracture (*arrow*) of the surgical neck of the humerus in a 3-year-old girl

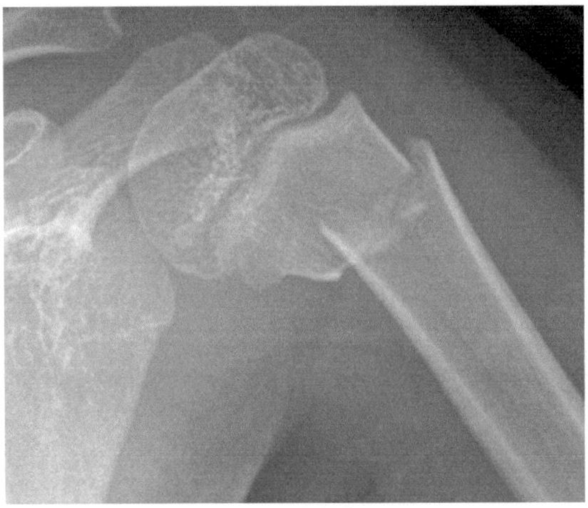

Fig. 6.12 Neer type I displaced and mildly comminuted fracture of the surgical neck of the humerus in a 5-year-old girl. There is less than 5 mm of lateral displacement of the distal fragment

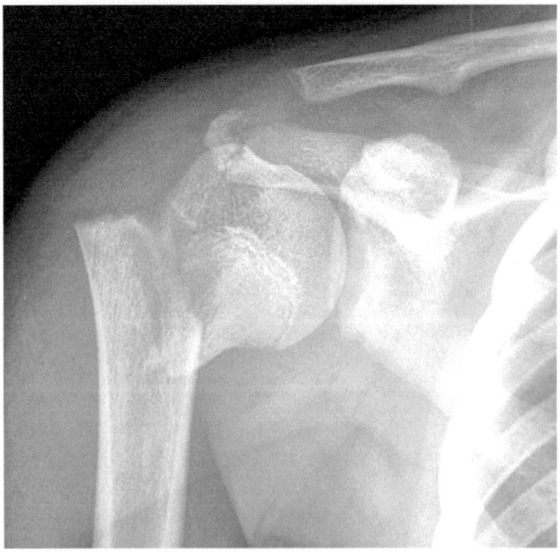

Fig. 6.14 Neer grade 4 proximal humeral fracture in a 13-year-old boy. The fracture extends from the lateral physis to the greater tuberosity and is displaced by more than two-third of the width of the shaft

comminution should be discussed, as with any fracture.

Radiography is almost always sufficient for imaging proximal humeral fractures. Occasionally, for complicated fractures, magnetic resonance imaging (MRI) may help identify tendon, periosteum, or muscle interposition at the fracture site [22], which could impede proper healing.

3 Little Leaguer's Shoulder (Box 6.2)

Box 6.2: Little Leaguer's Shoulder (Young Throwing Athlete)

Radiographs:

Proximal metaphyseal sclerosis, lateral metaphyseal fragmentation

Wide physis (resembles acute Salter-Harris I fracture)

MRI:

T1: Physeal widening

Fluid sensitive: metaphyseal edema, periosteal reaction, and juxtacortical soft tissue edema

Less common: epiphyseal edema, juxtaphyseal cysts, and periosteal edema

Little Leaguer's shoulder, seen in athletes who throw overhead, is an overuse injury of the proximal humeral physis and is most likely a chronic non displaced Salter Harris I fracture. The injury most commonly occurs during growth spurts in boys between 11 and 14 years of age [23]. Rotational torqueing generated during the acceleration phase of an overhead throw probably causes the injury.

The glenohumeral joint in childhood is quite lax. However, in early adolescence, a dramatic change in range of motion occurs, with decreased internal and external rotation, along with increased shoulder elevation. The decrease in rotational motion may contribute to excessive stress at the physis with throwing and thus predispose children to this injury [24].

A single acute event generally does not cause the injury; symptoms develop gradually and correlate with pitch count. Symptoms include pain during throwing, with palpation of the proximal humerus, and during resisted external rotation of the humerus [25].

The treatment for Little Leaguer's shoulder is rest from overhead throwing [23]. Surgery is not indicated. If the child returns to throwing too early, continued physeal damage may lead to displacement and eventual early physeal closure. Prevention of this injury is one of the reasons for pitch count regulations for Little League players.

Imaging

Little Leaguer's shoulder is usually diagnosed clinically. Radiographs can confirm the diagnosis or suggest alternative etiologies for symptoms. Findings include proximal metaphyseal sclerosis, lateral metaphyseal fragmentation, physeal widening, and demineralization (Fig. 6.15) [25, 26]. Note that this appearance is indistinguishable from an acute non-displaced Salter-Harris I fracture. The term Little Leaguer's shoulder should not be used when there is a displaced Salter-Harris I proximal humeral fracture (Fig. 6.16).

Distinguishing Little Leaguer's shoulder from normal variations of physeal widening is particularly challenging because the injury occurs during adolescent growth spurts when normal physiologic widening is present. Radiographs of the contralateral asymptomatic shoulder may be obtained to determine if the physeal widening is physiologic or due to chronic physeal injury (Fig. 6.17).

MRI demonstrates physeal widening, and there may be edema—usually in the metaphysis [27]. Less common findings include epiphyseal edema, juxtaphyseal cysts, and periosteal edema [28, 29]. T1-weighted (T1-W) sequences best evaluate physeal widening. Fluid-sensitive sequences help assess marrow edema, periosteal reaction, and juxtacortical soft tissue edema (Fig. 6.15). In the presence of physeal widening and/or juxtaphyseal cysts (but no edema), MRI may suggest chronic injury. However, if there are cysts and physeal widening along with juxtaphyseal and juxtacortical marrow edema, the process is likely acute superimposed on chronic.

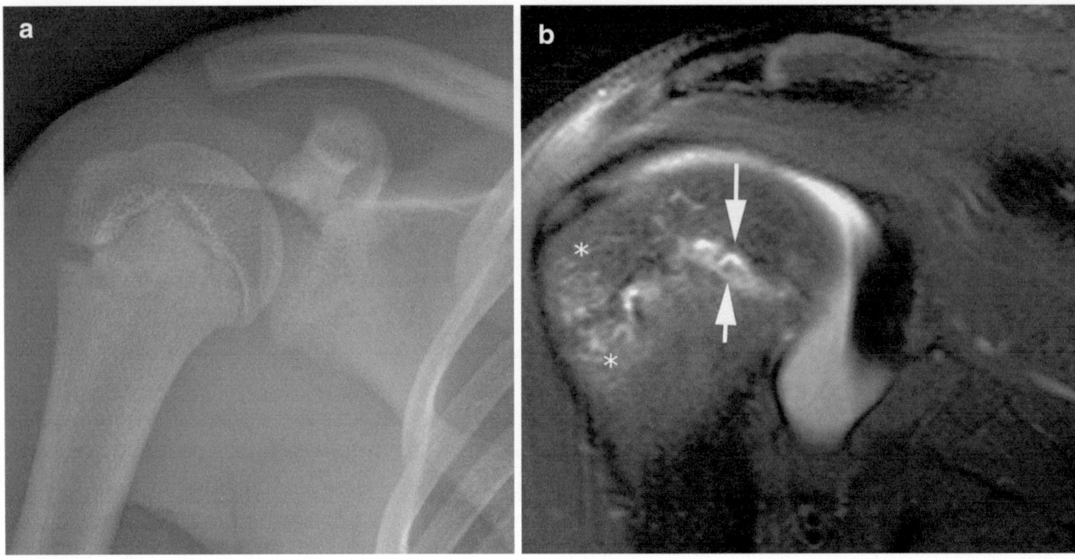

Fig. 6.15 Little leaguer's shoulder in a 14-year-old boy. (**a**) Widening of the proximal humeral physis. (**b**) Coronal T2-W FS MRA shows juxtaphyseal marrow edema (*) and physeal widening particularly along the medial physis (*between arrows*)

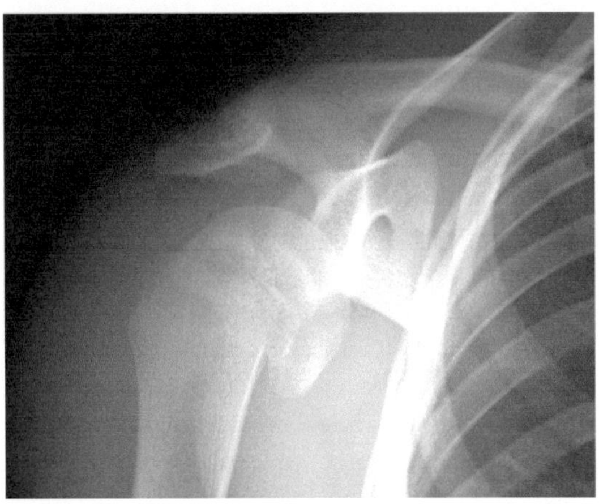

Fig. 6.16 Displaced Salter-Harris I fracture of the proximal humerus with glenohumeral dislocation in a 15-year-old boy

Differential Diagnosis

Little Leaguer's shoulder is indistinguishable from acute non-displaced Salter-Harris I fractures of the proximal humerus, and diagnosis is predicated on clinical history. The injury may also be difficult to distinguish from normal physiologic physeal widening, but imaging the asymptomatic shoulder should clarify this.

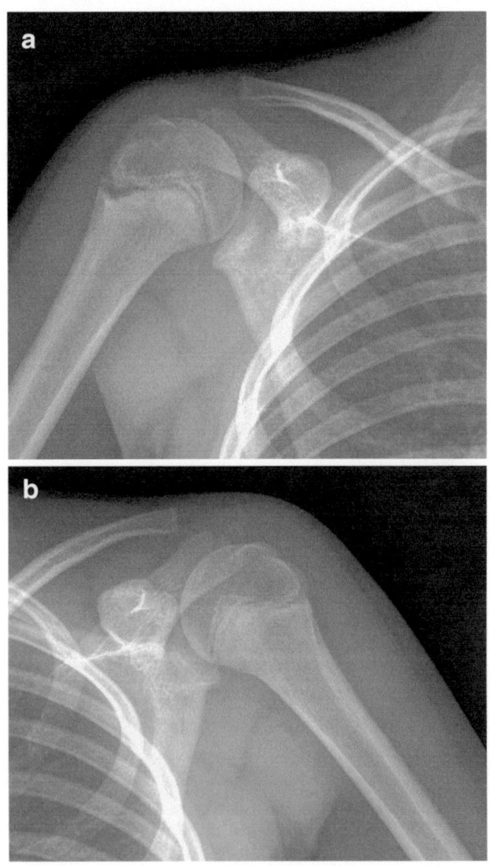

Fig. 6.17 Little leaguer's shoulder in a 13-year-old boy. (**a**) On the right, the proximal humeral physis is too wide. (**b**) Normal left shoulder (for comparison)

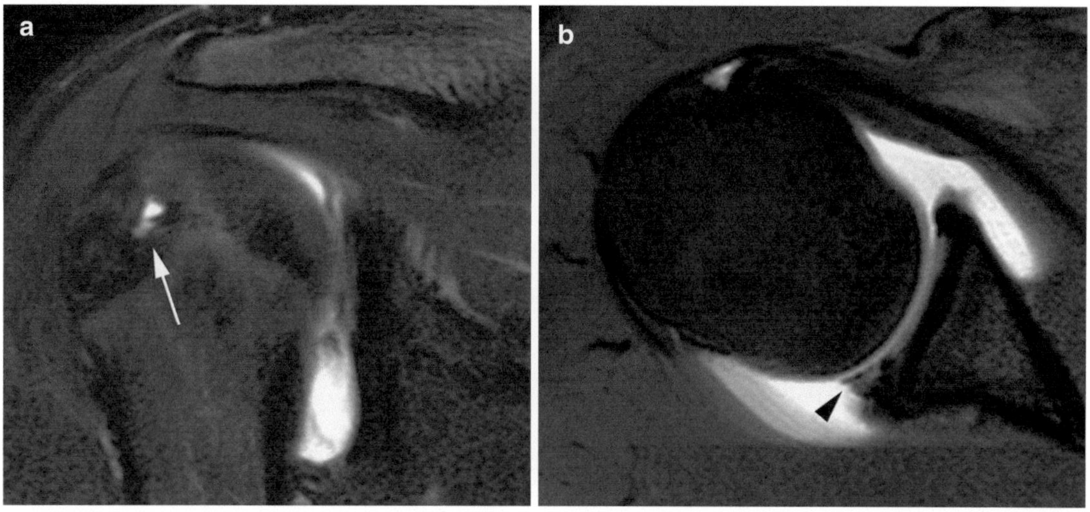

Fig. 6.18 Glenohumeral internal reduction deficit (*GIRD*) in a 17-year-old pitcher. (**a**) Coronal T2-weighted (*T2-W*) FS MRA shows posterolateral humeral head subchondral cysts (*arrow*). (**b**) Axial T1-W FS image shows a degenerative tear of the posterior labrum (*arrowhead*)

4 Glenohumeral Internal Rotation Deficit (GIRD)

Glenohumeral internal rotation deficit (GIRD) occurs in athletes who throw overhead, most commonly affecting baseball players but occasionally swimmers and tennis players. Repetitive overhead rotational motion causes anterior capsular laxity and posterior fibrosis of the glenohumeral joint, leading to reduced internal rotation [30]. Over time, the humeral head axis shifts posteriorly. Clinical GIRD is defined as loss of 25° of internal rotation in the affected shoulder.

If there are no associated labral or rotator cuff tears, treatment includes physical therapy to decrease muscle imbalance and capsular stiffness. If this is unsuccessful, posterior capsular release can be performed [30].

Imaging

Radiographs are often normal in the setting of GIRD. MRA optimally evaluates for GIRD, demonstrating undersurface tears of the posterior aspect of the supraspinatus, tears of the infraspinatus, posterosuperior labral tears, posterolateral humeral head cysts, and posterior capsular fibrosis (Fig. 6.18) [31, 32]. Posterolateral humeral head cysts are usually located at the site of attachment of the infraspinatus tendon and the posterior fibers of the supraspinatus tendon [31]. These cysts resolve after treatment.

Differential Diagnosis

Posterolateral humeral head cysts should not be confused with changes related to Hill-Sachs fractures from anterior glenohumeral dislocation. Unlike Hill-Sachs fractures, posterolateral humeral head cysts usually do not distort the spherical shape of the humeral head. These cysts should also not be confused with subchondral cysts related to osteoarthritis or with neoplastic entities such as giant cell tumor or chondroblastoma.

5 Clavicular Fractures (Box 6.3)

Box 6.3: Clavicular Fractures

Proximal and distal fractures are Salter-Harris equivalents

Distal fractures likely to be displaced if the fracture line is lateral to the coracoclavicular ligament

Floating shoulder is unstable: midclavicular fracture combined with glenoid neck fracture

Acromioclavicular or sternoclavicular dislocations are extremely rare in children/adolescents

Fractures of the clavicle may result from a direct blow while playing contact sports or from an indirect force transmitted across the shoulder, for instance, falling on an outstretched arm [33]. Contact sport injury is the most common cause of clavicular fracture in older children and adolescents. About one-third of clavicular fractures occur in preschool children who fall from a crib or bed. Only 4 % of all clavicular fractures result from birth trauma [34].

Several major ligaments and muscles attach to the clavicle; therefore, muscle spasm and/or unbalanced ligamentous retraction predisposes clavicular fractures to displacement and angulation. The coracoclavicular ligament, acromioclavicular capsule, and deltoid and trapezius muscles attach to the distal clavicle, and the acromioclavicular capsule, sternocleidomastoid muscle, and pectoralis major muscle attach proximally. The clavicle is located just above the subclavian artery and vein, and the brachial plexus is also nearby. Displaced fractures therefore carry significant risk of neurovascular injury.

Physeal and metaphyseal fractures are more likely to occur than are acromioclavicular or sternoclavicular capsular rupture, as these capsules are more resilient to biomechanical forces than are the adjacent physis and metaphysis. Pediatric clavicle fractures near the acromioclavicular or sternoclavicular joints are Salter-Harris equivalent fractures (the lateral clavicular physis fuses to the body of the clavicle at 19 years, and the medial physis fuses at 25 years) [35]. A so-called acromioclavicular pseudodislocation, or coracoclavicular periosteal sleeve fracture, may occur because the coracoclavicular ligament is more resilient than is the distal metaphysis [36].

Most clavicular fractures are treated nonoperatively, as even those with significant angulation or displacement remodel over time to a normal shape. Malalignment and nonunion are very rare in children. Midclavicular fractures are immobilized, and young children can usually return to their usual activities (including sports) within 6 weeks, although adolescents may need up to 10 weeks [33]. Particularly in younger patients, distal clavicle fractures near the acromioclavicular joint do not require surgery. However, patients older than 8 years with significantly displaced distal clavicular fractures may have a better cosmetic outcome if treated operatively [37].

Operative reduction is indicated if the fracture is open or severely displaced or if there is neurovascular injury. The latter complication is rare in distal and midclavicular fractures. However, medial clavicular fractures that are displaced posteriorly near the sternoclavicular joint may require surgical intervention due to mediastinal impingement [35]. Nonunion also mandates surgical reduction.

Imaging

Both frontal and angled frontal radiographs allow initial assessment of clavicular fractures. It is important to recognize that the mid-diaphysis of the normal clavicle may appear sharply angulated, especially on the angled view.

Midclavicular fractures are generally incomplete buckle fractures in younger children, whereas these fractures in adolescents tend to be complete. They may be displaced, angulated, or comminuted. If the major fracture fragments are near the coracoclavicular ligament and sternocleidomastoid muscle, angulation and displacement of the fracture fragments are common and may increase until healing supervenes (Fig. 6.19).

Proximal and distal clavicular fractures (Fig. 6.20) are usually Salter-Harris equivalent fractures, and extension to the physes of the associated ossification centers must be assessed. Since the medial and lateral apophyseal ossifica-

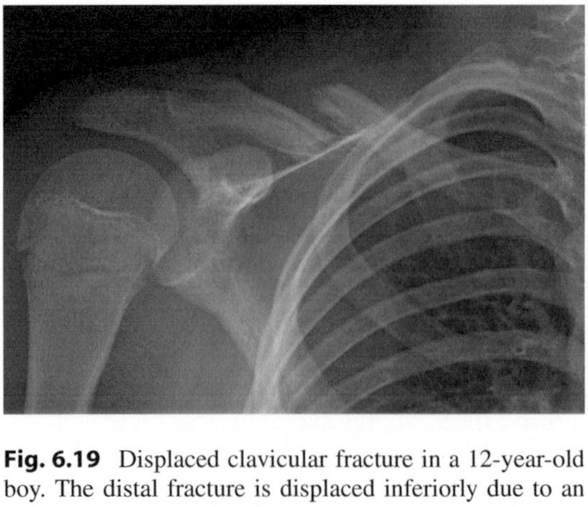

Fig. 6.19 Displaced clavicular fracture in a 12-year-old boy. The distal fracture is displaced inferiorly due to an intact coracoclavicular ligament. The proximal fracture fragment is displaced superiorly due to unbalanced force of the sternocleidomastoid muscle

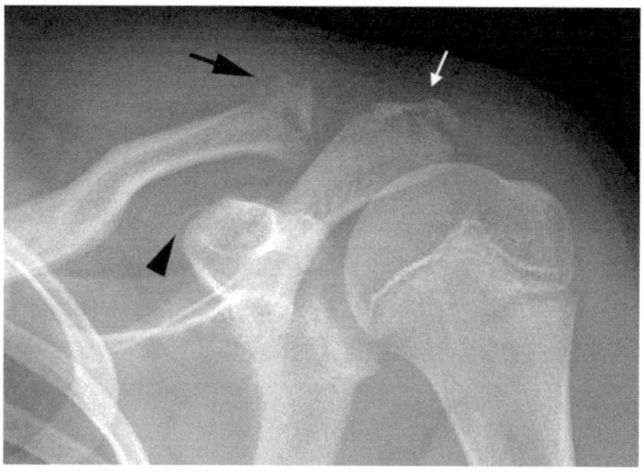

Fig. 6.20 Distal clavicular fracture in a 12 year-old boy. The clavicle fracture (*black arrow*) is a Salter-Harris II equivalent fracture since it extends to the distal clavicular physis. Normal fragmentary appearance of the acromial ossification center (*white arrow*) and apophysis of the coracoid at the level of the coracoclavicualr ligament (*black arrowhead*) should not be construed as fractures

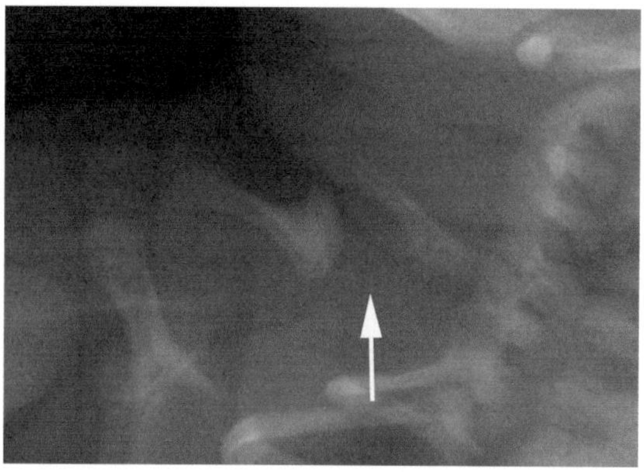

Fig. 6.21 Right clavicular pseudarthrosis (*arrow*) in a 6-day-old boy

tion centers do not appear until late adolescence [35], any fracture line extending to the medial or lateral clavicular end should be considered a Salter-Harris fracture.

Proximal clavicular fractures are easily missed on standard clavicular views due to the overlapping structures but are readily diagnosed by CT. CT is especially important for posteriorly displaced clavicular fractures since these may impinge upon the mediastinum.

The Neer and Rockwood classification system helps categorize distal clavicular fractures [38, 39]. Type 1 fractures are distal to the coracoclavicular ligaments, and therefore displacement is uncommon. Type 2 fractures are more medial, between the coracoclavicular ligaments. These fractures tend to be displaced because the distal component retains its alignment with the acromioclavicular joint, whereas the proximal component is aligned with the coracoid. Nonunion is more common with type 2 fractures. There may be coracoid avulsion injuries as well.

The floating shoulder, defined as a midclavicular fracture associated with a glenoid neck fracture, is considered unstable [40]. It is therefore important that clavicle radiograph series include the ipsilateral glenohumeral joint so that this fracture will be properly identified.

If acromioclavicular or coracoclavicular injury is suspected, it is essential to evaluate both the normal and the symptomatic shoulder with wide-view radiographs with and without weights. Views of the normal shoulder are important because normative adult measurements of the acromioclavicular and coracoclavicular distances on radiographs cannot be used in children, since the true ends of the acromion and coracoid are cartilaginous until late adolescence and even into early adulthood. For instance, the secondary ossification center of the acromion does not develop until between 15 and 18 years of age, and it does not fully fuse until age 22–25 [41]. The coracoid process has multiple ossification centers: the first appears by 1 year of age, the second at 10, and the third during puberty (Fig. 6.20). All three fuse by age 15 [42].

Differential Diagnosis

Midclavicular fractures should be distinguished from congenital pseudarthrosis of the clavicle (Fig. 6.21) (see Chap. 5), which almost always affects the right clavicle (except in cases of situs inversus). This results from failure of the medial and lateral clavicular mesenchymal primary centers to coalesce [43]. The ends of clavicular pseudarthrosis tend to be rounded and well corticated.

6 Scapular Fractures

Scapular fractures usually result from direct trauma related to either a motor vehicle accident in older patients or child abuse in infants and toddlers [44, 45]. Child abuse should always be suspected in infants and toddlers with scapular or acromial fractures (Fig. 6.22) [41, 45]. The scapula is also prone to avulsion fractures due to its numerous muscle attachments.

Direct trauma usually causes fractures of the lateral scapular body (Fig. 6.23), although occasionally greenstick fractures occur [46]. Athletes (especially those who throw a great deal) may

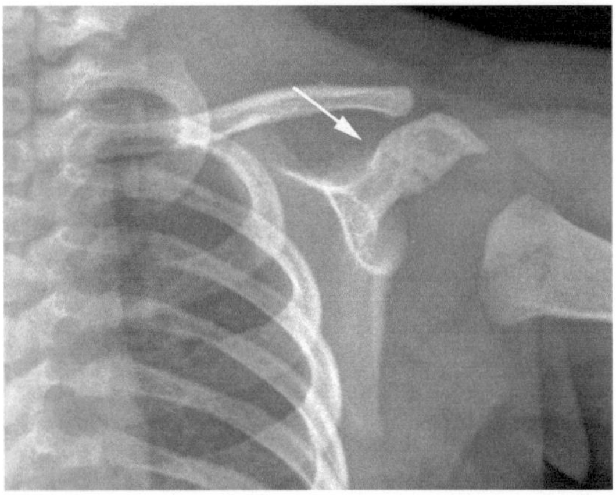

Fig. 6.22 Healing non-displaced acromion fracture (*arrow*) in a 5-month-old boy, a victim of non-accidental trauma

develop scapular stress fractures along the lateral border due to repetitive tug injury at the teres minor origin [47].

Avulsion fractures can occur at the many different sites of muscle attachment. Winging of the scapula—most often a result of injury to the long thoracic nerve—can result from avulsion fracture at the insertion of the serratus anterior muscle along the inferior angle of the scapula [48]. Additional sites for scapular avulsion fracture include the infraglenoid tubercle (the attachment site for the triceps muscle), acromion (the deltoid muscle), coracoid (the coracoclavicular ligament), and coracoid tip (the short head biceps and coracobrachialis muscles), among others.

Extra-articular scapular fractures are usually treated nonoperatively if there is less than 2 cm of displacement [49]. Nonoperative management of scapular fractures usually results in healing without complications because the adjacent muscle bulk helps stabilize the fracture fragments. Surgical reduction is recommended when fractures involve the glenoid fossa and are displaced more than 5 mm [50].

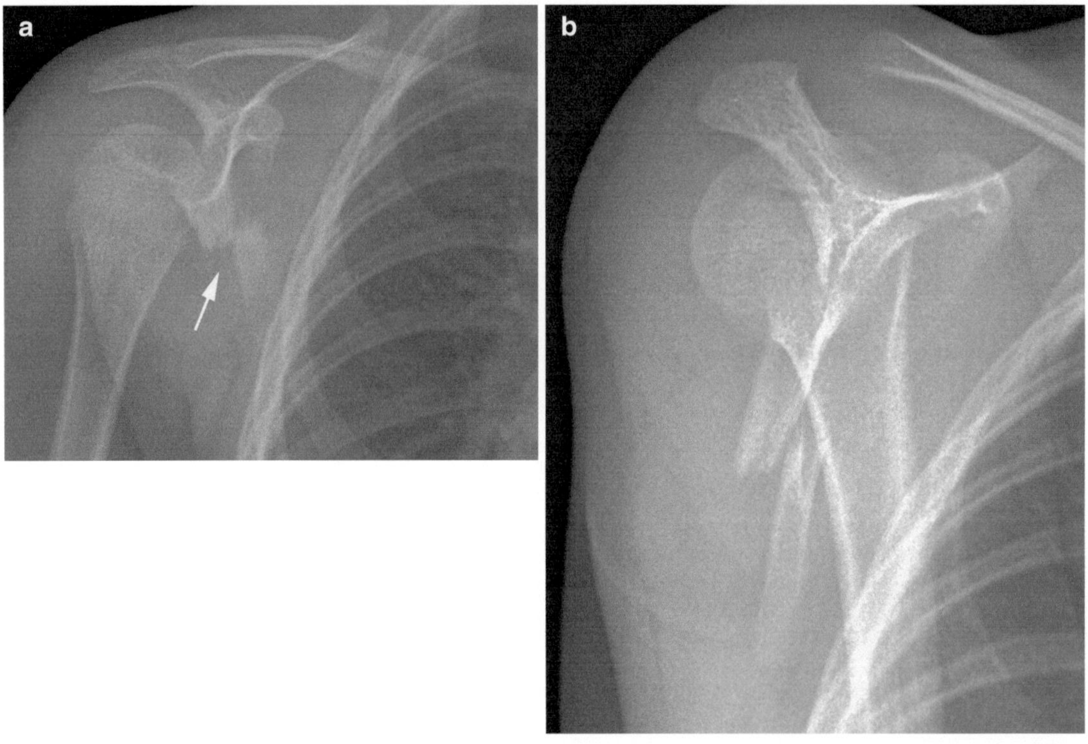

Fig. 6.23 Lateral scapular body fracture in a 4-year-old girl. Frontal view (**a**) shows medial displacement (*arrow*), and "Y" view (**b**) shows anterior displacement of the distal fragment

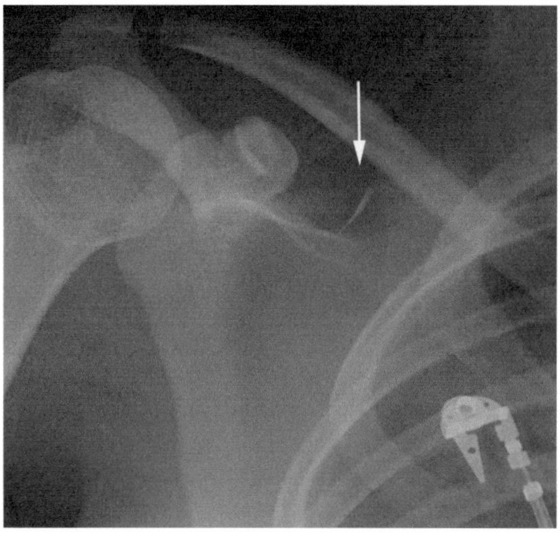

Fig. 6.24 Extra-articular superior scapular fracture (*arrow*) in a 13-year-old girl, a result of direct impaction injury

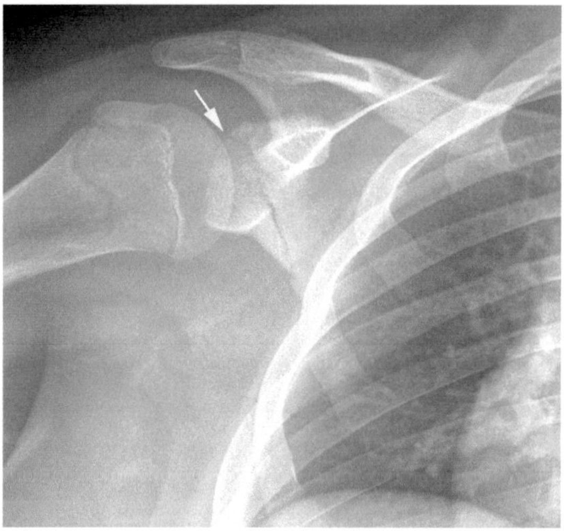

Fig. 6.25 Fractured scapular body and glenoid neck in a 10-year-old boy. There is intra-articular extension (*arrow*)

Imaging

If a fracture is suspected, the initial work-up includes shoulder and/or scapular radiographs (Fig. 6.24). It is important to address the degree of displacement, relationship of the scapular fracture to major muscle attachments, and involvement of the glenoid fossa (Figs. 6.24 and 6.25), since these factors affect management. If the fracture extends to the glenoid fossa, CT may help define the articular margin and determine displacement. However, the shoulder has often already been imaged in the course of a chest CT, as patients who suffer scapular fractures have usually sustained extensive additional trauma.

Differential Diagnosis

Scapular fractures should be differentiated from normal secondary ossification centers. These appear throughout the scapula during childhood and adolescence, as discussed above. They tend to have well-defined cortical margins and are rounded or ovoid, whereas true fracture lines have sharp non-corticated margins.

7 Chondral Injuries of the Glenohumeral Joint

Osteochondritis dissecans (OCD) most commonly occurs at the knee, usually during the second decade. Involvement of the glenohumeral joint is rare, but when OCD does affect the shoulder, it usually involves the anterosuperior humeral head [51]. Acute and/or repetitive microtrauma—both quite common in athletes—causes humeral head and glenoid OCD [52, 53]. Presenting symptoms include stiffness, locking, and clicking.

Stable OCD lesions are usually treated nonoperatively. If loose bodies or other features of instability are present, debridement, drilling, or allograft placement may be indicated [54]. As with OCD lesions elsewhere, severity of symptoms and the extent of physeal closure dictate the need for surgery. If the physis is still open, spontaneous healing is more likely. If an acute chondral or osteochondral fracture is unstable (discussed below), or if the patient experiences locking, debridement or possibly stabilization is generally advised.

Imaging

The appearance of glenohumeral OCD is similar to OCD elsewhere. If lesions are small, radiographs are usually normal. Larger lesions may demonstrate a subchondral lytic defect with or without underlying depression [51]. MRA best assesses these lesions, although they can usually be identified with routine shoulder MRI.

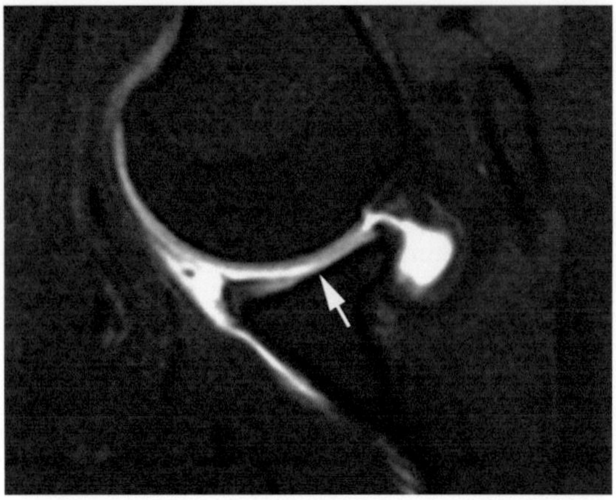

Fig. 6.26 The normal central bare area of the glenoid in a 16-year-old girl. Abduction external rotation (*ABER*) T1-W FS MRA shows typical smooth, tapering central bare area of the glenoid (*arrow*)

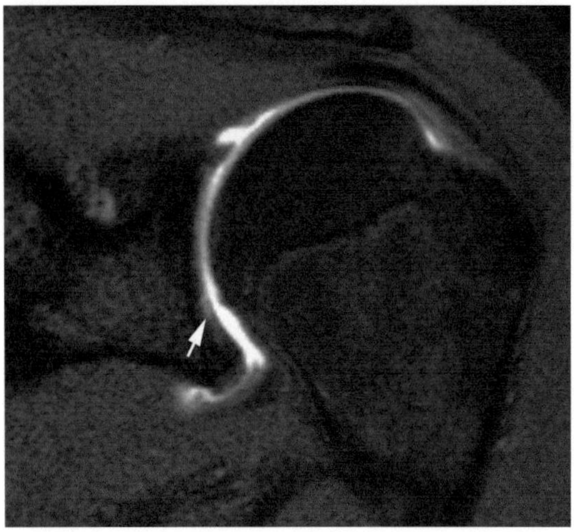

Fig. 6.27 Non-displaced delaminating chondral injury of the glenoid in a 16-year-old boy. Coronal T1-W FS MRA shows contrast insinuating (*arrow*) between the deep and superficial cartilage layers

Repeated insult, partial healing response, and remodeling result in MRA features that include overlying cartilage loss, cartilage fissuring, gadolinium insinuation between the cartilage fragment and parent bone, subchondral cysts, and loose body formation. Associated subchondral marrow edema and joint effusions may be seen. Any of these findings suggest the fragment is unstable.

Differential Diagnosis

Chondral injuries should be differentiated from the normal bare spot of the glenoid fossa [55]. On MRI, the normal glenoid bare spot is usually centrally located and has smoothly tapering margins without underlying cortical abnormality (Fig. 6.26). Alternative considerations for humeral head OCD include epiphyseal osteonecrosis, chondroblastoma, epiphyseal Brodie abscess related to osteomyelitis, and sequelae of prior shoulder dislocation with a depressed Hill-Sachs fracture. OCD injuries should be differentiated from acute cartilage and osteochondral fractures, which have more sharply demarcated margins (Fig. 6.27).

8 Soft Tissue Injuries About the Shoulder

Pediatric rotator cuff tears are extremely rare and occur in athletes suffering either acute injury or repetitive microtrauma [56]. Rotator cuff tears may also be seen in the setting of glenohumeral instability [17]. The scarcity of this injury has two causes: one, children have not lived long enough for repetitive microtrauma and overuse to compromise the rotator cuff, and, two, because the physis—not the tendon or myotendinous junction—is the weakest component of the musculoskeletal unit, biomechanical insult occurs at the physis before the rotator cuff is compromised.

References

1. Ecklund K. Magnetic resonance imaging of pediatric musculoskeletal trauma. Top Magn Reson Imaging. 2002;13(4):203–17.
2. Rowe CR. Prognosis in dislocations of the shoulder. J Bone Joint Surg Am. 1956;38-A(5):957–77.
3. Emery KH. Imaging of sports injuries of the upper extremity in children. Clin Sports Med. 2006;25(3):543–68, viii.
4. Davis KW. Imaging pediatric sports injuries: upper extremity. Radiol Clin North Am. 2010;48(6):1199–211.
5. Boone JL, Arciero RA. First-time anterior shoulder dislocations: has the standard changed? Br J Sports Med. 2010;44(5):355–60.

6. Omoumi P, et al. Glenohumeral joint instability. J Magn Reson Imaging. 2011;33(1):2–16.
7. Grahame R, Hakim AJ. Hypermobility. Curr Opin Rheumatol. 2008;20(1):106–10.
8. Macmahon PJ, Palmer WE. Magnetic resonance imaging in glenohumeral instability. Magn Reson Imaging Clin N Am. 2012;20(2):295–312, xi.
9. Jones KJ, et al. Functional outcomes of early arthroscopic Bankart repair in adolescents aged 11–18 years. J Pediatr Orthop. 2007;27(2):209–13.
10. Kirkley A, et al. Prospective randomized clinical trial comparing the effectiveness of immediate arthroscopic stabilization versus immobilization and rehabilitation in first traumatic anterior dislocations of the shoulder: long-term evaluation. Arthroscopy. 2005;21(1):55–63.
11. Chuang TY, Adams CR, Burkhart SS. Use of preoperative three-dimensional computed tomography to quantify glenoid bone loss in shoulder instability. Arthroscopy. 2008;24(4):376–82.
12. Burkhart SS, De Beer JF. Traumatic glenohumeral bone defects and their relationship to failure of arthroscopic Bankart repairs: significance of the inverted-pear glenoid and the humeral engaging Hill-Sachs lesion. Arthroscopy. 2000;16(7):677–94.
13. Paxinos A, et al. Advances in the management of traumatic anterior and atraumatic multidirectional shoulder instability. Sports Med. 2001;31(11):819–28.
14. Waldt S, et al. Anterior shoulder instability: accuracy of MR arthrography in the classification of anteroinferior labroligamentous injuries. Radiology. 2005;237(2):578–83.
15. Oh JH, et al. Effectiveness of multidetector computed tomography arthrography for the diagnosis of shoulder pathology: comparison with magnetic resonance imaging with arthroscopic correlation. J Shoulder Elbow Surg. 2010;19(1):14–20.
16. Beltran J, et al. Glenohumeral instability: evaluation with MR arthrography. Radiographics. 1997;17(3):657–73.
17. Yiannakopoulos CK, Mataragas E, Antonogiannakis E. A comparison of the spectrum of intra-articular lesions in acute and chronic anterior shoulder instability. Arthroscopy. 2007;23(9):985–90.
18. Pahlavan S, et al. Proximal humerus fractures in the pediatric population: a systematic review. J Child Orthop. 2011;5(3):187–94.
19. Neer 2nd CS, Horwitz BS. Fractures of the proximal humeral epiphysial plate. Clin Orthop Relat Res. 1965;41:24–31.
20. Bishop JY, Flatow EL. Pediatric shoulder trauma. Clin Orthop Relat Res. 2005;432:41–8.
21. Beringer DC, et al. Severely displaced proximal humeral epiphyseal fractures: a follow-up study. J Pediatr Orthop. 1998;18(1):31–7.
22. Lucas JC, Mehlman CT, Laor T. The location of the biceps tendon in completely displaced proximal humerus fractures in children: a report of four cases with magnetic resonance imaging and cadaveric correlation. J Pediatr Orthop. 2004;24(3):249–53.
23. Osbahr DC, Kim HJ, Dugas JR. Little league shoulder. Curr Opin Pediatr. 2010;22(1):35–40.
24. Meister K, et al. Rotational motion changes in the glenohumeral joint of the adolescent/Little League baseball player. Am J Sports Med. 2005;33(5):693–8.
25. Carson Jr WG, Gasser SI. Little Leaguer's shoulder. A report of 23 cases. Am J Sports Med. 1998;26(4):575–80.
26. Fleming JL, et al. Little Leaguer's shoulder. Skelet Radiol. 2004;33(6):352–4.
27. Obembe OO, et al. Little Leaguer's shoulder (proximal humeral epiphysiolysis): MRI findings in four boys. Pediatr Radiol. 2007;37(9):885–9.
28. Song JC, Lazarus ML, Song AP. MRI findings in Little Leaguer's shoulder. Skelet Radiol. 2006;35(2):107–9.
29. Hatem SF, Recht MP, Profitt B. MRI of Little Leaguer's shoulder. Skelet Radiol. 2006;35(2):103–6.
30. Kibler WB, Sciascia A, Thomas SJ. Glenohumeral internal rotation deficit: pathogenesis and response to acute throwing. Sports Med Arthrosc. 2012;20(1):34–8.
31. Giaroli EL, Major NM, Higgins LD. MRI of internal impingement of the shoulder. AJR Am J Roentgenol. 2005;185(4):925–9.
32. Tehranzadeh AD, Fronek J, Resnick D. Posterior capsular fibrosis in professional baseball pitchers: case series of MR arthrographic findings in six patients with glenohumeral internal rotational deficit. Clin Imaging. 2007;31(5):343–8.
33. Kocher MS, Waters PM, Micheli LJ. Upper extremity injuries in the paediatric athlete. Sports Med. 2000;30(2):117–35.
34. Soto F, et al. Presentation, evaluation, and treatment of clavicle fractures in preschool children presenting to an emergency department. Pediatr Emerg Care. 2009;25(11):744–7.
35. Kubiak R, Slongo T. Operative treatment of clavicle fractures in children: a review of 21 years. J Pediatr Orthop. 2002;22(6):736–9.
36. Black GB, McPherson JA, Reed MH. Traumatic pseudodislocation of the acromioclavicular joint in children. A fifteen year review. Am J Sports Med. 1991;19(6):644–6.
37. Nenopoulos SP, et al. Outcome of distal clavicular fracture separations and dislocations in immature skeleton. Injury. 2011;42(4):376–80.
38. Neer CS. Fractures of the distal third of the clavicle. Clin Orthop Relat Res. 1968;58:43.
39. Rockwood CA. Fractures of the outer clavicle in children and adults. J Bone Joint Surg Br. 1982;64B:642 (abstract).
40. Owens BD, Goss TP. The floating shoulder. J Bone Joint Surg Br. 2006;88(11):1419–24.
41. Currarino G, Prescott P. Fractures of the acromion in young children and a description of a variant in acromial ossification which may mimic a fracture. Pediatr Radiol. 1994;24(4):251–5.
42. Kim SJ, et al. Bilateral unfused coracoid process: report of a case. J Korean Med Sci. 1998;13(5):563–5.
43. Currarino G, Herring JA. Congenital pseudarthrosis of the clavicle. Pediatr Radiol. 2009;39(12):1343–9.

44. Wilber MC, Evans EB. Fractures of the scapula. An analysis of forty cases and a review of the literature. J Bone Joint Surg Am. 1977;59(3):358–62.
45. Kogutt MS, Swischuk LE, Fagan CJ. Patterns of injury and significance of uncommon fractures in the battered child syndrome. Am J Roentgenol Radium Ther Nucl Med. 1974;121(1):143–9.
46. Bowen TR, Miller F. Greenstick fracture of the scapula: a cause of scapular winging. J Orthop Trauma. 2006;20(2):147–9.
47. Herickhoff PK, et al. Scapular stress fracture in a professional baseball player: a case report and review of the literature. Am J Sports Med. 2007;35(7):1193–6.
48. Heyse-Moore GH, Stoker DJ. Avulsion fractures of the scapula. Skelet Radiol. 1982;9(1):27–32.
49. Jones CB, Sietsema DL. Analysis of operative versus nonoperative treatment of displaced scapular fractures. Clin Orthop Relat Res. 2011;469(12):3379–89.
50. Lantry JM, Roberts CS, Giannoudis PV. Operative treatment of scapular fractures: a systematic review. Injury. 2008;39(3):271–83.
51. Hamada S, et al. Osteochondritis dissecans of the humeral head. Arthroscopy. 1992;8(1):132–7.
52. Mahirogullari M, et al. Osteochondritis dissecans of the humeral head. Joint Bone Spine. 2008;75(2):226–8.
53. Chu PJ, et al. Osteochondritis dissecans of the glenoid: a rare injury secondary to repetitive microtrauma. J Trauma. 2009;67(3):E62–4.
54. Johnson DL, Warner JJ. Osteochondritis dissecans of the humeral head: treatment with a matched osteochondral allograft. J Shoulder Elb Surg. 1997;6(2):160–3.
55. Kim HK, Emery KH, Salisbury SR. Bare spot of the glenoid fossa in children: incidence and MRI features. Pediatr Radiol. 2010;40(7):1190–6.
56. Tarkin IS, et al. Rotator cuff tears in adolescent athletes. Am J Sports Med. 2005;33(4):596–601.

The Elbow and Forearm: Congenital and Developmental Conditions

7

Rebecca Stein-Wexler

Contents

R. Stein-Wexler, MD
Department of Radiology, University of California Davis Medical Center and UC Davis Children's Hospital, 4860 Y Street, Suite 3100, Sacramento, CA 95817, USA

Department of Diagnostic Imaging, Shriners Hospitals for Children Northern California, Sacramento, CA, USA
e-mail: rebecca.steinwexler@ucdmc.ucdavis.edu

Abstract

This chapter presents important normal anatomy and variants, including the supracondylar process and elbow fat pads. It then discusses a wide variety of congenital and developmental anomalies that affect the elbow, radius, and ulna. Several classification schemes of congenital developmental anomalies are presented. The more common entities, such as radial longitudinal deficiency, ulna dysplasia, elbow synostosis, and radial head dislocation, are presented. The chapter also discusses transverse deficiency, phocomelia, ulnar longitudinal deficiency, and Poland deformity. The associated syndromes are briefly discussed. Lastly, Madelung deformity is presented.

1 Normal Anatomy

Variant Ossification at the Elbow

Irregular ossification is typical of the lateral epicondyle of the humerus, often appearing as flake-like fragments that are displaced slightly from the shaft. These should not be misdiagnosed as avulsion injuries. The trochlear epiphysis is often granular and fissured (Fig. 7.1). Comparison with the opposite side is rarely helpful, since asymmetry is common [1, 2]. Occasionally apophyses ossify in aberrant order [2]. (See Chap. 8 for further discussion of the sequence of appearance of ossification centers.)

R. Stein-Wexler et al. (eds.), *Pediatric Orthopedic Imaging*,
DOI 10.1007/978-3-642-45381-6_7, © Springer-Verlag Berlin Heidelberg 2015

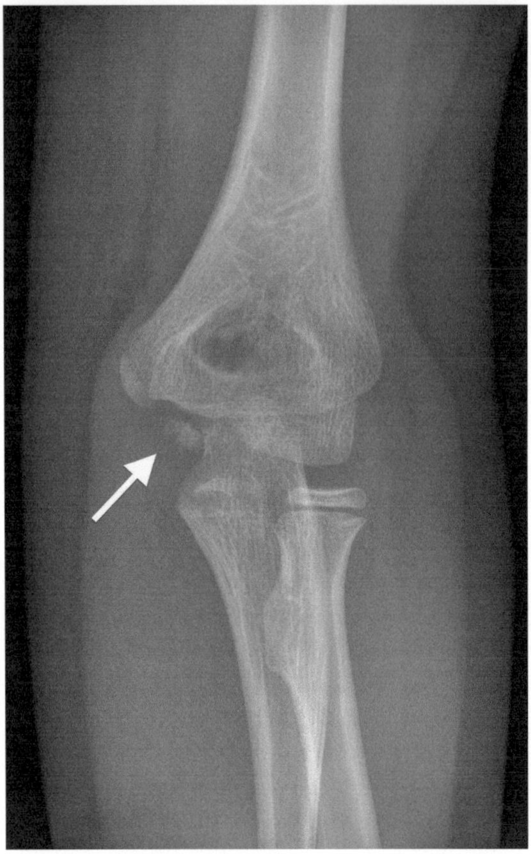

Fig. 7.1 Normal granular-appearing trochlear ossification center (*arrow*) in a 9-year-old boy

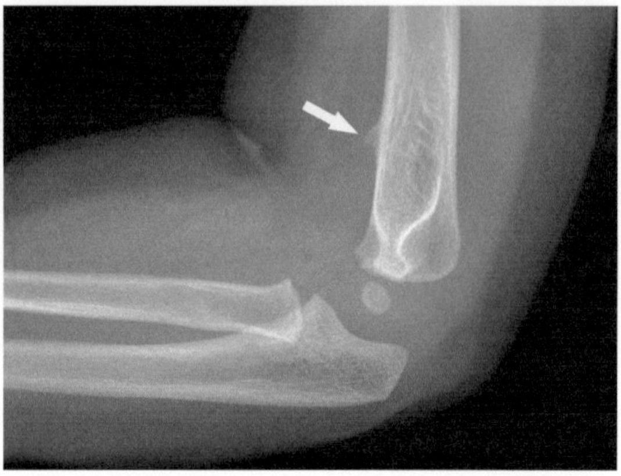

Fig. 7.2 Supracondylar process of the humerus (*arrow*), an uncommon normal variant

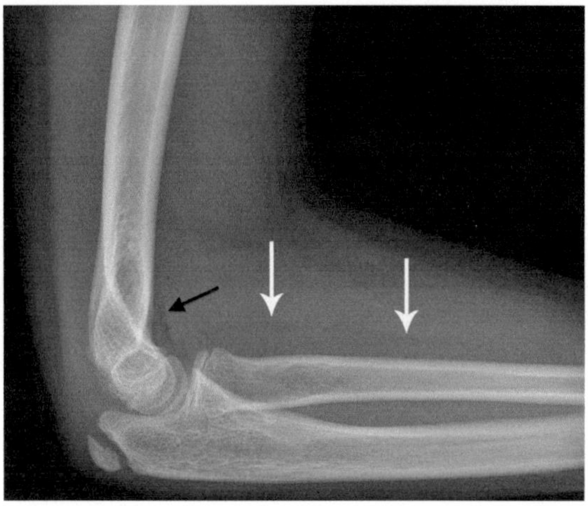

Fig. 7.3 Normal anterior fat pad (*black arrow*) in a 12-year-old boy. Also note the supinator fat plane (*white arrows*). No posterior fat pad is visible

Supracondylar Process

The supracondylar process of the humerus occurs in approximately one percent of patients. This bony spur projects anteriorly and toward the elbow, 5–7 cm above the medial epicondyle (Fig. 7.2). Unlike an osteochondroma, the supracondylar process arises directly from the cortex [1]. Occasionally a fibromuscular band connects this to the medial epicondyle, giving rise to an anomalous origin of the pronator teres muscle. Bone may form within this ligament, resulting in an osseous tunnel; the median artery and nerve may become compressed. The supracondylar process is more common in Cornelia de Lange syndrome.

Fat Pads

Fat pads at the elbow are well-recognized normal anatomic features that are useful for determining the presence of joint fluid. Two rest in the radial and coronoid fossae anterior to the distal humerus, and the third lies in the olecranon fossa posterior to the distal humerus. Enveloped by leaflets of the joint capsule, they are intracapsular but extrasynovial. They are evident in essentially all children 2 years of age or older, with the two anterior fat pads superimposed on the lateral projection of the humerus. In a right-angle flexion view of the elbow, the normal anterior fat pad has a triangular or teardrop shape, whereas the normal posterior fat pad is hidden within the olecranon fossa and therefore inapparent (Fig. 7.3). In extension, however, the anterior fat pad is flattened somewhat by the brachialis muscle, and the normal posterior fat pad may become visible as the muscles posterior to it relax.

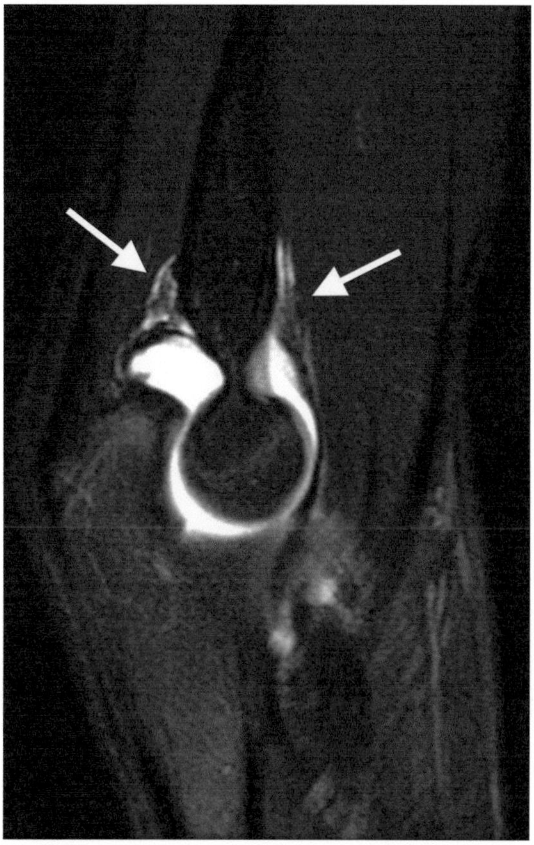

Fig. 7.4 Elevated fat pads. On this sagittal fast spin echo (FSE) fat-suppressed (FS) MR arthrogram of the elbow, the large amount of fluid within the joint elevates and clearly delineates the elevated and displaced anterior and posterior fat pads (*arrows*)

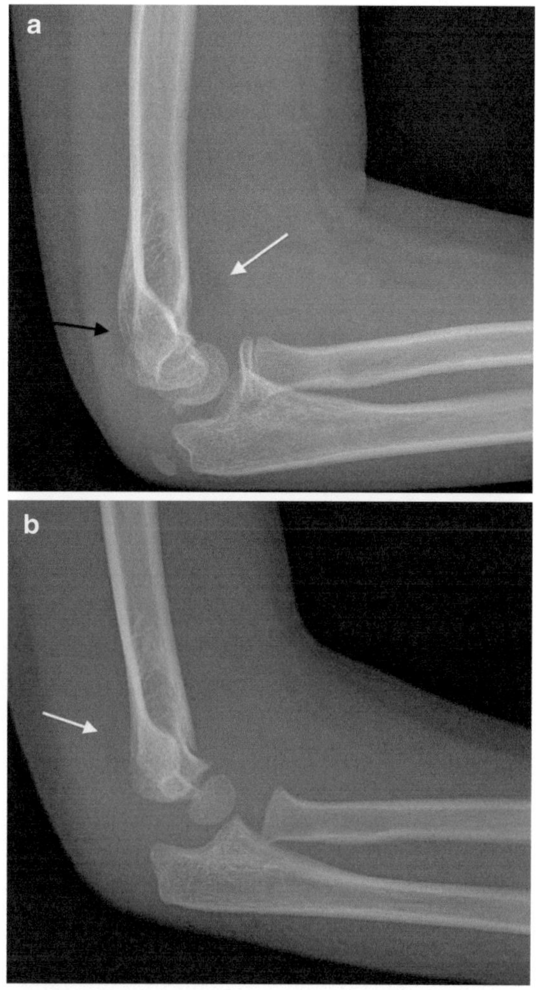

Fig. 7.5 Elevated fat pads at the elbow. (**a**) Anterior (*white arrow*) and posterior (*black arrow*) fat pads in a 10-year-old boy with a non-displaced supracondylar fracture. (**b**) Elevated posterior fat pad (*arrow*) in a 6-year-old boy with a supracondylar fracture and a hemorrhagic elbow effusion (note that the joint fluid is dense). The anterior fat pad has been pushed into the coronoid fossa

The application of the elbow fat pad signs in diagnosis should be restricted to non-rotated radiographs performed with the elbow flexed. In the case of elbow joint effusion or hemarthrosis, the anterior fat pad is elevated and sickle-shaped, whereas the posterior fat pad becomes visible as it is pushed from its fossa by fluid expanding the intra-articular space (Figs. 7.4 and 7.5).

The supinator fat plane in the upper forearm lies anterior to the supinator muscle and proximal radius and posterior to the pronator teres and brachioradialis muscles. This is normally slightly bowed anteriorly, running roughly parallel to the proximal one third of the radius (see Fig. 7.3). The fat plane is displaced if the radial head is fractured or if there is arthritis or regional edema.

2 Congenital Limb Deficiencies

Congenital limb deficiencies occur in about 0.5 per 1,000 live births and usually affect the upper extremity. As in all birth disorders, classification is difficult and can be mired in an attempt to devise an all-inclusive system. Swanson's classification system, adopted by the International

Table 7.1 Swanson's classification of congenital anomalies of the extremity

Failure of formation of parts/arrest of development
Transverse: congenital arrested formation (amputation appearance)
Longitudinal: deficiency in longitudinal axis
Phocomelia
Radial dysplasia
Ulnar dysplasia
Failure of differentiation or separation
Elbow synostoses
Radial head dislocation
Poland deformity
Sprengel deformity
Duplication
Overgrowth (gigantism)
Undergrowth (hypoplasia)
Congenital constriction band effects
Generalized skeletal abnormalities

Adapted from Swanson [3]

Federation of Societies for Surgery of the Hand (IFSSH) in 1976, presents broad categories that can be adapted to either extremity and even to portions of the axial skeleton (Table 7.1) [3]. A more recent classification takes into account advances in the understanding of the molecular mechanisms of limb development (Table 7.2) [4].

Ossified structures as well as nerves, vessels, muscles, capsule, ligaments, and cartilage must be evaluated in order to devise the best functional remedy [5]. Magnetic resonance imaging (MRI) as well as pre- and postnatal ultrasound contributes important information.

Transverse defects are very rare and result from arrested formation, perhaps a consequence of vascular interruption. They are different from intrauterine amputation due to amniotic band formation. The most common anomaly consists of unilateral amputation of the forearm below the elbow (Fig. 7.6). Rudimentary digits may be attached to the stump. Longitudinal defects are more common and include phocomelia as well as both radial deficiency and the much rarer ulnar deficiency. Longitudinal defects are named by the bones that are completely or partially absent.

Examples of failure of differentiation or separation include synostoses about the elbow (radioulnar being by far the most common) as well as radial head

Table 7.2 Classification of congenital anomalies of the hand and upper extremity based on developmental biology

Malformations
Failure of axis formation/differentiation—entire upper limb
Proximal-distal outgrowth
Brachymelia with brachydactyly
Symbrachydactyly
Transverse deficiency
Intersegmental deficiency
Radial-ulnar (anteroposterior) axis
Radial longitudinal deficiency
Ulnar longitudinal deficiency
Ulnar dimelia
Radioulnar synostosis
Humeroradial synostosis
Dorsal-ventral axis
Nail-patella syndrome
Failure of axis formation/differentiation—handplate
Radial-ulnar (anteroposterior) axis
Radial polydactyly
Triphalangeal thumb
Ulnar polydactyly
Dorsal-ventral axis
Dorsal dimelia (palmar nail)
Hypoplastic/aplastic nail
Failure of handplate formation/differentiation—unspecified axis
Soft tissue
Syndactyly
Camptodactyly
Skeletal deficiency
Brachydactyly
Clinodactyly
Kirner's deformity
Metacarpal and carpal synostoses
Complex
Cleft hand
Synpolydactyly
Apert hand
Deformation
Constriction ring sequence
Arthrogryposis
Trigger digits
Not otherwise specified
Dysplasias
Hypertrophy
Macrodactyly
Upper limb
Upper limb and macrodactyly
Tumorous conditions

Reprinted from Oberg et al. [4], with permission from Elsevier

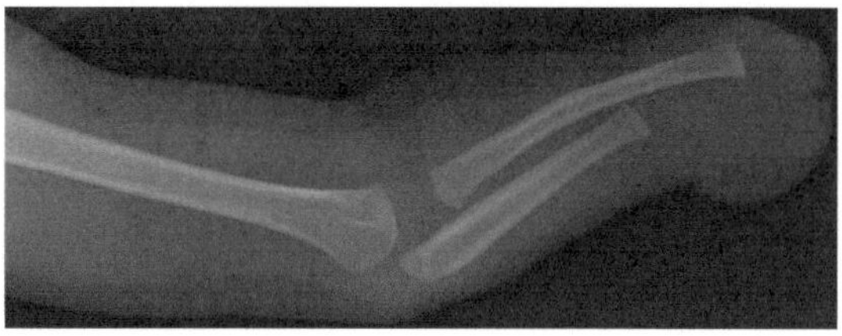

Fig. 7.6 Transverse deficiency. There is soft tissue distal to the hypoplastic radius and ulna and complete absence of formed osseous structures. As in this case, it is sometimes difficult to determine radiographically whether this appearance results from constriction bands or failure of formation, but the presence of fingernails is readily recognized clinically, helping differentiate transverse deficiency from amniotic bands (Image copyright Shriners Hospital for Children Northern California)

dislocation. Sprengel deformity (see Chap. 5) and Poland deformity (see Chap. 9) also fit this category.

Defects of duplication, overgrowth, undergrowth and constriction bands are most common in the hand (Chap. 9).

The more common entities are addressed here, and for those interested standard references can be consulted for more comprehensive analysis [3, 6, 7].

2.1 Phocomelia

Phocomelia refers to a flipper-like (Greek *phoke*, meaning "seal") anomaly with a distal part (also often abnormal) attached proximally with what grossly appears to be the absence of an intermediate segment [3] (Fig. 7.7). This denotation may

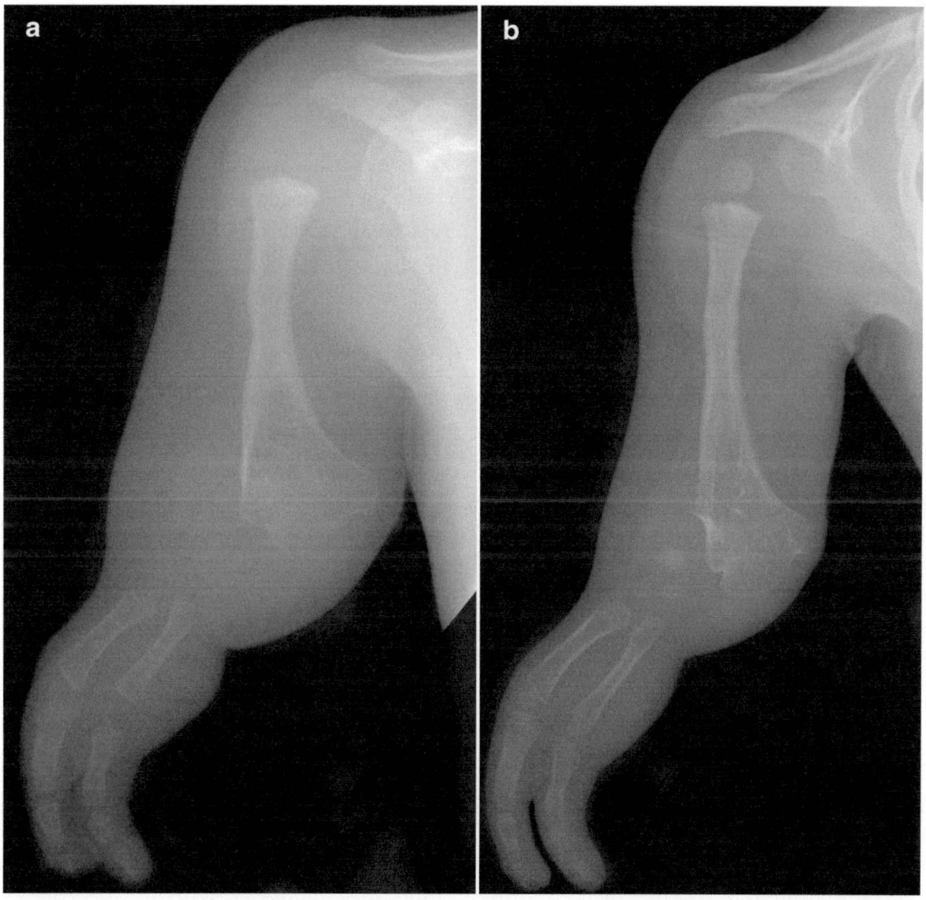

Fig. 7.7 Phocomelia. (**a**) The splayed distal humerus in this 2-year-old may represent a conglomeration of remnants of the proximal radius and ulna. Rays are deleted, and there is a large soft tissue gap between the bony mass and the two metacarpals. Note the flipper-like outline of the soft tissues. The parahumeral fat appears abnormal. (**b**) Four years later, three carpal bones have ossified, and the rays demonstrate further development. The parahumeral fat is more normal (Images copyright Shriners Hospital for Children Northern California)

be applied to both the upper and lower extremities. The hand may appear to be attached to the trunk, or there may be variable intervening segments of bone. Formerly considered a transverse intercalary segmental defect, phocomelia has recently been redefined as a subset of longitudinal deficiency [8]. Phocomelia is subdivided into three groups, based on whether there is proximal radial longitudinal dysplasia, proximal ulnar longitudinal dysplasia, or combined dysplasia, with an absent forearm or—occasionally—also an absent arm.

The digits are frequently abnormal or missing, and the joints are unstable owing to musculoligamentous relaxation or deficit. Other skeletal and systemic anomalies are frequently present (e.g., thalidomide embryopathy, thrombocytopenia-absent radius (TAR), Holt-Oram syndrome, and others [7]). Abnormalities of all four limbs (tetraphocomelia) are associated with facial dysmorphism in Roberts syndrome. Extreme cases of Poland syndrome may manifest phocomelia, further discussed in Chap. 9.

2.2 Radial Longitudinal Deficiency (or Radial Dysplasia, Radial Clubhand) (Box 7.1)

Box 7.1: Radial Longitudinal Deficiency

Complete or partial absence of the radius
Short, bowed ulna
Radioulnar synostoses common
Radial clubhand: hand at right angle to forearm
Navicular and thumb often absent

Several synonyms refer to radial longitudinal deficiency, stressing various aspects of the abnormality, such as its clinical appearance (radial clubhand) or the complete (radial aplasia) or partial (radial meromelia) absence of the radius. From a strictly anatomic point of view, this is an intercalary, longitudinal, radial meromelia, but the terms radial dysplasia or radial longitudinal deficiency are more appropriate, encompassing the accompanying abnormal nerves, blood vessels, muscles, and adjacent joint anomalies or fusion as well.

Radial longitudinal deficiency is often associated with other systemic or musculoskeletal abnormalities and is indeed isolated in only 33 % of patients [9]. Syndromes are present in about 33 %, usually thrombocytopenia-absent radius (TAR) syndrome or VACTERL association (vertebral-anal-cardiac-tracheo-esophageal-renal-limb anomalies) [9, 10]. Holt-Oram syndrome occurs in about 13 %. Cardiac lesions are usually ventricular or atrial septal defects, but pulmonary artery atresia and patent ductus arteriosus are also reported.

Two types of hematologic syndromes are associated with radial longitudinal deficiency. Fanconi anemia is an autosomal recessive aplastic anemia that presents between 2 and 15 years of age. It can be fatal if not treated by bone marrow transplantation. For this reason, all children with radial longitudinal deficiency should undergo a chromosomal breakage test, which can test for Fanconi anemia before the development of any symptoms. Second, congenital amegakaryocytic thrombocytopenia has been reported in frequent association with TAR syndrome. The TAR syndrome may also be associated with dysplastic genu varum, hooking of the lateral clavicle, and primary cranial synostosis (Baller-Gerold syndrome). This is probably an autosomal recessive disorder, and it may be diagnosed by fetal ultrasound. Children with TAR syndrome tend to have normal thumbs (Fig. 7.8), whereas the thumbs of most children with an absent radius (in the absence of TAR) are absent or hypoplastic.

Approximately 33 % of patients have nonsyndromic additional osseous abnormalities. Scoliosis is the most commonly associated abnormality; other associated abnormalities include humeral hypoplasia, proximal radioulnar synostosis, congenitally dislocated radial head, and stiff digits. The likelihood of having associated anomalies increases with the severity of radial longitudinal deficiency. If the radius is completely absent, additional anomalies are present in 80 %, whereas if the proximal humerus is also

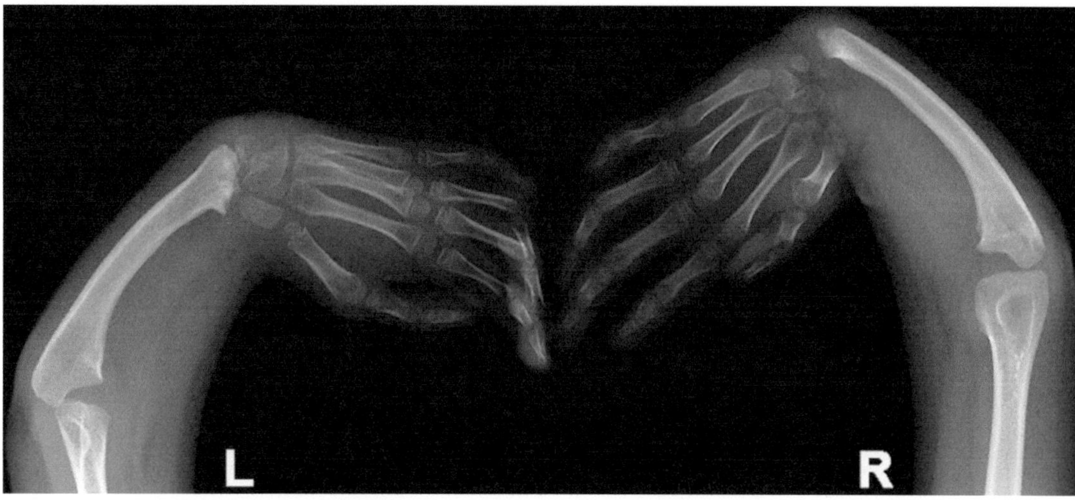

Fig. 7.8 Thrombocytopenia-absent radius (TAR). Neither radius is ossified. The ulnas are short and thick. The left carpus has been surgically centered on the distal ulna, whereas on the right there is still clubhand deformity. Both thumbs are present. Note the carpal bones on the left are more mature than those on the right (Image copyright Shriners Hospital for Children Northern California)

absent, essentially all children have additional anomalies. If only the thumb is hypoplastic, 35 % of children have additional anomalies [9].

Radial dysplasia occurs in 1 in 30,000 live births and is most common in boys. It is more often sporadic than inherited [11]. Up to 50 % are bilateral. When unilateral, the right side is affected twice as frequently as the left [12]. Radial longitudinal deficiency has been classified into six types based on the extent of radial shortening and the extent to which the thumb and carpus are involved [13] (Table 7.3). The radial anomaly takes three forms. Total aplasia is most common, occurring in 60 % (Fig. 7.9). Partial aplasia occurs in about 20 % and is usually characterized by absence of the distal growth plate and epiphysis, with deformity of the proximal portion (occasionally only the proximal radius is absent). Hypoplasia is defined as diminution in size without segmental absence. More mild deficiencies can present as absence or hypoplasia of the radial carpal bones or the thumb.

Stretching and corrective casting soon after birth may prevent further contracture. Centralization, the procedure to position the carpus on the ulna, is controversial, as it often leads to a stiff, albeit straighter, forearm and wrist, with a high likelihood of complications including growth arrest and recurrent contracture. Lengthening of the radius has been proposed but often requires several surgeries with a high risk of complications. Surgical treatment of the thumb deficiency, including tendon transfers and pollicization, is more commonly performed (Figs. 7.10 and 7.11). In pollicization, a digit (usually the second) is transferred to the position of the thumb and also rotated.

Imaging

Radiographs demonstrate complete or partial aplasia of the radius. The hand is positioned at a right angle to the forearm, angulated laterally due to the pull of abnormally positioned muscles or a fibrous band that may replace the radius (Fig. 7.12).

At birth, the ulna is short, typically 60 % of normal, and this relative deficiency persists. Ossification of the distal ulnar epiphysis may be delayed, and it may fuse prematurely. The ulna is bowed with convexity posterior and medial. The humeral-ulnar articulation is frequently abnormal, and the humerus may also be shortened. Both increased laxity and contractures occur. Proximal radioulnar synostosis and congenitally dislocated radial head are commonly associated with cases of relatively mild radial longitudinal deficiency [11].

Table 7.3 Classification of radial longitudinal deficiency

Type	Thumb	Carpus	Distal radius	Proximal radius
N	Hypoplastic or absent	Normal	Normal	Normal
0	Hypoplastic or absent	Absence, hypoplasia, or coalition	Normal	Normal, radioulnar synostosis, or congenital dislocation of radial head
1	Hypoplastic or absent	Absence, hypoplasia, or coalition	>2 mm shorter than ulna	Normal, radioulnar synostosis, or congenital dislocation of radial head
2	Hypoplastic or absent	Absence, hypoplasia, or coalition	Hypoplasia	Hypoplasia
3	Hypoplastic or absent	Absence, hypoplasia, or coalition	Physis absent	Variable hypoplasia
4	Hypoplastic or absent	Absence, hypoplasia, or coalition	Absent	Absent

Reprinted from James et al. [13], copyright 1999, with permission from Elsevier

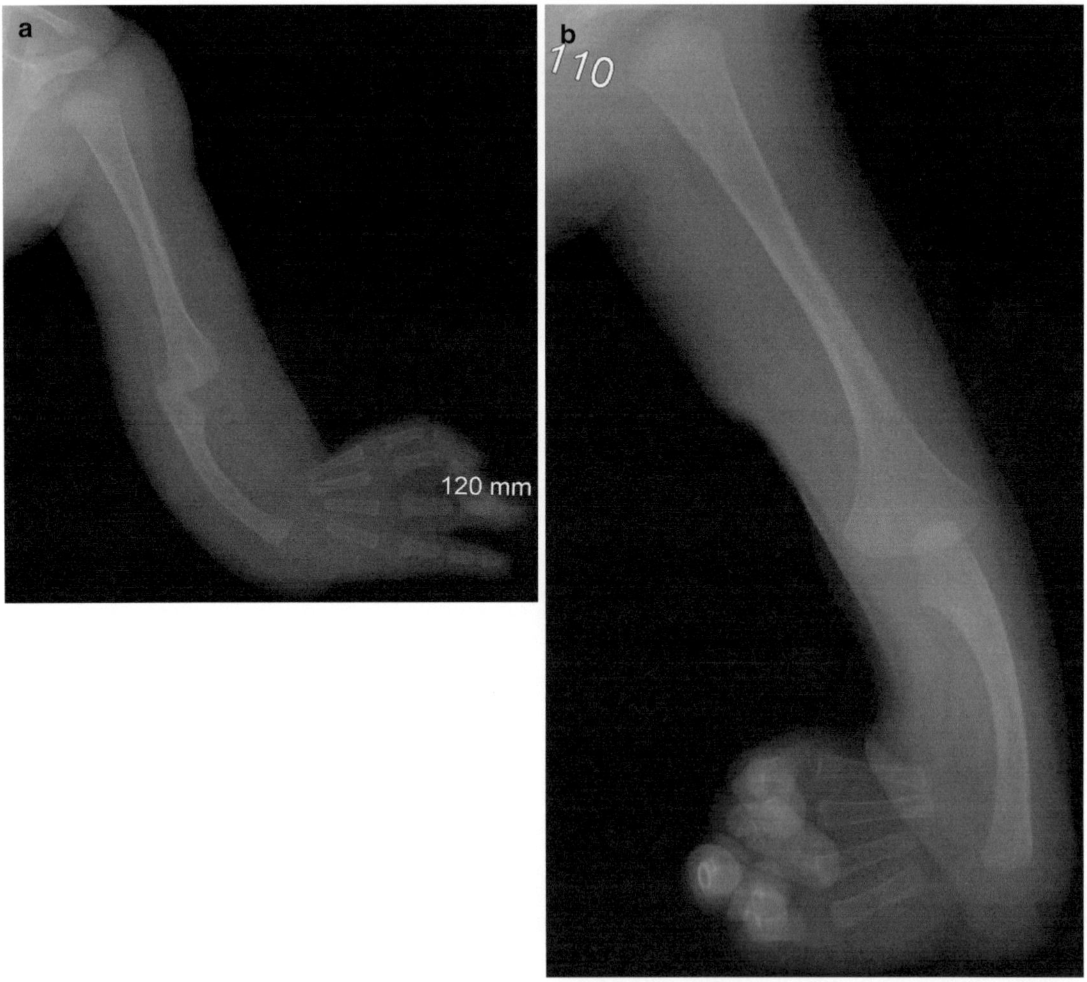

Fig. 7.9 Radial aplasia (same patient as Fig. 7.10). (**a**, **b**) There is radial aplasia with radial clubhand deformity and aplastic thumb. The ulna is hypoplastic and bowed (Images copyright Shriners Hospital for Children Northern California)

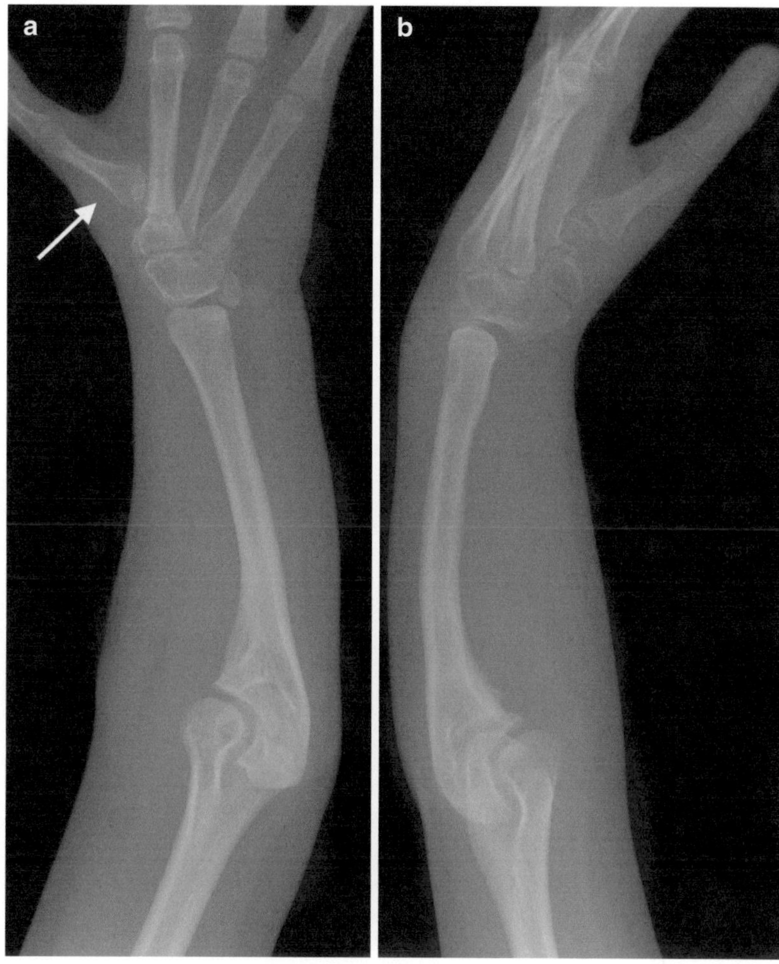

Fig. 7.10 Radial aplasia, after pollicization and centralization (same patient as Fig. 7.9). (**a**, **b**) The second finger has been transferred to the position of the thumb and rotated (*arrow*). Note carpal fusion (Images copyright Shriners Hospital for Children Northern California)

The wrist joint is often replaced by a mass of unorganized fibrous tissue. The navicular is almost always absent, and the trapezium is missing in about two thirds. However, the capitate, hamate, triquetrum, and ulnar four metacarpals and phalanges are almost always normal. The thumb is absent in up to 75 % of patients and hypoplastic in another 20 % (Fig. 7.13). Occasionally there is a fleshy rudimentary appendage.

Cross-Sectional Imaging

Prenatal ultrasound can identify radial dysplasia. MRI is useful for surgical planning, as it may allow identification of a radiologically occult cartilaginous anlage of the radius, and if not resected such a structure may tether the ulna's growth. MRI also allows characterization of the cartilaginous ends of the ulna.

2.3 Ulnar Longitudinal Deficiency (Ulnar Dysplasia)

Congenital ulnar longitudinal deficiency (ulnar dysplasia) is among the most uncommon congenital anomalies of the upper extremity and is encountered three to ten times less often than radial dysplasia. It occurs in 1–1.4/100,000 births [14]. Unlike its radial counterpart, the ulnar defect is rarely complete, and deviation of the hand is less severe. It is more common on the right and in males; in 25 % there is a bilateral abnormality.

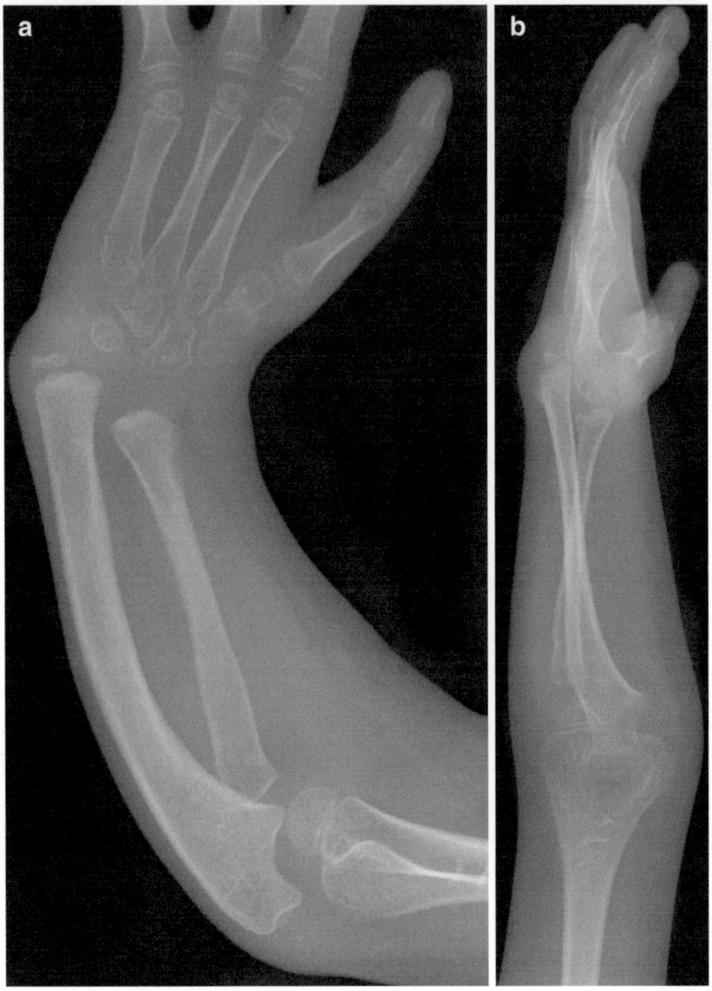

Fig. 7.11 Partial radial longitudinal deficiency. (**a**, **b**) The second ray has been pollicized and the carpal bones centralized (Images copyright Shriners Hospital for Children Northern California)

Accompanying skeletal abnormalities are common in the hand and wrist, and they are often more extensive than in radial dysplasia (Table 7.4) (Fig. 7.14). In up to 90 % of cases, digits are missing [11]. Anomalies occur on both the radial and ulnar sides; ectrodactyly and anomalies of the thumb and first web space are especially common [14]. The ulnar carpal bones may be missing or fused, and the ulnar metacarpals and phalanges may be absent or present with syndactyly (20 %) or symphalangism.

The radius and humerus are often abnormal [3]. The radial head is usually dislocated but may fuse with the distal humerus [15]. Elbow contractures are more common and more severe with ulnar longitudinal deficiency than with radial longitudinal deficiency [11]. Unlike in radial dysplasia, remote skeletal abnormalities are common, including anomalies of the other hand, phocomelia, proximal focal femoral deficiency, fibular deficiency, and scoliosis. Contralateral anomalies are seen in 29–47 % [14]. However, unlike radial dysplasia, nonskeletal abnormalities are rare. Ulnar dysplasia is usually sporadic but can occur in association with Cornelia de Lange, femur-fibula-ulna, and Schinzel syndromes.

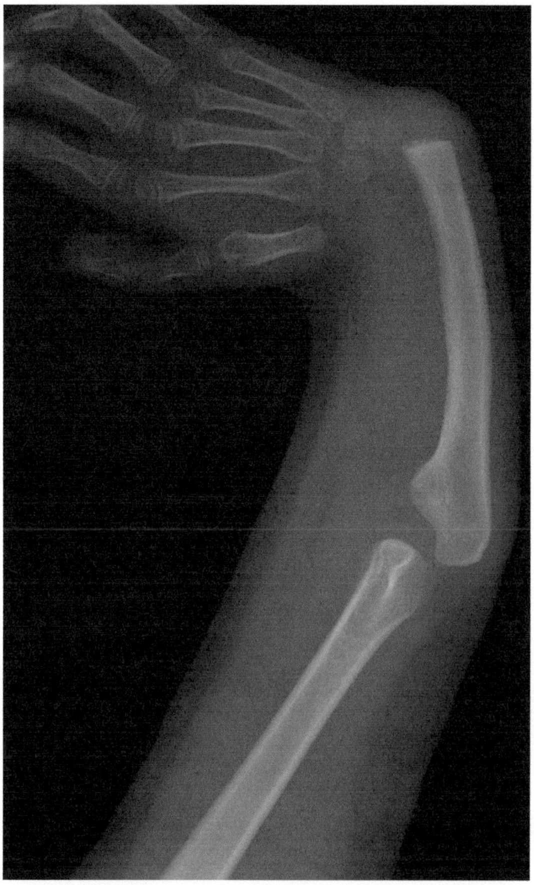

Fig. 7.12 Radial aplasia leading to radial clubhand deformity. The radius is absent, and the ulna is hypoplastic. The hand is positioned at a right angle to the forearm (Image copyright Shriners Hospital for Children Northern California)

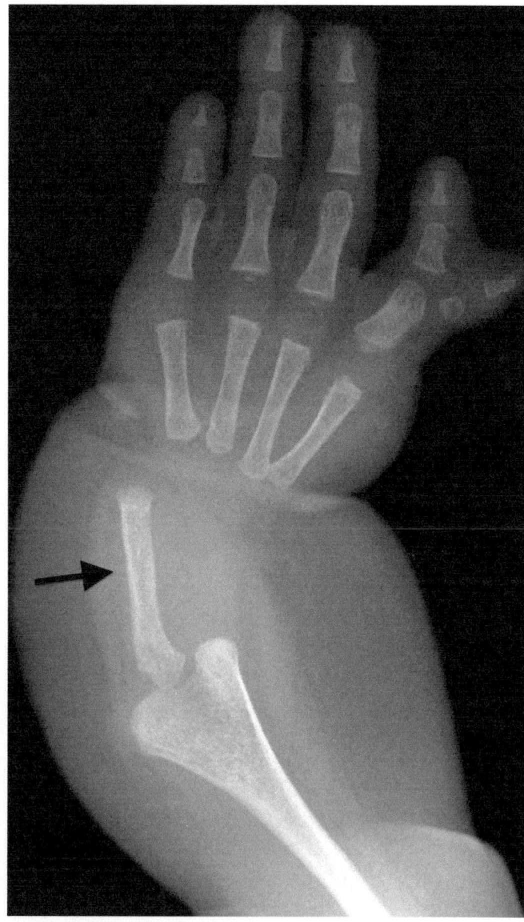

Fig. 7.13 Radial aplasia with absent thumb. The ulna is short and dysplastic (*arrow*), and the texture of the fat is abnormal. The middle and distal phalanges of the first ray are duplicated (Image copyright Shriners Hospital for Children Northern California)

Treatment of this forearm anomaly is controversial, but treatment of accompanying hand abnormalities and severe internal rotation of the forearm is generally advised (see Fig. 7.14) [14].

Radiology

Although the ulna can be absent, it is more often hypoplastic; its ossification center may ossify as late as 2 years of age. The radius is short and bowed, and the distal radial epiphysis deviates in an ulnar direction. The radial head is either normal, subluxated, dislocated, or fused to the humerus [14]. The radiological appearance of ulnar longitudinal deficiency has recently been classified as types 0–5 (Table 7.5) [11]. With type 0, the only abnormality is in the hand, where digits are absent or hypoplastic and carpal bones absent or fused. Types 1 through 3 involve progressively more extensive ulnar hypoplasia and elbow instability. Types 4 and 5 are accompanied with radiohumeral synostosis. If a cartilaginous or fibrous ulnar anlage is present

Table 7.4 Comparison of radial versus ulnar longitudinal deficiency

	Radial longitudinal deficiency	Ulnar longitudinal deficiency
	Common	Rare
	Complete in 60 %	Rarely complete
Associations	TAR, VACTERL	Remote skeletal abnormalities common
		Nonskeletal anomalies rare
Hand	Mild abnormalities	Extensive abnormalities of ipsilateral hand/arm common
Thumb	Absent in 75 % Hypoplastic in 20 %	Anomalies common

(types 2 and 4), radial bowing develops and may become severe; excision of the anlage improves both appearance and function. Ulnar anlage is absent in types 3 and 5, and the radius forms relatively straight. Ulnar deviation of the hand (with bowed radius) suggests a tethering force.

Magnetic Resonance Imaging and Ultrasound

Either MRI or ultrasound (US) can identify a tethering fibrocartilaginous band that connects the proximal ulnar primary ossification center with the carpus or distal radius; this may eventually ossify. MRI may also identify the ulnar neurovascular bundle, which is important for presurgical planning as the radial artery may be deficient. MRI also helps delineate musculature and cartilaginous anlage in young children [16].

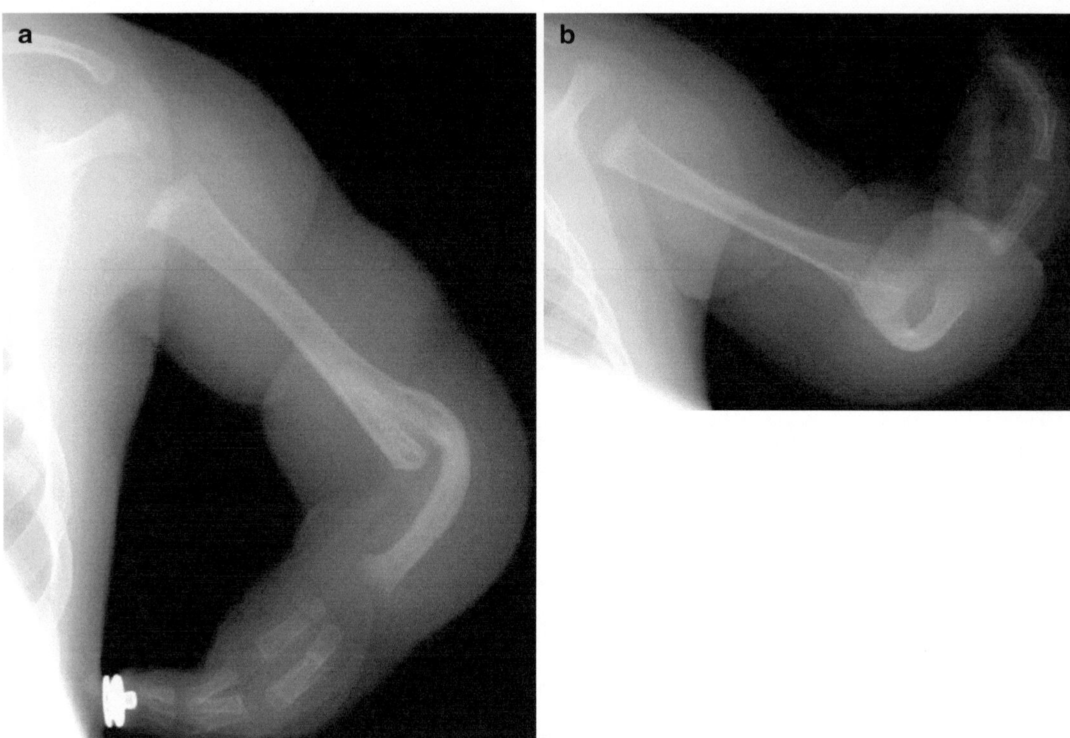

Fig. 7.14 (**a**, **b**) Ulnar longitudinal deficiency with radiohumeral synostosis in an infant. The radius is fused to the dysplastic distal humerus, and there may be a very short proximal ulna, also fused to the humerus. There are only three rays, which are dysplastic and demonstrate partial soft tissue syndactyly (Images courtesy of Michelle James, copyright Shriners Hospitals for Children Northern California)

Table 7.5 Classifications of ulnar longitudinal deficiency

Type	Ulna	Radius	Elbow	Wrist/hand
0	Normal	Normal	Stable	Absence/hypoplasia of digits Carpal bone absence or coalition
1	Hypoplasia Distal and proximal epiphyses present	Mild bowing	Stable	Mild ulnar wrist deviation Absence/hypoplasia of digits common
2	Partial aplasia Proximal ulna present Anlage tethers radius	Bowing	Stability variable Radial head may dislocate posterolaterally	Mild ulnar wrist deviation
3	Total absence No anlage	Straight	Unstable Posterolateral dislocation of radial head Severe elbow flexion deformity possible	Less ulnar wrist deviation Carpal/digital deficiencies severe
4	Usually completely absent Anlage present	Severe radial bowing	Radiohumeral synostosis Humeral internal rotation Forearm pronation	Ulnar wrist deviation
5	Total absence	Straight	Radiohumeral synostosis Humeral bifurcation or large medial condyle	Less ulnar wrist deviation Carpal/digital deficiencies severe

3 Synostosis of the Elbow (Box 7.2)

Box 7.2: Radioulnar Synostosis

Bony bar may be present in infancy
Distal radius bowed laterally or anteriorly
Radial head dislocation common
Distal ulna may be subluxated

Although any or even all of the bones about the elbow may fuse, radioulnar synostosis is by far the most common [17]. Fusion of the radius to the humerus is much less common and is generally accompanied by ulnar longitudinal deficiency (Figs. 7.15 and 7.16). Synostosis of the distal humerus, proximal radius, and proximal ulna is even more unusual. Humeroulnar synostosis is exceedingly rare [18].

Radioulnar synostosis is most common in males. Most patients present between 5 months and 6 years, but the bony connection may become evident only in later childhood [19, 20]. The radial head is often dislocated. Patients typically have difficulty performing tasks due to fixed pronation, although elbow flexion and extension are near normal. During adolescence, progressive radial head subluxation may result in pain. Tight fibrous tissue trapping the radial head may alternatively cause pain and/or a locking sensation [21]. Trauma may cause a superimposed acute elbow flexion contracture, presumably because the annular ligament slips off the radial head and becomes entrapped [22]. The literature is inconsistent regarding unilateral versus bilateral involvement [23].

The predilection for fusion at the proximal ends of the radius and ulna is best explained embryologically. These bones form as discrete cartilaginous rods in a single block of mesenchyme. Separation is initially distal, and the proximal ends remain connected until the end of the second fetal month. If this mesenchyme then fails to dissolve and form the proximal radioulnar joint, cartilage forms in the connection; ossification may become evident in later childhood.

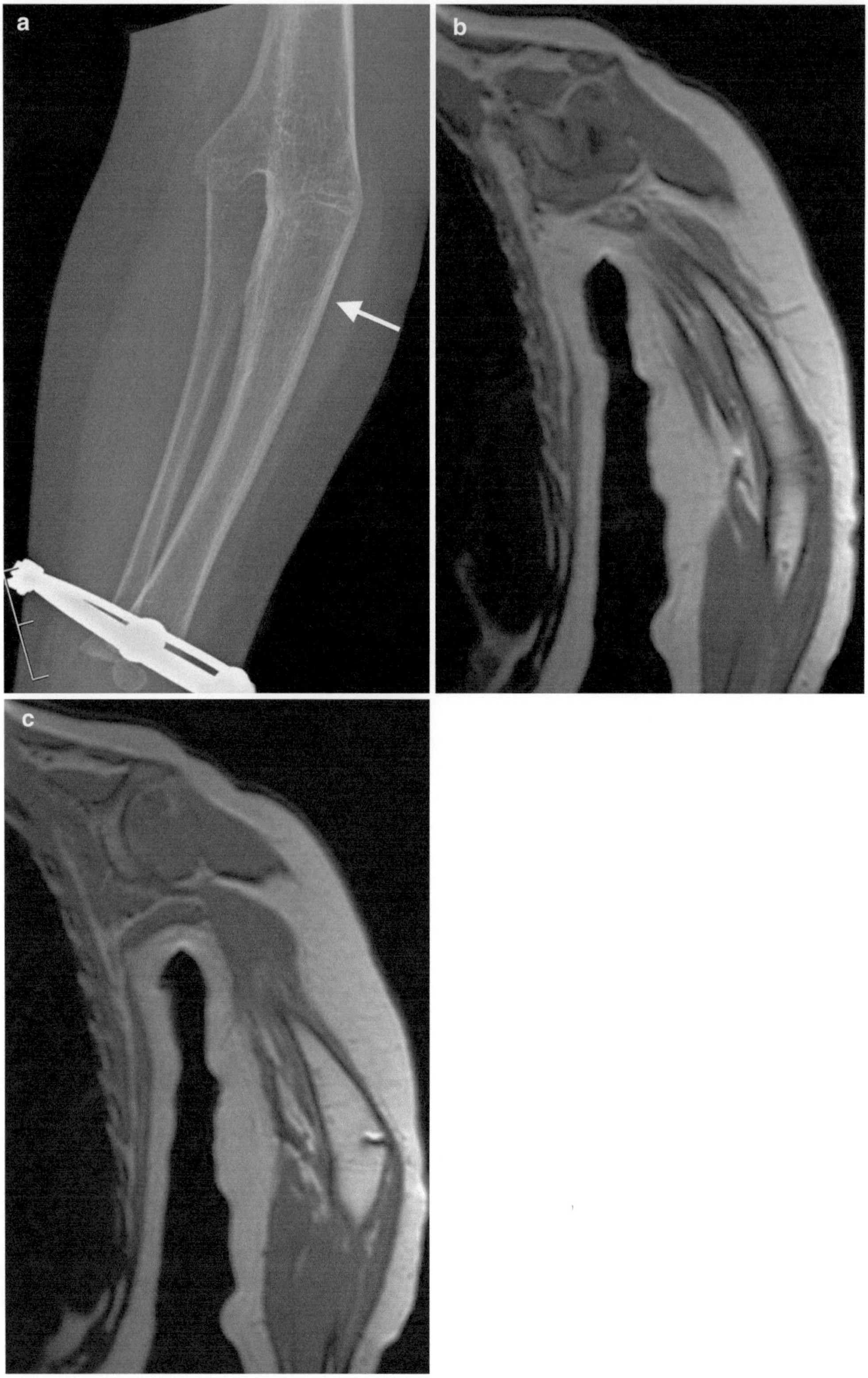

Fig. 7.15 Radiohumeral synostosis with ulnar hypoplasia. (**a**) Y-shaped deformity of the distal humerus, with fusion of its lateral portion to the adjacent, hypoplastic radius (*arrow*). The ulna is also hypoplastic (Image courtesy of Shriners Hospitals for Children Northern California). Coronal T1-weighted (T1-W) MRI (**b**, **c**) obtained several years earlier demonstrate osseous fusion of the humerus and radius with deficient biceps and triceps muscles

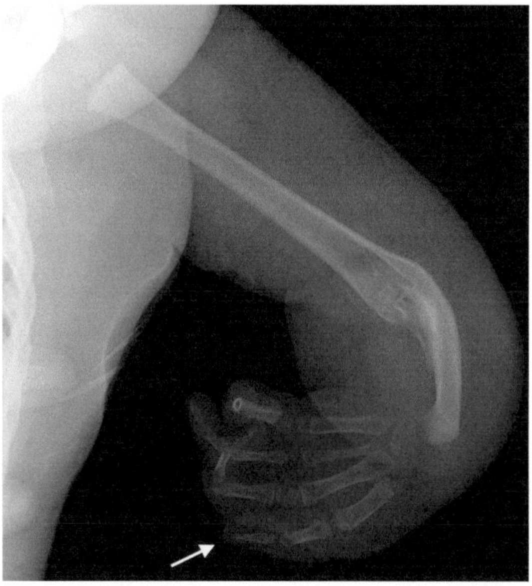

Fig. 7.16 Radiohumeral synostosis with absence of ulnar ossification indicating severe ulnar longitudinal deficiency. There are only four rays, with the thumb present (*arrow*) but an absent ulnar digit (Image copyright Shriners Hospital for Children Northern California)

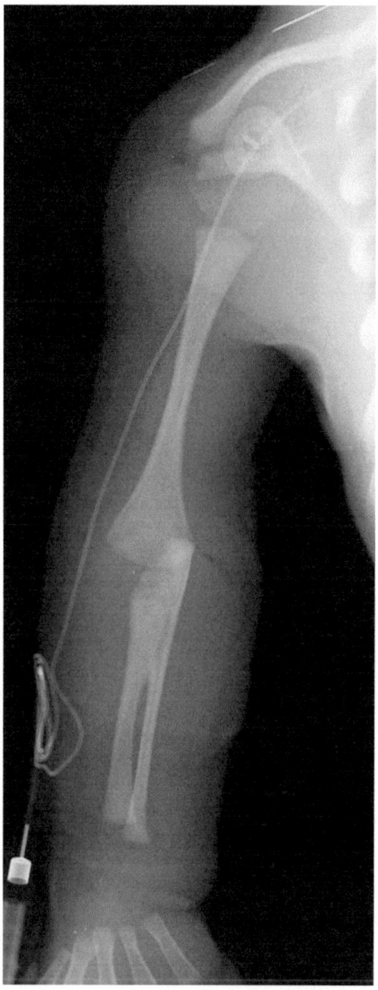

Fig. 7.17 Long-segment radioulnar synostosis in a newborn. The radial head has not yet ossified, but its proximity to the ulna indicates dislocation (Image copyright Shriners Hospital for Children Northern California)

Radioulnar synostosis is usually sporadic but is inherited in about 25 % of cases [20]. Sporadic cases that occur in isolation may result from a vascular insult [23]. It can be inherited as an autosomal dominant trait. However, chromosomal analysis frequently shows trisomy 18, trisomy 21, extra copies of the X chromosome in girls or boys, or multiple copies of the Y chromosome in boys. Common associated regional abnormalities include absent or rudimentary thumbs, symphalangism, carpal coalition, and abnormal musculature. Of other coexisting skeletal anomalies, Nievergelt syndrome (radioulnar synostosis, shortening and deformity of the tibia, and tarsal/carpal coalition) is the best known. There is also a high incidence of radioulnar synostosis in fetal alcohol syndrome. In patients with autosomal dominant amegakaryocytic thrombocytopenia and radioulnar synostosis, mutations in the homeobox A11 (HOXA11) gene have been reported. HOX genes play a critical role in limb development [23].

In the unusual case of synostosis involving the humerus (humeroradial, humeroradioulnar, or humeroulnar), the deformity is sporadic if there is also ulnar hypoplasia. However, if the ulna is normal, the disorder is likely to be familial and may be associated with multiple synostosis, Pfeiffer, Apert, or Antley-Bixler syndrome [18].

The extent of restricted pronation helps determine the need for surgery, such as a derotational osteotomy [20]. Surgery is generally only warranted in bilateral cases or those with hyperpronation. There is no current procedure to restore rotation, so surgical treatment focuses on achieving the best rotational position for function.

Imaging

An osseous bar is sometimes visible radiologically in infancy (Fig. 7.17), but even if fusion is only cartilaginous, tethering may produce secondary changes. The osseous coalition that eventually results may fully engulf the radial head, or the radial head may be identified as a separate entity (Figs. 7.18 and 7.19). Occasionally, a thin, nonossified septum divides the bony fusion. In general, the extent of fusion correlates with the severity of radial head dysplasia, and the configuration of the radial head may suggest the type of fusion before it has ossified. The distal radius is often bowed laterally or anteriorly, increasing the interosseous space (see Fig. 7.19) the distal ulna may be subluxated [20] or the entire forearm shortened. The thumb may be abnormal (Fig. 7.20) MRI depicts marrow continuity (Figs. 7.21 and 7.22) and may demonstrate an aberrant radial ligament.

Classification

Several classification schemes have been proposed. According to Cleary and Omer, type I (19 %) consists of a fibrous synostosis with normal configuration and position of the radial head. In type II (8 %), there is a visible bony synostosis, but the radial head is still normal. The most common form, type III (56 %), consists of a visible bony synostosis, accompanied with a hypoplastic and posteriorly dislocated radial head. A short osseous synostosis with anterior dislocation of a mushroom-shaped humeral head characterizes type IV (17 %). There is no relationship between pattern and function [24].

4 Congenital Dislocation of the Radial Head (Box 7.3)

Box 7.3: Congenital Radial Head Dislocation

Posterior 65 %, anterior 18 %, lateral 17 %
Small, dysplastic capitellum
Dome-shaped radial head and thin radial neck
Radioulnar synostoses may be associated
Differentiate from traumatic dislocation
  Radial head dysplastic: flat with central concavity

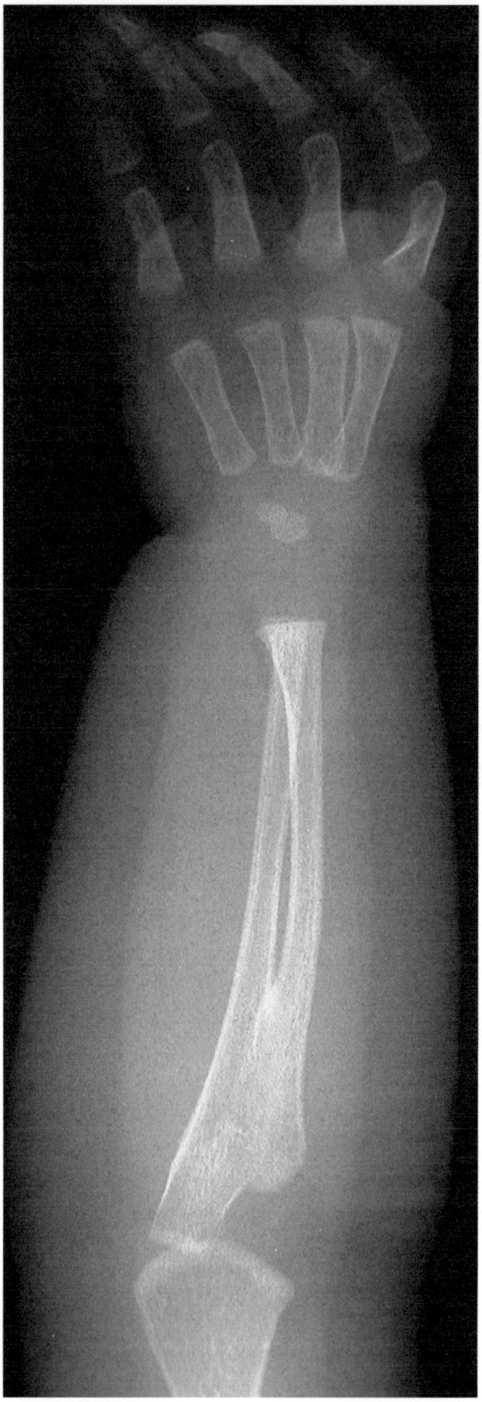

Fig. 7.18 Long-segment radioulnar synostosis, with mild displacement of the non-ossified radial head. The thumb is absent (Image copyright Shriners Hospital for Children Northern California)

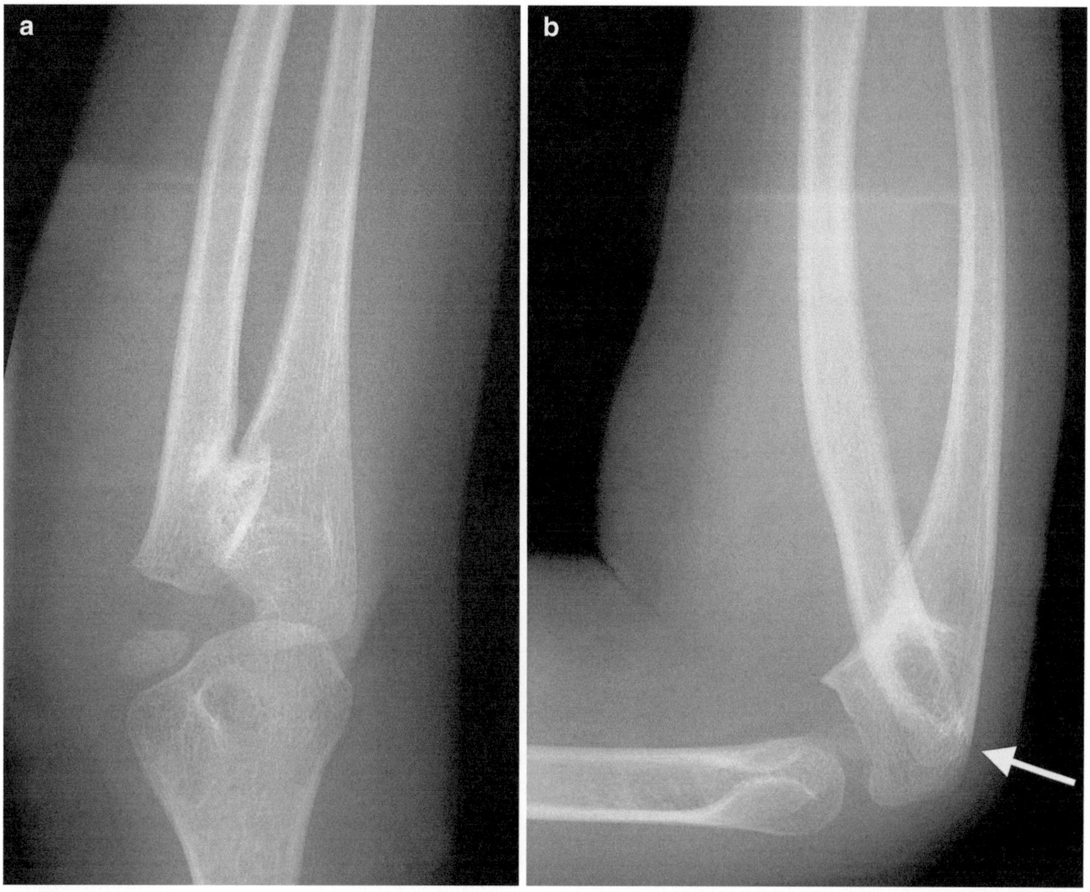

Fig. 7.19 Radioulnar synostosis. (**a**, **b**) Short-segment fusion with dorsal dislocation of the incorporated radial head (*arrow*). The radius is bowed with the apex anterior (Images copyright Shriners Hospital for Children Northern California)

Dislocation of the radial head is the most common congenital anomaly of the elbow. It is typically painless until adolescence, and presentation—due to deformity or restricted motion at the elbow—is often delayed. Clinically occult cases may present in the setting of trauma; differentiation from traumatic dislocation is important, as closed reduction succeeds only in the latter.

Congenital radial head dislocation may occur as an isolated defect or in association with other anomalies, though the literature is inconsistent about the frequency of associated anomalies. Between 35 and 60 % of cases are associated with such conditions as scoliosis, anomalous lower extremities, mental retardation, and numerous syndromes (such as nail-patella and Klippel-Feil) [19, 25, 26]. Whether the dislocation is isolated or associated with other anomalies, inheritance is usually autosomal dominant [26, 27]. Dislocation is most often posterior (65 %), but can be anterior (18 %) or lateral (17 %) [28]. The condition is often bilateral [28, 29]. The literature disagrees about whether isolated unilateral dislocations are congenital or secondary.

The normal radial head is relatively small and relatively poorly restrained by muscular and ligamentous structures, and the normal capitellum prevents dislocation in full extension. In cases of congenital dislocation of the radial head, the underlying abnormality is probably the formation of a hypoplastic and retroverted capitellum; the absence of normal pressure on the radial head results in an abnormal configuration of the radial head and radiocapitellar joint [26, 30, 31]. This is analogous to the sequence of events in developmental dysplasia of the hip. The annular ligament develops normally, but it does not contain the hypoplastic radial head [26].

Flexion and extension are usually unimpaired and, despite some limitation of rotation, children often have little functional impairment, as they tend to compensate well with wrist and shoulder movement. Standard treatment for painful congenital dislocation has been excision of the radial head, but complications abound, and so this is generally not attempted until skeletal maturity. More recently, open realignment at an early age has been suggested [31, 32].

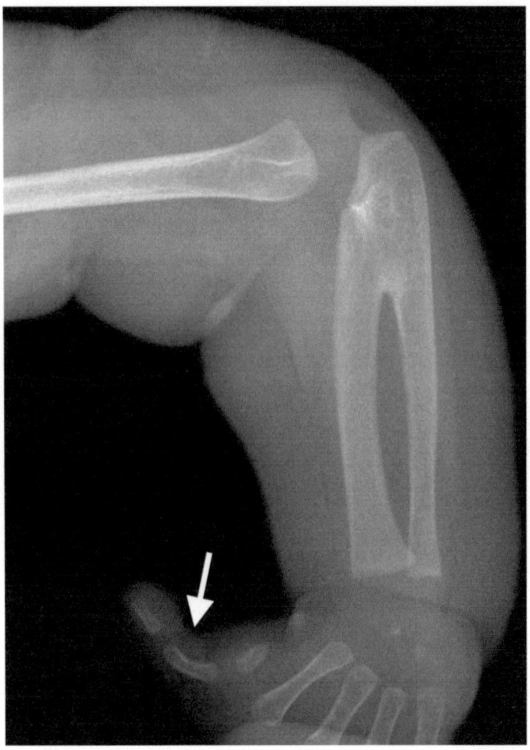

Fig. 7.20 Radiohumeral synostosis. The proximal radius and ulna are fused, and the thumb is hypoplastic (*arrow*) (Image copyright Shriners Hospital for Children Northern California)

Imaging

Diagnosis of congenital dislocation is straightforward if the condition is familial, present at birth, or bilateral; accompanying anomalies or syndromic features also facilitate diagnosis. Radiologic criteria include a small and dysplastic humeral capitellum, a dome-shaped radial head that lacks a normal central depression, and a thin radial neck (Fig. 7.23). There may be radioulnar synostosis and anomalies of the hand. Prior to age 5, when the radial head usually ossifies, its position can be deduced by noting whether a line drawn along the radial shaft bisects the capitellum (indicating normal radial head position) or whether it is directed anteriorly, posteriorly, or laterally. With posterior dislocation, the radius is often bowed with convexity anterior. The ulna is often bowed in the same direction as the radial head dislocation [31]; it may be short. Ultrasound or MRI can also demonstrate the position of the cartilaginous radial head (Fig. 7.24).

Differential Diagnosis

Congenital dislocation must be differentiated from posttraumatic dislocation, as clinically occult cases may come to attention in the setting of trauma. With traumatic dislocation, the radial head

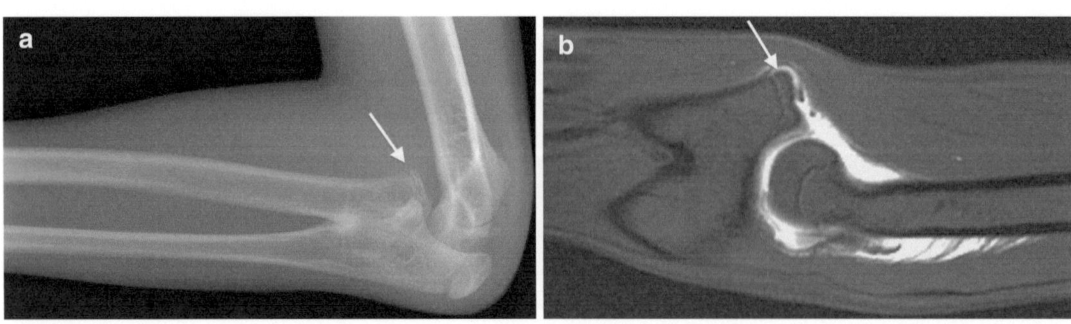

Fig. 7.21 Short-segment radioulnar synostosis. (**a**) The radial head (*arrow*) is anteriorly dislocated. (**b**) The sagittal T1-W FS arthrogram demonstrates marrow continuity in the synostosis, as well as the dislocated radial head (*arrow*)

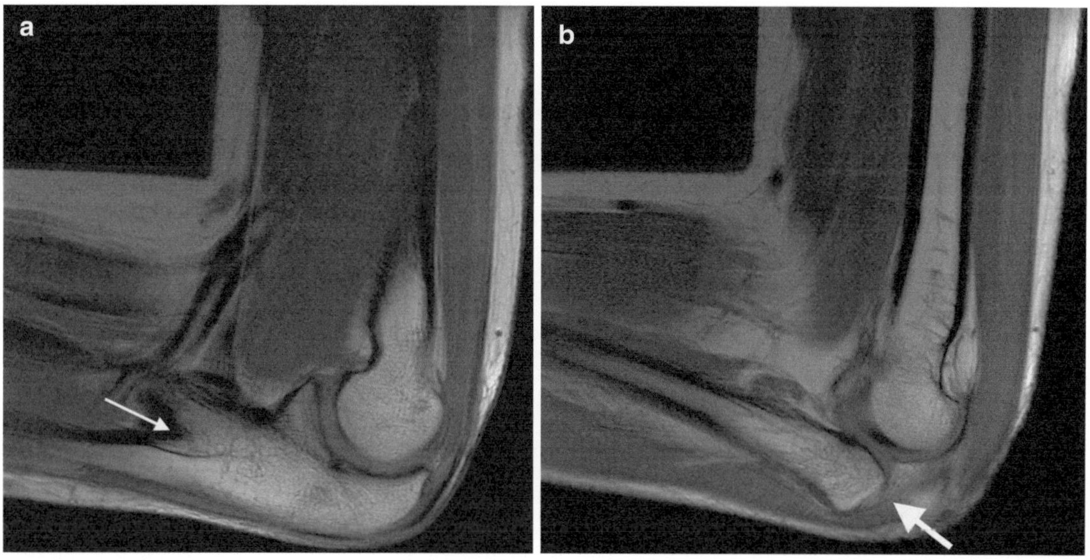

Fig. 7.22 Radioulnar synostosis. (**a**, **b**) Sagittal T1-W MRI images demonstrate close approximation of the proximal radius and ulna with suggestion of marrow continuity (*arrow*). The radial head is convex and dorsally dislocated (*arrow*)

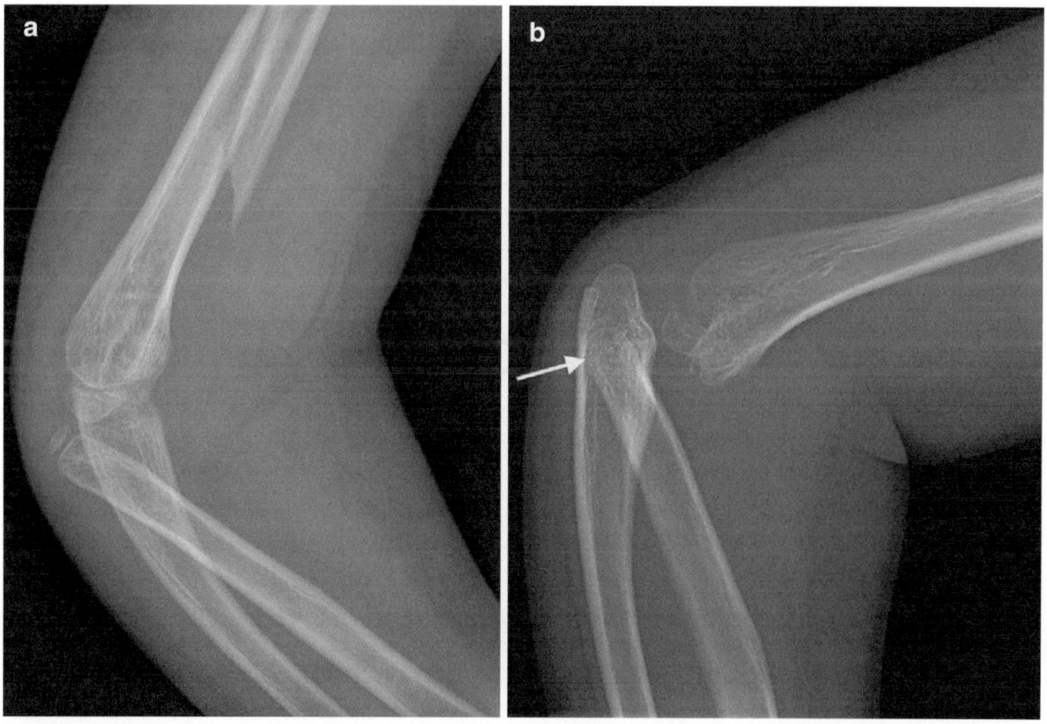

Fig. 7.23 Bilateral posterior congenital dislocation of the elbow in an 8-year-old boy presenting after trauma. (**a**) Acute humeral diaphyseal fracture with convex configuration of the radial head and small capitellum consistent with congenital dislocation. (**b**) Posterior dislocation (*arrow*) is also present on the contralateral asymptomatic side

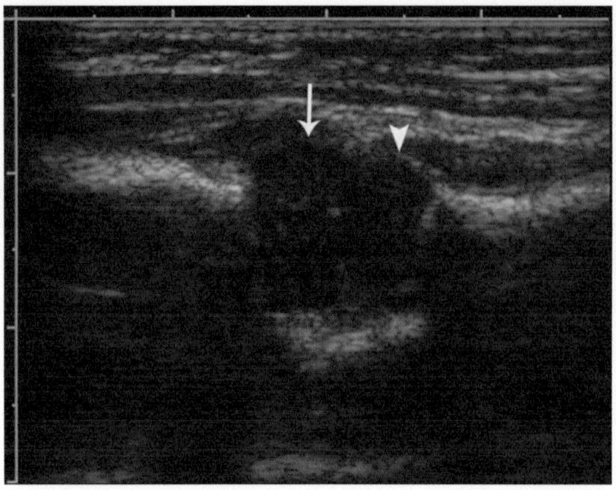

Fig. 7.24 Normal elbow in an 8-month-old boy with suspected radial head dislocation. Sagittal US from an anterior approach demonstrates a normal relationship between the nonossified capitellum (*arrow*) and radial head (*arrowhead*)

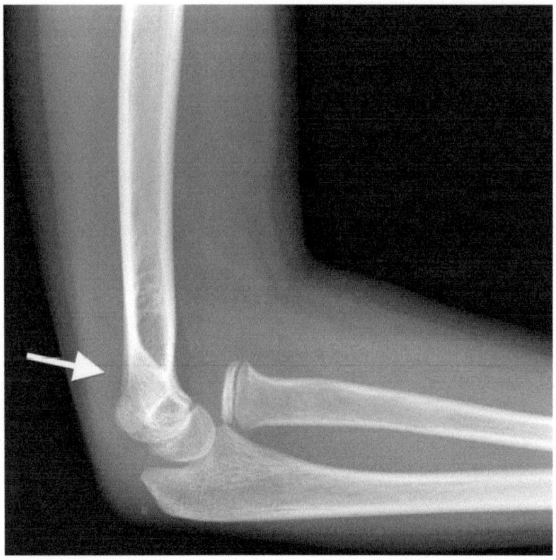

Fig. 7.25 Traumatic radial head dislocation. Note the normal configuration of the proximal radius despite its anterior dislocation. The posterior fat pad is elevated (*arrow*) due to a small joint effusion

has a normal flattened and centrally umbilicated configuration, and the capitellum is well developed (Fig. 7.25). The ulna is neither short nor bowed. Chronic dislocation of the radial head may also result from mass effect due to osteochondromas (Fig. 7.26) and tumors or from muscle imbalance in brachial plexus birth palsy (Fig. 7.27), arthrogryposis (Fig. 7.28), and cerebral palsy.

5 Madelung Deformity (Box 7.4)

Box 7.4: Madelung Deformity

Hyperangulation of distal radial articular surface

Proximal carpal row appears triangular (lunate at apex)

Radius bowed

Physeal bar bridges volar aspect of distal radial physis

MRI: Vickers ligament tethers lunate and/or triquetrum to radius

Madelung deformity of the wrist is a rare but well-defined clinical and radiological complex. A bayonet-like deformity of the wrist and hand is usually accompanied by decreased extension and supination; the distal ulna is prominent and dorsally dislocated, although reducible. Often bilateral, it is four times more common in girls. Patients typically present early in adolescence with progressive cosmetic deformity and decreased forearm rotation. Pain is thought to result from stretching of the ligaments [33].

The deformity may result from a bony bridge that traverses the ulnar aspect of the distal radial growth plate and causes tethering and asymmetric growth, although some favor a muscular disorder or vascular insufficiency as etiology [34–37]. There is relative shortening of the ulnar side of the radius and rotation of the articular surface. A thickened volar ligament, termed the Vickers ligament, tethers the lunate and/or triquetrum to the radius and may thin the distal radial epiphysis due to compression [36].

Madelung deformity may be idiopathic, secondary (due to damage from osteomyelitis or trauma or due to distortion resulting from multiple enchondromas or exostoses (see Fig. 7.26)), or genetic. The combination of Madelung deformity, short stature, and mesomelic shortening (forearms and tibias) constitutes Leri-Weill dyschondrosteosis [38]. This autosomal dominant disorder has variable penetrance and occurs predominantly in females. The incidence of dyschondrosteosis in patients with Madelung

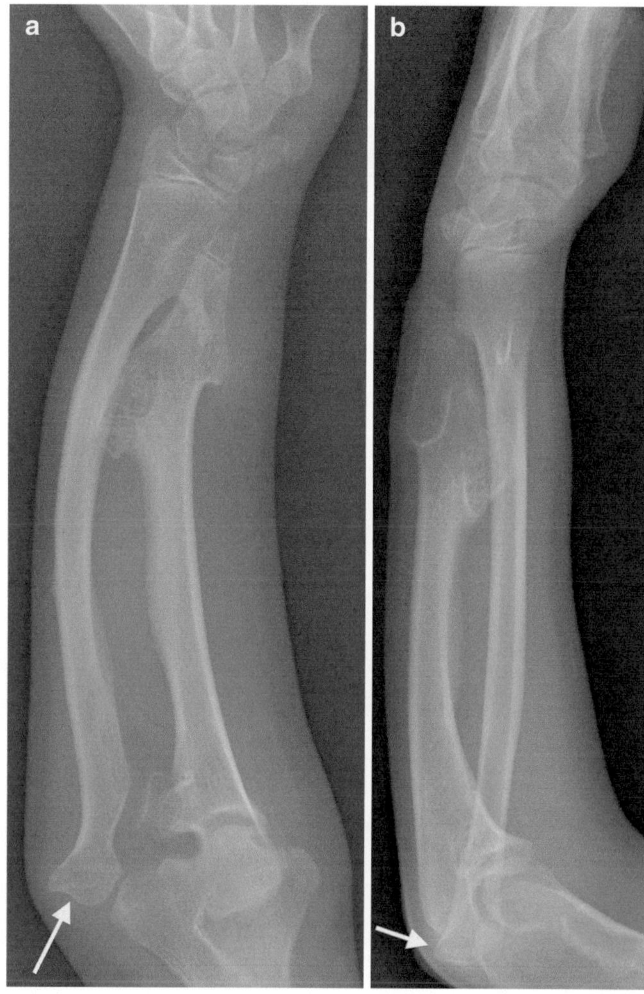

Fig. 7.26 Dislocation due to deformity secondary to multiple osteochondromas. (**a**) There are numerous osteochondromas, the largest at the distal ulna, with resultant ulnar foreshortening and dysplasia. The radius is elongated and bowed, and there is radial displacement of the dysplastic head (*arrow*). (**b**) There is also posterior dislocation of the radial head (*arrow*) (Images copyright Shriners Hospital for Children Northern California)

deformity is uncertain [34, 39–41]. A good but imperfect genetic test SHOX DNA DX can now identify the short stature homeobox genes in patients with this disorder. Madelung deformity is also associated with dysostosis multiplex and gonadal dysgenesis.

Treatment is usually unnecessary, but pain, severe cosmetic disturbance, and limited mobility may warrant intervention. Surgery is more likely to succeed when Madelung deformity is diagnosed before there is significant osseous distortion [39, 42].

Imaging

Radiographic findings are diagnostic but vary in degree (Figs. 7.29, 7.30, and 7.31). The major and primary change is in the radius; its carpal articular surface faces the ulna, hyperangulated to tilt 60° in a volar direction and up to 80° toward the ulna. The radius is short and bowed, with its convexity dorsal and lateral. Severe articular tilt, with accompanying ulnar shortening and dorsal dislocation, causes the proximal row of the carpal bones to assume a triangular configuration, with the lunate at the proximal apex and shifted volarly. The presence of abnormal ligaments may create a flame-shaped lucency at the distal radius adjacent to the ulna. The entire radial diaphysis may be bowed, and the radiocapitellar distance may be increased [40].

Several measurement techniques help quantify the extent of the abnormality [42]. Measurement of the lunate fossa angle (between a line parallel to the longitudinal axis of the ulna and a line

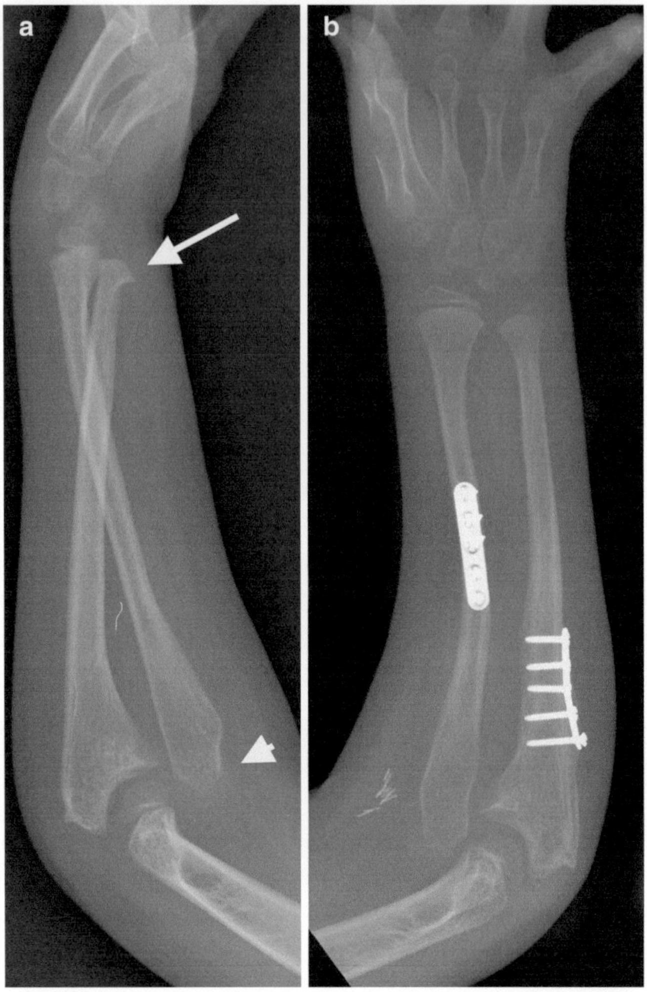

Fig. 7.27 Dislocated radial head in a patient with brachial plexus birth palsy. (**a**) Anterior dislocation of the radial head (*short arrow*) results from muscle imbalance. The distal ulna is also subluxated and hypoplastic (*long arrow*). (**b**) Alignment is improved after osteotomies (Images copyright Shriners Hospital for Children Northern California)

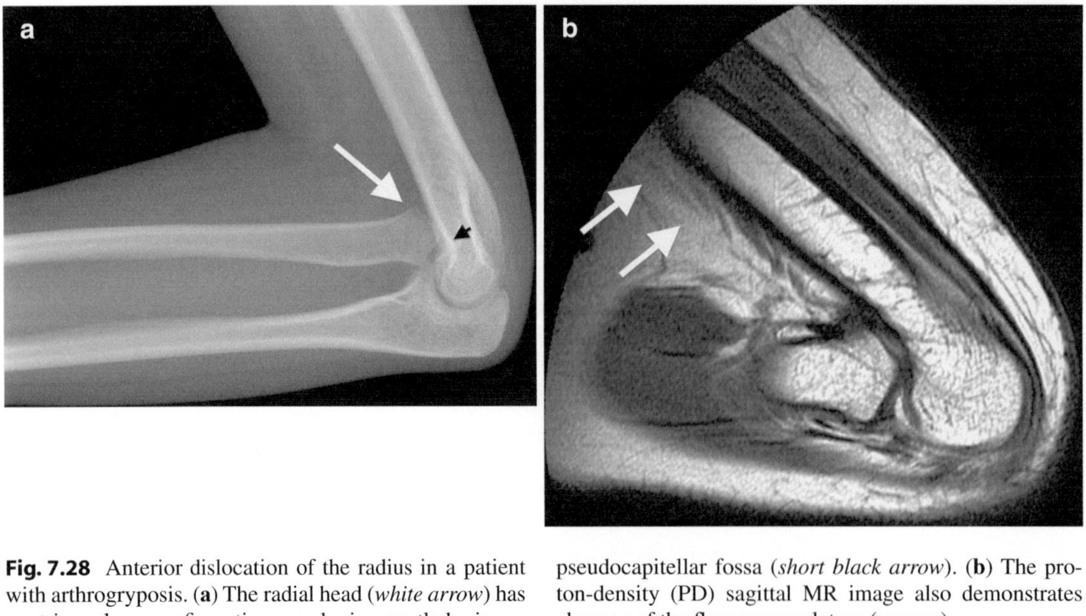

Fig. 7.28 Anterior dislocation of the radius in a patient with arthrogryposis. (**a**) The radial head (*white arrow*) has a triangular configuration and is nestled in a pseudocapitellar fossa (*short black arrow*). (**b**) The proton-density (PD) sagittal MR image also demonstrates absence of the flexor musculature (*arrows*)

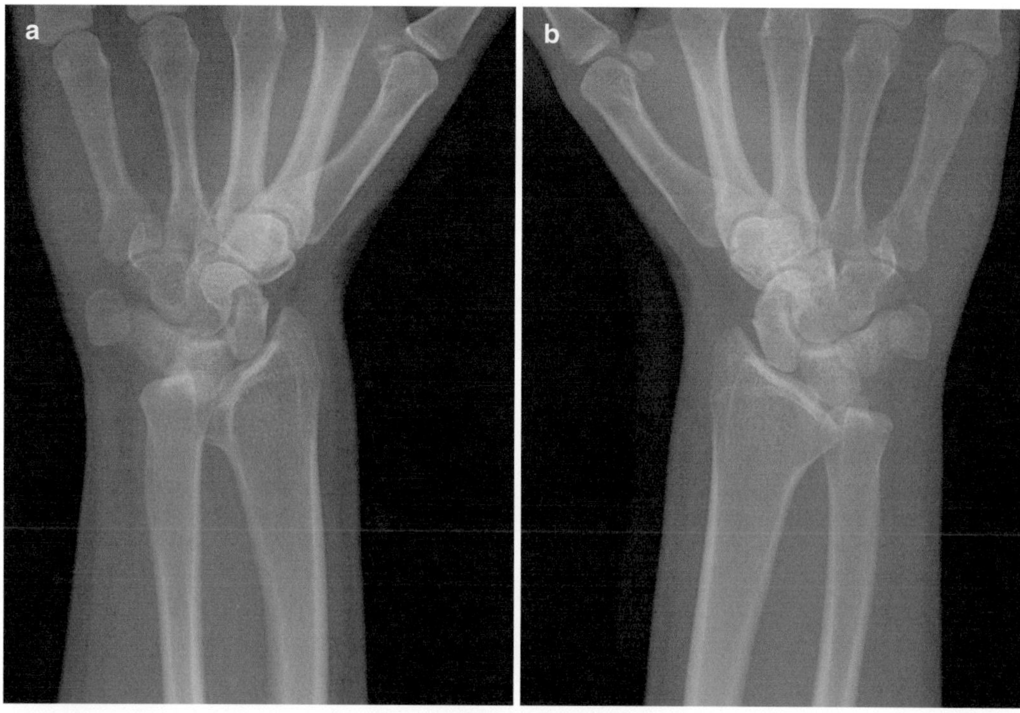

Fig. 7.29 Bilateral Madelung deformity in a 15-year-old boy. (**a**, **b**) The angulation of the distal articular surfaces induces a triangular orientation to the proximal carpal rows. The undulation of the ulnar cortex of the radius is relatively mild (Images copyright Shriners Hospital for Children Northern California)

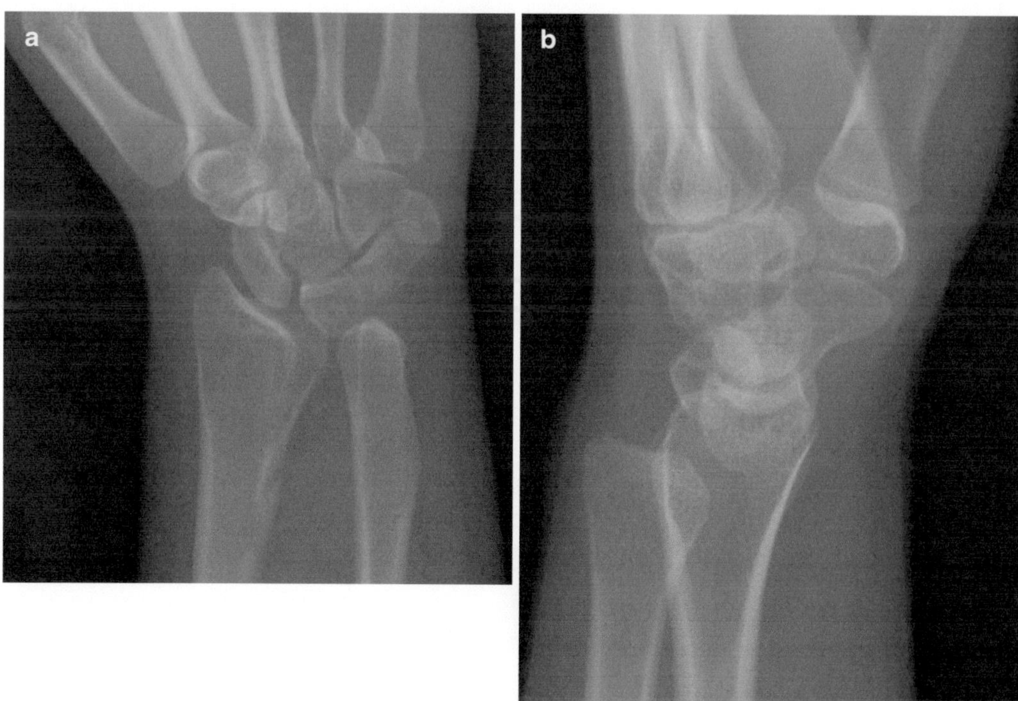

Fig. 7.30 Madelung deformity in a 16-year-old girl. On the frontal projection (**a**), the typical distal radial inclination is evident, as well as bowing deformity of the radius. The distal ulna is dorsally displaced on the lateral view (**b**) (Images copyright Shriners Hospital for Children Northern California)

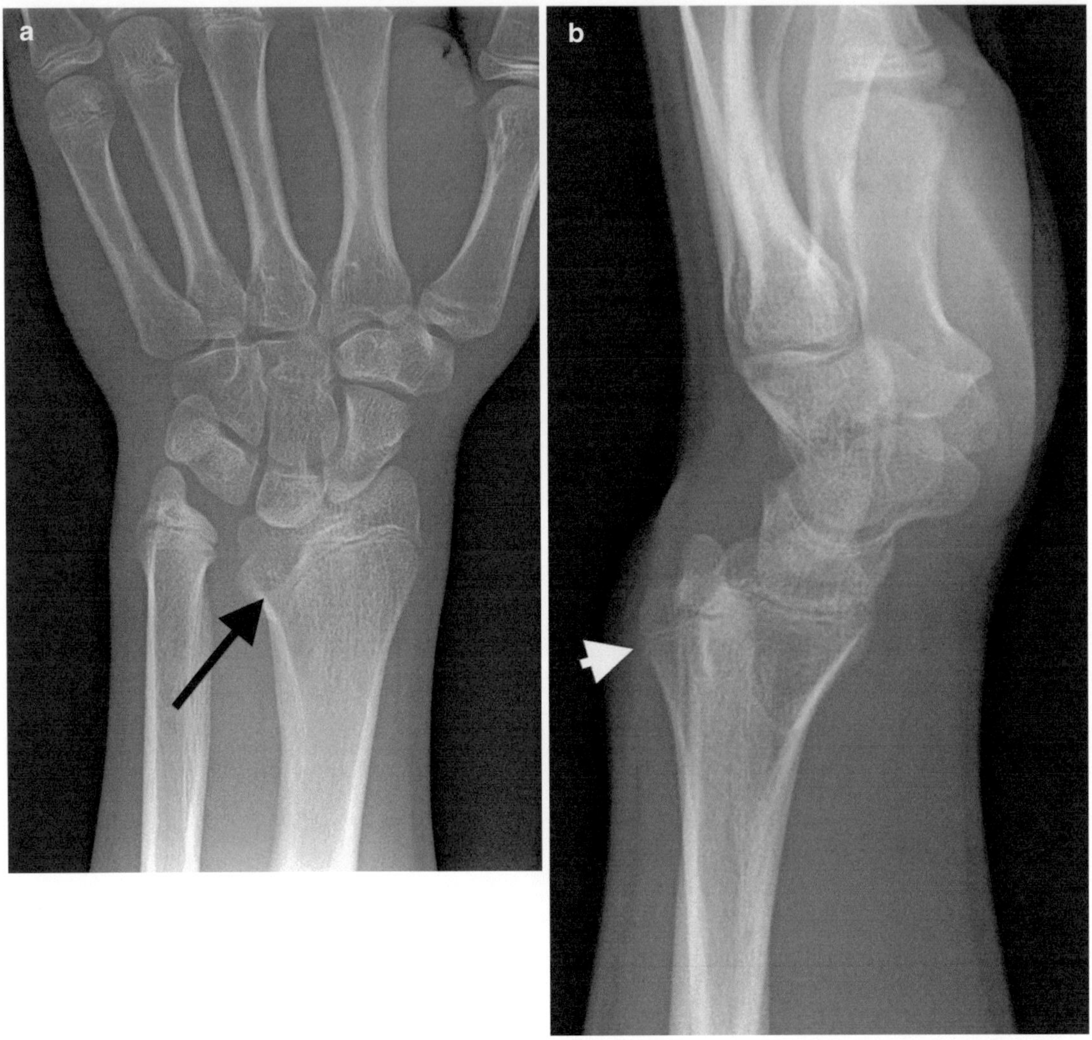

Fig. 7.31 Bilateral Madelung deformity (same patient as Fig. 7.32). The left (**a**, **b**) and right (**c**, **d**) wrists demonstrate typical distal radial angulation and triangular configuration of the carpal bones. The ulnar aspect of the distal radius on the left demonstrates striking flame-shaped lucency (*black arrow*). Dorsal dislocation of the distal ulna (*short white arrow*) is characteristic (Images copyright Shriners Hospital for Children Northern California)

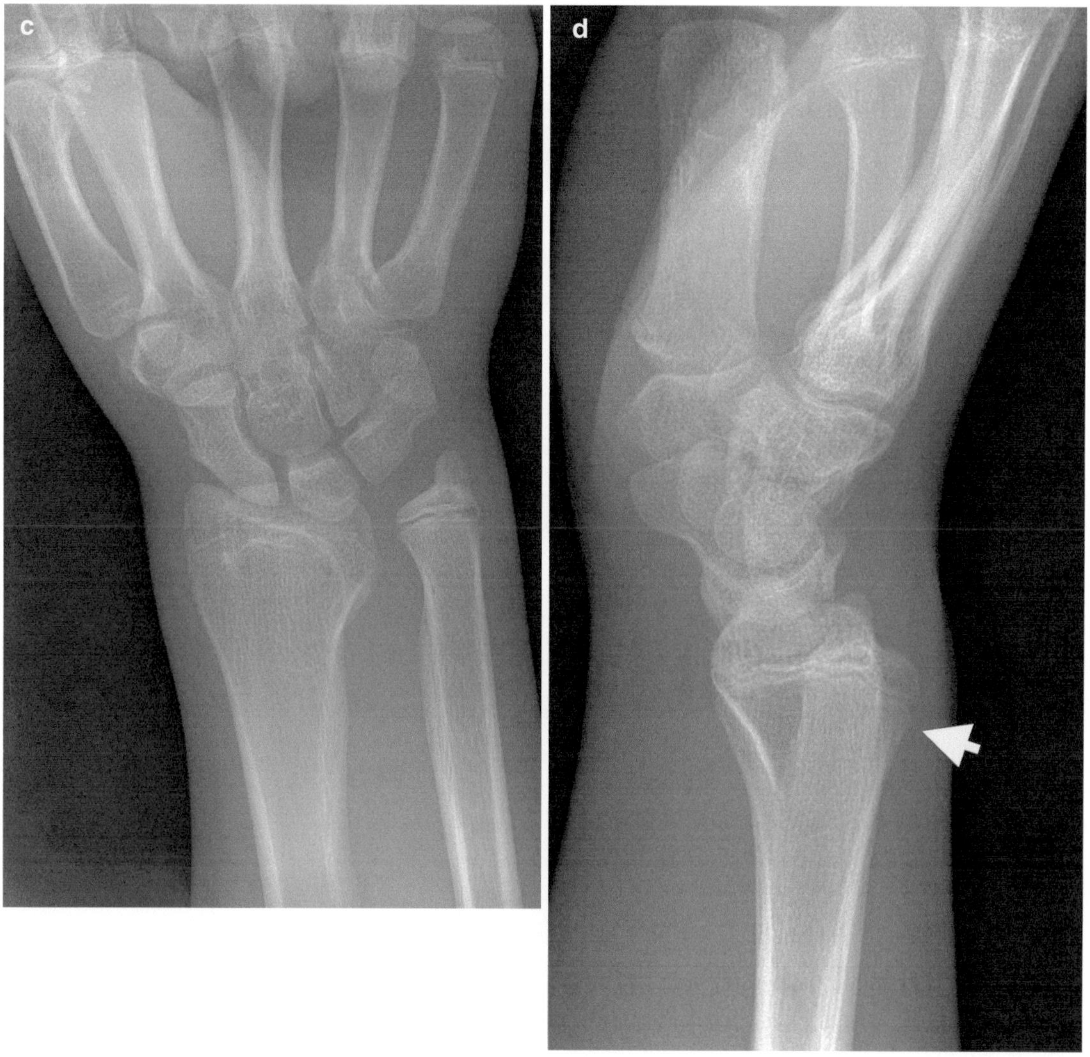

Fig. 7.31 (continued)

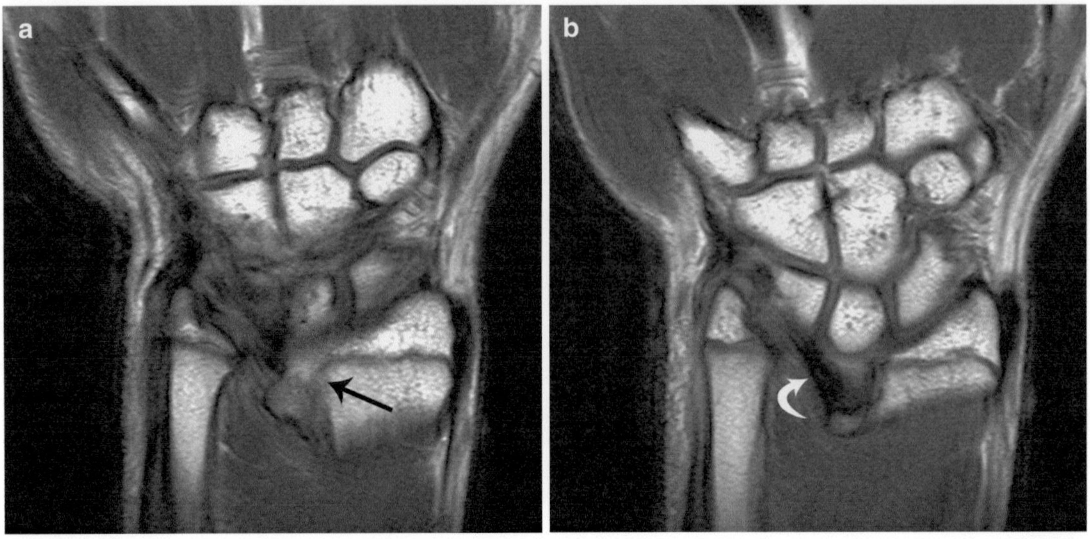

Fig. 7.32 Bilateral Madelung deformity on fast spin echo proton-density fat-suppressed (FSE PD FS) coronal MRI (same patient as Fig. 7.31). (**a**) The radial physis is wrapped over the metaphysis, and part of the osseous physeal bar (*arrow*) is evident. (**b**) A more posterior coronal image shows pronounced wrapping of the epiphysis, as well as the hypertrophied anomalous volar radiotriquetral ligament (*curved arrow*) between the radius and the triquetrum

across the lunate fossa of the radius, abnormal if greater than 40°) can diagnose early Madelung deformity in siblings or in the contralateral wrist, allowing early intervention. CT with 3D reconstruction is helpful for surgical planning.

MRI demonstrates a physeal bar bridging the volar aspect of the distal radial physis (Fig. 7.32); this may be more likely to be ossified in cases of dyschondrosteosis [43]. There are two anomalous ligaments: the hypertrophied radiolunate ligament (aka Vickers ligament) that may tether the lunate [36, 43] and the volar radiotriquetral ligament [35, 43]. These ligaments result in a lucent flame-shaped fossa in the distal radius. There is also notching of the distal radial articular surface [35].

References

1. Freyschmidt J, Brossmann J, Wiens J, Sternberg A. Koehler/Zimmer's borderlands of normal and early pathological findings in skeletal radiography. 5th ed. Stuttgart: Thieme; 2003.
2. Keats TL, Anderson MW. Atlas of normal roentgen variants that may simulate disease. 8th ed. Philadelphia: Mosby; 2006.
3. Swanson AB. Congenital limb defects classification and treatment. Clin Symp. 1981;33(3):1–32. PubMed PMID: 7344809, Epub 1981/01/01. eng.
4. Oberg KC, Feenstra JM, Manske PR, Tonkin MA. Developmental biology and classification of congenital anomalies of the hand and upper extremity. J Hand Surg Am. 2010;35(12):2066–76. PubMed PMID: 21134615, Epub 2010/12/08. eng.
5. Scotland TR, Galway HR. A long-term review of children with congenital and acquired upper limb deficiency. J Bone Joint Surg Br. 1983;65(3):346–9. PubMed PMID: 6841409, Epub 1983/05/01. eng.
6. Kelikian H. Congenital deformities of the hand and forearm. Philadelphia: WB Saunders; 1974.
7. Poznanski A. The hand in radiologic diagnosis. In: EJ P, editor. Philadelphia: WB Saunders and Company; 1984.
8. Goldfarb CA, Manske PR, Busa R, Mills J, Carter P, Ezaki M. Upper-extremity phocomelia reexamined: a longitudinal dysplasia. J Bone Joint Surg Am. 2005;87(12):2639–48. PubMed PMID: 16322613, Epub 2005/12/03. eng.
9. Goldfarb CA, Wall L, Manske PR. Radial longitudinal deficiency: the incidence of associated medical and musculoskeletal conditions. J Hand Surg Am. 2006;31(7):1176–82. PubMed PMID: 16945723, Epub 2006/09/02. eng.
10. Quan L, Smith DW. The VATER association. Vertebral defects, anal atresia, T-E fistula with esophageal atresia, radial and renal dysplasia: a spectrum of associated defects. J Pediatr. 1973;82(1):104–7. PubMed PMID: 4681850. Epub 1973/01/01. eng.

11. Bednar MS, James MA, Light TR. Congenital longitudinal deficiency. J Hand Surg Am. 2009;34(9):1739–47. PubMed PMID: 19896016, Epub 2009/11/10. eng.
12. Maschke SD, Seitz W, Lawton J. Radial longitudinal deficiency. J Am Acad Orthop Surg. 2007;15(1):41–52. PubMed PMID: 17213381, Epub 2007/01/11. eng.
13. James MA, McCarroll Jr HR, Manske PR. The spectrum of radial longitudinal deficiency: a modified classification. J Hand Surg Am. 1999;24(6):1145–55. PubMed PMID: 10584934, Epub 1999/12/10. eng.
14. Schmidt CC, Neufeld SK. Ulnar ray deficiency. Hand Clin. 1998;14(1):65–76. PubMed PMID: 9526157, Epub 1998/04/04. eng.
15. Ogden JA, Watson HK, Bohne W. Ulnar dysmelia. J Bone Joint Surg Am. 1976;58(4):467–75. PubMed PMID: 818089, Epub 1976/06/01. eng.
16. Azouz EM, Oudjhane K. Disorders of the upper extremity in children. Magn Reson Imaging Clin N Am. 1998;6(3):677–95. PubMed PMID: 9654591, Epub 1998/07/09. eng.
17. Makhoul IR, Goldstein I, Smolkin T, Avrahami R, Sujov P. Congenital limb deficiencies in newborn infants: prevalence, characteristics and prenatal diagnosis. Prenat Diagn. 2003;23(3):198–200. PubMed PMID: 12627419, Epub 2003/03/11. eng.
18. McIntyre JD, Brooks A, Benson MK. Humeroradial synostosis and the multiple synostosis syndrome: case report. J Pediatr Orthop B. 2003;12(3):192–6. PubMed PMID: 12703033, Epub 2003/04/19. eng.
19. Sachar K, Akelman E, Ehrlich MG. Radioulnar synostosis. Hand Clin. 1994;10(3):399–404. PubMed PMID: 7962146, Epub 1994/08/01. eng.
20. Yammine K, Salon A, Pouliquen JC. Congenital radioulnar synostosis. Study of a series of 37 children and adolescents. Chir Main. 1998;17(4):300–8.
21. Shinohara T, Horii E, Tatebe M, Yamamoto M, Okui N, Hirata H. Painful snapping elbow in patients with congenital radioulnar synostosis: report of two cases. J Hand Surg Am. 2010;35(8):1336–9. PubMed PMID: 20684930, Epub 2010/08/06. eng.
22. Wang E, Wenger DR, Zhang L, Zhao Q, Ji S, Li J. The mechanism of acute elbow flexion contracture in children with congenital proximal radioulnar synostosis. J Pediatr Orthop. 2010;30(3):277–81. PubMed PMID: 20357595. Epub 2010/04/02. eng.
23. Elliott AM, Kibria L, Reed MH. The developmental spectrum of proximal radioulnar synostosis. Skelet Radiol. 2010;39(1):49–54. PubMed PMID: 19669136, Epub 2009/08/12. eng.
24. Cleary JE, Omer Jr GE. Congenital proximal radioulnar synostosis. Natural history and functional assessment. J Bone Joint Surg. 1985;67(4):539–45. PubMed PMID: 3980498, Epub 1985/04/01. eng.
25. Lachman RS. Taybi and Lachman's radiology of syndromes, metabolic disorders and skeletal dysplasias. 5th ed. Philadelphia: Mosby; 2007.
26. Sachar K, Mih AD. Congenital radial head dislocations. Hand Clin. 1998;14(1):39–47. PubMed PMID: 9526155, Epub 1998/04/04. eng.
27. Cockshott WP, Omololu A. Familial congenital posterior dislocation of both radial heads. J Bone Joint Surg Br. 1958;40(3):483–6. PubMed PMID: 13575461, Epub 1958/08/01. eng.
28. Mardam-Bey T, Ger E. Congenital radial head dislocation. J Hand Surg Am. 1979;4(4):316–20. PubMed PMID: 469206, Epub 1979/07/01. eng.
29. Miura T. Congenital dislocation of the radial head. J Hand Surg Br. 1990;15(4):477–81. PubMed PMID: 2269842, Epub 1990/11/01. eng.
30. Wiley JJ, Loehr J, McIntyre W. Isolated dislocation of the radial head. Orthop Rev. 1991;20(11):973–6. PubMed PMID: 1749662, Epub 1991/11/01. eng.
31. Kim HT, Park BG, Suh JT, Yoo CI. Chronic radial head dislocation in children, part 2: results of open treatment and factors affecting final outcome. J Pediatr Orthop. 2002;22(5):591–7. PubMed PMID: 12198459. Epub 2002/08/29. eng.
32. Song KS, Ramnani K, Cho CH. Long term follow-up of open realignment procedure for congenital dislocation of the radial head. J Hand Surg Eur. 2011;36(2):161–2. PubMed PMID: 21285239, Epub 2011/02/03. eng.
33. Anderson BL, Lomasney LM, Demos TC, Bielski RJ. Radiologic case study. Madelung's deformity of the wrist. Orthopedics. 1997;20(6):576, 69-71. PubMed PMID: 9195641. Epub 1997/06/01. eng.
34. Schmidt-Rohlfing B, Schwobel B, Pauschert R, Niethard FU. Madelung deformity: clinical features, therapy and results. J Pediatr Orthop B. 2001;10(4):344–8. PubMed PMID: 11727381, Epub 2001/12/01. eng.
35. Stehling C, Langer M, Nassenstein I, Bachmann R, Heindel W, Vieth V. High resolution 3.0 Tesla MR imaging findings in patients with bilateral Madelung's deformity. Surg Radiol Anat. 2009;31(7):551–7.
36. Vickers D, Nielsen G. Madelung deformity: surgical prophylaxis (physiolysis) during the late growth period by resection of the dyschondrosteosis lesion. J Hand Surg Br. 1992;17(4):401–7. PubMed PMID: 1402266, Epub 1992/08/01. eng.
37. Aucourt J, Budzik JF, Manouvrier-Hanu S, Mezel A, Cotten A, Boutry N. Congenital malformations of the hand and forearm in children: what radiologists should know. Semin Musculoskelet Radiol. 2012;16(2):146–58. PubMed PMID: 22648430, Epub 2012/06/01. eng.
38. Langer Jr LO. Mesomelic dwarfism of the hypoplastic ulna, fibula, mandible type. Radiology. 1967;89(4):654–60. PubMed PMID: 6059604, Epub 1967/10/01. eng.
39. de Billy B, Gastaud F, Repetto M, Chataigner H, Clavert JM, Aubert D. Treatment of Madelung's deformity by lengthening and relaxation of the distal extremity of the radius by Ilizarov's technique. Eur J Pediatr Surg. 1997;7(5):296–8. PubMed PMID: 9402490, Epub 1997/12/24. eng.
40. Zebala LP, Manske PR, Goldfarb CA. Madelung's deformity: a spectrum of presentation. J Hand Surg Am. 2007;32(9):1393–401. PubMed PMID: 17996774, Epub 2007/11/13. eng.

41. Felman AH, Kirkpatrick Jr JA. Madelung's deformity: observations in 17 patients. Radiology. 1969;93(5):1037–42. PubMed PMID: 5350668, Epub 1969/11/01. eng.
42. McCarroll Jr HR, James MA, Newmeyer 3rd WL, Manske PR. Madelung's deformity: diagnostic thresholds of radiographic measurements. J Hand Surg Am. 2010;35(5):807–12. PubMed PMID: 20347533, Epub 2010/03/30. eng.
43. Cook PA, Yu JS, Wiand W, Lubbers L, Coleman CR, Cook 2nd AJ, et al. Madelung deformity in skeletally immature patients: morphologic assessment using radiography, CT, and MRI. J Comput Assist Tomogr. 1996;20(4):505–11. PubMed PMID: 8708046. Epub 1996/07/01. eng.

The Elbow and Forearm: Acquired Disorders

8

Markus Uhl

Contents

M. Uhl, MD, PhD
Department of Radiology, RKK Klinikum,
Sautierstr 1, Freiburg D-79104, Germany
e-mail: markus.uhl@rkk-sjk.de

Abstract

This chapter first discusses the timing of ossification of the apophyses and epiphyses at the elbow, as an understanding of the appearance of the normal elbow is essential to correct interpretation of the pediatric elbow radiograph. It then discusses fractures that are common in younger children, such as supracondylar, lateral condylar, and medial condylar fractures. It presents radial neck and olecranon fractures, generally encountered in the adolescent period. The many injuries that result from valgus stress are then discussed, including osteochondritis dissecans of the capitellum and medial epicondylar apophysitis. The chapter concludes with a presentation of osteochondrosis of the capitellum (Panner disease).

Fractures and overuse injuries are common in the pediatric elbow. Supracondylar, lateral condylar, and medial condylar fractures are especially common in younger children, often due to falls. After these centers fuse, physeal injuries no longer occur; radial neck fractures and olecranon fractures become more common in the adolescent period. Repetitive valgus stress—such as occurs in pitchers and other throwing athletes—may lead to osteochondritis dissecans of the capitellum, apophysitis of the medial epicondyle or olecranon, loose bodies, and growth disturbances. (Infection, neoplasia, and arthritis are addressed in Chaps. 19, 20, 21, and 22).

R. Stein-Wexler et al. (eds.), *Pediatric Orthopedic Imaging*,
DOI 10.1007/978-3-642-45381-6_8, © Springer-Verlag Berlin Heidelberg 2015

1 Normal and Variant Anatomy

The elbow joint is composed of three articulations—the radiocapitellar, ulnohumeral, and proximal radioulnar joints—all contained within a common joint cavity. The elbow is intrinsically stable due to the shape and congruence of its articular surfaces, and the ligaments provide additional extrinsic stability. The radial head rotates within the radial notch of the ulna, allowing supination and pronation. The proximal radius articulates with the capitellum of the distal humerus, and the proximal ulna articulates with the trochlea of the distal humerus. The olecranon and coronoid processes of the proximal ulna together form a pincerlike structure, allowing hinge-like flexion and extension of the elbow.

Thorough knowledge of the appearance of the multiple apophyses and epiphyses is essential to correct interpretation of the pediatric elbow radiograph in the setting of trauma. Six ossification centers (four in the distal humerus, one each in the proximal radius and ulna) develop in an orderly sequence: capitellum first, followed by the radial head, medial (or inner) epicondyle, trochlea, olecranon, and—finally—the lateral (or external) epicondyle (Fig. 8.1) (Box 8.1). The mnemonic "CRITOE" is helpful to remember the typical order of ossification. These centers infrequently ossify out of order. The capitellum contributes to the growth of the humerus and is therefore considered an epiphysis. The other ossification centers are apophyses.

> **Box 8.1: Typical Order of Ossification at the Elbow**
> C—capitellum
> R—radial head
> I—internal, or medial, epicondyle
> T—trochlea
> O—olecranon
> E—external, or lateral, epicondyle

Bone maturation is affected by genetic and racial variability as well as environmental factors and pathological processes that can affect bone growth and maturation [1, 2]. There is no significant difference in timing or ossification pattern between the right and left elbow [3]. However, the timing of appearance of the ossification centers varies widely (Table 8.1). All except the capitellum appear and fuse at least 1 year earlier in girls than in boys [1]. The capitellum ossifies at about 3 months in girls and 6 months in boys. The approximate age of ossification for the five

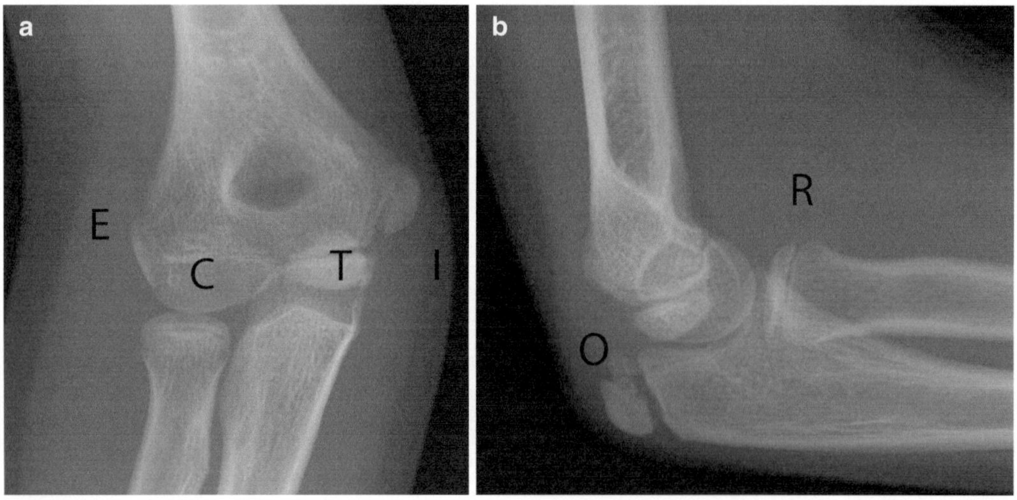

Fig. 8.1 (**a**, **b**) Six ossification centers of the distal humerus. *C* capitulum, *R* radial head, *M* medial epicondyle, *O* olecranon, *T* trochlea, *L* lateral epicondyle

Table 8.1 Reported ranges of appearance and fusion of ossification centers about the elbow

	Girls—age of appearance	Girls—age of fusion	Boys—age of appearance	Boys—age of fusion
Capitellum	0.33–1	9.4–15	0.08–1	12.4–17.5
Radial head	1.6–6.8	10.2–15	2.9–8.5	12.4–17.1
Medial epicondyle	1.3–7.1	11.5–15.3	3.5–9.7	13–16.8
Trochlea	5.7–11.1	9.2–13	7–12.5	11.6–15.2
Olecranon	6–11	10.8–14.8	7.6–12.2	12.4–16.5
Lateral epicondyle	7.3–11.6	9.5–13.3	8–14.4	12.1–15.9

Adapted from Ref. [1]

other centers in girls is 5 years for the radial head, 5 years for the medial epicondyle, 8–9 years for the trochlea, 8 years for the olecranon, and 9 years for the lateral epicondyle. In boys, the radial head ossification center appears at approximately 5–6 years, medial epicondyle at 7 years, trochlea at 9 years, olecranon at 10 years, and lateral epicondyle at 11 years. In general, the centers that ossify after the radial head appear about 2 years later in boys than in girls [1, 3–5].

The range of age of fusion of the elbow ossification centers is listed in Table 8.1. In general, girls fuse earlier than boys.

2 Distal Humeral Fractures

2.1 Supracondylar Fractures (Box 8.2)

Box 8.2: Supracondylar Fractures

Most common pediatric elbow fracture, age 5–9

Usually extension injury → posterior displacement of capitellum

Normally anterior humeral line should intersect posterior or middle one third capitellum

Disrupted hourglass or figure eight

Supracondylar fractures are the most common pediatric elbow fracture. The peak incidence is between 5 and 9 years of age, and boys are affected twice as often as girls [6]. The left elbow is affected more often than the right. These fractures usually result from a fall such as from a chair, crib, or playground equipment, and most are caused by hyperextension when the child falls on the outstretched extremity [7].

Supracondylar fractures are categorized according to mechanism of injury, which is determined by assessing the angulation of the distal fragment. The vast majority (95 %) result from extension injury. Only 5 % result from flexion, and these occur predominantly in older children. With the extension type of fracture, the capitellum is posteriorly displaced. Many systems have been developed for classifying these fractures. The Gartland system employs three categories, based on the degree of displacement [8]:

- Type 1: Nondisplaced or minimally displaced fracture (hairline fracture) (Fig. 8.2).
- Type 2: Partially displaced (posterior cortical hinge is intact (in extension-type fractures), fragments are nearly aligned, and some bony contact is present) (Fig. 8.3).
- Type 3: Completely displaced (no posterior cortical hinge (in extension-type fractures); fracture fragments are widely separated) (Fig. 8.4).

Numerous newer classification systems have been developed, but they offer neither more reproducibility nor better interobserver validity.

Compartment syndrome may develop at the flexor compartment if there is direct laceration or interruption, spasm, or intimal tear of the brachial artery [6] or even in the absence of these complications. The median and radial nerves are at risk for injury in an extension-type fracture, while the ulnar nerve is more vulnerable in a flexion-type fracture. These injuries are more likely with a Gartland Type 3 displaced fracture.

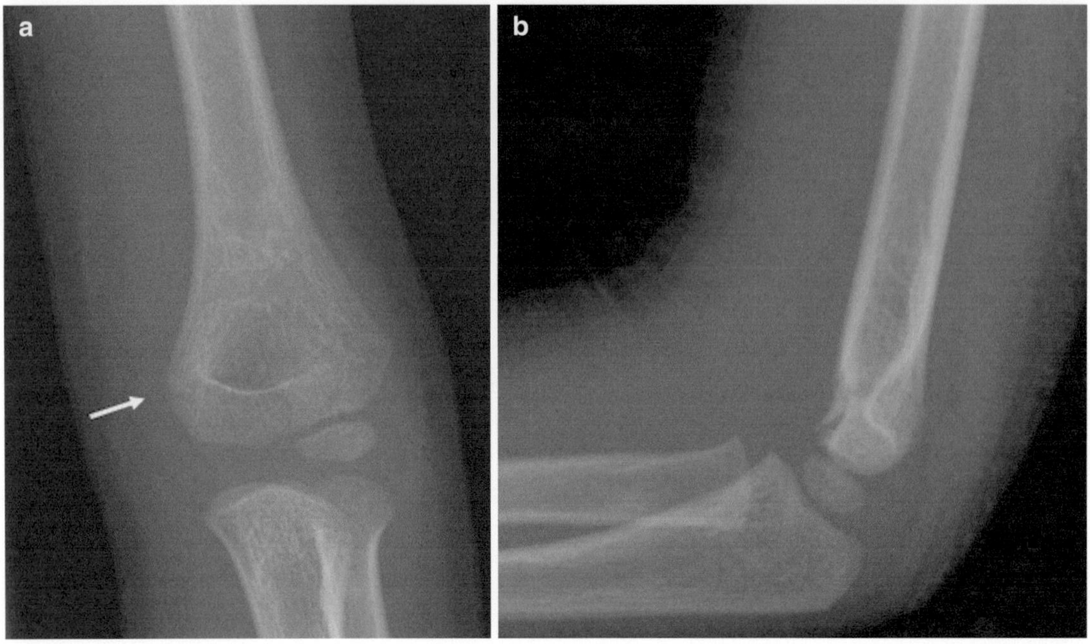

Fig. 8.2 Gartland type I minimally displaced supracondylar fracture. (**a**, **b**) There is subtle lucency, most obvious at the lateral supracondylar region (*arrow*). Alignment is normal

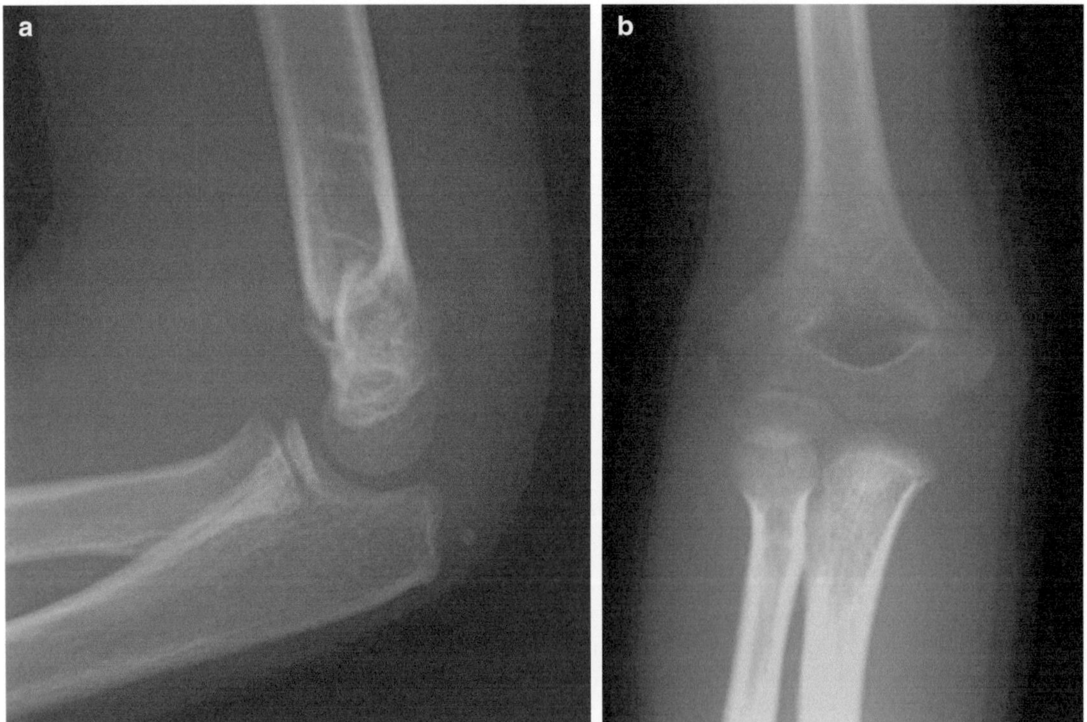

Fig. 8.3 Gartland Type II partially displaced supracondylar fracture. (**a**, **b**) The fracture line is more apparent at the lateral condyle. There is mild posterior displacement of the capitellum, but some bony contact is maintained

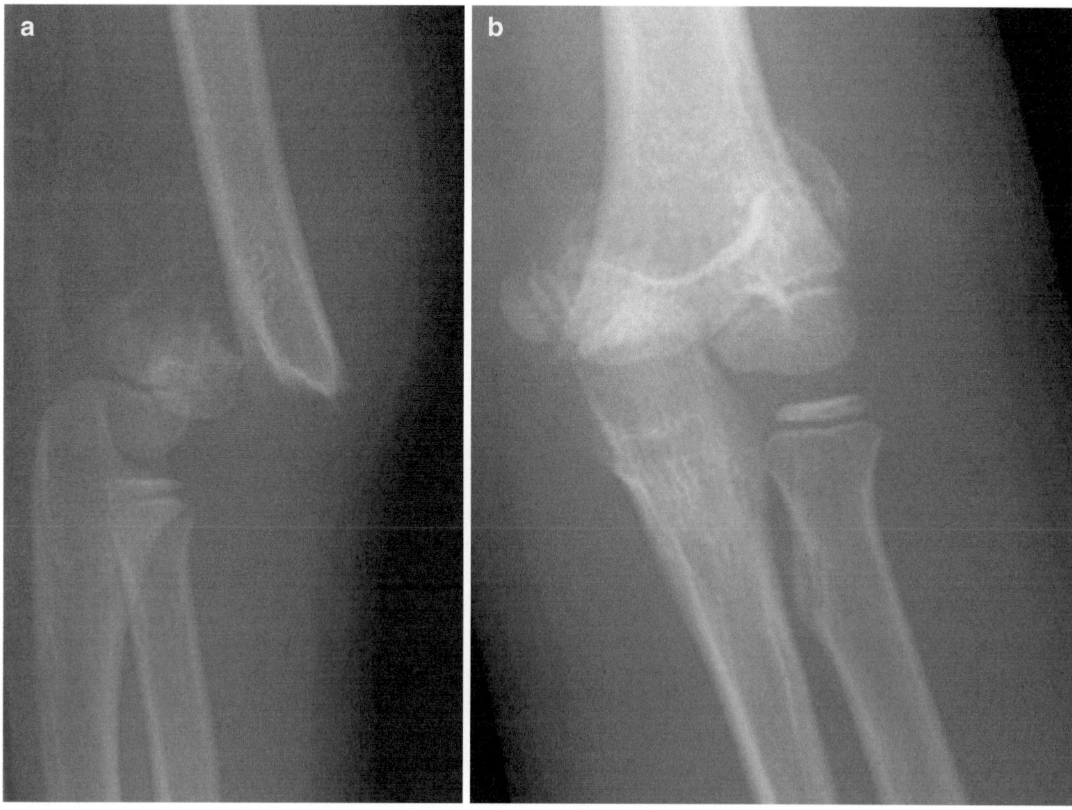

Fig. 8.4 Gartland Type III completely displaced supracondylar fracture. (**a**, **b**) The fracture is complete, and the distal fragment displaced by at least one bone width posteriorly. There is no contact between the fragments

The degree of displacement dictates the type of treatment. Type 1 Gartland extension fractures are immobilized without manipulation. Type 2 and Type 3 fractures require operative treatment. Closed reduction is attempted, stabilized by at least two crossed stainless steel Kirschner wires (K-wires). The conservative approach is less successful with the uncommon flexion fractures, as they are less stable.

Imaging

High-quality radiographic technique is essential for successful detection of subtle elbow fractures in children. The minimum standard examination for evaluating the injured elbow consists of a frontal view of the straight elbow and a lateral view of the flexed elbow [7]. Careful assessment of the soft tissues around the elbow joint can provide helpful clues about the presence and location of a fracture.

The vast majority of elbow fractures are accompanied by fluid within the elbow joint. An elbow effusion is easily detected on a well-positioned lateral view due to displacement of the anterior and posterior fat pads of the distal humerus. In the normal elbow, the anterior fat pad is partially visible extending from the coronoid fossa, but the posterior fat pad is hidden within the deeper olecranon fossa (Fig. 8.5). As fluid accumulates within the joint space, it displaces these fat pads upward and outward [7, 9, 10]. In the absence of a positive fat pad, significant intra-articular injury is unlikely but not impossible, as a capsular tear may allow fluid to leak into the surrounding soft tissues, preventing distension of the joint capsule (Fig. 8.6). A visible fat pad sign without a demonstrable fracture often (but does not absolutely [11]) indicates an occult fracture in the setting of trauma.

The anterior humeral line helps identify slight capitellar displacement, which in turn suggests a

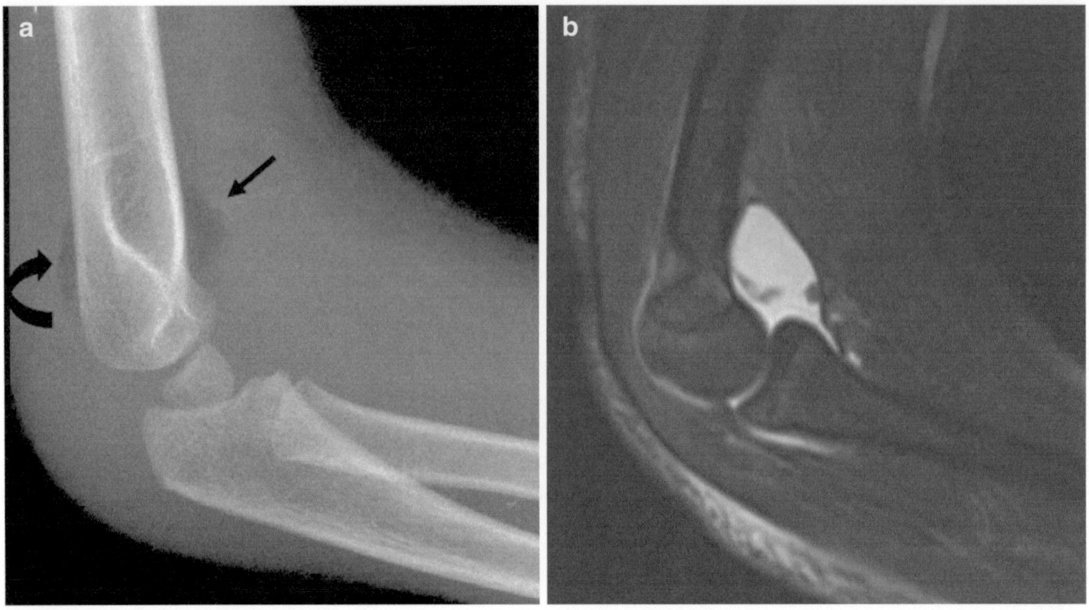

Fig. 8.5 Joint effusion. (**a**) The displaced anterior (*arrow*) and posterior (*curved arrow*) fat pads appear as lucent triangles extending from the bone margins. (**b**) T2-weighted (T2-W) fat-suppressed (FS) MRI shows hyperintense joint fluid elevating the soft tissues anterior to the joint

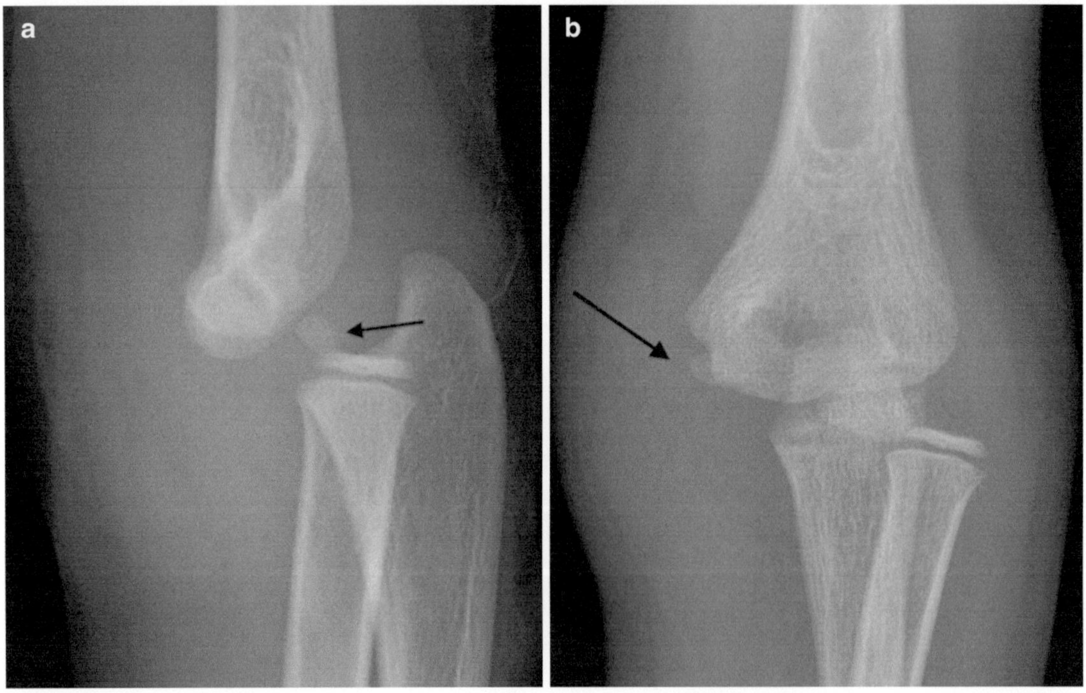

Fig. 8.6 Absence of a joint effusion despite severe injury. (**a**, **b**) The medial epicondyle is fractured and displaced (*arrow*), and the olecranon and radial head are also dislocated. Despite this severe trauma, there is no joint effusion. Increased density in the soft tissues probably results from extracapsular joint fluid due to capsular tear (Courtesy of Rebecca Stein-Wexler)

subtle distal humeral fracture may be present. This line is drawn along the anterior cortex of the humeral diaphysis on a well-positioned lateral view [7] and should intersect the posterior or middle third of the capitellum. If it crosses the capitellum more anteriorly, a supracondylar fracture is probably present (Fig. 8.7). The hourglass (or figure eight) sign is also useful (Fig. 8.8). Normal overlapping contours create an intact hourglass on the lateral view. In the presence of a supracondylar fracture, the hourglass may appear broken. However, in the absence of severe force, a supracondylar buckle or plastic bending fracture may occur, and these signs may be normal [7].

Ultrasound (US) is very sensitive for detecting joint effusions, which are best depicted by examining the olecranon fossa in the sagittal plane from a posterior approach (Fig. 8.9). Under normal conditions, only a small amount of fluid can be identified between the fat pad and the humerus. US can sometimes detect a fracture as an interruption of the cortical bone surface, and displaced fragments may be evident. Doppler US noninvasively assesses the integrity of the brachial artery.

Advanced imaging is generally not necessary in the diagnosis and treatment of supracondylar humerus fractures. However, computed tomography (CT) may be used to determine the position of displaced fragments in complex dislocation patterns.

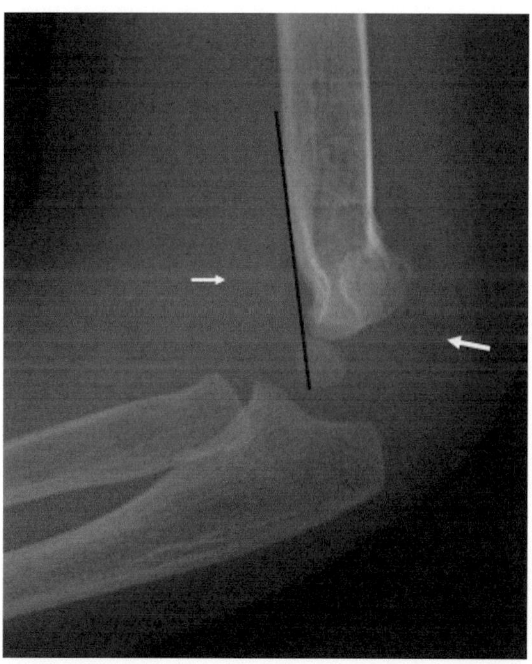

Fig. 8.7 Anterior humeral line with mildly displaced supracondylar fracture. The anterior humeral line intersects the anterior third of the capitellum, rather than the middle or posterior third. In addition, there is a large joint effusion, elevating both the posterior and anterior fat pads (*arrows*)

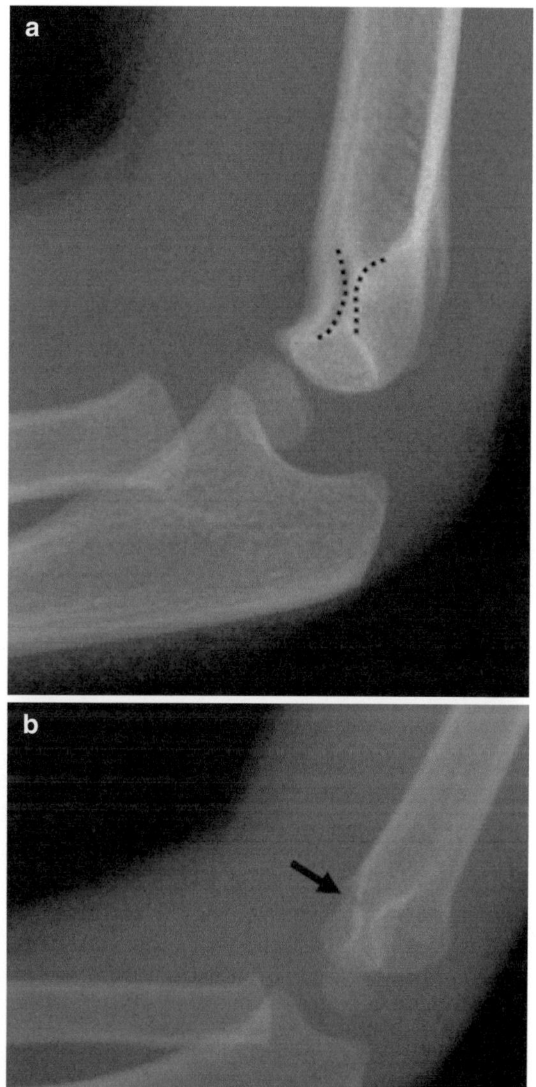

Fig. 8.8 Supracondylar fracture with broken hourglass sign (or figure eight). (**a**) Normal contralateral elbow for comparison shows intact hourglass. (**b**) Interrupted hourglass indicates supracondylar fracture, which in this case is also angulated (*arrow*)

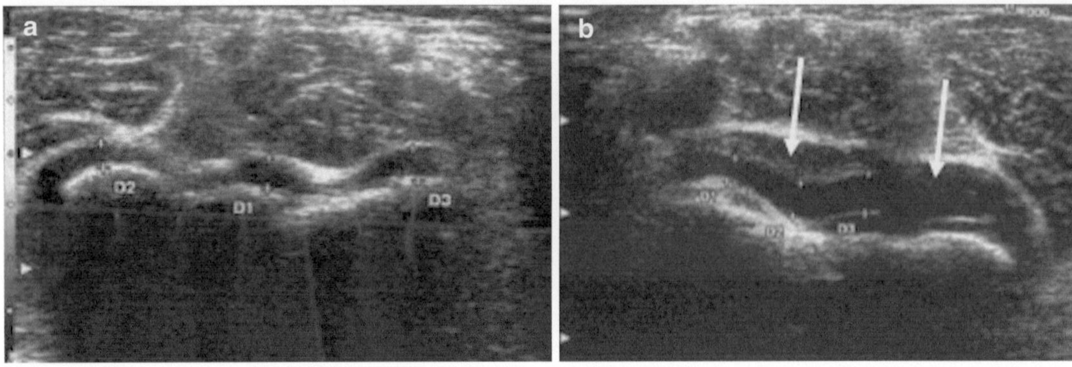

Fig. 8.9 Joint effusion demonstrated at ultrasound (US). (**a**) Transverse view of normal olecranon bursa for comparison showing minimal joint fluid. (**b**) Anechoic joint effusion (*arrows*) anterior to the surface of the humerus (D1-D3 label the measurements of the joint fluid)

2.2 Lateral Condylar Fracture (Box 8.3)

Box 8.3: Lateral Condylar Fractures

Second most common pediatric elbow fracture (20 %), age 4–10

Varus force to extended elbow in supination

Salter II or IV: unstable if extends through trochlear groove

- Traction from forearm extensors

Very subtle in young children as fracture predominantly involves cartilage

- Small bone flake
- Faint linear lucency between lateral condyle and trochlea

Sequelae
- Nonunion and cubitus varus deformity
- Avascular necrosis of trochlea or capitellum

Lateral condylar fractures are the second most common pediatric elbow fracture, accounting for 20 % of elbow fractures in children. They occur most often between ages 4 and 10 [12]. As with supracondylar fractures, the typical mechanism is a fall on an outstretched arm. This injury is caused by a varus force applied to an extended elbow while the forearm is supinated [13]. These fractures are usually Salter Harris Type II or IV: the fracture involves the metaphysis, physis, and the often incompletely ossified trochlea. Fractures of the lateral condyle are unstable and tend to become displaced even when immobilized because of traction from forearm extensors.

Several classification systems assess lateral condylar fractures. The amount of displacement can guide treatment (0–2 mm indicates casting, 2–4 mm indicates closed reduction and pinning, and >4 mm indicates open reduction and internal fixation). The Milch system determines stability by assessing whether the distal fracture extends to the trochlea. Type I fractures traverse the capitellar ossification center, passing lateral to the trochlear groove. They do not disrupt the trochlea, and therefore the elbow is stable. Type II fractures, which are most common, extend medial to the capitellum, sometimes passing through the trochlear groove, and pass through the physis and lateral trochlea, potentially allowing the ulna to subluxate [13]. Although commonly used in the USA, the Milch classification shows poor interobserver and only moderate intraobserver agreement [14] and in the majority of cases correlates poorly with intraoperative findings [15]. The Rutherford classification is also used to evaluate the stability of lateral condylar fractures, assessing whether the fracture line extends to the articular surface and whether the fragment is displaced [16].

The Weiss classification system, based on the amount of fracture fragment displacement and the presence of articular congruence, can direct surgery and predict likelihood of complications [17]. According to this system, a Type I fracture is displaced less than 2 mm. Type II and Type III fractures are displaced by 2 mm or more. The

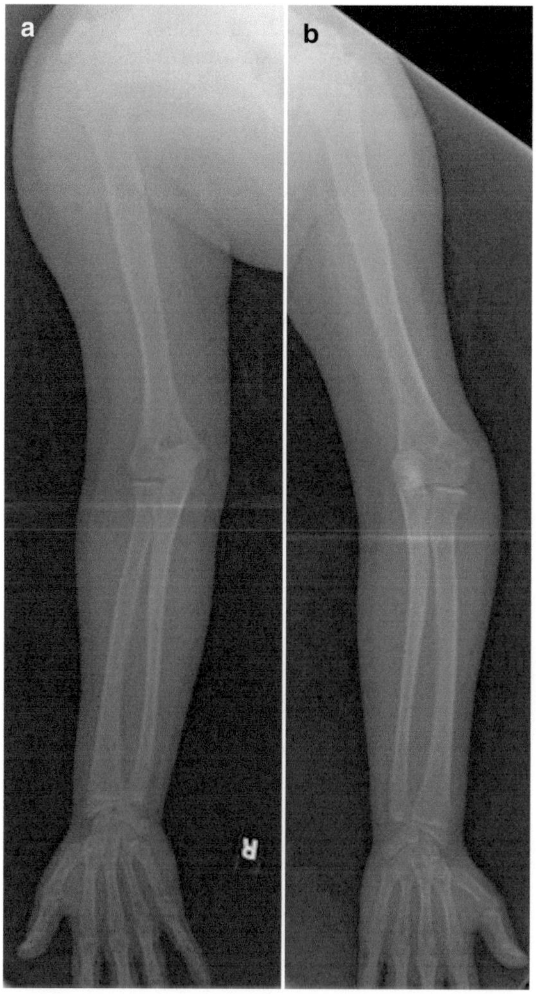

Fig. 8.10 Cubitus varus deformity. Frontal views of both arms with the forearm in supination show a normal right elbow (**a**). On the left (**b**), there is varus angulation at the elbow due to residual deformity after remote supracondylar fracture (Courtesy of Sandra L. Wootton-Gorges)

articular cartilage is intact with Type II fractures, whereas with Type III fractures, it is not. Both Types II and III require surgery, but surgical complications are more likely with Type III factures.

Nonunion is unfortunately relatively common with lateral condylar fractures. Residual deformity is common as well, most often cubitus varus due to progressive overgrowth of the lateral condyle [18] (the normal carrying angle is 15° of valgus). Occasionally, cubitus valgus (Fig. 8.10) due to lateral condylar growth arrest or delay and continued growth of the medial condyle occurs. In addition, in children, the vascular supply of the trochlea is vulnerable to injury [19], and resultant avascular necrosis may result in a fishtail deformity. Avascular necrosis of the capitellum may cause growth disturbance and deformity of the capitellum and radial head. Displaced lateral condylar fractures can result in both physeal and articular incongruity [20].

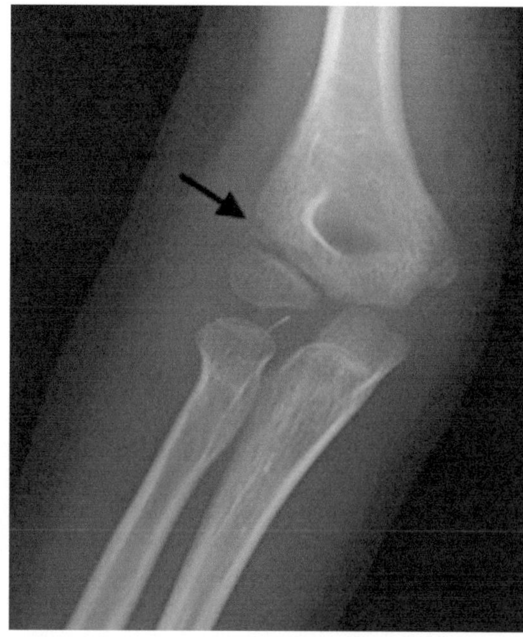

Fig. 8.11 Subtle lateral condylar fracture in an 8-year-old boy who fell on his outstretched arm. Subtle lucency proximal to the capitellum (*arrow*) may not extend to the trochlea. This fracture did not require fixation and is probably Milch Type I

Nondisplaced lateral condylar fractures with intact articular cartilage can be treated by immobilization and close follow-up. Displaced fractures should be stabilized with two divergent K-wires or screw fixation of the fracture through the metaphyseal fragment [12] and often require open reduction. Unlike most pediatric fractures, these heal slowly.

Imaging

Lateral condylar fractures can vary from a subtle cortical condylar avulsion to total lateral condylar avulsion and rotation. Subtle fractures may manifest only as a faint linear lucency between the lateral condyle and the trochlea (Fig. 8.11) or as a lateral metaphyseal flake with possible disruption of the radiocapitellar line. Especially in young children, the extent of the fracture may be grossly underestimated, as only a tiny flake may be evident, since the trochlear extent of the fracture traverses cartilage and is thus radiographically occult. Occasionally, only a cortical fragment of the capitellum is avulsed, which can be very difficult to detect [7]. Mild displacement may be evident, facilitating diagnosis.

This fracture may be much easier to appreciate on a lateral radiograph, as a large component can be directed posteriorly (Fig. 8.12). If the fracture extends to the articular surface, the joint becomes unstable, and the fragment is more likely to rotate (Figs. 8.13 and 8.14). Less commonly, the lateral condylar fracture extends through the capitellum itself. Isolated avulsion of the lateral epicondyle is a relatively rare injury, more often encountered in older children.

Because lateral condylar fractures can be difficult to identify, it is important to seek clues,

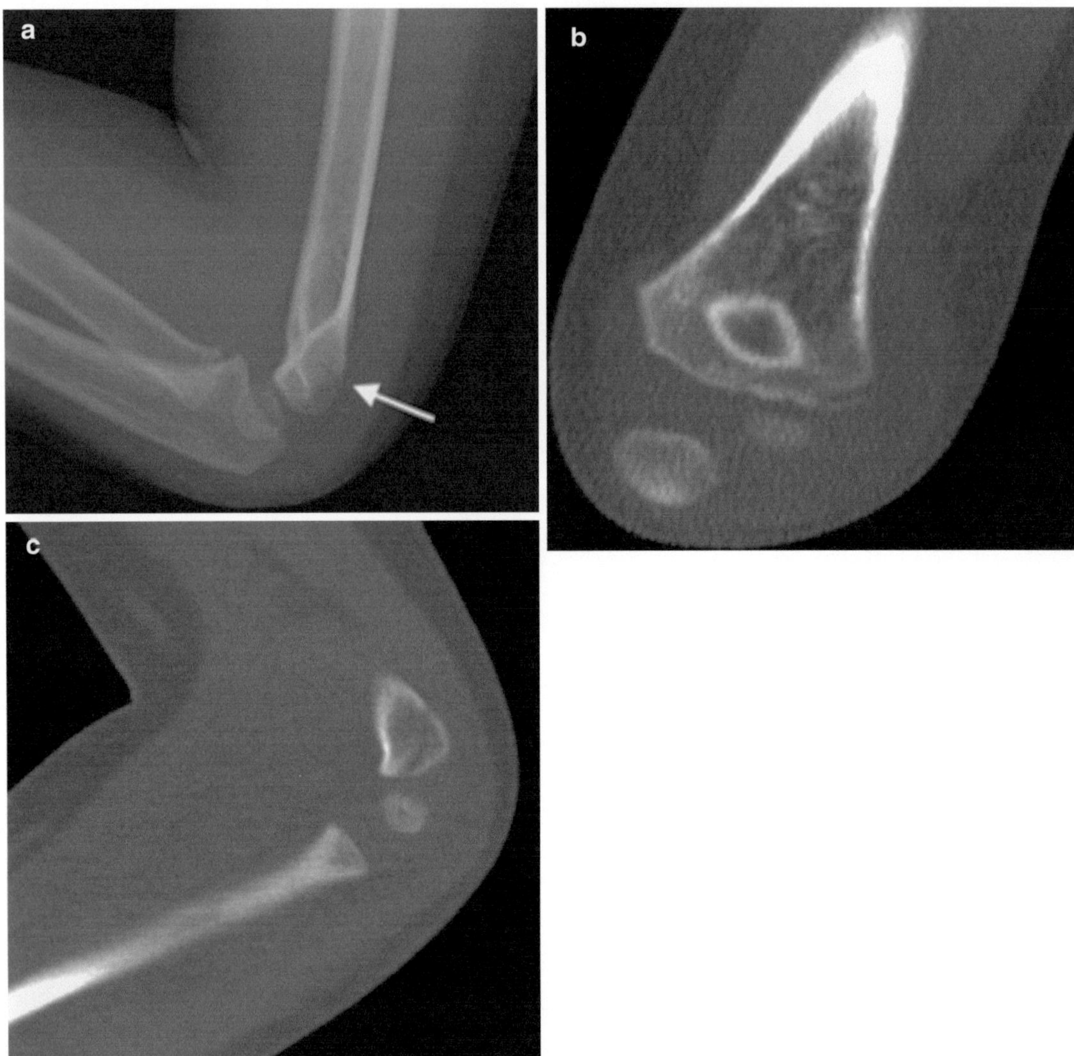

Fig. 8.12 Lateral condylar fracture seen on lateral radiograph. (**a**) Lateral view demonstrates subtle linear lucency (*arrow*) directed posteriorly. Coronal reformatted CT (**b**) shows lateral condylar location of fracture, which extends to the physis on the (**c**) sagittally reformatted CT (Courtesy of Rebecca Stein-Wexler)

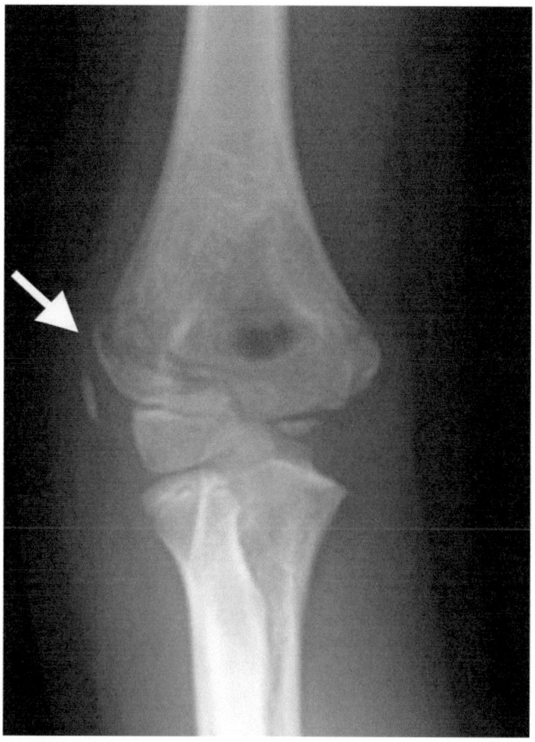

Fig. 8.13 Mildly displaced and rotated supracondylar fracture (*arrow*)

such as lateral soft tissue swelling on the frontal radiograph and a positive fat pad on the lateral (discussed in detail in the section on supracondylar fractures, above). An oblique radiograph with the arm internally rotated best demonstrates the amount of displacement and rotation of the lateral condylar fragment [21]. A significant gap in the lateral cortex may indicate articular discontinuity. It may take 4–14 days for the fracture line to appear, and the metaphyseal fragment can be very small and therefore overlooked. Furthermore, the diagnosis may be extremely difficult before the capitellum is ossified.

US can help establish the diagnosis of lateral condylar fracture by detecting joint fluid as well as cortical irregularity or an actual step-off at the lateral condylar bony or cartilaginous surface. CT may demonstrate the position of the displaced fragments in complex dislocation patterns (Fig. 8.15). Magnetic resonance imaging (MRI) can evaluate concomitant soft tissue injuries such as injury to the lateral collateral ligament complex, the muscles of supination, and/or the forearm extensors that are attached to the lateral condyle.

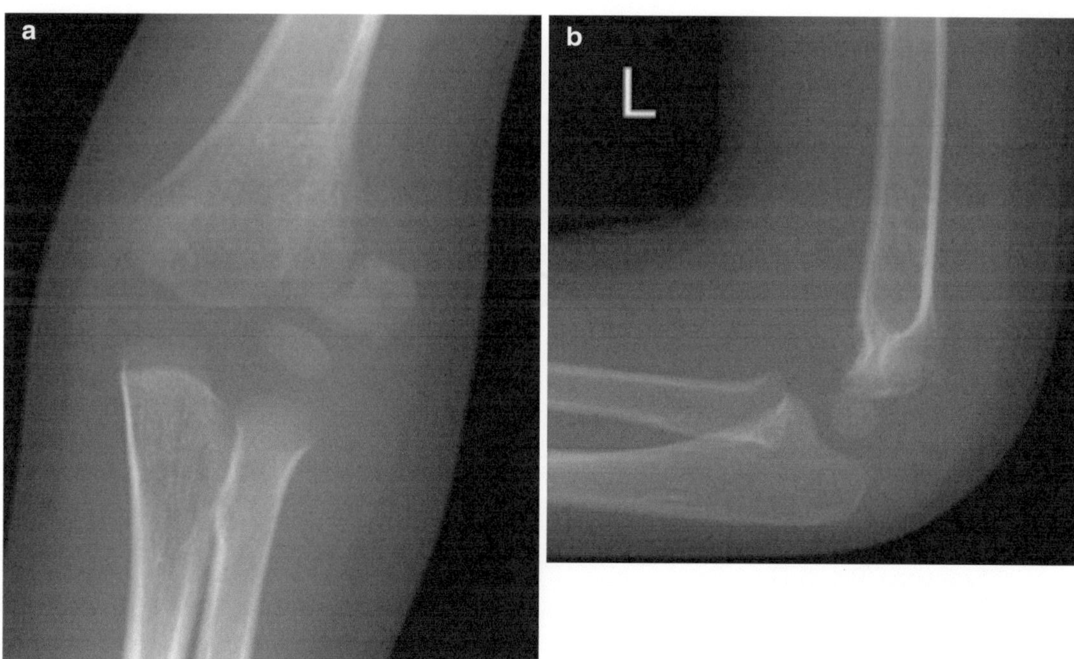

Fig. 8.14 Severely displaced and rotated lateral condylar fracture. (**a**, **b**) This is most likely a Salter Harris Type IV, with the fracture line crossing the physis and joint line

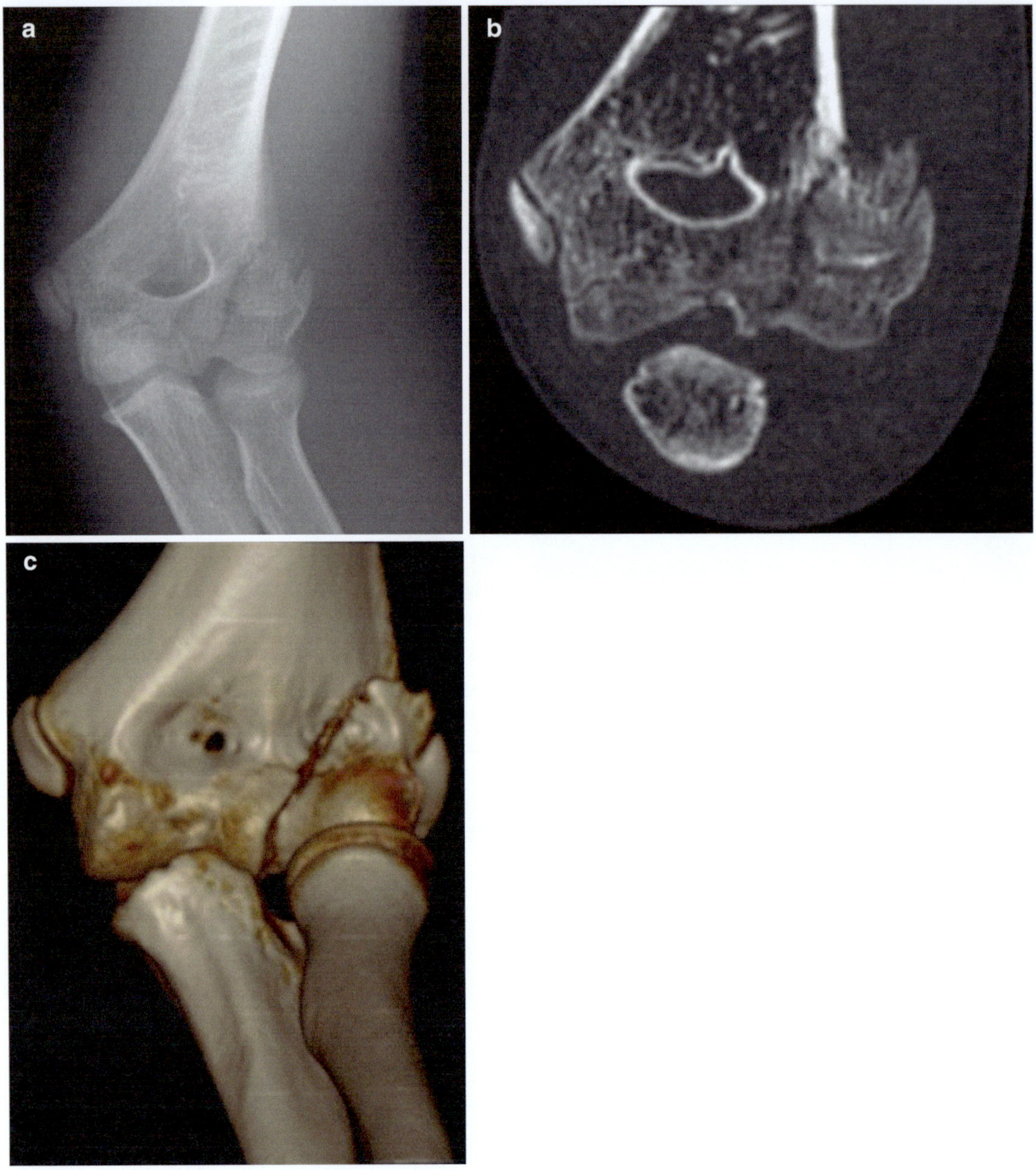

Fig. 8.15 Lateral condylar fracture. (**a**) The radiograph shows slight separation of the fragment at this Salter Harris IV fracture. Coronally reformatted CT (**b**) and 3D reconstruction (**c**) better define the extent of displacement

2.3 Medial Epicondylar Avulsion Fracture (Box 8.4)

Medial epicondylar avulsion fractures are less common and occur in older children, usually between 8 and 15 years [7]. Fractures of the medial epicondyle are associated with dislocation of the elbow joint at presentation in half of cases [6]. Both the radius and the ulna are usually posteriorly displaced [13]. The mechanism of injury is valgus strain to the joint, which causes the ulnar collateral ligament to exert traction on the medial epicondyle. This avulsive force causes the medial epicondyle to fail. The

Box 8.4: Medial Epicondylar Fractures

Less common, ages 8–15
Valgus strain causes ulnar collateral ligament and forearm flexors to pull on medial epicondyle
50 % also have dislocated elbow at presentation
  Radius and ulna posteriorly displaced
Fracture at cartilaginous physis (Salter I)
  Physis may appear wide
Fragment often displaced, may become trapped in joint near trochlea
  May mimic normal trochlear center
  Apply CRITOE to avoid mistakes—I before T

bone tends to separate at the cartilaginous physis—the weakest link in the pediatric skeleton. Another avulsion injury consists of purely muscular avulsion secondary to contraction of the forearm flexors when the elbow is flexed. This mechanism may be responsible for medial epicondylar fractures associated with arm wrestling and overhead throwing [22].

A displaced bony fragment can injure the ulnar nerve, which passes through a groove in the posterior aspect of the medial epicondyle. Furthermore, traction on the medial epicondyle secondary to contraction of forearm flexor muscles and tension from the medial collateral ligament may cause the fractured epicondyle to dislocate. In severe cases, the dislocated epicondyle may be trapped in the elbow joint, limiting joint mobility.

Nondisplaced fractures may be treated nonoperatively [6]. Open reduction (with K-wires for younger children, a screw for older) is usually performed if displacement exceeds 15 mm. However, such issues as hand dominance and whether the patient participates actively in sports affect the decision of whether to operate.

Imaging

The sequence and timing of ossification of the trochlea and medial epicondyle are important in interpreting medial elbow fractures. If the medial epicondyle is fractured and displaced, it may become entrapped between the trochlea and the coronoid process of the ulna (Fig. 8.16). In this position, it may be confused with the normal trochlear ossification center if that center has not yet ossified. However, that would imply that the trochlea had ossified before the medial epicondyle, which would be unusual. Infrequently, variant ossification order confounds this issue. In that case, imaging the contralateral elbow may help.

A lateral radiograph demonstrates a positive fat pad sign due to effusion, and a dislocated medial epicondyle may be apparent (see Fig. 8.6). On the frontal view, there is medial soft tissue swelling. Before ossification, radiographs can only suggest the possibility of fracture due to joint effusion or soft tissue swelling. If ossification has begun, the medial epicondylar physis may appear abnormally wide (Fig. 8.17).

US can assist with diagnosis prior to ossification of the medial epicondyle. MRI is usually not necessary but demonstrates physeal widening, bone contusion with edema on both sides of the physis, and possible dislocation of the medial epicondyle.

Differential Diagnosis

Fractures of the medial epicondyle may be mistaken for the very rare trochlear fracture. They may also be confused with medial condylar fractures that involve the medial column but are extra-articular. These two fracture patterns are treated differently and should not be mistaken. Elbow dislocation is very uncommon with medial condylar fractures but commonly encountered with fractures of the medial epicondyle.

2.4 T (or Y) Fracture

T- (or Y-) shaped fractures are intercondylar fractures with varying displacement between the condyles and the humerus. These fractures are uncommon in children and are generally caused by a blow to the elbow.

Imaging

Radiographs show that the intercondylar distance is increased, and there are displaced fracture fragments. These fractures require reconstruction of the articular surface and reattachment to the shaft [6]. CT or MRI helps with planning reconstruction.

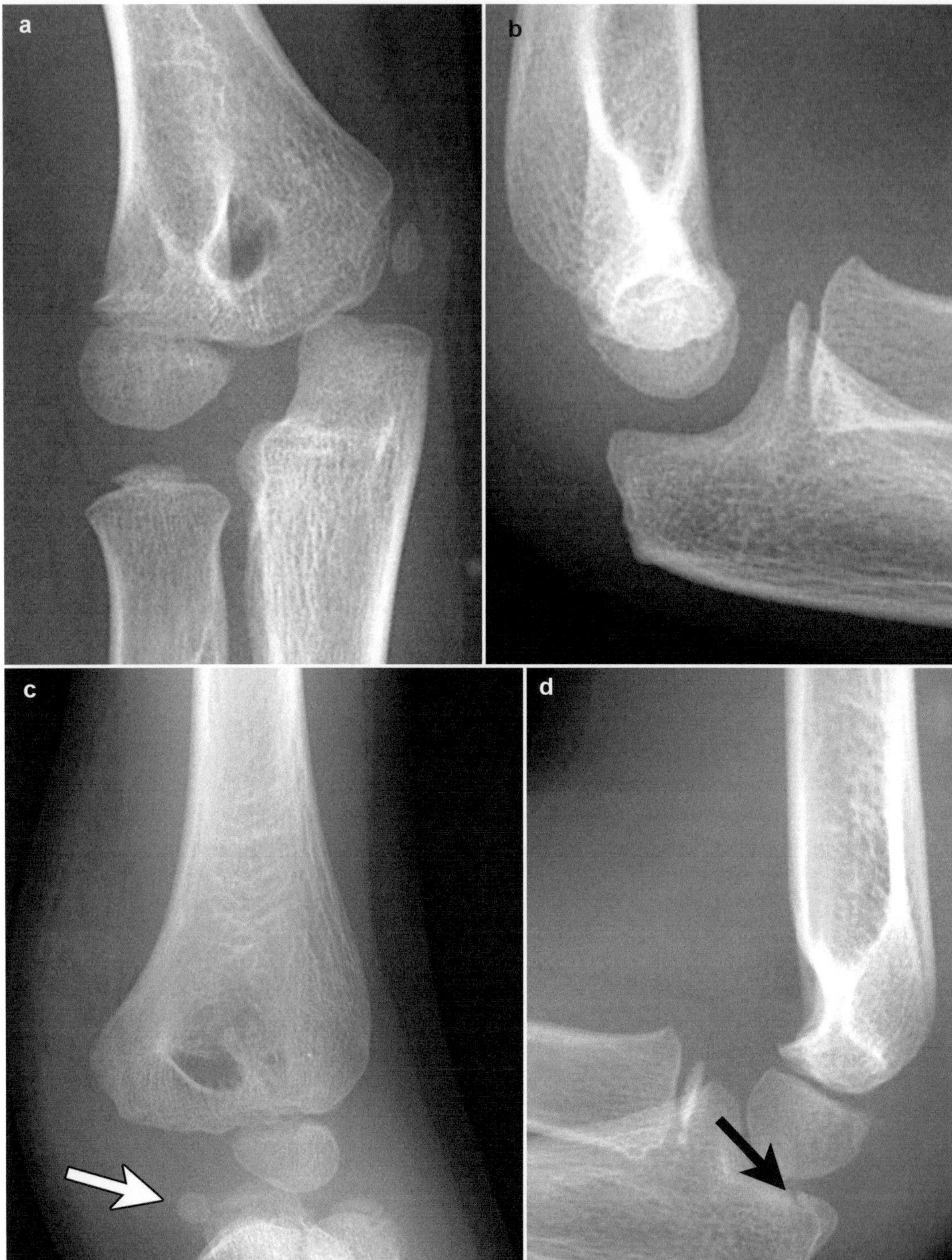

Fig. 8.16 Medial epicondylar fracture in a 6-year-old boy. (**a**, **b**) Normal right side for comparison. Note trochlear and olecranon apophyses have not yet ossified and normal position of the medial epicondyle. (**c**) The left medial epicondyle is displaced into the joint (*white arrow*). (**d**) There is also a nondisplaced olecranon fracture (*black arrow*) (Courtesy of Sandra L. Wootton-Gorges)

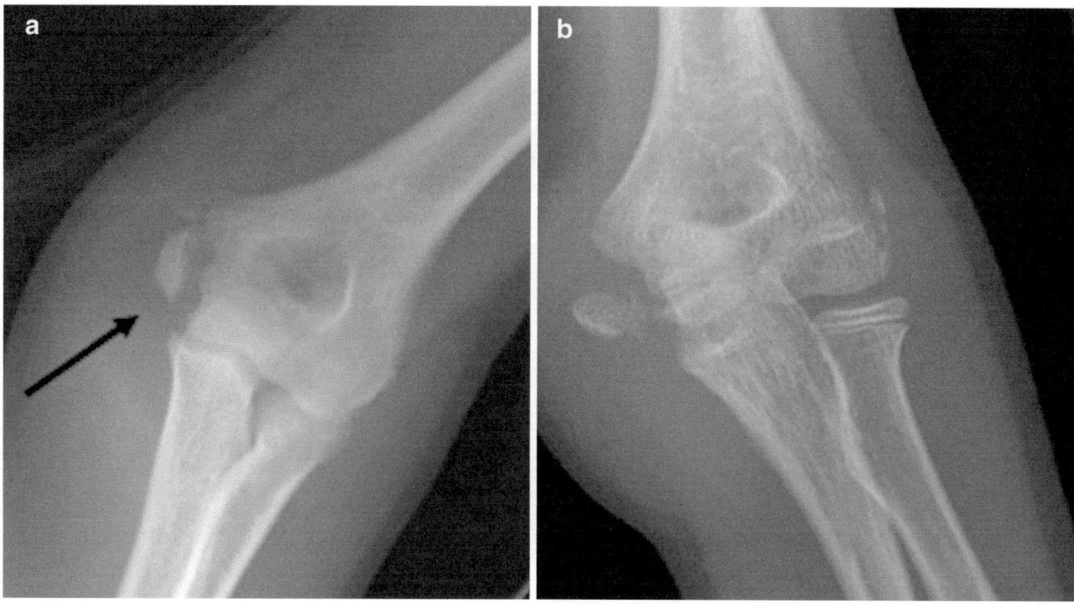

Fig. 8.17 (**a**) Medial epicondylar fracture in an 11-year-old girl. The physis at the medial epicondyle is abnormally wide (*arrow*), and the medial epicondyle slightly displaced. (**b**) Another child with a more displaced medial epicondylar fracture

2.5 Complete Physeal Displacement

Complete physeal displacement is a specific type of supracondylar fracture that generally occurs before age 2 [6]. As the name suggests, it is characterized by a fracture line that traverses the physes of the medial epicondyle, trochlea, capitellum, and lateral epicondyle, with displacement of this cartilaginous mass. The non-ossified epiphyses are markedly displaced but difficult to recognize, since the earliest to ossify—the capitellum—may ossify as late as 12 months. Delayed diagnosis increases the likelihood of avascular necrosis of the distal humerus. It is therefore important to maintain a high index of suspicion for this type of fracture in the infant who presents with a swollen elbow after birth or trauma. Treatment involves either closed reduction with a cast or pinning [6].

Imaging

On a frontal radiograph, the proximal radius and ulna appear displaced medially relative to the distal humerus, although they maintain a normal relationship to each other (Fig. 8.18). The radius and ulna appear posteriorly displaced on the lateral view.

Differential diagnosis includes elbow dislocation, but elbow dislocations in young children are exceedingly rare and generally show the proximal radius and ulna displaced posterolaterally instead of posteromedially, with disruption of the relationship between the proximal radius and the capitellum [23]. US or MRI successfully establish the diagnosis.

3 Fracture of the Radius and Ulna

3.1 Radial Neck Fractures

The radial neck is usually fractured during a fall on an outstretched arm. The compressive force causes the radius to impact upon the capitellum. Fractures in this area typically involve either the physis (Salter Harris I) or the metaphysis and physis (Salter Harris II) [6, 24]. Crepitus at the radial head and tenderness with gentle pronation and supination are common. In the acute setting, motion is usually limited by a painful hemarthrosis, rather than a true mechanical

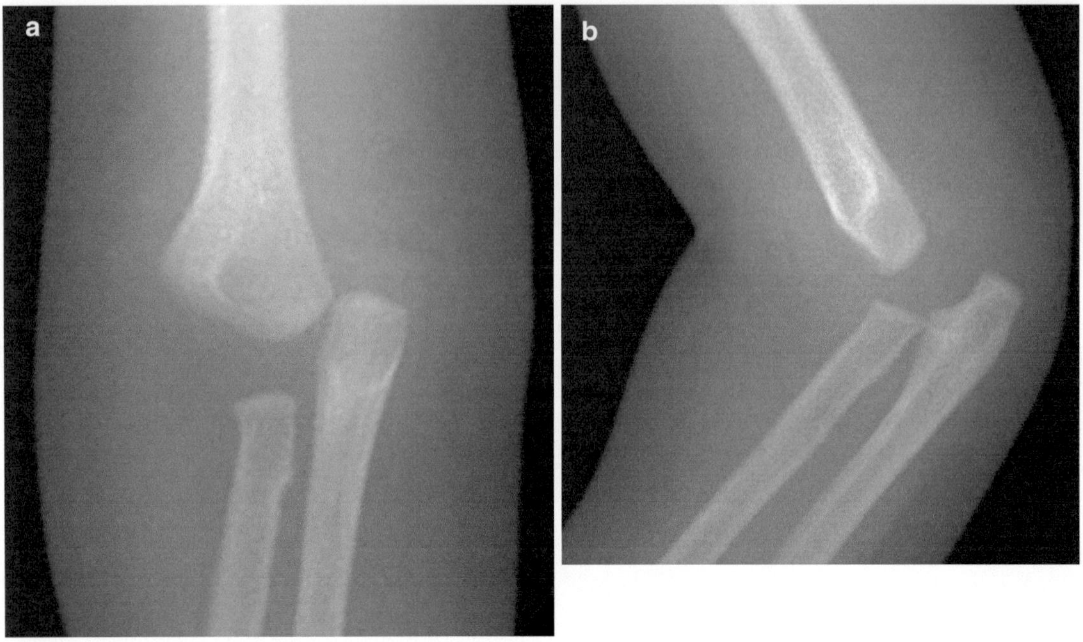

Fig. 8.18 Complete physeal displacement in an infant. (**a**, **b**) The radius and ulna maintain a normal relationship with each other but are displaced medially and posteriorly with respect to the distal humerus

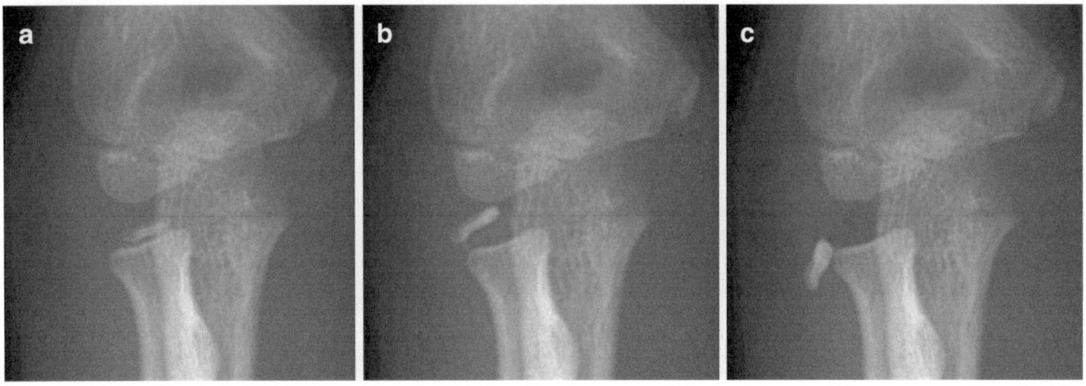

Fig. 8.19 AO classification of radial neck fractures. (**a**) With Type I, there is no angulation or displacement. (**b**) With Type II, the radial head is displaced less than 50 % of its diameter, and it appears angled. (**c**) Displacement more than 50 % (with angulation) constitutes Type III

block. However, displaced fracture fragments sometimes prevent forearm rotation.

The relationship between the radial head and the annular ligament determines the functional outcome of this fracture. The extent of angulation helps direct treatment; the AO classification scheme can be employed to describe fragment position (Fig. 8.19).

In general, any translation should be corrected, whereas angulation up to 30° (some suggest 50°) may be treated conservatively [6], depending on the age of the child. Displaced fractures require surgical stabilization with K-wires or an intramedullary elastic nail.

Imaging

As with all elbow fractures, injury to this area must be assessed with an understanding of when ossification centers ossify. Before radial head ossification, radiographs cannot differentiate radial head dislocation from physeal fracture with displacement. Frontal and lateral radiographs of the elbow are generally supplemented with either a radiocapitellar view or a Greenspan view (with the beam angled 45° cephalad and the elbow in neutral position).

The disk-shaped epiphysis at the proximal end of the radius articulates with the capitellum and with the lesser sigmoid notch of the ulna. Intra-articular in location, the radial head should point toward the capitellum on all views (Fig. 8.20). With injury, there may be a fracture line, abnormal alignment, angulation of the radial head, or depression, comminution, or displacement of the radial head or neck (Fig. 8.21). The fat pads are almost always elevated, indicating joint effusion. Small bony intra-articular fragments are infrequently present [25, 26].

As at the distal humerus, diagnosis is much more complex before epiphyseal ossification. In infants and young children, US may identify dislocations and joint effusion. It may also demonstrate gaps and irregularities in the cartilage surface, suggesting physeal injury [27, 28]. CT may assist with preoperative planning but is not indicated in the acute setting (Fig. 8.22). Although MRI can exquisitely delineate effusions, fractures,

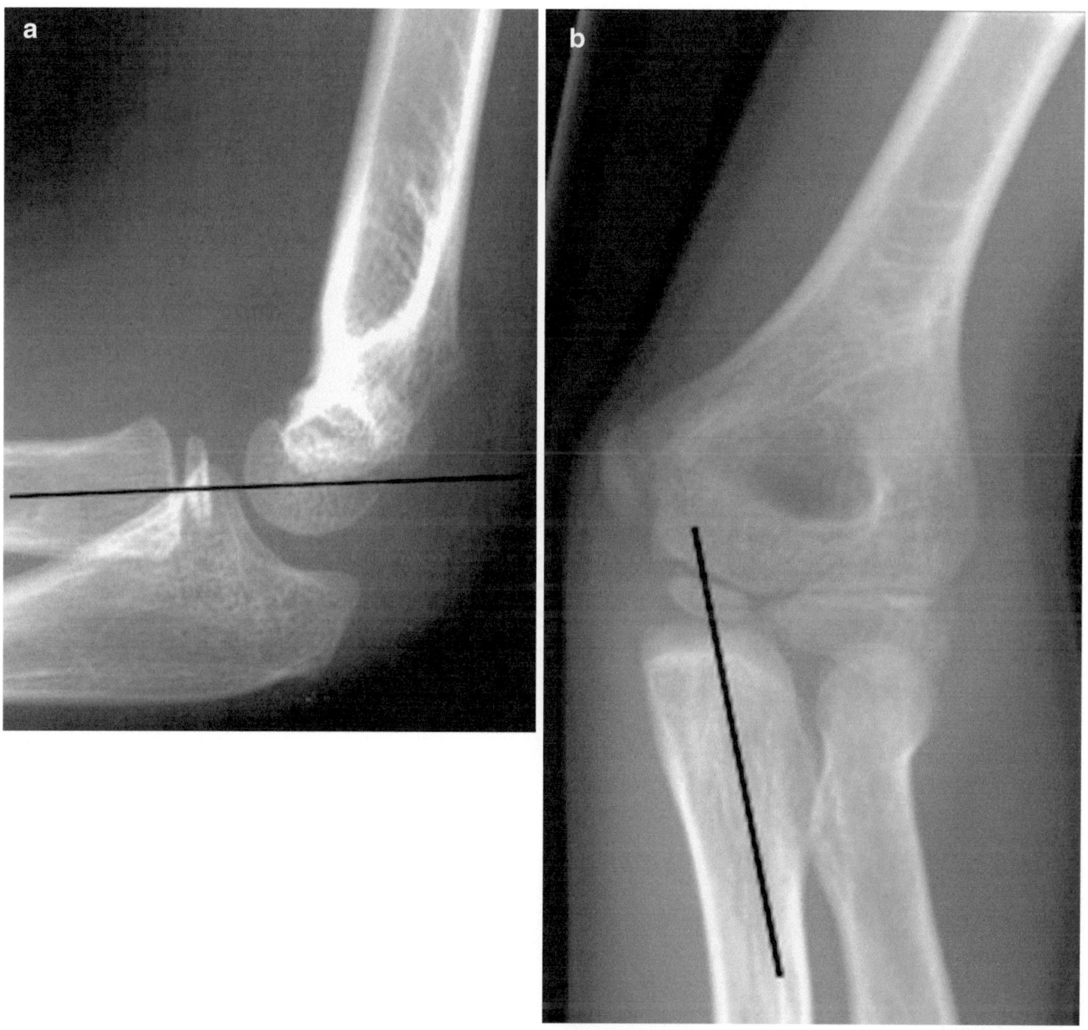

Fig. 8.20 (**a**, **b**) Radiocapitellar line. A line bisecting the proximal radius (and, if ossified, the radial head) should also pass through the capitellum

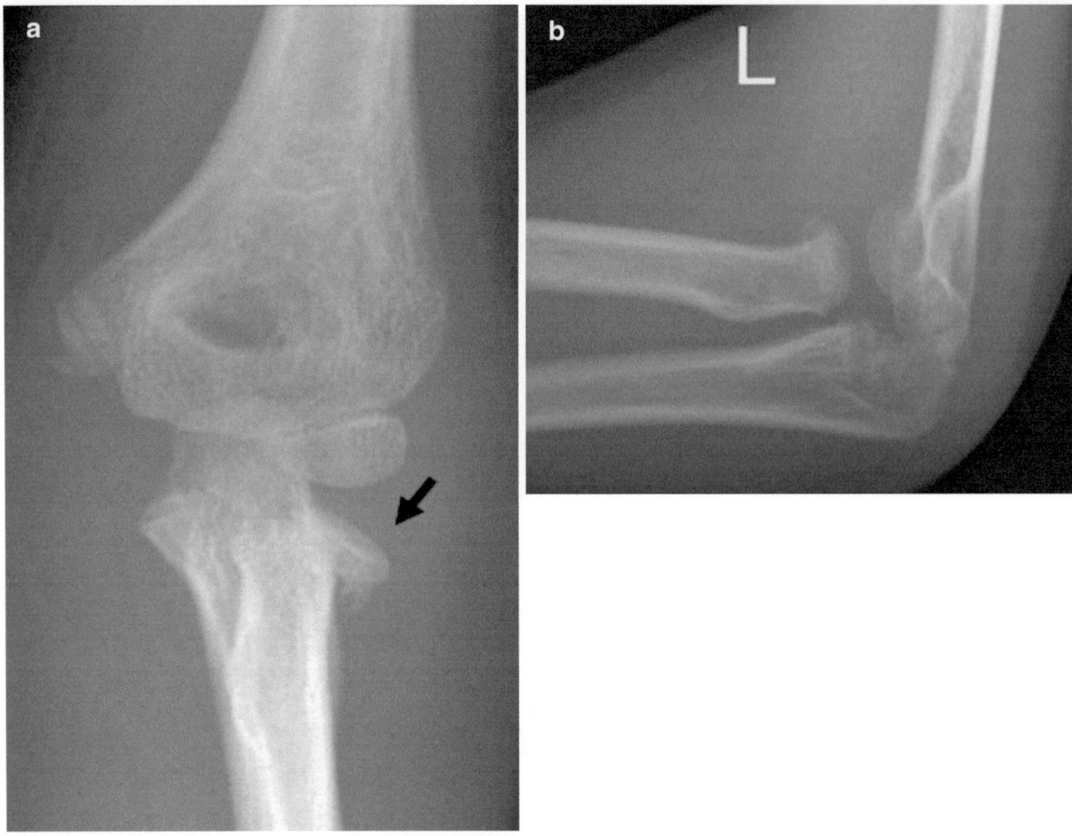

Fig. 8.21 Radial neck fracture in a 6-year-old boy. (**a**, **b**) There is a Salter Harris II fracture of the radial head and neck, and the radial head fragment (*arrow*) is angled and displaced slightly more than 50 % of the radius' diameter (grade III). Medial epicondyle is also fractured

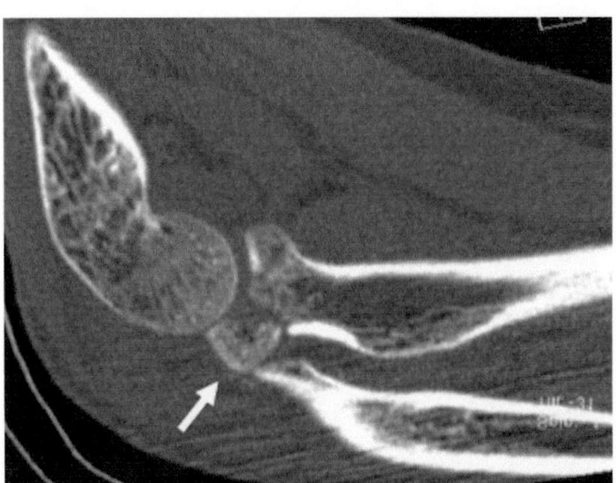

Fig. 8.22 Fracture dislocation of the radial head in a 16-year-old boy. The sagittal reformation from a CT shows a defect in the dorsal aspect of the radial head, with rotation of the fragment within the joint

and muscle/ligamentous injury not apparent on radiographs, the additional information provided generally has little bearing on treatment or clinical outcome [29].

Differential Diagnosis

Before ossification of the radial head, it is difficult to differentiate physeal fracture with dislocation from either congenital (see Chap. 7) or post-traumatic dislocation of the radial head. These entities are readily diagnosed after ossification.

3.2 Olecranon Fractures

Fractures of the olecranon represent approximately 4 % of fractures and dislocations at the elbow joint

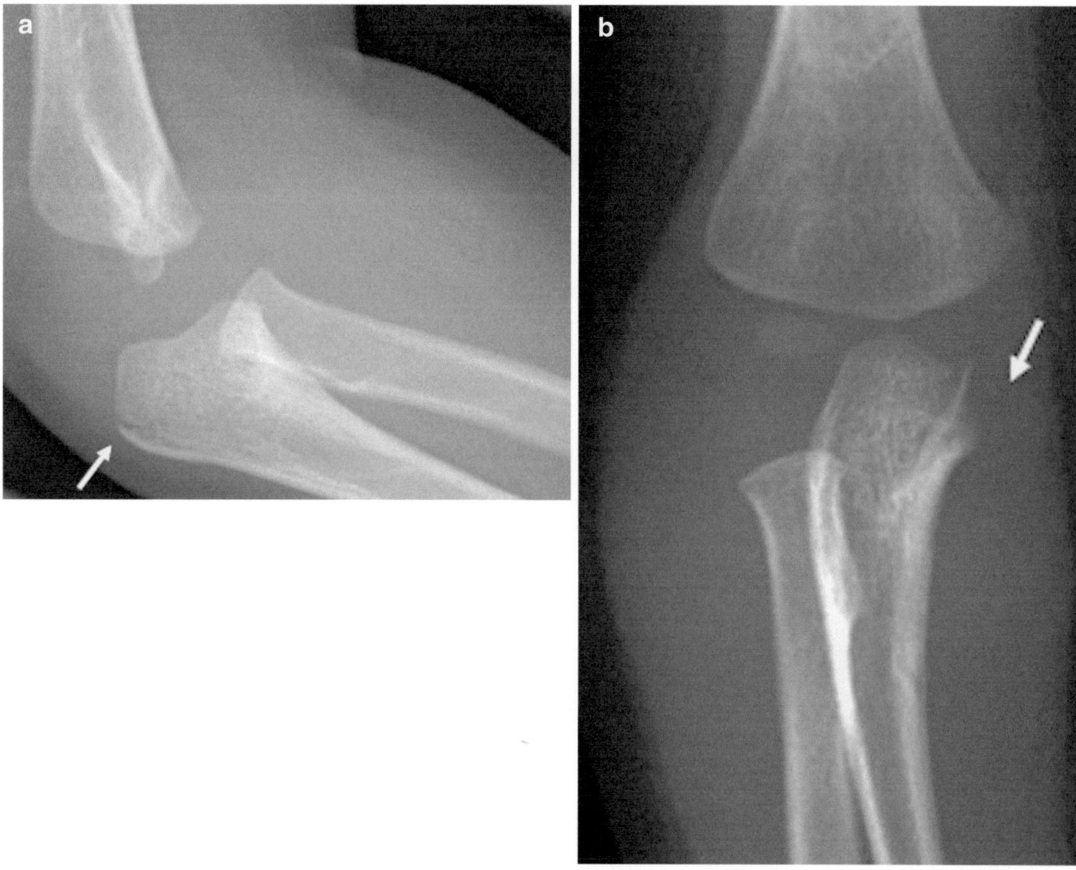

Fig. 8.23 Olecranon fracture in a 2-year-old boy. (**a**, **b**) The *white arrow* indicates the subtle fracture, reminiscent of a fish mouth in both projections

in children between the ages of 6 and 14 years [30]. After the olecranon fuses with the proximal ulna by age 14–16, the incidence of this fracture decreases further. One fifth of all olecranon fractures may be associated with a second elbow fracture, most often involving the medial epicondyle (Fig. 8.16) [31], although the coronoid process is sometimes fractured as well. (The Monteggia fracture/dislocation—ulnar fracture combined with radial head dislocation—is discussed in the following section.) Due to its position as the most exposed point of the elbow, the olecranon fracture typically results from high-energy injury, such as a direct blow [32]. Falls on the flexed forearm may also put tremendous strain on the olecranon, resulting in fracture.

Complex soft tissue injuries may accompany olecranon fractures. If the triceps muscle tears, the child may be unable to extend the elbow. Alternatively, the distraction force from the triceps may contribute to fracture displacement. The median, radial, or especially ulnar nerves may be injured.

Nondisplaced or minimally displaced fractures are immobilized in a long arm cast, whereas comminuted fractures or those with more than 2 mm displacement may require surgical intervention.

Imaging

Frontal and lateral radiographs usually allow diagnosis, but these fractures can be quite subtle and easily missed. Olecranon fractures are often oblique or transverse, crossing the olecranon and ending at the semilunar notch (Fig. 8.23). Traction from the triceps can cause obvious separation of fragments. An elbow effusion is usually present.

Differential Diagnosis

The secondary ossification center of the olecranon (bipartite olecranon) should not be misdiagnosed as fracture. The patella cubiti, sometimes confused with a fracture, is an uncommon accessory ossicle in the triceps tendon at its insertion in the olecranon.

3.3 Monteggia Fracture/Dislocation and Monteggia Variant Injuries (Box 8.5)

Box 8.5: Monteggia Fracture/Dislocation

- Fractured ulna (often proximal 1/3) and dislocated radial head
  - Radiocapitellar line (along center of radius) should intersect capitellum
- Direct blow, forceful hyper-pronation in extension, biceps contraction
- Ulnar injury commonly missed on initial radiographs
  - Isolated radial head dislocation very rare in children
    - If present, suspect Monteggia and seek ulnar bowing deformity
      - Posterior ulnar border should be straight on lateral view
- "Isolated" greenstick may have had spontaneously reduced radial head dislocation

The Monteggia fracture/dislocation is a fracture of the proximal third of the ulna accompanied with dislocation of the radial head. It was first described in 1814 by Giovanni Monteggia, an Italian surgeon who reported a proximal ulnar fracture in a young girl, which healed but was followed by radial head dislocation.

Various mechanisms of injury have been proposed. According to Monteggia, this fracture results from a direct blow to the back of the upper forearm. The other proposed mechanisms involve—as with many fractures of the upper extremity—a fall on an outstretched pronated arm. One theory suggests that forceful hyperpronation in extension causes the ulna to fracture and the radial head to dislocate [33]. Another suggests that sudden contraction of the biceps muscle causes dislocation of the radial head [34].

Classification of the Monteggia fracture/dislocation and its variants depends principally on the location and angulation of the ulnar fracture and on the direction of radial head dislocation [33]. Type I, which is most common (60 %), involves fracture or plastic deformation of the proximal or middle third of the ulna (with anterior angulation), along with dislocation of the radial head. For Type II, the location of the fracture is the same, but angulation is posterior and the radial head is posteriorly dislocated. Type III involves fracture of the proximal ulnar metaphysis and lateral dislocation of the radial head (often injuring the posterior interosseous nerve). Type IV is rare (5 %); the ulnar fracture resembles Type I or Type II, but the proximal third of the radius is also fractured, with anterior dislocation of the radial head.

The acute Monteggia injury is relatively benign in children, because the radial head pulls out of the annular ligament (which stabilizes the radial head) without tearing it. However, the posterior interosseous nerve, which lies close to the proximal radius, may be injured, with resultant paralysis of the forearm extensor musculature.

The goal of treatment of the acute Monteggia injury is restoration of anatomic length and alignment of the ulna, which facilitates reduction of the radial head. If the injury can be reduced closed, the patient is treated in a cast. Close follow-up is essential, as redislocation of the radial head is common. If the reduction cannot be maintained with casting, operative treatment is indicated. Chronic or "missed" Monteggia injuries may have significant consequences, including elbow pain, restricted forearm rotation, and valgus instability of the elbow. Treatment of these injuries involves corrective osteotomy of the ulna and can require open reduction of the ulna with reconstruction of the annular ligament.

Imaging

Monteggia injuries in children are among the most frequently missed injuries on initial radiographic evaluation. Much of the difficulty traditionally associated with managing Monteggia-type fracture/dislocations stems from the fact that ulnar injury can be very subtle. Since isolated radial head dislocations are very rare in older children, if initial elbow radiographs suggest radial head dislocation, ulnar injury should be suspected (Figs. 8.24 and 8.25). Additional imaging should then include bilateral full forearm radiographs to detect plastic deformation of the ulna. The posterior border of the ulna on a lateral view of the elbow should be straight, with no anterior bow [35].

The radial head dislocation is often initially unrecognized. Early recognition is facilitated by awareness of the normal radiocapitellar relationship, which is readily identified on radiographs (see Fig. 8.20). The radiocapitellar line, which is drawn along the center of the radial diaphysis and epiphysis, should intersect the capitellum, regardless of flexion, extension, or projection [36]. (However, the radiocapitellar relationship can be affected by bias, patient age, and forearm rotation [37]). Before initial ossification of the radial head, the line is based solely on the orientation of the diaphysis. Radiographs should include the distal radius since up to one quarter of Monteggia fracture/dislocations may be associated with a distal radius fracture [38]. Some cases of isolated bowing deformity of the ulna may actually have been accompanied with an unrecognized radial head dislocation that spontaneously reduced.

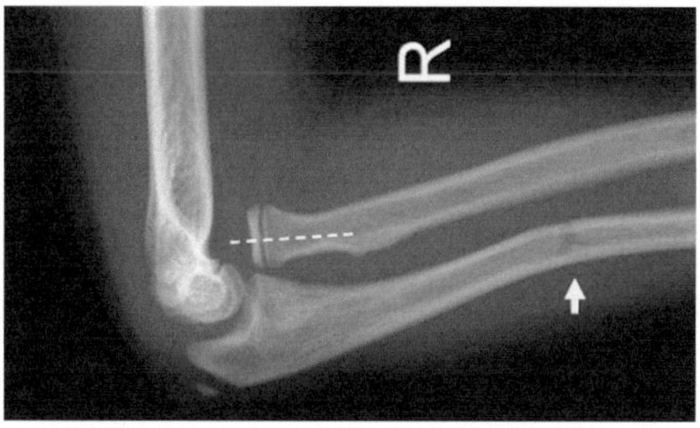

Fig. 8.24 Monteggia dislocation/fracture. The line bisecting the radial head and diaphysis does not align with the capitellum, as the radius is dislocated anteriorly. Nondisplaced fracture at proximal ulnar diaphysis (*arrow*)

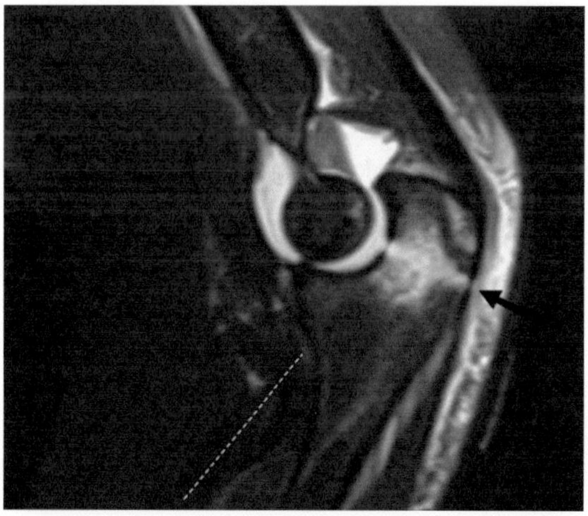

Fig. 8.25 Monteggia dislocation/fracture. Sagittal T2-W FS MRI shows posterior subluxation of the radius (*dotted line*) and a proximal ulnar fracture (*arrow*). Marrow edema and joint effusion

Differential Diagnosis

Congenital dislocations (see Chap. 7), with or without radioulnar synostosis, are often diagnosed quite late, after forearm rotation has become restricted (Fig. 8.26). However, the configuration of the radial head allows differentiation between traumatic and congenital dislocations. With traumatic dislocation, the radial head is concave, whereas with congenital dislocation, it is flat or convex, and the proximal radius is tapered. MRI shows the shape of the radial head more clearly, which helps differentiate between a chronic Monteggia injury and a congenital radial head dislocation in a young child.

3.4 Galeazzi Fracture/Dislocation (Box 8.6)

Box 8.6: Galeazzi Fracture/Dislocation

Fractured radial diaphysis, middle to distal third, with subluxation/dislocation of distal radioulnar joint (DRUJ)

Thirteen percent of forearm fractures

Adolescents, just before bony maturity

Forceful axial load to pronated forearm

Subluxation of ulna, dorsal > volar

- DRUJ widened on frontal view
- Possible ulnar styloid fracture

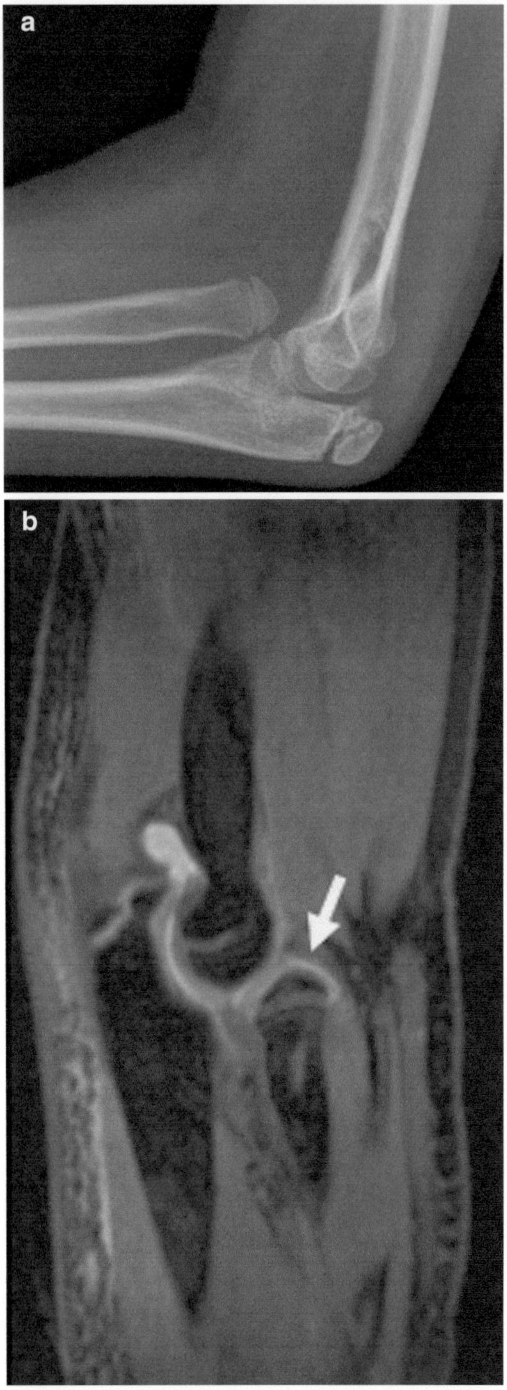

Fig. 8.26 Congenital radial head dislocation. (**a**) The dysplastic radial head has a triangular configuration and is displaced anteriorly. (**b**) Sagittal T2-W FS 3D gradient echo (GRE) MRI shows the displaced radial head (*arrow*)

The Galeazzi fracture/dislocation consists of a fracture of the radius combined with subluxation or dislocation of the distal radioulnar joint. This fracture complex is most common during adolescence, shortly before maturity, due to the extremely strong ligaments and joint capsule that characterize this period [6]. It results from a fall on an outstretched arm, in which the pronated forearm receives a forceful axial load. Galeazzi fractures account for 13 % of all forearm fractures and are less common than isolated fractures of the radius [39].

This fracture may result in compartment syndrome. Patients with crush or vascular injuries, open fractures, or coagulation disorders are at increased risk for this complication. Although a Galeazzi fracture rarely damages the anterior interosseus nerve, the radial nerve may be damaged, resulting in paralysis of the flexor pollicis longus and flexor digitorum profundus muscles and consequent wrist drop. Sometimes disruption of the triangular fibrocartilage complex, with or without an ulnar styloid fracture, occurs.

Closed reduction and casting in supination are usually adequate therapy in children, unlike in adults [39]. Even if a Galeazzi fracture/dislocation is not initially recognized, proper reduction of the radial fracture with concomitant reduction of the distal radioulnar joint and cast immobilization provides a good to excellent outcome [39]. If surgical stabilization of the radius is necessary, the approach and fixation type are determined by patient age and fracture location.

Imaging

Radiographs demonstrate a fracture of the radius, usually diaphyseal and involving the middle to distal third of the radius. Bayonet apposition may cause shortening (Fig. 8.27). Dislocation at the distal radioulnar joint is often manifested by subluxation of the ulna, usually in a dorsal but sometimes in a volar direction. The distal radioulnar joint may appear widened on the frontal projection, and there may be an ulnar styloid fracture or lysis of the distal ulnar epiphysis.

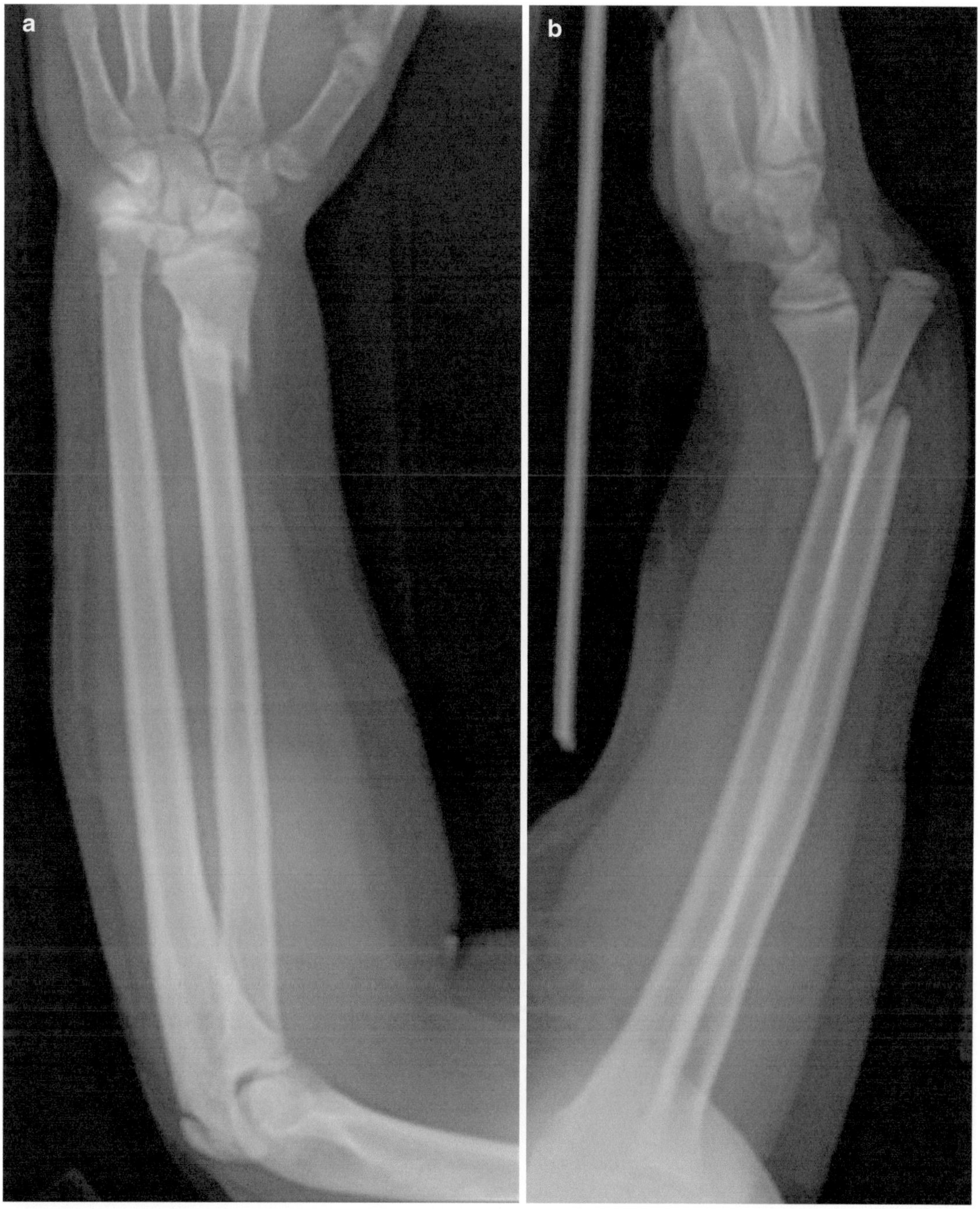

Fig. 8.27 Galeazzi fracture/dislocation in a 13-year-old boy. (**a**) Displaced distal radial fracture with bayonet apposition, dorsal dislocation of the distal ulna, and (**b**) disruption of the distal radioulnar joint (Courtesy of Tal Laor, Cincinnati Children's Hospital)

4 Transient Subluxation of the Radial Head (Nursemaid Elbow) (Box 8.7)

Box 8.7: Transient Subluxation of the Radial Head

Most common upper extremity injury in children <5 years old

Annular ligament slips or tears during pronation/supination

Radial head slips through defect

Radiograph to exclude effusion, fracture, dislocation

Transient subluxation of the radial head results from a sharp pull on a partially pronated forearm and is the most common musculoskeletal injury of the upper extremity in children younger than age 5. The annular ligament slips during pronation-supination maneuvers because of a variety of factors, but principally because the articular surface of the radial head is not perfectly perpendicular to the long axis of the radius, and the sides of the radial head are oblique [40]. As the child matures, the configuration of the radial head and neck does not change significantly [24, 41]. However, the annular ligament becomes less mobile and its site of insertion stronger, and

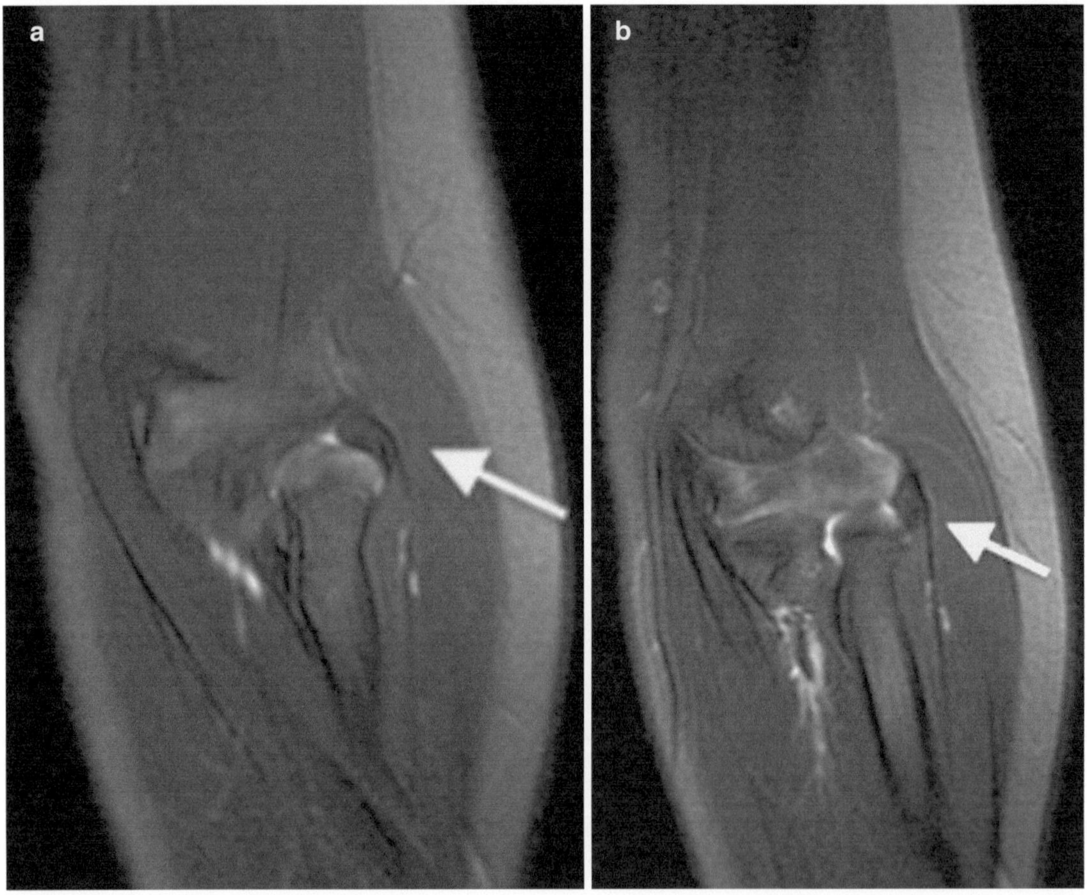

Fig. 8.28 Subluxated elbow in a toddler, with displaced annular ligament. (**a**, **b**) Coronal T2-W FS MRI images show the radial head is out-of-plane with the capitellum, indicating subluxation. The annular ligament (*arrow*) is displaced proximal to the radial head (Courtesy of Rebecca Stein-Wexler)

consequently radial head subluxation is relatively uncommon in older children.

An axial pull with the forearm in pronation results in tear or displacement of the mobile annular ligament. The radial head then slips through this aperture, and the ligament, capsule, or synovium becomes pinched between the radial head and the capitellum. This interposed soft tissue is usually too thin to significantly displace the radial head from the capitellum.

This injury is reduced by flexion and supination and requires no immobilization after reduction.

Imaging
It is debatable whether the typical "pulled elbow" needs radiological investigation. Radiographs are usually normal [6, 24, 42], and indeed the technologist often reduces radial head subluxation in the course of imaging. The main purpose of radiography is to exclude joint effusion, fracture, or dislocation. The displaced annular ligament can be identified at US [43] or MRI (Fig. 8.28).

5 Ligamentous Injuries

After physeal closure, when the physis no longer forms the weakest structure of the joint, ligamentous injury becomes more common. In late adolescence, therefore, acute trauma or repetitive stress is likely to damage ligaments and tendons, although of course fractures occur as well.

5.1 Ulnar Collateral Ligament Injury (Medial Collateral Ligament Injury) (Box 8.8)

Box 8.8: Ulnar Collateral Ligament Injury

- Valgus stress (repetitive or sudden/severe): throwing athlete
  - UCL and common flexor tendon stabilize flexed elbow medially
- MRI: coronal PD
  - Proximal/distal avulsion, midportion rupture
  - Medial epicondyle avulsion
  - Partial tear: focal thickening/T2 signal
    - Caveat: before physeal fusion, slightly high signal is normal at epicondylar insertion

The ulnar collateral ligament (UCL), sometimes referred to as the medial collateral ligament (MCL), is composed of two separate bundles or bands. Both have a triangular configuration, fanning out for their distal attachments. The proximal part of the anterior band attaches to the inferior aspect of the medial epicondyle, and its broad distal portion attaches to the sublime tubercle at the medial aspect of the ulna's coronoid process. The apex of the posterior band extends from the inferoposterior medial epicondyle to the medial margin of the olecranon. The UCL and common flexor tendon (the conjoined tendon of the flexor carpi radialis, flexor carpi ulnaris, flexor digitorum superficialis, palmaris longus, and pronator teres) form the primary medial stabilizer of the flexed elbow joint.

Valgus stress may injure the UCL. Sudden severe trauma can cause a complete tear, but repetitive stress—such as occurs in the pitcher or other overhead-throwing athlete—is more common, resulting in tendinosis or partial tear. Patients complain of medial pain that is accentuated during the late cocking and acceleration stages of throwing. Valgus instability can be evident at physical examination.

Imaging
Radiographs are typically normal, but stress views may show slightly increased separation between the trochlea and the olecranon. Heterotopic calcification within the ligament is unusual in the pediatric age group.

US can be employed to evaluate the UCL, especially its anterior band. The proximal attachment can be identified in 94 % of asymptomatic people and the distal attachment in 90 % [44]. The normal ligament should be more echogenic than muscle; tears appear hypoechoic (the contralateral side can also be studied to clarify questionable cases). Dynamic evaluation with valgus stress and at rest

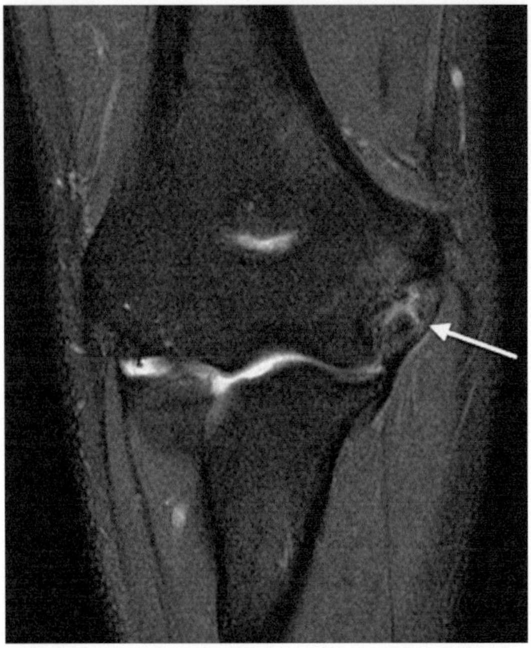

Fig. 8.29 Partial avulsion of the ulnar collateral ligament in a 15-year-old boy. Coronal PD FS MRI shows partial avulsion of the proximal aspect of the UCL, and the high-signal tear extends into the substance of the ligament (*arrow*). There is also subtle marrow edema (Courtesy of Jasjeet Bindra)

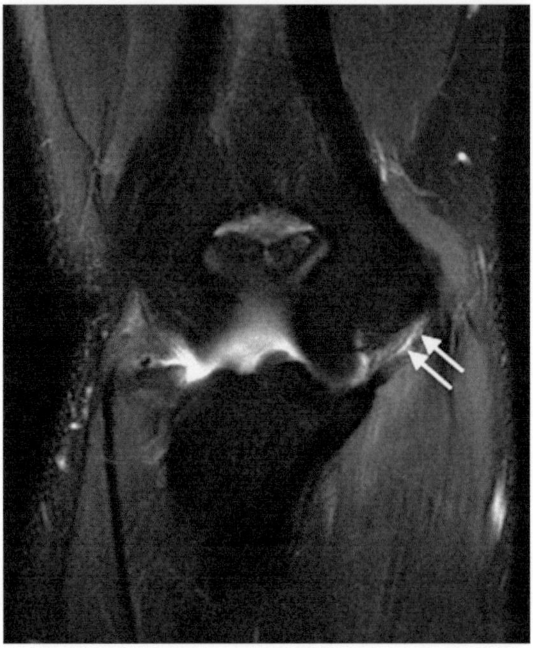

Fig. 8.30 Longitudinal partial-thickness tear of the ulnar collateral ligament in a 19-year-old pitcher. Coronal PD FS image shows longitudinal hyperintense signal in the UCL (*arrows*) (Courtesy of Jasjeet Bindra)

helps assess integrity or laxity of the ligament and is especially useful if there is a partial tear [45, 46].

MRI evaluates elbow ligaments in exquisite anatomic detail. The UCL is best visualized on coronal proton-density (PD) images. Ligament rupture appears as focal, complete discontinuity and may result from either proximal or distal avulsion or from midportion rupture. There may be laxity, as well as increased T2-signal within and around the ligament. The medial epicondyle may be avulsed, and the brachialis muscle may appear edematous. If there is an effusion and the joint capsule is torn, extravasation will be evident (this can also be seen at arthrography or magnetic resonance arthrography (MRA)). Focal thickening or increased T2 signal characterizes partial tears (Figs. 8.29 and 8.30). An undersurface partial tear of the anterior bundle may result in the T-sign, characterized by the extension of fluid (or contrast-medium in arthrography) between the UCL undersurface and the adjacent coronoid (Fig. 8.31). In uncertain cases, MRA has the greatest ability to identify ligamentous injuries [47].

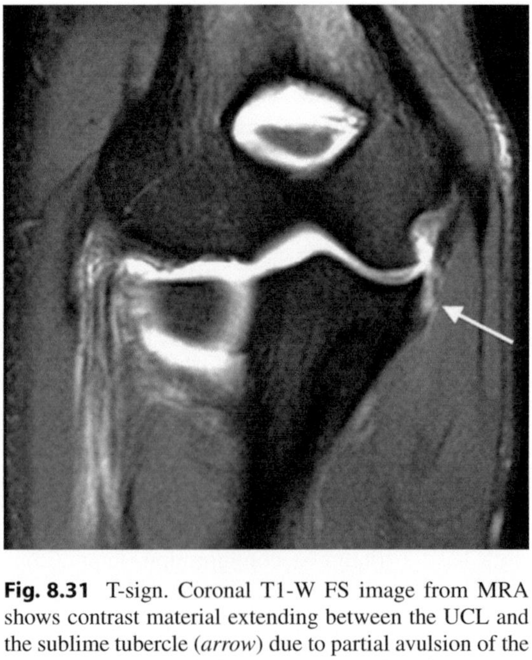

Fig. 8.31 T-sign. Coronal T1-W FS image from MRA shows contrast material extending between the UCL and the sublime tubercle (*arrow*) due to partial avulsion of the distal attachment of the anterior bundle of the UCL (Courtesy of John Hunter)

It is important to recognize that in the skeletally immature elbow, before physeal fusion, slightly high T1 and T2 signal in the MCL at its epicondylar insertion is normal. This may be due to increased elastin and decreased type I collagen at the enthesis [48].

5.2 Injuries Affecting the Lateral Ligaments of the Elbow

Three key ligaments stabilize the lateral aspect of the elbow:

- The annular ligament (AL) encircles the radial head, tapering distally over the proximal portion of the radial neck. It attaches to the posterior and anterior margins of the radial notch of the ulna.
- The radial collateral ligament extends from the lateral epicondyle to the AL, deep to the common extensor tendons.
- The lateral ulnar collateral ligament (LUCL) extends from the lateral epicondyle to the supinator crest at the dorsal aspect of the ulna, merging with the posterior aspect of the radial collateral ligament (RCL). The LUCL also swings around the posterior portion of the radial head, forming a posteromedial sling before inserting on the supinator crest of the lateral ulna.

The RCL and LUCL constitute capsular thickenings that originate from a common origin at the lateral epicondyle. The attachment site measures approximately 5 mm. At their origin, the LUCL and RCL are deep and slightly distal to the common extensor tendon origin.

Rupture of these ligaments causes either posterior dislocation of the radius and ulna or posterolateral rotatory instability [49]. With posterior dislocation of the elbow, which is the most common dislocation in children, the RCL and LUCL may rupture. The UCL may rupture as well, but this usually occurs only with extreme dislocation. Posterolateral rotatory instability results from capsular weakness or rupture of the proximal portions of the LUCL and RCL and possibly the posterior bundle of the UCL as well. The proximal LUCL and RCL are the most important stabilizers, restraining rotatory and posterior motion. If ruptured, they allow the proximal radius and ulna to shift posteriorly with respect to the humerus, and if injury is severe, they can result in multidirectional instability.

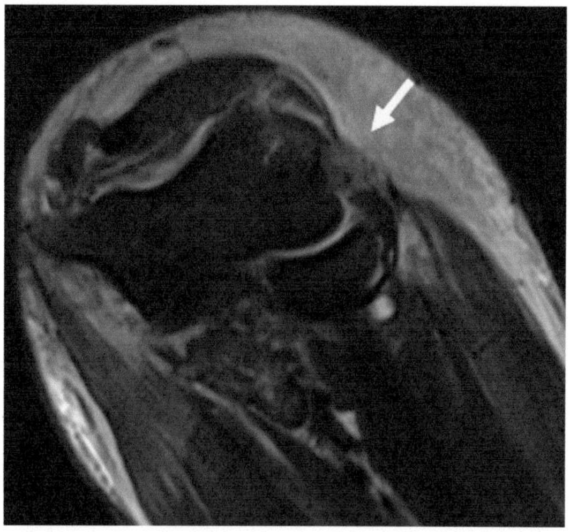

Fig. 8.32 Rupture of radial collateral ligament in an 18-year-old boy. Coronal PD MRI with elbow bent shows thickening and increased signal (*arrow*) at the proximal attachment of the RCL, consistent with tear (Courtesy of Rebecca Stein-Wexler)

Imaging

Radiography offers little in the evaluation of lateral ligament injury, but MRI is essential. The appearance of the RCL and LUCL varies significantly between individuals. However, proximal to the annular ligament, they generally appear inseparable [50]. Coronal and transverse proton-density-weighted (PD-W) MRI show focal ligament discontinuity (Fig. 8.32). If the tear is complete, joint fluid extravasation results. Tears of the LUCL usually occur at the humeral attachment and allow the radial head to move posteriorly.

Coronoid fractures in children may occur in association with posterior elbow subluxation or dislocation, often due to a fall on the outstretched arm. The coronoid process is key to bony stability, and if a fracture heals with malunion, this predisposes the elbow to recurrent posterior subluxation, especially if the lateral stabilizing ligaments are torn. Small shear fractures generally heal without complication. However, fractures that are not successfully reduced or that involve more than 50 % of the coronoid process heal poorly and may result in repeat episodes of subluxation or dislocation.

6 Little Leaguer's Elbow

This extension overload injury results in chronic traction injury to the medial epicondyle and compression injury at the radiocapitellar joint. It is common in young baseball players and other overhead throwers, who experience overuse with repetitive valgus stress. About 20 % of pitchers aged 10–14 years have experienced elbow pain [51], resulting in overuse injuries of the medial epicondyle in 2–8 % of all juvenile pitchers in this age group [13].

6.1 Medial Epicondylitis and Avulsion (Box 8.9)

Box 8.9: Medial Epicondylitis/Avulsion

Valgus stress (contraction of flexor-pronators) in overhead thrower/gymnast
Chronic stress reaction
Wide epicondylar physis
Apophysis sclerotic, irregular, fragmented
Severe injury: avulsion/displacement of epicondyle
MRI: wide physis, edema in apophysis/along physis

Traction apophysitis develops in response to chronic submaximal force that causes microavulsions at the bone-cartilage interface, resulting in a chronic stress reaction at the growth plate. Valgus stress in the throwing athlete is due to contraction of the flexor-pronator muscle group, which inserts in the medial epicondyle. As the physis is weaker than either bone or the myotendinous unit, the apophysis is especially vulnerable to stress during periods of rapid growth [52]. Overuse injury can also result in traction apophysitis at the olecranon, especially in young gymnasts [53].

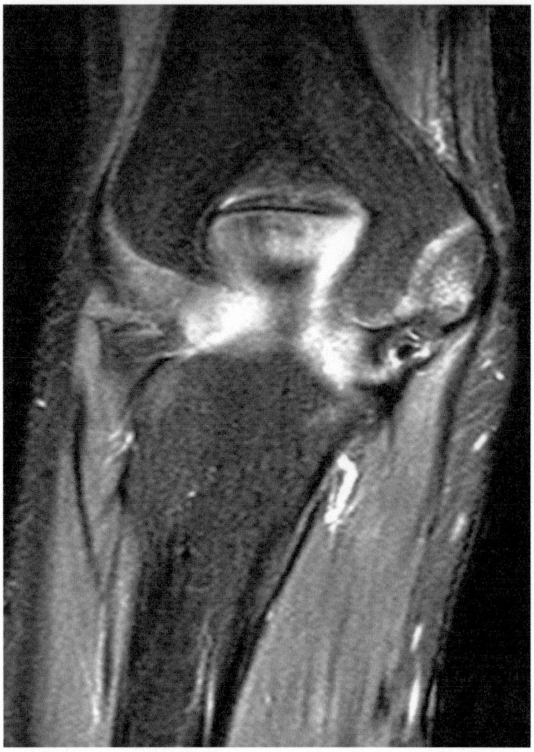

Fig. 8.33 Medial epicondylitis in an 11-year-old pitcher. Coronal PD FS image shows edema within the medial epicondyle and along both sides of the physis (Courtesy of Rebecca Stein-Wexler)

Imaging

On a frontal radiograph, the medial epicondylar physis may appear wide and indistinct. The apophysis may appear sclerotic, irregular, and fragmented. MRI (especially PD and fat-suppressed (FS) T2-weighted (T2-W) coronal and transverse sequences) depicts a wide physis. There is also soft tissue and bone marrow edema within and around the medial epicondylar apophysis, along with abnormal high-T2 signal along the physis (Fig. 8.33). With severe injury, there may be avulsion of the ossification center (Fig. 8.34), and it may even separate completely and displace into the joint.

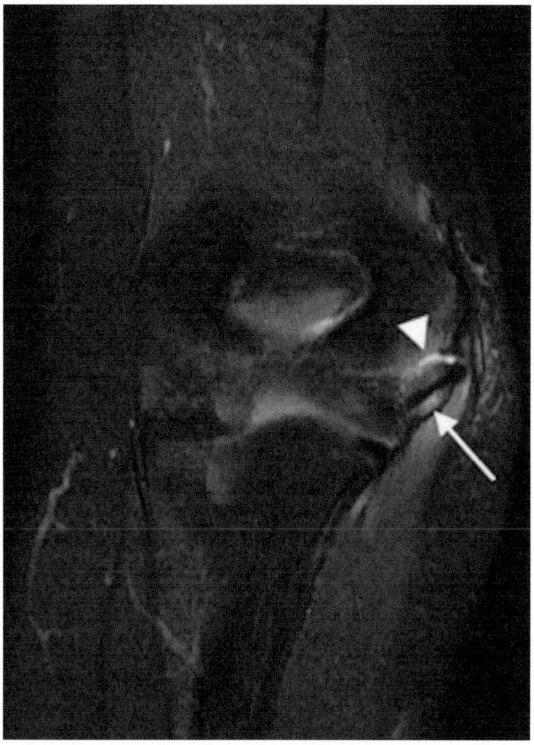

Fig. 8.34 Avulsion of the medial epicondyle in a 12-year-old pitcher. Coronal PD FS image shows a hyperintense fracture line (*arrowhead*) disrupting the hypointense cortex of the medial epicondyle. There is also a partial tear of the UCL at its proximal attachment (*arrow*). Note edema within the common flexor tendon (partially obscured by *arrow*) (Courtesy of Jasjeet Bindra)

Box 8.10: Osteochondritis Dissecans

Osteochondral lesion, usually anterolateral capitellum

Baseball pitchers, 10–15 years old

Repetitive valgus extension overload causes impaction

X-ray	Rarefaction of capitellar epiphysis near radial head
	Fraying, sclerosis, variable bony flake
MRI	Stable if cartilage intact, no surrounding high-T2 signal
	Unstable if fluid separates fragment from adjacent bone

Pseudodefect of capitellum: absent cartilage at posterolateral capitellum

6.2 Osteochondritis Dissecans (Box 8.10)

Osteochondritis dissecans (OCD) describes a condition in which a saucerlike piece of subchondral bone, sometimes along with its overlying cartilage, becomes damaged and possibly separated from the adjacent bone. This is considered an osteochondral lesion, although its name derives from the dissecting appearance of the condition. The pathophysiology is incompletely understood but presumed to be valgus extension overload that causes impaction at the radiocapitellar articulation. Increased incidence in pitchers and gymnasts between the ages of 10 and 15 supports this theory. Growing cartilage is especially vulnerable to repetitive microtrauma, rendering the cartilage at joint surfaces more prone to shear injuries and consequent detachment. The occasional occurrence of similar abnormalities in other joints raises the possibility that defective cartilage, blood supply, or repair mechanisms may contribute to this disorder. Apparently familial cases may actually represent cases of epiphyseal dysplasia.

The capitellum is consistently involved, and the radial head is occasionally affected. OCD at the elbow is more common in males and primarily affects the right side, although it is occasionally bilateral. Patients present with dull ache, effusion, restricted extension, and locking. Satisfactory healing with conservative management is likely for localized stable lesions in patients whose capitellar growth plate is open and whose elbow motion is not limited [54]. The prognosis for more advanced cases is guarded, as many progress to fragmentation and loose body formation with eventual osteoarthritis.

Imaging

Radiographs initially demonstrate mild rarefaction of the capitellar epiphysis adjacent to its articulation with the radial head. The contour

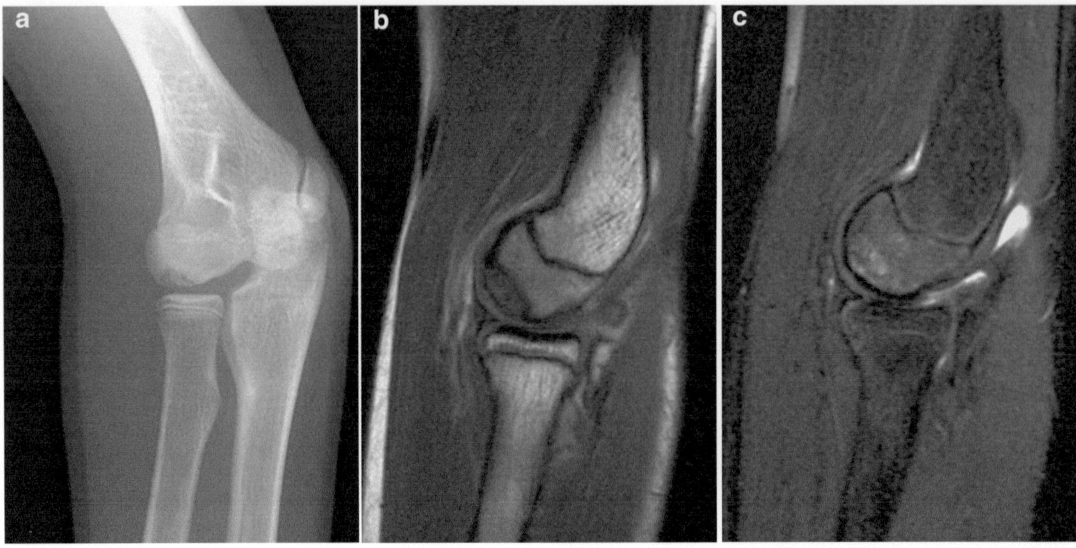

Fig. 8.35 Stable osteochondritis dissecans (OCD) in a 14-year-old pitcher. (**a**) Sclerosis with surrounding lucency at the capitellum. (**b**) Sagittal T1-W MRI shows intermediate signal at the subchondral capitellum, with an irregular hypointense line at the interface with normal bone. Cartilage appears thinned. (**c**) Corresponding sagittal inversion recovery (IR) image shows that there is edema, but high signal does not undercut the defect, and there are no cysts (Courtesy of Rebecca Stein-Wexler)

becomes frayed and the bone faintly sclerotic. A variably sized bony flake may be seen within a saucerlike defect. This is not necessarily a loose body, although if significantly displaced from the bone, it can be assumed to be free within the joint space.

MRI reliably detects osteochondritis dissecans. Early on, the superficial lesion appears normal on T2-W imaging but demonstrates low signal on T1. As disease progresses, increased T2 signal becomes apparent. OCD can be classified as grades 1–4 [55]:

- Grade 1: Hyaline cartilage covering the lesion is intact.
- Grade 2: There is an enhancing zone of separation (these lesions are still considered stable).
- Grade 3: Fluid is evident in the zone of separation (these lesions are unstable).
- Grade 4: There is a loose or displaced bone fragment.

In the pediatric age group, OCD lesions without surrounding high-T2 signal and with an intact cartilaginous surface are stable (Fig. 8.35) [52]. However, if there are multiple underlying cysts or a large (>5 mm) single cyst, if fluid signal separates the fragment from adjacent bone, if there are breaks in the subchondral bone, or if there is a fluid-filled osteochondral defect or a linear T2-hyperintense osteochondral fracture line, the fragment is likely to be unstable [56]. MRA improves staging of capitellar osteochondral lesions. Unstable lesions are characterized by fluid or contrast agent encircling the osteochondral fragment (Fig. 8.36) or by a cystic lesion subjacent to the fragment [13].

It is important not to confuse the relatively common pseudodefect of the capitellum (absence of cartilage at the posterolateral capitellum) (Fig. 8.37) with OCD, which occurs anterolaterally [57].

Loose bodies within the joint are usually of decreased signal intensity on both T1-weighted (T1-W) and T2-W imaging, although sometimes they contain fatty marrow and therefore appear bright on T1. They are most common in the anterior joint space (Fig. 8.38) or within the olecranon fossa but may lie anywhere within the joint capsule (Fig. 8.39). In the presence of a joint effusion, loose bodies are surrounded by fluid and therefore easier to appreciate. MRA assists with

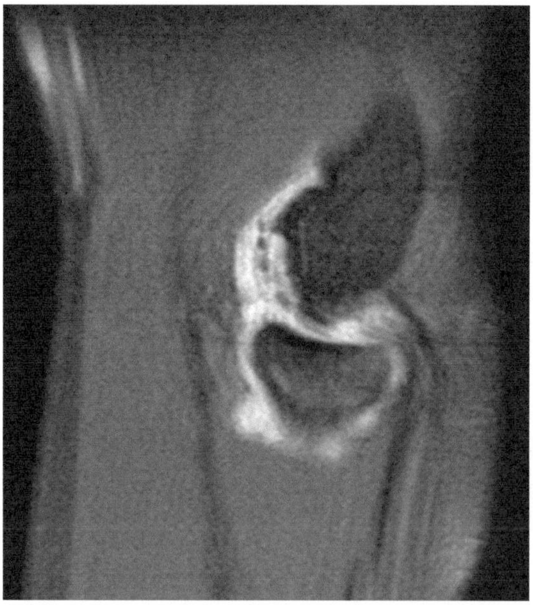

Fig. 8.36 OCD with unstable in situ fragments in a 14-year-old. Sagittal T1-W FS image from MRA shows hyperintense contrast material undercutting three separate hypointense fragments. Since contrast insinuates between them and adjacent bone, they are considered unstable (Courtesy of Rebecca Stein-Wexler)

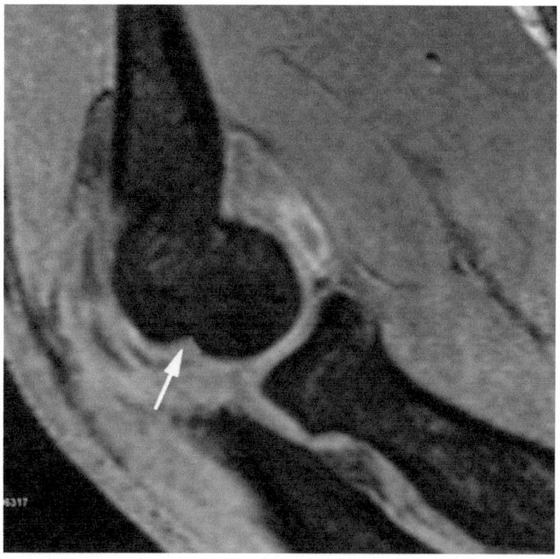

Fig. 8.37 Typical pseudodefect (*arrow*) at the posterolateral region of the capitellum on sagittal T1-W GRE MRI

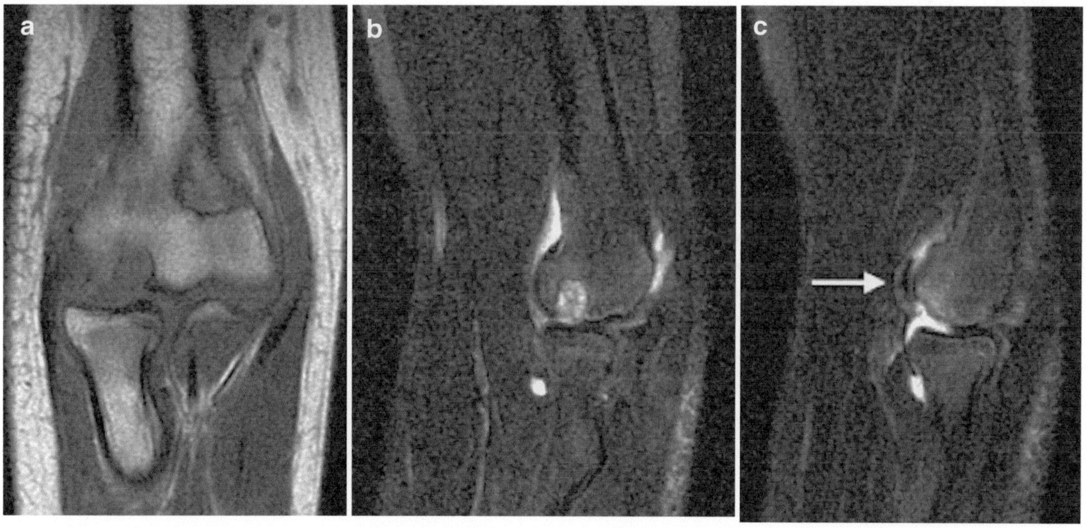

Fig. 8.38 Osteochondritis dissecans with loose body in anterior joint space. (**a**) Coronal T1-W image shows a smoothly marginated defect in the capitellum. (**b**) Sagittal T2-W FS image shows a small joint effusion, with high signal filling the bony defect. (**c**) Another sagittal T2-W FS image demonstrates marrow edema in the capitellum. A loose body (*arrow*) has rotated into the anterior joint compartment (Courtesy of Rebecca Stein-Wexler)

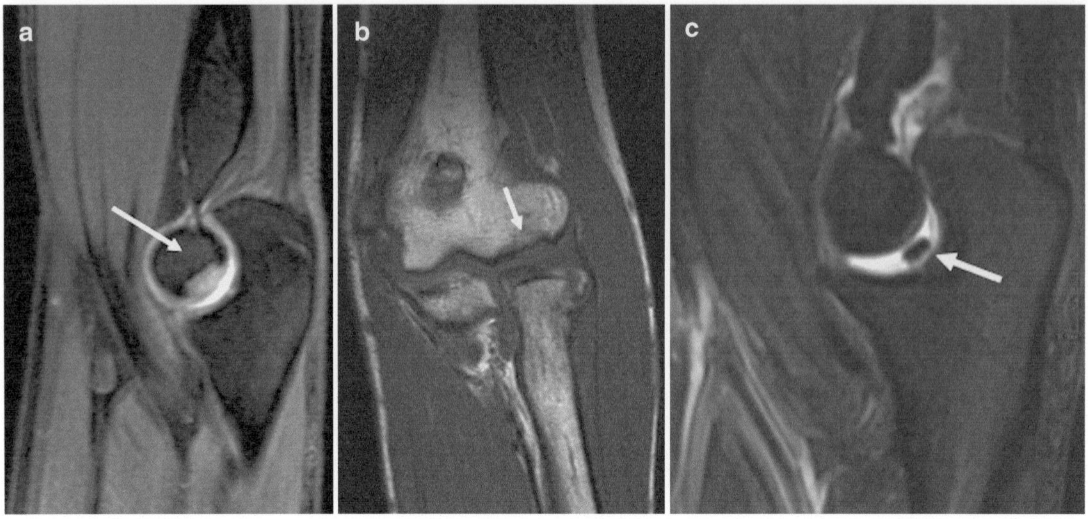

Fig. 8.39 Osteochondrosis dissecans in a 14-year-old boy with loose body between the olecranon and trochlea. Sagittal PD FS (**a**) and coronal T1-W (**b**) images demonstrate a broad-based defect in the capitulum (*arrow*) without marrow edema. (**c**) Sagittal T2-W FS image shows the loose body (*arrow*) wedged next to the sigmoid notch of the olecranon

identification, helps determine mobility, and better evaluates cartilage thinning at the bony defect.

If the OCD lesion heals, radiographs may become normal. However, there may be residual flattening, overgrowth, secondary reactive sclerosis, and cystic changes at the capitellum. The radial head and neck may enlarge, but some speculate that this contributes to, rather than results, from the process [58]. The physes of the distal humerus and radial neck may close prematurely.

Differential considerations are presented at the end of the next section, since they are similar for both osteochondritis dissecans and osteochondrosis.

Box 8.11: Osteochondrosis of Capitellum (Panner Disease)

Boys younger than 10 years
Repetitive trauma, compression loading: avascular necrosis
Involves entire capitellum (not just subcartilaginous bone)
- Fissures/irregular contour
- Fragmentation, flattening
- Eventual restoration of contours
- No loose bodies

MRI T1 hypointense; fragmented

7 Osteochondrosis of the Capitellum (Panner Disease) (Box 8.11)

Osteochondrosis of the capitellum, or Panner disease, is often confused with OCD. Like OCD, Panner disease is more common in boys. However, Panner disease occurs in younger children, before ossification of the capitellum is complete—most are under age 10. Furthermore, it characteristically involves the entire ossification center, rather than just the subcartilaginous bone. Also related to repetitive trauma and compression loading, Panner disease is thought to result from avascular necrosis. The adjacent radial head may demonstrate accelerated maturation [59].

The prognosis is much better than for OCD. Clinical series report self-limited disease with

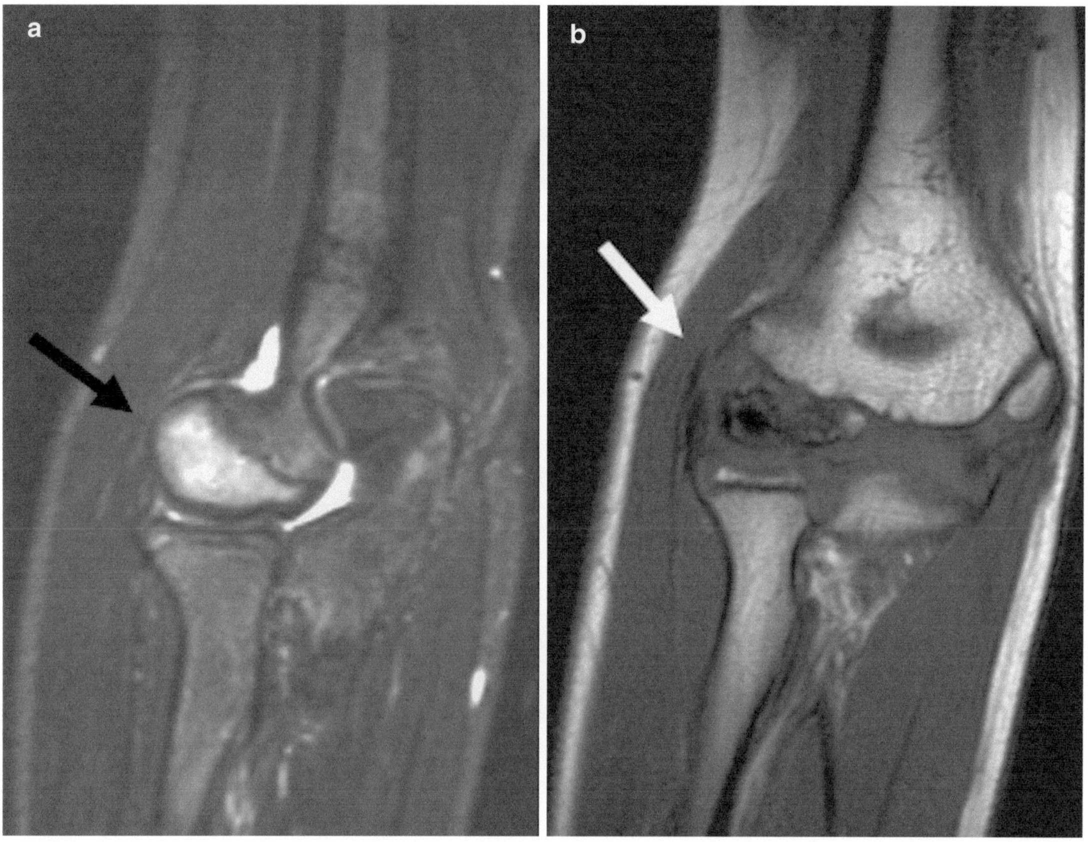

Fig. 8.40 Panner disease in a 9-year-old boy. (**a**) Sagittal T2-W image shows diffuse increased signal in the capitellum (*black arrow*). (**b**) The coronal T1-W image shows marked hypointensity involving the entire capitellum (*white arrow*)

good long-term results in the vast majority of patients treated without surgery [60].

Imaging

Unlike osteochondritis dissecans, with Panner disease the entire epiphysis is usually affected. The ossification center goes through the typical stages of necrosis and healing. As in the hip with Legg-Perthes disease, fissures and irregular contour develop, with subsequent fragmentation and flattening. In the elbow, contours are usually restored as the lesion heals and re-ossifies. MRI of course provides greater detail. The capitellum appears fragmented and hypointense at T1-W imaging (Fig. 8.40). The articular surface is usually intact, and therefore loose bodies do not usually develop.

Differential Diagnosis

Both OCD and Panner disease resemble multiple epiphyseal dysplasia, which may temporarily demonstrate similar-appearing irregular ossification. However, multiple epiphyseal dysplasia is not limited to the elbow. Synovial chondromatosis can also occasionally be confused with these disorders, but MRI demonstrates characteristic multiple rounded ossicles within the joint. Ossification variants should be considered, especially if the capitellum does not show typical progression and healing. The pseudodefect of the capitellum, which occurs at its posterolateral margin, may mimic Panner disease or OCD. Small air bubbles in MRA may resemble loose bodies, but bubbles demonstrate typical magnetic susceptibility artifact along their margin, most prominent on T2-W images.

References

1. Patel B, Reed M, Patel S. Gender-specific pattern differences of the ossification centers in the pediatric elbow. Pediatr Radiol. 2009;39(3):226–31. PubMed PMID: 19125245. Epub 2009/01/07. eng.
2. Cheng JC, Wing-Man K, Shen WY, Yurianto H, Xia G, Lau JT, et al. A new look at the sequential development of elbow-ossification centers in children. J Pediatr Orthop. 1998;18(2):161–7. PubMed PMID: 9531396. Epub 1998/04/08. eng.
3. Girdany BR, Golden R. Centers of ossification of the skeleton. Am J Roentgenol Radium Ther Nucl Med. 1952;68(6):922–4. PubMed PMID: 12996717.
4. Bajaj ID, Bhardwaj OP, Bhardwaj S. Appearance and fusion of important ossification centres: a study in Delhi population. Indian J Med Res. 1967;55(10): 1064–7. PubMed PMID: 5594378.
5. Garn SM, Rohmann CG, Silverman FN. Radiographic standards for postnatal ossification and tooth calcification. Med Radiogr Photogr. 1967;43(2):45–66. PubMed PMID: 6056078.
6. Hunter JB. Fractures around the shoulder joint and humerus. In: Bensom MFJ, Parsch K, editors. Children's orthopaedics and fractures, vol. 3. New York: Springer; 2010.
7. John SD, Wherry K, Swischuk LE, Phillips WA. Improving detection of pediatric elbow fractures by understanding their mechanics. RadioGraphics. 1996;16(6):1443–60. PubMed PMID: 8946546. quiz 63–4; Epub 1996/11/01. eng.
8. Gartland JJ. Management of supracondylar fractures of the humerus in children. Surg Gynecol Obstet. 1959;109(2):145–54. PubMed PMID: 13675986. Epub 1959/08/01. eng.
9. von Laer L. The supracondylar fracture of the humerus in children (author's transl). Arch Orthop Trauma Surg Archiv fur orthopadische und Unfall-Chirurgie. 1979;95(1–2):123–40. PubMed PMID: 526123. Die supracondylare Humerusfraktur im Kindesalter.
10. Webb AJ, Sherman FC. Supracondylar fractures of the humerus in children. J Pediatr Orthop. 1989; 9(3):315–25. PubMed PMID: 2656758.
11. Al-Aubaidi Z, Torfing T. The role of fat pad sign in diagnosing occult elbow fractures in the pediatric patient: a prospective magnetic resonance imaging study. J Pediatr Orthop B. 2012;21(6):514–9. PubMed PMID: 22735922. Epub 2012/06/28. eng.
12. Badelon O, Bensahel H, Mazda K, Vie P. Lateral humeral condylar fractures in children: a report of 47 cases. J Pediatr Orthop. 1988;8(1):31–4. PubMed PMID: 3335619. Epub 1988/01/01. eng.
13. Iyer RS, Thapa MM, Khanna PC, Chew FS. Pediatric bone imaging: imaging elbow trauma in children–a review of acute and chronic injuries. AJR Am J Roentgenol. 2012;198(5):1053–68. PubMed PMID: 22528894.
14. Pennington RG, Corner JA, Brownlow HC. Milch's classification of paediatric lateral condylar mass fractures: analysis of inter- and intraobserver reliability and comparison with operative findings. Injury. 2009;40(3):249–52. PubMed PMID: 19193372.
15. Mirsky EC, Karas EH, Weiner LS. Lateral condyle fractures in children: evaluation of classification and treatment. J Orthop Trauma. 1997;11(2):117–20. PubMed PMID: 9057147.
16. Rutherford A. Fractures of the lateral humeral condyle in children. J Bone Joint Surg Am. 1985;67(6):851–6. PubMed PMID: 4019532. Epub 1985/07/01. eng.
17. Weiss JM, Graves S, Yang S, Mendelsohn E, Kay RM, Skaggs DL. A new classification system predictive of complications in surgically treated pediatric humeral lateral condyle fractures. J Pediatr Orthop. 2009;29(6):602–5. PubMed PMID: 19700990.
18. Koh KH, Seo SW, Kim KM, Shim JS. Clinical and radiographic results of lateral condylar fracture of distal humerus in children. J Pediatr Orthop. 2010; 30(5):425–9. PubMed PMID: 20574257.
19. Wattenbarger JM, Gerardi J, Johnston CE. Late open reduction internal fixation of lateral condyle fractures. J Pediatr Orthop. 2002;22(3):394–8. PubMed PMID: 11961463. Epub 2002/04/19. eng.
20. Bernthal NM, Hoshino CM, Dichter D, Wong M, Silva M. Recovery of elbow motion following pediatric lateral condylar fractures of the humerus. J Bone Joint Surg Am. 2011;93(9):871–7. PubMed PMID: 21543677.
21. Song KS, Kang CH, Min BW, Bae KC, Cho CH. Internal oblique radiographs for diagnosis of nondisplaced or minimally displaced lateral condylar fractures of the humerus in children. J Bone Joint Surg Am. 2007;89(1):58–63. PubMed PMID: 17200311. Epub 2007/01/04. eng.
22. Ip D, Tsang WL. Medial humeral epicondylar fracture in children and adolescents. J Orthop Surg (Hong Kong). 2007;15(2):170–3. PubMed PMID: 17709855. Epub 2007/08/22. eng.
23. Gruber HE, Phieffer LS, Wattenbarger JM. Physeal fractures, part II: fate of interposed periosteum in a physeal fracture. J Pediatr Orthop. 2002;22(6):710–6. PubMed PMID: 12409893.
24. Salter RB, Zaltz C. Anatomic investigations of the mechanism of injury and pathologic anatomy of "pulled elbow" in young children. Clin Orthop Relat Res. 1971;77:134–43. PubMed PMID: 5140442. Epub 1971/01/01. eng.
25. Uptodate [Internet]. Wolters Kluwer health 2012. Available from: http://www.uptodate.com/home/about/index.html.
26. Arner O, Ekengren K, Von Schreeb T. Fractures of the head and neck of the radius; a clinical and roentgenographic study of 310 cases. Acta Chir Scand. 1957;112(2):115–34. PubMed PMID: 13402366. Epub 1957/02/19. eng.
27. Davidson RS, Markowitz RI, Dormans J, Drummond DS. Ultrasonographic evaluation of the elbow in infants and young children after suspected trauma. J Bone Joint Surg Am. 1994;76(12):1804–13. PubMed PMID: 7989385. Epub 1994/12/01. eng.
28. Zuazo I, Bonnefoy O, Tauzin C, Borocco A, Lippa A, Legrand M, et al. Acute elbow trauma in children: role of ultrasonography. Pediatr Radiol. 2008;38(9):982–8. PubMed PMID: 18626636. Epub 2008/07/16. eng.

29. Griffith JF, Roebuck DJ, Cheng JC, Chan YL, Rainer TH, Ng BK, et al. Acute elbow trauma in children: spectrum of injury revealed by MR imaging not apparent on radiographs. AJR Am J Roentgenol. 2001;176(1):53–60. PubMed PMID: 11133538.
30. Matthews JG. Fractures of the olecranon in children. Injury. 1980;12(3):207–12. PubMed PMID: 7228373. Epub 1980/11/01. eng.
31. Landin LA, Danielsson LG. Elbow fractures in children. An epidemiological analysis of 589 cases. Acta Orthop Scand. 1986;57(4):309–12.
32. Wheeless CR I. Wheeless' textbook of orthopaedics; 2011 [updated 13 Sept 2011]. Available from: http://www.wheelessonline.com/ortho/elbow_joint_menu.
33. Bado JL. The Monteggia lesion. Clin Orthop Relat Res. 1967;50:71–86. PubMed PMID: 6029027.
34. Tompkins DG. The anterior Monteggia fracture: observations on etiology and treatment. J Bone Joint Surg Am. 1971;53(6):1109–14. PubMed PMID: 5092801.
35. Lincoln TL, Mubarak SJ. "Isolated" traumatic radial-head dislocation. J Pediatr Orthop. 1994;14(4):454–7. PubMed PMID: 8077426.
36. Ring D, Jupiter JB, Waters PM. Monteggia fractures in children and adults. J Am Acad Orthop Surg. 1998;6(4):215–24. PubMed PMID: 9682084.
37. Kunkel S, Cornwall R, Little K, Jain V, Mehlman C, Tamai J. Limitations of the radiocapitellar line for assessment of pediatric elbow radiographs. J Pediatr Orthop. 2011;31(6):628–32. PubMed PMID: 21841436. Epub 2011/08/16. eng.
38. Kay RM, Skaggs DL. The pediatric Monteggia fracture. Am J Orthop (Belle Mead NJ). 1998;27(9):606–9. PubMed PMID: 9758451. Epub 1998/10/03. eng.
39. Eberl R, Singer G, Schalamon J, Petnehazy T, Hoellwarth ME. Galeazzi lesions in children and adolescents: treatment and outcome. Clin Orthop Relat Res. 2008;466(7):1705–9. PubMed PMID: 18443894. Pubmed Central PMCID: 2505249. Epub 2008/04/30. eng.
40. McCarthy SM, Ogden JA. Radiology of postnatal skeletal development. VI. Elbow joint, proximal radius, and ulna. Skelet Radiol. 1982;9(1):17–26.
41. Ryan J. The relationship of the radial head to radial neck diameters in fetuses and adults with reference to radial-head subluxation in children. J Bone Joint Surg Am. 1969;51(4):781–3. Pubmed Central PMCID: 5783859.
42. Ogden JA. Skeletal injury in the child. 2nd ed. Philadelphia: Saunders; 1990. p. 442–5.
43. Kim MC, Eckhardt BP, Craig C, Kuhns LR. Ultrasonography of the annular ligament partial tear and recurrent "pulled elbow". Pediatr Radiol. 2004;34(12):999–1004. PubMed PMID: 15517238.
44. Stewart B, Harish S, Oomen G, Wainman B, Popowich T, Moro JK. Sonography of the lateral ulnar collateral ligament of the elbow: study of cadavers and healthy volunteers. AJR Am J Roentgenol. 2009;193(6):1615–9. PubMed PMID: 19933656.
45. Finlay K, Ferri M, Friedman L. Ultrasound of the elbow. Skelet Radiol. 2004;33(2):63–79. PubMed PMID: 14714145.
46. Lee KS, Rosas HG, Craig JG. Musculoskeletal ultrasound: elbow imaging and procedures. Semin Musculoskelet Radiol. 2010;14(4):449–60. PubMed PMID: 20827626.
47. Carrino JA, Morrison WB, Zou KH, Steffen RT, Snearly WN, Murray PM. Noncontrast MR imaging and MR arthrography of the ulnar collateral ligament of the elbow: prospective evaluation of two-dimensional pulse sequences for detection of complete tears. Skelet Radiol. 2001;30(11):625–32. PubMed PMID: 11810154. Epub 2002/01/26. eng.
48. Sugimoto H, Ohsawa T. Ulnar collateral ligament in the growing elbow: MR imaging of normal development and throwing injuries. Radiology. 1994;192(2):417–22. PubMed PMID: 8029407.
49. O'Driscoll SW, Bell DF, Morrey BF. Posterolateral rotatory instability of the elbow. J Bone Joint Surg Am. 1991;73(3):440–6. PubMed PMID: 2002081.
50. Hannouche D, Begue T. Functional anatomy of the lateral collateral ligament complex of the elbow. Surg Radiol Anat. 1999;21(3):187–91. PubMed PMID: 10431332. Epub 1999/08/04. eng.
51. DaSilva MF, Williams JS, Fadale PD, Hulstyn MJ, Ehrlich MG. Pediatric throwing injuries about the elbow. Am J Orthop (Belle Mead NJ). 1998;27(2):90–6. PubMed PMID: 9506193.
52. Davis KW. Imaging pediatric sports injuries: upper extremity. Radiol Clin N Am. 2010;48(6):1199–211. PubMed PMID: 21094406.
53. Maffulli N, Chan D, Aldridge MJ. Overuse injuries of the olecranon in young gymnasts. J Bone Joint Surg. 1992;74(2):305–8. PubMed PMID: 1544975.
54. Takahara M, Mura N, Sasaki J, Harada M, Ogino T. Classification, treatment, and outcome of osteochondritis dissecans of the humeral capitellum. Surg Tech J Joint Surg Am Vol. 2008;90(Suppl 2 Pt 1):47–62. PubMed PMID: 18310686.
55. Stoller DW. Magnetic resonance imaging in orthopaedics and sports medicine. 3rd ed. Philadelphia: Lippincott Williams & Wilkins; 2007. 2336 p.
56. Jans LB, Ditchfield M, Anna G, Jaremko JL, Verstraete KL. MR imaging findings and MR criteria for instability in osteochondritis dissecans of the elbow in children. Eur J Radiol. 2012;81(6):1306–10. PubMed PMID: 21353415.
57. Tuite MJ, Kijowski R. Sports-related injuries of the elbow: an approach to MRI interpretation. Clin Sports Med. 2006;25(3):387–408. PubMed PMID: 16798134.
58. Smillie IS, Smillie IS. Osteochondritis dissecans; loose bodies in joints: etiology, pathology, treatment. Edinburgh: Livingstone; 1960.
59. Smith MG. Osteochondritis of the humeral capitulum. J Bone Joint Surg. 1964;46:50–4. PubMed PMID: 14126237. Epub 1964/02/01. eng.
60. Bowen RE, Otsuka NY, Yoon ST, Lang P. Osteochondral lesions of the capitellum in pediatric patients: role of magnetic resonance imaging. J Pediatr Orthop. 2001;21(3):298–301. PubMed PMID: 11371809.

The Hand and Wrist: Congenital and Developmental Conditions

9

Rebecca Stein-Wexler

Contents

R. Stein-Wexler, MD
Department of Radiology,
University of California Davis Medical Center and UC Davis Children's Hospital,
4860 Y Street, Suite 3100, Sacramento, CA 95817, USA

Department of Diagnostic Imaging,
Shriners Hospitals for Children Northern California,
Sacramento, CA, USA
e-mail: rebecca.steinwexler@ucdmc.ucdavis.edu

Abstract

This chapter discusses the common and uncommon forms of carpal coalition and then presents a variety of manifestations of amniotic bands. Following split-hand anomaly, macrodystrophia lipomatosa is discussed, followed by a brief discussion of symphalangism. Poland syndrome is discussed in greater depth. Four digital curvatures (clinodactyly, camptodactyly, Kirner deformity, longitudinal epiphyseal bracket) are presented. The chapter concludes with a discussion of thumb malformations, including those that are accompanied with potentially serious systemic manifestations (VACTERL association, Holt-Oram syndrome, Fanconi anemia, erythrogenesis imperfecta, and thrombocytopenia-absent radius).

The wrist and hand are affected by a variety of congenital and developmental disorders. Some of these are severely disfiguring and critically affect hand function, such as amputations due to amniotic bands, macrodystrophia lipomatosa, split hand, and symphalangism. Thumb malformations can be the first clue to the presence of a serious systemic disease. Some anomalies are asymptomatic or just mildly disfiguring, such as carpal coalition, clinodactyly or delta phalanx.

R. Stein-Wexler et al. (eds.), *Pediatric Orthopedic Imaging*,
DOI 10.1007/978-3-642-45381-6_9,

1 Normal Variants

Lucencies caused by soft tissues may project across the phalangeal epiphyses owing to slight flexion of the fingers or toes, simulating fractures. Thin developmental fissures in the navicular have been misinterpreted as fractures; such lines are usually more prominent on the ulnar side of the bone [1].

The pronator fat plane is located posterior to the flexor digitorum profundus tendons and anterior to the pronator quadratus muscle (Fig. 9.1). With almost all fractures at this level, it appears effaced, displaced anteriorly by joint effusion, or abnormally bowed. However, it may be normal if there is a buckle fracture limited to the posterior cortex.

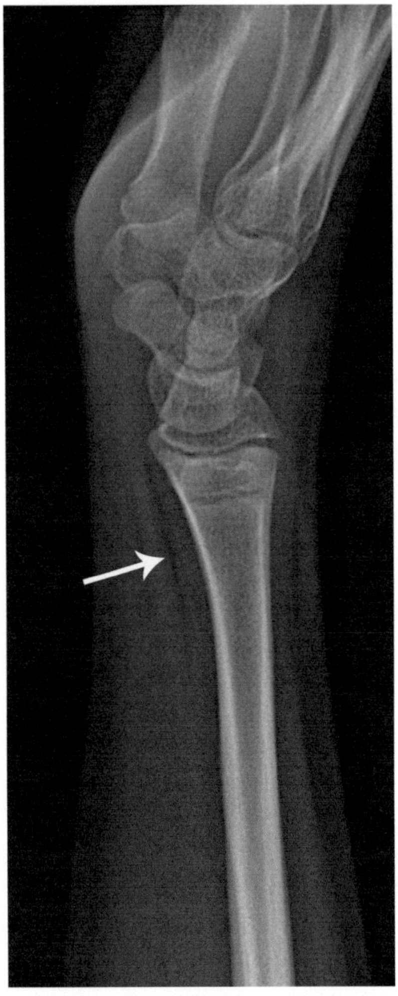

Fig. 9.1 Pronator fat plane in a 9-year-old girl. The fat that lies volar to the pronator quadratus muscle is well shown (*arrow*)

2 Carpal Coalition

Carpal fusion or coalition results from failure of normal segmentation of primitive embryologic mesenchyme. Usually asymptomatic, this occurs in up to 3.6 % of the white American population and is even more common in those of West African descent [2]. It is often familial and bilateral [3]. At times, overlap on radiographs simulates carpal fusion, but evaluation in other projections should clarify this issue. Magnetic resonance imaging (MRI) is rarely necessary. Patients rarely complain of pain or dysfunction unless the fusion is fibrous or crosses carpal rows.

Complete fusion with trabeculae connecting adjacent bones is observed in late childhood or adolescence, but earlier radiographs may demonstrate separate bone nuclei that gradually fuse during maturation. Incomplete fusion has been described in adults, with diminished joint space and small cystic lucencies in the subcortical regions of adjacent bones.

Isolated carpal fusion involves the same row and occurs by far most commonly between the lunate

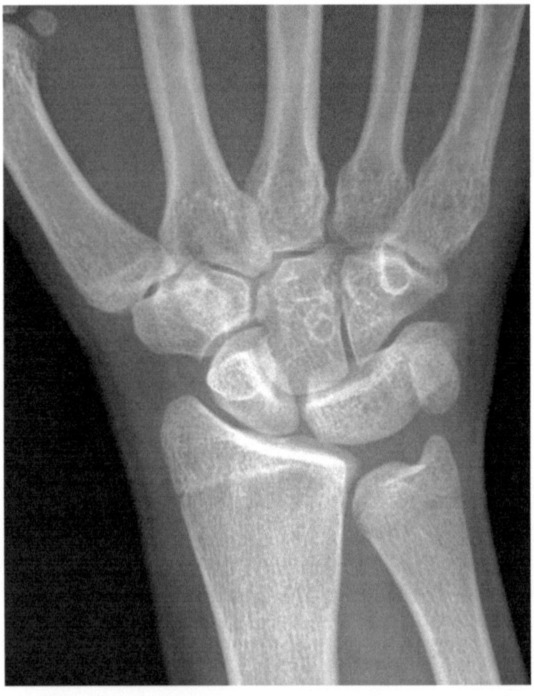

Fig. 9.2 Lunatotriquetral fusion in a 15-year-old girl. There is solid osseous fusion between the lunate and triquetrum (Courtesy of J. Herman Kan)

and triquetrum (Fig. 9.2), although occasionally the capitate and hamate fuse [3]. Fusion of other centers, or between carpal bones in different rows, should raise concern for prior infection, an associated systemic disorder (such as Turner's syndrome, arthrogryposis, or Ellis-van Creveld), or a skeletal dysplasia [4]. In the latter case, brachydactyly, symphalangism, or other anomalies may also be present. Acquired coalition usually indicates prior infection or, more commonly, juvenile idiopathic arthritis (JIA); severe JIA is frequently complicated by multicenter carpal fusion (see Chap. 20).

3 Amniotic Bands

Congenital amputations may occur when strands of amniotic tissue entrap and constrict fetal parts. The timing determines clinical findings—when early, there is amputation or complete syndactyly, and there may be severe accompanying multisystem involvement. A late event disrupts limb formation to a lesser extent, resulting in fewer amputations and fenestrated syndactyly [5]. Vascular congestion and hemorrhage occur distal to the bands [6], and various malformations result. Incidence is sporadic and varies between 1:1,200 and 1:150,000 births [7, 8]. There is no gender predilection.

Amniotic bands may be completely circumferential or segmental, and they may be shallow or deep enough to cause distal edema or ischemia; occasionally a distal fragment is delivered separately at birth. Defects are usually transverse and unilateral—if bilateral, they are rarely symmetric (Fig. 9.3). If the bands are deep, there may be accompanying vascular abnormalities [7]. MRI delineates soft tissue anomalies as well as vessels and nerves, which can assist surgical planning. Prenatal ultrasound (US) may identify defects and demonstrate bands of amniotic tissue.

Constriction defects are most common in the distal extremities, especially the hand. The middle digit is involved most often, and the thumb tends to be spared, perhaps due to fetal positioning (Fig. 9.4) [8]. Severity varies from cutaneous or osseous syndactyly to complete transverse

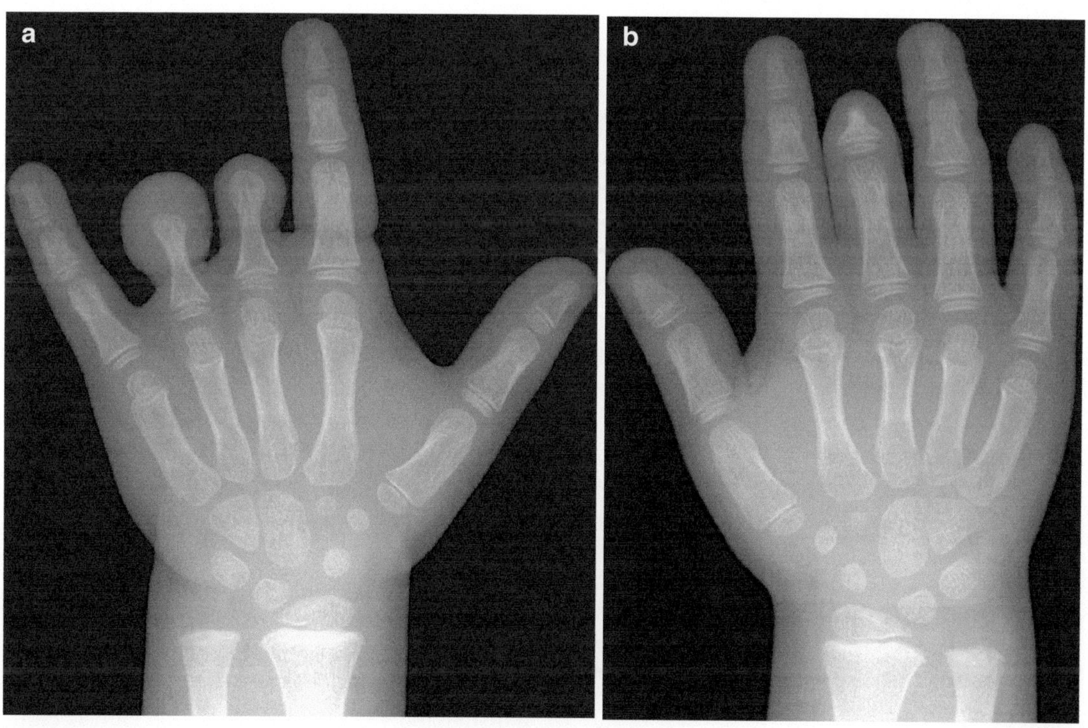

Fig. 9.3 Bilateral congenital amniotic bands. (**a**) (*left*) and (**b**) (*right*) hands demonstrate bilateral amputations that are more severe on the left (Images copyright Shriners Hospital for Children Northern California)

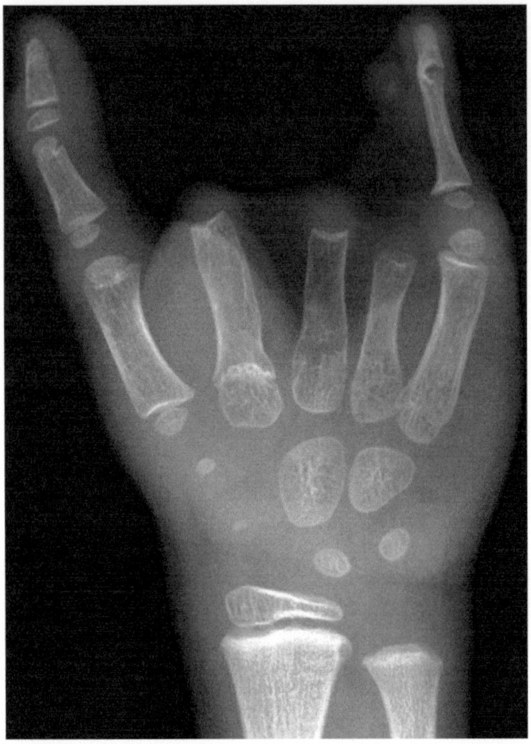

Fig. 9.4 Congenital amniotic bands. The second through fourth rays are amputated at the distal metacarpals, with dysplasia of the fifth finger (Image copyright Shriners Hospital for Children Northern California)

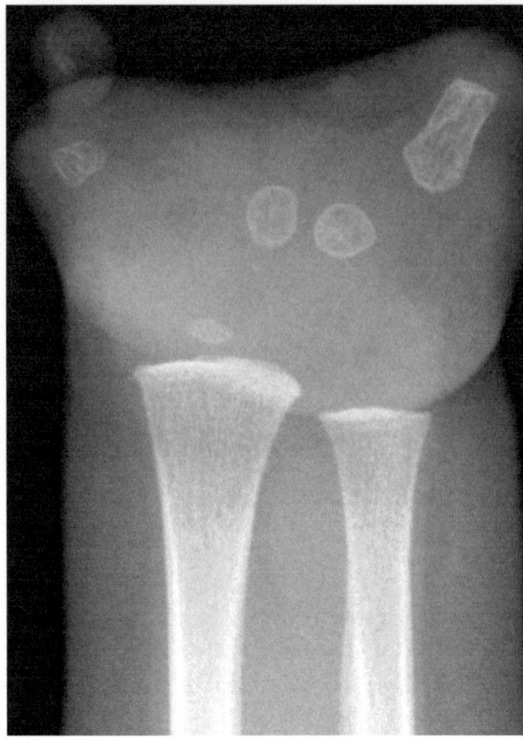

Fig. 9.5 Severe amputation, with minimal first and fifth rays present (Image copyright Shriners Hospital for Children Northern California)

terminal defects (Fig. 9.5). The distal portions of the digits may both amputate and fuse, resulting in acrosyndactyly (Fig. 9.6). Deformed digits may contain complete or incomplete bony units; stubby fleshy rudiments are common. Proximal fusion is often incomplete, resulting in epithelium-lined clefts between the proximal portions of digits [8]. Anencephaly and multiple asymmetric encephaloceles may accompany this abnormality. Clubfoot has been reported in more than one third of cases.

Differential Diagnosis

Transverse deficiency resembles amniotic band constriction defects. However, transverse deficiency of the hand (symbrachydactyly) is differentiated by the presence of nails and the absence of syndactyly (Figs. 9.7 and 9.8). Similarly, the presence of vestigial digits differentiates transverse deficiency of the forearm from amniotic bands [9] (see Chap. 7).

4 Split Hand

Split-hand defect, also known as cleft hand, may involve all four extremities and is inherited in an autosomal dominant pattern, occasionally skipping generations. Unilateral or sporadic cases are less common (Fig. 9.9). The term ectrodactyly, formerly used synonymously, is not specific for split hand but refers generally to total or partial hand/finger aplasia [4]. Deficiency of radial digits usually accompanies split hand; a strictly median split with all five digits present is rare. Syndactyly or symphalangism is common, and two digits may articulate with one forked metacarpal. A strut-like bone resembling a phalanx may cross from one metacarpal to another (Fig. 9.10). Carpal bones may be fused or absent, and the ulna is occasionally abnormal. The hand tends to function well but is aesthetically quite unusual and so surgery to close the cleft is com-

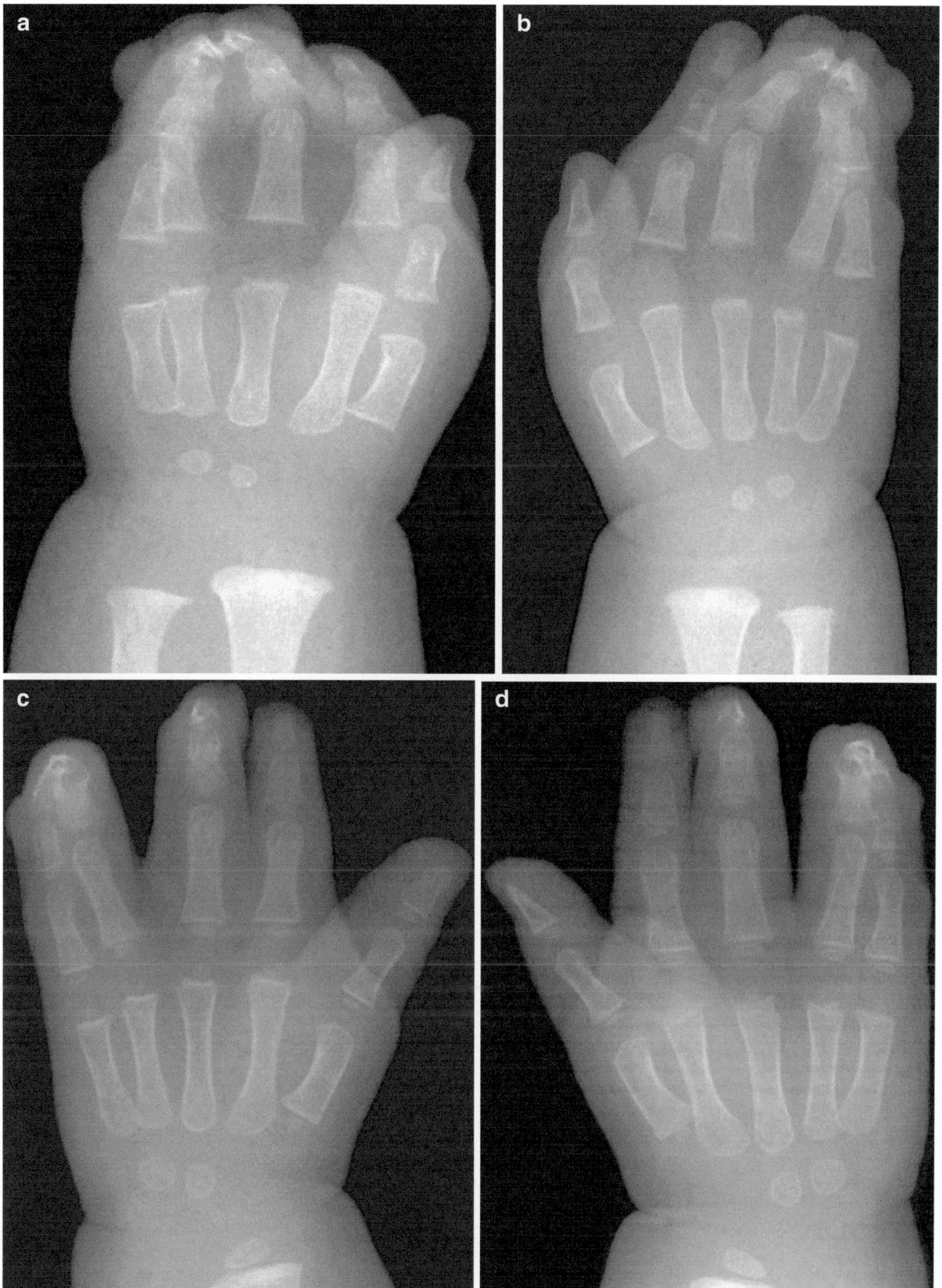

Fig. 9.6 Congenital amputations in a 1-month-old. (**a, b**) At presentation, there is typical mitten-like syndactyly. (**c, d**) Two years after surgical separation. (**e, f**) Three years later, after additional intervention, syndactyly is no longer present (Images copyright Shriners Hospital for Children Northern California)

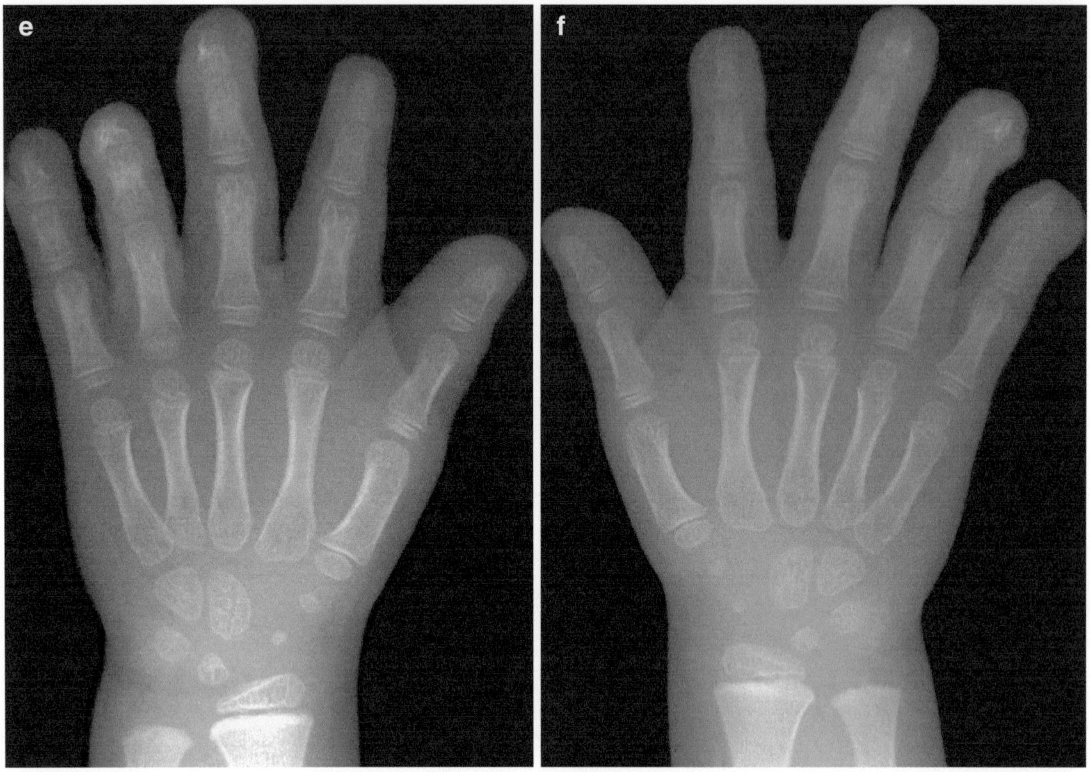

Fig. 9.6 (continued)

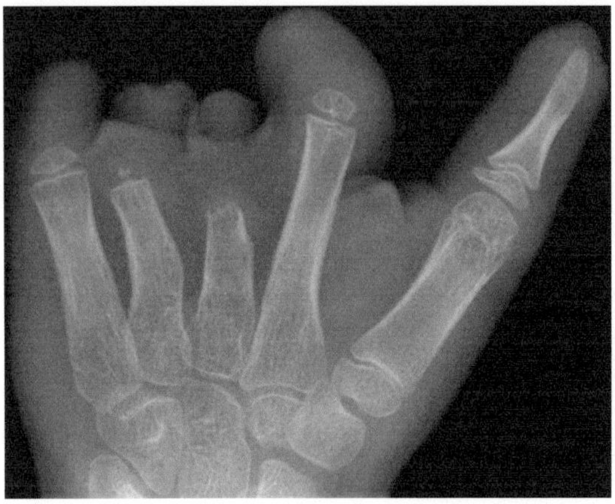

Fig. 9.7 Symbrachydactyly. There are varying degrees of hypoplasia of the metacarpals, a single phalanx at the thumb, and soft tissue nubbins representing the second through fourth digits. Well-formed nails can be appreciated at the first and third digits and are suggested at the other digits (Image copyright Shriners Hospital for Children Northern California)

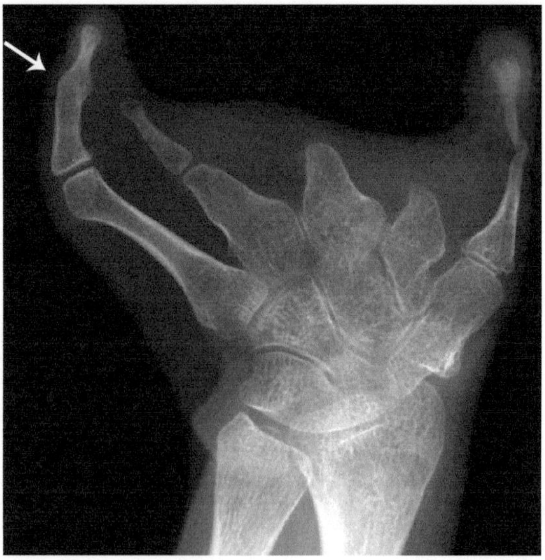

Fig. 9.8 Symbrachydactyly in a patient with Poland syndrome. The first through fourth metacarpals are hypoplastic and deformed, and there is symphalangism (*arrow*) at the fifth ray, as well as syndactyly between the fourth and fifth rays. The first ray is deformed and partially fused (Image copyright Shriners Hospital for Children Northern California)

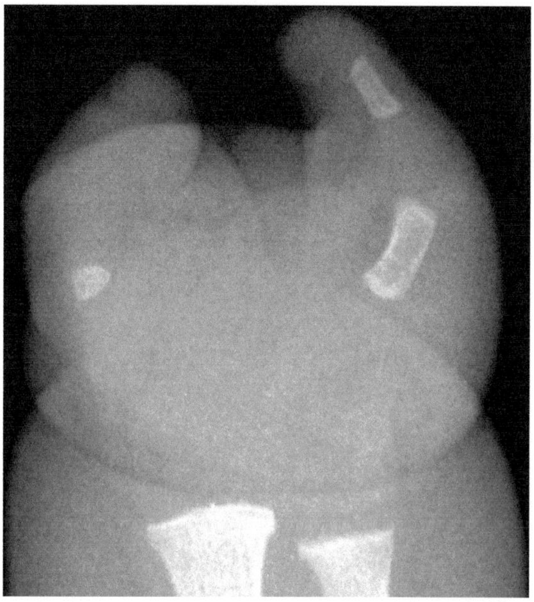

Fig. 9.9 Severe split hand, with markedly diminished ossification. There are only two ossified metacarpals, and both are severely hypoplastic (Image copyright Shriners Hospital for Children Northern California)

monly performed (Fig. 9.10). In addition, any transverse bones should be removed to prevent widening of the cleft, and finger deformities may be treated with rotation osteotomy.

5 Macrodystrophia Lipomatosa (Box 9.1)

Macrodystrophia lipomatosa—hamartomatous overgrowth of all mesenchymal elements of the digit including adipose tissue, phalanges, tendons, nerves, and vessels—presents at birth [10]. It is usually unilateral; if bilateral, rarely symmetric. Severe cases may also affect the more proximal portion of the extremity.

Etiology is obscure. Macrodystrophia lipomatosa may result from alteration in somatic cells during limb bud development as well as disturbed fetal circulation [11]. It can be considered to be a localized form of Proteus syndrome, in part because in both conditions PTEN (phosphatase and tensin homolog) is deleted from chromosome 10 [12]. However, although all elements of the finger (blood vessels, tendons, bones, nails) are overgrown, adipose tissue and nerves are especially affected. The adipose tissue is distributed in a mesh of fibrous tissue, involving marrow, periosteum, muscles, nerve sheaths, and subcutaneous tissues. When encountered in the hand, it typically occurs in the distribution of the median nerve, and there may be palmar neuromas or fibrolipomatous hamartomas of the nerve, suggesting it represents a neural disorder, probably related to the sensory nerve distribution pattern. Macrodystrophia lipomatosa does not appear to be inherited and is almost always isolated [13].

Macrodystrophia lipomatosa in the foot is more likely to involve only the phalanges and to demonstrate disproportionate growth; it other wise behaves and appears similar to the hand [13]. The plantar nerves are often enlarged.

In the hand, multiple osteotomies and debulking procedures can be performed with the goal of cosmesis and good function. However, stiffness almost always eventually develops in the affected digits. If only one digit is involved, ray amputation can be a good option (Fig. 9.11). Additionally, multiple epiphysiodeses can be considered in an attempt to stop longitudinal growth. Amputation is often performed in the foot, with the goal of symmetric shoe size. Premature osteoarthritis may develop in late adolescence.

Imaging

The involved digit is enlarged at birth and may develop proportionately or disproportionately. If more than two fingers are involved, syndactyly may be present as well. The second and third digits are affected most often, whereas the fifth is rarely involved (Figs. 9.12 and 9.13). A rare type has associated hyperostosis and apparent osteochondromatous masses [14]. The metacarpals are frequently normal, but may grow disproportionately. The distal ends of the phalanges are splayed, and the phalanges are broad and elongated. Soft tissues are obviously enlarged, with fatty proliferation most pronounced at the palmar/plantar and lateral regions. This contributes to apparent hyperextension and ulnar deviation [13]. Fatty infiltration is visible radiographically and can be confirmed with MRI (Fig. 9.14).

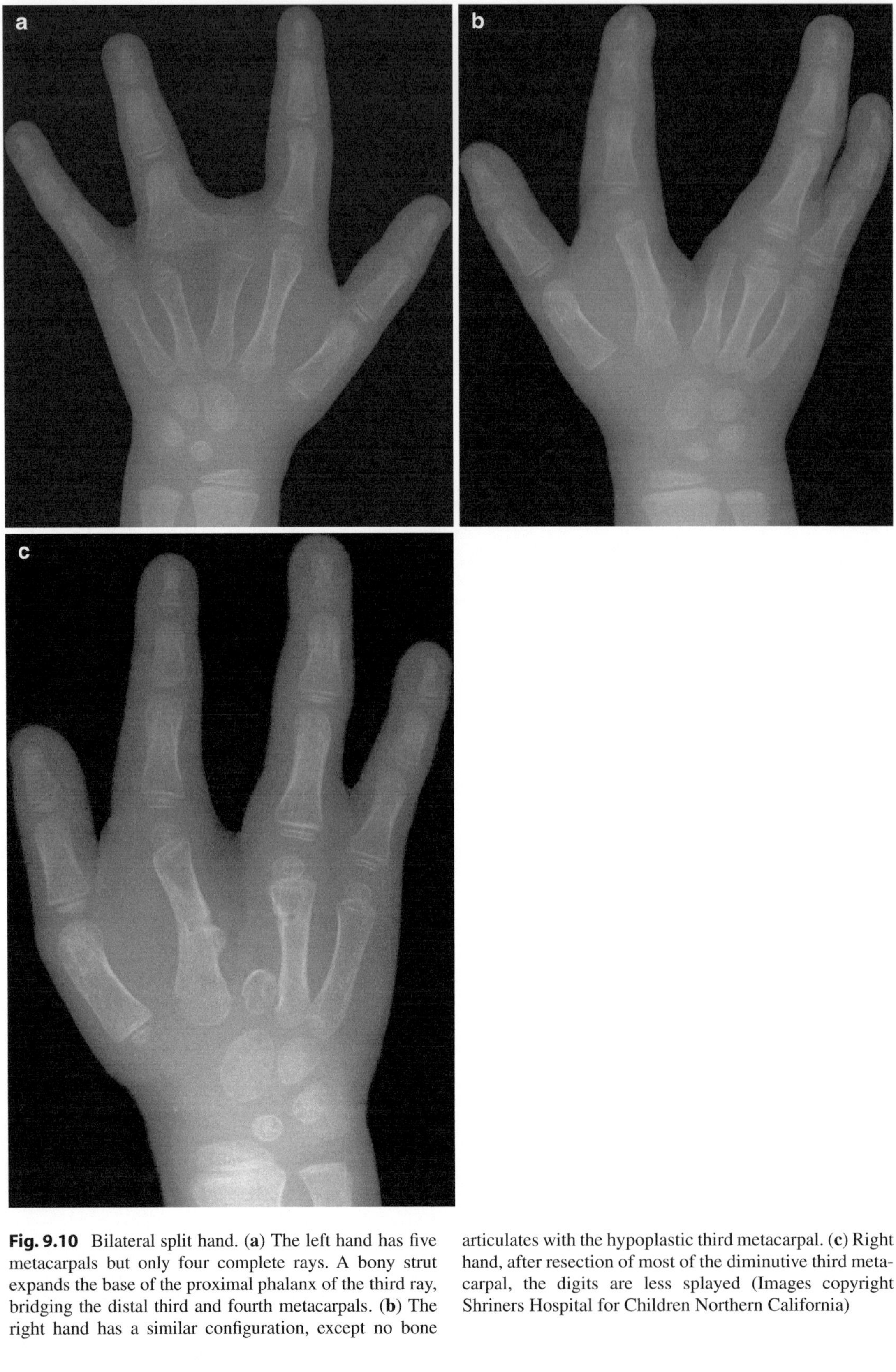

Fig. 9.10 Bilateral split hand. (**a**) The left hand has five metacarpals but only four complete rays. A bony strut expands the base of the proximal phalanx of the third ray, bridging the distal third and fourth metacarpals. (**b**) The right hand has a similar configuration, except no bone articulates with the hypoplastic third metacarpal. (**c**) Right hand, after resection of most of the diminutive third metacarpal, the digits are less splayed (Images copyright Shriners Hospital for Children Northern California)

At magnetic resonance imaging (MRI), T1-weighted (T1-W) images show hyperintense fat signal interspersed between linear fibrous hypointense bands; at T2-weighted (T2-W) imaging, most of the tissue demonstrates intermediate signal intensity, following that of fat [15]. The fatty tissue, lacking encapsulation, is less defined than typical lipomas [16]. There may be accompanying fibrolipomatous hamartomas of the nerve, resulting in fusiform enlargement due to fat interspersed between nerve bundles [17]. If there is severe fatty infiltration of the nerve, it may be difficult to differentiate from the surrounding adipose tissue.

Box 9.1: Macrodystrophia Lipomatosa

Hamartomatous overgrowth of mesenchymal elements

Second and third digits most often

T1-W: hyperintense fat between linear fibrous hypointense bands

T2-W: intermediate signal

Lacks encapsulation, less defined than lipomas

Differential Diagnosis

Congenital enlargement of one or several digits may be a local manifestation of a more extensive disease, such as hemangiomatosis, lymphangiomatosis, arteriovenous malformation, Klippel-Trenaunay syndrome, neurofibromatosis, or congenital lymphedema.

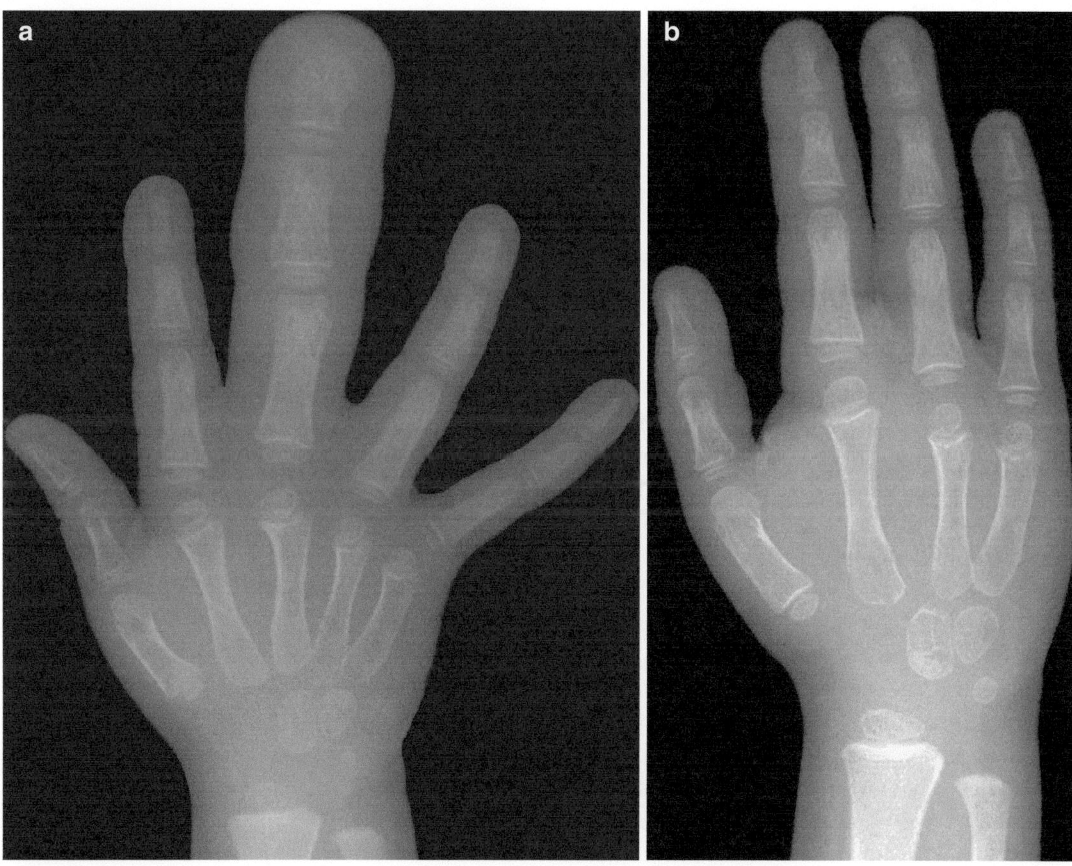

Fig. 9.11 Macrodystrophia lipomatosa in a 3-year-old girl, before and after treatment. (**a**) The third ray is markedly enlarged, with overgrowth of the bones and soft tissues. Debulking procedures had been unsuccessful. (**b**) Several months later, it has been resected (Images copyright Shriners Hospital for Children Northern California)

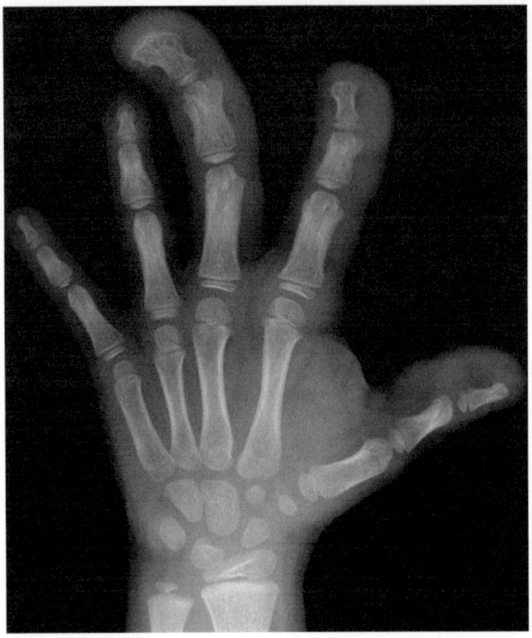

Fig. 9.12 Macrodystrophia lipomatosa in a 6-year-old boy. The phalanges of the third digit (and to a lesser extent the second) are broad and elongated. There is fatty infiltration, with ulnar deviation of the overgrown third ray (Image copyright Shriners Hospital for Children Northern California)

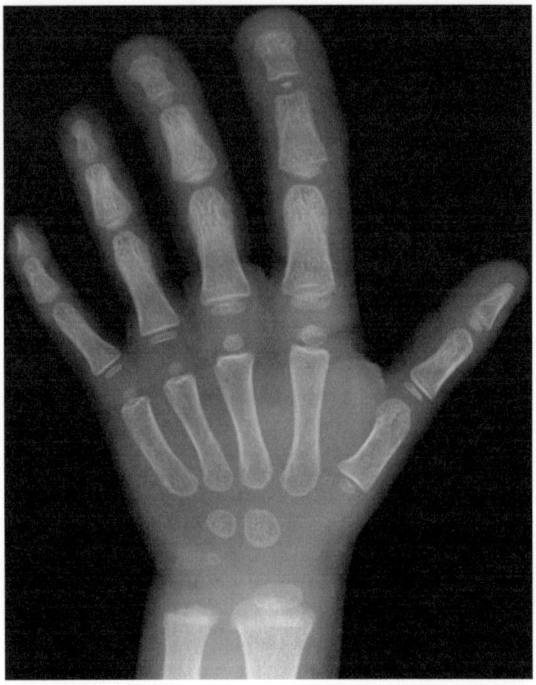

Fig. 9.13 Macrodystrophia lipomatosa involving the second and third rays, with relatively mild bone and soft tissue overgrowth (Image copyright Shriners Hospital for Children Northern California)

6 Symphalangism

Symphalangism refers to the fusion of one phalanx to another within the same digit and presumably results from failure of the joint segment to differentiate (Fig. 9.15). Since this area is cartilaginous in infancy, the lack of segmentation may not be evident radiographically until later, although the interphalangeal space or the physis of the middle phalanx may be narrowed [4]. Clinically, the normal flexion and extension creases in the skin overlying the affected joint are absent from birth. The middle phalangeal physis may fuse prematurely, or the epiphysis may first fuse with the phalanx just proximal to it. Symphalangism is distinguished from syndactyly, which refers to cutaneous or osseous fusion between adjacent digits.

Frequently inherited as an autosomal dominant trait, symphalangism can affect both hands and both feet in a bilaterally symmetric pattern. In the hands it characteristically affects the proximal interphalangeal joint (Fig. 9.15), whereas in the feet the distal interphalangeal joint is usually involved. The fifth finger is affected most often, and the thumb is rarely abnormal. The proximal and middle phalanges may be linked by a smooth continuum of bone, but there is frequently expansion at the expected level of the joint, and a partial cleft or irregular lucency may be present. The distal phalanges are often hypoplastic, and the metacarpal heads slightly flattened. The skin around the joint is smooth due to lack of flexion.

Carpal and tarsal fusions accompany symphalangism in many families. In the hand, triquetral-hamate and capitate-hamate fusions are most common; in the foot, talonavicular or calcaneocuboid fusions occur. Syndactyly is often associated, and syndromic cases often have associated acrocephalosyndactyly. Elbow dysplasia may coexist.

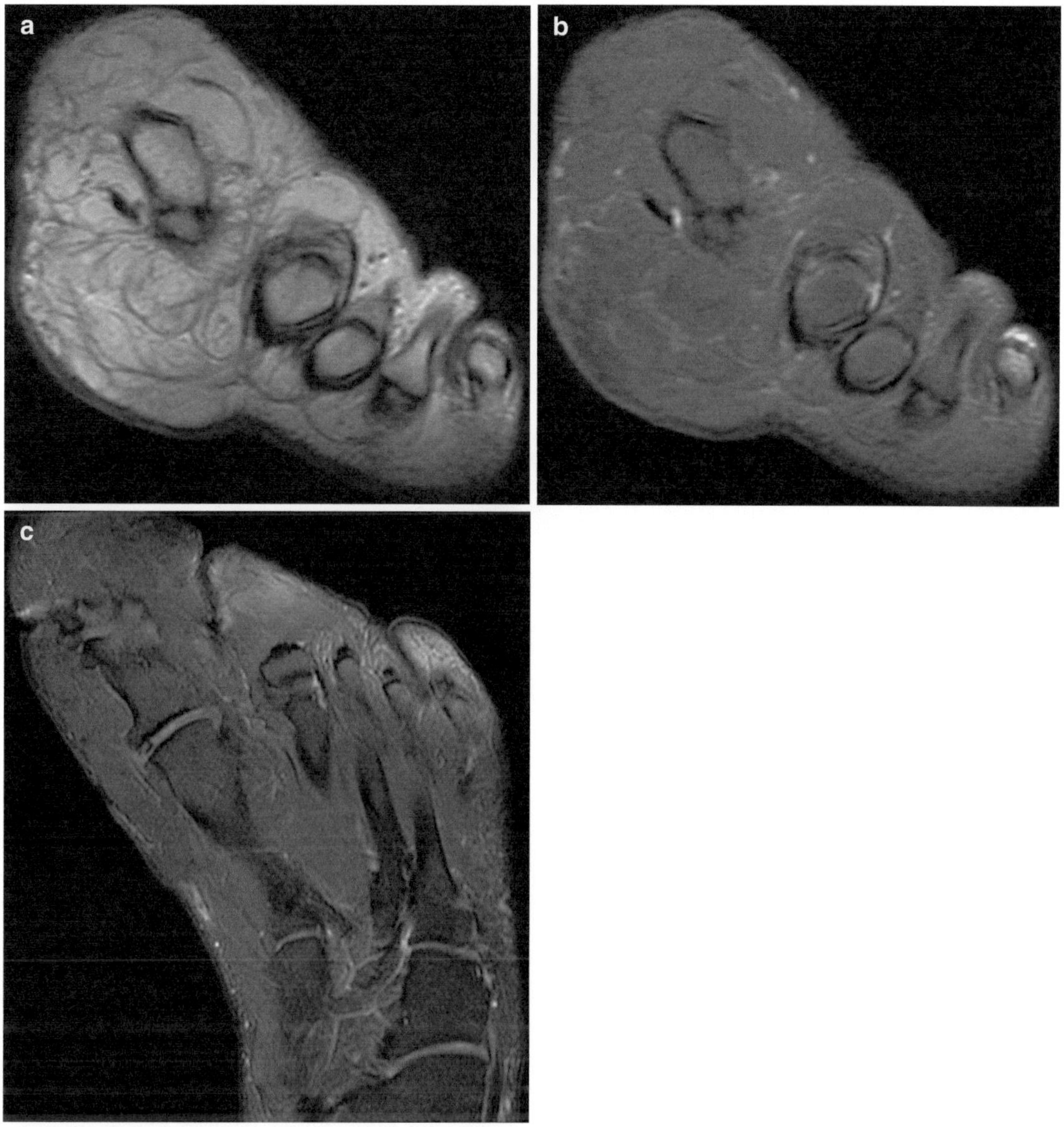

Fig. 9.14 Macrodystrophia lipomatosa in a 17-year-old boy. (**a**) Coronal proton density (PD) MRI through the distal metatarsals demonstrates fatty infiltration of the interosseous spaces; this is hypointense on the corresponding coronal PD fat-suppressed (FS) image (**b**). An axial PD FS image (**c**) through the foot demonstrates both osseous and soft tissue hypertrophy

7 Pectoral Aplasia-Dysdactyly (Poland Syndrome) (Box 9.2)

Poland syndrome consists of unilateral anomalies of thoracic musculature, sometimes accompanied with ipsilateral hypoplasia of the hand. The most common muscular abnormality is aplasia of the sternocostal head of the pectoralis major muscle, but sometimes the entire muscle is missing and—rarely—the pectoralis minor and latissimus dorsi muscles are absent as well. Mammary hypoplasia is common.

Local pressure or damaged mesoderm probably leads to temporary or permanent disruption of

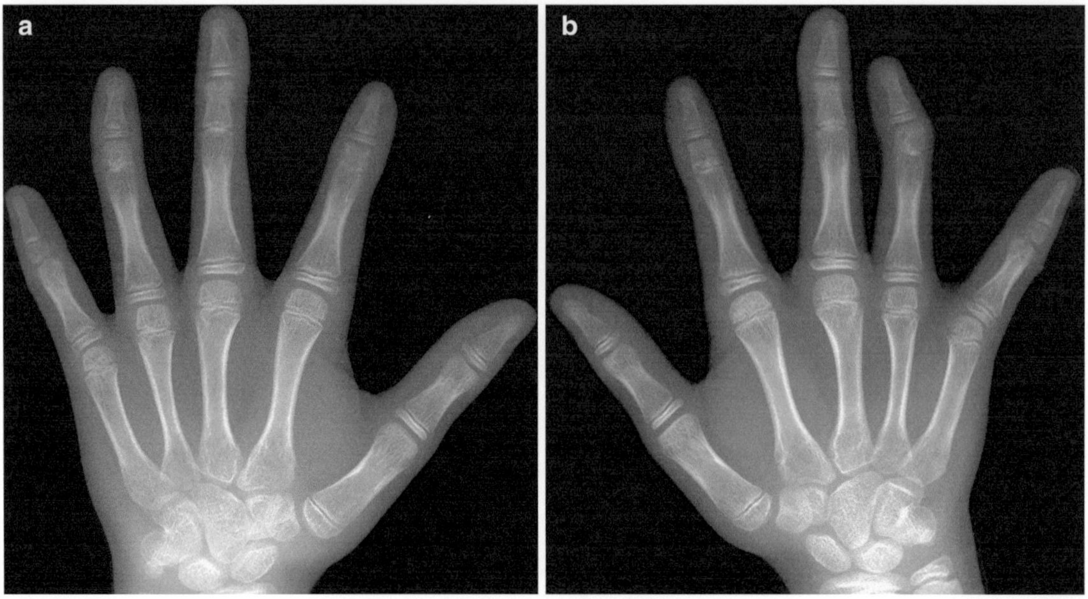

Fig. 9.15 Symphalangism in a 12-year-old girl. (**a**) (*left*) and (**b**) (*right*) radiographs show the proximal interphalangeal joints of the second through fourth digits are fused to a variable but symmetric extent, with partial clefts evident in the third and fourth digits. The middle phalanges are hypoplastic, and the heads of the metacarpals are flattened (Courtesy of Tal Laor, Cincinnati Children's Hospital)

Box 9.2: Poland Syndrome

Unilateral anomaly of thoracic musculature and sometimes hand

Hypoplastic hand, especially middle phalanges

Split hand possible

Hypoplastic ribs, especially third through fifth

MRI: aplasia of sternocostal head of pectoralis major muscle most common

the subclavian artery, vertebral artery, and their branches; exposure to ergot alkaloids during the first trimester is also associated [18, 19]. Poland syndrome is a predominantly sporadic lesion that occurs in one in 50,000 newborns [18]. Moebius, Klippel-Feil, and Adams-Oliver syndrome rarely accompany this syndrome [19]. Eight percent of patients with syndactyly have Poland syndrome [20], but only 12 % of patients with Poland syndrome have an abnormal hand [19]. Usually found in boys, it is most common on the right. In girls, there is no side predilection [2]. Deformities are rarely bilateral. Accompanying abnormalities of the feet are infrequent.

Imaging

If the hand is affected, the entire hand is usually hypoplastic, typically with short fingers and the absence or hypoplasia of the middle phalanges (especially on the ulnar side) (Fig. 9.16). Syndactyly is often present, potentially involving all fingers but in milder cases limited to the index and middle fingers [21]. Often the thumb and fifth finger are spared. Brachysyndactyly, split hand, and congenital amputations may occur. Carpal bones—usually the scaphoid and trapezium—are often fused; delayed carpal ossification is common, often disharmonious compared with the phalanges [2]. These carpal abnormalities are best appreciated before 10 years of age. Hypoplasia of the forearm is proportional to the extent of the hand anomaly.

A chest radiograph reveals increased lucency on the affected side, secondary to absent musculature and in some cases breast tissue. The clavicular segment of the pectoralis major muscle may be identified as a faintly dense band. Ribs—especially the third through fifth—may be missing or hypoplastic, and the sternum may be rotated or otherwise abnormal. The scapula may be elevated,

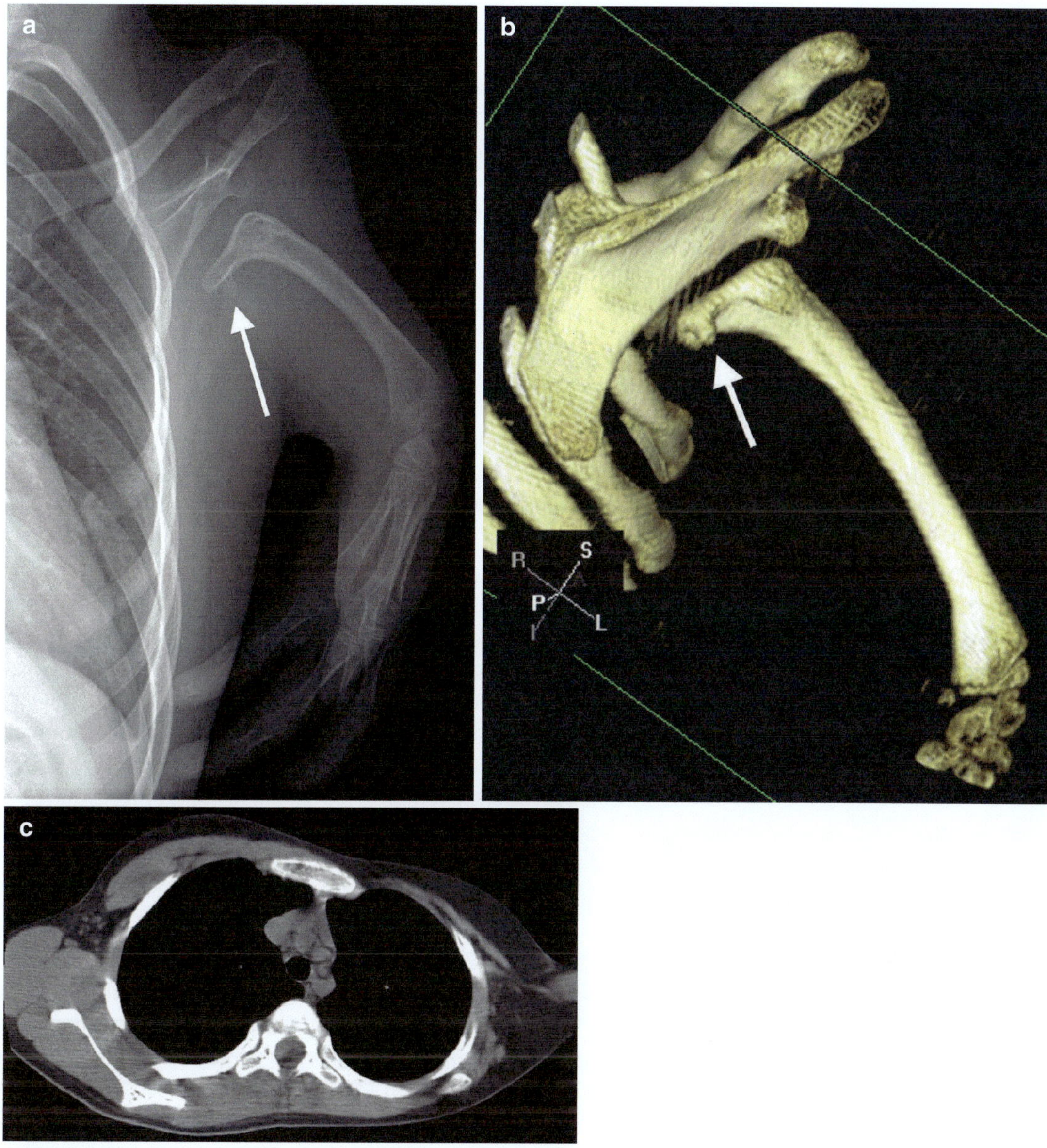

Fig. 9.16 Phocomelia and Poland syndrome in a 10-year-old girl. (**a**) The upper extremity consists of a large osseous structure, principally the radius, fused to a very hypoplastic humerus. Note the hypoplastic ulna (*arrow*). There are four rays. (**b**) Three-dimensional reformatted CT (3D CT) image also demonstrates the rudimentary ulna (*arrow*). (**c**) Axial CT shows the absence of the sternal head of the pectoralis major muscle as well as atrophic bones and musculature of the entire left side of the thorax

and there may be scoliosis [19]. Radiographs of the upper extremity and hand delineate a wide variety of abnormalities as described above.

Color Doppler ultrasound (US) of the interdigital arteries may reveal decreased velocity and resistive index [18].

Computed tomography with three-dimensional reconstruction (3D CT) is especially useful if surgery is being considered (usually for cosmetic reasons). 3D CT delineates both soft tissue and osseous chest wall abnormalities and assists with planning (Figs. 9.17 and 9.18) [19, 22].

Magnetic resonance imaging (MRI) of the chest characterizes muscular abnormalities. Hand and wrist MRI may demonstrate absence of flexor and extensor tendons along with anomalous musculature [2, 23]. Magnetic resonance angiography demonstrates narrowed vessels.

8 Digital Curvatures (Box 9.3)

Positional artifact is the most common cause of digital deviation, and especially in infants and uncooperative children, it is important to ascertain that an apparent deformity persists. Growth alteration following epiphyseal damage in cases of trauma, burn, frostbite, osteomyelitis, and sensory loss or paralysis may cause phalangeal deformity (see Chap. 10). Once these and other primary conditions have been excluded, a group of uncommon but distinctive isolated digital deformities should be considered.

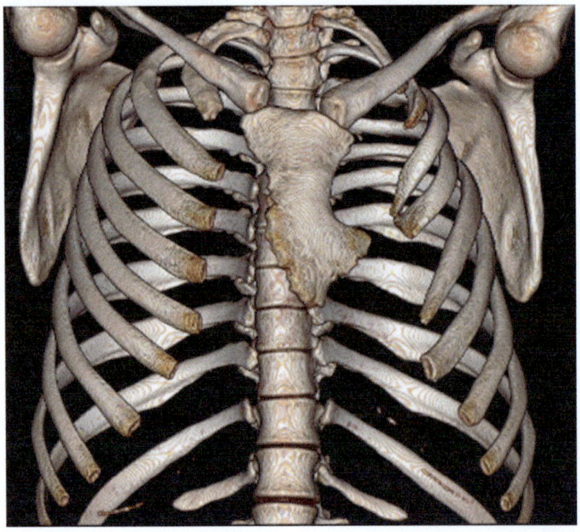

Fig. 9.17 Poland syndrome in a 17-year-old female. 3D CT shows sternal deviation toward the dysplastic left ribs

8.1 Clinodactyly

Clinodactyly usually affects the fifth digit and results from an abnormal middle phalanx that causes the distal phalanx to tilt laterally in the coronal plane. The middle phalanx is often hypoplastic, with an inclined distal articular surface (Fig. 9.19). There may be a longitudinally bracketed epiphysis, with growth restricted on the side of the bone with the C-shaped epiphysis (further discussed below) [24]. A distal pseudoepiphysis with a radially open cleft is characteristic at an early age. Often bilateral, this occurs as a sporadic variant in up to one percent of some populations or can be inherited as an autosomal dominant trait. It often occurs in trisomy 21 and is also encountered in many other conditions [4]. Function is rarely impaired. Surgical correction involves osteotomy and/or resection of a portion of the abnormal epiphysis [25].

8.2 Camptodactyly

This permanent dorso-volar flexion of the digit usually occurs at the proximal interphalangeal joint of the fifth finger (Fig. 9.20). It probably results from an abnormal fascia or insertion of

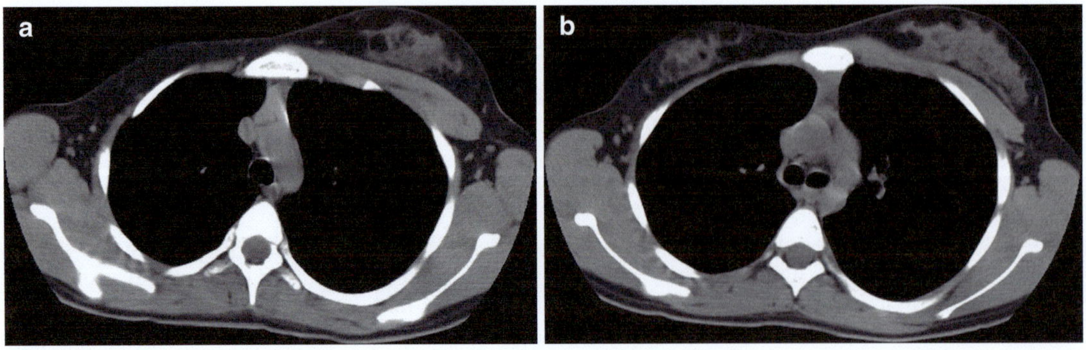

Fig. 9.18 Poland syndrome in a 13-year-old female. Axial CT images (**a, b**) demonstrate hypoplastic right hemithorax with aplasia of the right pectoralis major muscle and hypoplastic breast tissue

the flexor digitorum sublimis tendon. Although some children can present with camptodactyly at birth, others do not develop the condition until adolescence. It may be sporadic or inherited as an autosomal dominant trait, sometimes associated with clinodactyly. If digits other than the fifth are affected, an accompanying syndrome is likely [24].

Box 9.3: Fifth Digit Curvatures

Clinodactyly: hypoplastic middle phalanx causes distal phalanx to tilt laterally

Camptodactyly: dorso-volar flexion at PIP joint

Kirner deformity: distal phalanx curves in radial and volar direction

8.3 Kirner Deformity (Dystelephalangy)

In this rare but characteristic anomaly, the distal phalanx of the fifth digit curves in a radial and volar direction, and the growth plate is often abnormally thick (Fig. 9.21). The epiphysis may be enlarged and demonstrate a steplike profile. There may be osteolysis between the diaphysis and the epiphysis [24]. Kirner deformity is often bilaterally symmetric though more severe on the right, and it is more frequent in girls.

Different etiologies have been proposed, including abnormal insertion of the flexor digitorum profundus tendon, unusual vascular pattern, or chronic inflammation. However, recent work utilizing MRI has demonstrated no evidence of these pathological processes, and etiology

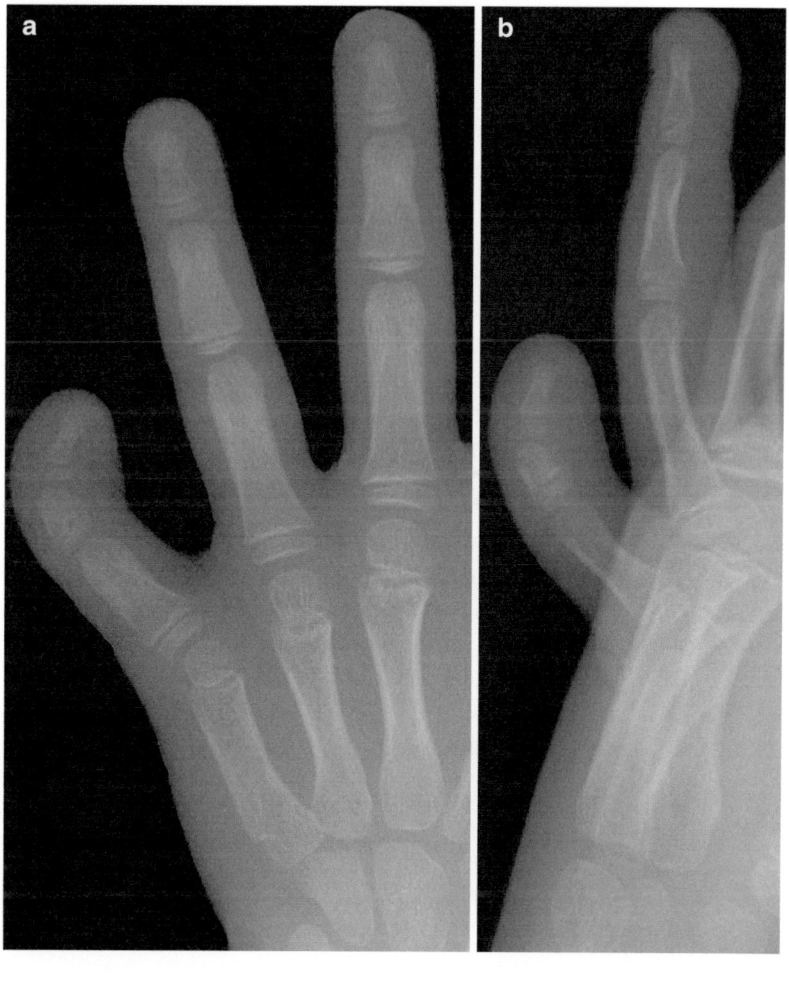

Fig. 9.19 Clinodactyly. (**a, b**) The middle phalanx is shortened, and the growth plate is inclined. There is radial angulation at the distal interphalangeal joint (Images copyright Shriners Hospital for Children Northern California)

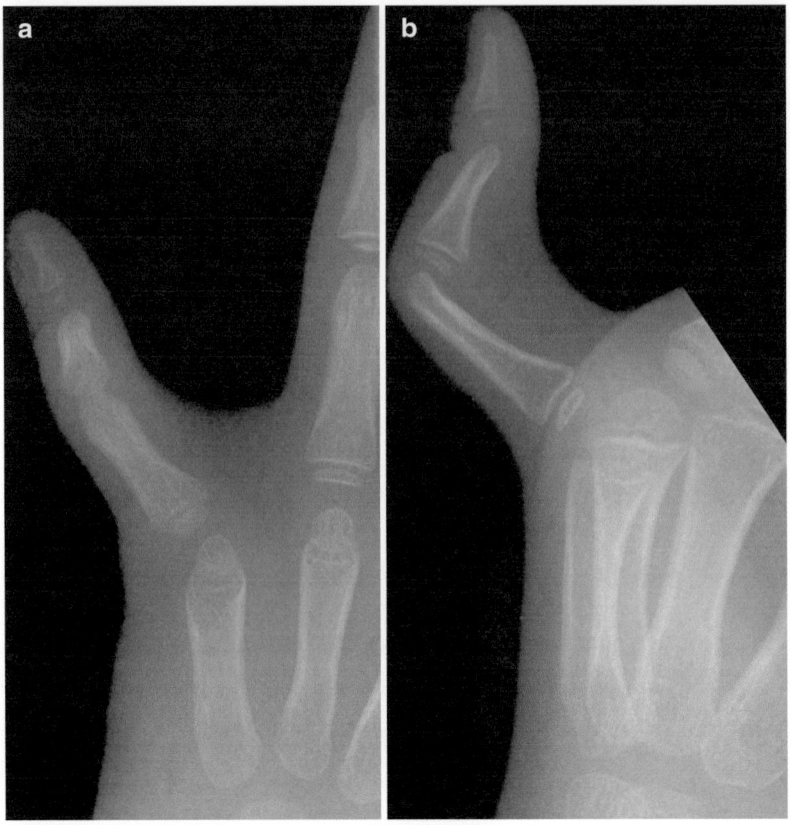

Fig. 9.20 Camptodactyly. (**a, b**) There is flexion of the proximal interphalangeal joint and asymmetric growth plate fusion (Images copyright Shriners Hospital for Children Northern California)

remains obscure [26]. Kirner deformity is sporadic or inherited in an autosomal dominant pattern with variable penetrance [26]

8.4 Longitudinal Epiphyseal Bracket (Delta Phalanx)

A specific triangular phalangeal deformity causing angulation of a finger has been termed delta phalanx or longitudinal epiphyseal bracket [27, 28]. Restricted to bones with a proximal epiphysis (the phalanges and first metacarpal and metatarsal), it is most common in the thumb (Fig. 9.22). There are often associated digital anomalies, such as overt or abortive duplication of the same ray. The epiphysis is frequently so large and deformed that it dwarfs the phalangeal shaft; the complex of these two parts has a deltoid shape (Fig. 9.23).

Rarely, the longitudinal bracketed epiphysis is duplicated, resulting in a "kissing delta" phalanx (Fig. 9.24). These patients are very likely to have an accompanying syndrome, such as central polydactyly, Carpenter syndrome, or Cenani-Lenz syndrome [29, 30]. Partial or complete duplication is postulated to tether one side of the affected epiphysis, causing the epiphysis to assume a proximal-distal vertical rather than mediolateral horizontal orientation. The abnormality may alternatively arise from fusion between the normal and an accessory ossification

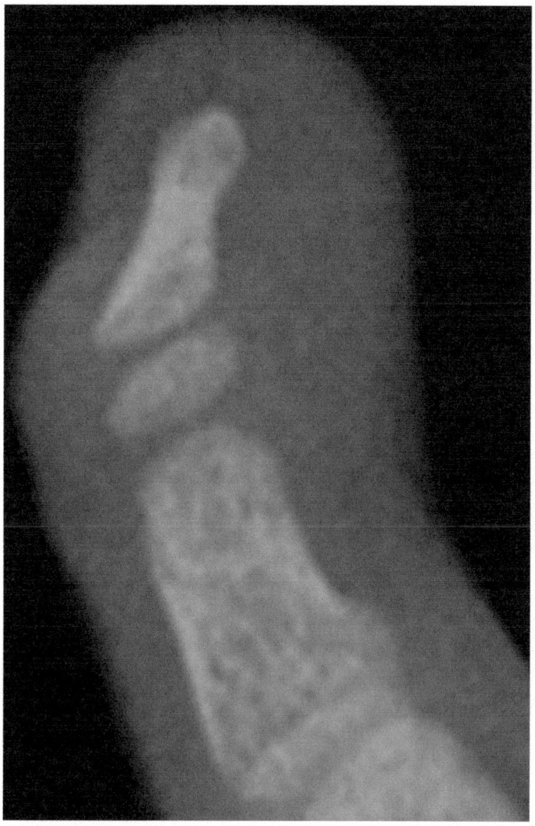

Fig. 9.21 Kirner deformity in a 10-year-old boy. The shaft of the distal phalanx is bent in a volar direction, and the epiphysis is relatively large (Courtesy of Tal Laor, Cincinnati Children's Hospital)

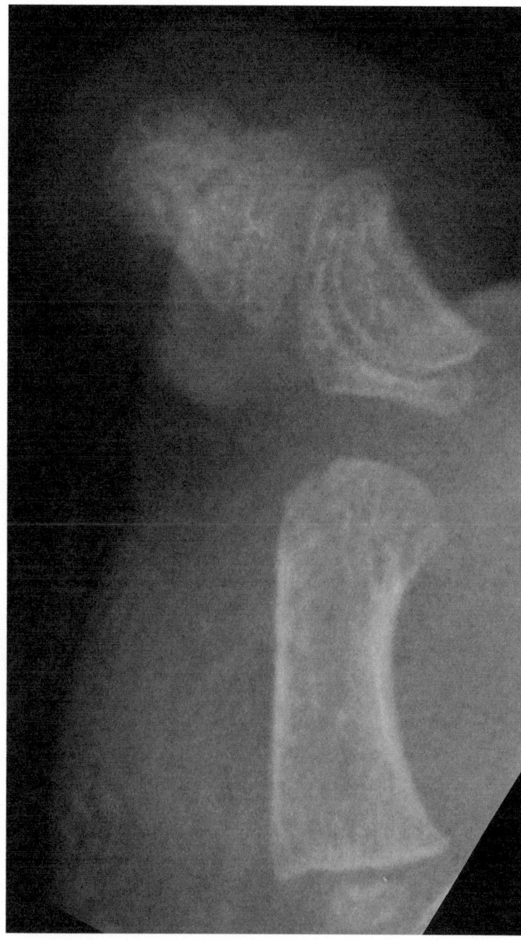

Fig. 9.22 Longitudinal epiphyseal bracket. The proximal phalanx of the thumb demonstrates a typical longitudinal bracket (Image copyright Shriners Hospital for Children Northern California)

center [28]. In early childhood, MRI can delineate an epiphyseal bracket before it ossifies. MRI can also assist with surgical planning by demonstrating vascular abnormalities [31].

9 Thumb Malformation in Systemic Disease

Congenital abnormality of the thumb may be characterized by complete absence or hypoplasia of either the entire ray (Figs. 9.25 and 9.26) or specific phalangeal segments, an extra phalanx (triphalangealism), duplication (Figs. 9.27 and 9.28), malposition, or enlargement. Absence or hypoplasia of the first metacarpal with hypoplasia of the proximal phalanx produces a "floating thumb" (*pouce flottant*) (Fig. 9.29). The scaphoid and trapezium are almost always absent if the bones of the thumb are missing. It may be necessary to measure the phalangeal and metacarpal segments and compare them with normal hand structures to identify the

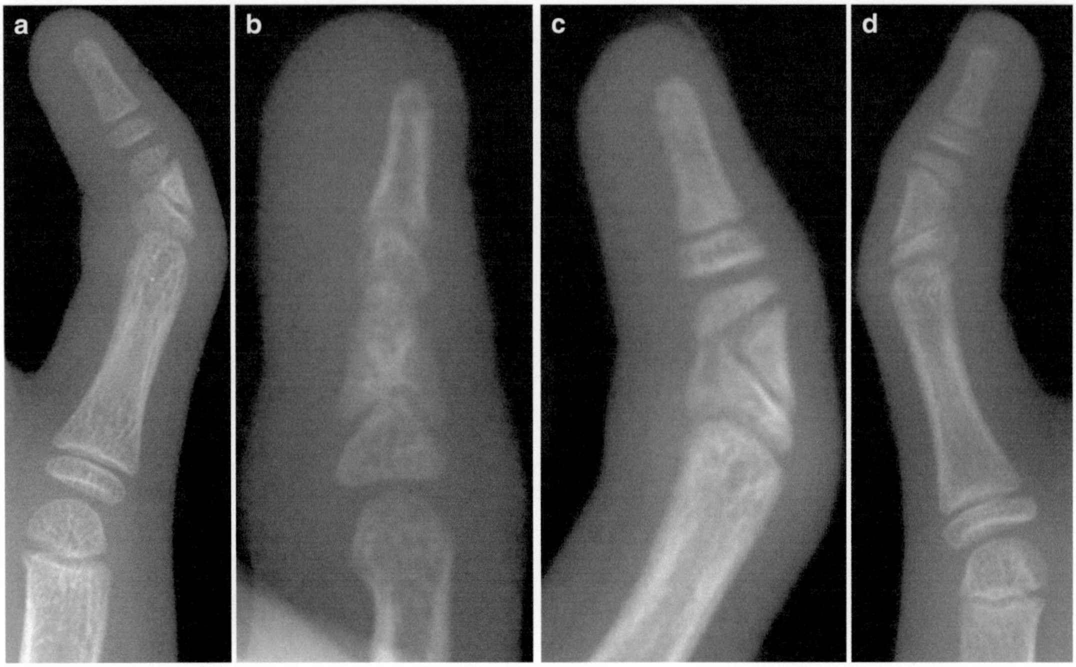

Fig. 9.23 Longitudinal epiphyseal bracket at the middle phalanx of the fifth digit in a 10-year-old boy. (**a, b**) At presentation. (**c**) Two years later, the longitudinal bracket is fusing. (**d**) There is a pseudoepiphysis on the other side (Images copyright Shriners Hospital for Children Northern California)

problem. This is important, since specific phalangeal abnormalities can suggest or confirm the presence of a syndrome. For further reference, tables are available that list these values and their differential diagnostic significance [32].

Thumb hypoplasia is bilateral in 63 % of patients and more common in males. About 60 % of cases are accompanied with radial longitudinal deficiency alone; 86 % are accompanied with other anomalies as well. VACTERL (vertebral, anal, cardiac, tracheoesophageal, renal, limb anomalies) association and Holt-Oram syndrome are encountered most often, with Fanconi anemia, Nager syndrome, and thrombocytopenia-absent radius (Fig. 9.30) occurring less frequently [33]. Congenital heart disease is common. The thumb is also malformed in trisomy 18 and other syndromes, such as myositis ossificans congenita, arthrogryposis, neural crest anomalies, and erythrogenesis imperfecta, as well as with maternal use of teratogens [4, 32]. Significant problems that accompany Fanconi anemia, erythrogenesis imperfecta, and Holt-Oram syndrome may be occult or manifest only in later childhood.

The surgical approach to thumb malformations varies depending on the size of the thumb, the presence or absence of carpals and metacarpals, the position and tightness of the first web, and the status of musculature and ligaments (characterized by the "Blauth" classification) [33]. Reconstruction is possible if the thumb and first metacarpal are reasonably well formed and the first carpometacarpal joint is stable (about 20 %). If the thumb is extremely hypoplastic or

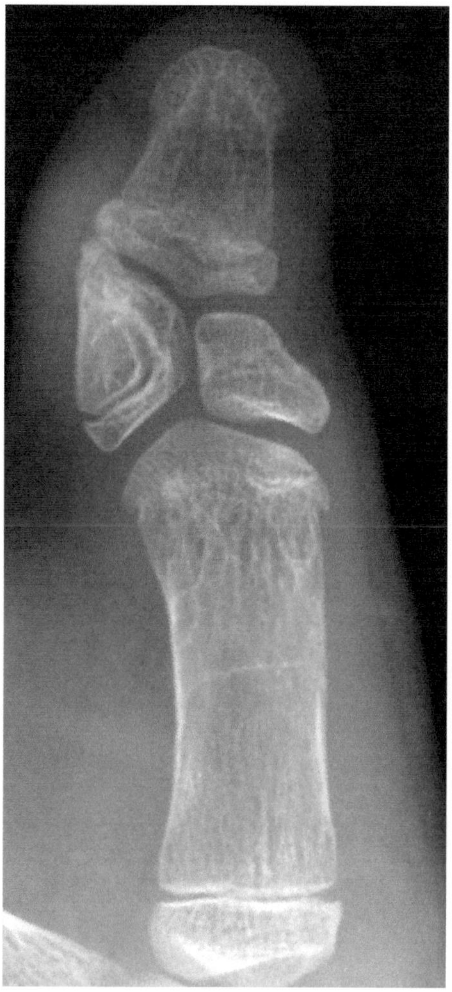

Fig. 9.24 "Kissing delta" phalanx in a patient with Carpenter syndrome. The proximal phalanx of the thumb is duplicated. The more medial of the two phalanges has an obvious longitudinal epiphyseal bracket, whereas the more lateral has a triangular configuration that suggests an incompletely visualized longitudinal bracket (Image copyright Shriners Hospital for Children Northern California)

absent (about 60 %), pollicization is usually performed, based on reconstruction of the index finger [33] (Fig. 9.31). Triphalangeal thumb is treated by resection of the extra phalanx and also possibly shortening of the first metacarpal, which is usually elongated [34].

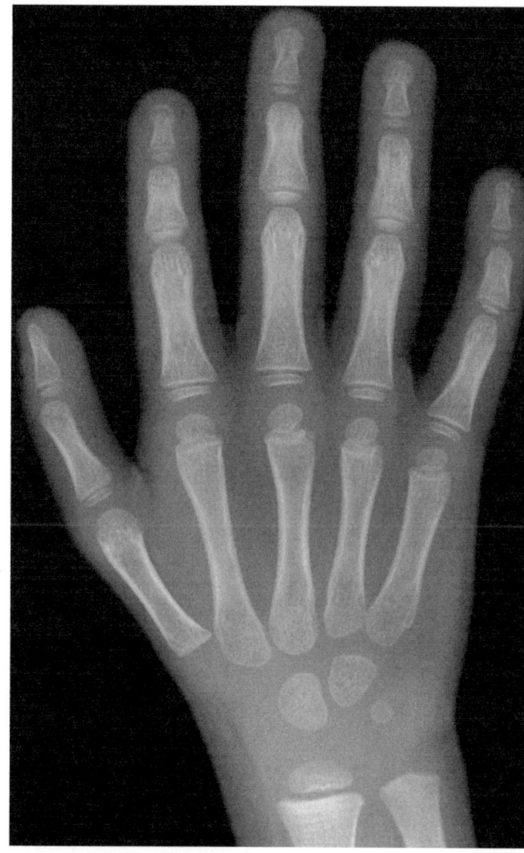

Fig. 9.25 Mild hypoplasia of the thumb and first metacarpal (Image copyright Shriners Hospital for Children Northern California)

9.1 Fanconi Anemia

This consists of a constellation of symptoms including pancytopenia with marrow hypoplasia, skin bronzing, and small stature. Microcephaly and hypoplastic genitalia are often present in this autosomal recessive aplastic anemia. Expression varies, and only the skeletal or only various degrees of the hematologic abnormality may occur in different members of the same kindred. The pancytopenia does not become manifest until mid-childhood (typically 4–10 years), and the disease is usually fatal within 5 years owing to anemia, hemorrhage,

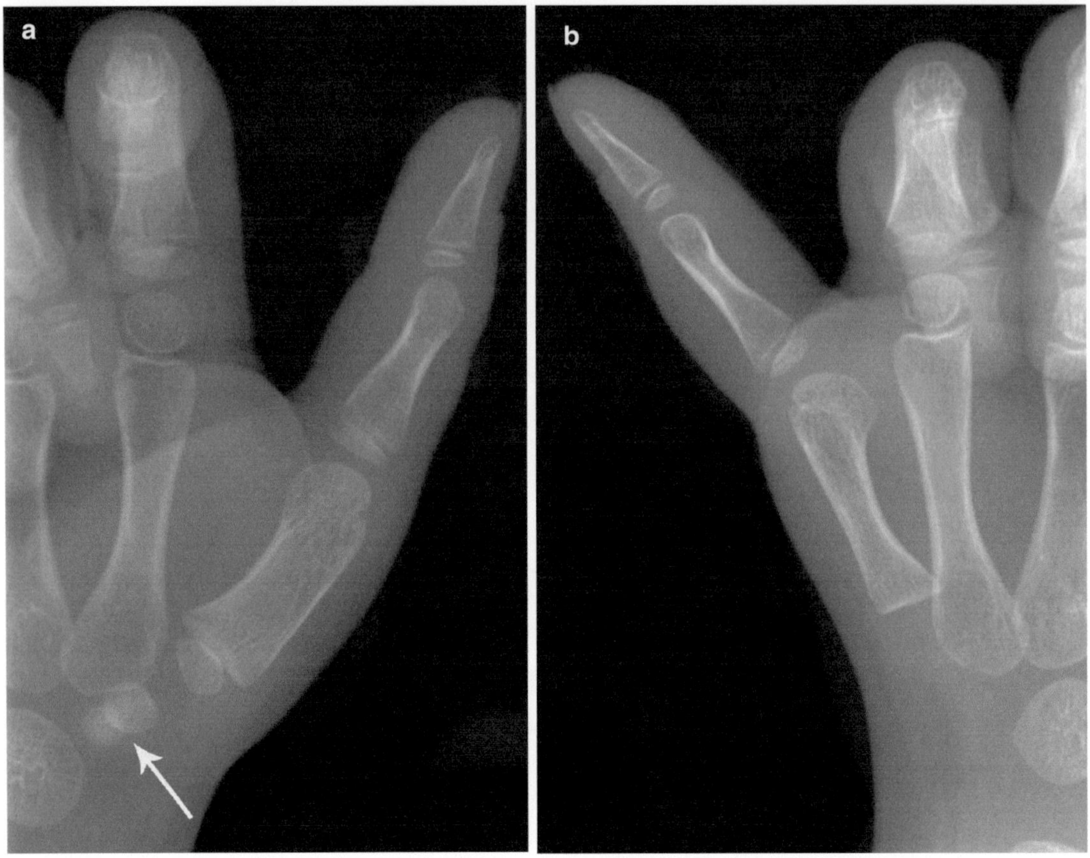

Fig. 9.26 Hypoplastic right thumb. (**a**) Normal left thumb, with ossified trapezium and trapezoid (*arrow*). (**b**) The right thumb is hypoplastic, and the radial carpal bones have not ossified (Images copyright Shriners Hospital for Children Northern California)

leukemia, or sepsis. However, bone marrow transplantation can be curative, and therefore children with thumb anomalies should undergo chromosomal breakage test to diagnose presymptomatic Fanconi anemia.

Some type of skeletal abnormality is present in more than two thirds of patients; of these, about 75 % have thumb anomalies. Usually the thumb is completely absent or—almost as often—hypoplastic (especially the distal phalanx). Duplication of the thumb also occurs. The entire or only the proximal first metacarpal may be slender, and the proximal epiphysis is often absent. The radius is absent in 20 % of patients. Renal anomalies are common, and hip dislocation and cervical spine fusion occasionally occur.

9.2 Erythrogenesis Imperfecta (Congenital Hypoplastic Anemia)

This slowly progressive purely red-cell anemia manifests during the first 18 months of age. It is less often fatal than the Fanconi syndrome. The most common associated abnormality is triphalangeal thumb, occasionally with duplication. Skeletal maturation is delayed. One third of patients have some other cardiac, renal, or skeletal abnormality.

9.3 Holt-Oram Syndrome

Thumb and other skeletal malformations are associated with congenital heart disease in Holt-Oram

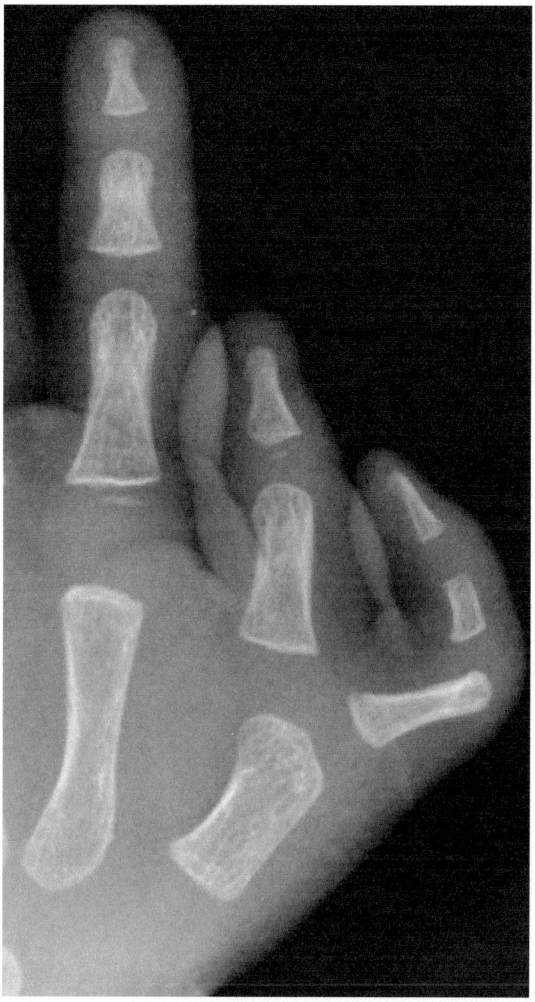

Fig. 9.27 Duplicated thumb. The duplicated ray is triphalangeal. The head of the fifth metacarpal is angled, each surface articulating with its respective proximal phalanx (Image copyright Shriners Hospital for Children Northern California)

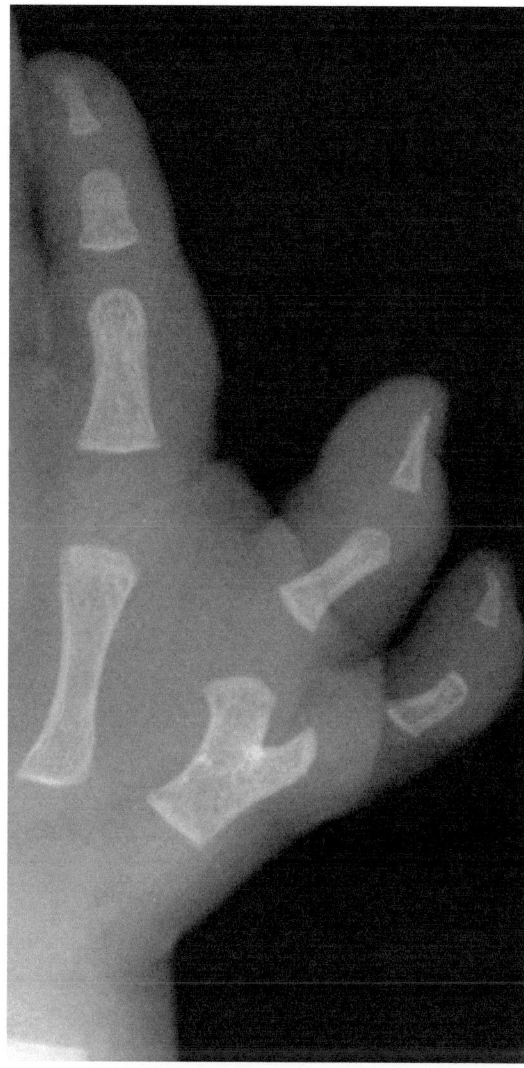

Fig. 9.28 Duplicated thumb. The distal portion of the first metacarpal is also duplicated (Image copyright Shriners Hospital for Children Northern California)

syndrome (Fig. 9.32). This autosomal dominant trait has considerable intra- and interfamilial variability. Thumb abnormalities are frequently bilateral but asymmetric; they may be fingerlike, absent, or triphalangeal. One or all three segments of the first ray may be duplicated. The first metacarpal may be elongated and slender. The left side is more severely affected. Carpal anomalies take the form of persistent primitive central carpal row, with an accessory bone ulnar to the navicular (os centrale).

Some form of congenital heart disease, usually atrial or ventricular septal defect, is almost always present in this syndrome; the unusual patient with only skeletal defects may transmit both osseous and cardiac defects to their offspring. Other skeletal anomalies include scapular tilt, coracoclavicular joint abnormality, and clavicular, medial humeral epicondyle, and sternal deformity. Phocomelia, absent radius, and sacral agenesis have been reported. Mutations in the T-box transcription factor gene (TBX5) result in the wide range of upper limb anomalies that are seen in Holt-Oram syndrome [35].

Fig. 9.29 Floating thumb ("pouce flottant"). The first metacarpal is absent and the thumb hypoplastic in this patient with radial aplasia (Image copyright Shriners Hospital for Children Northern California)

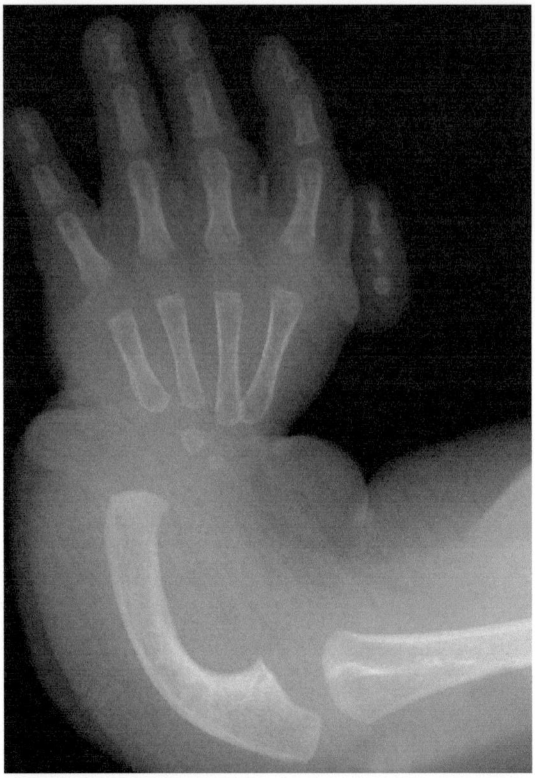

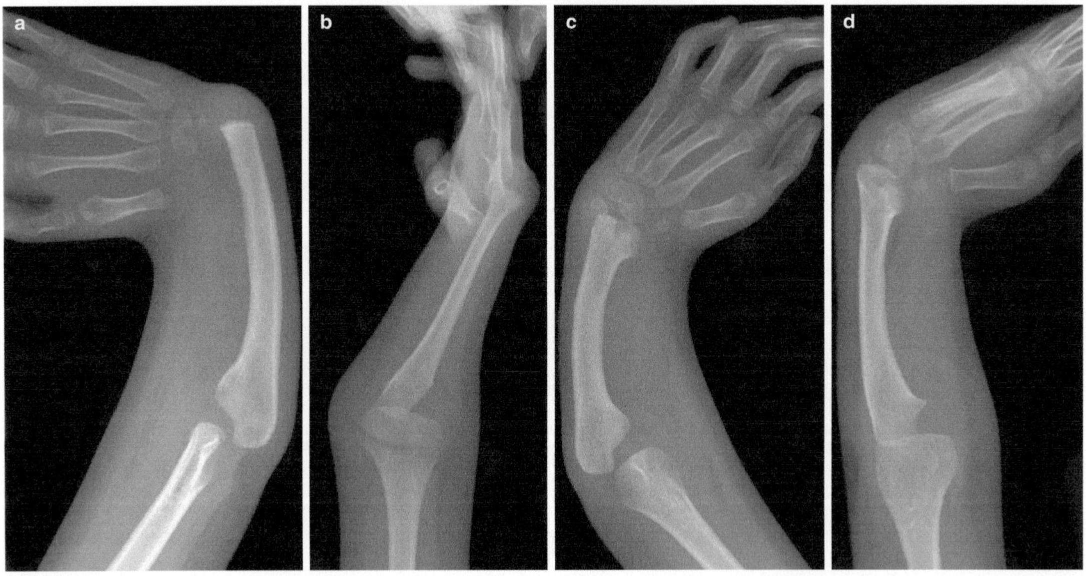

Fig. 9.30 Thrombocytopenia-absent radius. Both radii are absent, and the ulnas are dysplastic. Views of the right hand (**a, b**) demonstrate clubhand with dislocated carpus and a hypoplastic thumb. On the left (**c, d**), centralization has been performed (Images copyright Shriners Hospital for Children Northern California)

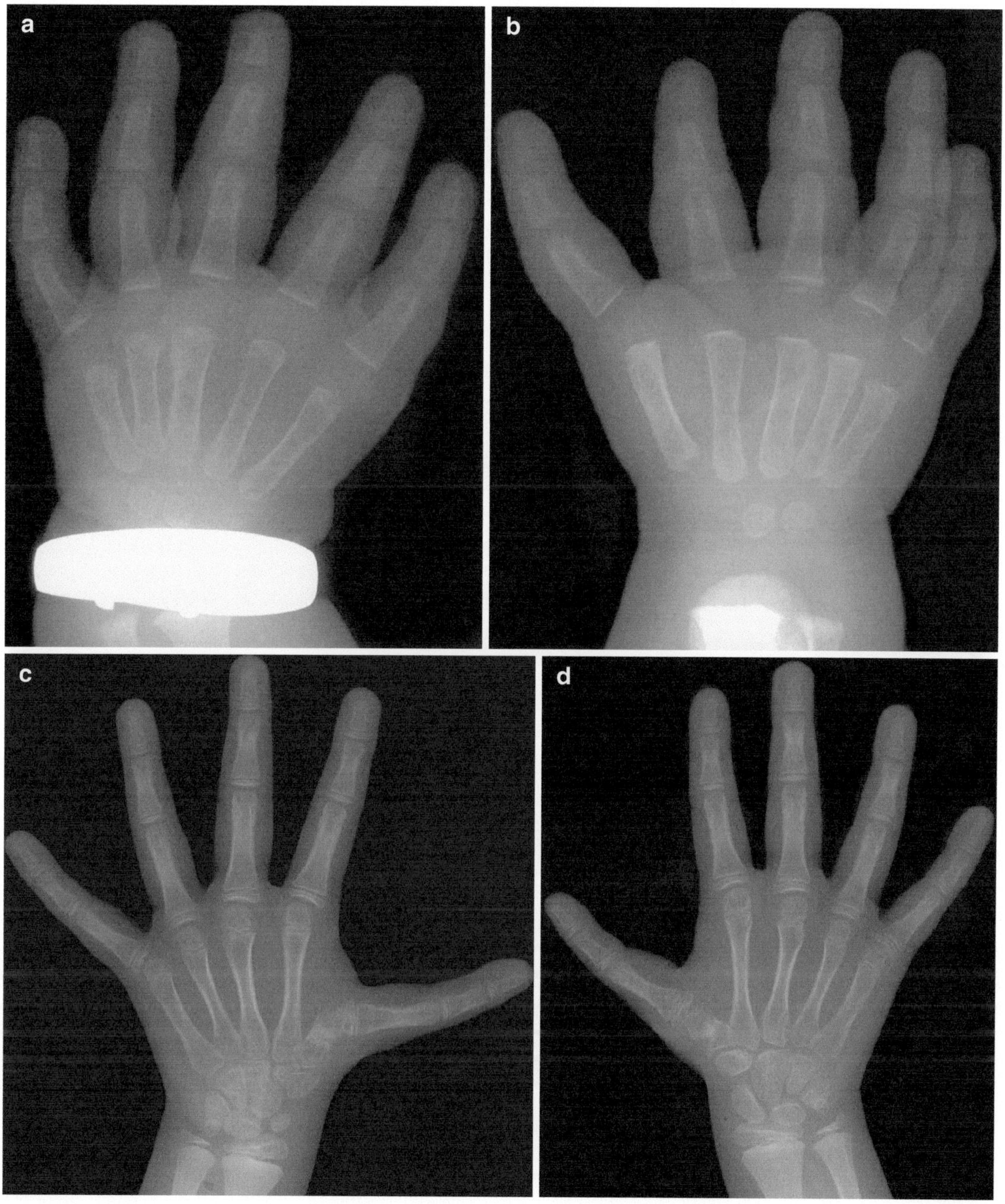

Fig. 9.31 A 10-month-old girl with bilateral triphalangeal thumbs. (**a**) and (**b**) demonstrate symmetric abnormalities. (**c, d**) Polliciziation was performed, and 8 years later the first metacarpal has been shortened, as have the rays of the first digit (Images copyright Shriners Hospital for Children Northern California)

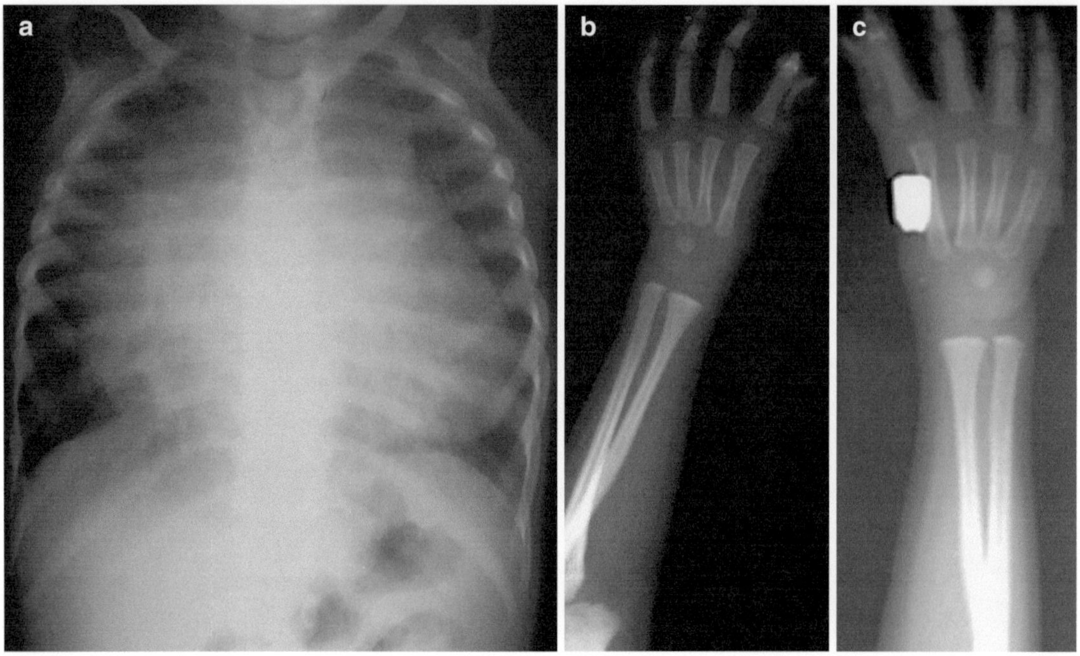

Fig. 9.32 Holt-Oram syndrome. (**a**) Severe cardiomegaly secondary to a large atrial septal defect. (**b, c**) Views of both forearms and hands demonstrate absent thumbs and decreased carpal ossification (Images copyright Shriners Hospital for Children Northern California)

References

1. Keats TL, Anderson MW. Atlas of normal roentgen variants that may simulate disease. 8th ed. Philadelphia: Mosby; 2006.
2. Friedman T, Reed M, Elliott AM. The carpal bones in Poland syndrome. Skelet Radiol. 2009;38(6):585–91. PubMed PMID: 19183988. Epub 2009/02/03. eng.
3. Delaney TJ, Eswar S. Carpal coalitions. J Hand Surg (Am). 1992;17(1):28–31. PubMed PMID: 1538108. Epub 1992/01/01. eng.
4. Poznanski A. In: EJ P, editor. The hand in radiologic diagnosis. Philadelphia: W B Saunders and Company; 1984.
5. Higginbottom MC, Jones KL, Hall BD, Smith DW. The amniotic band disruption complex: timing of amniotic rupture and variable spectra of consequent defects. J Pediatr. 1979;95(4):544–9. PubMed PMID: 480028. Epub 1979/10/01. eng.
6. Goldfarb CA, Sathienkijkanchai A, Robin NH. Amniotic constriction band: a multidisciplinary assessment of etiology and clinical presentation. J Bone Joint Surg Am. 2009;91 Suppl 4:68–75. PubMed PMID: 19571071. Epub 2009/07/11. eng.
7. Daya M. Amniotic band syndrome with persistent sciatic artery: a case report. Ann Plast Surg. 2008;61(5):549–51. PubMed PMID: 18948784. Epub 2008/10/25. eng.
8. Moran SL, Jensen M, Bravo C. Amniotic band syndrome of the upper extremity: diagnosis and management. J Am Acad Orthop Surg. 2007;15(7):397–407. PubMed PMID: 17602029. Epub 2007/07/03. eng.
9. Reed MH. Radiologic features of congenital transverse deficiency of the forearm. Can Assoc Radiol J. 1991;42(5):345–8. PubMed PMID: 1933502. Epub 1991/10/01. eng.
10. Goldman AB, Kaye JJ. Macrodystrophia lipomatosa: radiographic diagnosis. AJR Am J Roentgenol. 1977;128(1):101–5. PubMed PMID: 401563. Epub 1977/01/01. eng.
11. Gupta SK, Sharma OP, Sharma SV, Sood B, Gupta S. Macrodystrophia lipomatosa: radiographic observations. Br J Radiol. 1992;65(777):769–73. PubMed PMID: 1393412. Epub 1992/09/01. eng.
12. Rohilla S, Jain N, Sharma R, Dhaulakhandi DB. Macrodystrophia lipomatosa involving multiple nerves. J Orthop Traumatol. 2012;13(1):41–5. PubMed PMID: 21948052: Pubmed Central PMCID: 3284677. Epub 2011/09/29. eng.
13. Kalen V, Burwell DS, Omer GE. Macrodactyly of the hands and feet. J Pediatr Orthop. 1988;8(3):311–5.
14. Kelikian H. Congenital deformities of the hand and forearm. Philadelphia: WB Saunders; 1974.
15. Soler R, Rodriguez E, Bargiela A, Martijnez C. MR findings of macrodystrophia lipomatosa. Clin Imaging. 1997;21(2):135–7.

16. Wang YC, Jeng CM, Marcantonio DR, Resnick D. Macrodystrophia lipomatosa. MR imaging in three patients. Clin Imaging. 1997;21(5):323–7. PubMed PMID: 9316750. Epub 1997/10/08. eng.
17. Boren WL, Henry Jr RE, Wintch K. MR diagnosis of fibrolipomatous hamartoma of nerve: association with nerve territory-oriented macrodactyly (macrodystrophia lipomatosa). Skelet Radiol. 1995;24(4):296–7. PubMed PMID: 7644945. Epub 1995/05/01. eng.
18. Mentzel HJ, Seidel J, Sauner D, Vogt S, Fitzek C, Zintl F, et al. Radiological aspects of the Poland syndrome and implications for treatment: a case study and review. Eur J Pediatr. 2002;161(8):455–9. PubMed PMID: 12172832. Epub 2002/08/13. eng.
19. Stylianos K, Constantinos P, Alexandros T, Aliki F, Nikolaos A, Demetriou M, et al. Muscle abnormalities of the chest in Poland's syndrome: variations and proposal for a classification. Surg Radiol Anat. 2012;34(1):57–63. PubMed PMID: 21800018. Epub 2011/07/30. eng.
20. Beals RK, Crawford S. Congenital absence of the pectoral muscles. A review of twenty-five patients. Clin Orthop Relat Res. 1976;119:166–71. PubMed PMID: 954307. Epub 1976/09/01. eng.
21. Powell CV, Coombs RC, David TJ. Poland anomaly with contralateral ulnar ray defect. J Med Genet. 1993;30(5):423–4. PubMed PMID: 8320708: Pubmed Central PMCID: 1016383. Epub 1993/05/01. eng.
22. Hurwitz DJ, Stofman G, Curtin H. Three-dimensional imaging of Poland's syndrome. Plast Reconstr Surg. 1994;94(5):719–23. PubMed PMID: 7938299. Epub 1994/10/01. eng.
23. Senrui H, Egawa T, Horiki A. Anatomical findings in the hands of patients with Poland's syndrome. J Bone Joint Surg Am. 1982;64(7):1079–82. PubMed PMID: 7118976. Epub 1982/09/01. eng.
24. Aucourt J, Budzik JF, Manouvrier-Hanu S, Mezel A, Cotten A, Boutry N. Congenital malformations of the hand and forearm in children: what radiologists should know. Semin Musculoskelet Radiol. 2012;16(2):146–58. PubMed PMID: 22648430. Epub 2012/06/01. eng.
25. Caouette-Laberge L, Laberge C, Egerszegi EP, Stanciu C. Physiolysis for correction of clinodactyly in children. J Hand Surg (Am). 2002;27(4):659–65. PubMed PMID: 12132092. Epub 2002/07/20. eng.
26. Lee J, Ahn JK, Choi SH, Koh EM, Cha HS. MRI findings in Kirner deformity: normal insertion of the flexor digitorum profundus tendon without soft-tissue enhancement. Pediatr Radiol. 2010;40(9):1572–5. PubMed PMID: 20336287. Epub 2010/03/26. eng.
27. Ogden JA, Light TR, Conlogue GJ. Correlative roentgenography and morphology of the longitudinal epiphyseal bracket. Skelet Radiol. 1981;6(2):109–17. PubMed PMID: 7256305. Epub 1981/01/01. eng.
28. Theander G, Carstam N. Longitudinally bracketed diaphysis. Ann Radiol (Paris). 1974;17(4):355–60. PubMed PMID: 4217116. Epub 1974/05/01. Eng fre.
29. Wood VE, Shuren N. Duplicated longitudinal bracketed epiphysis 'kissing delta phalanx' in the hand. J Hand Surg (Br). 2002;27(3):249–52. PubMed PMID: 12074612. Epub 2002/06/21. eng.
30. Yucel A, Kuru I, Bozan ME, Acar M, Solak M. Radiographic evaluation and unusual bone formations in different genetic patterns in synpolydactyly. Skelet Radiol. 2005;34(8):468–76. PubMed PMID: 15947976. Epub 2005/06/11. eng.
31. Johnson JM, Higgins TJ, Lemos D. Appearance of the delta phalanx (longitudinally bracketed epiphysis) with MR imaging. Pediatr Radiol. 2011;41(3):394–6. PubMed PMID: 20972673. Epub 2010/10/26. eng.
32. Poznanski AK, Garn SM, Holt JF. The thumb in the congenital malformation syndromes. Radiology. 1971;100(1):115–29. PubMed PMID: 5147019. Epub 1971/07/01. eng.
33. James MA, McCarroll Jr HR, Manske PR. Characteristics of patients with hypoplastic thumbs. J Hand Surg (Am). 1996;21(1):104–13. PubMed PMID: 8775204. Epub 1996/01/01. eng.
34. Zuidam JM, Dees EE, Selles RW, Hovius SE. Implications for treatment of variations in length of the first metacarpal in different types of triphalangeal thumbs. J Hand Surg Eur. 2010;35(1):65–9. PubMed PMID: 20100712. Epub 2010/01/27. eng.
35. Oberg KC, Feenstra JM, Manske PR, Tonkin MA. Developmental biology and classification of congenital anomalies of the hand and upper extremity. J Hand Surg (Am). 2010;35(12):2066–76. PubMed PMID: 21134615. Epub 2010/12/08. eng.

The Hand and Wrist: Acquired Disorders

10

Deepa R. Pai, Ethan A. Smith, and Peter J. Strouse

Contents

D.R. Pai, MD, MHSA (✉)
Department of Radiology, C.S. Mott Children's Hospital, 1540 E. Hospital Drive,
Ann Arbor, MI 48109, USA
e-mail: dpai@med.umich.edu

E.A. Smith, MD • P.J. Strouse, MD, FACR
Section of Pediatric Radiology,
Department of Radiology,
C.S. Mott Children's Hospital,
University of Michigan Health System,
1540 E. Hospital Dr., SPC 4252,
Ann Arbor, MI 48109-4252, USA
e-mail: ethans@med.umich.edu;
pstrouse@umich.edu

Abstract

This chapter discusses the clinical and imaging characteristics of acquired lesions that are encountered in the pediatric hand and wrist. The first section addresses three categories of fractures: radial and ulnar fractures, carpal bone fractures, and hand fractures. The second section focuses on overuse injuries including Kienböck osteonecrosis, gymnast wrist, and ulnocarpal impaction. Disorders involving tendons and ligaments are then discussed, addressing tendon pathology in the extensor compartments, trigger thumb, carpal instability, the ulnar collateral ligament of the thumb, and the triangular fibrocartilage complex. Following this in-depth section on tendons and ligaments, imaging of neurovascular injuries and ganglion cysts is addressed. The chapter closes with a discussion of burns and frostbite.

1 Fractures

1.1 Radial and Ulnar Fractures

The distal radius and ulna are affected in 25–33 % of pediatric fractures [1–3]. Interestingly, the incidence of these fractures has increased over the last several decades, a phenomenon which some authors attribute to increasing participation in organized sports [1–4]. Distal radial and ulnar fractures are more common in school-aged

R. Stein-Wexler et al. (eds.), *Pediatric Orthopedic Imaging*,
DOI 10.1007/978-3-642-45381-6_10, © Springer-Verlag Berlin Heidelberg 2015

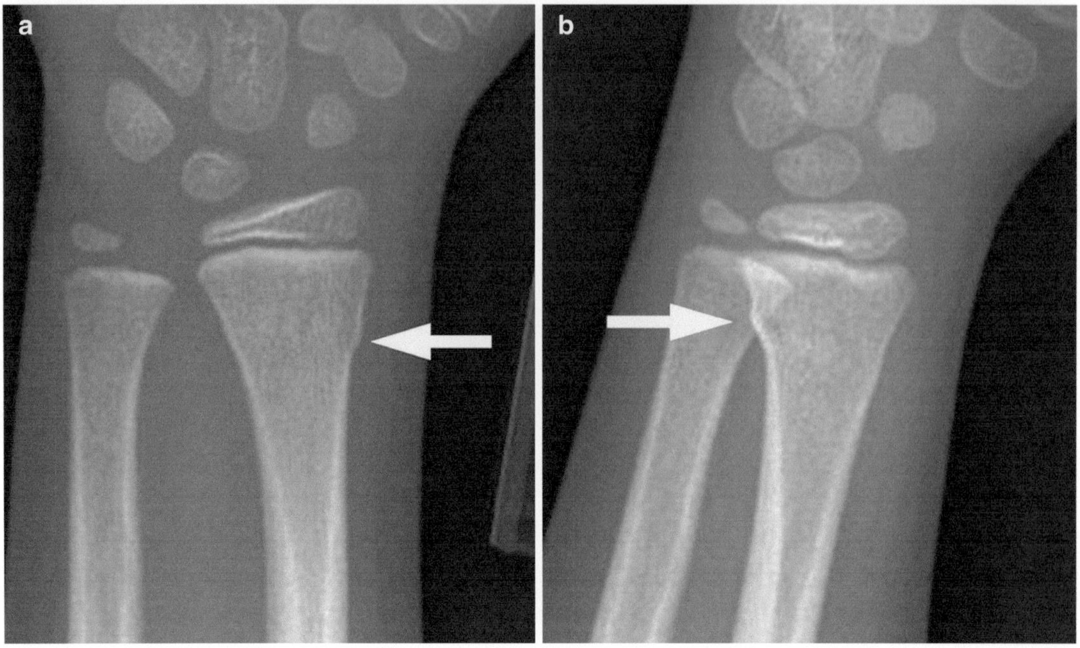

Fig. 10.1 Distal radial buckle fracture in a 6-year-old boy. (**a**, **b**) There is angulation of the distal radial metaphyseal cortex (*arrows*)

children than in younger children, probably due to increased activity levels. However, across all age groups, a fall onto an outstretched hand is the most common mechanism of injury [3]. In younger children, these fractures tend to result from accidental falls, while in older children sports-related injuries are more common [4].

Treatment depends on a variety of factors, including the type, location, pattern, displacement, and angulation of the fracture [5]. Fractures are classified as either buckle (also called torus, or incomplete) or bicortical (or complete). Buckle fractures are caused by a compression injury and involve only one portion of the cortex, most commonly the dorsal (Fig. 10.1). These fractures are inherently stable and can be treated with either a removable splint or a cast [6]. Once immobilized, they do not generally require radiographic follow-up unless there is specific clinical concern or the initial diagnosis is in question [5, 6].

Bicortical and more complex fractures are the result of bending—rotation or shear—and involve both cortices [5]. With regard to displacement, in general, angulation of less than 20° in the anteroposterior (AP) plane and 10° in the transverse plane is considered adequate for remodeling [5]. The remodeling potential of the fracture will be greatest in young children, in fractures that are close to the physis, and in fractures which are angulated in the AP plane. Rotational misalignment will not remodel [5]. Depending on the alignment, reducibility, and the presence of associated neurovascular injuries, these fractures may be treated with closed reduction and casting, open reduction, or surgical fixation.

Unique to pediatrics, involvement of the physis does sometimes precipitate disturbed growth. Approximately 20 % of distal radial fractures involve the physis (most commonly Salter-Harris type II fractures) [5]. However, the risk of physeal growth arrest for a distal radial fracture is relatively small, approximately 4 % [7]. A smaller proportion of distal ulnar fractures involve the physis, but the risk of physeal growth arrest is high—up to 50 % [7].

Imaging

Radiographs are generally sufficient for imaging distal radial and ulnar fractures. With a buckle fracture, radiographs demonstrate angulation of the cortical margin, commonly at the metaphysis. By definition, the opposite cortex is intact and the degree of displacement minimal. Adjacent soft tissue swelling, evidenced by obscuration of the fat planes, is usually present. The most easily visualized fat plane is the pronator fat pad, located volar to the distal radial and ulnar metaphyses. The pronator fat pad (Fig. 10.1) often becomes indistinct or completely obscured when there is significant soft tissue edema. Bicortical fractures manifest radiographically with or without displacement of the fracture fragments. Distal radial fractures commonly have an associated distal ulnar fracture, often involving the styloid process. Computed tomography (CT) or magnetic resonance imaging (MRI) is used for more complex fractures or if there is concern for soft tissue impingement and other complications.

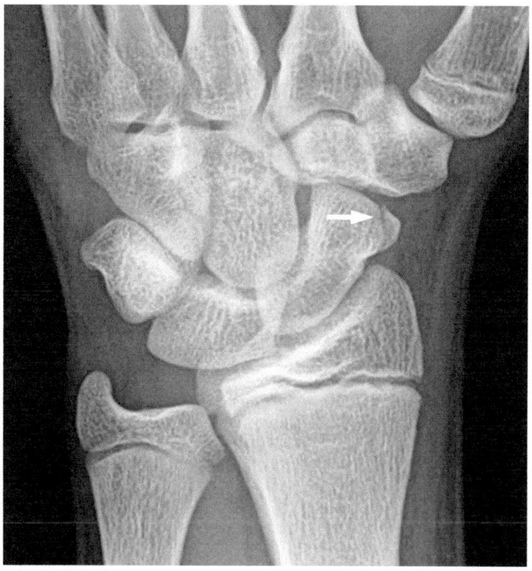

Fig. 10.2 Fracture through distal scaphoid in a 16-year-old boy (*arrow*)

1.2 Carpal Bone Fractures

Carpal bone fractures are infrequent in children, accounting for less than 1 % of all pediatric fractures [8, 9]. One proposed explanation is that the non-ossified cartilage surrounding the ossification centers of the carpal bones acts as a shock absorber, protecting the ossification center from impact and fractures [10]. The incidence of carpal bone fractures is highest in the teenage years and is extremely low in patients under age 8 [9].

Scaphoid Fractures (Box 10.1)

Box 10.1: Scaphoid Fractures

Most common carpal fracture (but unusual in children)

Low incidence of nonunion in children

Scaphoid waist is the most often fractured

Fractures of the scaphoid waist and especially the proximal pole most often lead to distal avascular necrosis

In children as in adults, the scaphoid is by far the most commonly fractured carpal bone [9, 11]. For example, in one series, scaphoid fractures accounted for approximately 89 % (33/37) of carpal fractures [9]. The peak incidence of scaphoid fractures is between the ages of 11 and 15 [9, 12]. Patients typically present with a history of fall on outstretched hand and pain localized to the anatomic snuffbox.

In the past, scaphoid fractures in children differed from those in adults, more likely to occur at the distal third of the scaphoid [9, 11, 12], possibly due to early ossification of the distal scaphoid and the protective effect of thicker soft tissues over the proximal pole [11] (Fig. 10.2). However, this pattern appears to have changed, with altered patient characteristics and activities. Acute scaphoid fractures in children now most often involve the scaphoid waist, as in adults [13] (Fig. 10.3). Most fractures are non-displaced, and incomplete fractures also occur [8]. Nonunion is less common in appropriately treated pediatric patients than in adults [9]. Since most of the blood supply to the scaphoid is distal, transverse fractures of the proximal or mid-scaphoid often result in avascular necrosis of the distal pole.

Scaphoid fractures in the acute setting are usually immobilized with either a short- or long-arm thumb-spica cast [8, 9]. In rare cases with significant displacement, acute operative management is required. More often, surgical treatment is

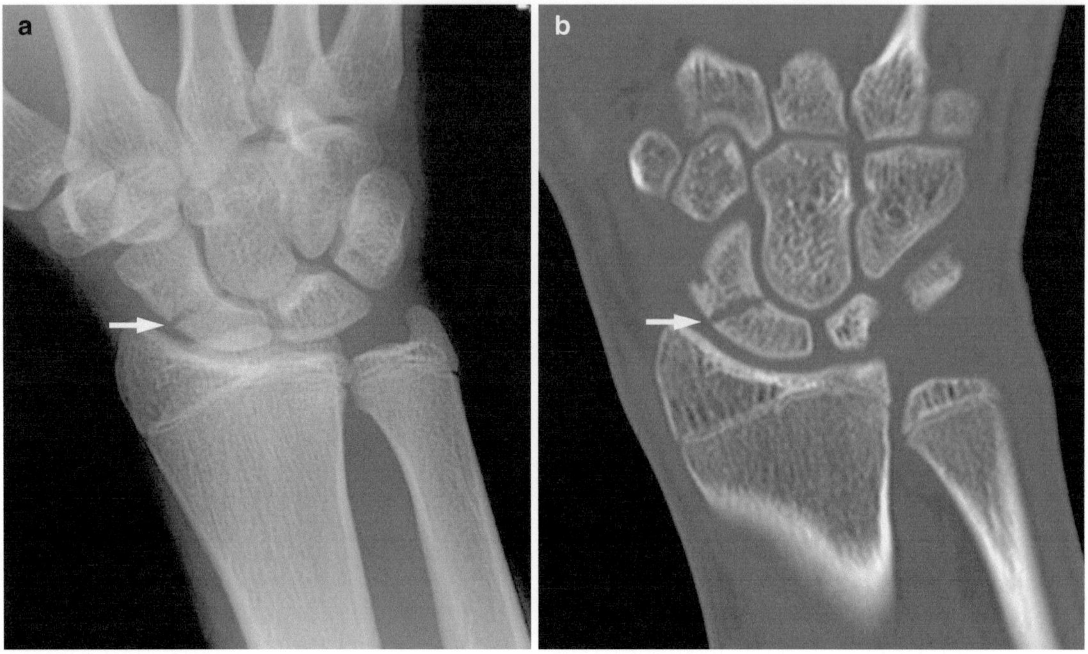

Fig. 10.3 Scaphoid fracture in a 17-year-old boy. (**a**) Transverse fracture through the waist of the scaphoid (*arrow*). (**b**) CT confirms transverse fracture (*arrow*)

reserved for cases of nonunion after failed nonoperative management. The relatively low incidence of nonunion, coupled with the more distal location of the fractures, makes the serious complication of avascular necrosis of the proximal polc of thc scaphoid rarc [14].

Imaging

If there is suspicion of a scaphoid fracture, a dedicated "scaphoid view" with the hand in ulnar deviation should be included, along with standard hand or wrist radiographs. CT may be helpful in selected cases to confirm the presence of a fracture. MRI has been shown to be more sensitive than radiographs in equivocal or clinically discrepant cases [15]. Findings on MRI include focal bone marrow edema, a low signal fracture line on T1-weighted (T1-W) images, and cortical disruption [15].

In the non-acute setting, CT is useful to evaluate nonunion and for subtle evidence of healing. MRI is helpful for suspected cases of avascular necrosis. Findings include low signal on both T1- and T2-weighted (T2-W) images and a lack of enhancement after intravenous contrast administration.

Other Carpal Bone Fractures

Fractures of the other carpal bones are extremely rare in children. Fractures of the capitate, triquetrum, hamate, trapezoid, and pisiform have been reported [16] (Figs. 10.4 and 10.5). Most often, thcsc fracturcs arc thc rcsult of a fall or a dircct blow [9, 16]. Carpal fractures are typically managed nonoperatively and have an excellent prognosis [9].

Imaging

The most common radiographic findings are a lucent fracture line or cortical disruption. Some fractures have more unique patterns; for example, a fracture of the triquetrum often manifests as a small osseous fragment posterior to the proximal carpal row on the lateral radiograph [16]. Most fractures do not demonstrate significant displacement [9]. MRI can be used in difficult cases and is more sensitive to bone marrow edema and non-displaced fractures [16]. Findings on MRI include increased T2 signal in the bone marrow, cortical disruption, and visualization of a discrete low T1 signal fracture line.

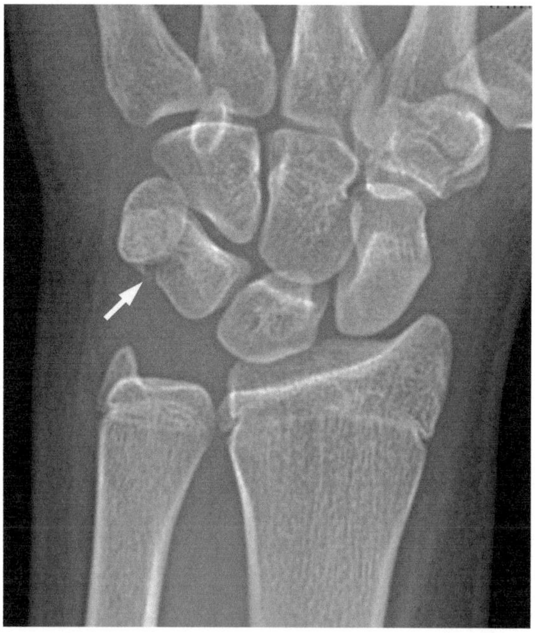

Fig. 10.4 Triquetral fracture in a 15-year-old girl that occurred during a softball injury. There is focal disruption of the triquetrum (*arrow*)

1.3 Hand Fractures

The hand is the most commonly injured part of the pediatric skeleton [11, 17, 18]. The phalanges are more frequently injured than the metacarpals. Injuries are also more common in the so-called border digits—the thumb and fifth finger [17, 18]. Fractures of the hand are most common in older children with a reported peak incidence between ages of 9 and 13 years [17, 18]. The radiographic evaluation of suspected fractures of the hand should include posteroanterior (PA), oblique, and lateral projections with the fingers fanned.

Metacarpals

Although fractures of the metacarpals usually involve the shaft or neck, periarticular and periphyseal fractures are also relatively frequent [11]. Metacarpal fractures typically occur as the result of a crush injury or a compressive force, such as

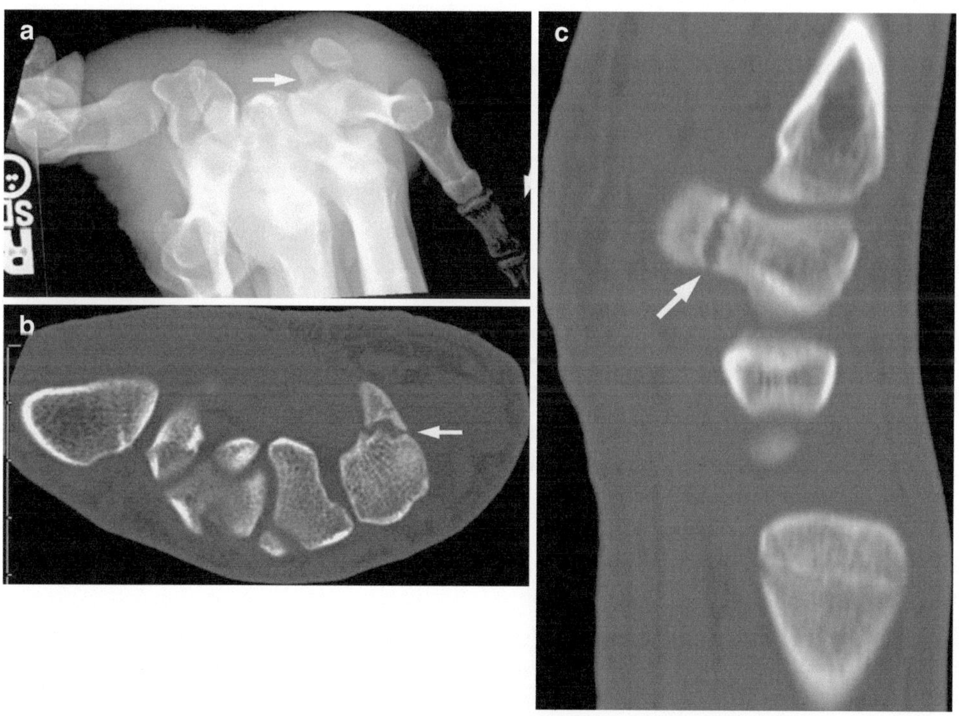

Fig. 10.5 Fractured hook of the hamate in a 17-year-old hockey player injured 2 weeks earlier. (**a**) Carpal tunnel view demonstrates questionable lucency through the hook of the hamate. Axial (**b**) and sagittal reformatted (**c**) CT images demonstrate a non-displaced fracture of the hook of the hamate (*arrows*). Sclerosis along the fracture line suggests the injury is beginning to heal

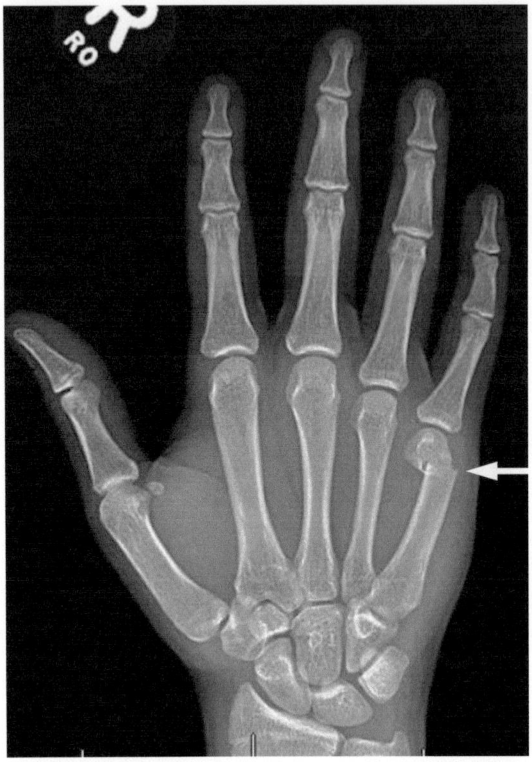

Fig. 10.6 Fifth metacarpal fracture after a 16-year-old boy punched a wall. Note the characteristic apex dorsal angulation (*arrow*)

punching a hard object (Fig. 10.6). The first and fifth metacarpals are most frequently injured [17]. Radiographs are usually sufficient for diagnosing a metacarpal fracture. The degree of displacement and angulation across the fracture site varies with mechanism of injury. Treatment depends on the degree of displacement and any associated injuries. Most fractures are treated with immobilization, although some require closed reduction or even surgical management. The prognosis is generally excellent.

Phalanges

The majority of phalanx fractures are periphyseal or periarticular [18]. The most common is a Salter-Harris type II fracture of the proximal phalanx [17–19]. This type of injury is often secondary to rotation or shearing [18]. Buckle fractures of the phalangeal metaphyses are also common. Fractures of the phalangeal neck are unique to children and can be difficult to visualize on radiographs.

Distal phalangeal fractures are usually secondary to a crush injury. In younger children, this usually results from an accident, such as catching a finger in a closing door [18]. In older children, these injuries are often related to participation in sports [17]. Crush injuries that involve the nail bed may require prophylactic antibiotics due to a relatively high incidence of osteomyelitis [11]. Of special importance is the Seymour fracture, a physeal fracture of the distal phalanx which is open through the nail bed. Clinically this will present as a subungual hematoma with a displaced physeal fracture on radiographs. Removal of the nail plate and irrigation of the fracture are required to prevent infection.

In general, the treatment of most phalangeal fractures is nonsurgical. In one series, almost 90 % were managed solely by immobilization. Surgical treatment was reserved for fractures which were unstable or had significant intra-articular involvement, rotation, or shortening [18]. The prognosis for most phalangeal fractures is excellent. Despite the periphyseal predominance, associated growth disturbances are rare [17].

Imaging

Radiographs typically demonstrate a lucent fracture line. Incomplete and buckle fractures also occur. The degree of displacement varies with the mechanism of injury, although two-thirds are displaced either minimally or not at all [17]. Cross-sectional imaging with CT or MRI is reserved for cases with complex fracture patterns or when associated soft tissue injury is suspected. Salter-Harris II fractures are the most common, although other Salter-Harris fractures also occur [18]. Ligament or tendon injury can be associated with Salter-Harris III fractures [11]. For example, mallet finger occurs with a fracture of the base of the distal phalanx and disruption of the extensor digitorum tendon, resulting in the inability to extend the finger at the distal interphalangeal joint. Another specific injury that deserves mention is a Salter-Harris III fracture of the proximal phalanx of the thumb. As in adults, this fracture can be associated with ulnar collateral ligament injuries and may require surgical correction [11].

2 Kienböck Osteonecrosis (Box 10.2)

Box 10.2: Kienböck Osteonecrosis

Associated with negative ulnar variance
Four radiographic stages
 I = normal
 II = sclerosis
 III = lunate collapse
 IV = carpal instability
MRI most sensitive for early stages

Kienböck osteonecrosis (also known as Kienböck disease or malacia, lunatomalacia, and osteonecrosis of the lunate) was first described by the Austrian radiologist Robert Kienböck in 1910. Commonly seen in young adults, the peak age incidence is 20–40 years [20]. The disorder does occur in pediatric patients, usually in mid to late adolescence [21, 22]; however, it has been reported in patients as young as 6 years of age [23].

The etiology is unknown and thought to be multifactorial, but the most widely accepted theory is that vascular perfusion of the lunate is ultimately altered [24]. One potentially important anatomic consideration in Keinböck disease is that of negative ulnar variance. Negative ulnar variance describes a relative foreshortening of the ulna in relation to the radius. Some studies have shown a correlation between negative ulnar variance and an increased incidence of Kienböck disease, but others have shown no association [20]. It is proposed that negative ulnar variance alters the mechanics of the radiolunate joint and results in increased mechanical stress. Interestingly, this association has not been found in patients with negative ulnar variance after ulnar shortening procedures [20].

The treatment of Kienböck disease varies with patient age, severity of symptoms, and the extent to which function is impaired. Various treatments, including supportive measures, ulnar lengthening, radial shortening, revascularization of the lunate, and arthrodesis with carpal fusion have been employed. The most commonly described treatments in children are supportive therapy and radial shortening surgery [21, 22, 25]. With treatment, the radiographic abnormalities of the lunate may completely normalize [25].

Imaging

Radiographs demonstrate varying degrees of lunate abnormality, ranging from mild to complete collapse; with advanced disease, secondary degenerative changes may develop. Lichtman radiographic staging system is most widely used and classifies the appearance as I (normal), II (sclerosis), III (lunate collapse), and IV (carpal instability) [24]. MRI is more sensitive to early stages of Kienböck disease [26, 27]. Early disease (Lichtman stage I on radiographs) manifests as decreased T1 signal and increased T2 signal, reflecting bone marrow edema. The imaging appearance at this stage is nonspecific, resembling edema secondary to trauma. As the disease progresses (Lichtman stage II on radiographs), there will be low signal on both T1- and T2-W images, reflecting increased sclerosis [26]. More advanced stages of the process (Lichtman stages III and IV on radiographs) will manifest as diffuse T1 and T2 hypointense signal changes throughout the lunate, coupled with alterations in lunate shape (i.e., collapse) and bone marrow edema in the adjacent carpus. CT, with its excellent spatial resolution, can be a useful tool both for evaluating subtle findings of sclerosis and collapse and for evaluating associated perilunate degenerative changes [26] (Fig. 10.7).

3 Overuse Injuries

3.1 Gymnast Wrist (Box 10.3)

Box 10.3: Gymnast Wrist

Overuse leads to chronic physeal injury
Radius much more common and severe than the ulna
 Distal physeal widening, irregularity, and haziness
 Cystic change in distal metaphysis
 Premature closure of distal physis
MRI T2 hyperintense cartilage extends into metaphysis
 Edema, premature physeal closure, and bone bridging

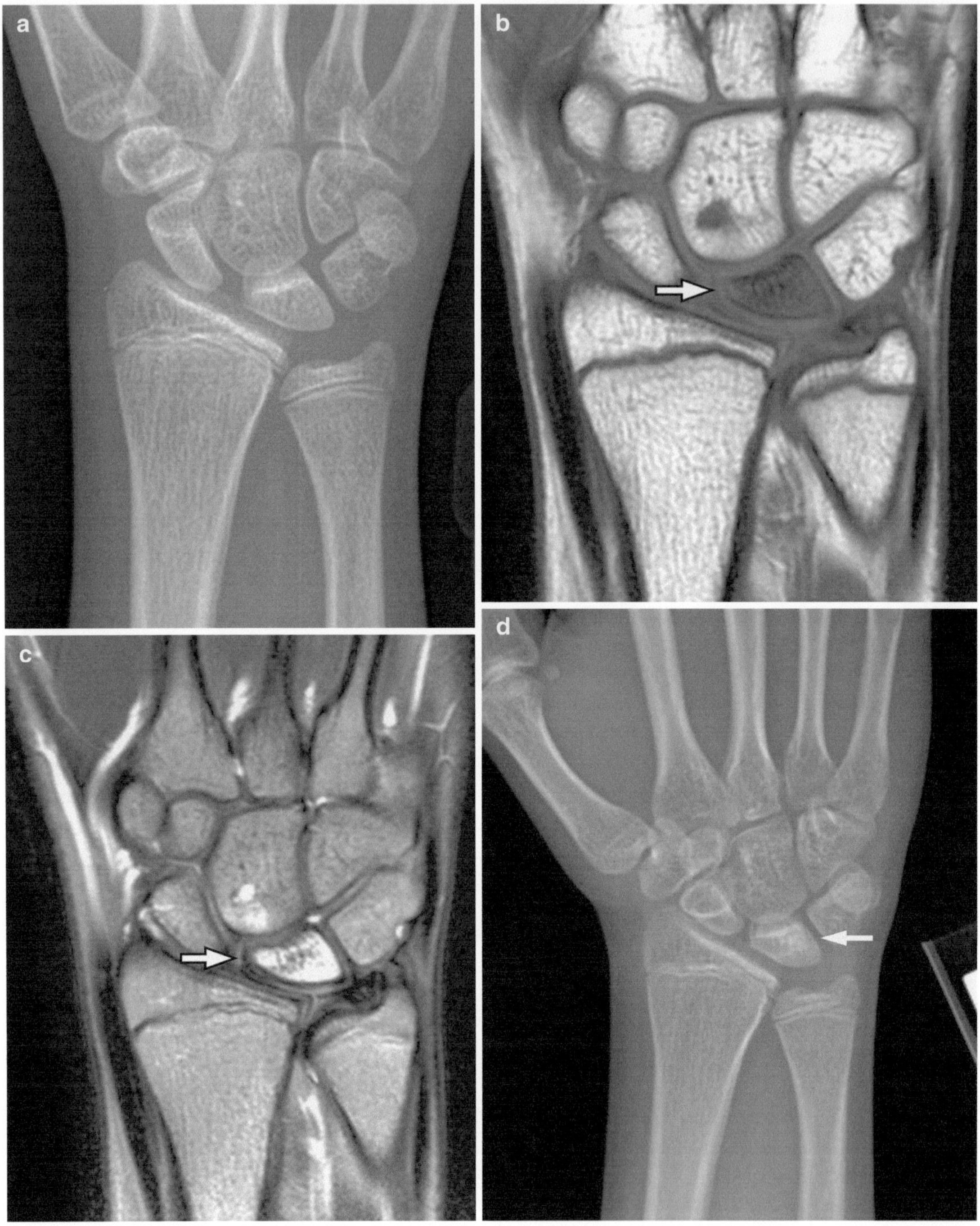

Fig. 10.7 Keinböck osteonecrosis in a 13-year-old girl. (**a**) Initial radiographs were normal except for negative ulnar variance. Coronal T1-W (**b**) and T2-W fat-suppressed (**c**) images show diffuse low T1 signal and corresponding high T2 signal (*arrows*). Similar abnormal marrow signal in the capitate is likely secondary to altered mechanical stress related to the abnormal lunate. (**d**) One month later, there is sclerosis and mild collapse of the lunate

Growing bones are uniquely susceptible to injury from repetitive stress or loading. For example, injury to the distal radial physis occurs in young gymnasts. Wrist pain is common in competitive and elite gymnasts, with an estimated prevalence of 46–79 % [28, 29]. Up to half of beginner or mid-level gymnasts report wrist pain as well [30].

Due to the nature of several of the maneuvers performed in competitive gymnastics, the wrist, which is normally not a weight-bearing structure, commonly supports the athlete's entire weight [28]. The distal radius, in particular, bears the brunt of the injury as it supports approximately 80 % of the wrist's axial load [31, 32]. In younger children, in whom there is typically a degree of negative ulnar variance [33], the radius can be called upon to support up to 96 % of the load [32].

Chronic mechanical stress decreases the vascular supply to the metaphysis, inhibiting ossification of chondrocytes at the zone of provisional calcification [34, 35]. The radiographic findings of growth plate widening and cystic changes in the metaphysis result from the accumulation of these non-ossified chondrocytes at the metaphyseal margin of the growth plate and within partially ossified portions of the metaphysis. This correlates with the histopathological findings seen in animal models [35]. Excessive mechanical stress to the physis has also been linked to premature physeal closure [36]. Stress fractures of the distal radial metaphysis can also be seen. Occasionally, in the setting of an acute injury, a Salter-Harris type I fracture of the distal radius with physeal widening and displacement of the epiphysis may occur.

A clinical and radiographic correlation has been found between gymnasts and positive ulnar variance, or relative increased length of the ulna in relation to the radius. As mentioned above, negative ulnar variance occurs in the skeletally immature wrist [33]. However, in competitive gymnasts, even those that have not yet reached skeletal maturity, there is an increased rate of positive ulnar variance [37, 38]. This may be secondary to growth disturbance of the distal radius resulting in relative overgrowth of the ulna. However, no direct evidence links distal radius stress and growth disturbance to wrist pain and positive ulnar variance [32].

Clinical management of a young gymnast with wrist pain is generally supportive. Imaging is usually performed in order to characterize the injury and to exclude acute fractures or soft tissue injuries. In general, treatment consists of rest and cessation of load-bearing activities. Gradual return to activities is recommended, with routines altered to minimize the load on the wrists [32]. The efficacy of bracing, either prophylactically or as treatment, has not been well established [32].

Imaging

Radiographic findings in these patients vary. In some patients, radiographs are normal; however, the distal radial physis is often widened [39]. Additional radiographic findings may include cystic changes in the distal radial metaphysis, beaking of the epiphysis, and haziness of the normally radiolucent physis (Fig. 10.8) [40]. Premature closure of the distal radial physis has also been reported [41]. Pseudo-Madelung appearance has been described, secondary to premature closure of the ulnar aspect of the radial physis [42]. Acute Salter-Harris type I fractures manifest as displacement of the epiphysis in relation to the metaphysis. In patients undergoing MRI, findings include physeal widening, abnormal T2 hyperintense cartilage extending proximally into the distal radial metaphysis, T2 hyperintense bone marrow edema, and premature physeal closure with bridging (Fig. 10.9) [43]. Similar changes can also be seen in the ulna but are less common and are often less pronounced [39, 43, 44].

3.2 Ulnocarpal Impaction (Box 10.4)

Box 10.4: Ulnocarpal Impaction

Degeneration due to abutment of distal ulna into proximal carpal row

Early findings:

Radiographs–usually normal

MRI–T1 hypointense and T2 hyperintense signal (edema) within lunate and occasionally within triquetrum

Late findings:

Radiographs–lunate sclerosis and (with advanced disease) collapse and fragmentation; secondary degenerative changes of the carpus.

MRI–T1 and T2 hypointense signal in lunate (sclerosis), along with fragmentation and collapse

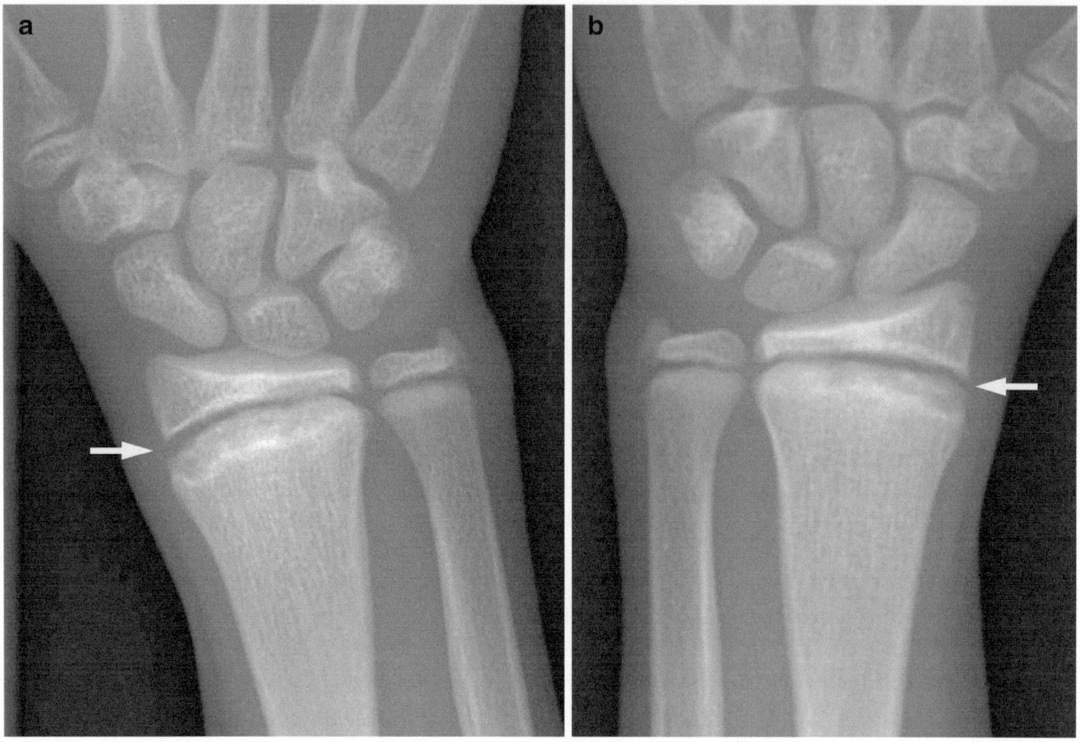

Fig. 10.8 Gymnast wrist in a 13-year-old girl. (**a**, **b**) There is bilateral metaphyseal irregularity and sclerosis with widening of the distal radial physes

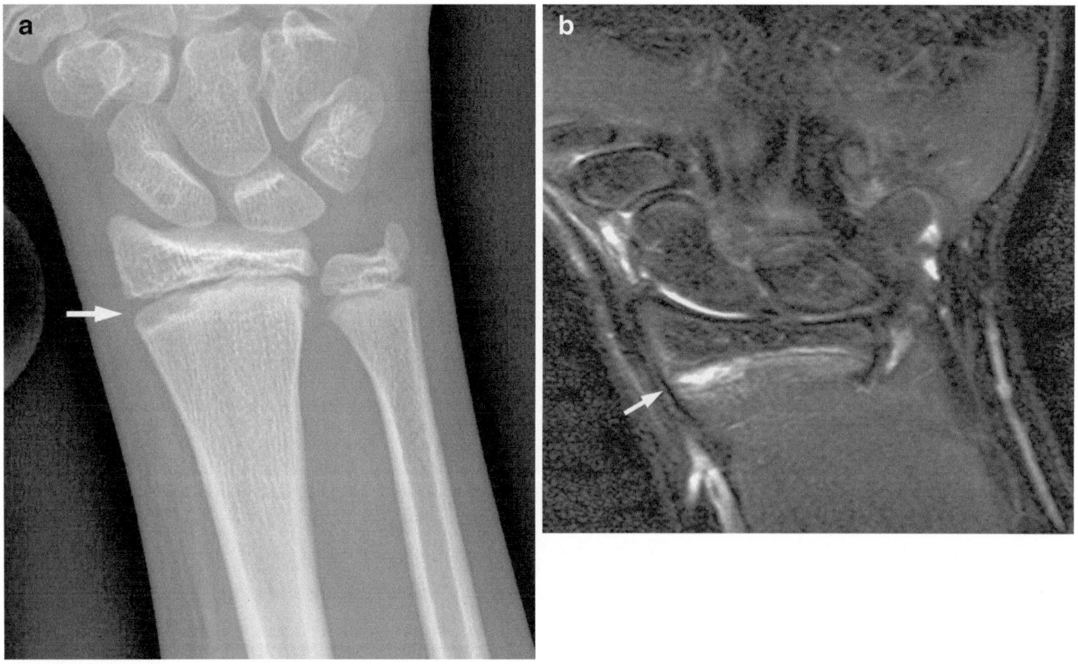

Fig. 10.9 Gymnast wrist in a teenager. (**a**) Asymmetric widening of the distal radial physis (*arrow*). (**b**) Coronal short tau inversion recovery MRI shows corresponding increased thickness and high T2-W signal at distal radial physeal cartilage (*arrow*), with adjacent marrow edema (Courtesy of Diego Jaramillo, Philadelphia, PA)

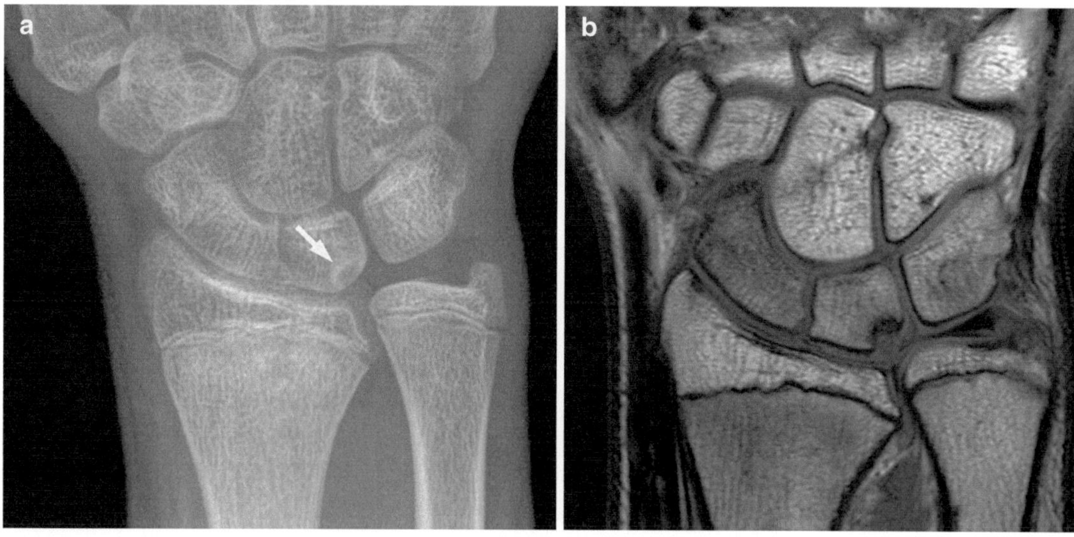

Fig. 10.10 Ulnocarpal impaction in a 14-year-old girl. (**a**) There is positive ulnar variance and cystic change along the ulnar aspect of the lunate (*arrow*). (**b**) Coronal proton density MRI confirms ulnocarpal impaction

Patients with ulnocarpal impaction syndrome present with slow-onset wrist pain exacerbated by pronation and ulnar deviation. Causes include congenital ulnar positive variance, trauma that affects relative growth of the distal radius or ulna, Madelung deformity, and elbow trauma [45]. Abutment of the distal ulna into the proximal carpal row causes degeneration.

Treatment for ulnocarpal impaction syndrome is based on the patient's symptoms and can be conservative or surgical [45]. Corticosteroid injections and nonsteroidal anti-inflammatory medications can provide symptomatic relief. Surgical options include either ulnar shortening osteotomy or a wafer procedure, which removes a portion of the ulnar head while preserving the radioulnar ligaments, fovea, triangular fibrocartilage complex (TFCC), and articular surface of the distal radioulnar joint (DRUJ) [45].

Imaging

Early MRI shows ulnocarpal impaction syndrome while radiographs are still normal (Fig. 10.10). Edema is seen in the lunate, most commonly followed by edema within the radial portion of the triquetrum. According to one study, only 10 % of patients demonstrated edema within the ulnar head [46]. Late MRI shows decreased signal intensity on T1- and T2-W images, suggesting subchondral sclerosis; radiographs show sclerosis of the involved osseous structures and subchondral cystic change. Ulnar impaction can also result in degeneration of the TFCC. This can progress to complete tears, best identified with MR arthrography.

Differential Diagnosis

Differential diagnosis of ulnar impaction syndrome includes other causes of ulnar-sided wrist pain including TFCC tears and lunotriquetral ligament injury.

4 Pathology of Tendons and Ligaments

4.1 Tendons

Overuse injuries such as tendonosis are generally more common in adolescents than in younger children. Risk factors include a change in training intensity, muscle-tendon imbalance, poor conditioning prior to training, nutritional deficiencies, and rapid growth [47, 48]. Tendonosis and tendon injuries typically occur with repetitive motion or impact, such as in gymnastic and racquet sports. The most common tendon pathology in the wrist occurs in the first and sixth extensor compartments.

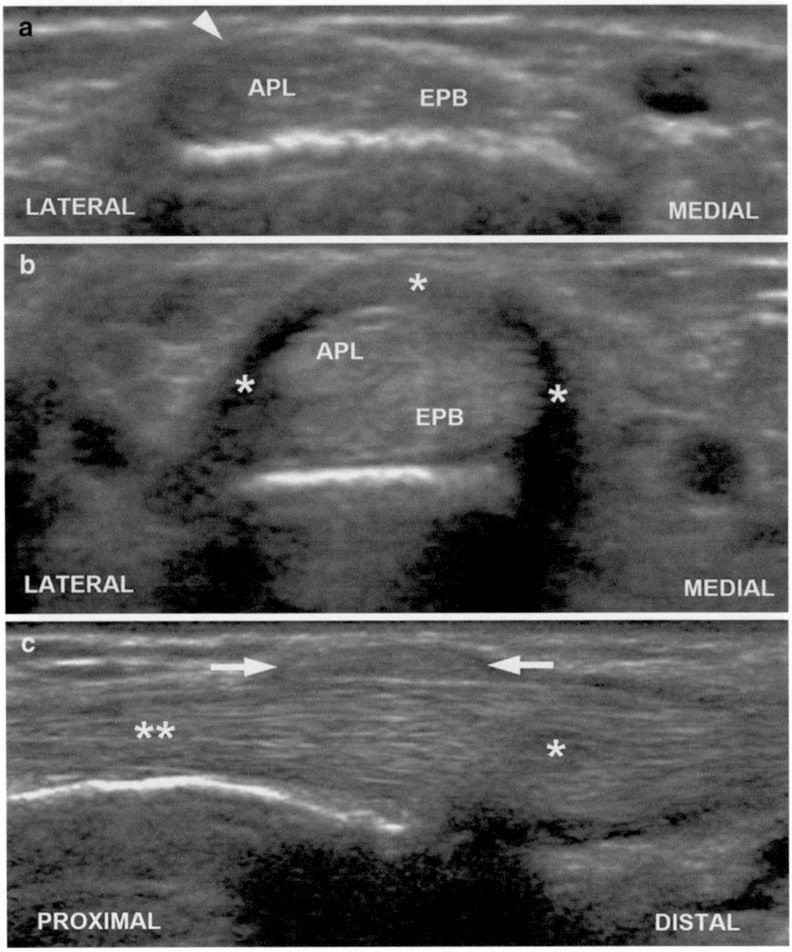

Fig. 10.11 de Quervain tenosynovitis in a 17-year-old girl. (**a**) Normal side. Transverse US through the first extensor compartment of the wrist demonstrates the normal appearance of the abductor pollicis longus (*APL*) and extensor pollicis brevis (*EPB*) tendons with overlying barely perceptible retinaculum (*arrowhead*). (**b**) Symptomatic side. Transverse US through the first extensor compartment shows the heterogeneous and thickened APL and EPB tendons along with a thickened extensor retinaculum (*asterisks*). (**c**) Longitudinal US of symptomatic side shows heterogeneity and thickening of the distal APL tendon (*single asterisk*) with thickening of the overlying extensor retinaculum (*arrows*) consistent with tenosynovitis. Note the more normal appearance of the proximal tendon (*double asterisk*)

First Extensor Compartment

de Quervain tenosynovitis is a stenosing tenosynovitis involving the first extensor compartment of the wrist. It presents with pain and functional impairment. Generally, females are more affected than males. This condition is more commonly seen in active children.

This tenosynovitis is caused by repetitive microtrauma at the level of the extensor retinaculum. Inflammation of the tendon sheaths of the extensor pollicis brevis (EPB) and abductor pollicis longus (APL) results in fibrotic changes [49]. There is anatomic variability in the first dorsal compartment tendons—some people have more than one slip of the APL tendon, while some may also have a separate tendon sheath for the EPB. These anatomic differences may increase the risk of developing de Quervain.

Ultrasound has been used to guide corticosteroid injections into the tendon sheath, resulting in decreased fluid within the sheath as well as rapid clinical improvement [50, 51].

Imaging

Although the diagnosis of de Quervain tenosynovitis is mostly clinical, both ultrasound (US) and MRI can be used to investigate this condition. In acute cases, US demonstrates fluid surrounding the tendon, causing distension of the tendon sheath; the synovial fluid appears as a hypoechoic collection surrounding a hyperechoic tendon [52]. Thickening of the tendon sheath may also be seen (a normal tendon sheath appears as a thin, circumferential hypoechoic rim measuring less than 1 mm) [52]. In chronic cases, the tendon itself may appear thick and demonstrate abnormal echogenicity (Fig. 10.11). There may be hyperemia of

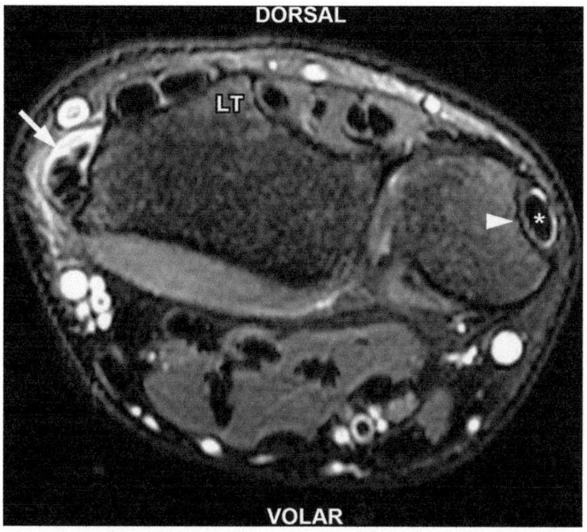

Fig. 10.12 de Quervain tenosynovitis in a 17-year-old girl. Axial T2-W fat-suppressed MRI shows abnormal fluid (*arrow*) surrounding the abductor pollicis longus and extensor pollicis brevis tendons of the first extensor compartment consistent with tenosynovitis. Mildly increased T2 signal within the tendons indicates tendinosis. There is mild adjacent subcutaneous edema. Note the normal position of the extensor carpi ulnaris (*asterisk*) tendon within its groove (*arrowhead*). *LT* Lister's tubercle

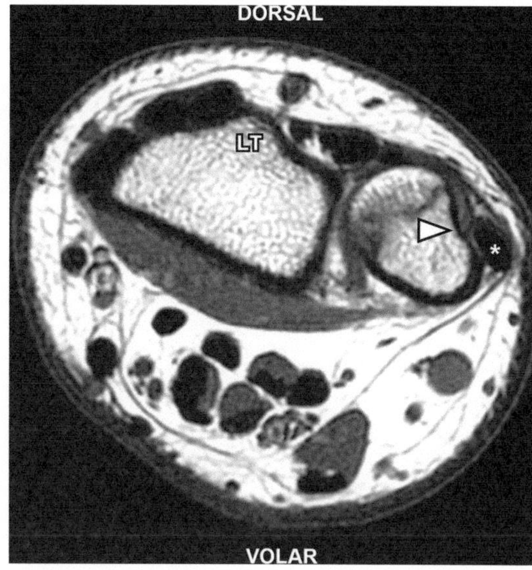

Fig. 10.13 Extensor carpi ulnaris subluxation in a 15-year-old boy after punching a wall. Axial T1-W image demonstrates subluxation of the extensor carpi ulnaris tendon (*asterisk*) from its groove (*arrowhead*). Compare this to the normal position of the extensor carpi ulnaris (*ECU*) shown in Fig. 10.12

the adjacent bone [52]. A study focusing on MRI evaluation of de Quervain tenosynovitis reported that increased tendon thickness and peritendinous edema are the most reliable findings [53] (Fig. 10.12).

Differential Diagnosis

Other pathologic findings in the region of the first extensor compartment, such as intersection and Wartenberg syndromes, must be differentiated from de Quervain tenosynovitis.

Sixth Extensor Compartment

Disruption of the extensor carpi ulnaris tendon has been observed in more athletic populations, particularly with racquet sports [54].

Disorders of the extensor carpi ulnaris tendon include tendinosis, tenosynovitis, subluxation, dislocation, or rupture. This tendon lies within the sixth extensor compartment of the wrist and passes through a fibro-osseous sheath formed by the distal ulna and an overlying extensor retinaculum. The anatomical features of this compartment make the tendon less mobile than other extensor tendons, thereby predisposing it to injury particularly during supination and ulnar deviation [54].

Imaging

Tendon subluxation or dislocation is best detected with dynamic ultrasound demonstrating abnormal excursion of the tendon with certain maneuvers. MRI may demonstrate nonspecific synovitis of the extensor carpi ulnaris but cannot demonstrate dynamic instability [55] (Fig. 10.13). The remaining pathologies, including tendinosis, tenosynovitis, and rupture, are clearly demonstrated by both MRI and US [55].

Trigger Thumb

Patients typically present around age two with the thumb fixed in either extension or flexion. A volar mass or knot is palpable corresponding to the focally thickened flexor pollicis longus tendon and sheath. Pediatric trigger thumb is approximately ten times more common than trigger finger [56]. Approximately 25 % have bilateral involvement [56]. Evidence suggests that trigger thumb varies depending on ethnicity. The incidence in the United States is unknown [56].

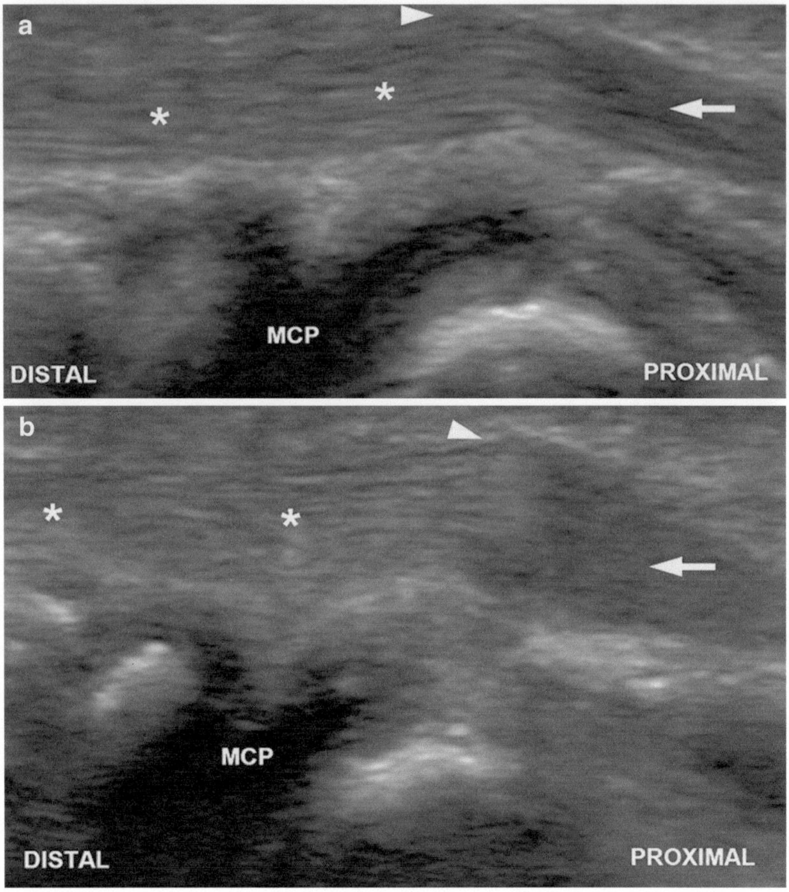

Fig. 10.14 Flexion deformity due to trigger thumb in a 3-year-old. (**a**) Normal longitudinal US appearance of flexor pollicis longus tendon (*asterisks*) and barely perceptible A1 pulley (*arrowhead*). Relatively hypoechoic appearance of the proximal tendon (*arrow*) is due to artifact (anisotropy). (**b**) Longitudinal US of symptomatic side shows that the flexor pollicis longus tendon proximal to the MCP joint (*arrow*) is t hick and heterogeneous. The A1 pulley (*arrowhead*) is prominent. Note the normal appearance of the tendon distally (*asterisks*). *MCP* metacarpophalangeal joint

Pediatric trigger thumb is caused by a discrepancy in size between the flexor pollicis longus tendon and the A1 pulley. This leads to inhibition of normal tendon gliding at the thumb's metacarpophalangeal joint. The exact etiology of this discrepancy in size is unknown. However, multiple studies suggest that trigger thumb is not congenital, but rather degenerative, infectious, or perhaps inflammatory.

Management of trigger thumb can be surgical or nonsurgical. Spontaneous resolution has been reported to range from zero to 66 % [56]; however, studies are limited. Spontaneous recovery after 2 years of age is unusual. Nonsurgical management includes passive thumb extension exercises and extension splinting. However, published outcomes are inconclusive [56]. Operative management involves open surgical release of the A1 pulley restoring interphalangeal joint motion. The risks of neurovascular injury, infection, and persistent or recurrent triggering are minimal [56].

Imaging

Trigger thumb is a clinical diagnosis that does not require routine imaging. If the diagnosis is in question, ultrasound is the preferred imaging modality. The flexor pollicis longus tendon is imaged in longitudinal and transverse planes proximal to the level of the thenar eminence and distal to the interphalangeal joint. Uniformity, echogenicity, and motion of the tendon are assessed with dynamic maneuvers. The A1 pulley is also evaluated for thickening. In most cases, the contralateral thumb is imaged for comparison.

The echogenicity of the flexor pollicis longus tendon is usually normal, but it is often focally thickened, and it may be too large to fit within the A1 pulley (Fig. 10.14). The A1 pulley itself is usually thickened as well. The flexed or extended position of the thumb depends on the location of the focal thickening (Notta's node) in relation to the A1 pulley.

4.2 Ligaments

Carpal Instability

Both intrinsic and extrinsic ligaments contribute to carpal instability. The scapholunate ligament and lunotriquetral ligaments (both intrinsic ligaments) along with the triangular fibrocartilage cartilage complex (TFCC) are injured most often and therefore associated with carpal instability.

Both the scapholunate and lunotriquetral ligaments have three portions: dorsal, volar, and membranous. The dorsal band of the scapholunate ligament and the volar band of the lunotriquetral ligament are the most mechanically important structures. Tears are classified as complete if all three portions of either the scapholunate or the lunotriquetral ligaments are disrupted. Most patients with partial tears can be treated conservatively and have no sign of wrist instability [57]. Tears of the dorsal and volar components are usually posttraumatic and associated with wrist pain, whereas central (membranous) tears are usually due to degeneration and can be asymptomatic [58].

Imaging

The dorsal and volar components are best seen with axial imaging. At MRI, fluid-like signal intensity within the ligament and irregularity or the absence of the ligament are direct signs of injury (Fig. 10.15). Indirect signs of scapholunate injury include scapholunate dissociation (increased scapholunate distance), avulsive cystic changes at the osseous attachment of the scapholunate ligament, disruption of the carpal arch, and ganglion cyst formation [58]. Tears of the scapholunate ligament are associated with dorsal intercalated segmental instability, in which the scaphoid flexes and the lunate extends. Scapholunate ligament distance should be interpreted with caution as this space may appear widened due to incomplete ossification of the carpus.

Tears of the lunotriquetral ligament are associated with lunate osteonecrosis (Kienböck disease), volar intercalated segmental instability (in which the lunate flexes, rare in children), and ulnar impaction. Ulnar impaction is associated

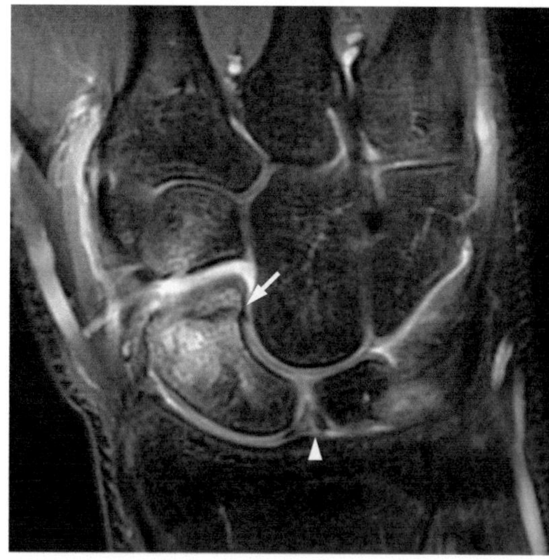

Fig. 10.15 Scapholunate ligament tear after a 16-year-old boy falls from a dirt bike. Coronal T2-W fat-suppressed image demonstrates a vertically oriented band of high signal within the dorsal band of the scapholunate ligament consistent with a tear (*arrowhead*). The patient also has edema and hypointense linearly oriented signal alteration within the distal pole of the scaphoid (*arrow*) consistent with a fracture

with degenerative tears of the membranous component. The prognosis is worse and management affected if a lunotriquetral and a TFCC tear occur together [58].

Ulnar Collateral Ligament of the Thumb

The ulnar collateral ligament and base of the thumb's proximal phalanx resist valgus stress at the metacarpophalangeal joint. Injury to the ulnar collateral ligament is caused by hyperextension and hyperabduction of the metacarpophalangeal joint. If not appropriately treated, ulnar collateral ligament injuries can lead to degenerative changes and chronic pain [52].

Ulnar collateral ligament injuries range from sprains to partial- and full-thickness tears. For full-thickness tears, the greater the degree of displacement, the more likely the injury will be treated surgically. Also surgically managed, a Stener lesion is a displaced full-thickness ulnar collateral ligament tear with the adductor aponeurosis interposed between the retracted ligament and its insertion site at the base of the

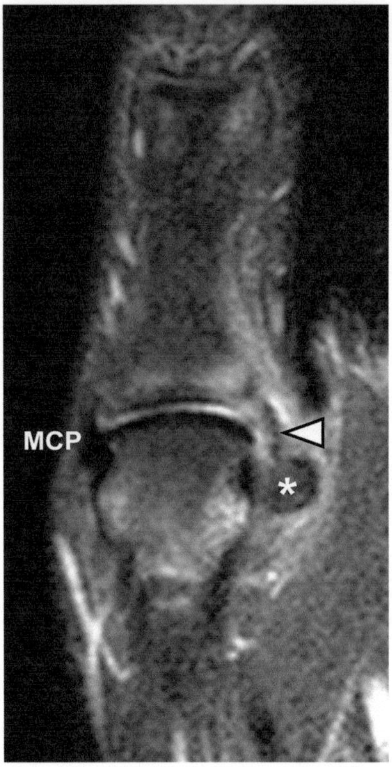

Fig. 10.16 Stener lesion in a 17-year-old boy after falling on outstretched hand. Coronal T2-W fat-suppressed image through the thumb along the expected plane of the ulnar collateral ligament at the level of the metacarpophalangeal (*MCP*) joint demonstrates a round hypoechoic mass-like abnormality (*asterisk*) representing a completely torn, proximally retracted ulnar collateral ligament. Note the linear hypointense structure (*arrowhead*) extending to the torn ligament, which is the interposed adductor aponeurosis

proximal phalanx [52], so that the ligament is actually superficial to the adductor aponeurosis, making spontaneous healing impossible.

Imaging

Both MRI and US allow adequate visualization of the ulnar collateral ligament and surrounding structures (Figs. 10.16, 10.17, and 10.18). US allows for dynamic evaluation as well as longitudinal and transverse imaging. Ligamentous disruption and degree of retraction should be assessed. A normal tendon appears hyperechoic, whereas a non-displaced tendon tear demonstrates focal hypoechoic clefts. Integrity of the thin overlying hyperechoic adductor aponeurosis should also be assessed. Associated findings include osseous avulsion, joint effusion, and volar plate injury [52].

Differential Diagnosis

Other causes of thumb pain such as tendinosis, tenosynovitis, joint pathology, and disorders of the thenar region can be assessed.

Triangular Fibrocartilage Complex

Triangular fibrocartilage complex (TFCC) injuries can be caused by compression, acute trauma, repetitive motion such as twisting, or ulnar deviation or impaction.

The TFCC can be divided into two portions: proximal and distal. Tears of the proximal portion are associated with instability of the distal radioulnar joint (DRUJ); instability and tears of the distal portion can cause subluxation of the ulnar carpus but do not affect the stability of the DRUJ [59]. The Palmer classification can help determine treatment of TFC complex tears, which are divided into two main categories: traumatic or degenerative [59].

Treatment is partially determined by the vascular anatomy of the TFCC. Because the peripheral ulnar portion of the TFCC is supplied by penetrating vessels, tears in this region can heal without surgical intervention. Cast immobilization is initially attempted, but subacute tears of the TFCC or those that fail cast immobilization may require arthroscopic or open surgical repair. However, the central and radial portions of the TFCC are avascular, and therefore tears in these areas do not heal [60]. Treatment includes arthroscopy and debridement; ulnar shortening is performed in cases of ulnar impaction [61].

Imaging

Radiography will not demonstrate TFCC abnormalities but will show the osseous abnormalities that may be associated. These include positive ulnar variance, ulnar styloid process fractures, and avulsion fractures of the ulnar fovea [55]. Magnetic resonance (MR) arthrography is considered most accurate for evaluating the TFCC; findings, however, can be nonspecific. In fact, findings

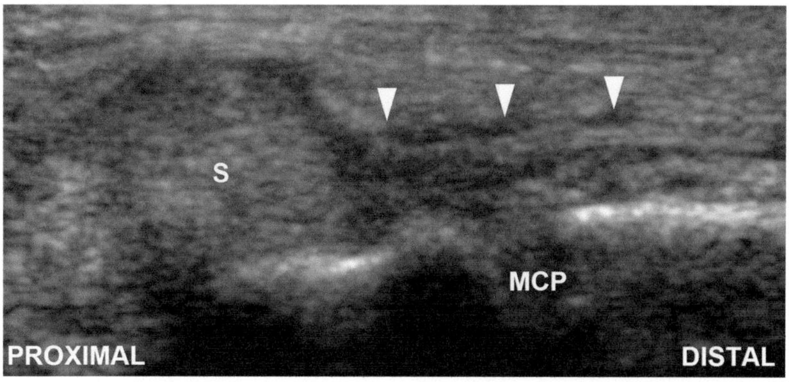

Fig. 10.17 Stener lesion after a 17-year-old boy suffers snowboarding accident. Longitudinal US of the thumb including the collateral ligament at the level of the metacarpophalangeal (*MCP*) joint demonstrates a mass-like appearance of the completely torn and retracted ligament (*S*). The linear hypoechoic structure (*arrowheads*) extending to the retracted tissue is the interposed adductor aponeurosis

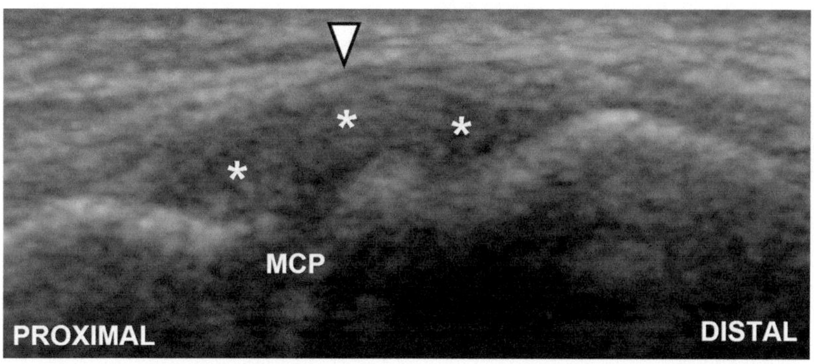

Fig. 10.18 Sprain of the ulnar collateral ligament of the thumb after a 17-year-old girl suffers a skiing accident. Longitudinal US of the ligament at the level of the meta carpophalangeal (*MCP*) joint demonstrates thickening and heterogeneity of the ligament (*asterisks*) without retraction or defect consistent with a sprain. *Arrowhead* denotes the intact overlying adductor aponeurosis

are commonly present on the contralateral asymptomatic side [55]. With improvement in imaging, some advocate 3T non-arthrogaphic MR to demonstrate clinically significant tears [58].

The ulnar attachment of the TFCC can be obscured by adjacent connective tissue in conventional MRI (Fig. 10.19). Thus, MR arthrography is particularly useful for detecting peripheral ulnar-sided tears. T1-W fat-suppressed multiplanar imaging demonstrates abnormal fluid perforating the TFCC. With full-thickness tears, contrast crosses from the radiocarpal compartment into the distal radioulnar joint (Fig. 10.20). Depending on the site of injection, noncommunicating partial-thickness tears can be demonstrated proximal or distal to the TFCC [55].

5 Neurovascular Injuries

After the elbow, the wrist is the most common location for ulnar neuropathy. The ulnar nerve can become entrapped in Guyon canal. Ulnar neuropathy often affects athletes who perform repetitive wrist motion: impaction, as in racquet sports, or pressure, as in biking (handlebar palsy) [62]. Continuous exposure of this area to vibratory forces (e.g., from frequent use of a drill) increases risk of ulnar neuropathy [62].

Guyon canal, also known as the pisohamate tunnel, is a fibro-osseous canal along the ulnar and volar aspects of the wrist. The ulnar nerve and artery usually pass through this canal; however, variations in normal anatomy or pathology involving the canal may lead to extrinsic compression of the artery and nerve [63]. The most common causes are ganglion cysts, lipomas, accessory muscles, ulnar artery aneurysms, fractures (radius, pisiform, and hook of hamate), and repetitive trauma [55, 58, 62]. Nerve entrapment may cause loss of motor and/or sensory function depending on the site of compression.

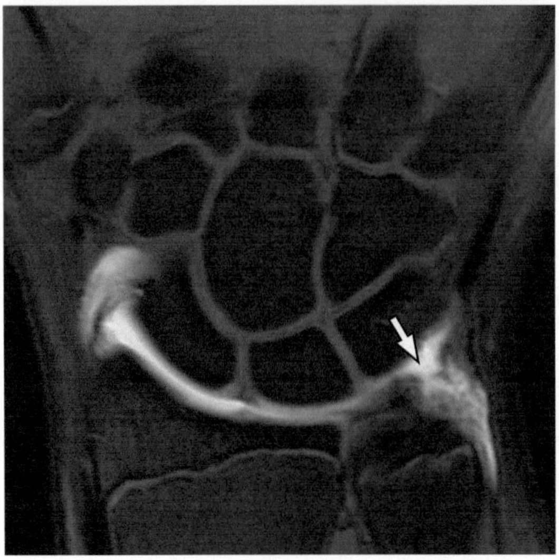

Fig. 10.19 Ulnar-sided triangular fibrocartilage tear in a 14-year-old gymnast. Coronal T1-W fat-suppressed image from an MR arthrogram after a radiocarpal joint injection demonstrates irregularity and a high signal cleft (*arrow*) along the ulnar attachment of the triangular fibrocartilage, consistent with a tear

Carpal tunnel syndrome results from compression of the medial nerve by the transverse ligament. Causes range from infection, inflammation, trauma, masses, and repetitive friction to congenital, idiopathic, and metabolic [58, 64]. Children with mucopolysaccharidoses, such as Hunter and Hurler syndromes, are especially prone to carpal tunnel syndrome, as deposits accumulate within the carpal tunnel causing a mass effect. Symptoms in children may go unrecognized for years. Children often present with complaints of hand pain, stiffness, and thenar atrophy, rather than the numbness and tingling described by adult patients.

Imaging

Ultrasound, MRI, or CT can be used to evaluate the canal and assess for possible causes of compression. A normal nerve should appear ovoid, isointense on T1-W imaging, and iso- to mildly hyperintense on T2-W imaging when compared to skeletal muscle. In peripheral neuropathy, the nerve demonstrates abnormally hyperintense T2-W signal and appears swollen proximal to

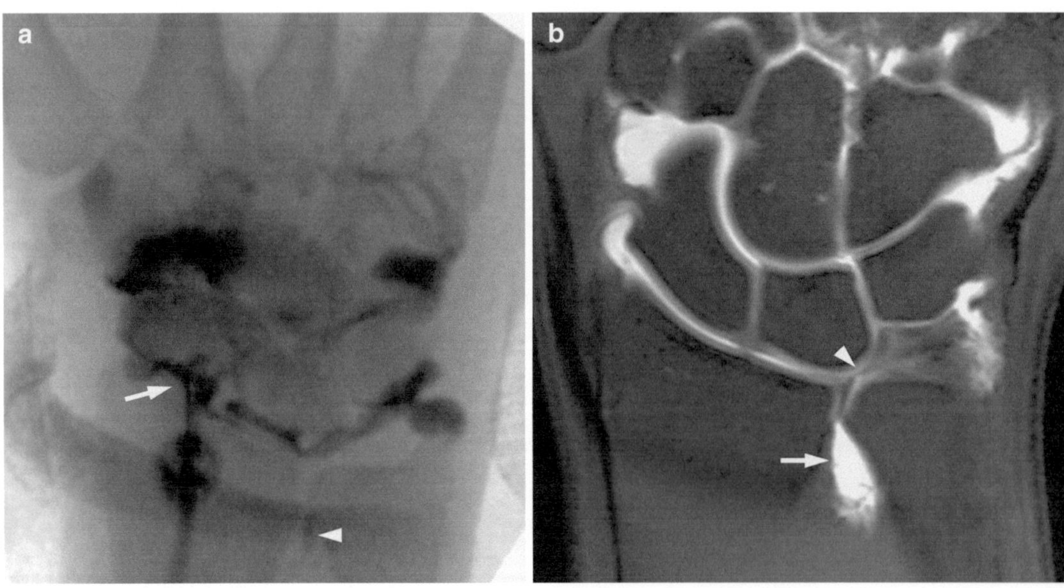

Fig. 10.20 Central triangular fibrocartilage tear in a 15-year-old girl. (**a**) Fluoroscopic image during an arthrogram with radiocarpal joint injection (*arrow*) shows abnormal extension of contrast proximally into the radioulnar joint (*arrowhead*). (**b**) Coronal T1-W fat-suppressed MRI shows abnormal contrast within the radioulnar joint (*arrow*) and thinning of the central triangular fibrocartilage (*arrowhead*)

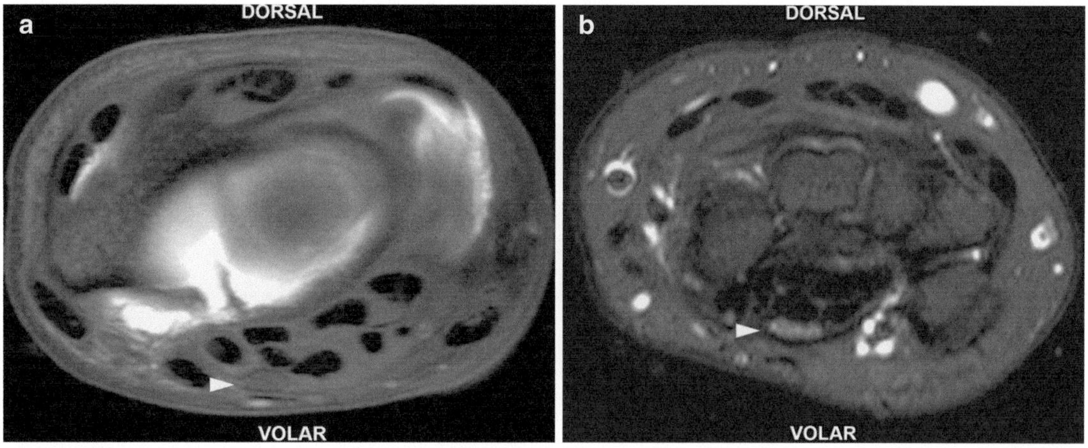

Fig. 10.21 Carpal tunnel syndrome. (**a**) Normal appearance of median nerve (*arrowhead*) on axial T2-W fat-suppressed MRI. (**b**) Axial T2-W fat-suppressed image in 17-year-old girl with carpal tunnel syndrome shows abnormally increased T2 signal within the median nerve (*arrowhead*) without significant change in caliber of the nerve itself

the canal but flattened within the canal [55, 58] (Fig. 10.21). With carpal tunnel syndrome, MRI may demonstrate effacement of fat within the carpal tunnel and outward bowing of the flexor retinaculum; this is best seen at the level of the pisiform [58]. MRI can also assess the surrounding soft tissue structures and allow characterization of anomalous musculature or masses. Alternatively, dynamic US may identify compression of the nerve due to such structures [55].

The ulnar artery, which also resides within Guyon canal, is at risk for mechanical injury. Hypothenar hammer syndrome (aneurysm formation and possible thrombosis) has been described but is generally uncommon in the pediatric population [62]. These injuries generally occur in athletes, particularly those who play racquet sports, along with baseball catchers, martial artists, and breakdancers [62]. CT angiography best evaluates this condition [62].

6 Ganglion Cysts (Box 10.5)

Ganglion cysts are the most common mass in the hand and wrist. Patients present with a palpable abnormality or pain. Although ganglion cysts typically arise in older patients, they are also common in children. Approximately 10 % of all reported cases occur in patients younger than 20 years of age, and less than 2 % in patients younger than 10 years of age [65]. A small percentage of patients report a history of trauma, but the pathogenesis of ganglion cysts is usually unclear [66].

Box 10.5: Ganglion Cyst

- Most common mass in the hand and wrist
- Often dorsal near scapholunate ligament (volar if <10 years old)
- Assess communication with joint for surgical planning (must resect neck)
- MRI: homogeneously T1 hypointense, T2 hyperintense, without central or nodular enhancement
- US: variable, often complex with variable echogenicity, loculated, thick walled

A ganglion cyst is a sac filled with mucin surrounded by fibrous tissue without synovial lining. It usually communicates with a joint or tendon sheath. Ganglion cysts are commonly found dorsally at the level of the scapholunate ligament. The second most common location is along the volar aspect of the wrist, adjacent to the radial artery and flexor carpi radialis [67]. In patients younger than 10 years of age, the majority of ganglion cysts are located on the volar side of the hand and wrist [65].

Imaging

Either MRI or US can demonstrate the cystic nature of ganglia and establish involvement of adjacent anatomy, such as communication with the joint. This information is particularly helpful for surgical planning. A stalk extending to the joint must be

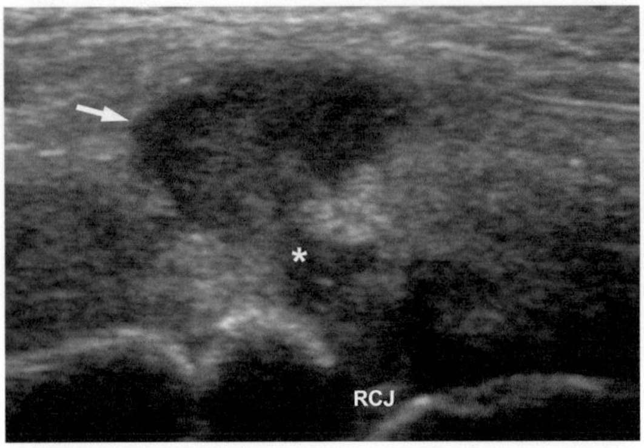

Fig. 10.22 Ganglion cyst in a 14-year-old girl presenting with a painless volar wrist mass. Longitudinal US along the volar aspect of the radiocarpal joint (*RCJ*) demonstrates an oval hypoechoic lesion (*arrow*) with thin neck (*asterisk*) communicating with the RCJ. This lesion was avascular upon Doppler interrogation

resected to minimize the risk of recurrence. MRI will typically show a homogeneous T1 hypointense and T2 hyperintense well-defined round, oval, or lobulated lesion; there should be no central or nodular enhancement [58]. The ultrasound appearance varies, but ganglia usually appear complex with locules, variable echogenicity, and thick walls (Fig. 10.22) [66]. Unlike in adults, ganglion cysts in children often resolve spontaneously.

7 Thermal Injury

The hand and wrist are relatively exposed and are thus susceptible to thermal injury. Children are particularly at risk because they tend to explore their environment using tactile stimulation [68, 69]. Younger children are at especially increased risk as they may be unable to escape from dangerous situations and potential sources of thermal injury.

7.1 Burns

The majority of burns in pediatric patients are thermal (caused by a heat source); electrical and chemical burns are much less common [68]. While most burns occur at home and are accidental [69], certain patterns of burns should raise the suspicion for non-accidental trauma. For instance, a glove-like distribution of burns could result from a child's hand being forced into hot water [69].

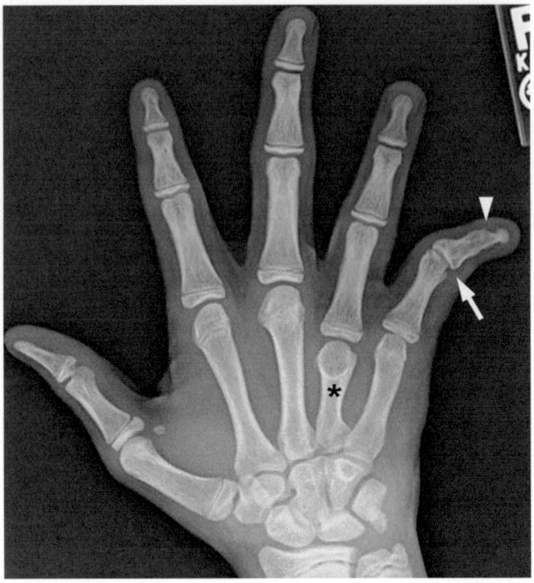

Fig. 10.23 Chronic changes due to prior burn injury in a 13-year-old boy. There is ulnar deviation of the fifth digit at the proximal interphalangeal joint (*arrow*), likely due to a combination of joint space loss and growth disturbance of the middle phalanx. The distal interphalangeal joint is fused (*arrowhead*). The fourth metacarpal is also foreshortened (*asterisk*), likely secondary to post-injury growth disturbance (this finding could be incidental and unrelated to the prior injury given the more normal appearance of the distal portions of the digit)

Imaging

Radiographic assessment plays a limited role in the care of acute hand and wrist burns. However, late complications can be seen, including soft tissue syndactyly, palmar flexion contractures, boutonniere deformity of the fingers, and an absence of the distal portions of the digits [70] (Fig. 10.23). Periarticular heterotopic ossification is a rare sequela [71].

7.2 Frostbite

Prolonged exposure to cold temperatures can also lead to severe tissue damage. This is likely due to a variety of pathophysiologic alterations, including ice crystal formation in the tissues, cellular dehydration, and microvascular occlusion [72]. This type of injury is rare in children, but can be seen in those who are accident victims or those who have become lost outdoors or are unable to escape a cold environment.

The clinical manifestations of frostbite can be divided into acute and late findings. Acutely, the

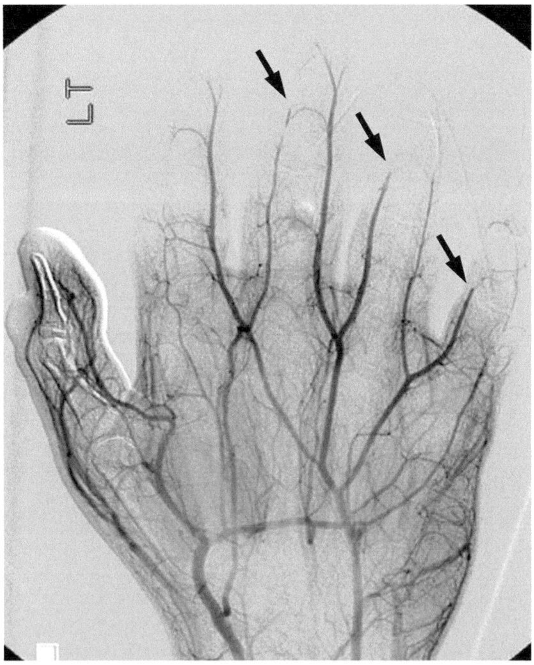

Fig. 10.24 Frostbite in a 17-year-old college freshman who fell asleep in the snow while intoxicated. An angiogram was performed for both diagnosis and potential thrombolytic therapy. Digital subtraction angiography of the right hand demonstrates abrupt cutoff of the digital arteries in multiple digits (*arrows*). Note the relative sparing of the thumb

affected extremity can demonstrate hyperemia, edema, freezing, or frank necrosis [72, 73]. In the acute setting, rapid rewarming may prevent further damage [73]. The thumb is often spared as the child may shelter it with the other digits [73, 74] (Fig. 10.24). Late clinical findings are mainly related to tissue ischemia, including necrosis and mummification. Secondary soft tissue infection is also an important clinical consideration. Treatment focuses on debridement or amputation of necrotic tissue and prevention or management of infection [72].

Imaging

In the acute setting, radiographic findings are limited to the soft tissues and include swelling and—if there is necrosis—soft tissue gas [73]. Technetium 99m methylene diphosphonate (MDP) three-phase bone scan has been used to evaluate tissue perfusion [75]. MRI assesses the extent of soft tissue injury, and MR angiography allows detailed evaluation of vascular changes [72].

Radiographs may demonstrate osseous findings in the late phase. In skeletally immature individuals, the physis and epiphysis are particularly susceptible to injury, and disturbed growth may result [73, 74, 76]. Radiographs obtained months to years after injury may show premature physeal closure with short, thick phalanges [73, 76]. Resorption or erosion of the distal phalangeal tuft [77], periarticular bone destruction, and early degenerative changes may also be seen [73, 76, 77].

References

1. Cooper C, Dennison EM, Leufkens HG, Bishop N, van Staa TP. Epidemiology of childhood fractures in Britain: a study using the general practice research database. J Bone Miner Res. 2004;19(12):1976–81. PubMed PMID: 15537440, Epub 2004/11/13. eng.
2. Lyons RA, Delahunty AM, Kraus D, Heaven M, McCabe M, Allen H, et al. Children's fractures: a population based study. Inj Prev. 1999;5(2):129–32. PubMed PMID: 10385833. Pubmed Central PMCID: 1730475. Epub 1999/07/01. eng.
3. Rennie L, Court-Brown CM, Mok JY, Beattie TF. The epidemiology of fractures in children. Injury. 2007;38(8):913–22. PubMed PMID: 17628559. Epub 2007/07/14. eng.
4. de Putter CE, van Beeck EF, Looman CW, Toet H, Hovius SE, Selles RW. Trends in wrist fractures in children and adolescents, 1997–2009. J Hand Surg Am. 2011;36(11):1810–5 e2. PubMed PMID: 22036281. Epub 2011/11/01. eng.
5. Bae DS. Pediatric distal radius and forearm fractures. J Hand Surg Am. 2008;33(10):1911–23. PubMed PMID: 19084202. Epub 2008/12/17. eng.
6. Plint AC, Perry JJ, Correll R, Gaboury I, Lawton L. A randomized, controlled trial of removable splinting versus casting for wrist buckle fractures in children. Pediatrics. 2006;117(3):691–7. PubMed PMID: 16510648. Epub 2006/03/03. eng.
7. Cannata G, De Maio F, Mancini F, Ippolito E. Physeal fractures of the distal radius and ulna: long-term prognosis. J Orthop Trauma. 2003;17(3):172–9; discussion 9-80. PubMed PMID: 12621255. Epub 2003/03/07. eng.
8. Christodoulou AG, Colton CL. Scaphoid fractures in children. J Pediatr Orthop. 1986;6(1):37–9. PubMed PMID: 3941178. Epub 1986/01/01. eng.
9. Wulff RN, Schmidt TL. Carpal fractures in children. J Pediatr Orthop. 1998;18(4):462–5. PubMed PMID: 9661853. Epub 1998/07/14. eng.
10. Grundy M. Fractures of the carpal scaphoid in children. A series of eight cases. Br J Surg. 1969;56(7):523–4. PubMed PMID: 5794969. Epub 1969/07/01. eng.
11. Nofsinger CC, Wolfe SW. Common pediatric hand fractures. Curr Opin Pediatr. 2002;14(1):42–5. PubMed PMID: 11880732. Epub 2002/03/07. eng.

12. Vahvanen V, Westerlund M. Fracture of the carpal scaphoid in children. A clinical and roentgenological study of 108 cases. Acta Orthop Scand. 1980;51(6):909–13.
13. Gholson JJ, Bae DS, Zurakowski D, Waters PM. Scaphoid fractures in children and adolescents: contemporary injury patterns and factors influencing time to union. J Bone Joint Surg Am. 2011;93(13):1210–9. PubMed PMID: 21776574. Epub 2011/07/22. eng.
14. Waters PM, Stewart SL. Surgical treatment of nonunion and avascular necrosis of the proximal part of the scaphoid in adolescents. J Bone Joint Surg Am. 2002;84-A(6):915–20. PubMed PMID: 12063324. Epub 2002/06/14. eng.
15. Johnson KJ, Haigh SF, Symonds KE. MRI in the management of scaphoid fractures in skeletally immature patients. Pediatr Radiol. 2000;30(10):685–8. PubMed PMID: 11075601. Epub 2000/11/15. eng.
16. Goldfarb CA, Yin Y, Gilula LA, Fisher AJ, Boyer MI. Wrist fractures: what the clinician wants to know. Radiology. 2001;219(1):11–28. PubMed PMID: 11274530. Epub 2001/03/29. eng.
17. Hastings 2nd H, Simmons BP. Hand fractures in children. A statistical analysis. Clin Orthop Relat Res. 1984;188:120–30. PubMed PMID: 6467708. Epub 1984/09/01. eng.
18. Mahabir RC, Kazemi AR, Cannon WG, Courtemanche DJ. Pediatric hand fractures: a review. Pediatr Emerg Care. 2001;17(3):153–6. PubMed PMID: 11437136. Epub 2001/07/05. eng.
19. Fischer MD, McElfresh EC. Physeal and periphyseal injuries of the hand. Patterns of injury and results of treatment. Hand Clin. 1994;10(2):287–301. PubMed PMID: 8040207. Epub 1994/05/01. eng.
20. Schuind F, Eslami S, Ledoux P. Kienbock's disease. J Bone Joint Surg Br. 2008;90(2):133–9. PubMed PMID: 18256076. Epub 2008/02/08. eng.
21. Ferlic RJ, Lee DH, Lopez-Ben RR. Pediatric Kienbock's disease: case report and review of the literature. Clin Orthop Relat Res. 2003;408:237–44. PubMed PMID: 12616065. Epub 2003/03/05. eng.
22. Matsuhashi T, Iwasaki N, Oizumi N, Kato H, Minami M, Minami A. Radial overgrowth after radial shortening osteotomies for skeletally immature patients with Kienbock's disease. J Hand Surg Am. 2009;34(7):1242–7. PubMed PMID: 19700072. Epub 2009/08/25. eng.
23. Docquier PL, Traore A, Hugon S. Kienbock's disease in a 6-year-old boy. Acta Orthop Belg. 2009;75(6):832–5. PubMed PMID: 20166368. Epub 2010/02/20. eng.
24. Lesley N, Lichtman D. Classification and treatment of Kienbock disease: a review of the past 100 years, and a look at the future. Handchir Mikrochir Plast Chir. 2010;42(3):171–6. PubMed PMID: 20446244. Epub 2010/05/07. Klassifikation und Behandlung des Morbus Kienbock: Eine Ubersicht uber die vergangenen 100 Jahre und ein Blick in die Zukunft. ger.
25. Beredjiklian PK. Kienbock's disease. J Hand Surg Am. 2009;34(1):167–75. PubMed PMID: 19121745. Epub 2009/01/06. eng.
26. Kazuki K, Uemura T, Okada M, Egi T. Time course of magnetic resonance images in an adolescent patient with Kienbock's disease treated by temporary scaphotrapezoidal joint fixation: a case report. J Hand Surg Am. 2006;31(1):63–7. PubMed PMID: 16443106. Epub 2006/01/31. eng.
27. Schmitt R, Heinze A, Fellner F, Obletter N, Struhn R, Bautz W. Imaging and staging of avascular osteonecroses at the wrist and hand. Eur J Radiol. 1997;25(2):92–103. PubMed PMID: 9283837. Epub 1997/09/01. eng.
28. Caine D, Roy S, Singer KM, Broekhoff J. Stress changes of the distal radial growth plate. A radiographic survey and review of the literature. Am J Sports Med. 1992;20(3):290–8. PubMed PMID: 1636860. Epub 1992/05/01. eng.
29. Mandelbaum BR, Bartolozzi AR, Davis CA, Teurlings L, Bragonier B. Wrist pain syndrome in the gymnast. Pathogenetic, diagnostic, and therapeutic considerations. Am J Sports Med. 1989;17(3):305–17. PubMed PMID: 2729480. Epub 1989/05/01. eng.
30. DiFiori JP, Puffer JC, Aish B, Dorey F. Wrist pain, distal radial physeal injury, and ulnar variance in young gymnasts: does a relationship exist? Am J Sports Med. 2002;30(6):879–85. PubMed PMID: 12435656. Epub 2002/11/19. eng.
31. af Ekenstam FW, Palmer AK, Glisson RR. The load on the radius and ulna in different positions of the wrist and forearm. A cadaver study. Acta Orthop Scand. 1984;55(3):363–5. PubMed PMID: 6741492. Epub 1984/06/01. eng.
32. DiFiori JP, Caine DJ, Malina RM. Wrist pain, distal radial physeal injury, and ulnar variance in the young gymnast. Am J Sports Med. 2006;34(5):840–9. PubMed PMID: 16493174. Epub 2006/02/24. eng.
33. Hafner R, Poznanski AK, Donovan JM. Ulnar variance in children–standard measurements for evaluation of ulnar shortening in juvenile rheumatoid arthritis, hereditary multiple exostosis and other bone or joint disorders in childhood. Skeletal Radiol. 1989;18(7):513–6. PubMed PMID: 2588029. Epub 1989/01/01. eng.
34. Ecklund K, Jaramillo D. Patterns of premature physeal arrest: MR imaging of 111 children. AJR Am J Roentgenol. 2002;178(4):967–72. PubMed PMID: 11906884. Epub 2002/03/22. eng.
35. Jaramillo D, Laor T, Zaleske DJ. Indirect trauma to the growth plate: results of MR imaging after epiphyseal and metaphyseal injury in rabbits. Radiology. 1993;187(1):171–8. PubMed PMID: 8451408. Epub 1993/04/01. eng.
36. Matsuda JJ, Zernicke RF, Vailas AC, Pedrini VA, Pedrini-Mille A, Maynard JA. Structural and mechanical adaptation of immature bone to strenuous exercise. J Appl Physiol. 1986;60(6):2028–34. PubMed PMID: 3722069. Epub 1986/06/01. eng.

37. De Smet L, Claessens A, Lefevre J, Beunen G. Gymnast wrist: an epidemiologic survey of ulnar variance and stress changes of the radial physis in elite female gymnasts. Am J Sports Med. 1994;22(6):846–50. PubMed PMID: 7856811. Epub 1994/11/01. eng.
38. Lishen Q, Jianhua O. Epiphyseal injury in gymnasts. Chin J Sports Med. 1983;2:7–12.
39. Liebling MS, Berdon WE, Ruzal-Shapiro C, Levin TL, Roye Jr D, Wilkinson R. Gymnast's wrist (pseudorickets growth plate abnormality) in adolescent athletes: findings on plain films and MR imaging. AJR Am J Roentgenol. 1995;164(1):157–9. PubMed PMID: 7998530. Epub 1995/01/01. eng.
40. Roy S, Caine D, Singer KM. Stress changes of the distal radial epiphysis in young gymnasts. A report of twenty-one cases and a review of the literature. Am J Sports Med. 1985;13(5):301–8. PubMed PMID: 4051086. Epub 1985/09/01. eng.
41. Albanese SA, Palmer AK, Kerr DR, Carpenter CW, Lisi D, Levinsohn EM. Wrist pain and distal growth plate closure of the radius in gymnasts. J Pediatr Orthop. 1989;9(1):23–8. PubMed PMID: 2915034. Epub 1989/01/01. eng.
42. Brooks TJ. Madelung deformity in a collegiate gymnast: a case report. J Athl Train. 2001;36(2):170–3. PubMed PMID: 12937458. Pubmed Central PMCID: 155529. Epub 2003/08/26. Eng.
43. Shih C, Chang CY, Penn IW, Tiu CM, Chang T, Wu JJ. Chronically stressed wrists in adolescent gymnasts: MR imaging appearance. Radiology. 1995;195(3):855–9. PubMed PMID: 7754021. Epub 1995/06/01. eng.
44. Dwek JR, Cardoso F, Chung CB. MR imaging of overuse injuries in the skeletally immature gymnast: spectrum of soft-tissue and osseous lesions in the hand and wrist. Pediatr Radiol. 2009;39(12):1310–6. PubMed PMID: 19847413. Pubmed Central PMCID: 2776148. Epub 2009/10/23. eng.
45. Sachar K. Ulnar-sided wrist pain: evaluation and treatment of triangular fibrocartilage complex tears, ulnocarpal impaction syndrome, and lunotriquetral ligament tears. J Hand Surg Am. 2012;37(7):1489–500. PubMed PMID: 22721461. Epub 2012/06/23. eng.
46. Imaeda T, Nakamura R, Shionoya K, Makino N. Ulnar impaction syndrome: MR imaging findings. Radiology. 1996;201(2):495–500. PubMed PMID: 8888248. Epub 1996/11/01. eng.
47. Gill TJ, Micheli LJ. The immature athlete. Common injuries and overuse syndromes of the elbow and wrist. Clin Sports Med. 1996;15(2):401–23. PubMed PMID: 8726322. Epub 1996/04/01. eng.
48. O'Neill DB, Micheli LJ. Overuse injuries in the young athlete. Clin Sports Med. 1988;7(3):591–610. PubMed PMID: 3042161. Epub 1988/07/01. eng.
49. Giovagnorio F, Andreoli C, De Cicco ML. Ultrasonographic evaluation of de Quervain disease. J Ultrasound Med. 1997;16(10):685–9. PubMed PMID: 9323674. Epub 1997/11/05. eng.
50. Kamel M, Moghazy K, Eid H, Mansour R. Ultrasonographic diagnosis of de Quervain's tenosynovitis. Ann Rheum Dis. 2002;61(11):1034–5. PubMed PMID: 12379534. Pubmed Central PMCID: 1753934. Epub 2002/10/16. eng.
51. McDermott JD, Ilyas AM, Nazarian LN, Leinberry CF. Ultrasound-guided injections for de Quervain's tenosynovitis. Clin Orthop Relat Res. 2012;470(7):1925–31. PubMed PMID: 22552767. Pubmed Central PMCID: 3369070. Epub 2012/05/04. eng.
52. Ebrahim FS, De Maeseneer M, Jager T, Marcelis S, Jamadar DA, Jacobson JA. US diagnosis of UCL tears of the thumb and Stener lesions: technique, pattern-based approach, and differential diagnosis. Radiographics. 2006;26(4):1007–20. PubMed PMID: 16844929. Epub 2006/07/18. eng.
53. Glajchen N, Schweitzer M. MRI features in de Quervain's tenosynovitis of the wrist. Skeletal Radiol. 1996;25(1):63–5. PubMed PMID: 8717121. Epub 1996/01/01. eng.
54. Montalvan B, Parier J, Brasseur JL, Le Viet D, Drape JL. Extensor carpi ulnaris injuries in tennis players: a study of 28 cases. Br J Sports Med. 2006;40(5):424–9. PubMed PMID: 16632573. Pubmed Central PMCID: 2577486. discussion 9; Epub 2006/04/25. eng.
55. Watanabe A, Souza F, Vezeridis PS, Blazar P, Yoshioka H. Ulnar-sided wrist pain. II. Clinical imaging and treatment. Skeletal Radiol. 2010;39(9):837–57. PubMed PMID: 20012039. Pubmed Central PMCID: 2904904. Epub 2009/12/17. eng.
56. Shah AS, Bae DS. Management of pediatric trigger thumb and trigger finger. J Am Acad Orthop Surg. 2012;20(4):206–13. PubMed PMID: 22474090. Epub 2012/04/05. eng.
57. Moser T, Dosch JC, Moussaoui A, Buy X, Gangi A, Dietemann JL. Multidetector CT arthrography of the wrist joint: how to do it. Radiographics. 2008;28(3):787–800; quiz 911. PubMed PMID: 18480484. Epub 2008/05/16. eng.
58. Chhabra A, Soldatos T, Thawait GK, Del Grande F, Thakkar RS, Means Jr KR, et al. Current perspectives on the advantages of 3-T MR imaging of the wrist. Radiographics. 2012;32(3):879–96. PubMed PMID: 22582365. Epub 2012/05/15. eng.
59. Cerezal L, de Dios B-MJ, Canga A, Llopis E, Rolon A, Martin-Oliva X, et al. MR and CT arthrography of the wrist. Semin Musculoskelet Radiol. 2012;16(1):27–41. PubMed PMID: 22447235. Epub 2012/03/27. eng.
60. Vezeridis PS, Yoshioka H, Han R, Blazar P. Ulnar-sided wrist pain. Part I: anatomy and physical examination. Skeletal Radiol. 2010;39(8):733–45. PubMed PMID: 19722104. Pubmed Central PMCID: 2895881. Epub 2009/09/02. eng.
61. Lee JI, Suh DH, Byun JS, Bae JH, Hong JY, Park JH, et al. Radiographic appearance and patient outcome after ulnar shortening osteotomy for idiopathic ulnar impaction syndrome. J Hand Surg Am.

2012;37(5):975–81. PubMed PMID: 22541154. Epub 2012/05/01. eng.
62. Blum AG, Zabel JP, Kohlmann R, Batch T, Barbara K, Zhu X, et al. Pathologic conditions of the hypothenar eminence: evaluation with multidetector CT and MR imaging. Radiographics. 2006;26(4):1021–44. PubMed PMID: 16844930. Epub 2006/07/18. eng.
63. Pierre-Jerome C, Moncayo V, Terk MR. The Guyon's canal in perspective: 3-T MRI assessment of the normal anatomy, the anatomical variations and the Guyon's canal syndrome. Surg Radiol Anat. 2011;33(10):897–903. PubMed PMID: 21695542. Epub 2011/06/23. eng.
64. Wilson D, Allen GM. Imaging of the carpal tunnel. Semin Musculoskelet Radiol. 2012;16(2):137–45. PubMed PMID: 22648429. Epub 2012/06/01. eng.
65. Simon Cypel TK, Mrad A, Somers G, Zuker RM. Ganglion cyst in children: reviewing treatment and recurrence rates. Can J Plast Surg. 2011;19(2): 53–5. PubMed PMID: 22654533. Pubmed Central PMCID: 3328107. Epub 2012/06/02. eng.
66. Teefey SA, Dahiya N, Middleton WD, Gelberman RH, Boyer MI. Ganglia of the hand and wrist: a sonographic analysis. AJR Am J Roentgenol. 2008;191(3):716–20. PubMed PMID: 18716098. Epub 2008/08/22. eng.
67. Wang G, Jacobson JA, Feng FY, Girish G, Caoili EM, Brandon C. Sonography of wrist ganglion cysts: variable and noncystic appearances. J Ultrasound Med. 2007;26(10):1323–8; quiz 30–1. PubMed PMID: 17901135. Epub 2007/09/29. eng.
68. Choi M, Armstrong MB, Panthaki ZJ. Pediatric hand burns: thermal, electrical, chemical. J Craniofac Surg. 2009;20(4):1045–8. PubMed PMID: 19634213. Epub 2009/07/28. eng.
69. Mok JY. Non-accidental injury in children–an update. Injury. 2008;39(9):978–85. PubMed PMID: 18656192. Epub 2008/07/29. eng.
70. Smith MA, Munster AM, Spence RJ. Burns of the hand and upper limb–a review. Burns. 1998;24(6):493–505. PubMed PMID: 9776087. Epub 1998/10/17. eng.
71. Price CE, Guggenheim M, Rode H. Heterotopic para-articular ossification in a child following flame burns. Eur J Pediatr Surg. 2010;20(5):351–3. PubMed PMID: 20383823. Epub 2010/04/13. eng.
72. Barker JR, Haws MJ, Brown RE, Kucan JO, Moore WD. Magnetic resonance imaging of severe frostbite injuries. Ann Plast Surg. 1997;38(3):275–9. PubMed PMID: 9088467. Epub 1997/03/01. eng.
73. Crouch C, Smith WL. Long term sequelae of frostbite. Pediatr Radiol. 1990;20(5):365–6. PubMed PMID: 2349021. Epub 1990/01/01. eng.
74. Carrera GF, Kozin F, Flaherty L, McCarty DJ. Radiographic changes in the hands following childhood frostbite injury. Skeletal Radiol. 1981;6(1):33–7. PubMed PMID: 7466414. Epub 1981/01/01. eng.
75. Mehta RC, Wilson MA. Frostbite injury: prediction of tissue viability with triple-phase bone scanning. Radiology. 1989;170(2):511–4. PubMed PMID: 2911677. Epub 1989/02/01. eng.
76. Selke Jr AC. Destruction of phalangeal epiphyses by frostbite. Radiology. 1969;93(4):859–60. PubMed PMID: 5824241. Epub 1969/10/01. eng.
77. Vinson HA, Schatzki R. Roentgenologic bone changes encountered in frostbite, Korea 1950–51. Radiology. 1954;63(5):685–95. PubMed PMID: 13215798. Epub 1954/11/01. eng.

The Pelvis and Hip: Congenital and Developmental Conditions

11

Leslie E. Grissom

Contents

L.E. Grissom, MD
Department of Medical Imaging, Nemours/AI duPont Hospital for Children, 1600 Rockland Road, Wilmington, DE 19803, USA

Departments of Radiology and Pediatrics, Thomas Jefferson University, Philadelphia, PA, USA
e-mail: lgrissom@nemours.org

Abstract

The chapter begins with a section on the normal development of the pelvis, acetabulum, and femoral neck, head, and epiphysis. Discussion of congenital and developmental abnormalities follows. Proximal focal femoral deficiency is described first. This is followed by a discussion of both intrauterine hip dislocation and a lengthy discussion of developmental dysplasia of the hip (DDH). Within this section, many different imaging techniques are broken down, the treatment of DDH by osteotomies is discussed, and postoperative complications as well as differential diagnosis are explained. Sections on coxa vara and acetabular protrusion follow. Femoral head dysplasia is broken down into both localized and generalized disorders: microepiphyseal dysplasia, Meyer dysplasia, osteochondritis dissecans-like femoral head dysplasia, multiple epiphyseal dysplasia, and epiphyseal dysgenesis in hypothyroidism.

R. Stein-Wexler et al. (eds.), *Pediatric Orthopedic Imaging*,
DOI 10.1007/978-3-642-45381-6_11, © Springer-Verlag Berlin Heidelberg 2015

1 Normal Development and Variant Ossification

Knowledge of normal development and its variants is essential to accurate diagnosis in pediatrics. Understanding the embryology of the hips and pelvis helps us interpret congenital abnormalities. In the growing child, variations in outline, symmetry, time of appearance, and ossification pattern are common in the pelvis and hip. Many normal variants can simulate disease, and some normal variants can be symptomatic, so it is important to be able to recognize and differentiate these entities. The more common variants are discussed below, after a brief review of relevant embryology.

The femoral head, neck, greater trochanter, and acetabulum form by 11 fetal weeks as one solid mesenchymal and cartilaginous block. A fissure in this block becomes the future joint line. Perfect congruence results and any incongruity present at or beyond birth must be secondary to abnormal development. At 4 fetal months, the femur is ossified up to the lesser trochanter. The primary ossification centers in the ilium, ischium, and pubis are seen by 2, 3, and 4 fetal months, respectively. By 5 months, the hip joint and its supporting ligamentous, capsular, and muscular structures are all completely developed. Orientation of the femoral head during the fetal period ranges from 30° of retroversion to 40° of anteversion; however, by birth, it averages 35° of anteversion.

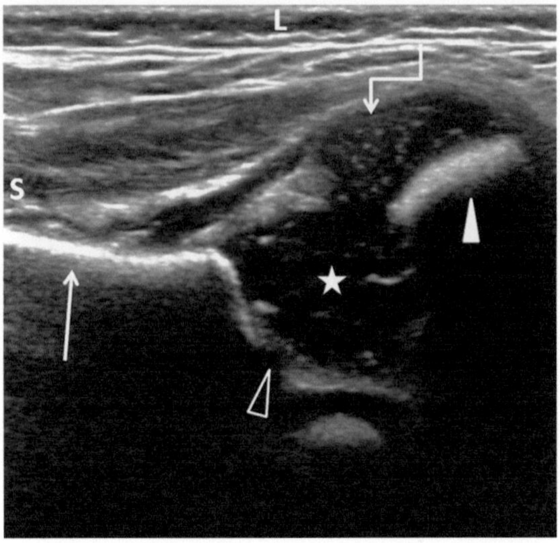

Fig. 11.1 Cartilage between the femoral head and greater trochanter is continuous in this 3-months-old, as they develop from one block of cartilage (coronal US). Ilium (*arrow*), triradiate cartilage (*open arrowhead*), femoral head (*asterisk*), greater tuberosity (*crooked arrow*), and metaphysis (*white arrowhead*). Note the specular foci of echogenicity in the femoral head and greater tuberosity, due to blood vessels viewed in cross section. *S* superior, *L* lateral

1.1 Proximal Femur

The neonatal proximal femur is one continuous block of cartilage from which both the femoral head and greater trochanteric epiphyses develop (Fig. 11.1) [1, 2]. The lower edge of the cartilage mass is the functional growth plate, producing linear elongation of the proximal femur. Although this growth plate is an anatomically continuous line across the entire femur, the growth rate varies in different sections [3]. Differential growth (the central segment grows faster than the medial, and lateral growth under the future greater trochanter is slowest) elongates the diminutive neonatal femoral neck. This process also changes the orientation of the relatively horizontal neonatal growth plate: the segments under the femoral head and greater trochanter separate and angulate toward each other. The rapid growth of the central plate brings this segment from its neonatal extracapsular location into an intra-capsular position.

The medial and lateral femoral circumflex branches of the common or deep femoral arteries supply the developing femoral head and neck; the femoral ligament artery is a branch of the obturator artery but is inconstant. The pattern of vascular supply to the head is thought to change during the first 3 years of age such that a few discrete branches of the medial circumflex artery supply the epiphysis, and the lateral circumflex artery supplies the greater trochanter region. The femoral and gluteal veins drain the femoral head and neck [4].

At birth, the ossific pattern of the femoral neck is a meshwork of uniformly distributed fine trabeculae. The adult pattern develops slowly; in one half of children between 12 and 18 months, the principal medial and lateral arching pattern is faintly evident [5]. These linear condensations are well developed by age 5; trabeculae aligned with the medial pattern are eventually seen as extensions on the epiphyseal side of the growth plate adjacent to the ossification center. By adolescence, short secondary medial and lateral arches develop inferior to the major lines of force. These trabeculae, with a large surface area-to-volume ratio, are more sensitive than cortical bone to systemic (endocrine, genetic, metabolic, nutritional, toxic) or local (trauma, infection) factors [6].

Both the timing and the symmetry of ossification of the femoral head vary. As with many structures, the proximal femoral epiphysis ossifies earlier in girls (2–6 months versus 3–7 months in boys). Ossification is seen in the femoral head in one half of all infants by 4 months and in more than 90 % by 7 months (200 days) [7]. With so broad a normal range, great variability is possible, and one must be cautious about labeling absent or decreased ossification as pathologic.

During infancy, the ossific center usually mineralizes and grows uniformly. However, it may appear crenulated, stippled, or granular, and multiple separate centers may be seen. These typically become homogeneous by mid-childhood, but occasionally a granular appearance or even a vertical cleft may persist. The medial portion of the epiphysis may appear relatively dense due to the superimposed lower acetabular wall.

Discrete notches at the vertex are common; these represent ossific defects only, since the contour of the epiphyseal cartilage over the notch is smooth [8]. This defect should not be confused with the fovea centralis at the insertion of the ligamentum teres, located in the medial aspect of the epiphysis, just above the femoral head equator (Fig. 11.2).

Multiple ossification centers are infrequently seen at the greater trochanter (Fig. 11.3). The absence of symptoms distinguishes these normal variants from bursitis with calcific fragments or a “tug” lesion.

1.2 Pelvis

Variations in contour and symmetry are frequent in the pelvis, as they are elsewhere. Numerous apophyses contribute to formation of the pelvis,

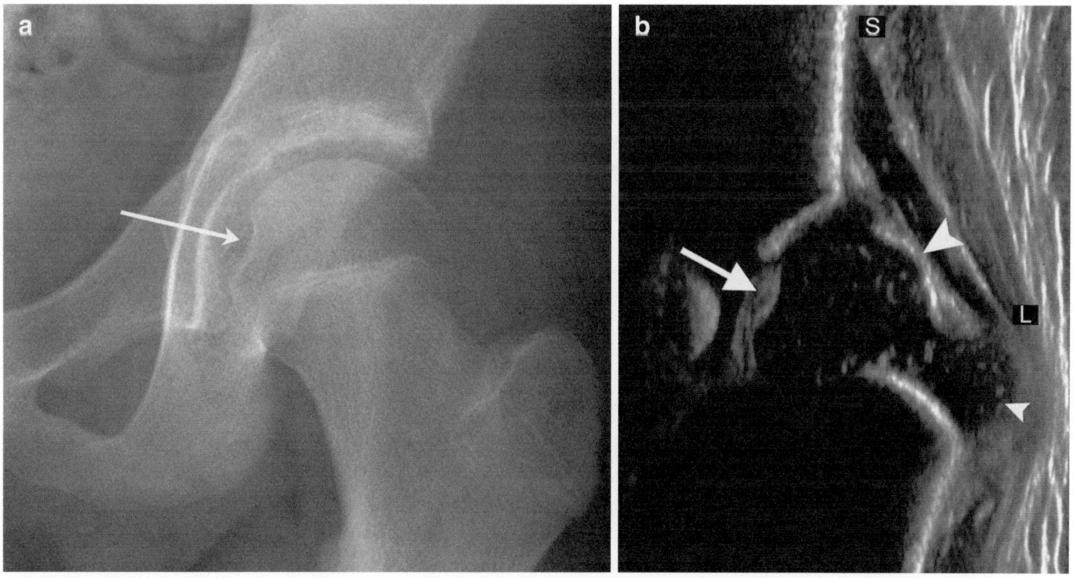

Fig. 11.2 Normal fovea (*arrow*) on (**a**) radiograph and (**b**) coronal neutral US. *S* superior, *L* lateral. The *small arrowhead* indicates the greater tuberosity, and the large arrowhead indicates the femoral head

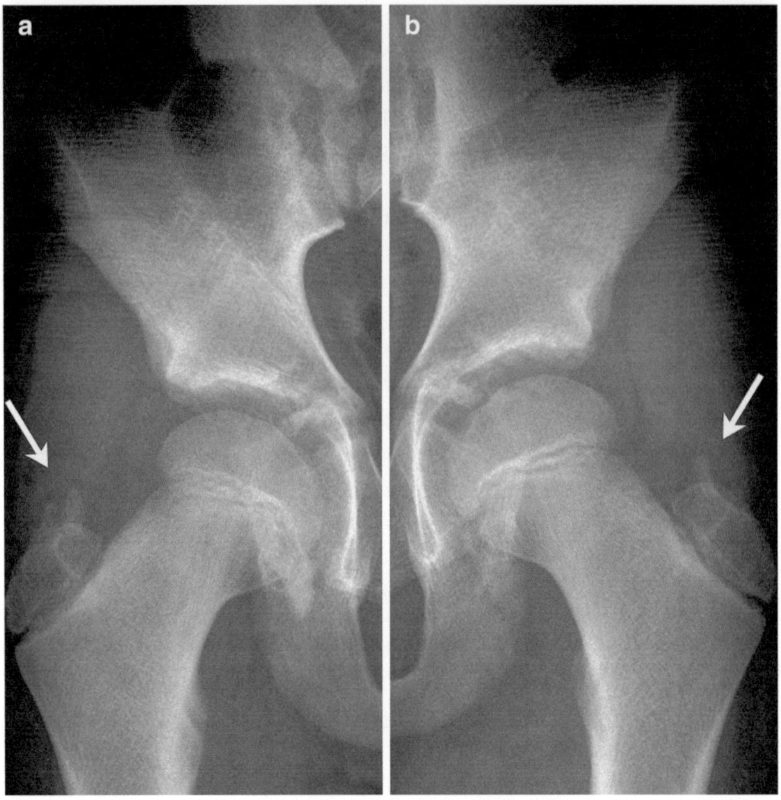

Fig. 11.3 (**a**, **b**) Normal irregular ossification centers (*arrows*) of greater trochanters in an asymptomatic 10-year-old boy

and the timing of their appearance and fusion varies, as does their appearance during ossification. Some can be confused with avulsion fractures and even with tumors. The more common radiographic features are discussed below.

A secondary ossification center forms in the anterior superior iliac spine at age 13–15, fusing to the ilium by age 16–18. It is usually seen well only in slightly oblique projections. Although avulsion of this center may occur during vigorous activity, it may normally be separated from the body of the ilium by a substantial layer of cartilage. As at other apophyses, the diagnosis of traumatic separation should be made only if there is adequate clinical correlation. Ossification centers are also present at the iliac crest and at the anterior inferior iliac spine.

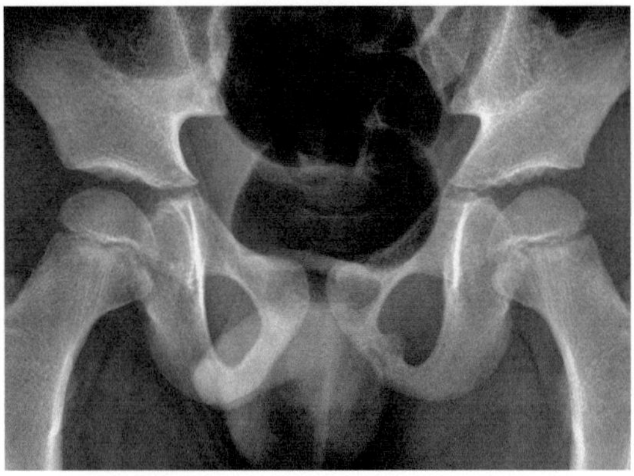

Fig. 11.4 Normal asymmetric closure of the ischiopubic synchondrosis in a 7-year-old boy. The *right* has closed, but the *left* is bubbly and expanded

The timing of closure of the ischiopubic synchondrosis is extremely variable, closing as early as 3 years of age, but incomplete in 18 % of children at age 12. The lucent cartilaginous component often enlarges before closure and may appear swollen or bubbly for up to 3 years (Fig. 11.4). Occasionally, there is cyclic swelling, bone union, reopening, swelling, and repeat closure, sometimes associated with pain. Unilateral synchondrosis expansion can be found in 57 % of

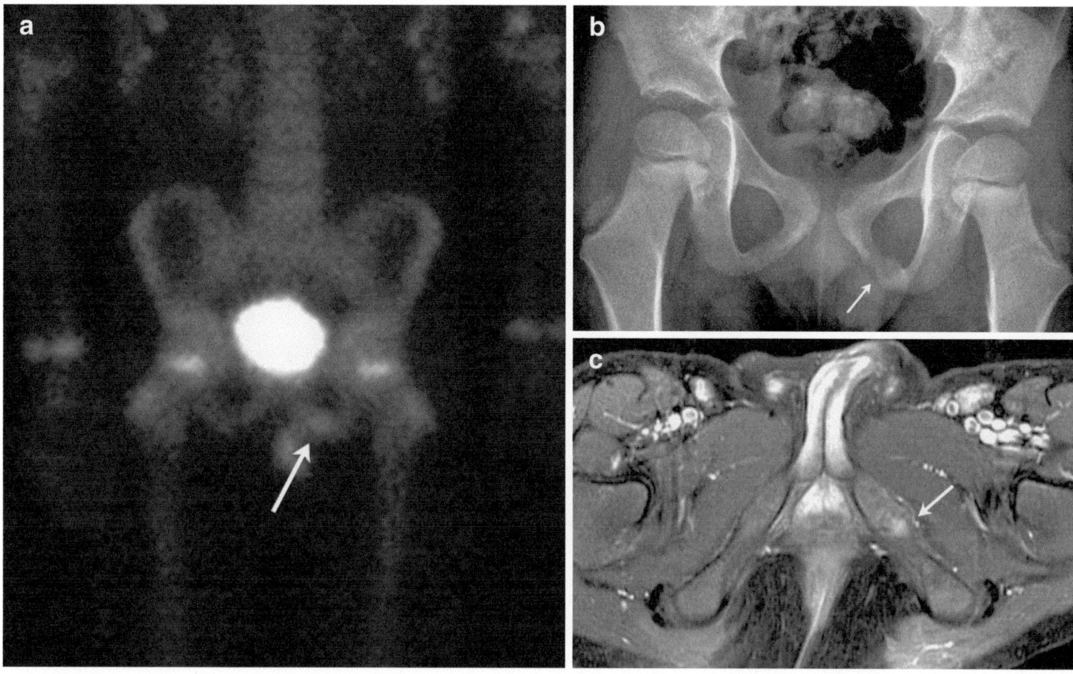

Fig. 11.5 Normal asymmetry in the ischiopubic synchondrosis in a 5-year-old boy with an adrenal tumor. (**a**) Asymmetric increased uptake at the left ischiopubic synchondrosis (*arrow*) is less intense than at the physeal cartilage. (**b**) Expansion, sclerosis, and lucency (*arrow*) on the left. (**c**) T1-weighted (T1-W) fat-suppressed (FS) gadolinium-enhanced (GE) MRI shows mildly increased signal intensity (*arrow*) but no mass

children at age 7 [9]. In almost one half of patients, scintigraphy reveals bilateral but unequal uptake in this area. This asymmetry is well defined, does not extend into adjacent bone, and is never more active than that adjacent to the triradiate cartilage (Fig. 11.5). Magnetic resonance imaging (MRI) can be misleading, as increased asymmetric signal makes distinguishing between normal variation and pathology difficult [10]. Clinical correlation is extremely important, as young athletes often experience muscle strain in this region, and this may not necessarily correlate with radiographic asymmetry (see Chap. 12).

The appearance of the pubic bones varies. The pubic symphysis is not always perfectly symmetric, and variant ossification centers infrequently develop in this area (Fig. 11.6). Vertical clefts and multiple centers of ossification are occasionally noted in the superior pubis at birth [11, 12]. During adolescence, accessory ossification centers may be seen in or just below the pubic symphysis. Irregularity of the lateral borders of the ischium may be quite striking in mid-childhood just before secondary ossification centers appear.

The os acetabuli is a well-demarcated ossicle just below the anterior-inferior iliac spine, at the most lateral margin of the acetabular cartilage rim. Uncommonly seen, this structure ossifies as a discrete triangular body between the ages of 11 and 20 (Fig. 11.7). Usually fusing to the acetabular margin by age 30, it may remain unfused through adulthood, when it is sometimes mistaken for an avulsion fracture. A similar ossification center may be present at the roof of the acetabulum.

Variant ossification at the acetabulum can cause confusion. A well-defined but wavy outline of the superior posterior acetabular margin is common. Sharp beaking of the medial intrapelvic portion of the acetabular triradiate synchondrosis is often prominent between ages 10 and 12 (Fig. 11.8). This is associated with inward bulging of the medial acetabular wall, producing a

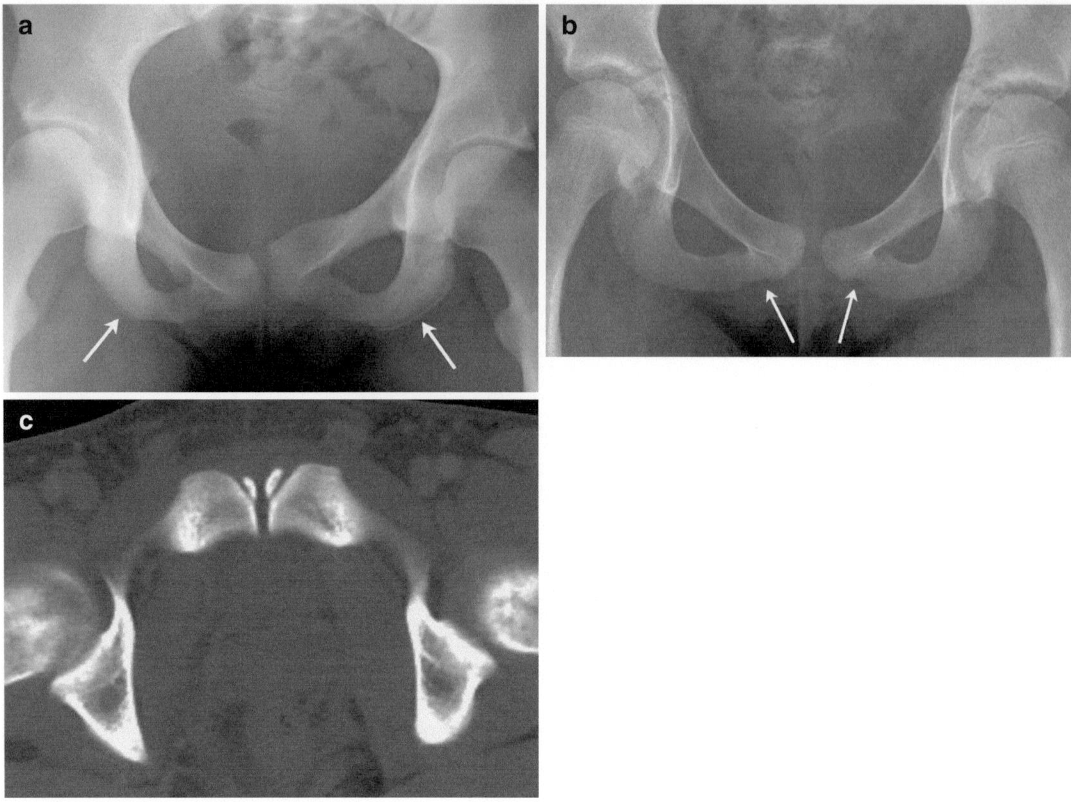

Fig. 11.6 Normal variation of the pubic bones. (**a**) Asymmetric ischial ossification centers (*arrows*), along with asymmetric pubic bones and symphysis. (**b**) Undulating margins of the inferior pubic rami (*arrows*) (there was no history of trauma). (**c**) Normal ossification centers adjacent to the symphysis in a 17-year-old boy (axial CT)

transitory relative acetabular protrusion that disappears by the end of puberty. Although rarely apparent on radiographs, multiple bone fragments are apparent on computed tomography (CT) in and around the triradiate cartilage in the adolescent prior to growth plate closure (Fig. 11.9).

2 Proximal Focal Femoral Deficiency (PFFD)

PFFD is a rare, nonhereditary defect of the femur, defined by defective development of the proximal femur and iliofemoral articulation, limb malrotation, and leg length discrepancy. The lower extremity typically appears short and thick, held in abduction, flexion, and external rotation [13]. It ranges in severity from mild dysgenesis of the proximal femur (Fig. 11.10) to almost complete absence of the femur, with only a small distal stub (Fig. 11.11). The defect is usually isolated and unilateral, although it may be a component of the caudal regression syndrome in infants of diabetic mothers. Incidence is about 1 in 52,000 births [13]. Total femoral agenesis, phocomelia, simple leg-length discrepancy without a proximal focal abnormality, and congenital femoral neck varus without shortening are not included in the definition of PFFD.

Associated anomalies of the distal bones and musculoligamentous structures as well as secondary effects on articulating structures at the hip and knee are common. Tibial and especially fibular hypoplasia can occur. Femoral shortening averages 60 %; tibial and fibular length discrepancies average 7 % and 28 %, respectively.

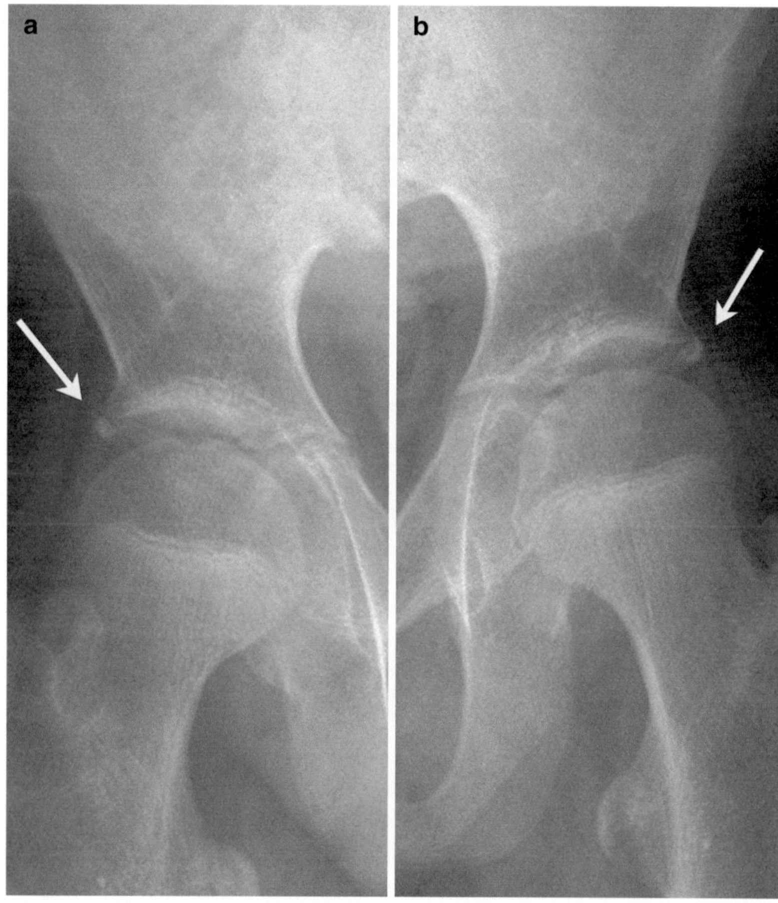

Fig. 11.7 (**a**, **b**) Bilateral os acetabuli (*arrows*) in a 14-year-old boy

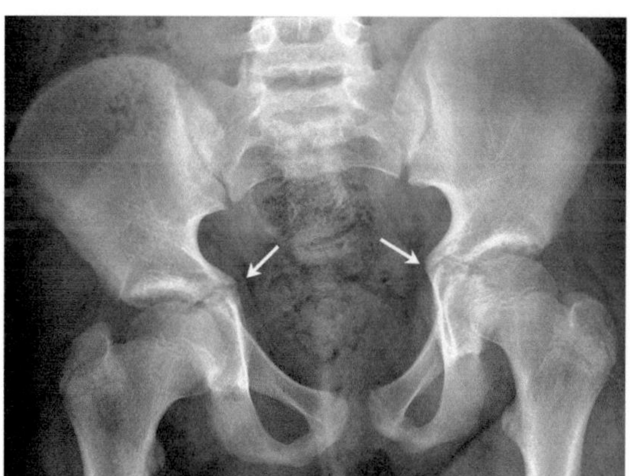

Fig. 11.8 Normal bilateral beaking and medial protrusion of the triradiate cartilage (*arrows*) in an 11-year-old boy

Accurate prediction of ultimate discrepancy is possible due to the linear nature of growth impairment [14] (see Chap. 2).

Treatment aims to maximize function and stability and varies depending on the severity of the defect. For milder PFFD, treatment may consist solely of femoral lengthening. In more severe forms, amputation and prostheses may be required (Fig. 11.12). Van Ness rotationplasty—fusion of the distal tibia to the short femur with 180° rotation of the tibia—is used to gain flexion at the rotated ankle joint and prepare a stump for prosthesis, essentially transforming the ankle into a knee [15].

Imaging

While PFFD may be difficult to classify at an early stage, doing so improves prognosis by helping to direct appropriate therapy. Of the many classification systems available, the Aitken and the Amstutz [16] are often employed. The Aitken system (Fig. 11.13) (Table 11.1) divides PFFD

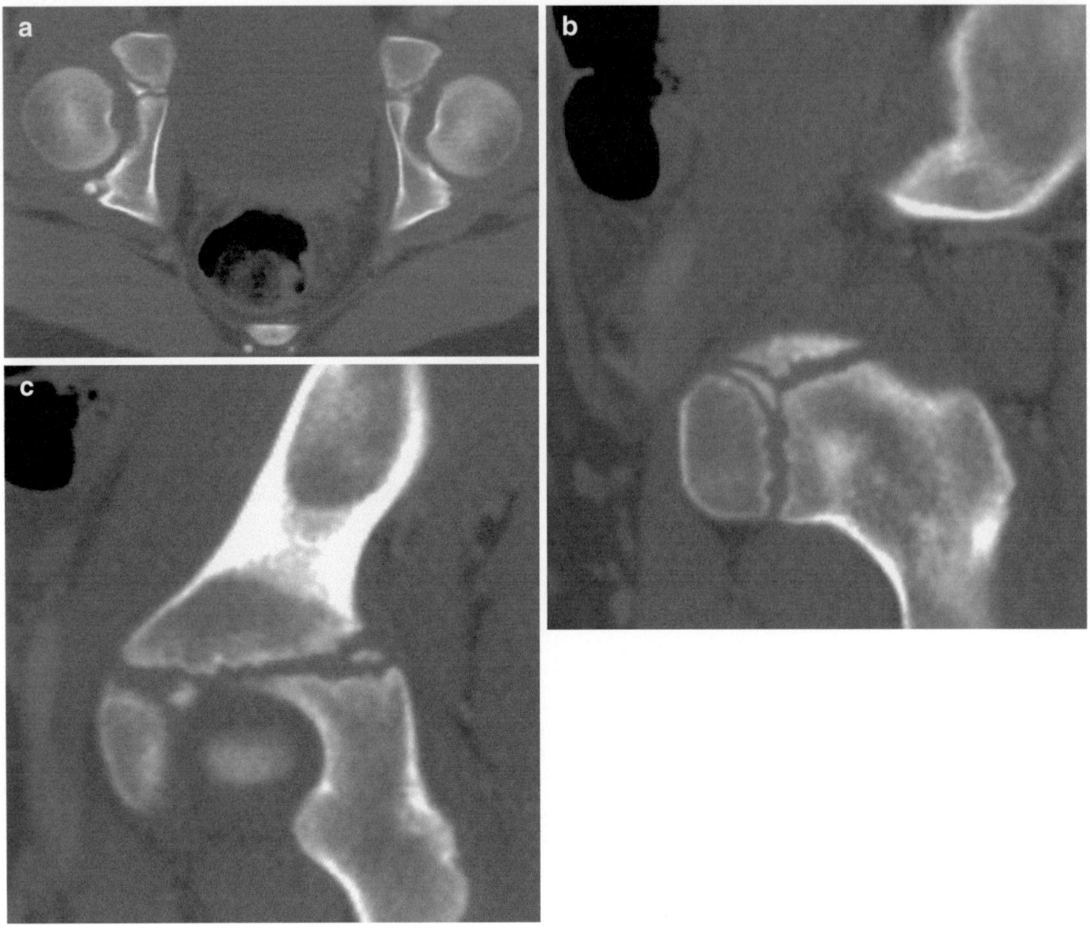

Fig. 11.9 Multiple normal ossification centers in the triradiate cartilage in a 10-year-old girl. Axial (**a**) and sagittal reformatted (**b**, **c**) CTs

into four classes [17]. In class A, the femoral head is well formed and attached to a short but otherwise well-formed femur; the acetabulum is normal. A bony connection eventually forms between the proximal femur and the shaft, but often with a pseudarthrosis. In class B, the femoral head is also present, but there is no bony connection between it and the femoral shaft at maturity; there may be no cartilaginous connection either. The acetabulum is either adequate or moderately dysplastic. Class C is defined by complete absence of ossification of a femoral head. A short femur tapers proximally and has a small proximal tuft. The acetabulum is severely dysplastic. Both the femoral head and the acetabulum are absent in class D, and the femoral segment is even shorter and more deformed, often pointed proximally. The Amstutz system further divides Aitken A into types 1 and 2, based on characteristics of the femoral neck (cartilaginous in type 1; pseudarthrosis in type 2); Aitken B through D are termed Amstutz 3–5. These systems predict femoral head development and its relation to the acetabulum and femoral neck. However, prediction of the final relationships is not always possible. More complex systems are also available (Fig. 11.14).

Ultrasound (US) offers a relatively simple initial evaluation of femoral head and acetabular development prior to ossification (Fig. 11.15) [19]. However, severe coxa vara can limit the sonographic window. MRI (Fig. 11.16) provides

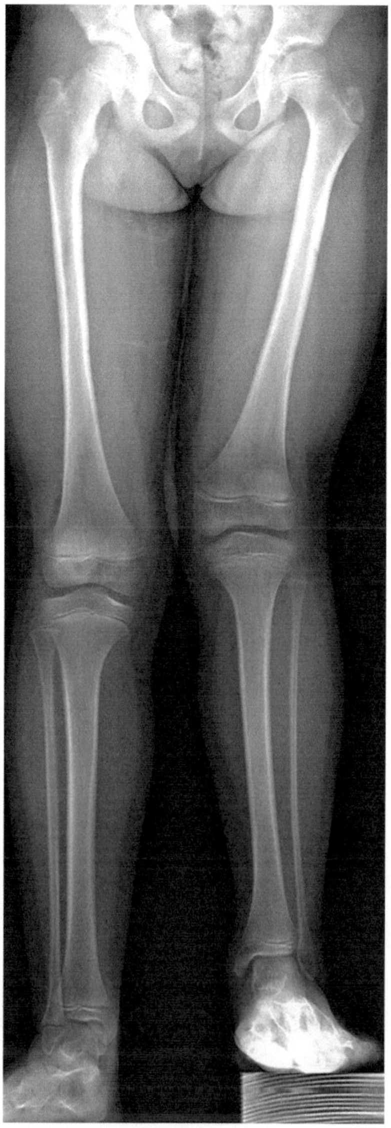

Fig. 11.10 Very mild PFFD. The left femur is short, but the acetabulum and femoral head/neck are well formed. The left fibula is mildly hypoplastic but the tibia essentially normal. This is Pappas Class IX, which is essentially a congenitally short femur. The Aitken system does not classify this appearance

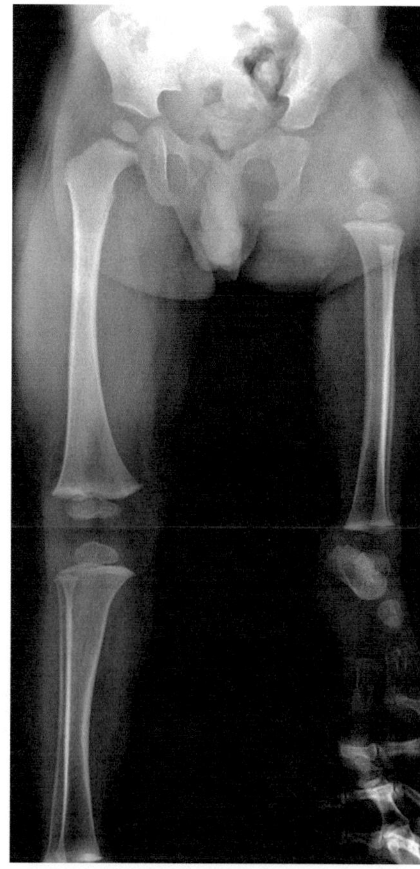

Fig. 11.11 Aitken Class D PFFD (Pappas Class 2). The femoral fragment is very small, and there is no ossified femoral head. The acetabulum has not formed. Note the thick soft tissues about the hip. The fibula is hypoplastic

more detailed evaluation of non-ossified structures, and this can help the orthopedic surgeon determine treatment. It can determine whether a cartilaginous femoral head is present and characterize growth plate abnormalities. It also evaluates acetabular contour and the presence of an osseous, cartilaginous, or fibrous connection between the proximal and distal femur. It characterizes ligaments and muscles and if extended to include the knee, can identify the accompanying ligamentous abnormalities that are common there. All this information assists in determining surgical treatment [13, 20]. Intraoperative arthrography may also be used to assess hip mobility and guide treatment.

Differential Diagnosis

Congenital short femur is the mildest form of PFFD (see Chap. 13). The proximal femur in developmental coxa vara appears similar to the milder forms of PFFD but lacks bone shortening. Dysplasias with proximal shortening as well as those with delayed proximal femoral ossification are in the differential.

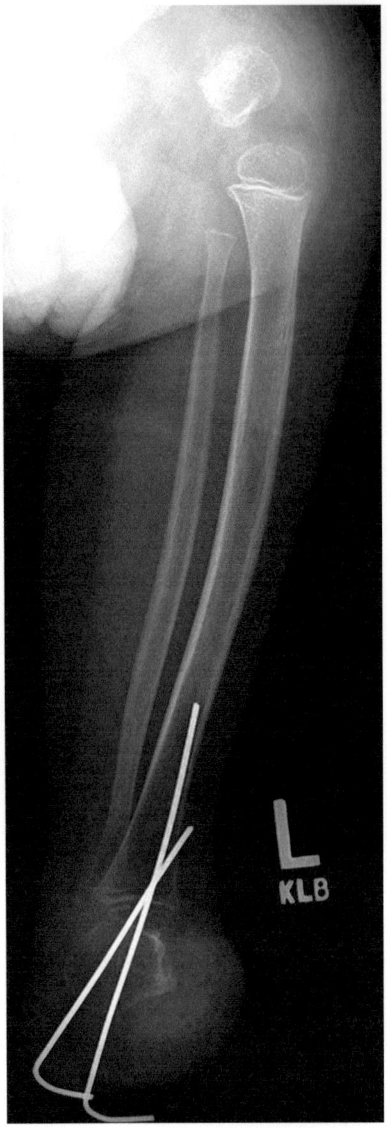

Fig. 11.12 PFFD treated with partial amputation of the foot and fusion of the ankle joint (same patient as Fig. 11.11)

3 Intrauterine Hip Dislocation

When associated with other congenital abnormalities, prenatal hip dislocation is considered teratologic, with multiple anomalies resulting from a common insult. Children born with hip dislocation along with, for example, arthrogryposis (Fig. 11.17) or cranio-carpal-tarsal dysplasia have primary teratologic dislocations. However, use of this term should be restricted to these complex situations, as simple prenatal dislocations can also occur. In either case, by the time of birth, prenatal dislocations are often firmly fixed by articular adhesions and secondary adaptive musculoligamentous changes and thus are difficult to reduce. Avascular necrosis (AVN) is a frequent treatment complication [21]. In general, intrauterine hip dislocation is unlikely to resolve completely without complications.

Prenatal dislocation can also result from paralytic states, such as myelomeningocele and other neuromuscular disorders. Many of these cases represent intrauterine postural deformity rather than true malformations. Flexion contracture of the knees and severe rigid varus and valgus deformity of the hindfoot may be present as well. This condition is associated with multiple gestations, breech presentation, and oligohydramnios.

4 Developmental Dysplasia of the Hip (DDH) (Box 11.1)

Box 11.1: Developmental Dysplasia of the Hip

Exam maneuvers	
Barlow: detects displacement by pistoning flexed hip	
Ortolani: attempts to reduce dislocated hip by flexion and abduction	
Ultrasound	
Dynamic examination	
Coronal	Acetabular depth
	Labral configuration
	Femoral head position
Transverse	Position of femoral head (resting and stressed)
Static examination	
Alpha angle	>/= 60° normal
Beta angle	</= 55° normal

This relatively common condition arises during the perinatal period and refers to the musculoligamentous, capsular, cartilaginous, and osseous changes that result from subluxation or dislocation

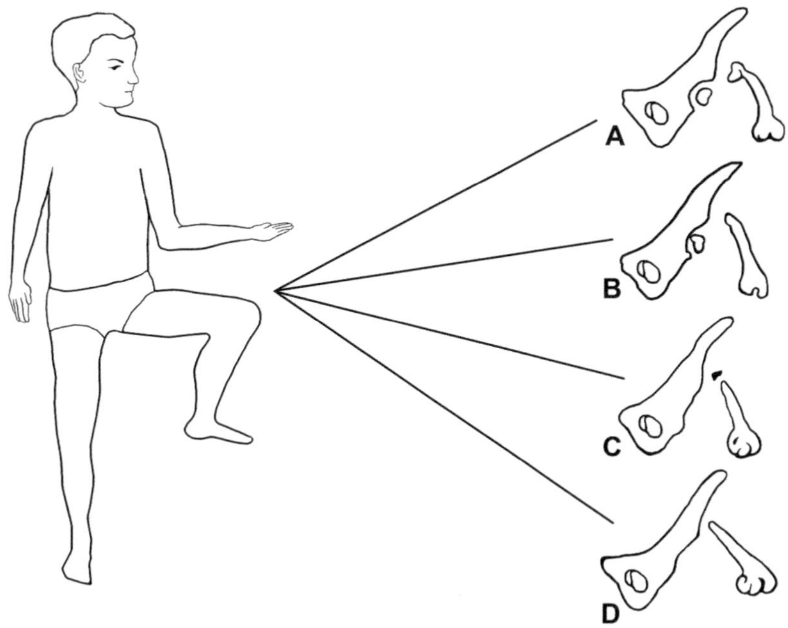

Fig. 11.13 The four categories of the Aitken PFFD classification system

Table 11.1 Aitken classification of proximal femoral focal deficiency (Fig. 11.13)

Class	Femoral head	Acetabulum	Femoral segment	Relationship among components of femur and acetabulum at skeletal maturity
A	Present	Normal	Short	Bony connection between components of femur Femoral head in acetabulum Subtrochanteric varus, often with pseudarthrosis
B	Present	Adequate or moderately dysplastic	Short, usually proximal bony tuft	No osseous connection between head and shaft Femoral head in acetabulum
C	Absent or represented by ossicle	Severely dysplastic	Short, usually proximally tapered	Possible osseous connection between shaft and proximal ossicle No articular relation between femur and acetabulum
D	Absent	Absent Obturator foramen enlarged Pelvis squared in bilateral cases	Short, deformed	None

Adapted from Aitken [17]

of the femoral head. Although most dislocations occur during the perinatal period, dislocations do occur up to 1 year of age, often in patients documented to be normal before this time. Initial dislocation in later childhood is rare and generally results from abnormal muscular forces, trauma, or effusion.

In newborns, some degree of instability occurs in approximately 55 per 1,000 births, but most cases resolve within the first month without treatment, and the incidence of instability after that time is closer to 5 per 1,000 births [22]. The etiology and pathogenesis of infantile hip instability and displacement are subject to debate, but the

a **Congenital Abnormalities of the Femur**

	Class I	Class II	Class III	Class IV
	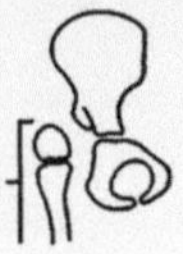	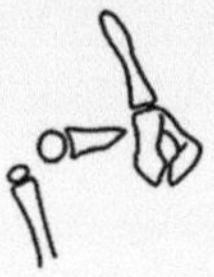	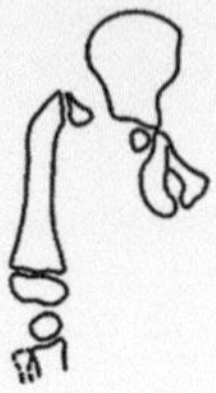	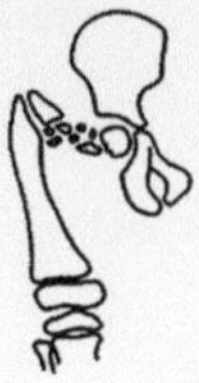
Femoral shortening		70 - 90%	45 - 80%	40 - 67%
Femoral pelvic abnormalities	Femur absent Ischiopubic bone structures underdeveloped and deficient Lack of acetabular development	Femur head absent Ischiopubic bone structures delayed in ossification	No osseous connection between femoral shaft and head Femoral head ossification delayed Acetabulum may be absent Femoral condyles maldeveloped Infrequent irregular tuft on proximal end of femur	Femoral head and shaft joined by irregular calcification in a fibrocartilaginous matrix
Associated abnormalities	Fibula absent	Tibia shortened Fibula, foot, knee joint, and ankle-joint abnormal	Tibia shortened 0-40% Fibula shortened 5-100% Patela absent or small and high riding Knee joint instability frequent Foot malformed	Tibia shortened 0-20% Fibula shortened 4-60% Knee joint instability frequent Foot small with infrequent malformations
Treatment objectives	Prosthetic management	Pelvic-femoral stability through prosthetic management	Union between femoral shaft and hip for hip stability Prosthetic management	Union between femoral head, neck, and shaft Prosthetic management

Fig. 11.14 (**a**, **b**) The nine categories of Pappas PFFD classification system (Adapted from Pappas [18])

b

Congenital Abnormalities of the Femur

	Class V	Class VI	Class VII	Class VIII	Class IX
	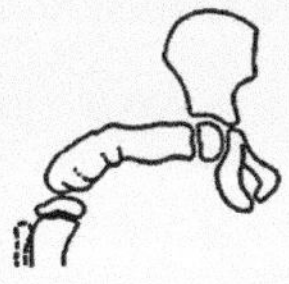	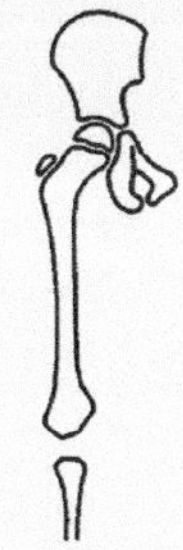	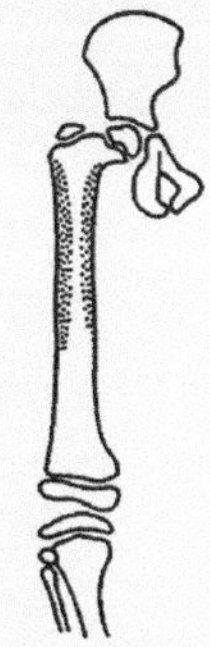	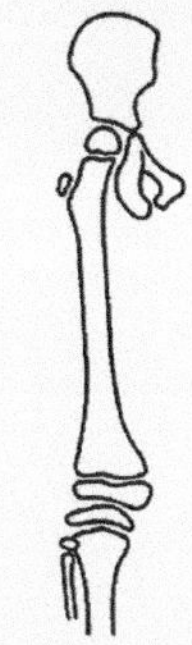	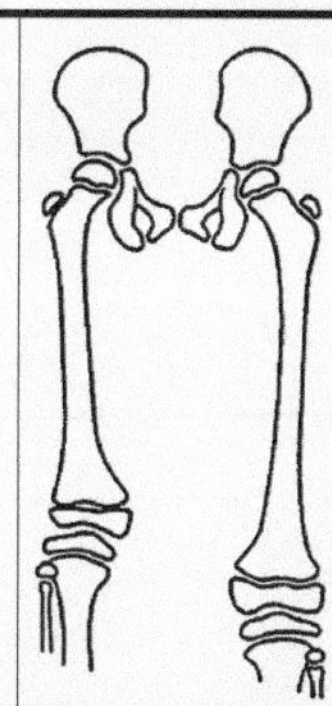
Femoral shortening	48 - 85%	30 - 60%	10 - 50%	10 - 41%	6 - 20%
Femoral pelvic abnormalities	Femur incompletely ossified, hypoplastic, and irregular Midshaft of femur abnormal	Distal femur short, irregular, and hypoplastic Irregular distal femoral diaphysis	Coxa vara Hypoplastic femur Proximal femoral diaphysis irregular with thickened cortex Lateral femoral condyle deficiency frequent Valgus distal femur	Coxa valga Hypoplastic femur Femoral head and neck smaller Proximal femoral physis horizontal Abnormality of femoral condyles frequent with associated bowing of shaft and valgus of distal femur	Hypoplastic femur
Associated abnormalities	Tibia shortened 4-27% Fibula shortened 10-100% Knee joint instability frequent Severe malformations of the foot frequent	Single bone lower leg Patella absent Foot malformed	Tibia shortened < 10-24% Fibula shortened < 10-100% Lateral and high riding patella frequent	Tibia shortened 0-36% Fibula shortened 0-100% Lateral and high riding patella frequent Foot malformed	Tibia shortened 0-15% Fibula shortened 3-30% Additional ipsilateral and contralateral malformations frequent
Treatment objectives	Prosthetic management	Prosthetic management	Extremity length equality Improved alignment of (a) proximal and (b) distal femur	Extremity length equality Improved alignment of (a) proximal and (b) distal femur	Extremity length equality

Fig. 11.14 (continued)

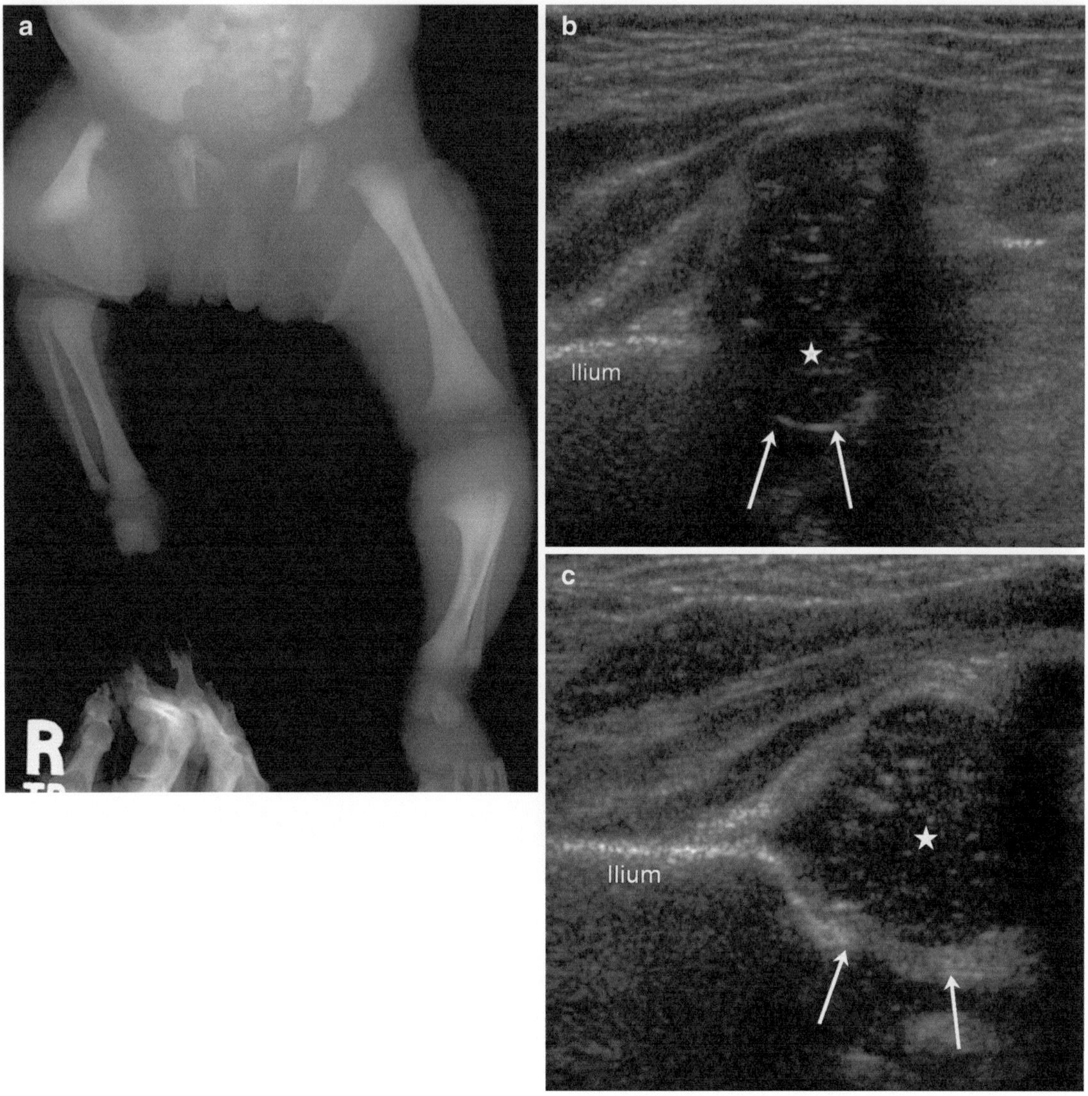

Fig. 11.15 Aitken Class A PFFD (Pappas Class 3) in an infant. (**a**) The right femur is short. Although the distal contour is fairly well formed, the proximal femur is hypoplastic, with a pointed upper end. Note coxa vara. The acetabulum is well formed, suggesting the presence of a femoral head. The tibia and fibula are small. (**b**) Coxa vara on coronal flexion US. The femoral head (*) is small but well positioned. The acetabulum (*arrows*) is small. Hypoechoic cartilage lateral to the femoral head indicates varus configuration of the femoral neck. (**c**) Normal contralateral hip with the same notations

origin of most dislocations seems to be multifactorial. Breech positioning and family history of joint laxity predispose to DDH, but many patients have none of these risk factors. Gender plays a role in this condition, which is four to eight times more common in female than in male infants.

Abnormal laxity is important in the development of femoral-acetabular incompetence. However, the degree of laxity that is considered abnormal is open to debate. In the first few days after birth, an ultrasound performed with stress can reveal as much as 6 mm of posterolateral displacement of the femoral head, but this usually resolves within a few weeks [23]. A hormonal contribution to ligamentous laxity has been suggested [24, 25].

The common intrauterine position of hip flexion plays an important role in maintaining proper

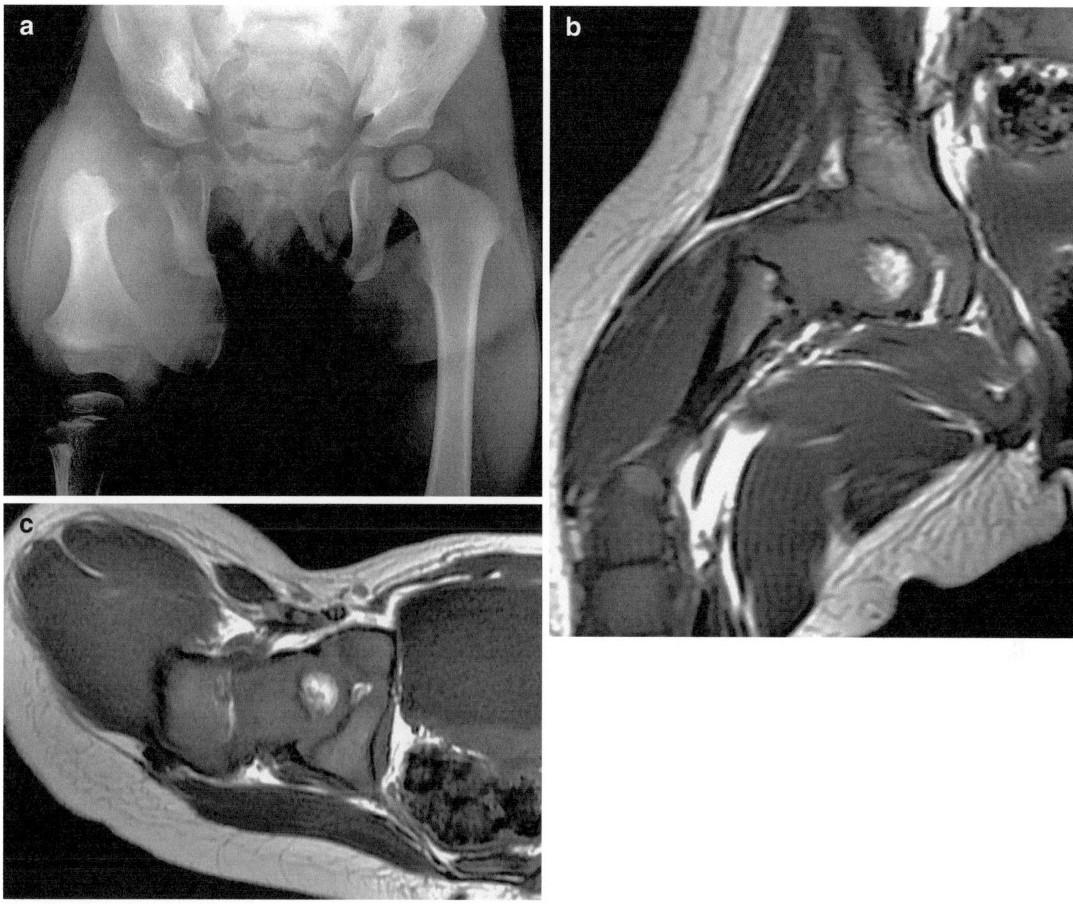

Fig. 11.16 Aitken Class B PFFD (Pappas Class 4). (**a**) Hypoplastic femur with ossification defect in femoral neck. T1-W coronal (**b**) and axial (**c**) MRIs show satisfactory positioning of femoral head and focal bone defect

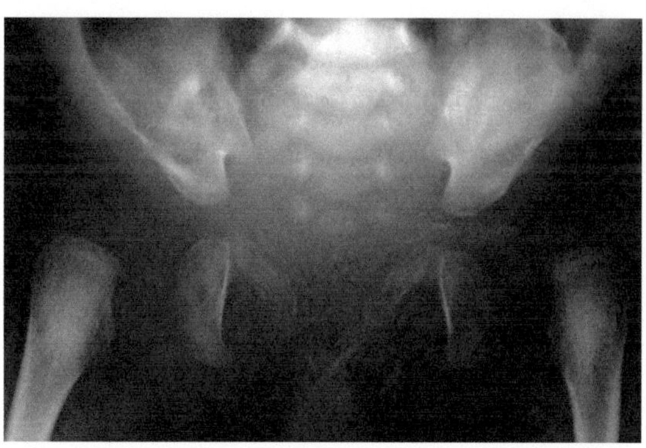

Fig. 11.17 Bilateral hip dislocation in a 1-month-old with arthrogryposis. Note steep obliquity of the exceedingly shallow acetabula. The left proximal femur is small

position of the femoral head, and this in turn allows normal acetabular development. The hyperflexion of breech positioning leads to shortening and contraction of the iliopsoas muscle, predisposing to hip dislocation. Infants that have developed in the breech position are six times more likely to have DDH. In addition, the position of the fetus relative to the uterus and of one leg to the other probably account for what some studies have found to be increased involvement of the left hip.

Almost two thirds of infants with hip instability are firstborn. The maternal uterus and abdominal wall in a first pregnancy likely confine the infant, preventing the full intrauterine motion that is needed for normal femoroacetabular development. Associated conditions such as congenital torticollis [26] and congenital foot deformities such as metatarsus adductus and calcaneovalgus [27, 28] are also attributed to this "packaging" problem.

Although many patients with DDH have no affected family members, genetic factors play a role in hip dislocation [29]. If a parent has DDH, the risk to the child is 12 %. The risk to a younger sibling of a child with DDH and normal parents is 6 %. If one parent and one child are affected, a second child's risk is 36 % [30]. In addition, DDH is more common in Caucasians than in those of African descent, and it is more common in Eastern Europe than in Africa and Asia. Infants who are swaddled with their legs in extension have increased risk of DDH; this is a common practice in certain populations, including some Native American cultures.

The significance of anatomic variation in the acetabulum or femoral neck is not settled, but the acetabulum tends to become shallower and the femoral head more hemispheric in late fetal life, perhaps promoting dislocation under appropriate conditions (e.g., breech positioning). The parents of children with DDH have been shown to have less acetabular coverage, suggesting that anatomic factors, possibly heritable, may be significant.

DDH is diagnosed by Barlow and Ortolani maneuvers, which are performed routinely on infants in the first few months of life. The Barlow maneuver pistons the flexed hip to detect displacement; the Ortolani maneuver assesses the dislocated hip with flexion and abduction to determine if it is reducible. Limited or asymmetric abduction of the hip is another sign of DDH and typically occurs after 2–3 months of age as the hip capsule tightens. Asymmetric thigh folds are neither sensitive nor specific for DDH. An audible clunk may occur as the hip dislocates or reduces, but clicks may be heard in normal hips. Leg-length discrepancy and limping are late signs.

When the clinical exam is abnormal or if there is a risk factor for DDH, US is performed to diagnose and determine the severity of the condition. The range of abnormalities found by US is extensive. The hip can be lax, mildly displaced with stress, dislocatable with stress, or dislocated at rest. In the latter case, the hip is positioned completely outside the acetabulum and may or may not be reducible. Laxity typically resolves within the first month. Subluxation may also resolve without treatment but must be monitored either clinically or by US. Dislocation is often treated at diagnosis with a flexion/abduction brace. Unsuccessful treatment usually necessitates intraoperative closed reduction and subsequent immobilization.

Clinical screening of all newborns by a skilled examiner has led to earlier diagnosis and better prognosis. Despite this, late diagnosis does occur in infants who were normal during the immediate postnatal period [31, 32]. It is possible that multiple examinations increase the instability of the hip [33]. In order to avoid late diagnosis, there has been considerable interest in sonographic screening. Some countries have instituted universal sonographic screening, whereas others only screen high-risk infants and those with a positive physical examination. The former approach is costly and some believe results in overdiagnosis and unnecessary treatment [34]. The more limited approach fails to diagnose DDH in infants who lack risk factors [35].

The American Academy of Pediatrics has recommended that all infants be screened by physical examination. If at any time there are positive physical findings (positive Ortolani or Barlow test), the patient should be referred to an orthopedist. If the physical examination is inconclusive, the infant should be reexamined in 2 weeks. If the examination is still inconclusive, orthopedic consult or US is recommended. Breech babies and female babies with a positive family history should have hip US at 6 weeks of age or a radiograph of the pelvis and hips at 4 months even if the physical exam is negative. Infants without risk factors or initial positive physical exam should be clinically monitored [36].

4.1 Imaging to Diagnose DDH

US of the hips has become the imaging standard in infants up to 6 months of age. The cartilage of the femoral head and acetabulum is readily depicted, whereas it cannot be seen on radiographs in young infants [37]. Hip US also benefits from real-time evaluation of hip motion.

The cartilaginous femoral head is recognized as a hypoechoic rounded structure with specular internal echoes that allow transmission of the sound wave to the acetabulum and the triradiate cartilage. Before it is visible radiographically, a small focus of echogenicity representing the nidus for the ossification center can be seen in most infants [38]. Like the femoral head, the hyaline cartilage of the acetabulum and the labrum is hypoechoic, whereas the fibrocartilaginous tip of the labrum is hyperechoic. The bony components of the acetabulum are brightly echogenic and prevent sound transmission. The joint space is clearly identified with movement of the femoral head and sometimes made more conspicuous by the presence of gas bubbles induced by examination maneuvers. The relationship of the femoral head to the acetabulum, the depth and configuration of the latter, and the position and morphology of the labrum are easily shown. Ultrasound can thus diagnose instability and cartilage abnormalities that are clinically and radiographically occult, and this has led to earlier diagnosis and treatment of DDH. Specular echogenic structures in the femoral head are caused by microvasculature. Doppler interrogation can demonstrate these vessels as curvilinear echogenic lines. However, this is primarily a research tool and not part of the routine exam [39, 40].

There are two popular methods of US examination, the dynamic and the Graf static technique. The dynamic technique [37, 38] emphasizes hip position and stability, with stress maneuvers that simulate Barlow and Ortolani maneuvers, whereas the static method is based on morphology as a reflection of hip position and stability [41]. Either method is suitable when used correctly. The American College of Radiology has established practice guidelines that recommend that both hips be examined in two orthogonal planes, including a coronal view at rest and a transverse view with and without stress [42].

Dynamic Hip Ultrasound

Standardized coronal and transverse images are obtained with hips in neutral and flexed positions. Scanning is performed over the lateral aspect of the hip joint with the patient supine or in shallow decubitus position, using a high-resolution linear transducer. The scan may be performed by a physician or technologist and with static images or stored clips. Experience is required to obtain diagnostic images. During treatment with an abduction brace such as a Pavlik harness, only coronal and transverse flexion views are performed. The harness should be removed and stress applied only at the request of the orthopedic surgeon. Ultrasound monitors improvement and helps guide adjustment of the device.

Coronal Views

The coronal views, performed with a neutral (Fig. 11.18) and with a flexed (Fig. 11.19) hip, show the femoral head and acetabulum as they appear on a frontal radiograph. Acetabular coverage of the femoral head should be 50 % or more. The normal osseous acetabulum should have a concave surface, and there should be a well-defined superolateral acetabular lip or margin. The labrum should resemble a sickle extending laterally over the femoral head with an echogenic tip at the outer margin.

Transverse Views

Performed posterolaterally in the axial plane, these are obtained according to the Harcke technique in both neutral (Fig. 11.20) and flexed (Fig. 11.21) positions. In the neutral position, the hypoechoic femoral head rests on the ischium posteriorly and on the pubic bone anteriorly, with the triradiate cartilage between these two echogenic structures. Aside from a thin layer of intervening hyaline cartilage, the femoral head should be positioned against these bones, with no intervening soft tissue. When flexed, the femoral head rests on the ischium with the triradiate cartilage and pubic bone seen medially and anteriorly, forming the acetabulum.

Similar to the Barlow maneuver, the Harcke technique uses pistoning and adduction stress in the flexion view to detect instability. With stress, the unstable hip migrates away from the acetabulum laterally and posteriorly to a variable degree. Echogenic soft tissue then fills the space between the acetabulum and the femoral head. In subluxation, the femoral head remains in partial contact with the acetabulum (Fig. 11.22), whereas in dislocation, it is entirely outside the acetabulum (Fig. 11.23). It is important to examine the abnormal hip at rest and then with stress in order to determine the severity of displacement. If the hip is abnormal, it should be

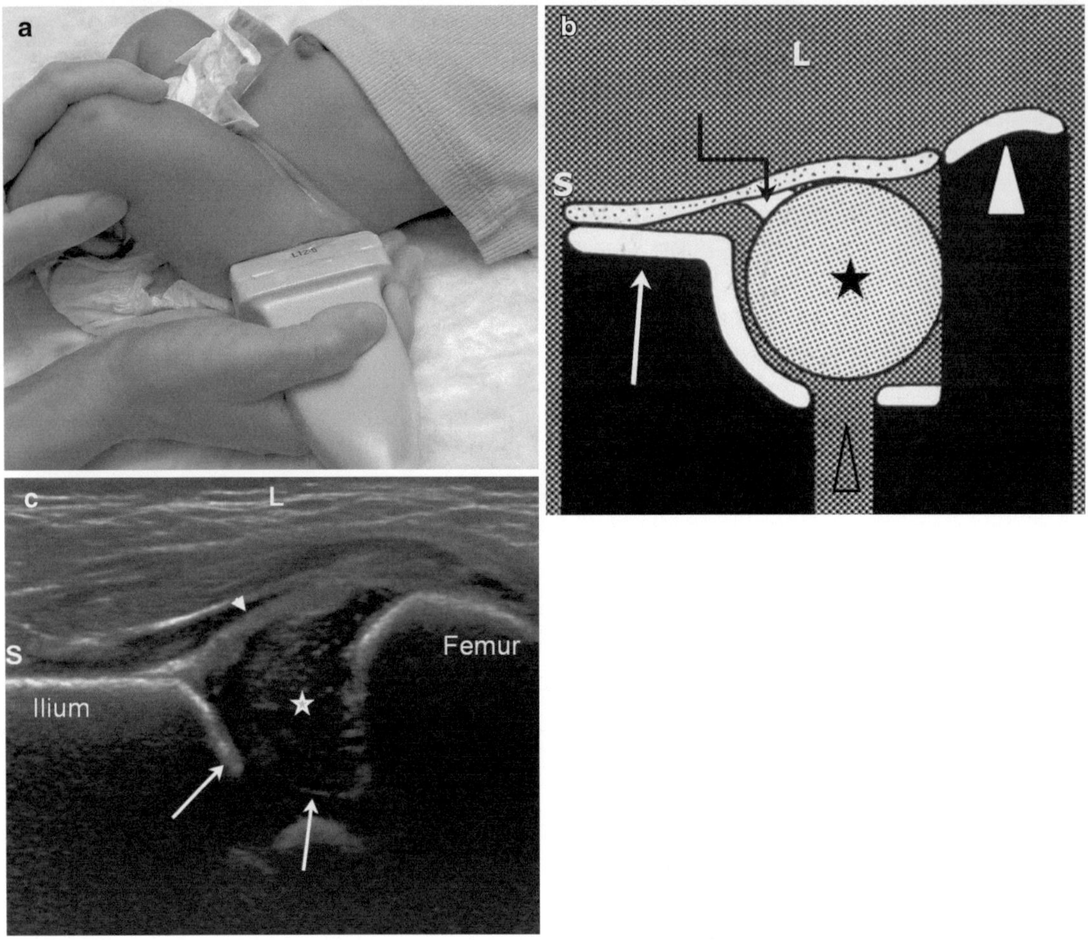

Fig. 11.18 Normal coronal neutral hip US. (**a**) The leg is in a physiologic neutral position (relaxed) with the transducer in the coronal plane. The Graf view is also obtained in this plane, but with the patient in the decubitus position and immobilized in a holder. (**b**) Diagram shows ilium (*arrow*), labrum (*crooked arrow*), femoral head (*asterisk*), triradiate cartilage (open *arrowhead*), and femoral shaft (*white arrowhead*). (**c**) Coronal neutral US shows the femoral head (*star*) positioned deep in the acetabulum (*arrows*) with no echoes between the femoral head and the medial acetabular wall. The iliac bone forms an echogenic structure superiorly, the femur, inferiorly. The labrum (*arrowhead*) curves over the femoral head. *S* superior, *L* lateral

flexed and abducted to determine reducibility. Mild displacement with or without stress is normal in the first 3–4 weeks of life, but after this period, such movement is considered abnormal (although laxity may persist for a few more weeks in breech babies).

The acetabular d/D measurement, obtained in the coronal plane, evaluates acetabular coverage; the appearance is comparable to a frontal radiograph (Fig. 11.24) (Table 11.2) [43, 44]. The d/D measurement also correlates with the Graf alpha angle [45].

Graf Static Hip Ultrasound

Coronal views are obtained with the patient in the decubitus position, typically in an immobilizing device. Landmarks that must be included are the straight lateral margin and inferior tip of the ilium, as well as the fibrocartilaginous tip of the labrum. The slope of the acetabulum, the alpha and beta angles, and the labral coverage are measured. The normal alpha angle is 60° or more, and the normal beta angle is less than 55° (Fig. 11.25) (Table 11.3). The Graf classification system primarily uses the alpha angle for prognosis and

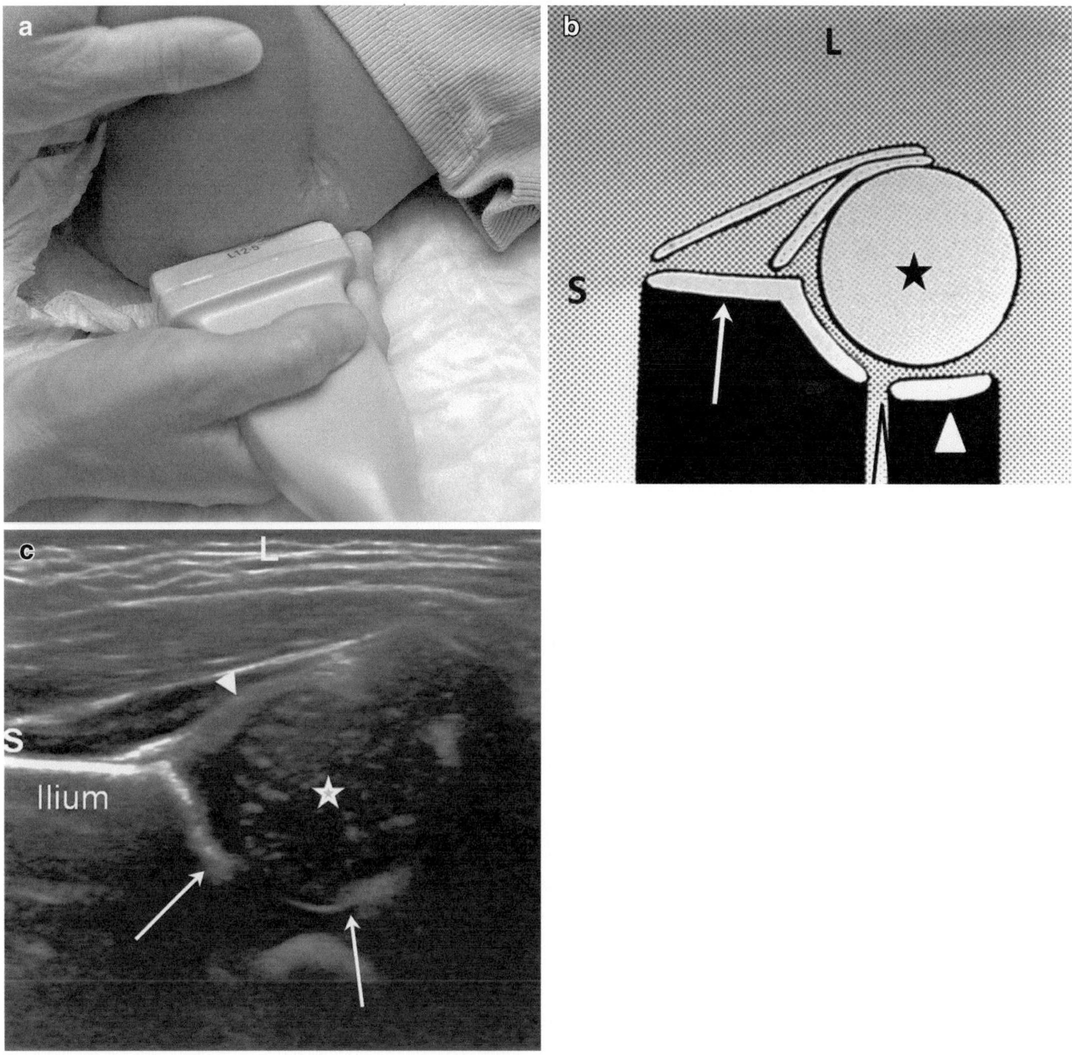

Fig. 11.19 Normal coronal flexion view. (**a**) The hip is flexed to approximately 90° with the transducer in the coronal plane. (**b**) Diagram shows the ilium (*arrow*), femoral head (*asterisk*), and ischium (*white arrowhead*). (**c**) The metaphysis and shaft are not visible. The femoral head (*star*) is well positioned within the acetabular fossa (*arrows*) without intervening echoes. *S* superior, *L* lateral

treatment. This method is employed extensively in Europe and in many centers in the United States as well.

Radiography

Although US plays a very important role in infancy, radiographs are useful after 6 months of age, when the ossification center of the femoral head has developed. However, secondary capsular, ligamentous, muscular, and cartilaginous changes, which occur soon after persistent instability or dislocation has been established, cannot be appreciated. Osseous changes happen relatively late, implying substantial cartilage loss and soft tissue deformation.

A frontal radiograph of the pelvis is preferred, with hips in neutral position. For accurate assessment of hip position and acetabular development, it is important that the legs are symmetrically positioned with the patellae facing forward or, if necessary, rotated symmetrically. The pelvis should not be tilted; this can be confirmed by checking that

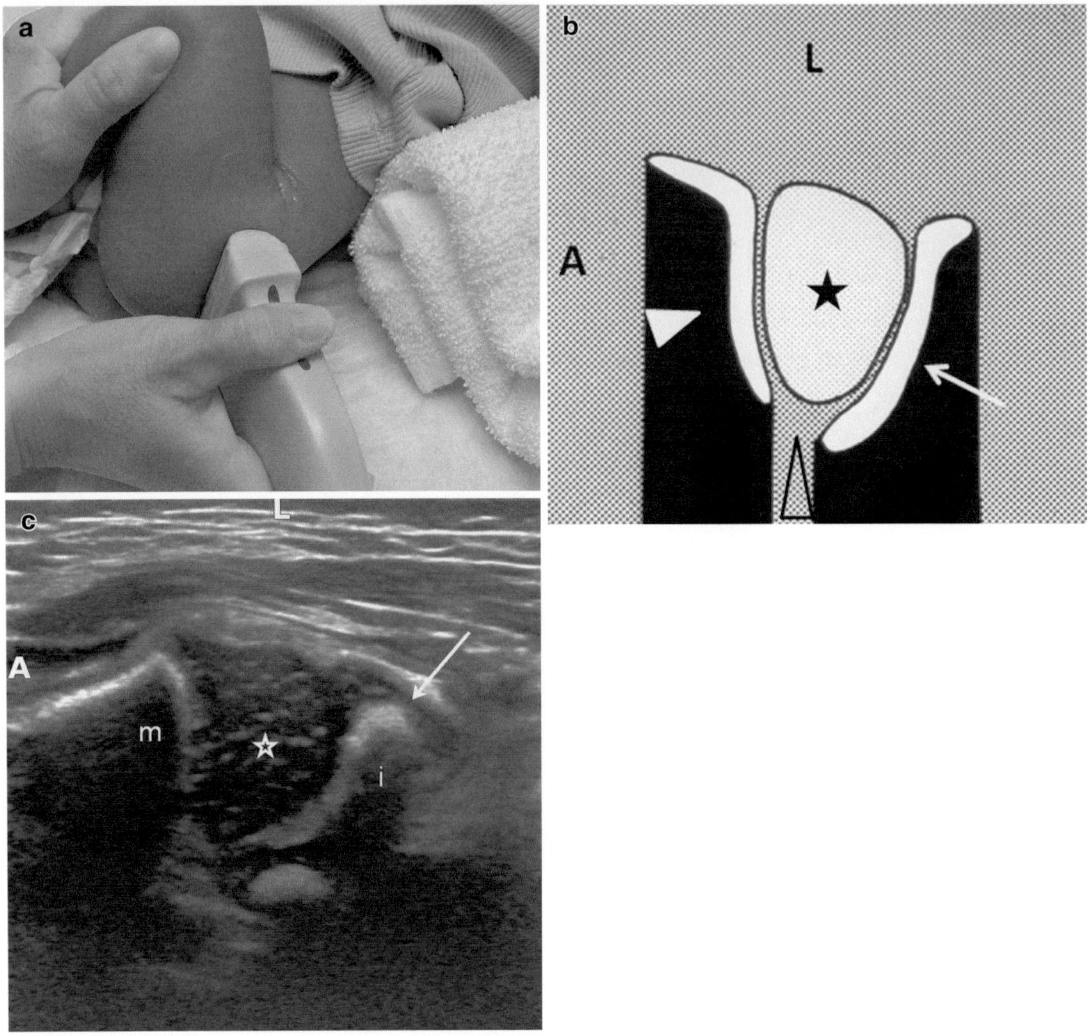

Fig. 11.20 Normal transverse (axial) flexion US. (**a**) The hip is flexed and the transducer rotated approximately 90°, parallel to the femoral shaft, posterolateral to the hip. (**b**) Diagram shows femoral metaphysis (*white arrowhead*), femoral head (*asterisk*), triradiate cartilage (*open arrowhead*), and acetabulum (*arrow*). (**c**) US shows the femoral head (*star*) with the metaphysis anterior (*m*) and the ischium (*i*) posterior without significant echoes deep in the acetabulum. The *arrow* indicates the posterior lip of the acetabulum. *A* anterior, *L* lateral

the coccyx is centered over the pubic symphysis and that the obturator foramina are symmetric (Fig. 11.26). A second frontal radiograph of the pelvis with the thighs in abduction, flexion, and external rotation (the frog lateral projection) is performed to determine if a displaced or questionably displaced hip is reducible. In this position, the femur is viewed in lateral profile, but the acetabulum remains in coronal projection.

The pelvis and both hips are included on both radiographs, allowing the opposite hip to serve as a comparison in evaluating expected femoral head and acetabular growth, maturation, and relative position. Gonadal shielding can be used on all radiographs in boys, with adequate care being taken to ensure that the pubic symphysis is not obscured. In girls, one of the initial radiographs should have pelvic shielding, but it may be omitted on the second of the pair. If US is not available, additional views can be obtained, with maneuvers designed to produce and document the dislocation.

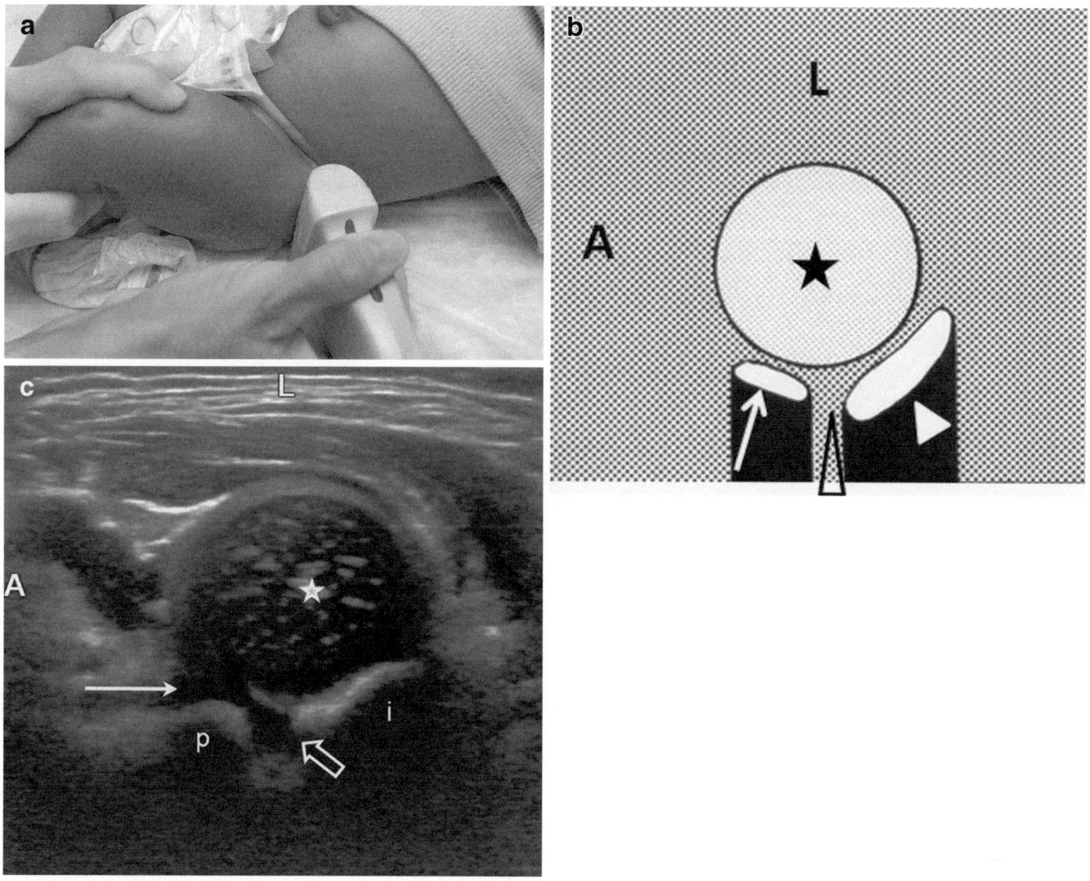

Fig. 11.21 Normal transverse neutral view. (**a**) The leg is now in the physiologic neutral position with the transducer positioned laterally over the hip. (**b**) Diagram shows the femoral head (*asterisk*), pubis (*arrow*), triradiate cartilage (*open arrowhead*), and ischium (*white arrowhead*). (**c**) On the US, the femoral head (*star*) is centered over the triradiate cartilage (*open arrow*) with the ischium (*i*) posterior and the pubis (*p*) anterior. Note the cartilage overlying the pubic bone is thicker (*arrow*) than that overlying the ischium. The triradiate cartilage allows through transmission of sound. *A* anterior, *L* lateral

The radiographic hallmarks of DDH are displacement of the femoral head, delayed ossification of the cartilaginous femoral epiphysis, and dysplasia (loss of concavity, increased angulation, irregularity) of the acetabular roof (Fig. 11.27). Lines and angles help localize the femoral head in relation to the osseous portion of the acetabulum before the femoral ossification center appears at 3–4 months of age. The visible osseous structures should be examined to determine the probable location of the cartilaginous femoral epiphysis before performing these measurements. The width of the cartilaginous femoral head is at least equal to the linear measurement of the femoral neck segment. Drawing a circle that touches the neck on a well-positioned neutral view provides a fairly accurate estimate of the normal cartilaginous femoral head. This anatomic projection should prevent complete dependency on lines and angles. As a general guideline, the normal non-ossified femoral head is largely confined to the area below the Y-synchondrosis and medial to the lateral edge of the acetabulum.

Evaluation of the acetabular side of the joint is difficult, since the actual contact surface is a thick layer of cartilage. The acetabula should be examined for bilateral symmetry in regard not only to angulation but also to the details of size, concavity of the acetabular roof, and distinctness of the outer margin. Too often, a measurement line obscures important signs of femoral head-acetabular contact and development. If bilateral disease exists, side-to-side comparison is obviously limited.

After examining the morphology of the osseous structures, femoral head position and acetabular configuration are measured. The most commonly used measurements are summarized

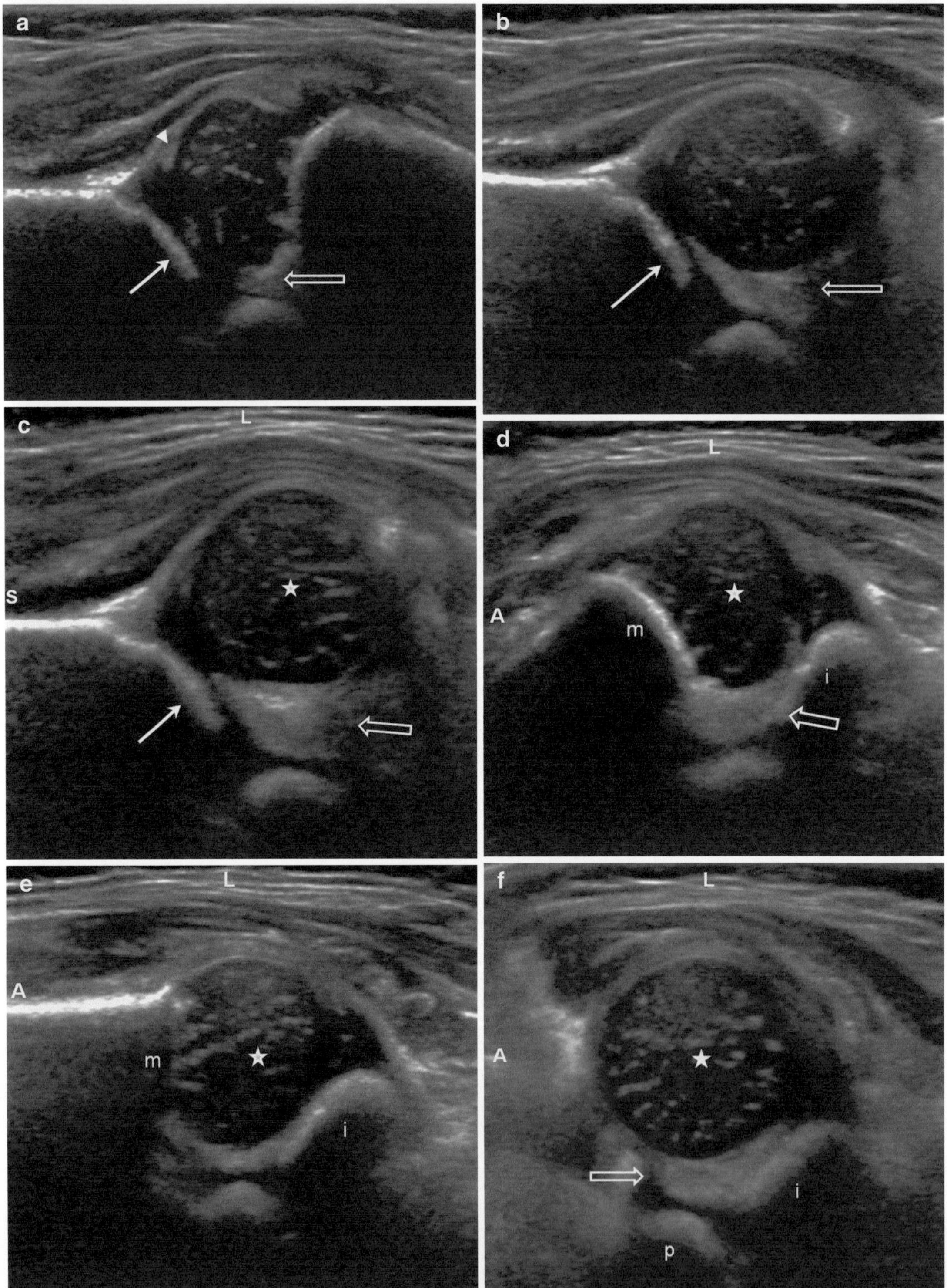

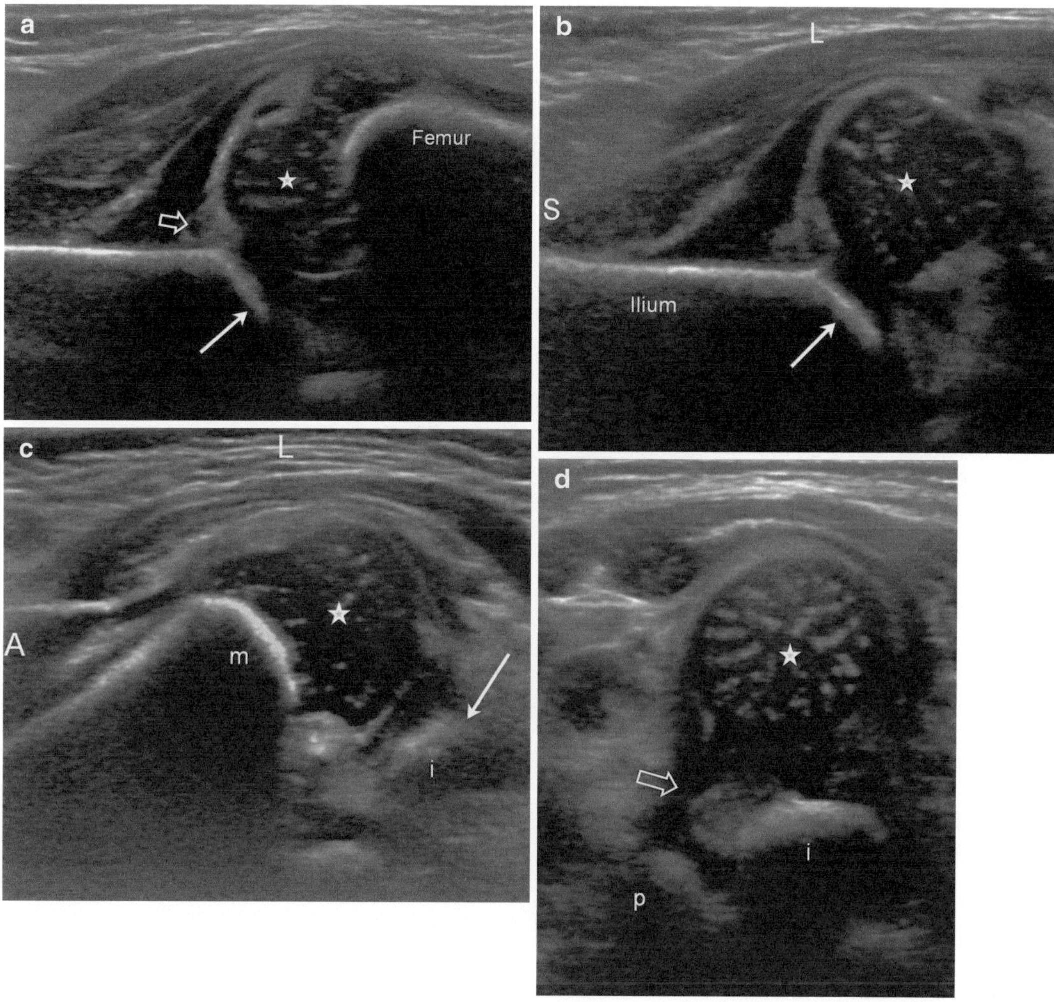

Fig. 11.23 US of dislocation (*S* superior, *L* lateral, *A* anterior). (**a**) Coronal neutral view shows the femoral head (*star*) lateral to the acetabulum (*arrows*). The labrum (*open arrow*) is echogenic and thickened; the acetabulum is angled and incompletely seen. (**b**) Coronal flexion view. The femoral head (*star*) is displaced laterally and uncovered by the acetabulum (*arrow*). The labrum again appears abnormal, and the shallow acetabulum is angled (*arrow*). (**c**) Transverse flexion view. The femoral head (*star*) is displaced laterally, perched on the margin of the posterior acetabulum, or "posterior lip" (*arrow*) formed by the ischium (*i*) (*m* metaphysis). (**d**) Transverse neutral view. The femoral head (*star*) is laterally displaced well away from the acetabulum, composed of the ischium (*i*) and pubis (*p*). Abundant echogenic soft tissue intervenes (*open arrow*)

Fig. 11.22 US of subluxation (*S* superior, *L* lateral, *A* anterior). (**a**) Coronal neutral view shows mild lateral displacement of the femoral head with echogenic fibrofatty tissue (*open arrow*) between the femoral head and the acetabulum (*arrow*). The acetabular roof is angled and irregular consistent with dysplasia. Note the echogenic tip of the labrum (*arrowhead*). (**b**) Coronal flexion view, without stress. The femoral head subluxates laterally, creating space lateral to the acetabulum (*arrow*), which fills with echogenic fibrofatty tissue (*open arrow*). Again, note the irregularity of the acetabular roof. (**c**) Coronal flexion view with adduction stress. The gap and echogenic material (*open arrow*) between the femoral head (*star*) and the acetabulum (*arrow*) are further increased, but the femoral head still contacts the acetabulum. (**d**) Transverse flexion view in adduction. The femoral head (*star*) is displaced laterally with echogenic material (*open arrow*) between the femoral head and the medial acetabulum (*open arrow*). The ischium (*i*) is posterior and metaphysis (*m*) anterior. (**e**) Transverse flexion view in abduction. The femoral head (*star*) is now reduced, resting on the ischium (*i*) with no material intervening between the femoral head and the medial acetabulum (*m* metaphysis). (**f**) Transverse neutral view. The femoral head (*star*) is mildly laterally displaced with space and echogenic material (*open arrow*) between the head and the acetabulum, composed of the ischium (*i*) posteriorly and the pubis (*p*) anteriorly

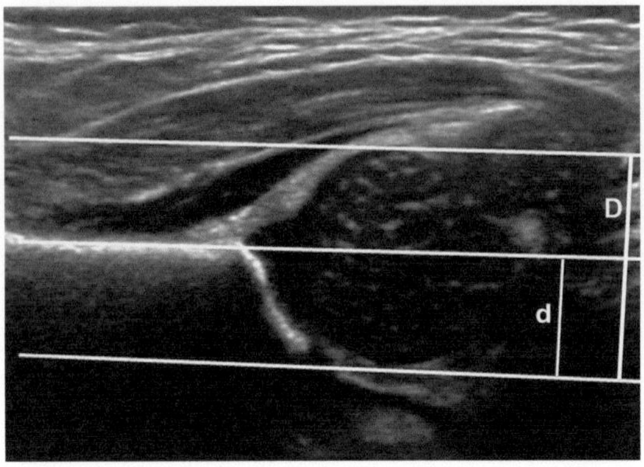

Fig. 11.24 Normal coronal flexion US showing d/D ratio. Three lines parallel to the iliac wing define the depth of the acetabulum (d, *short line*) and the diameter of the femoral head (D, *long line*). The most lateral is tangent to the lateral margin of the femoral head. The middle line runs along the edge of the straight, echogenic iliac bone. The most medial line is tangent to the medial margin of the femoral head. The d/D ratio is normally over 58 %

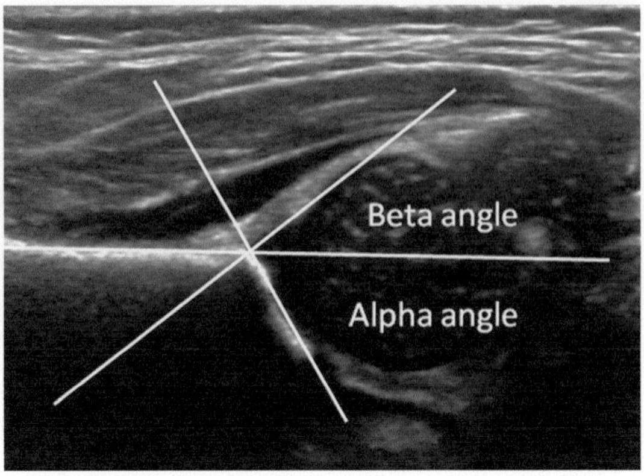

Fig. 11.25 Normal coronal neutral US shows Graf angles. The alpha angle is normally greater than 60°

Table 11.2 Ultrasound measurements. Acetabular (d/D ratio)

Acetabular coverage (d/D ratio) (Fig. 11.24)	
Purpose	To estimate the acetabular coverage by comparing the diameter of the femoral head to the depth of the acetabular cup
Definition	In the coronal flexion view, with the hip normally positioned in the acetabulum, three parallel lines are drawn, one along the ilium (iliac line) and the other 2 parallel to it, one tangent to the lateral aspect of the femoral head, and one tangent to the junction of the medial femoral head and the acetabular fossa. The distance from the medial line and the iliac line is d, and the distance from the medial line and the lateral line is D. The d/D ratio is multiplied by 100 and represents the percentage of the femoral head covered by the bony acetabulum
Note	When the hip is not well positioned in the acetabulum or the acetabulum is dysplastic, 4 parallel lines must be drawn, one along the ilium and one parallel to it in the deepest portion of the acetabulum, representing d, the depth of the acetabulum, and the other two tangential to the medial and lateral aspects of the femoral head, representing D, the width of the femoral head
Values	Greater than 58° is normal, less than 33° is abnormal, and between 33 and 58 are "borderline" [43, 44, 45]

in Tables 11.4, 11.5, and 11.6 (Figs. 11.28, 11.29, and 11.30). However, there is considerable intra- and interobserver variability.

The acetabular angle measures between 18 and 36° at birth [48] and decreases by 5° during the next 6 months. Because of this wide variability, simple measurement of this angle is usually not helpful unless it is markedly increased or unquestionably normal. Determining the position of the femoral ossific nucleus in relation to the acetabulum and noting the intrinsic character of the acetabular margin is more important. A normally located femoral head causes a congruent impression on the acetabular surface; its presence indicates a normal and stable relationship. Therefore, the normal acetabulum has slight central concavity and a distinct lateral edge (although neither may be visible if the patient is improperly positioned). Absence of either finding, as well as persistent increased obliquity of the bony edge, indicates an abnormal femoral-acetabular relationship. Abnormal sclerosis of the outer portion of the acetabulum suggests increased lateral stress. If any of these acetabular changes is encountered in a newborn, persistent dislocation occurred prenatally. Although normal asymmetry of the femoral ossification centers can occur in up to 25 % of infants, this (or unilateral absence) is another important sign of potentially abnormal development, provided that one or more of the other signs is also present. However, asymmetry alone

Table 11.3 Graf classification system (Fig. 11.25)

Purpose	To measure the development of the acetabulum as a guide for treatment and prognosis of DDH
Definition	A coronal view is obtained in the neutral position with the critical landmarks of the straight iliac line, the fibrocartilaginous tip of the labrum, and the inferior tip of the ilium. A line is drawn along the straight portion of the iliac bone (iliac line). A line is then drawn connecting the inferior margin of the ilium and the lateral margin of the acetabular roof to create the alpha angle. A second line can be drawn connecting the fibrocartilaginous tip of the labrum and the lateral margin of the acetabulum, forming the beta angle
Note	All landmarks must be present on the same image to ensure that the measurements are in the correct plane

Graf type	Values [46, 47]	
	Alpha angle	Beta angle
I	≥60° (normal)	
Ia		<55°
Ib		>55°
IIa	50–59°	
IIb	50–59°	
IIc	43–49°	
D ("about to decenter")	43–49°	<77°
III (types IIIa and IIIb are distinguished on the grounds of structural alteration of the cartilaginous roof)	<43°	>77°
IV (dislocated with labrum interposed between the femoral head and acetabulum)	<43°	

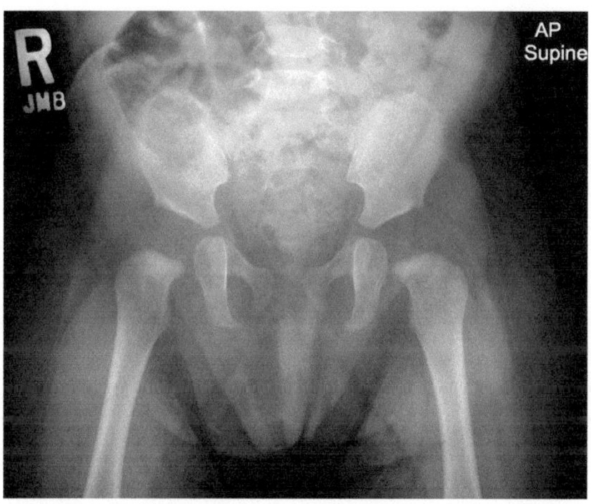

Fig. 11.26 Neutral normal pelvis in a 2-month-old girl. Note the sacrum centered above the symphysis pubis and symmetric obturator foramina. Slightly asymmetric ossification of the femoral heads, as in this case, is common

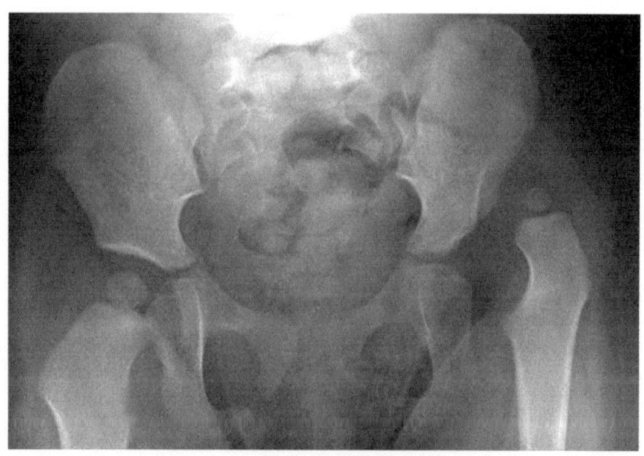

Fig. 11.27 DDH on the left, diagnosed late. The femur is displaced superolaterally. The left femoral head ossification center and femoral neck are smaller than that on the right. The acetabulum is angled and shallow; increased curvature of the iliac bone results from a pseudoacetabulum

is quite common, and in the absence of other features, this should not lead to diagnosis of DDH.

With appropriate treatment, these secondary changes should reverse and result in a normal acetabulum. It can take 6–12 months for delayed ossification in a dislocated femoral head to catch up with that of the opposite normal hip.

4.2 Imaging of DDH During Nonoperative Treatment

If the hip has been shown to be dislocatable or completely dislocated by clinical Ortolani or Barlow maneuvers, the infant is usually placed in a flexion-abduction harness (e.g., Pavlik), splint, or cast. Sequential clinical, US, and radiographic

Table 11.4 Acetabular angle (Fig. 11.28)

Purpose	To measure the angulation of the acetabulum on a radiograph of the infant pelvis and thus estimate acetabular development
Definition	Anteroposterior (AP) neutral radiograph. Baseline connects the Y-synchondroses. A second line connects the superolateral and inferomedial points of the iliac portion of the acetabular roof
Note	This is only an estimate, since the true boundaries of the acetabulum are cartilaginous. Only the upper portion of the acetabulum is measured. The baseline is difficult to delineate once the synchondrosis begins to close, age 6 years or later. A false low value is seen with severe pelvic tilt. (This is called *acetabular index* by orthopedists)
Normal [48, 49]	Newborn female, 28.8 ± 4.8°; male, 26.4 ± 4.4°
	3 m/o female, 25 ± 3.5°; male, 22 ± 4°
	6 m/o female, 23.2 ± 4.0°; male, 20.3 ± 3.7°
	1 y/o female, 21.2 ± 3.8°; male, 19.8 ± 3.6°
	2 y/o female 18 ± 4°; male 19 ± 3.6°

m/o month(s) old, *y/o* year(s) old

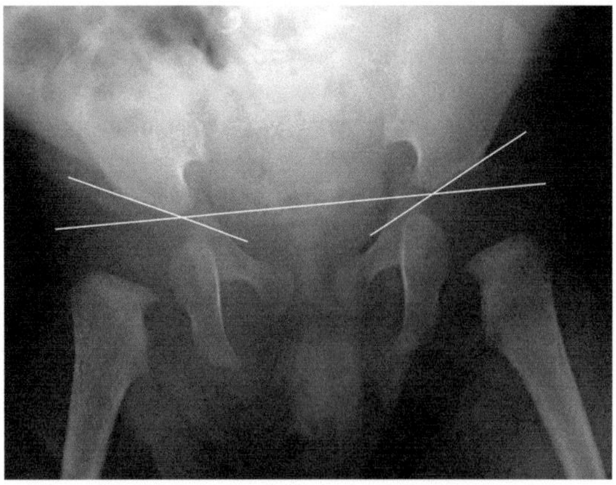

Fig. 11.28 Acetabular angles in a normal patient. A horizontal line (*Hilgenreiner line*) joins the inferior tips of the iliac bones, and angled lines parallel the acetabular roofs to form the acetabular angles

examinations usually show satisfactory acetabular-femoral relationships and subsequent acetabular development. The typical case is diagnosed with US, treated with an abduction brace, followed with sequential sonography during and at conclusion of treatment, and evaluated with a radiograph at completion of treatment [53, 54]. Orthopedic surgeons usually follow patients to maturity and may obtain additional radiographs. If treatment with an abduction brace is unsuccessful, arthrography with closed or open reduction and casting is indicated. Whether the hip is reduced or not, pelvic reconstruction may ultimately be required to improve acetabular containment.

Table 11.5 Hilgenreiner and Perkins lines (Figs. 11.28 and 11.29)

Purpose	To determine whether the cartilaginous femoral head is in satisfactory position prior to ossification
Definition	On an AP neutral view of the pelvis, Hilgenreiner line connects the inferior tips of the ilia. Perkins line is drawn perpendicular to Hilgenreiner line at the outer acetabular margin
Note	It may be difficult to determine exactly where the acetabular margin is
Normal [50, 51]	Perkins line should intersect the femoral metaphysis in its central portion if the femoral head is within the acetabulum

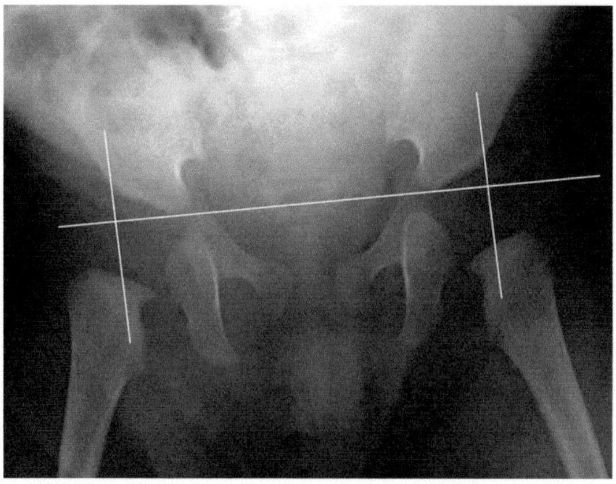

Fig. 11.29 Perkins line in a normal patient. Perkins line is perpendicular to the horizontal Hilgenreiner line and intersects the most lateral ossified portion of the acetabular roof. In a normal patient, Perkins line also approximately bisects the proximal femoral metaphysis

Early diagnosis and treatment allow congruent, concentric reduction, which in turn leads

Table 11.6 Shenton line (Fig. 11.30)

Purpose	To determine whether the cartilaginous or ossified femoral head is in satisfactory position
Definition	On an AP neutral view of the pelvis, a curved line is drawn along the inferior cortex of the superior pubic ramus, and a second curved line is drawn on the medial cortex of the femoral neck
	These lines should connect in the shape of a circle without a step off
Normal	
Notes [52]	Sometimes the lines form more of an oval than a circle even though the hip is in good position
	This line can appear abnormal if there is valgus configuration of the femoral neck, even if the femoral head is correctly positioned within the acetabulum

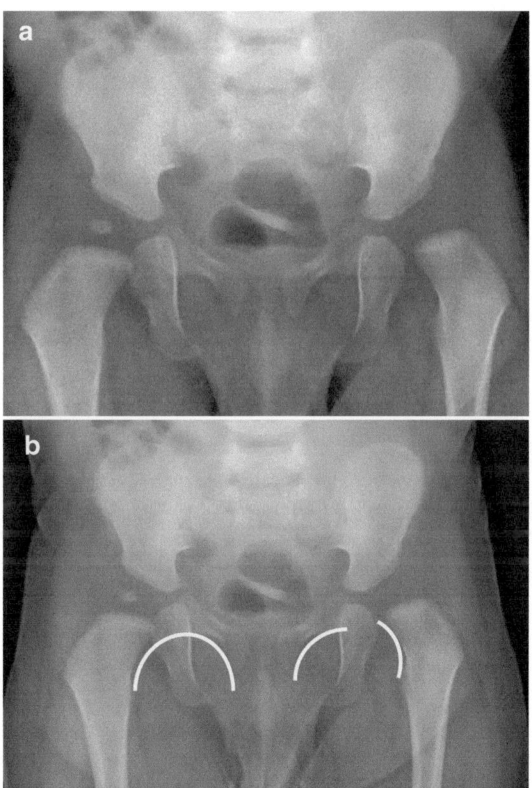

Fig. 11.30 Shenton line, with DDH on the left. (**a**) There is delayed ossification of the left femoral head, and the metaphysis is displaced superolaterally. Increased angulation of the acetabulum. (**b**) Shenton lines in the same patient. The intact smooth arc on the right connects the normally positioned medial femoral neck and the superior aspect of the obturator foramen. On the left, it is disrupted

to normal hip development and function. US has helped facilitate this by decreasing the age at diagnosis [36, 55]. If subluxation or dislocation is not treated, dysplasia will progress and lead to premature degenerative disease and disability.

Positive Contrast Arthrography

This is a technically simple procedure when performed under fluoroscopic control and can be used during operative reduction [56, 57]. It is not indicated in the usual case of easily reducible neonatal hip instability but should be performed without hesitation if concentric reduction seems questionable or difficult to maintain. It is advised when dislocation is discovered late or when sequential examination does not show satisfactory change. Note that too much contrast will distend the joint capsule and simulate pooling of contrast seen in subluxation.

The normal cartilaginous femoral head is spherical, regular, and smooth, outlined by a uniformly thin line of contrast in all projections. The surface of the normal acetabular cartilage is smooth and congruous with that of the head. The labrum is the triangular extension of the acetabular cartilage and is often outlined by contrast within the joint (Fig. 11.31). The term "limbus" denotes a labrum that is deformed by malposition of the femoral head. The femoral head ligament (ligamentum teres) can sometimes be seen medial to the femoral head, extending from the inferior recess of the capsule. Its diameter varies, and it is more easily seen when there is capsular laxity. Contrast-filled lymphatic vessels and venous channels are occasionally shown with arthrography. Visualization of lymphatic drainage only persists for a few minutes. Draining veins are rarely seen except when synovial permeability is increased or the lymphatic vessels are increased in size or number, as occurs with synovitis. They are larger than lymphatic vessels and are not opacified unless the contrast injection is at least partly intraosseous. Opacification of veins usually ceases immediately after contrast injection.

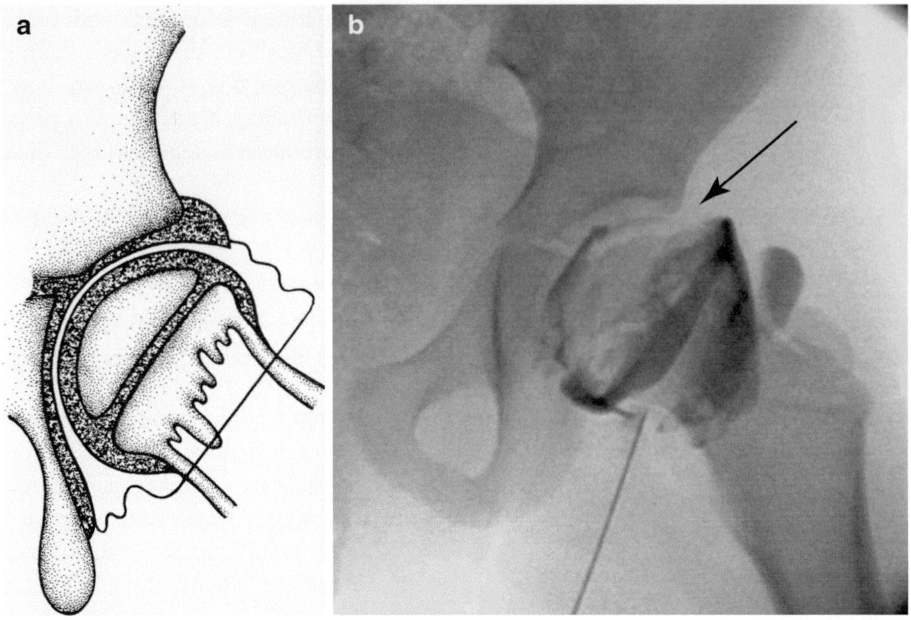

Fig. 11.31 Arthrogram of a normal hip. (**a**) Drawing of normal hip arthrogram (Reprinted from Ozonoff [56], copyright 1987 with permission from Elsevier). (**b**) Intraoperative image shows a thin layer of contrast surrounding the femoral head contained by the normal acetabular roof. The cartilaginous labrum (*arrow*) extends laterally from the acetabulum over the femoral head

The position of the femoral head with respect to the acetabulum can be defined as normal, subluxated, or dislocated. In *subluxation*, the femoral head lies lateral to its normal contact with the medial acetabular cartilage surface but is still below the margin of the labrum. A medial pool of contrast medium is present, rather than the thin rim that normally coats all surfaces (Fig. 11.32). A stretched ligamentum teres can be outlined in the medial pool of contrast. When stress is applied, the femoral head may push the labrum superiorly, but the head will always lie below or lateral to its underside. The labrum itself may be elevated and flattened against the capsule. The capsule is usually loose and more capacious than normal, and reduction is easy to perform but often difficult to maintain.

With complete *dislocation*, the femoral head has lost all contact with the central portion of the acetabulum and instead lies superior and lateral to the edge of the acetabular labrum. Reduction can be prevented by a variety of anatomic features. These include the presence of a deformed, adherent labrum (the limbus) interposed between the head of the femur and the acetabulum, capsular constriction (resulting in figure-of-eight capsular configuration), and thickened ligamentum teres. In addition, hyperplastic intra-articular synovium, fat (pulvinar), and a tight iliopsoas muscle can prevent reduction (Fig. 11.33). Care must be taken to ensure that the reduced femoral head is not pressed against an infolded labrum and capsule (Fig. 11.34), as this type of incomplete reduction is believed to lead to late complications [58]. Although there is evidence that continued pressure in a harness or cast may cause atrophy or displacement of blocking structures and lead to normal seating of the femoral head [59], total reduction without interposed tissues should be the goal.

CT and MRI

Following reduction, CT or MRI is performed in the cast and can usually be accomplished without sedation. Either study can confirm reduction in the axial plane; this is important because the hip tends to re-dislocate posteriorly. If the hip has not

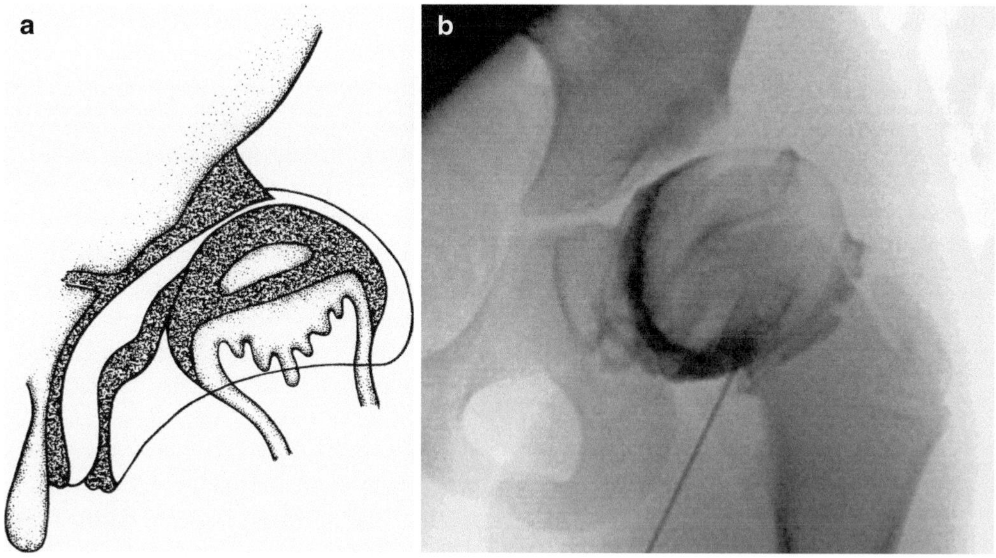

Fig. 11.32 Arthrogram of hip subluxation. (**a**) Drawing of hip arthrogram showing subluxation (Reprinted from Ozonoff [56], copyright 1987 with permission from Elsevier). (**b**) Intraoperative image shows medial pooling of contrast indicating displacement of the hip and capsular laxity. The acetabulum is angled, and the femoral head is slightly ovoid. The labrum extends laterally over the femoral head, but coverage is decreased

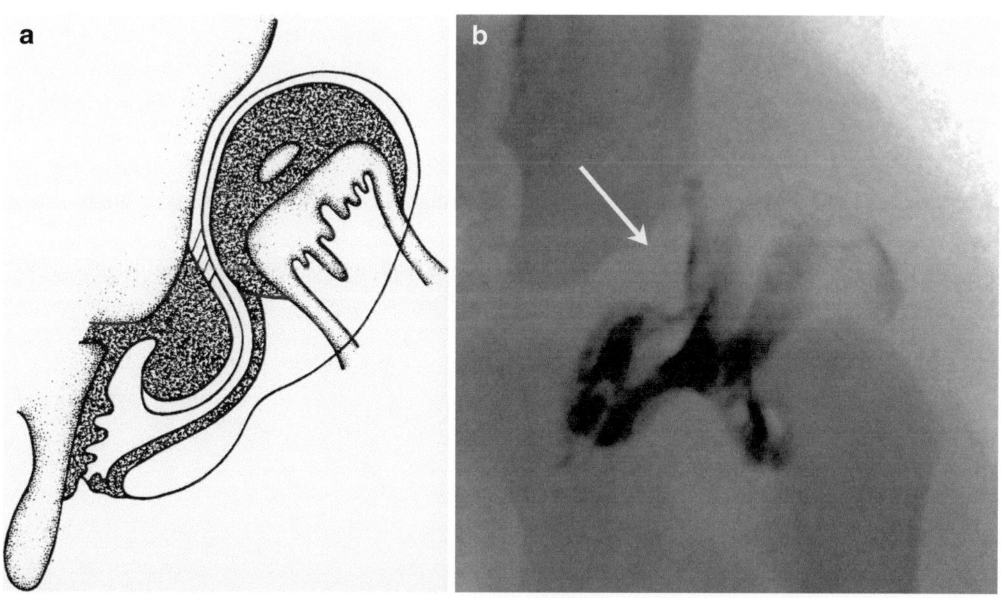

Fig. 11.33 Arthrogram of hip dislocation. (**a**) Drawing of hip arthrogram shows dislocated hip (Reprinted from Ozonoff [56], copyright 1987 with permission from Elsevier). (**b**) Intraoperative image shows superior and lateral dislocation of the femoral head. The mid-portion of the capsule is stretched and narrowed by the inverted thickened labrum (*arrow*), and the labrum is interposed between the femoral head and the acetabulum. Adhesions are evident between the femoral head, capsule, and labrum, and the acetabular capacity is small. Contrast pools in the medial portion of the acetabulum, indicating loss of contact with the femoral head

been successfully reduced, repeat reduction is necessary, often surgical. With low-dose CT in a cast (Fig. 11.35), the radiation dose per tomographic slice is similar to that of frontal and lateral radiographs [60]. Sagittal and coronal reformatted images along with three-dimensional (3D) CT reconstructions demonstrate anterior and posterior acetabular coverage, but this degree of detail requires more cuts (and more radiation). MRI (Fig. 11.36) is particularly attractive because of its multiplanar capability and lack of ionizing radiation [61]. Furthermore, it can identify soft tissue structures interposed within the joint (such as the ligamentum teres and hypertrophied pulvinar), along with surrounding musculature. The nonossified femoral head is readily defined. MRI can distinguish the labrum from the capsule and the acetabular cartilage and can also detect the presence of joint fluid and epiphyseal ischemia.

Avascular necrosis can occur during treatment of DDH due to traction on the vessels supplying the femoral head. This can potentially be diagnosed with contrast-enhanced MRI or with diffusion-weighted imaging. Both methods have been used experimentally [62, 63].

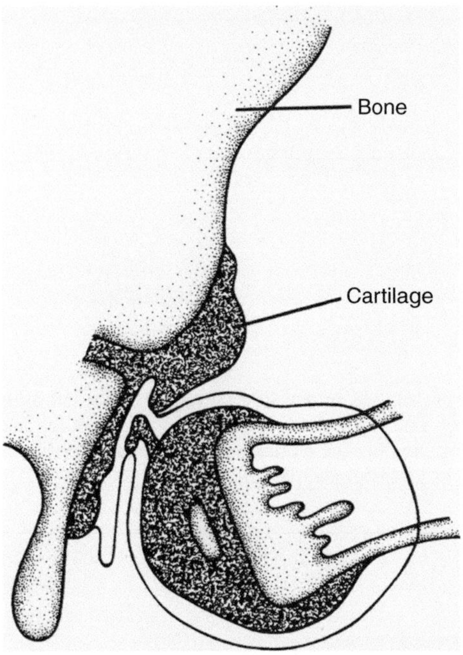

Fig. 11.34 Drawing of incompletely reduced hip with flattening of the abnormal interposed labrum. This is not an acceptable complete reduction, as the infolded labrum (limbus) and capsule prevent the femoral head from contacting the central acetabulum (Reprinted from Ozonoff [56], copyright 1987 with permission from Elsevier)

4.3 Imaging of DDH in Planning and Following Operative Treatment

Pelvic or femoral surgery is often needed if satisfactory acetabular development and hip stability have not been achieved. These procedures attempt to provide better acetabular coverage,

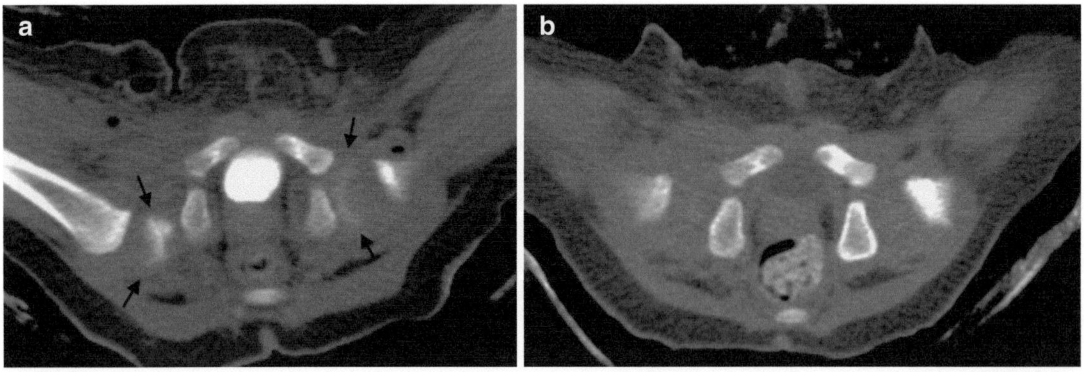

Fig. 11.35 Postoperative low-dose CTs of patient with DDH on the right. (**a**) Initial postoperative study shows dislocated right hip. On the *left*, the normal anterior femoral neck forms a smooth arc with the anterior pubic bone, whereas this line is disrupted on the *right*. Note arthrographic contrast material (*arrows*) in both hip joints and a small amount of gas in the soft tissues. (**b**) After repeat surgery, a second study shows that both hips are positioned normally. Intra-articular contrast material is no longer present

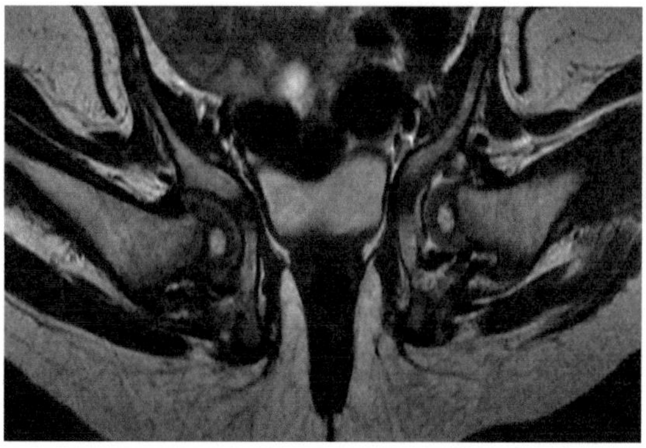

Fig. 11.36 Postreduction coronal T1-W MRI in an older patient (note the ossific nuclei). Both hips are well positioned. Compared to the normal right side, the left shows a shallow, angled bony acetabulum, inverted labrum, thickened joint capsule, and smaller ossific nucleus

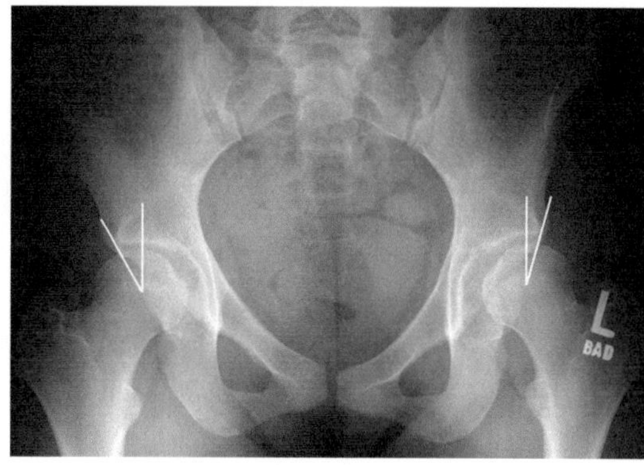

Fig. 11.37 Residual decreased acetabular coverage and lateralization of the left femoral head in a 16-year-old with a history of treated DDH. The center-edge angle of Wiberg is decreased

more normal femoral head-acetabular congruence, decreased pressure loading on the femoral head, and increased efficiency of the hip musculature. These objectives can be met by many procedures; the most commonly used are the Dega acetabuloplasty, Salter osteotomy, and triple innominate osteotomy. In skeletally mature patients, periacetabular osteotomies are often performed.

The hips are evaluated radiographically with various views in addition to the routine frontal and frog lateral views. These views are somewhat institution/practitioner-specific, based on orthopedist preference and patient anatomy. The center-edge angle evaluates acetabular coverage in the coronal plane (Fig. 11.37) (Table. 11.7). The false profile view assesses anterior acetabular development in suspected acetabular impingement (Fig. 11.38) (Table 11.8) [67]. At times, a horizontal or cross-table true lateral view of the pelvis may be necessary to demonstrate the anatomy of and relationship between the femoral articulation and acetabulum. Abduction radiographs may be obtained preoperatively if a varus derotational osteotomy is contemplated. Internal rotation demonstrates the best centralization available if excessive valgus, anteversion, or subluxation is present. The Dunn view, performed with 45° hip flexion and 20° abduction, demonstrates sphericity of the femoral head. Various lines and angles are used to analyze the hips and determine which procedure is optimal.

Table 11.7 Center edge (CE) angle (Wiberg) (Fig. 11.37)

Purpose	To evaluate the relation of the femoral head to the acetabulum and the coverage of the femoral head in the coronal plane
Definition	On an AP radiograph of the pelvis, a baseline connects the centers of the femoral heads. The CE angle is then formed by the intersection of two lines: one through the center of the femoral head, perpendicular to the baseline and the other from the center of the femoral head to the edge of the acetabulum
Note	This method has limited applicability if the femoral head is deformed (and its center not reliably determined) or if the ossific center is small or eccentrically located
Normal range [49, 64]	3 months, 18–20° 2 years, 30° Lowest limit of normal, age 5–8, 19; age 9–12, 25; age 13–20, 26–30° [65]

In older children, preoperative CT or MRI assesses residual displacement of the femoral head and acetabular dysplasia and also helps plan acetabular reconstruction. Bone detail is superior in CT. Multiplanar reformatted and 3D CT enable interactive visualization of spatial relationships (Fig. 11.39). Several angles can be measured on axial CT images [68]. These measurements are affected by pelvic tilt in the coronal or sagittal planes, so careful positioning is important. Bony landmarks are used to measure the anterior and

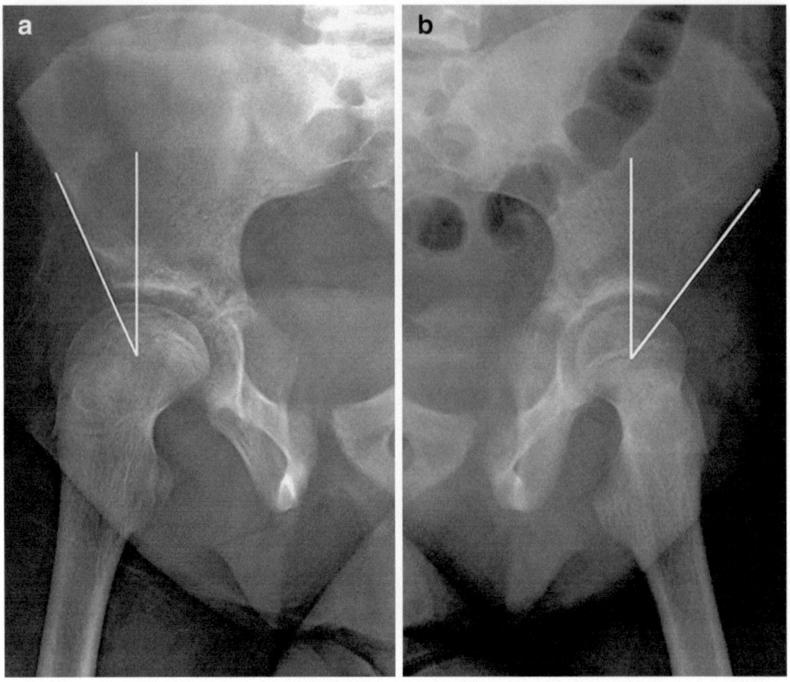

Fig. 11.38 Late deformity following avascular necrosis on the right after treatment for DDH. False profile view with anterior center edge angle abnormally low on the right (**a**), normal on the left (**b**)

Table 11.8 Vertical center anterior margin angle (VCA): false profile view (Fig. 11.38)

Purpose	To evaluate the anterior acetabular coverage of the femoral head
Definition	On a standing AP radiograph, obtained at an angle of 65° between the pelvis and the recording cassette, the VCA angle is formed by the intersection between a vertical line from the center of the femoral head and a second line connecting the center of the femoral head and the acetabular edge
Note	If the femoral head is deformed, this angle is less accurate, and a different angle can be used, the anterior acetabular head index, using the same view
Normal [66]	Greater than 25°

posterior acetabular indices, the axial acetabular index, the acetabular version angle, the anterior and posterior center edge angles, and the acetabular anteversion angle [69–71]. 3D CT can eliminate pelvic positioning issues but requires additional software and time [72]. These measurements inform the orthopedist about acetabular development as well as version/depth, which are important for surgery. Abnormalities of acetabular version are seen in DDH as well as other hip conditions and are associated with subsequent development of osteoarthritis [73].

Imaging

Imaging provides important information during and after operative treatment of DDH (see Chap. 27 for more detailed discussion). Dega osteotomy consists of an incomplete transverse iliac osteotomy performed anteriorly and laterally just above the acetabular roof. Graft insertion decreases the acetabular angle and improves coverage of the femoral head. This is usually performed with a shortening osteotomy of the proximal femur in patients with late-diagnosed dislocations (more than 2–3 years of age) [74]. The Salter osteotomy is a complete transiliac osteotomy indicated for remote persistent subluxation with mild to moderate acetabular dysplasia. It effectively redirects the acetabulum without changing its size or shape. The osteotomy is made between the anterior superior and anterior inferior iliac spines and exits in the sciatic notch in a horizontal plane across the pelvis,

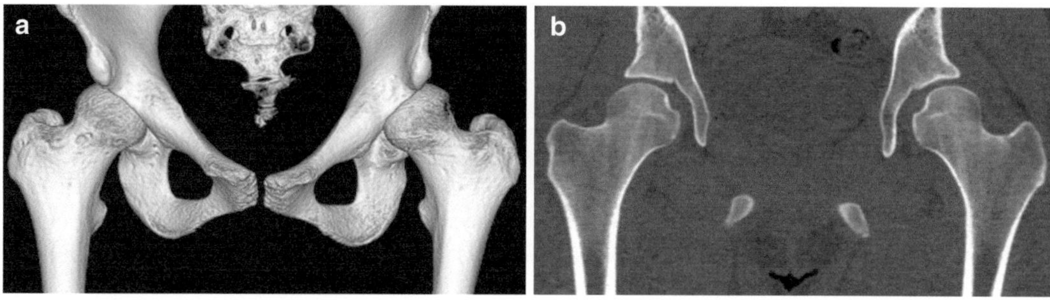

Fig. 11.39 Residual decreased acetabular coverage of the left hip on coronal reformatted (**a**) and 3D reconstructed CT (**b**). There is also slight widening of the left hip joint (same patient as in Fig. 11.37)

above the acetabulum, and higher than the Dega procedure. The distal fragment is rotated anteriorly and laterally to provide more coverage, and the resultant gap is filled with graft material. This may be combined with open reduction of the hip and/or an intertrochanteric osteotomy.

In older children, triple innominate osteotomies, including osteotomies of the iliac bone, the pubic bone, and the ischium, can be performed to provide adequate coverage for a congruous but dysplastic hip by rotating, grafting, and pinning the mobile acetabular segment (Fig. 11.40). Concomitant open hip reduction may be necessary. Postoperative radiographs show marked asymmetry of the two iliac wings and obturator foramina, but this usually resolves with subsequent remodeling.

After the triradiate cartilage is closed, periacetabular osteotomies are performed. These are similar to the triple innominate osteotomies and are accompanied with femoral osteotomies. Though technically demanding, this procedure has the advantage of preserving part of the posterior column for better postoperative stability. (See Chap. 27 for additional information about the surgical treatment of DDH.)

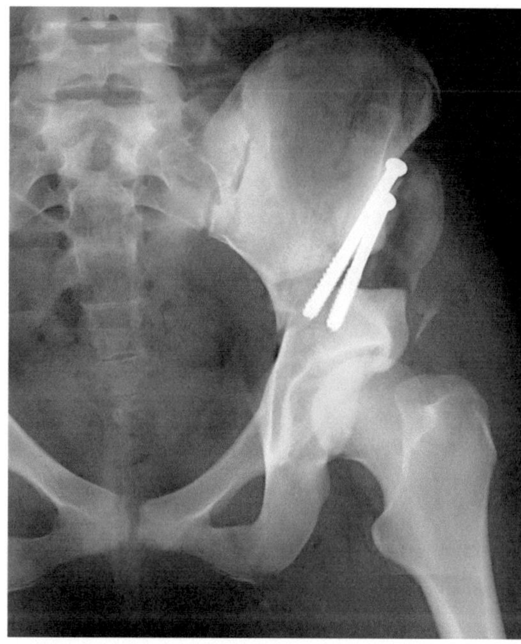

Fig. 11.40 Triple osteotomy with pins transfixing the iliac osteotomy and improved coverage of the femoral head (same patient as in Fig. 11.37)

4.4 Complications of Treatment for DDH

Avascular Necrosis (AVN)

Of the possible complications following DDH, AVN and premature osteoarthritis are the most common. In the setting of DDH, AVN of the femoral head usually occurs only after treatment and is generally considered iatrogenic [75]. Earlier treatment decreases the likelihood of occurrence. Reported incidence varies, but several researchers have reported AVN in 3–14 % of treated hips [76, 77]. This complication can develop after all types of immobilization (pillow, harness, splint, cast) or after surgical intervention [78, 79]. It can also be seen in the contralateral normal hip if both are immobilized [80].

Rigid immobilization in extreme positions of abduction or manipulation/traction can cause vascular impairment. It is uncertain whether the occlusion occurs in vessels along the femoral neck or in the enchondral circulation. It is possible that many changes ascribed to infarction are really caused by abnormal growth processes or interference with the physiology of the epiphyseal and growth plate germinal cartilage and bone cells; an identifiable vascular occlusion is therefore not always necessary.

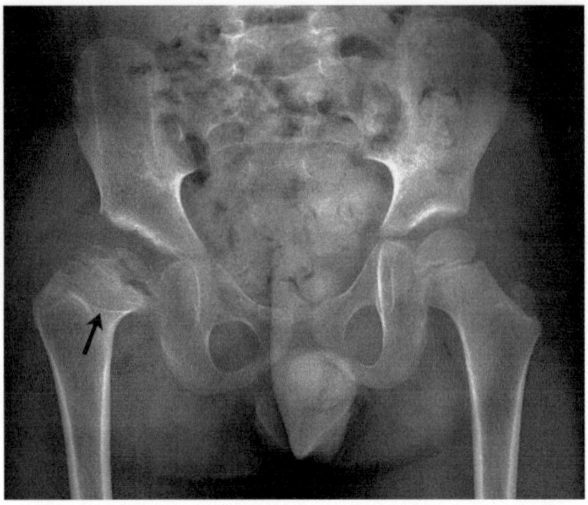

Fig. 11.41 Advanced AVN in a 6-year-old treated for bilateral DDH. Right hip shows typical findings of small, fragmented epiphysis, wide metaphysis, and coxa vara, along with the sagging rope sign (*arrow*). The acetabulum is dysplastic

Imaging

Radiographic identification of early femoral head necrosis is rarely easy, and continued observation is usually necessary. Sequelae of epiphyseal and growth plate damage have been classified [81, 82]. A completely cartilaginous femoral head may begin to ossify soon after reduction; if the ossification appears as several granular foci rather than the usual homogeneous single ossification center, this may represent a transient growth disturbance resulting from extracapsular damage to the main medial circumflex artery. It does not necessarily lead to significant, if any, later deformity, although late follow-up may reveal minor but definite changes. Failure of the femoral ossification center to appear or—if already established—to grow during the first year after reduction is evidence of avascular necrosis. In addition, characteristic signs of femoral head AVN, such as broadening of the femoral neck, may become evident at this time or later.

The type of deformity of the femoral head and neck (femoral neck shortening, rotational abnormalities, coxa magna) depends on which vessel is compromised or whether there has been excessive compression. Growth arrest lines in the femoral neck following treatment help predict future angular deformity [83, 84].

Enlargement of the femoral head does not necessarily indicate previous AVN; it can follow the hyperemia induced by surgery [85]. Segmental necrosis occasionally occurs and may be difficult to recognize. Although preliminary traction, gentle reduction, and avoidance of extreme immobilization position significantly decrease the incidence of total femoral head necrosis, these maneuvers do not seem to affect the occurrence of segmental necrosis.

Although growth of the femoral neck is slowed, that of the greater trochanter is usually unaffected. This results in apparent overgrowth of the greater trochanter, although the pathologic process is actually decreased growth of the femoral neck. As a consequence of appositional bone deposition and normal growth plate function, the position of the superior tip of the greater trochanter becomes abnormal. Instead of its normal position well below the articular surface of the femoral head, the greater trochanter may tower above it. The relatively low position of the femoral neck gives the appearance of coxa vara, but close inspection reveals that the neck-shaft angle is normal: the coxa vara is functional or effective, but not a true varus (Fig. 11.41). In any case, the deformity leads to inefficient abductor muscular force. It may be prevented by trochanteric epiphysiodesis or treated by moving the greater trochanter inferiorly.

Radiographic abnormalities in the metaphysis are frequently associated with growth plate dysfunction or damage. The femoral neck becomes broad, due to a relatively ovoid and

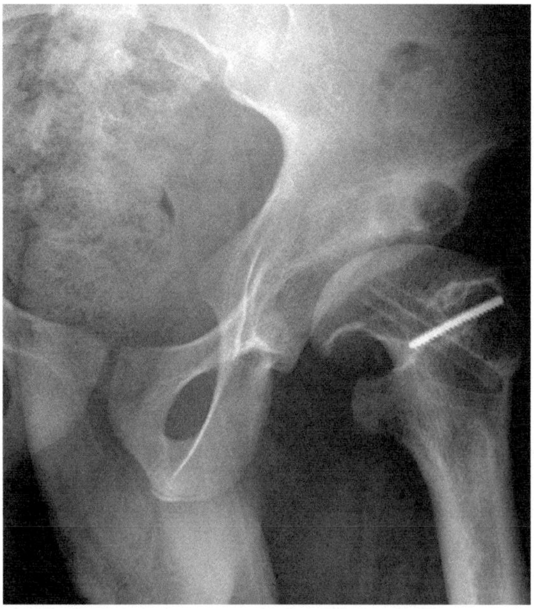

Fig. 11.42 Avascular necrosis and subsequent severe osteoarthritis in a 16-year-old treated for DDH. Note the narrow superior joint space, lateral focal acetabular sclerosis, and cysts as well as broad flattening of the lateralized femoral head

wide femoral epiphysis. The growth plate may become irregular, and cyst-like lucencies may form in the metaphysis. A sharply defined convex-downward line projected across the metaphysis (sagging rope sign) is formed either by the edge of the femoral head cortex seen tangentially or as the result of epiphyseal cartilage cutting into the neck with a resultant reactive bony ridge. As this is not a growth arrest line, it indicates a significant deformity of the femoral head.

Acetabular dysplasia may persist or worsen if residual subluxation allows abnormal lateral pressure from a dysmorphic femoral head to further deform the acetabulum. The lateral acetabular margin may be deficient after excision of the limbus during earlier operative intervention [86].

Secondary degenerative osteoarthritis may develop at an early age, caused by acetabular dysplasia, femoral head deformity, and persistent subluxation (Fig. 11.42). Osteoarthritis induced by DDH is more severe and occurs at a younger age than that induced by an apparently comparable case of Legg-Perthes disease. Severe degenerative changes may be seen as early as 12 years of age. In a large group of patients followed for an average of 39 years after developing DDH-induced AVN, 80 % developed degenerative changes by age 42 [87]. (See Chap. 12 for further discussion of AVN.)

4.5 Differential Diagnosis of DDH

Lateral displacement of the femoral metaphysis may occur in septic arthritis and in other causes of hip effusion (see Chap. 19). Superior and lateral displacement of the femoral head is a common finding in myelomeningocele and may occur in infancy. The acetabulum may be shallow, subject to unusual stress in utero. Spinal dysraphism should be readily apparent on the pelvic radiograph.

Inadequate acetabular coverage of the ossific epiphysis is often erroneously assumed to be evidence of lateral subluxation of the femoral head. This is not always the correct explanation. Lateral uncovering may occur not only in subluxation but also when the acetabulum is normally shaped but developmentally smaller (as in cerebral palsy) or when the femoral head is too large (as in Legg-Perthes disease). In the latter case, the size of the ossification center may be normal but the cartilage overgrown, a frequent concomitant of AVN. Pelvic rotation, common in severe neuromuscular disease, causes further uncovering of the femoral head on the high side of the rotated pelvis. Finally, femoral neck valgus, increased anteversion, and femoral adduction (all present in severe cerebral palsy) rotate the femoral head outward and thus contribute to poor coverage.

Hip subluxation in cerebral palsy (CP) and other spastic conditions develops gradually and is rarely present during infancy (see Chap. 24). Subluxation, often progressing to complete dislocation, is rare in diplegia but can be present in over 60 % of those with severe upper and lower extremity involvement. Pelvic obliquity and scoliosis are commonly associated, and the combination of dislocation with these abnormalities is almost pathognomonic for a neuromuscular

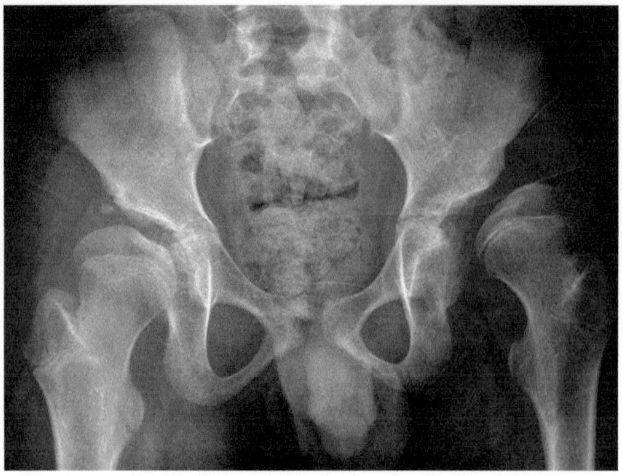

Fig. 11.43 Long-standing cerebral palsy in a teenager with hip subluxation, acetabular dysplasia, and coxa valga, left greater than right

etiology. The acetabulum becomes oblique and shallow (Fig. 11.43). At CT, there is no abnormal acetabular anteversion. The femoral ossific epiphysis is often deformed. Medial flattening of the head has been attributed to pressure deformity by the ligamentum teres and acetabular margin; this occurs only with subluxation. Lateral flattening is less common and may occur without subluxation, probably caused by capsular or psoas pressure. If both surfaces are flattened, an arrowhead deformity may result.

With CP, femoral neck anteversion is usually increased at least two standard deviations above the age-appropriate mean (see Chap. 13 for discussion of femoral anteversion measurement techniques). An increased femoral neck angle, often erroneously attributed to valgus angulation, results from this increased anteversion. Bilateral femoral adduction is common, but occasionally adduction on one side is associated with abduction on the other, causing a "windswept" appearance (see Chap. 24). Flexion contracture is recognized by characteristic apparent femoral neck bowing into varus and increased soft tissue density on the flexed side.

Traumatic hemarthrosis and epiphyseal slip may result from severe trauma, child abuse, or birth injury. If the epiphyseal ossification center has not ossified, lateral shift of the femoral shaft may be misinterpreted as a dislocation rather than a shearing fracture, in which case US or MRI can assist with diagnosis.

4.6 Hip Dysplasia in Generalized Syndromes

The role of increased joint laxity or hypermobility as a complicating factor in hip dislocation is uncertain. However, increased joint laxity is found in those with DDH and their close relatives [30, 88]. Familial joint laxity has been shown in several kindreds, but most of this group is asymptomatic. Hypotonia and joint laxity are common in Down syndrome, and the incidence of recurrent hip dislocation or subluxation in ambulatory children is as high as 5 % [89].

Patients with Ehlers-Danlos syndrome have hyperlaxity of skin and joints, as well as other connective tissue problems. Multiple subtypes of this syndrome have variable expression [90]. Skeletal abnormalities include hyperextensibility, instability and dislocations of the joints, joint effusions, and enlarged bursae over the olecranon and in the prepatellar region. The degree of hyperextensibility varies. If hip dislocation occurs, reduction is easy but difficult to maintain. Radiographs can be difficult to interpret, as they demonstrate considerable lateral subluxation with relatively normal acetabula. Arthrography, however, demonstrates large, lax, redundant capsular structures within which the femoral head can be easily manipulated. Acetabular reconstruction may successfully maintain hip position.

In Larsen syndrome, early joint laxity leads to multiple dislocations (especially in the hips, elbows, and knees); these joints later become stiff. A typical flat facies with saddle-nose deformity is characteristic. Some patients have a distinctive juxtacalcaneal ossification center.

5 Coxa Vara (Box 11.2)

Box 11.2: Coxa Vara

Varus present if femoral neck/shaft angle
- <150° in early childhood
- <120° in adults

Growth plate more vertical than 30° to horizontal

Medial triangular buttressing fragment

Femoral retroversion common

The angle between the femoral neck and shaft varies with age, measuring about 150° at birth and decreasing to between 120 and 130° at maturity. The term coxa vara denotes a neck-shaft angle of less than 120°. However, this value is based on the appearance of the adult hip, and in early childhood, when 150° can be normal, a neck-shaft angle greater than 120° may constitute abnormal varus. In addition, the final angle of the growth plate itself should be less than 30° to the horizontal.

Normal infantile femoral neck valgus results from relatively more growth of the medial portion of the subcapital growth plate during the perinatal period. The shift toward varus during childhood is due to a corresponding growth in the lateral portion of the growth plate. Weight bearing, erect posture, and normal gait probably affect this process. In cases of severe cerebral palsy, diminished weight bearing and upright position contribute to persistent femoral neck valgus.

If the appearance of the hip suggests coxa vara, it is necessary both to separate true coxa vara from apparent (or functional) coxa vara and to distinguish primary (or developmental) coxa vara from that caused by a disease process. Apparent (functional) coxa vara due to femoral neck shortening and relative trochanteric overgrowth is often confused with true coxa vara. In apparent coxa vara, the greater trochanter towers over the femoral neck, but the actual angle that the neck makes with the shaft appears normal. This commonly results from growth plate dysfunction due to trauma, infection, AVN (especially following reduced hip dislocation), and other problems (Fig. 11.44). The term trochanteric overgrowth is frequently yet misleadingly used, but the situation actually reflects femoral neck underdevelopment and normal greater trochanteric growth.

In true coxa vara, the neck-shaft angle actually approaches a right angle, and the proximal femoral growth plate thus becomes more vertical. The coxa vara angulation results from relatively more growth in the lateral aspect of the growth plate than in the medial portion, with resultant tilt of the growth plate to an abnormally oblique angle. Congenital coxa vara without femoral shortening is rare and diagnosed by clinical examination, confirmed radiographically. Developmental coxa vara is an uncommon, possibly hereditary condition that usually presents around 2 years of age as a painless limp or waddling gait [91]. The sexes are equally affected. The condition is bilateral in one third to one half of patients [92].

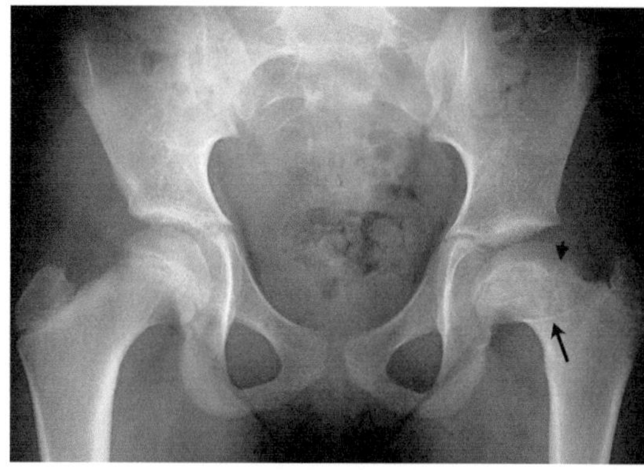

Fig. 11.44 Apparent coxa vara on the left, secondary to Legg-Perthes disease that caused premature fusion of the lateral growth plate (*short arrow*). Note the broad and relatively flat femoral head as well as the sagging rope sign (*long arrow*)

It is important to recognize that this process is developmental, not congenital. Both traumatic and vascular causes have been suggested. Abnormal transition of resting to proliferating cartilage cells has been noted in the medial growth plate [93]. Asymmetric growth may cause the growth plate to become more oblique than usual, resulting in increased shearing force. Disruption of the degenerative zone of the growth plate probably produces multiple small epiphyseal slips.

A metaphyseal triangular fragment is typically positioned under the femoral head, inferomedial to the growth plate. This probably occurs as the displaced growth plate attempts to buttress the slipping epiphysis (a reaction similar to that of other epiphyseal slips). Once the orientation of the growth plate has changed, subsequent weight bearing and growth perpetuate the varus angle and contribute to further abnormal cortical modeling. Eventually, the acetabulum becomes dysplastic, growth of the femoral neck slows, and relative trochanteric overgrowth occurs.

Imaging

The radiographic diagnosis is based on the sequence of events just described. The growth plate is wide, and its alignment is more vertical than normal, more than 30° to the horizontal pelvic baseline (Fig. 11.45). From a prognostic point of view, angles in the 30–45° range tend to eventually resolve, and those over 60° usually continue to slip [94]. The characteristic medial triangular metaphyseal fragment is almost always present in patients less than 9 years old, but in older patients, the fragment usually fuses with the femoral neck and cannot be identified. The neck-shaft angle is more varus than normal for age. In late stages, secondary remodeling thickens the medial cortex of the neck and upper shaft, the trochanter overgrows, and abnormal weight bearing changes the orientation of the acetabulum, perhaps inducing secondary degenerative changes. Valgus osteotomy improves the alignment of the femoral head and acetabulum and prevents impingement as the child matures (Fig. 11.46). Femoral retroversion is common in coxa vara and can be assessed with CT or MRI [95].

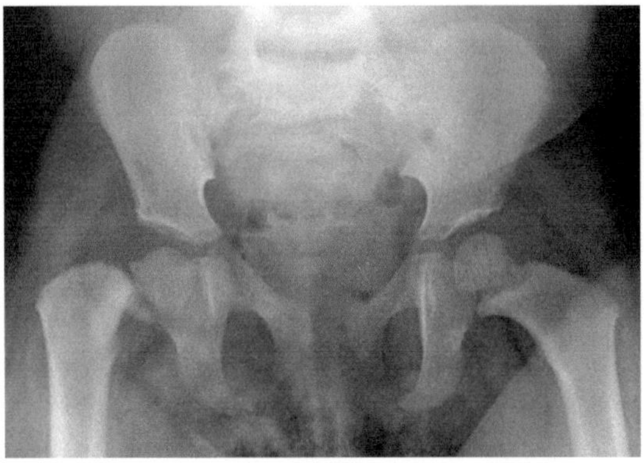

Fig. 11.45 Bilateral developmental coxa vara in a 28-month-old with a triangular buttressing medial fragment. Note the growth plate on the right is more vertical than that on the left and that the right femoral head has slipped

Differential Diagnosis

Secondary coxa vara may be due to a congenital anomaly (congenital short femur with coxa vara), bone softening (osteogenesis imperfecta, fibrous dysplasia, renal osteodystrophy, rickets) (Fig. 11.47), or abnormal growth processes in systemic disease (spondyloepiphyseal dysplasia, cleidocranial dysplasia, metaphyseal chondrodysplasia, spondylometaphyseal dysplasia-corner fracture type). Myelomeningocele, birth trauma, or child abuse may result in significant epiphyseal slip in infants, simulating coxa vara. The coxa vara following AVN from previously treated hip dislocation, Gaucher disease, Legg-Perthes disease, growth plate trauma, or infection is usually an apparent rather than true coxa vara, as discussed above.

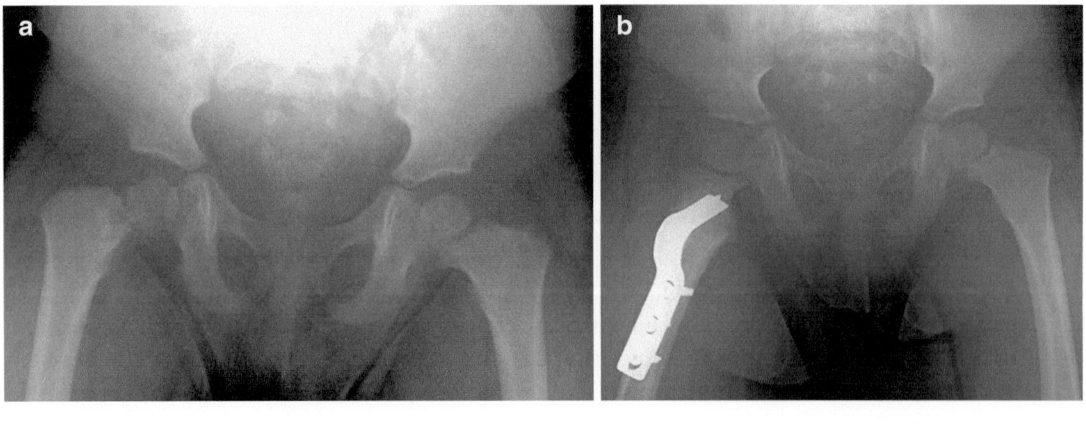

Fig. 11.46 Bilateral developmental coxa vara in a 19-month-old. (**a**) There is medial buttressing and a near-vertical proximal femoral growth plate. (**b**) After valgus osteotomy, right femoral configuration is markedly improved, but coxa vara persists on the left

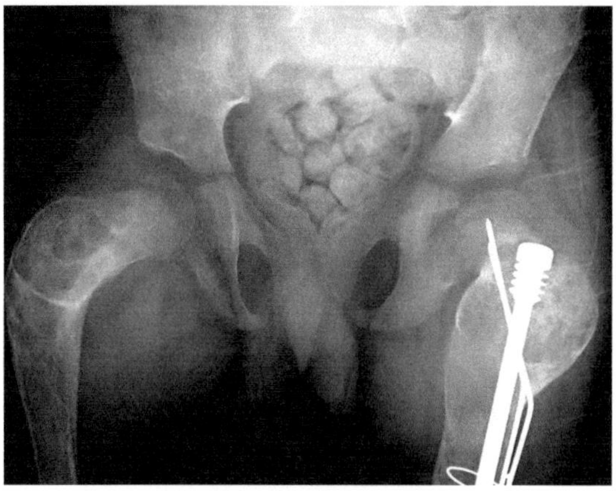

Fig. 11.47 Coxa vara on the right, caused by fibrous dysplasia. There is expansion of the proximal femur, with both ground glass density and cystic lucencies. Intramedullary nail and wires support the left femur

6 Increased Femoral Anteversion

Femoral neck anteversion normally decreases from 30 to 50° at birth to measure 8–15° by skeletal maturity (see Chap. 13 for discussion of measurement technique). Increased anteversion may persist in otherwise normal children, leading to decreased range of lateral rotation in extension. This forces the child to walk with the femurs internally rotated (and the feet turned in) to achieve a satisfactory gait. The tibias then develop lateral torsion, which straightens the position of the feet, but this causes foot eversion and valgus, and the patellas remain medially displaced. Persistent anteversion is usually bilateral and is most common in girls. Whether increased anteversion is associated with any physical or psychological deficit is debatable, as is the necessity for correction in an otherwise normal child.

Increased femoral anteversion is also seen in a variety of disorders. Patients treated for DDH can develop anteversion measuring 17–20° above normal in both the treated hip and in the normal opposite hip. In Legg-Perthes disease, femoral anteversion is initially near normal, but it increases slightly by age 12 in some patients, clearly a secondary change and not causative. Patients with cerebral palsy and myelomeningocele often have increased anteversion (see Chap. 24).

7 Acetabular Protrusion (Protrusio Acetabuli)

Severe medial displacement of the acetabulum's inner wall threatens normal obstetrical delivery and can develop into degenerative osteoarthritis, but fortunately this is uncommon. Minor acetabular protrusion is common in preadolescents and is not necessarily significant. A variable degree of acetabular protrusion accompanies the well-known normal beaking of the inner margin of the acetabular Y-synchondrosis. This is seen in more than half of all children, peaking at ages 8–11. Beaking probably results from medial displacement of the Y-synchondrosis due to normal weight bearing and ambulation. Later development remodels the area and reverses the minor acetabular protrusion.

Pathologic acetabular protrusion can be primary or secondary. The etiology of primary acetabular protrusion is unknown [96]. Usually bilateral, it is up to five times more common in females and often not detected until adulthood, at which time secondary osteoarthritic or obstetric complications may ensue. Familial cases have been described. Marked beaking and possible early fusion of the Y-synchondrosis along with abnormal varus angulation of the femoral neck inhibit normal remodeling, and primary acetabular protrusion results [97]. Potential causes of secondary acetabular protrusion include conditions that cause local or generalized bone softening (particularly osteogenesis imperfecta) (Fig. 11.48). It may follow infection, trauma, arthritis, and other processes that displace the hip or decrease resistance to normal weight bearing. It also occurs in Marfan syndrome and sickle cell anemia, the latter probably caused by osteopenia rather than AVN and marrow hypertrophy [98, 99].

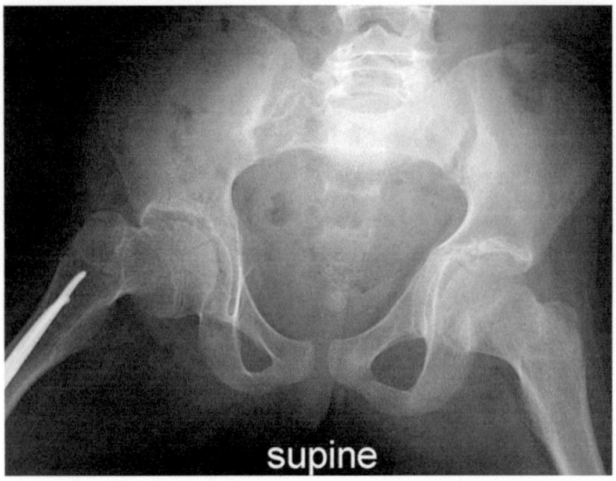

Fig. 11.48 Secondary acetabular protrusion in a patient with osteogenesis imperfecta. Intramedullary nails on the right traverse a pathologic fracture. Note asymmetric deformation of the pelvic basin

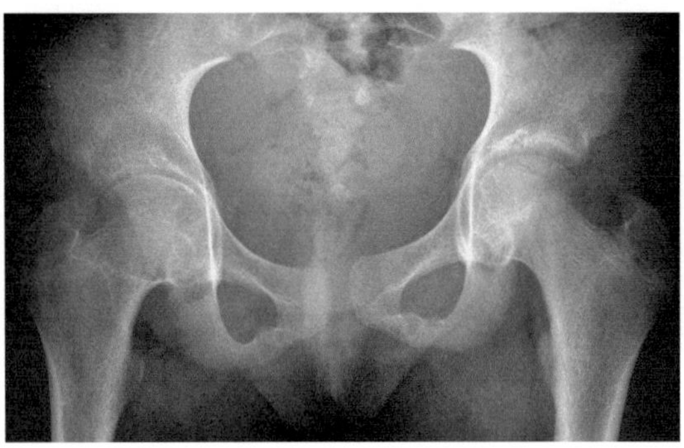

Fig. 11.49 Primary acetabular protrusion in a 13-year-old girl. On both sides, the acetabular line is medial to the ilio-ischial line

Imaging

The femoral head migrates medially, and the medial wall of the acetabulum bulges inward (Fig. 11.49). Abnormal acetabular protrusion is diagnosed if the medial wall of the acetabulum projects medial to the lateral pelvic wall. Several measurements can assess this, such as the center-edge angle (see Figs. 11.37 and 11.38). This is established by determining the angle between two lines that radiate from the center of the femoral head: one vertical and the other intersecting with the lateral edge of the acetabulum. However, slight pelvic rotation can lead to incorrect values, and the more reliable method to evaluate protrusion is measuring the distance between the lateral pelvic wall (ilio-ischial line) and the medial wall of the acetabulum (measured at a right angle to the ilio-ischial line). This should measure at least 1 mm in girls and at least 3 mm in boys [100]. CT or MRI can supply more accurate measurements [101].

It is uncertain at what stage medial migration leads to osteoarthritic changes. Classic severe acetabular protrusion ("Otto pelvis"), especially if associated with pain, limited motion, and bony erosion, is unlikely to result simply from poor adolescent remodeling and is usually secondary, often due to juvenile idiopathic arthritis (see Chap. 20). Treatment consists of femoral osteotomy in younger patients and total hip replacement in older patients [96].

8 Femoral Head Dysplasias (Box 11.3)

Box 11.3: Femoral Head Dysplasias

Microepiphyseal dysplasia	Very delayed ossification (beyond 11 years old)
	Small epiphyses, bilaterally symmetric
	MRI: cartilage size normal
Meyer	Ossification delayed to 2 years old
	Single or multiple ossific granules
	Coalesce by 6 years old
Osteochondritis dissecans-like	Multiple epiphyses or only femoral head
	Saucer-like defect superolateral to fovea
Multiple epiphyseal dysplasia	Irregular, delayed ossification of many epiphyses
	Two forms
	Mild with flat epiphyses
	Severe with small, irregular centers

Dysplasia of the proximal femoral epiphysis may be either isolated to this area or a component of a multiple epiphyseal dysplasia syndrome. Femoral head dysplasia is easily mistaken for Legg-Perthes disease or secondary AVN if the examination is limited to the hip or if this area is examined only once (see Chap. 12). In addition, Legg-Perthes disease-like avascular changes can complicate multiple epiphyseal dysplasia, further confusing the situation. Since some dysplasias have a strong hereditary tendency as well as specific treatment and prognosis, distinguishing them from idiopathic Legg-Perthes disease is essential.

Although femoral head and multiple epiphyseal dysplasias are reported as distinct entities, categorization is difficult. One type can seem to morph into another during a child's development. In some cases, different family members may have different forms of epiphyseal dysplasia. In addition, one family member may have only femoral head involvement, whereas another may have multiple epiphyseal involvement. Finally, distinguishing between minor normal ossification variants and mild epiphyseal dysplasia is often arbitrary, and only serial examination allows a definitive diagnosis. These caveats must be considered when reviewing the following processes.

8.1 Microepiphyseal Dysplasia

This condition, also known as "bilateral hereditary microepiphyseal dysplasia," is apparently autosomal dominant. In one family, 17 of 37 members of four generations were affected when initially evaluated; more recently, 54 members of 6 generations have been shown to be affected [102, 103]. These patients are healthy and of normal intelligence, but somewhat short. The diagnosis is usually made before age 4. Severe early degenerative osteoarthritis affects young adults with this dysplasia.

The hips resemble those of multiple epiphyseal dysplasia. The femoral head ossification centers are small, bilaterally symmetric, triangular, and positioned relatively lateral in the cartilaginous epiphysis. The ossification pattern may be coarse, but it is not sclerotic. Initial ossification is markedly delayed, even past 11 years of age. Arthrography demonstrates normal cartilaginous head size with lateral positioning of the ossification centers; similar findings should be evident at MRI. The epiphyses of the proximal humeri are small, as are those about the knee. Small carpal centers may mature late. After ossification, the medial aspect of the femoral head appears relatively flat, with valgus deformity of a short, thick femoral neck and a dysplastic acetabulum [102]. Severe osteoarthritis develops early.

8.2 Meyer Dysplasia

This dysplasia affects the femoral head almost exclusively in boys and is bilateral in 42 % [104]. There is often a family history of hip disease (labeled though possibly misdiagnosed as Legg-Perthes disease or congenital hip dislocation). Diagnosis is usually made before age 5, as an incidental finding. Meyer dysplasia is usually asymptomatic [105], although patients with bilateral involvement may have a mild and inconsistent waddling gate. Pain, limping, or limitation of movement is rare and usually transient [106]. This condition is easily confused with Legg-Perthes disease, and many patients have been misdiagnosed and treated as such [107]. Infrequently—but more often than in the general population—Legg-Perthes disease-like AVN develops in the affected or contralateral hip.

Delayed ossification is the defining rule, and the femoral head may begin to ossify as late as age 2 years. Initial ossification appears abnormal. There may be a single granular focus of ossification, or there may be several overlapping clusters of nodules or granules that cause uneven density (Fig. 11.50) [105]. However, unlike with true Legg-Perthes disease, there is no epiphyseal sclerosis or fissuring. The only possible metaphyseal change appears as faint sclerosis below the growth plate. Differentiation from Legg-Perthes disease may be difficult, however, with serial radiography often necessary. The separate ossific nodules coalesce and become homogeneous as ossification increases. Resorption, sclerosis, fissuring, and other changes of AVN do not occur. After initial delayed ossification, the epiphyseal ossification centers usually coalesce within 3 years, by about age 6. Mild flattening of the femoral head on follow-up can be attributed to hypoplasia. Triple phase bone scan is normal.

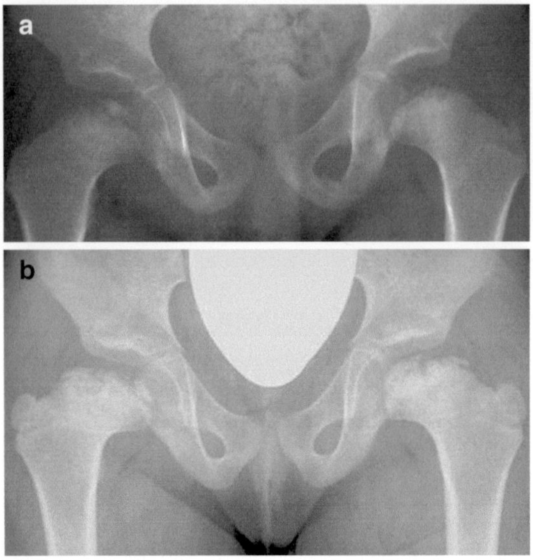

Fig. 11.50 Meyer dysplasia in a 3-year-old girl presenting with mild waddling gait. (**a**) Delayed appearance of the ossification centers of both femoral heads initially. (**b**) At follow-up, 2 years later, the presumed femoral head contour is ovoid, and the femoral heads are enlarged. Positive sagging rope sign (Case courtesy of Karen Rosendahl)

At MRI, the osseous nuclei appear fragmented and the height of the cartilaginous epiphysis is short. Signal intensity, however, is normal, as contrasted with Legg-Perthes disease [105].

Differential Diagnosis

Legg-Perthes disease is the principal differential diagnosis for unilateral Meyer dysplasia and is characterized by both abnormal bone marrow signal in the femoral head on MRI and an abnormal bone scan. Although the radiographic appearance of Meyer dysplasia can resemble early Legg-Perthes disease, the latter demonstrates distinct epiphyseal sclerosis when advanced. If bilateral abnormalities are present, multiple epiphyseal dysplasia and hypothyroidism should be excluded.

8.3 Osteochondritis Dissecans-Like Femoral Head Dysplasia

This epiphyseal abnormality may affect only the femoral head or may be a feature of some cases of multiple epiphyseal dysplasia. Its inheritance and prognosis have not been elucidated, and it is not certain that this is actually a separate form of dysplasia. The superior aspect of the femoral head has a sharply marginated and saucer-like ossification defect that is superolateral to the normal fovea centralis. Arthrography may show an uninterrupted, smooth cartilaginous epiphysis. Presumably, the defect is one of resorption or non-ossification rather than transchondral fracture. It should not be confused with the notch that can normally be present at the apex of the femoral head [8].

8.4 Multiple Epiphyseal Dysplasia (MED)

Multiple epiphyseal dysplasia is an autosomal dominant short-limbed disproportionate dwarfism, and in this disorder, femoral head dysplasia is usually associated with irregular, delayed ossification of many other epiphyses (see Chap. 23). However, as discussed above, there may be overlap between the appearance of limited MED, isolated femoral head dysplasia, and microepiphyseal dysplasia. Chromosomal analysis allows diagnosis, as a defect in the COMP (cartilage oligomeric matrix protein) gene on chromosome 19 is often present. Mutations in this gene lead to dysfunction of Type II collagen and consequent abnormal epiphyseal ossification. The abnormalities in MED may be so mild that they are equivocal. In such subtle cases, it can be helpful to determine the ratio between the height of the distal femoral epiphyseal and its epiphyseal/metaphyseal width, which is decreased in MED. Values can be compared to established norms [108].

This dysplasia usually become apparent after 2 years of age, and mild cases can manifest in adulthood merely with relatively short stature. MED is usually recognized when a child or family member is diagnosed with classic epiphyseal changes. Epiphyseal abnormalities become less obvious as the child matures, and cases suspected late are difficult to confirm radiographically. Eventually, the articular surface is just slightly flattened and the remainder of the epiphysis is

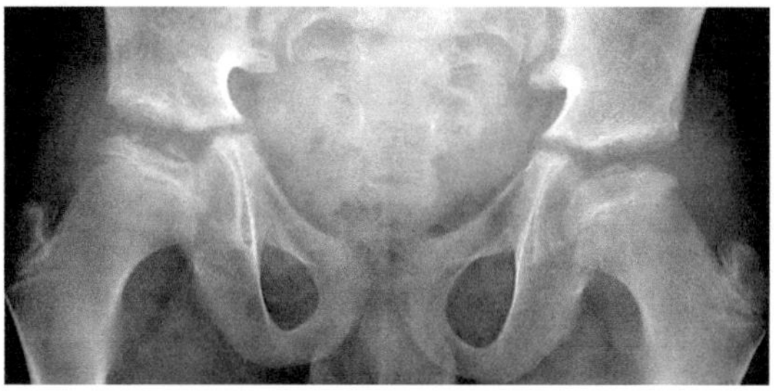

Fig. 11.51 Fragmentation of the femoral heads in an 11-year-old with the osteochondritis dissecans-like form of multiple epiphyseal dysplasia

relatively normal. However, premature osteoarthritis is common [109].

Generally, MED takes two forms: (1) mild with flat epiphyseal centers (Ribbing type) or (2) severe with small, irregular centers as well as late-ossifying and irregular carpal bones (Fairbank type). It is uncertain whether these are separate entities, as a patient may have mild changes in one area and severe changes in another. Additionally, members of an affected family may demonstrate similar variability [110]. Abnormal ossification is most severe in the hips, knees, and wrists (Fig. 11.51). Lateral wedging of the distal tibial epiphysis may be the only abnormality at the ankle. Some families exhibit mild vertebral flattening, which may suggest spondyloepiphyseal dysplasia. Legg-Perthes disease-like AVN with femoral head collapse may develop [111]. Small ossification centers may hinder evaluation with radionuclide imaging. However, MRI demonstrates typical osteonecrosis affecting fragmented but otherwise normal bony centers [112].

8.5 Epiphyseal Dysgenesis in Hypothyroidism

Although characteristic of hypothyroidism, epiphyseal dysgenesis also develops in panhypopituitarism. Both are marked by delayed epiphyseal ossification. The ossific nucleus eventually demonstrates separate nodular or lamellar foci, so-called epiphyseal dysgenesis. The dysgenesis is indistinguishable from some epiphyseal dysplasias and may mimic the intermediate stage of Legg-Perthes disease, especially when the abnormality is unilateral. Skeletal age determination shows extreme delay, usually at least four standard deviations below the mean. Rapid recovery to normal epiphyseal shape and maturation may occur promptly after thyroid hormone therapy.

References

1. Petterson H, Theander G. Ossification of femoral head in infancy. I Normal standards. Acta Radiol Diagn (Stockh). 1979;20:170–9.
2. Johnson ND, Wood BP, Noh KS, Jackman KV, Westesson P-L, Katzberg RW. MR imaging of the infant hip. AJR Am J Roentgenol. 1989;53:127–33.
3. Ogden JA. Changing patterns of proximal femoral vascularity. J Bone Joint Surg Am. 1974;56(5):941–50.
4. Keats TE, Anderson MW. Atlas of normal roentgen variants that may simulate disease. Philadelphia: Elsevier Saunders; 2013.
5. Osborne D, Effmann E, Broda K, Harrelson J. The development of the upper end of the femur, with special reference to its internal architecture. Radiology. 1980;137:71–6.
6. Osborne D, Effmann E. Disturbances of trabecular architecture in the upper end of the femur in childhood. Skelet Radiol. 1981;6:165–73.
7. Stewart RJ, Patterson CC, Mollan RAB. Ossification of the normal femoral capital epiphysis. J Bone Joint Surg. 1986;68B:653–6.
8. Ozonoff MB, Ziter Jr FMH. The femoral head notch. Skelet Radiol. 1987;16:19–22.
9. Caffey J, Ross SE. The ischiopubic synchondrosis in healthy children: some normal roentgenologic findings. Am J Roentgenol Radium Ther Nucl Med. 1956;76:488–94.
10. Hemeth AM, Trattnig S, Bader TR, Ba-Ssalamah A, Ponhold W, Wandl-Vergesslick K, et al. MR imaging of the ischiopubic synchondrosis. Magn Reson Imaging. 2000;18:519–24.
11. Caffey J, Madell SH. Ossification of the pubic bones at birth. Radiology. 1956;67:346–50.
12. Perez-Rosello JM, Connolly SA, Newton AW, Thomason M, Jenny C, Sugar NF, Kleinman PK. Pubic ramus radiolucencies in infants: the good, the bad, and the indeterminate. AJR Am J Roentgenol. 2008;190:1481–6.
13. Biko DM, Davidson R, Pena A, Jaramillo D. Proximal focal femoral deficiency: evaluation by MR imaging. Pediatr Radiol. 2012;42:50–6.
14. Shapiro F. Developmental patterns in lower-extremity length discrepancies. J Bone Joint Surg. 1982;64A:639–51.
15. Tachdjian MO. Limb deficiencies. In: Herring JA, editor. Tachdjian's paediatric orthopaedics. 4th ed. Philadelphia: W. B. Saunders; 2007. p. 1983–2054.

16. Amstutz HC. The morphology, natural history, and treatment of proximal femoral focal deficiencies. In: Aitken GT, editor. Proximal femoral focal deficiency, a congenital anomaly. A symposium. Washington: National Academy of Sciences; 1969.
17. Aitken GT. Proximal femoral focal deficiency: definition, classification, and management. In: Aitken GT, editor. Proximal femoral focal deficiency, a congenital anomaly. A symposium. Washington, DC: National Academy of Sciences; 1969.
18. Pappas AM. Congenital abnormalities of the femur and related lower extremity malformations: classification and treatment. J Pediatr Orthop. 1983;3:45–60.
19. Grissom LE, Harcke HT. Sonography in congenital deficiency of the femur. J Pediatr Orthop. 1994;14:29–33.
20. Maldjian C, Patel TY, Klein RM, Smith RC. Efficacy of MRI in classifying proximal focal femoral deficiency. Skelet Radiol. 2007;36:215–20.
21. Gruel CR, Birch JG, Roach JW, Herring JA. Teratologic dislocation of the hip. J Pediatr Orthop. 1986;6:693–702.
22. Bialik V, Bialik GM, Blazer S, Sujov P, Wiener F, Berant M. Developmental dysplasia of the hip: a new approach to incidence. Pediatrics. 1999;103:93–9.
23. Keller MS, Weltin GG, Rattner Z, Taylor KJ, Rosenthal NS. Normal instability of the hip in the neonate: US standards. Radiology. 1988;169:733–9.
24. Theime WT, Wynne-Davies R, Blair HAF, Bell ET, Loraine JA. Clinical examination and urinary oestrogen assays in newborn children with congenital dislocation of the hip. J Bone Joint Surg. 1968;50B:546–50.
25. Vogel I, Andersson JE, Uldbjerg N. Serum relaxin in the newborn is not a marker of neonatal hip instability. J Pediatr Orthop. 1998;18:535–7.
26. von Heideken J, Green DW, Burke SW, Sindle K, Haglund-Akerlind Y, Widmann RF. The relationship between developmental dysplasia of the hip and congenital muscular torticollis. J Pediatr Orthop. 2006; 26:805–8.
27. Kumar SJ, MacEwen GD. Incidence of hip dysplasia with metatarsus adductus. Clin Orthop. 1982;164:234–5.
28. Paton RW, Choudry Q. Neonatal foot deformities and their relationship to developmental dysplasia of the hip: an 11-year prospective, longitudinal observational study. J Bone Joint Surg. 2009;91:655–8.
29. Hoaglund FT, Healey JH. Osteoarthrosis and congenital dysplasia of the hip in family members of children who have congenital dysplasia of the hip. J Bone Joint Surg. 1990;72A:1510–8.
30. Wynne-Davies R. Acetabular dysplasia and familial joint laxity: two etiological factors in congenital dislocation of the hip: a review of 589 patients and their families. J Bone Joint Surg. 1970;52B:704–16.
31. Yngve D, Gross R. Late diagnosis of hip dislocation in infants. J Pediatr Orthop. 1990;10:777–9.
32. Macnicol MF. Results of a 25-year screening programme for neonatal hip instability. J Bone Joint Surg. 1990;72B:1057–60.
33. Moore FH. Examining infant's hips—can it do harm? J Bone Joint Surg. 1989;71B:4–5.
34. Lee J. Developmental dysplasia of the hip: universal or selective ultrasound screening. Ann Acad Med. 2008;37:101–3.
35. Clarke NMP, Clegg J, Al-Chalabi AN. Ultrasound screening of the hips at risk for CDH: failure to reduce the incidence of late cases. J Bone Joint Surg. 1989;71B:9–12.
36. Committee on Quality Improvement, Subcommittee on Developmental Dysplasia of the Hip. American Academy of Pediatrics. Pediatrics. 2000;105: 896–905.
37. Grissom LE, Harcke HT. The pediatric hip and musculoskeletal ultrasound. In: Rumack CM, Wilson SR, Charboneau JW, Levine E, editors. Diagnostic ultrasound. 4th ed. Philadelphia: Elsevier; 2011. p. 1982–2005.
38. Harcke HT, Lee MS, Sinning L, Clarke NMP, Borns PF, MacEwen GD. Ossification center of the infant hip: sonographic and radiographic correlation. AJR Am J Roentgenol. 1986;147:317–21.
39. Bearcraft PW, Berman LH, Robinson AH, Butler GJ. Vascularity of the neonatal femoral head: in vivo demonstration with power Doppler US. Radiology. 1996;200:209–11.
40. Barnewolt CE, Jaramillo D, Taylor GA, Dunning PS. Correlation of contrast-enhanced power Doppler sonography and conventional angiography of abduction-induced hip ischemia in piglets. AJR Am J Roentgenol. 2003;180:1731–5.
41. Graf R. Hip sonography. Diagnosis and management of infant hip dysplasias. New York: Springer; 2006.
42. American College of Radiology. ACR-AIUM practice guideline for the performance of the ultrasound examination for detection and assessment of developmental dysplasia of the hip. 2008. http://www.acr.org/~/media/ACR/Documents/PGTS/guidelines/US_Hip_Dysplasia.pdf. Accessed 30 Aug 2012.
43. Morin C, Harcke HT, MacEwen GD. The infant hip: real-time US assessment of acetabular development. Radiology. 1985;157:673–7.
44. Morin C, Zouaoui S, Delvalle-Fayada A, Delforge PM, Leclet H. Ultrasound assessment of the acetabulum in the infant hip. Act Orthop Belgica. 1999;65:261–5.
45. Gunay C, Atalar H, Dogruel H, Yavuz OY, Uras I, Sayh U. Correlation of femoral head coverage and Graf alpha angle in infants being screened for developmental dysplasia of the hip. Int Orthop. 2009;33:761–4.
46. Czubak J, Kotwicki T, Piontek T, Skrzypek H. Ultrasound measurements of the newborn hip. Comparison of two methods in 657 newborns. Acta Orthop Scand. 1998;69(1):21–4.
47. Gaillard F, et al. Ultrasound classification of DDH. Available at: www.radiopaedia.org/articles/ultrasound-classification-of-ddh. Accessed 5 Jul 2012.
48. Caffey J. Contradiction of the congenital dysplasia-predislocation hypothesis of congenital dislocation of the hip through a study of the normal variation in acetabular angles at successive periods in infancy. Pediatrics. 1956;17(5):632–41.

49. Scoles PV, Boyd A, Jones PK. Roentgenographic parameters of the normal infant hip. J Pediatr Orthop. 1987;7:656–63.
50. Classic HH. Translation: Hilgenreiner on congenital hip dislocation. J Pediatr Orthop. 1986;6:212–4.
51. Perkins G. Signs by which to diagnose congenital dislocation of the hip. Lancet. 1928;214:648–50.
52. Parvizi J. Radiographic features: DDH. Wheeless' textbook of orthopaedics. Available at: www.wheelssonline.com/ortho/radiographic_features_ddh. Accessed 28 Jul 2012.
53. Harcke HT. The role of ultrasound in diagnosis and management of developmental dysplasia of the hip. Pediatr Radiol. 1995;25:225–7.
54. Harding MG, Harcke HT, Bowen JR, Guille JT, Glutting J. Management of dislocated hips with Pavlik harness treatment and ultrasound monitoring. J Pediatr Orthop. 1997;17(2):189–98.
55. Zdravkovic N, Stojanovic S. Early diagnosis of developmental hip dysplasia in the district of Pirot, Serbia. Med Biol. 2004;11:26–30.
56. Ozonoff MB. The radiological assessment of congenital dislocation of the hip. Curr Orthopaed. 1987;1(3):258–66.
57. Kotnis R, Spiteri V, Little C, Theologis T, Wainwright A, Benson MK. Hip arthrography in the assessment of children with developmental dysplasia of the hip and Perthes' disease. J Pediatr Orthop B. 2008;17(3):114–9.
58. Renshaw TS. Inadequate reduction of congenital dislocation of the hip. J Bone Joint Surg. 1981;63A:1114–21.
59. Dahlstrom H, Friber S, Oberg L. Stabilisation and development of the hip after closed reduction of late CDH. J Bone Joint Surg. 1990;72B:186–9.
60. Eggli KD, King SH, Boal DK, Quique T. Low-dose CT of developmental dysplasia of the hip after reduction: diagnostic accuracy and dosimetry. AJR Am J Roentgenol. 1994;163:1441–3.
61. Gould SW, Grissom LE, Niedzielski A, Kecskemethy HH, Bowen JR, Harcke HT. Protocol for MRI of the hips after spica cast placement. J Pediatr Orthop. 2012;32:504–9.
62. Tiderius C, Jaramillo D, Connolly S, Griffey M, Rodriguez DP, Kasser JR, Millis MB, Zurakowski D, Kim YJ. Post-closed reduction perfusion magnetic resonance imaging as a predictor of avascular necrosis in developmental hip dysplasia: a preliminary report. J Pediatr Orthop. 2009;29:14–20.
63. Jaramillo D, Connolly SA, Vajapeyam S, Robertson RL, Dunning PS, Mulkern RV, Hayward A, Maier SE, Shapiro F. Normal and ischemic epiphysis of the femur: diffusion MR imaging: study in piglets. Radiology. 2003;227:825–32.
64. Tonnis D. Normal values of the hip joint for the evaluation of x-rays in children and adults. Clin Orthop. 1976;119:39–47.
65. Wiberg G. A measuring method for distinguishing between a normal and maldeveloped acetabulum. Acta Chir Scand Suppl. 1939;58:28.
66. Chosa E, Tajima N. Anterior acetabular head index of the hip on false-profile views. New index of anterior acetabular cover. J Bone Joint Surg. 2003; 85B:826–9.
67. Crockarell Jr JR, Trousdale RT, Guyton JL. The anterior centre-edge angle. A cadaver study. J Bone Joint Surg. 2000;82B:532–4.
68. Bowen RJ, Kotzias-Neto J. Developmental dysplasia of the hip. Brooklandville: Data Trace Publishing Company; 2006.
69. Kotzias Neto A. Estudo dos valores angulares em toografia axial computadorizada de criancas com quadric normais. Master's thesis, Ortopedia e Traumatologia de Escola Paulista de Medicina, Universidade Federal de Sao Paulo, 1997.
70. Anda S, Terjesen T, Kvistad KA. Computed tomography measurements of the acetabulum in adult dysplastic hips: which level is appropriate. Skelet Radiol. 1991;20:267–71.
71. Anda S, Terjesen T, Kvistad KA, Svenningsen S. Acetabular angles and femoral anteversion in dysplastic hips in adults: CT investigation. J Comput Assist Tomogr. 1991;15:115–20.
72. Perreira AC, Hunter JC, Laird T, Jamali AA. Multilevel measurement of acetabular version using 3-D CT-generated models. Implications for hip preservation surgery. Clin Orthop Relat Res. 2011;469:552–61.
73. Tonnis D, Dortmund MD, Heinecke A. Acetabular and femoral anteversion: relationship with osteoarthritis of the hip. J Bone Joint Surg. 1999;81A:1747–70.
74. Grudziak JS, Ward T. Dega osteotomy for the treatment of congenital dysplasia of the hip. J Bone Joint Surg. 2001;83:845–54.
75. Salter RB, Kostuik J, Dallas S. Avascular necrosis of the femoral head as a complication of treatment for congenital dislocation of the hip in young children: a clinical and experimental investigation. Can J Surg. 1969;12:44–61.
76. Kruczynski J. Avascular necrosis of the proximal femur in developmental dislocation of the hip. Incidence, risk factors, sequelae and MR imaging for diagnosis and prognosis. Acta Orthop Scand Suppl. 1996;268:1–48.
77. Senaran H, Bowen JR, Harcke HT. Avascular necrosis rate in early reduction after failed Pavlik harness treatment of developmental dysplasia of the hip. J Pediatr Orthop. 2007;27:192–7.
78. Hadley NA, Brown TD, Weinstein S. The effects of contact pressure elevations and aseptic necrosis on the long-term outcome of congenital hip dislocation. J Orthop Res. 1990;8(4):504–13.
79. Kim YM, Oh HC, Kim HJ. The pattern of bone marrow oedema on MRI in osteonecrosis of the femoral head. J Bone Joint Surg. 2000;82B:837–41.
80. Gore DR. Iatrogenic avascular necrosis of the hip in young children: a review of six cases. J Bone Joint Surg. 1974;56A:493–502.
81. Bucholz RW, Ogden JA. Patterns of ischemic necrosis of the proximal femur in non-operatively treated congenital hip disease. In: The hip: Proceedings of

the sixth open scientific meeting of the Hip Society, pp 43–63. St Louis: CV Mosby, 1978.
82. Thomas CL, Gage JR, Ogden JA. Treatment concepts for proximal femoral ischemic necrosis complicating congenital hip disease. J Bone Joint Surg. 1982;64A:817–28.
83. O'Brien T. Growth-disturbance lines in congenital dislocation of the hip. J Bone Joint Surg. 1985;67A:626–32.
84. O'Brien T, Millis MB, Griffin PP. The early identification and classification of growth disturbances of the proximal end of the femur. J Bone Joint Surg. 1986;68A:970–80.
85. O'Brien T, Salter RB. Femoral head size in congenital dislocation of the hip. J Pediatr Orthop. 1985;5:299–301.
86. O'Hara JN. Congenital dislocation of the hip: acetabular deficiency in adolescence (absence of the lateral acetabular epiphysis) after limbectomy in infancy. J Pediatr Orthop. 1989;9:640–8.
87. Cooperman DR, Wallensten R, Stulberg SD. Postreduction avascular necrosis in congenital dislocation of the hip: long-term follow-up study of twenty-five patients. J Bone Joint Surg. 1980;62A:247–58.
88. Carter C, Wilkinson J. Persistent joint laxity and congenital dislocation of the hip. J Bone Joint Surg. 1964;46B:40–5.
89. Bennet GC, Rang M, Roye DP, Aprin H. Dislocation of the hip in trisomy 21. J Bone Joint Surg. 1982;64B:289–94.
90. Giunta C, Superti-furga A, Spranger S, Cole WG, Steinmann B. Ehlers-Danlos syndrome type VII: clinical features and molecular defects. J Bone Joint Surg. 1999;81A:225–38.
91. Cordes S, Dickens DRV, Cole WG. Correction of coxa vara in childhood. The use of Pauwels' y-shaped osteotomy. J Bone Joint Surg. 1991;73B:3–6.
92. Pavlov H, Goldman AB, Freiberger RH. Infantile coxa vara. Radiology. 1980;135:631–40.
93. Bos CF, Sakkers RJ, Bloem JL, van Stadt RJ, van Kamp JJ. Histological, biochemical, and MRI studies of the growth plate in congenital coxa vara. J Pediatr Orthop. 1989;9(6):660–5.
94. Weinstein JN, Kuo KN, Millar EA. Congenital coxa vara: a retrospective review. J Pediatr Orthop. 1984;4:70–7.
95. Kim HT, Chambers HG, Mubarak SJ, Wenger DR. Congenital coxa vara: computed tomographic analysis of femoral retroversion and the triangular metaphyseal fragment. J Pediatr Orthop. 2000;20(5):551–6.
96. Leunig M, Shane J, Turchetto L, Ganz R. New insights and experience with joint preservation. Protrusio acetabuli. Clin Orthop Relat Res. 2009;467:2241–50.
97. Alexander C. The aetiology of primary protrusion acetabuli. Br J Radiol. 1965;38:567–80.
98. Martinez S, Apple JS, Baber C, Putman CE, Rosse WF. Protrusio acetabuli in sickle-cell anemia. Radiology. 1984;151:43–4.
99. Rijke A, Pope TL, Keats T. Bilateral protrusion acetabuli in sickle cell anemia. Southern Med J. 1990;83:328–9.
100. Gusis SE, Babini JC, Garay SM, Morteo OG, Maldonado C, Occo JA. Evaluation of the measurement methods for protrusion acetabuli in normal children. Skelet Radiol. 1990;19:279–82.
101. Richards PJ, Pattison JM, Belcher J, Decann RW, Anderson S, Wynn-Jones C. A new tilt on pelvic radiographs: a pilot study. Skelet Radiol. 2009;38:113–22.
102. Mostert AK, Dijkstra PF, Jansen BR, van Horn JR, de Graaf B, Heutink P, Lindhout D. Familial multiple epiphyseal dysplasia due to a matrilin-3 mutation: further delineation of the phenotype including 40 years follow-up. Am J Med Genet A. 2003;120A:490–7.
103. Elsbach L. Bilateral hereditary micro-epiphyseal dysplasia of the hips. J Bone Joint Surg. 1959;41B:514–23.
104. Meyer J. Dysplasia epiphysealis capitis femoris: a clinical-radiological syndrome and its relationship to Legg-Calve-Perthes disease. Acta Orthop Scand. 1964;34:183–97.
105. Khermosh O, Wientroub S. Dysplasia epiphysealis capitis femoris. Meyer's dysplasia. J Bone Joint Surg Br. 1991;73:621–5.
106. Harel L, Kornreich L, Ashkenazi S, Rachmel A, Karmazyn B, Amir J. Meyer dysplasia in the differential diagnosis of hip disease in young children. Arch Pediatr Adolesc Med. 1999;153:942–5.
107. Muzaffar N, Song H, Devmurari K, Modi H. Meyer's dysplasia: delayed ossification of the femoral head as a differential diagnosis in Perthes' disease. Acta Orthop Belg. 2010;76:608–12.
108. Schlesinger AE, Poznanski AK, Pudlowski RM, Millar EA. Distal femoral epiphysis: normal standards for thickness and application to bone dysplasias. Radiology. 1986;159:515–9.
109. Treble NJ, Jenson FO, Bankier A, Rogers JG, Cole WG. Development of the hip in multiple epiphyseal dysplasia. Natural history and susceptibility to premature osteoarthritis. J Bone Joint Surg. 1990;72B:1061–4.
110. Spranger JW, Langer Jr LO, Weidemann HR. Bone dysplasias: an atlas of constitutional disorders of skeletal development. Philadelphia: WB Saunders; 1974.
111. Ozonoff MB. The diagnosis of femoral head dysplasia in children: isolated and generalized forms. Presented before the ninth annual refresher course in musculoskeletal disorders. San Francisco: International Skeletal Society; 1982.
112. Mandell GA, Mackenzie WG, Scott Jr CI, Harcke HT, Wills JS, Bassett GS. Identification of avascular necrosis in the dysplastic proximal femoral epiphysis. Skelet Radiol. 1989;18:273–81.

The Pelvis and Hip: Acquired Disorders

12

Lauren W. Averill and Mihir M. Thacker

Contents

L.W. Averill, MD (✉)
Department of Medical Imaging, Nemours/AI duPont Hospital for Children, 1600 Rockland Road, Wilmington, DE 19803, USA

Department of Radiology, Sidney Kimmel Medical College of Thomas Jefferson University, Philadelphia, PA, USA
e-mail: lauren.averill@nemours.org

M.M. Thacker, MD
Department of Orthopaedic Surgery, Nemours/AI duPont Hospital for Children, 1600 Rockland Road, Wilmington, DE 19803, USA

Department of Orthopedic Surgery, Sidney Kimmel Medical College of Thomas Jefferson University, Philadelphia, PA, USA
e-mail: mihir.thacker@nemours.org

Abstract

This chapter first presents the general pathophysiology of avascular necrosis (AVN) of the femoral head. Extensive discussion of different manifestations of AVN follows, including Legg Perthes disease, Gaucher disease, sickle cell disease and other hemoglobinopathies, corticosteroid-induced osteonecrosis, avascular necrosis in treated developmental hip dislocation, posttraumatic femoral head necrosis, avascular necrosis in osteomyelitis and septic arthritis, and femoral head dysplasia. Femoral acetabular impingement is then reviewed. Sections on slipped capital femoral epiphysis, traumatic hip fracture and dislocation, and apophyseal injuries of the adolescent hip follow. The chapter concludes with brief discussions of transient synovitis, septic arthritis, juvenile idiopathic arthritis, and synovial chondromatosis.

R. Stein-Wexler et al. (eds.), *Pediatric Orthopedic Imaging*,
DOI 10.1007/978-3-642-45381-6_12, © Springer-Verlag Berlin Heidelberg 2015

Hip pain is a relatively common and nonspecific complaint in childhood. The most common acquired causes of hip pain are stratified by age: Legg-Perthes disease is most common between the ages of 4 and 8, whereas slipped capital femoral epiphysis predominates in pre- and early adolescence. However, other entities span all ages, and although clinical factors often help differentiate, imaging plays a crucial role in establishing these diagnoses.

1 Traumatic Hip Fracture and Dislocation

Both fractures and traumatic dislocations of the femoral head and neck are uncommon in children. Femoral neck fractures are estimated to occur 130 times more often in adults than in children. Although in most parts of the body, trauma usually produces a growth plate fracture, most hip fractures in children occur through the mid-portion or occasionally base of the femoral neck [1]. Residual deformity occurs in more than 80 %, including avascular necrosis (20 %), femoral head enlargement (10 %), and coxa vara (10 %) [2].

Traumatic hip dislocation is uncommon. Likely a result of relative joint laxity in young children, the prognosis is excellent in patients younger than 5 years of age. Young children also have a lower incidence of associated acetabular or femoral head fractures. However, avascular necrosis is seen in about 10 % of patients and is usually associated with severe regional trauma, proximal femoral or pelvic fractures, and delay in reduction. Almost one-half eventually develop relative coxa magna of 2 mm. Even when suspected, associated labral tears are difficult to demonstrate with arthrography and magnetic resonance imaging (MRI).

Hip fractures and dislocation are most commonly caused by high-energy trauma such as motor vehicle accidents and falls from a height. Approximately 30 % of cases are associated with other major injuries, including abdominopelvic visceral injury and head injury. Underlying bone pathology, such as simple or aneurysmal bone cyst, osteogenesis inperfecta, fibrous dysplasia, or osteopenia, increases susceptibility to hip fracture.

Imaging

Frontal and cross-table lateral radiographs are usually sufficient to diagnosis hip fractures. The Delbet system classifies traumatic pediatric hip fracture [3]. Type I fractures (transepiphyseal separations) are the least common and occur primarily in young children; they are similar to Salter-Harris Type I epiphyseal fractures. Delbet Type II fractures (transcervical) are the most common hip fractures in older children and adolescents. Delbet Type III fractures (cervicotrochanteric) are the second most common. Delbet Type IV fractures (intertrochanteric) have the best overall outcome and lowest risk for avascular necrosis (Fig. 12.1). Incidence of avascular necrosis is highest with Delbet Type I and II injuries.

Femoral head dislocations are largely posterior (Fig. 12.2). Most hip dislocations in children can be treated with closed reduction. However, post-reduction radiographs should be evaluated for joint space asymmetry, as soft-tissue interposition may prevent congruous hip reduction and

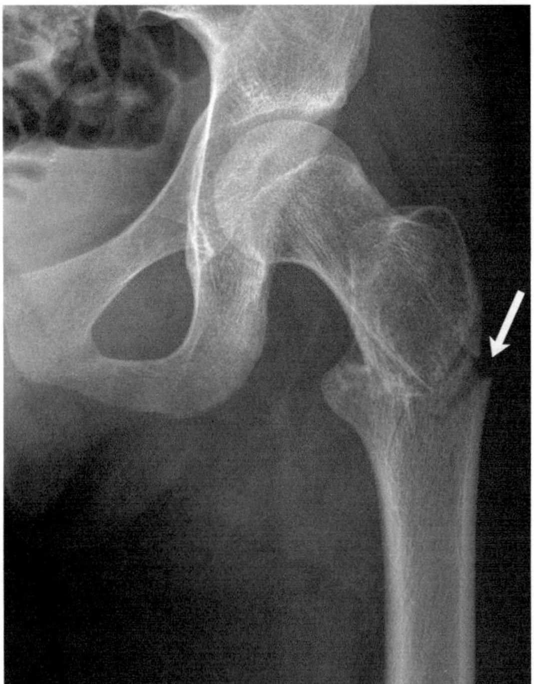

Fig. 12.1 Intertrochanteric fracture in a 15-year-old girl whose leg tangled in a swing as she fell. The fracture (*arrow*) required plate and screw fixation

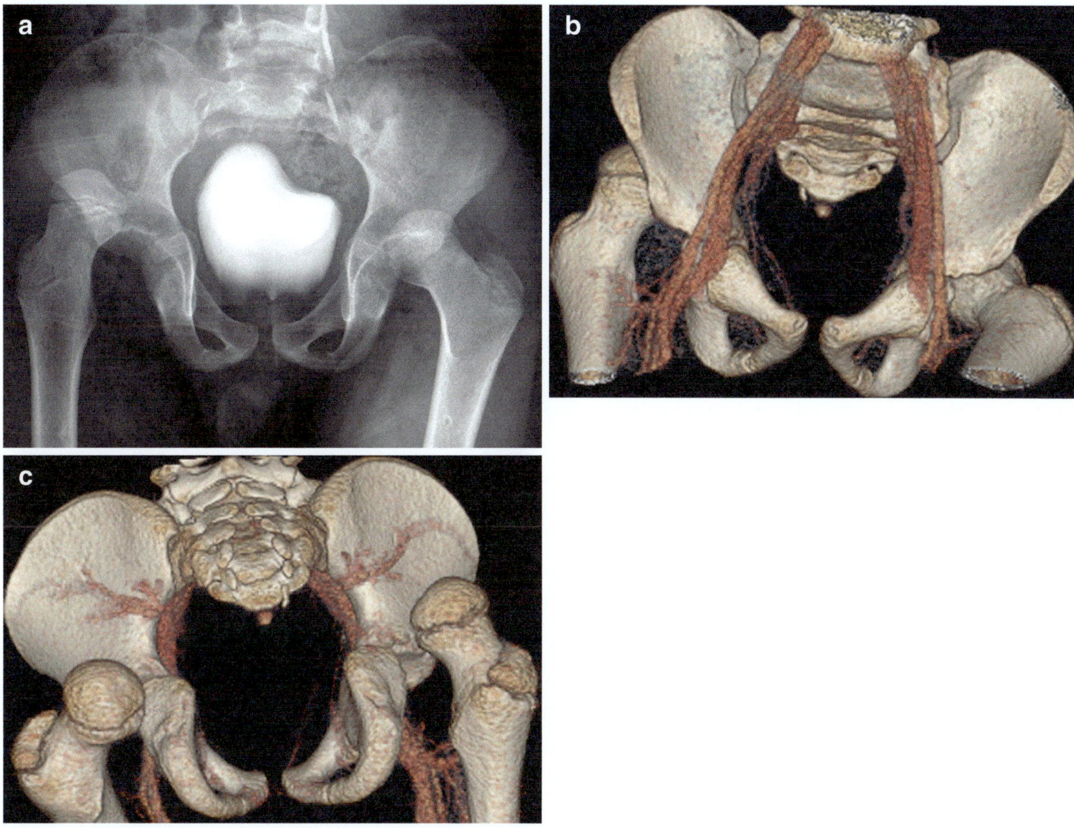

Fig. 12.2 Bilateral acute posterior hip dislocations in a 6-year-old boy after a motor vehicle accident. (**a**) Both hips are dislocated, and there is no obvious fracture. Anterior (**b**) and posterior (**c**) views from contrast-enhanced three-dimensional (3D) computed tomography (CT) reformation with surface rendering more clearly display the relationship of the dislocated femoral heads to their respective acetabula

necessitate open reduction. The labrum, capsule, lateral acetabular apophysis, avulsed ligamentum teres, and osteochondral fragments may become entrapped [4]. If there is joint space asymmetry after closed reduction of hip dislocation, computed tomography (CT) can help evaluate for intraarticular osteochondral fragments and subtle acetabular fractures, whereas MRI best evaluates soft-tissue interposition. Although MRI cannot predict avascular necrosis, it can help characterize this after hip fracture or dislocation [5].

2 Apophyseal Injuries

Overuse injuries of the hip are increasing as more adolescents become involved in year-round competitive sports. Apophyseal injury around the hip is most commonly encountered in the mid- to late teen period, after the long bone growth spurt. At this time, the physis is the most biomechanically vulnerable component of the muscle-tendon-bone axis (whereas in skeletally mature individuals, similar stress typically leads to injury of the tendon or the myotendinous junction instead). The ischial tuberosity at the hamstring tendon attachment site is most often affected [6] (Fig. 12.3). Other apophyses that may be injured include the anterior inferior iliac spine (insertion site for the rectus femoris); the anterior superior iliac spine (sartorius); the iliac crest (abdominal oblique); and the lesser trochanter (iliopsoas) (Figs. 12.4, 12.5, and 12.6). Chronic repetitive stress may lead to apophyseal strain, presenting as dull, activity-related pain near the hip. An acute apophyseal avulsion fracture, on the other hand, presents as acute, localized pain and swelling, exacerbated by palpation or stretching.

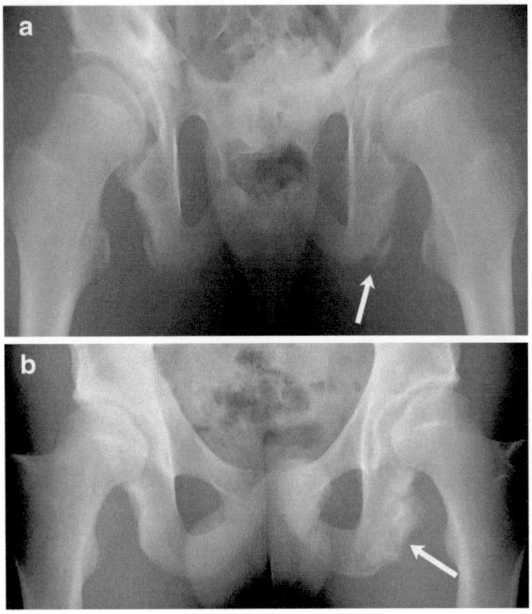

Fig. 12.3 Avulsion of the ischial tuberosity in a 14-year-old soccer player with left hamstring pain for 3 months. (**a**) Outlet view shows avulsion of the left ischial tuberosity (*arrow*) with irregularity and indistinctness of the underlying bone margin. Ossification center on the right is normal. (**b**) Three years later, frontal radiograph shows mature exuberant bone production at the avulsion site (*arrow*), whereas the ossification center on the right has fused

Chronic repetitive stress at the apophyseal growth plates about the hip may cause microfractures and secondary inflammation, akin to a Salter-Harris I stress fracture. However, an acute apophyseal avulsion fracture is caused by sudden eccentric muscle contraction, often during deceleration or landing. This leads to fracture through the growth plate and separation of the apophysis. These injuries are most commonly seen in adolescent athletes whose sports involve kicking, jumping, and rapid acceleration/deceleration such as soccer, football, gymnastics, sprinting, and ice hockey.

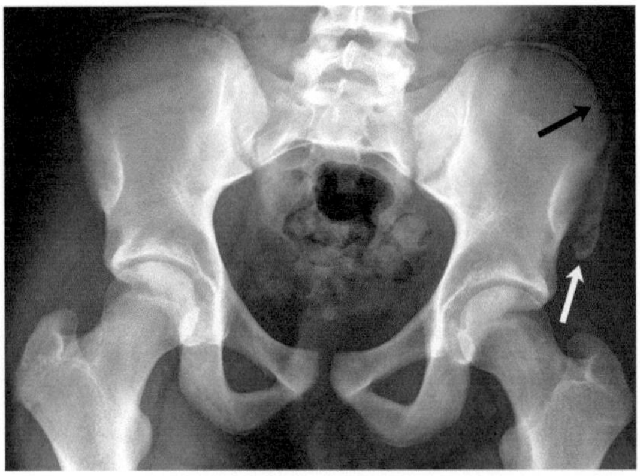

Fig. 12.4 Acute avulsion of the anterior superior iliac spine in a 15-years-old who developed sudden, excruciating left hip pain while playing football. There is acute avulsion of the left anterior superior iliac spine (*white arrow*) as well as the lateral aspect of the iliac crest apophysis (*black arrow*)

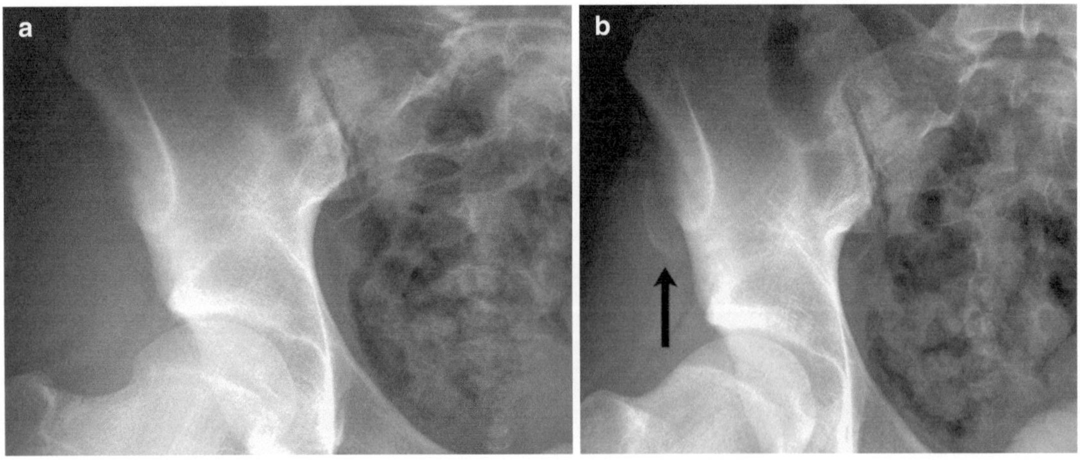

Fig. 12.5 Avulsion of the anterior superior iliac crest in a 16-year-old boy who developed severe right hip pain and heard a "pop" while sprinting. The avulsion is hidden on the straight frontal neutral view (**a**) but is clearly seen (*arrow*) with frog lateral positioning and slight tilt of the pelvis (**b**)

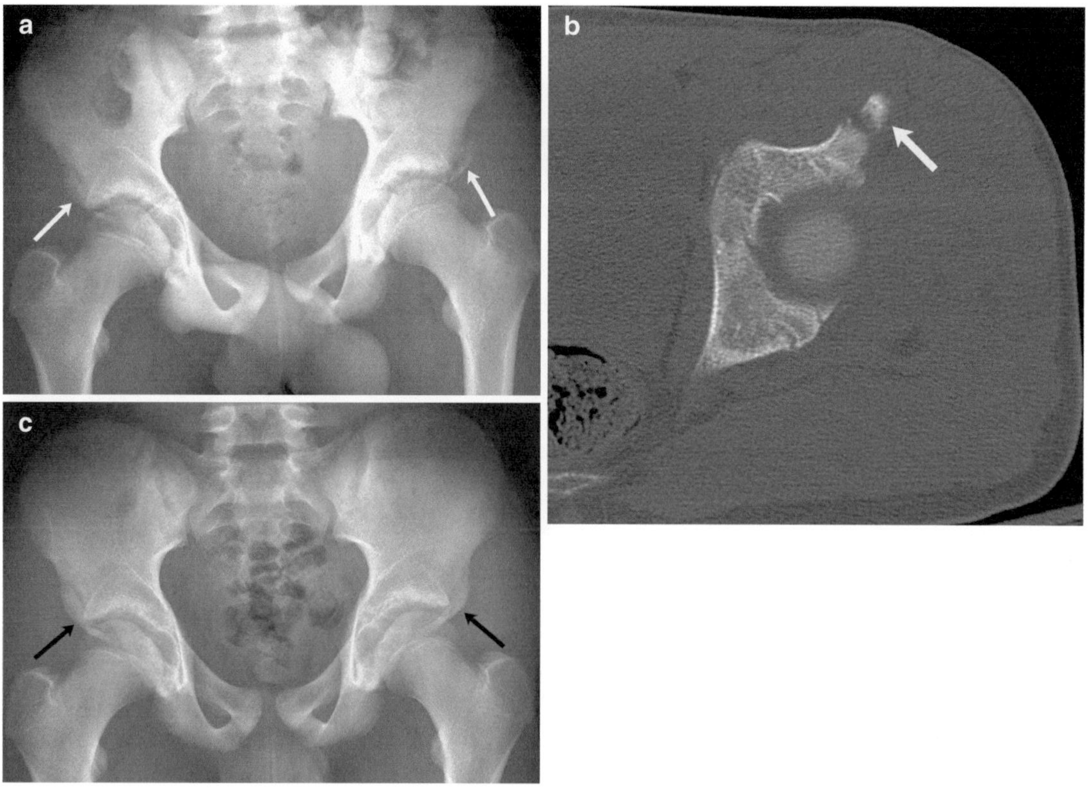

Fig. 12.6 Bilateral fractures of the anterior inferior iliac spine (AIIS) in a 13-year-old boy with sudden hip pain while playing soccer. (**a**) There is an acute avulsion fracture of the left AIIS and a healed avulsion fracture of the right AIIS as well (*arrows*). (**b**) CT at the time of injury shows mild displacement of the apophysis (*arrow*). (**c**) Four months later, bilateral AIIS fractures have healed and appear symmetric (*arrows*)

Apophyseal injuries are treated conservatively with rest and ice followed by gradual return to weight bearing and physical therapy. Surgical intervention is rarely needed but may be undertaken if a large, displaced fragment causes ongoing pain or if there is unstable nonunion.

Imaging

In chronic apophyseal strain, the physis may appear normal or mildly wide and irregular, but the apophysis is not displaced. If the ischial tuberosity has not yet fully ossified at the time of stress, a fracture fragment may not be evident but the bone margin may appear sclerotic and irregular, suggesting infection or tumor. With acute apophyseal avulsion, the apophysis is variably displaced. If the acute event is missed and imaging performed later, then well-rounded soft-tissue ossification may be seen near the expected location of the apophysis.

Ultrasound (US) can demonstrate tendonopathy associated with apophyseal strain, with a thickened and echogenic tendon insertion. CT is rarely needed for diagnosis or treatment planning, but it can clearly show the pelvic avulsion fracture. Especially in cases that are unclear clinically, MRI may be useful to demonstrate edema in the apophysis and adjacent bone and sometimes in the enthesis as well (Fig. 12.7).

Although overuse injuries are more common in adults, they are also seen in athletic adolescents. These include femoral neck or pelvic stress fractures (Fig. 12.8), tendonosis involving the iliopsoas and adductor tendons, the iliotibial band "snapping hip" syndrome, athletic pubalgia (Fig. 12.9), and labral tears.

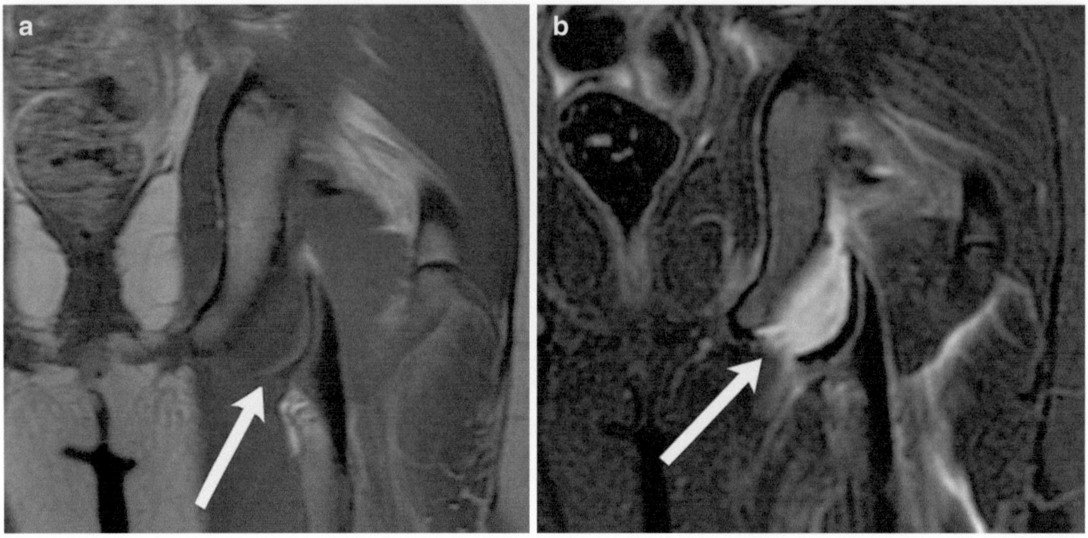

Fig. 12.7 Avulsion fracture of the left ischial tuberosity. (**a**) Coronal T1-weighted (T1-W) magnetic resonance image (MRI) demonstrates separation of the cortex (*arrow*) at the left ischial tuberosity from the underlying bone. (**b**) Coronal short tau inversion recovery (STIR) image shows fluid in the gap between the two bone fragments (*arrow*), along with edema in the surrounding musculature (Courtesy of J. Herman Kan)

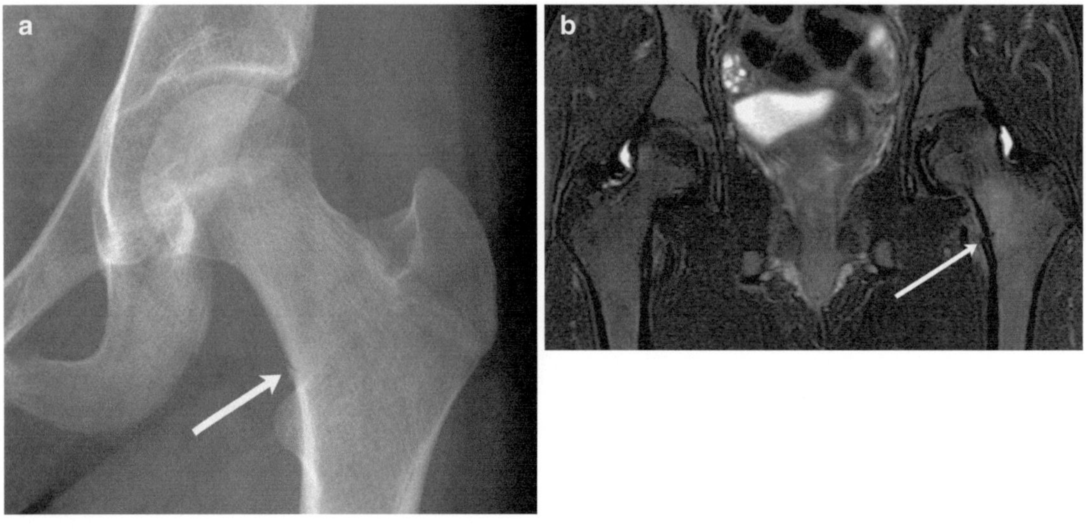

Fig. 12.8 Stress fracture in a 15-year-old girl with history of an eating disorder, who presented with left hip pain after increasing the intensity of her cross-country training. (**a**) There is a stress fracture (*arrow*) in the medial cortex of the base of the femoral neck. (**b**) Coronal T2-weighted (T2-W) fat-suppressed (FS) magnetic resonance (MR) image shows mild cortical offset at the fracture site (*arrow*) with surrounding bone marrow and soft-tissue edema

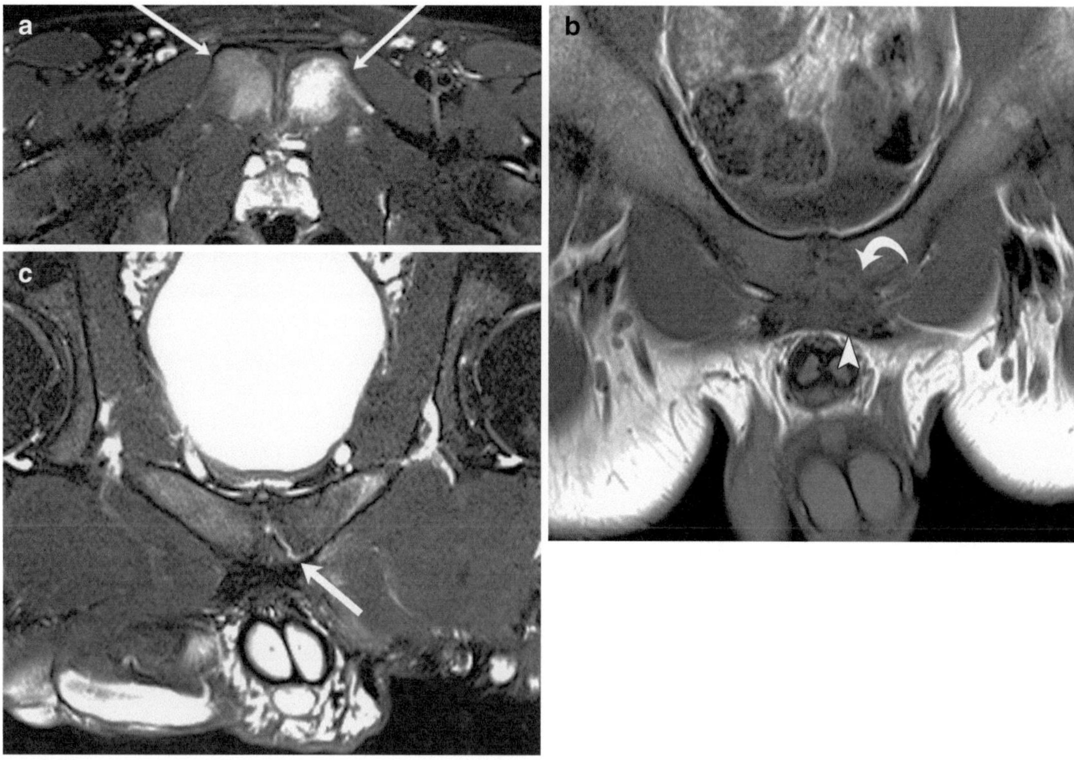

Fig. 12.9 Athletic pubalgia in two teenage male soccer players with groin pain. Axial T2-W FS (**a**) and coronal oblique T1-W (**b**) images of a 14-year-old boy show severe osteitis pubis (*arrows*), with midline pubic plate injury involving detachment of the left side of the rectus aponeurosis (*arrowhead*) and pubic apophysis (*curved arrow*). Coronal oblique T2-W FS image (**c**) in a 19-year-old man shows a left-sided sub-apophyseal aponeurosis injury, with fluid cleft (*arrow*). Athletic pubalgia is seen in young adult high-level athletes (Courtesy of Adam Zoga)

3 Slipped Capital Femoral Epiphysis

3.1 Epidemiology

Slipped capital femoral epiphysis (SCFE) typically develops in obese young adolescents, and, although it can result from local infection or trauma, it usually occurs in response to routine activity. This shearing disruption of the growth plate and subsequent slip of the femoral head is most often encountered during periods of rapid growth. The epiphyseal slip thus affects boys about 2 years later (age 12–15, median 13 years) than girls, who generally exhibit symptoms before menarche. SCFE is the most common hip abnormality of adolescence, with an annual incidence of approximately 11 per 100,000 [7]. The condition occurs almost twice as often in boys as in girls, possibly due to their more vigorous activity and a longer and more intense growth spurt. Incidence increases in warm weather, suggesting that environmental trauma may be a factor. One-half of patients have a history of significant injury antecedent to diagnosis of the epiphyseal slip. At presentation, approximately 10 % of slips are bilateral.

Several other demographic features are of interest. For unknown reasons, SCFE is nearly four times more common in black children than in white children in the United States [7]. The condition is also more frequently seen in Native Americans, Hispanics, and Asian/Pacific Islanders compared to white children. Regardless of race, incidence is much higher in those who are overweight, with more than 80 % of children diagnosed with SCFE having a body mass index greater than the 95th percentile [8]. The incidence of SCFE has increased over the past 40 years, mirroring the trend of childhood obesity [9]. In addition, skeletal maturity is often mildly delayed. Although 40 % have a bone age within one standard deviation above the mean, few are more mature than this and 60 % are below the mean. The combination of being overweight and skeletally immature means children with SCFE are often both short and heavy. SCFE in a tall, thin child is quite unusual.

3.2 Etiology

Although the predisposing factors are known, the actual precipitating event and pathogenesis of epiphyseal slip are not well understood. Because SCFE is often linked to the adolescent growth spurt, a hormonal etiology or substrate is likely, but investigation has found that growth hormone levels in these patients are normal. Nonetheless, there is a substantial increased risk for SCFE in children with endocrinopathies, especially those with hypothyroidism and those treated with growth hormone. SCFE occasionally appears to be familial [10].

During adolescence, the shear strength of the upper femoral growth plate increases and becomes more dependent on the internal anatomy of the growth plate than on the perichondral complex. In overweight children, forces generated by usual activity (which can be up to six to ten times body mass) are sufficient to produce shear fracture of the proximal femoral growth plate experimentally. After epiphyseal slip, the otherwise normal growth plate shows a fracture-like cleft meandering through the degenerative zone and the cartilage-bone junction [11].

The biomechanical stresses that most likely produce growth plate shear are abduction and external rotation, especially in extension; decreased femoral anteversion may also play a role. The muscles around the hip insert into the region below the greater trochanter laterally and in a spiral fashion. All but the adductors pull the shaft anterolaterally and encourage external rotation. If a shear fracture occurs through the growth plate, the femoral epiphysis will remain within the acetabulum, appearing to be displaced posterior and medial with respect to the upper femur. However, it is actually the femoral shaft that has moved anterolaterally.

Idiopathic SCFE must be distinguished from the pathologic growth plate and metaphyseal fractures that occur in renal osteodystrophy with secondary hyperparathyroidism and that follow radiation therapy. Careful evaluation will show the actual slip in these cases to be within the metaphysis, not at the growth plate.

3.3 Presentation

Diagnosis of idiopathic SCFE can be difficult, as early symptoms are often vague, including mild weakness, fatigue, or limp. About one-half of children with SCFE present with hip pain, while one-fourth complain of knee pain. Onset of symptoms can be abrupt or insidious, developing over several months, and it is common for diagnosis to be delayed by several months. In cases that progress slowly, the child may walk with a limp, hold the leg in external rotation, and have limited, painful internal rotation. If onset of symptoms is sudden (in the setting of acute athletic trauma), pain is usually severe, and there is often marked epiphyseal displacement.

3.4 Prognosis

With subacute to chronic symptoms, diagnosis may be delayed, especially if the child is initially evaluated in the primary care setting. This is unfortunate, since delayed diagnosis may result in increased slippage (Fig. 12.10). Once identified, the child with SCFE needs to be closely evaluated for bilateral disease. Both hips will eventually be involved in 20–80 % of cases [8]. Most contralateral slips develop within 1 year of diagnosis. Contralateral slip is most common in younger children and has been found in all children whose SCFE occurred before age 10. Girls less than 12 years old and boys less than

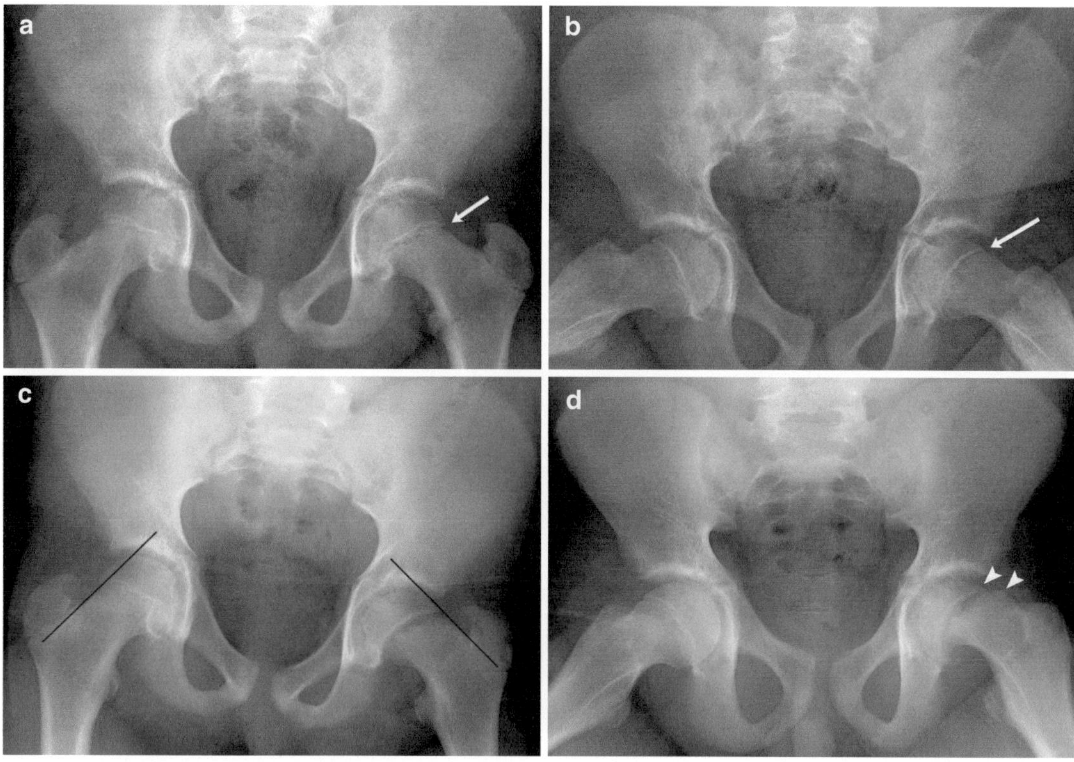

Fig. 12.10 Slipped capital femoral epiphysis (SCFE) in a 14-year-old boy with intermittent hip pain for several months, presenting with increased left hip pain after falling off his bicycle. (**a**) (neutral), (**b**) (frog lateral). Subtle left hip physeal widening without femoral head offset (*arrows*) was initially missed. (**c**) (neutral), (**d**) (frog lateral). Eleven days later, after another bicycle fall and increased left hip pain, the slip is much more evident. No portion of the left femoral head lies lateral to a line drawn along the femoral neck tangent, but a small amount of the normal right femoral head does. There is now approximately 25 % offset of the left femoral head and neck (*arrowheads*), still mild according to the Wilson grading method

14 are also at increased risk [12]. The modified Oxford bone age score, based on features of the proximal femur and acetabulum, can more reliably predict risk of subsequent contralateral slip, with less skeletally mature children at greater risk (Table 12.1) [13, 14]. For example, the risk of a subsequent contralateral slip in a child with a modified Oxford score of 16 is about 85 %. Postoperative weight loss in obese children can reduce the risk of contralateral slip [15].

Depending on their ability to bear weight and/or the results of orthopedic manipulation on evaluation, hips are considered either "stable" (able to walk with/out crutches) or "unstable" (unable to walk). Treatment, as described below, consists primarily of in situ stabilization with a screw across the physis. For unstable hips presenting less than 24 h after onset of symptoms, gentle repositioning can be attempted prior to fixation. Early complications include slip progression, hardware failure, avascular necrosis, and chondrolysis. Unstable SCFE has a much higher incidence of avascular necrosis (up to 50 % in some series) compared with stable SCFE (nearly 0 %), likely due to retinacular vascular injury at the time of initial displacement [16]. Other risk factors for the development of avascular necrosis include (a) over-reduction of an acute (unstable) SCFE or attempting reduction of a chronic SCFE, (b) placement of pins in the superolateral femoral head, or (c) performing a femoral neck osteotomy for correction of SCFE [17]. Avascular necrosis is radiographically evident within 1 year after the slip [17].

Table 12.1 Modified Oxford method of assessing skeletal maturity

Location	Point score	Determining features
Femoral head	5	Proximal femoral neck straight
		Fovea poorly defined
		Beak at distal medial epiphysis
	6	Epiphysis wider than neck
		Fovea clearly defined
	7	Physis closing
Greater trochanter	4	Peak or nodule tops greater trochanter
	5	Space between nodule and femoral neck smoothly filled with bone
	6	Physis closing
Lesser trochanter	3	Physis open
	4	Physis closing
	5	Physis closed
Triradiate cartilage	1	Open
	2	Partially closed
	3	Closed
Ilium	3	No ossification of iliac crest apophysis
	4	Apophysis beginning to ossify

Adapted from Stasikelis et al. [14]
Point score from each of the five locations is summed to give the modified Oxford score

Chondrolysis, a rapid loss of cartilage in the hip joint, follows SCFE in a small minority of patients (see section below). Although not etiologically related, chondrolysis can coincide with avascular collapse of the femoral head and usually occurs within 1 year of the epiphyseal slip. Chondrolysis is common after severe epiphyseal slips but sometimes occurs in the immobilized normal hip during treatment of the opposite side. It occurs in untreated as well as surgically operated hips, especially if fixation hardware penetrates the cartilage. The etiology of chondrolysis with SCFE is unknown. Synovial and capsular fibrosis and adhesions could potentially lead to a decrease or alteration in the synovial fluid with subsequent impairment of cartilage nutrition. Immunologic changes have been documented but may be secondary rather than causative.

Late complications of SCFE include osteoarthritis, "pistol-grip" deformity leading to femoroactabular impingement (see section below) (Fig. 12.11), and limb length discrepancy due to premature closure of the growth plate. Epiphyseal slip during adolescence is thought to predispose adults to osteoarthritis. For chronic slips in general, approximately three-fourths of patients will have good outcomes, whereas one-fourth will progress to premature osteoarthritis. However, the long-term prognosis for pinned mild chronic slip is excellent.

3.5 Treatment

Treatment of SCFE attempts to stabilize slip and prevent further displacement, stimulate early growth plate closure, and prevent complications such as avascular necrosis, chondrolysis, and osteoarthritis [18]. Manipulation and attempted reduction are associated with an increased incidence of avascular necrosis, although this approach may be considered in acute, unstable SCFE presenting less than 24 h after onset of symptoms. At least in theory, relieving acute kinking of epiphyseal blood vessels may restore blood flow.

Further slip is generally prevented by mechanical fixation of the femoral epiphysis relative to the femoral neck (see Fig. 12.11). A single cannulated screw is employed most often, though occasionally a second pin is placed if the slip is very unstable. Care should be taken to ensure that all stabilizing devices are in fact within the bone, not protruding through the femoral head into the joint space. Even with biplane right angle radiographs, this can be difficult due to the spherical nature of the femoral head. Sometimes CT is helpful, but artifact from hardware may limit its utility.

For severe SCFE with a high likelihood of developing femoroacetabular impingement, slip reduction using the modified Dunn procedure can be considered [19]. In this newer surgical technique, the hip is dislocated via greater trochanter osteotomy, preserving the blood supply to the femoral head to reduce the risk for avascular necrosis. Femoral neck osteotomies may also be performed at the time of original surgery or afterwards to realign the hip, but these are associated with increased incidence of avascular necrosis.

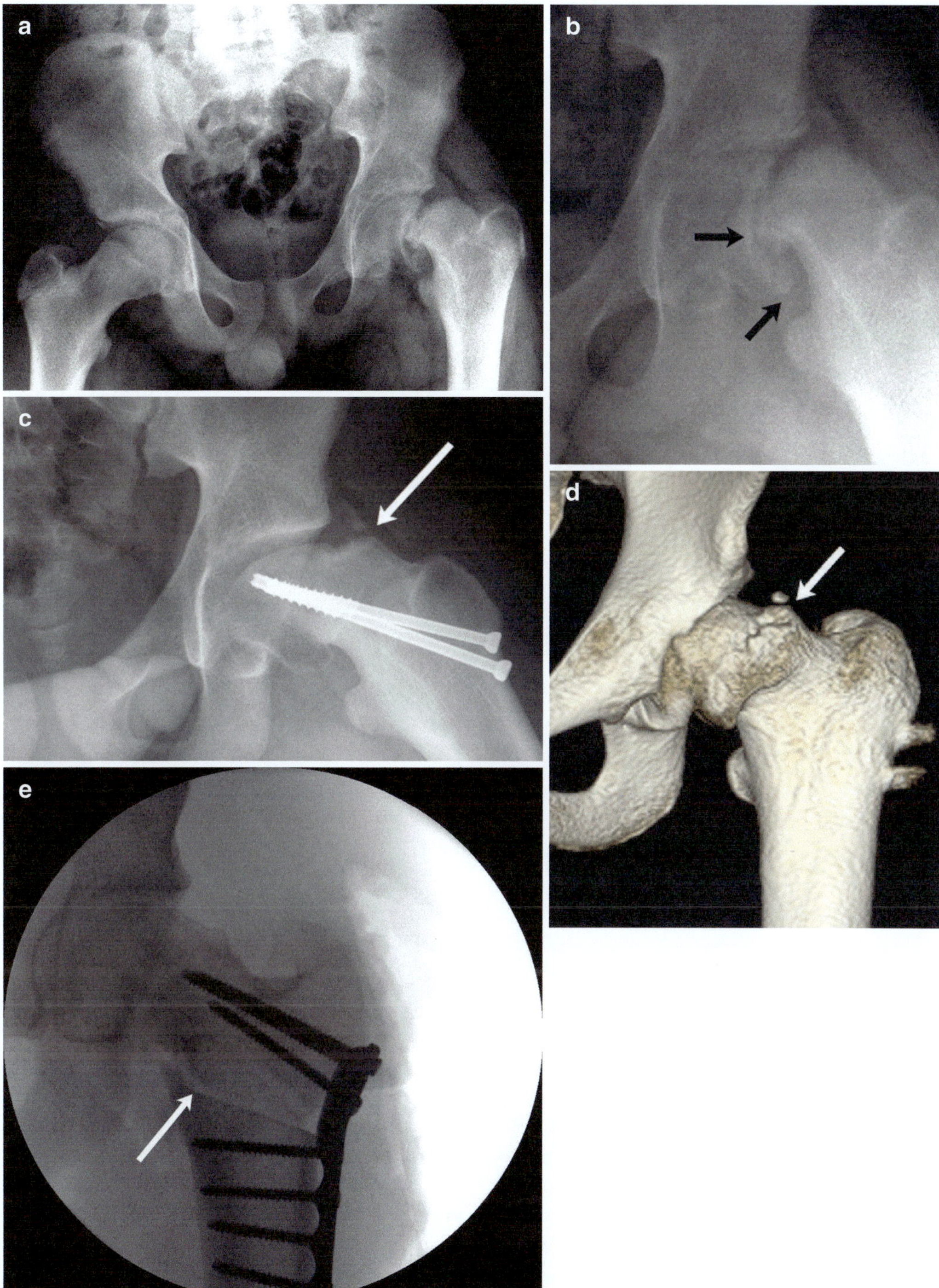

Fig. 12.11 SCFE and resultant femoroacetabular impingement in a 15-year-old boy complaining of left hip and knee pain 3 months after falling off a porch. (**a**) (neutral), (**b**) (frog lateral). There is approximately 50 % slip of the femoral head in relation to the neck (*small arrows*), moderate to severe according to the Wilson grading method. The patient underwent immediate screw fixation (**c**, frog lateral). At 1.5 years follow-up, there is significant pistol-grip deformity of the femoral head and neck with a large bony bump along the lateral femoral neck (*arrow*), resulting in limited range of motion. (**d**) Preoperative 3D-CT also shows the bony bump (*arrow*) causing femoroacetabular impingement. (**e**) After proximal femoral osteotomy (*arrow*), alignment is improved

Prophylactic contralateral pinning is commonly employed, especially if patients have known endocrinopathy, are young, or are likely to be lost to follow-up.

3.6 Imaging (Box 12.1)

Radiography

It is difficult to confirm mild epiphyseal slips solely with a frontal projection. Demineralization of the femoral head and neck is usually evident. The growth plate may appear wide, probably owing in part to angulation following the slip (see Fig. 12.10). Increased opacity, generally below the growth plate, results from density caused by either the slipped and superimposed base of the epiphysis or by reactive sclerosis in the metaphysis. While a line drawn along the lateral femoral neck (Klein line) in a normal patient will intercept the epiphyseal ossification center so that a small portion of femoral head lies lateral to this line, with SCFE there is either no femoral head ossification center lateral to the line or the amount is less than on the normal side (see Fig. 12.10). In addition, rotation may make the height of the epiphysis appear smaller than on the unaffected side. These signs are often quite helpful but may be equivocal, and a frog or true lateral projection may be necessary to confirm the diagnosis.

Box 12.1: Imaging Features of Slipped Capital Femoral Epiphysis

Frontal radiographs	Wide physis
	No femoral head lateral to Klein line
	Smaller femoral head due to rotation
Lateral radiographs (frog or true lateral)	Offset of femoral head relative to neck
MRI	Wide physis
	Increased signal on fluid-sensitive sequences
	Periphyseal edema
	Joint effusion
Nuclear scintigraphy	Increased proximal femoral physeal activity

If an acute slip is suspected, a true lateral projection of the hip and pelvis avoids the stress of positioning the patient for the frog lateral position, which may increase slippage. Unfortunately the resultant radiograph is often suboptimal in obese children. A modified rolled lateral hip view may be useful, as it is less painful than performing the frog lateral. In any of these lateral projections, the anterior and posterior corners of the epiphysis and metaphysis should closely match. Consistent displacement of these points indicates an epiphyseal slip. Occasionally, a second image with a rotated thigh is needed to confirm osseous offset.

If the epiphyseal slip is not recent, reactive bone will have formed along the medial and posterior femoral neck, buttressing the posteriorly and medially displaced femoral epiphysis. With very severe slips, the lateral portion of the femoral neck articulates with the acetabulum, and remodeling generally incorporates this into the functional femoral head. Premature fusion of the growth plate may result in femoral shortening.

Frog lateral radiographs can be employed to grade the severity of chronic slips [18] (Box 12.2). The Wilson method calculates the degree of femoral head displacement relative to the metaphysis (see Fig. 12.11). Less than one-third displacement is considered mild, one-third to one-half displacement moderate, and greater than one-half displacement severe. The Southwick method compares the angle between the femoral head and shaft on both hips in the frog lateral view. Subtraction of the head-shaft angle of the uninvolved hip from the head-shaft angle of the involved hip calculates the slip angle. Less than a 30° difference is mild, 30–60° moderate, and greater than 60° severe.

Nuclear Scintigraphy

In cases of hip pain with negative or equivocal radiographs, a technetium-99m methylene diphosphonate (Tc-99m MDP) bone scan can demonstrate early SCFE and increased proximal femoral physeal activity (Fig. 12.12). Pre- and postsurgical Tc-99m MDP bone scans can occasionally help

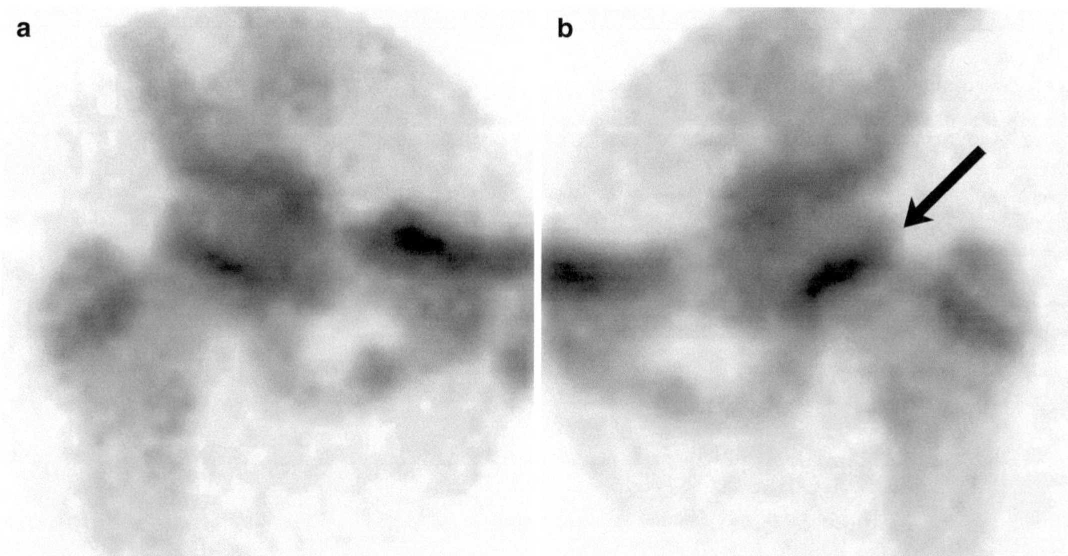

Fig. 12.12 SCFE in an 11-year-old girl with left hip pain. Pinhole images of the normal right (**a**) and symptomatic left (**b**) hips from Tc-99 MDP bone scan show asymmetrically increased activity in the left proximal femoral physis (*arrow*) compared to the right. Subsequent evaluation confirmed the diagnosis of SCFE on the left

Box 12.2: Grading of Slipped Capital Femoral Epiphysis Using Frog or True Lateral Hip Radiographs

Grade	Wilson method: amount of femoral head displacement	Southwick method: slip angle
Mild	Less than 1/3	0–30°
Moderate	1/3 to 1/2	30–60°
Severe	Greater than 1/2	Greater than 60°

predict development of avascular necrosis (AVN), as patients with decreased femoral head uptake are more likely to progress to AVN [20].

CT

CT is generally not employed for diagnosis, although it can be used to measure hip angles, to assess hardware position, and to aid in preoperative planning before capital realignment or femoral neck osteotomy [21].

MRI

MRI can be useful in cases with negative or equivocal radiographs [22, 23]. In such cases, MRI may demonstrate distortion of the physis as well as periphyseal bone marrow edema (Fig. 12.13). In both acute and chronic cases, coronal or axial T1-weighted (T1-W) images best demonstrate focal or diffuse widening of the physis along with globular or diffuse intermediate T1 signal in the growth plate. Hyperintensity of the physis on short tau inversion recovery (STIR) imaging is inconsistently seen. Joint effusion and synovitis are common. MRI can also help detect occult contralateral SCFE and assess later complications, especially labral injury related to femoroacetabular impingement (discussed below). Chondrolysis and AVN can also be characterized on MRI, despite susceptibility artifact from fixation hardware [24].

3.7 Differential Diagnosis

Early changes on radiographs may be subtle, so high suspicion for SCFE is necessary in any adolescent or preadolescent with hip or knee pain; a frog lateral or true lateral view of the hip is indispensible. The differential diagnosis

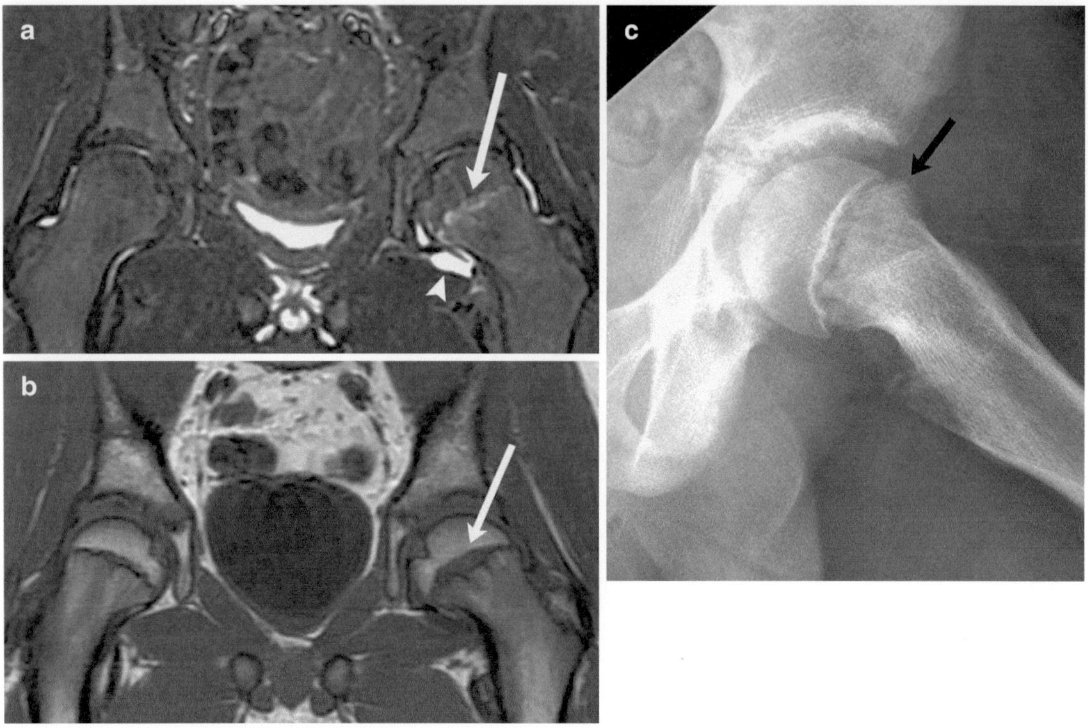

Fig. 12.13 Minimally displaced SCFE in an 11-year-old with left hip pain. (**a**) Coronal STIR image shows increased signal in the left proximal femoral physis (*arrow*) and a joint effusion (*arrowhead*). (**b**) Coronal T1-W MR image more clearly depicts physeal widening (*arrow*). (**c**) Subsequent radiograph confirms subtle femoral head and neck offset (*arrow*)

for this pathology includes synovitis, arthritis, infection, early-stage AVN, myotendinous injury, and labral tear. However, imaging features are characteristic once the slip has progressed.

4 Avascular Necrosis

Ischemic osteonecrosis is usually referred to as avascular necrosis (AVN). However, circulatory disturbance is not necessarily complete and may only cause isolated osteocyte death, possibly preserving some marrow viability. Although it follows a similar reparative course in all epiphyseal areas, local factors and treatment will affect the rate and radiographic manifestations of healing. The basic etiology of ischemia may be unknown, as in Legg-Perthes (LP) disease, or well understood, as in the hemoglobinopathies and Gaucher disease. Either the major vascular supply or small intraepiphyseal vessels may be affected.

The pattern and development of the arterial supply to the femoral head helps elucidate the etiology of idiopathic AVN. Vessels originate from the medial and lateral femoral circumflex arteries, which form an anastomotic ring at the base of the capsule [25]. Those that penetrate the capsular attachment run sub-synovially along the neck of the femur to form an intracapsular network; several well-defined ascending cervical vessels supply the metaphysis and then pass peripherally to the growth plate and then the femoral head chondroepiphysis. The most important blood supply to the epiphysis comes from a single lateral ascending cervical branch (also called the lateral epiphyseal artery). This artery passes through a narrow interval between the greater trochanter and femoral neck, a prime location for potential compression and occlusion. A variable and small portion of the femoral head blood supply comes from the foveolar (ligamentum teres) artery.

Up to the age of 15–18 months, abundant arteriosinusoidal vessels pass through—rather than around—the growth plate. After this time, the bony plate of the ossification center creates a barrier, and vessels no longer penetrate the physis [26]. The vascular supply changes in other ways as well during early development. By age 2–3 years, the growth plate has become intracapsular, the lateral circumflex artery has assumed the role of supplying the greater trochanteric region, and the femoral head relies on the medial circumflex artery alone. Thus, the infantile pattern of multiple small vessels originating from both the lateral and medial circumflex arteries changes to a childhood pattern, in which a few large ascending cervical arteries (the posterosuperior and posteroinferior epiphyseal vessels) arise without significant anastomotic connections. In infancy, AVN generally requires occlusion of one large extracapsular vessel. This might result from compression in the treatment of infantile hip dislocation. Later in childhood, occlusion of a smaller—but relatively more important intracapsular branch—can produce AVN.

The actual occlusive event and ensuing bone death may be clinically unapparent. However, histologic changes are seen almost immediately as osteocytes disappear, leaving empty lacunae. Note that the process of bone infarction is radiographically occult and that radiographic changes actually reflect healing (with the exception of ossification center fractures). Epiphyseal resorption is not a sign of destruction but rather a sign of repair.

Imaging (Box 12.3)

Dead bone has no distinctive radiographic appearance and is indistinguishable in form and density from live bone [27]. Therefore, any change in appearance means that the process of healing has begun. As new bone lamellae are laid down over the dead trabeculae, a slight but definite increase in the opacity of the epiphysis develops; this is the first radiographic change in the femoral head (Fig. 12.14).

Lack of vascular supply to the ossification center prevents its continued normal growth. Growth of the cartilaginous epiphysis, however, is unimpaired, since it is nourished by synovial fluid. In fact, cartilage growth is stimulated by the insult at the ossification center, and hyperplasia

Box 12.3: Radiographic Changes of Avascular Necrosis of the Femoral Head

Phase	Pathology	Radiology
Initial	Vascular occlusion and osteocyte death	Normal
Early	Necrotic bone with beginning revascularization	Increased bone density
	Ossific growth impairment	Small ossific epiphysis
	Cartilaginous epiphysis continues to grow	Increased medial joint space
	Subchondral fracture of necrotic bone	Subchondral fissure
Early intermediate	Dead bone resorption Fibroblast ingrowth	Intermixed lucencies (sequestra and immature bone)
	Early new bone deposition	Resorption dominates
Late intermediate	Resorption slows	Gradual reconstitution of outline and integrity of ossification center
	Deposition predominant	Bone of mixed maturity
Late	Formation of mature Haversian systems	Remodeling of amorphous bone into mature trabeculae

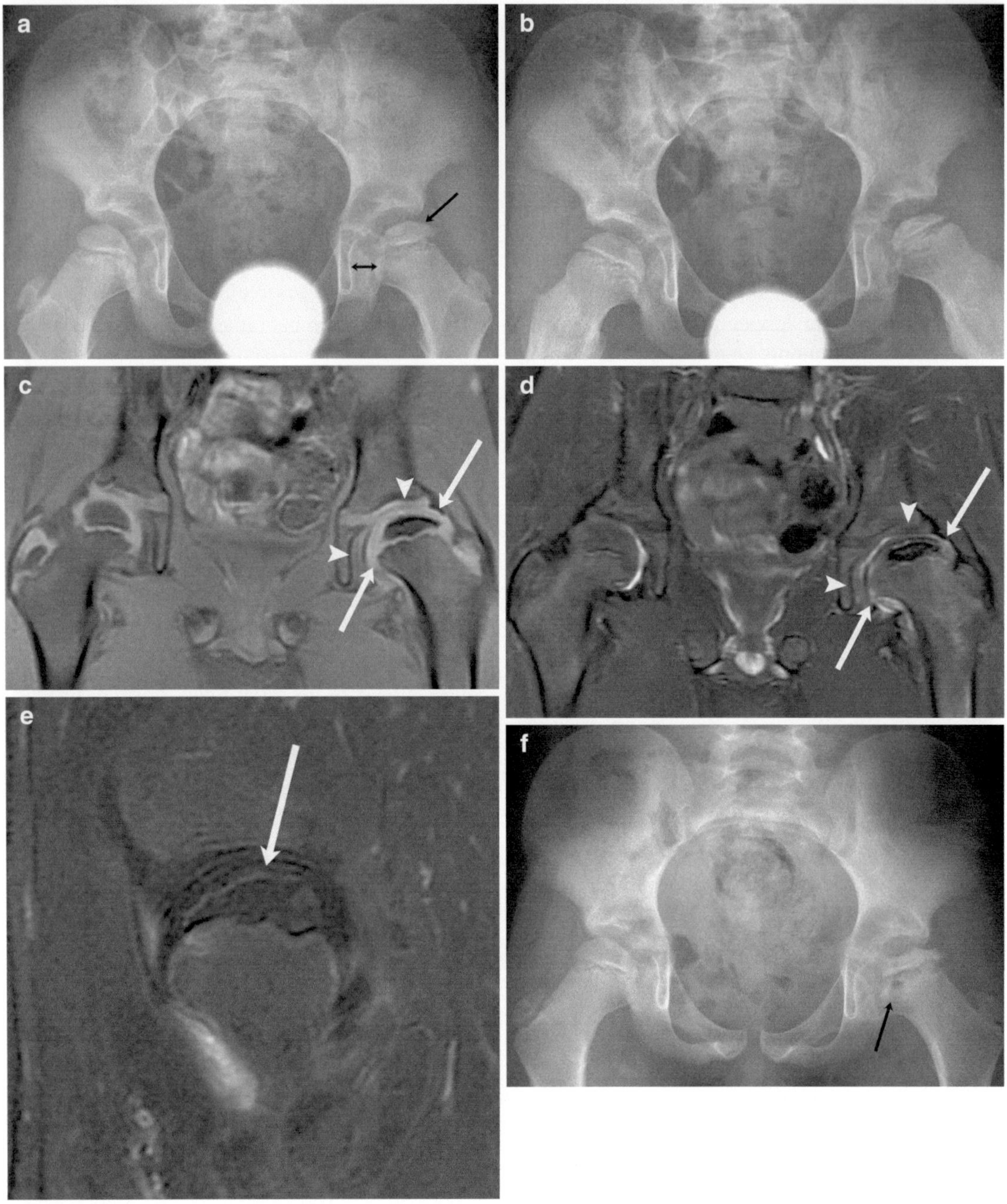

Fig. 12.14 Progressive findings of LP disease in a 7-year-old boy who presented with hip pain. At presentation (**a** (neutral), **b** (frog lateral)), there is mild flattening of the relatively dense left femoral epiphysis (*arrow*, **a**) and mild widening of the medial joint space (*double arrow*, **a**). Subtle fissuring is evident on the frog lateral view (**b**). Coronal T1-W (**c**) and T2-W (**d**) images 6 weeks later show no significant joint effusion, but acetabular (*arrowheads*) and femoral head (*arrows*) cartilage overgrowth accounts for joint space widening, and the epiphysis is small and diffusely hypointense. (**e**) Sagittal T1-W FS gadolinium-enhanced subtraction MRI shows the femoral head (*arrow*) does not enhance. (**f**) Four months later, at stage of intermediate healing, there is progressive flattening and early fragmentation of the femoral head. Multiple fracture lines are evident. Note metaphyseal lucency (*arrow*)

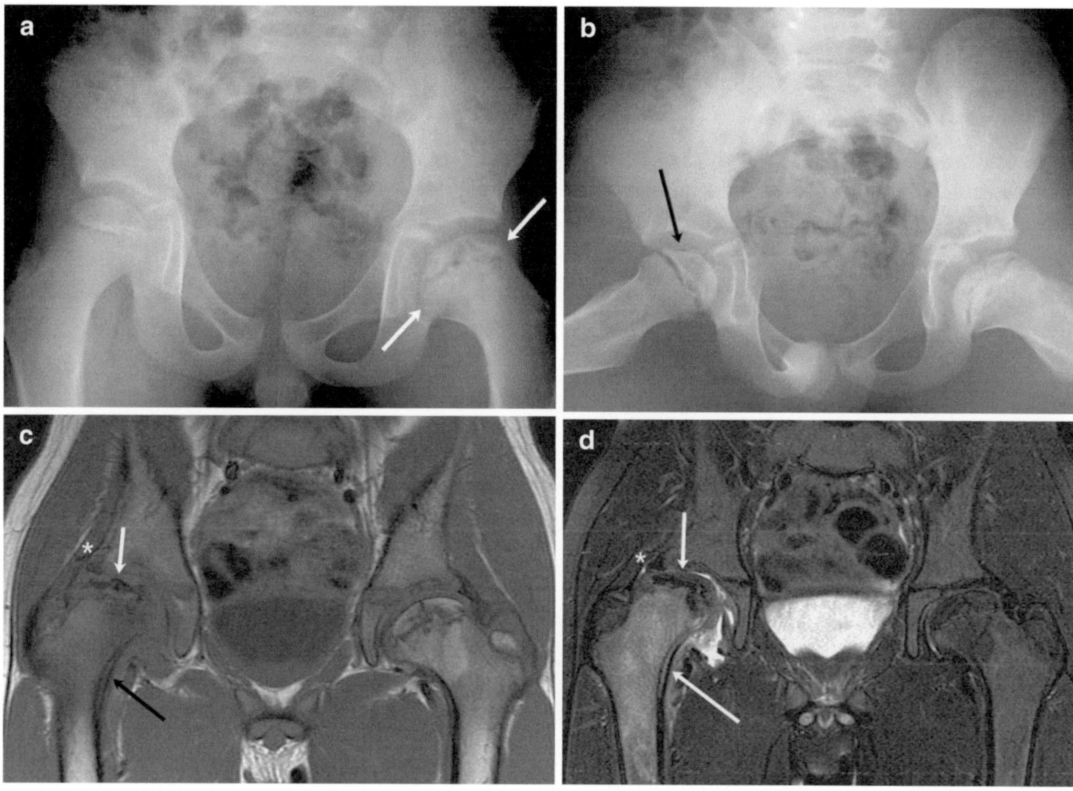

Fig. 12.15 Old left-sided and acute right-sided LP disease in a 6-year-old boy with 1 week of limp and right knee pain. (**a**) At presentation, the left femoral head is broad (*arrows*) and the femoral neck is short and wide, indicating previous LP disease. (**b**) The crescent sign of acute right-sided LP disease is seen only on the frog lateral (*arrow*), since it is in the anterior portion of the femoral head. Ten months later, coronal T1-W (**c**) and T2-W FS (**d**) MR images show marked fragmentation of the right femoral head (*short arrows*) with edema and periosteal thickening of the femoral neck (*black arrow* (**c**), *long arrow* (**d**)), indicating intermediate stage of healing. Also note deformed labrum (*asterisk*) as the femoral head is extruded. In contrast, the left hip is in the late stage, with normal fatty marrow signal in the remodeled femoral head

of both epiphyseal and acetabular cartilage takes place. MRI or arthrography of both hips may demonstrate this cartilaginous overgrowth (Fig. 12.15). Increased cartilage along the medial aspect of the femoral head displaces the small ossification center laterally, increasing the distance to the bony acetabulum (the medial joint-cartilage space). Thus, although AVN is itself radiographically occult, secondary signs may be evident.

A fissure fracture is another common relatively early finding in AVN. The fracture occurs in necrotic bone rather than at the interface between dead and live bone. In the hip, the fissure is located anterolaterally in the epiphysis and is thus best shown on the frog lateral projection (see Fig. 12.15) (note that orthopedic surgeons usually refer to this as the “crescent” rather than “fissure”). It usually appears as a single thin, linear lucency extending over the lateral one-third of the epiphysis; it may extend in an arcuate fashion over most of the periphery of the ossification center. The fissure may vary in width, or it may spread, forming several fissures. It is often more lucent than a simple linear fracture, probably because the fracture line contains gas induced by the vacuum phenomenon. If this is the case, the fissure may seem to lie between the ossification center and the overlying cartilage. This type of fissure fracture line is a moderately early sign of AVN and becomes apparent only when other signs of osteonecrosis are present. Resorption often starts peripheral to this fissure, and, as the adjacent bone is removed, the line quickly disappears.

The vascular and fibroblastic ingrowth that supplied the osteoblasts for the new bone lamellae is also the source for the osteoclasts that begin the resorption of the necrotic bone marrow and trabeculae. The resorptive process starts anterolaterally and is seen as a gradual disappearance of bony trabeculae as they are replaced with fibrous material. Since the process is temporally and spatially both irregular and unpredictable, islands of bone may persist adjacent to large areas of fibrosis, leading to a granular, fragmented radiographic appearance. Large sections of normal or dense bone surrounded by lysis represent sequestra; these may persist unchanged for months or years.

Bone deposition follows resorption, but the rate is unpredictable. In some cases, resorption and re-ossification are so closely allied that they cannot be differentiated, whereas in others resorption is so complete that the ossific epiphysis vanishes before new bone formation becomes evident. The immature bone appears clumped and amorphous and is eventually replaced with mature bone trabeculae. The process from bone death to complete remodeling can be quite rapid in the very young (less than age 4 years) but typically lasts 2 or more years. It is not uncommon to find a saucerlike osseous deficiency at the vertex of the femoral head more than 5 years after the initial necrosis.

4.1 Legg-Perthes Disease

Legg-Perthes (LP) disease is an idiopathic osteonecrosis of the proximal femoral epiphysis. Sufficient evidence from both pathologic and nuclear imaging studies indicates that this is an AVN, but until the precipitating cause is recognized LP disease will remain a puzzling condition, distinct from well-understood avascular necroses. However, the arterial caliber in these children is unusually small; they also demonstrate an impaired hyperemic response when exposed to an ischemic stimulus [28]. LP disease may result from a hypercoagulable state.

Legg and Waldenström reported the disease in 1909, and in 1910 the descriptions of Legg, Calvé, and Perthes were published [29–32]. LP disease has been labeled "coxa plana" in an attempt to avoid eponyms, but this term is inaccurate, as progression to a flat femoral head is often avoidable with current treatment. "Femoral head osteochondrosis" or "idiopathic osteonecrosis of the femoral head epiphysis" are acceptable synonyms but are infrequently used. Legg-Perthes disease seems to be the most common eponym, but other permutations are employed.

Epidemiology

The epidemiology of LP disease is characteristic and suggests strong environmental factors in addition to genetic predisposition. Its incidence ranges from 5 to 15 cases per 100,000. Although bilateral in 13 % of cases, the likelihood of involvement of the second hip decreases if disease onset is after age 6 or 7. The disorder is four times more common in boys than in girls. LP disease is much more common in Caucasian children than in other ethnic groups. It is uncommon enough in children of African descent that investigation for underlying disorders is warranted. Independent of race, the disease is more prevalent in northern latitudes, with each 10° increase in latitude associated with an incidence increase of 1.44 [33]. LP disease is also associated with Down syndrome and minor birth defects. There is a strong correlation between LP disease and lower socioeconomic status and markers of deprivation such as low birth weight, short stature, and small foot size [34]. Maternal smoking and exposure to secondhand smoke have also been implicated.

The age range of LP disease is 3–12 years, with few patients seen at either age extreme and most first seeking treatment around age 5–8. Girls tend to present younger than boys. Markedly delayed skeletal maturation is common in both sexes and may be seen in siblings. It is very rare to have a bone age equal to or greater than the chronologic age, and almost three-fourths of boys studied have bone ages more than two standard deviations below the mean [35]. Maturation can plateau for as many as 3 years in some patients [36].

Presentation

While the appearance is distinctive, signs and symptoms of LP disease are not different from most afflictions of the hip. Groin pain, limp, spasm, decreased internal rotation, and thigh and buttock atrophy are characteristic. An early history of transient hip pain (but not toxic synovitis) may be found in less than 5 % of cases [37, 38].

In most, one or more of the initial episodes of infarction are neither clinically nor radiographically detectable. Instead, imaging findings are based on the reestablishment of the vascular supply, resorption of necrotic bone trabeculae and marrow, and subsequent re-ossification. Revascularization can occur within weeks by recanalization of the occluded vessel. However, the process of neovascularization sometimes takes months to years. The complete healing process typically occurs over a period of 2–4 years.

Prognosis

Prognosis depends on age at presentation. Children who are diagnosed before the age of 5–7 years have a significantly better outcome than those who present after eight or nine, likely because they have a longer time before maturity in which to heal and remodel. In general, the prognosis for girls is worse than for boys. Poor outcome is associated with being overweight and having progressive loss of hip movement, adduction contracture, longer duration from onset to completion of the healing phase, and worse clinical symptoms. Partial epiphyseal necrosis heals with less femoral head deformity and incongruity that do cases with total femoral head involvement.

Multiple classification systems for disease severity have been proposed over the years. The Catterall classification [39] divides the process into four categories:

(i) Anterior involvement only, without collapse or sequestrum formation
(ii) Greater involvement, with some collapse or sequestrum formation but with viable medial and lateral bony segments supporting normal epiphyseal height
(iii) Large central sequestrum with collapse, but viable posterior segment and small medial and lateral supports
(iv) Total or nearly complete collapse and resorption of the bony epiphysis

The problem with this classification is that 16–40 months must pass before a case can be assigned to a category. Indeed, if classification is attempted too early, 40 % of patients change category. In addition, considerable interobserver error is encountered with this system [40].

The lateral pillar classification system [41] is more reproducible (more than 80 % interobserver agreement) and has more prognostic value [42]. Similar to the Catterall system, this imaging scheme is applied only after the disease has progressed to fragmentation. The revised system uses the following groups, based on the loss of height observed in the lateral quarter of the femoral head or the lateral pillar:

Group A. Lateral pillar is normal.
Group B. Loss of lateral pillar height up to 50 %.
Group B/C border. Loss of lateral pillar height of 50 %.
Group C. Loss of lateral pillar height greater than 50 %.

A study evaluating outcomes for these different groups found that the prognosis for all lateral pillar group A hips and two-thirds of group B hips is excellent. However, the prognosis for group C and the group B/C border hips is generally poor. Only one in four group B/C border and only one in eight group B hips had good result [43].

The ultimate shape of the femoral head after reconstitution of the bony nucleus depends not only on the initial amount of necrosis but also on the intensity and direction of forces acting on the epiphysis during healing, when it is biologically plastic. The final result ranges from a round femoral head indistinguishable from the normal side to a grossly flattened, enlarged, and deformed articular segment (coxa plana and magna). The extent of deformity results from unusual growth patterns caused by muscular and weight-bearing forces acting on a weakened structure. The lateral portion of a subluxated femoral head is subject to increased pressure, resulting in deformity of both the osseous and cartilaginous components of the epiphyseal head. Lateral growth of epiphyseal cartilage also causes an increase in the growth plate's circumference, widening the femoral neck in continuity with the enlarged head. In addition, periosteal new bone laid down along the femoral neck widens the proximal femur. Lateral extrusion of femoral head cartilage is easily detected on arthrography or MRI but may not be recognized on radiographs until epiphyseal ossification begins to appear superolateral to the outer edge of the femoral neck.

Injury to the vascular supply of the dividing cartilage cells at the growth plate may slow or completely halt growth, leading to premature fusion and resultant shortening of the femoral neck. The greater trochanter, with its separate blood supply, continues to grow by enchondral and appositional processes, shortening the normal articular-trochanteric distance (see Fig. 12.18 below). Thus, what appears as overgrowth of the trochanter is actually caused by lack of growth of the femoral neck. This configuration contributes to a Trendelenburg gait. Greater trochanter epiphysiodesis in younger children or distal transfer of the greater trochanter in skeletally mature children addresses this problem.

Separation of an osteochondral fragment at the vertex can occur as late as 18 years after treatment. This is an uncommon problem, encountered in only 2–4 % of patients. The mechanism is uncertain—perhaps a segment of bone never united with the main center or a late shear fracture occurred through a weak and partially ossified zone at the vertex. Separation is more likely with late-onset disease. One-third of the reported cases have been bilateral, suggesting that these cases may actually represent femoral head dysplasia of the osteochondritis dissecans type. There is both histologic and scintigraphic evidence that second episodes of infarction occur, but—unlike with AVN due to Gaucher disease—clinically apparent recurrence is uncommon.

Several different classification systems describe the radiographic appearance of late LP disease, all with the goal of predicting the likelihood of premature osteoarthritis. These include epiphyseal-femoral neck-acetabular measurements as well as various quotients, relationships, and tests for symmetry and roundness [44–47]. Catterall's grading is usually adequate [39]:

Good: head essentially round, slight decrease in height acceptable

Fair: femoral head broadened, up to one-fifth uncovered

Poor: more than one-fifth uncovered, increased medial joint space, short neck

Complete coverage of the femoral head is not necessary for an acceptable outcome, since 80 % of normal children have some uncovering of the femoral head.

Overall, two thirds of patients are symptom-free about 30–40 years later, despite the presence of residual radiographic abnormalities in almost all patients treated with older modes of therapy. Those with residual effects may have mild limp, minimal leg shortening, and little or no pain or functional impairment. However, premature osteoarthritis may develop in some patients who have significant abnormal findings, such as aspherical femoral head with incongruent acetabulum, osteochondral fragment, labral tear, or trochanteric overgrowth. This is in marked contrast to patients with a history of developmental hip dysplasia, who may have severe symptoms despite relatively mild radiographic abnormalities.

Etiology

It is uncertain what causes interruption of blood supply to the femoral epiphysis in LP disease, but genetic and environmental factors probably contribute to the process. Thrombophilias such as protein-C, protein-S, or antithrombin III deficiencies, or Factor V Leiden mutations, have been inconsistently linked to LP disease. Abnormalities in the insulin-like growth factor I pathway may be associated as well. A type II collagen mutation has been identified in Asian families with multiple members affected by AVN of the femoral head and no other detectable skeletal abnormalities. This gene mutation has not been identified in sporadic cases, however. There is an increased incidence of both major and minor birth defects in children with LP disease, suggesting that genetic or early developmental problems may be a factor.

Of the numerous possible environmental factors, subclinical trauma to the vessels supplying the femoral head seems to be the most likely cause. Several anatomic areas supplied by key vessels are especially vulnerable (as described earlier for AVN in general). Mechanisms can include traumatic compression of intraepiphyseal vessels or tamponade of extraepiphyseal vessels due to increased intraarticular pressure in the setting of joint effusions, but a universally applicable etiology has not been determined. In addition to arterial insufficiency, abnormal venous drainage has been demonstrated, and increased bone marrow pressures have been found in cases of osteonecrosis in adults. Regardless of the etiologic factors at play, infarction—perhaps multiple times—and subsequent repair lead to disease [48, 49].

Treatment

The treatment of LP disease invokes a great deal of controversy. Children who are less than 6 years old at onset are often not treated, regardless of the severity of femoral head involvement. Similarly, children of any age with minimal segmental necrosis may not be treated. Early in the course of disease, the goal of treatment is to prevent deformity of the femoral head by maintaining or improving its containment within the acetabulum, thus providing a template for cartilage shape. Improved alignment encourages normal development of the biologically plastic cartilaginous epiphysis while reducing pressure on the lateral segment of the epiphyseal cartilage. Containment strategies include ambulatory abduction bracing, varus femoral osteotomy, innominate osteotomy, and labral support shelf acetabuloplasty. Surgical intervention significantly improves the outcome in children with lateral pillar B hips who are older than 8—for those treated with surgery, 73 % will have spherical femoral heads (versus 44 % without surgery) [43]. However, early surgical intervention appears to neither prevent progression nor accelerate healing. Previous misguided attempts at surgical revascularization with bone grafting have led to premature fusion of the growth plate.

Late in the course of disease, treatment focuses on minimizing deformation of the femoral head caused by extrusion. If there is femoral head extrusion, hinged abduction may occur—the femoral head hinges instead of rotating within the acetabulum, resulting in a medial gap. This hinged abduction may be treated with excision of lateral head extrusion (cheilectomy or partial capitectomy) as a salvage procedure. In adolescents or young adults with healed LP disease, treatment depends on the specific causes of pain, dysfunction, or deformity. Gait abnormalities from femoral neck shortening and pain from femoroacetabular impingement (FAI) may need to be addressed surgically (see below for discussion of FAI, and see Chap. 27 for further discussion of surgical techniques and associated radiographic findings).

Imaging

Radiography

In general, LP disease is best imaged with radiographs, both for initial evaluation and for follow-up. Both frontal and frog lateral views of the hips and pelvis contribute useful information, but the lateral projection is almost always the most informative, since much of the resorption process is anterior. This area is superimposed on the more normal posterior epiphysis on the frontal view but is shown in profile on the lateral.

Examinations at 3–4-month intervals usually suffice, although in the later stages of repair, there is frequently little change between sequential studies and frequency of imaging may be reduced. Simultaneous evaluation of both hips helps track progress and also enables detection of asymptomatic bilateral disease. The usual gonadal shielding pertains.

Radiographic evaluation of other epiphyses (to investigate the possibility of other epiphyseal dysplasia, hematologic disease, etc.) is not advised unless unusual familial, age, or racial factors so indicate or if there is symmetric bilateral hip involvement that suggests multiple epiphyseal dysplasia. In case of questionable diagnosis, a bone age above the chronologic age may dictate further workup.

Subtle but definite radiographic abnormalities are commonly evident shortly after patients become symptomatic. Considering the time that must elapse between a vascular insult and the development of radiographic findings, it is likely that the vascular insult of LP disease is silent and that the blood supply has already been restored by the time of presentation.

Early Stage

Both height and transverse diameter of the affected ossific epiphysis are smaller than on the other side; diminished size implies that growth ceased or slowed several months earlier (Fig. 12.16). In addition, the distance between the inner margin of the acetabulum and the femoral metaphysis is larger on the abnormal side. Although this increase has been attributed to lateral displacement due to synovial swelling or effusion, arthrography generally does not demonstrate true subluxation, synovial hypertrophy, or synovial fluid under pressure. Rather, the acetabular cartilage is thickened, and there is overgrowth of the cartilage of the femoral head (see Fig. 12.14). These two radiolucent structures conspire to shift the observable epiphyseal ossification center laterally, although the medial joint space is not actually increased. Cartilage overgrowth along with the small size of the ossification center further indicates that the vascular insult or insults occurred long before the patient became symptomatic.

As with all types of AVN, early generalized increased density and subchondral fissure(s) accompany decreased epiphyseal size and apparent lateral shift of the ossification center. Sclerosis of the ossification center is in part due to early new bone formation, which sheaths the necrotic trabeculae well before resorption begins. However, sclerosis can be exaggerated by its contrast with the adjacent metaphysis, which is often demineralized due to disuse or hyperemia.

The subchondral fissure fracture usually appears as a fine arc that parallels the outer and anterior periphery of the ossification center. It may vary in width along its course, ramify, or extend across the vertex of the ossified epiphysis (see Fig. 12.15). The fissure is an almost constant feature of early LP disease, best seen on the frog lateral projection. It is often quite lucent, presumably due to incorporated gas released from the synovial fluid by the vacuum phenomenon. The fissure is usually evanescent, since the initial resorptive process subsequently removes the small segment of bone just superior to the fracture line.

Cyst-like areas of demineralization in the metaphysis are seen in about one-third of patients (Figs. 12.14, 12.16, and 12.17). These are rarely present in the early stages of necrosis but accompany the process of epiphyseal resorption. They are most often located in the anterior metaphysis just under the physis, where the sometimes multiple lucencies often appear as sharply demarcated lucent foci. Occasionally they appear as an irregularly marginated and broad band of demineralization, running across the entire femoral neck below the physis.

Metaphyseal lucencies appear quickly but ossify and disappear long before the epiphyseal ossification center fully reconstitutes. Large areas of demineralization confer a worse prognosis for complete restoration of the epiphysis. These lucencies may represent true metaphyseal cysts (located within the metaphysis only) or false cysts (extending from the epiphysis and physis) [50]. They are generally thought to result

Fig. 12.16 LP disease in a 7-year-old boy with pain and limping. (**a**, **b**) There is mild loss of height of the right femoral epiphysis and a subtle lucency in the anterior aspect of the metaphysis (*arrow*). The articular-trochanteric distance is demonstrated on the normal left hip on image (**a**). (**c**) Coronal T1-W MRI shows decreased marrow signal in the subcortical femoral head (*arrow*) and neck (*arrowhead*). (**d**) Sagittal STIR image shows crescentic high signal in the anterosuperior aspect of the femoral head (*arrow*), representing a subchondral fracture. (**e**) Slightly more medial, another sagittal STIR image shows the metaphyseal lucency (*arrow*) with surrounding bone marrow edema and a joint effusion. Shelf acetabuloplasty was performed 3 months later, and after one more month (**f**) loss of height and sclerosis of the femoral head have progressed (*arrow*). Graft material appears dense and cloudlike (*arrowheads*). (**g**) One year later, femoral head fragmentation has progressed (graft is incorporated into iliac bone). (**h**) Four years later, after remodeling, the femoral neck is broad and short, and the femoral head sclerotic, wide, and flat. Note decreased distance between acetabulum and greater trochanter

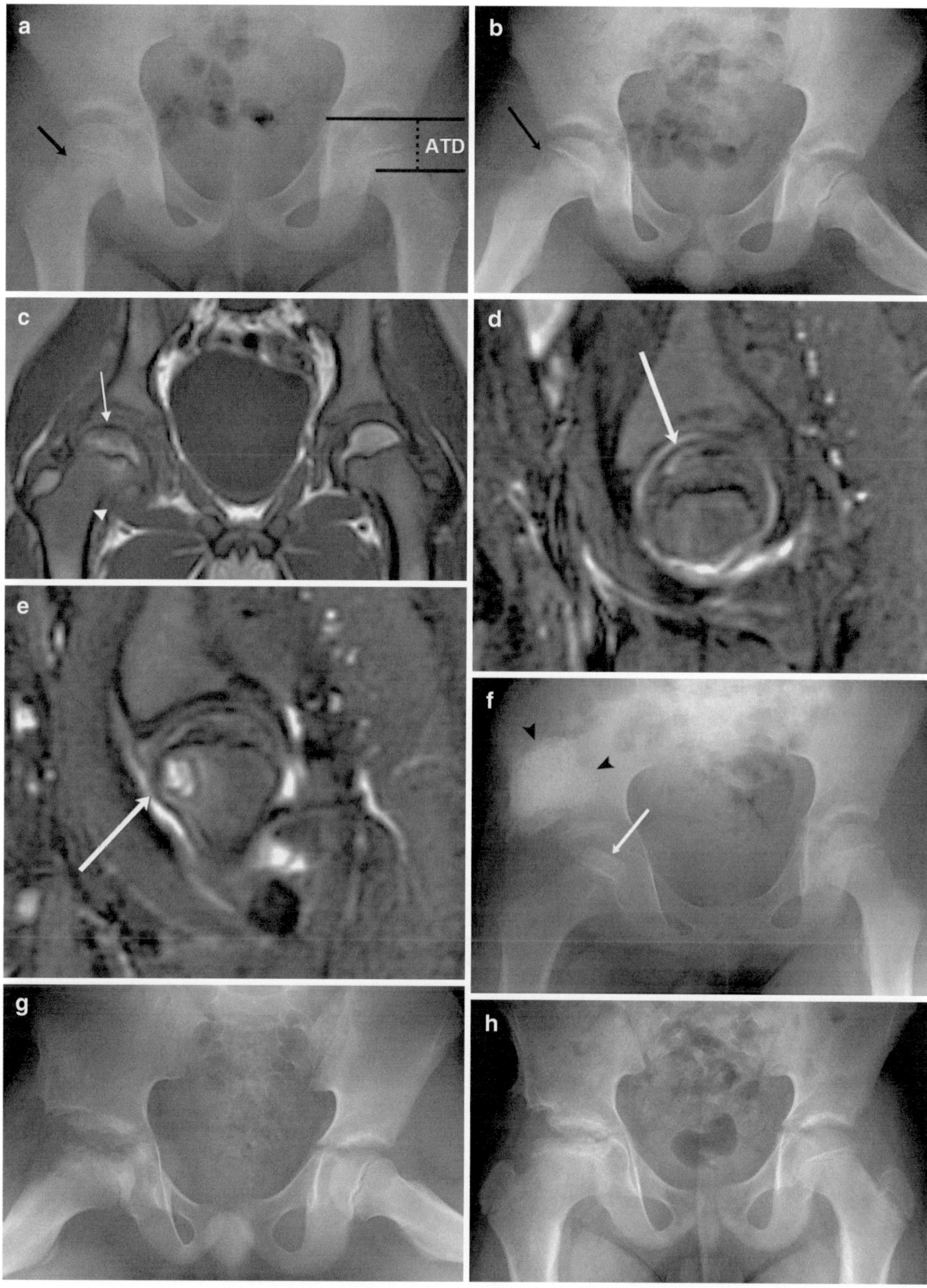
a
ATD
b
c
d
e
f
g
h

from growth plate disturbance, with secondary tonguelike extensions of cartilage into the metaphysis. Limited pathologic studies have found that these lucencies may represent blood cavities and fibrous walled cysts, as well as foci of cartilage, granulation tissue, and hyperemic immature bone [51].

Early Intermediate Stage

In the intermediate and longest phase of repair, the bony epiphysis may be almost completely resorbed before re-ossification begins. However, resorption and re-ossification usually proceed together, either in different zones of the ossification center or admixed throughout the bony epiphysis, resulting in a granular or fragmented appearance. The apparent lateralization of the ossification center usually persists and sometimes becomes permanent. The bony acetabulum often de-ossifies along its superior margin; this is associated with increased scintigraphic activity, implying generalized hyperemia. Although the irregular contour and shallow enlargement of the acetabulum may remodel, these changes may also persist. Premature fusion of the triradiate cartilage predicts a worse outcome.

Late-Intermediate Stage

If the epiphysis is not protected from deleterious force vectors during the resorption phase and support for cartilage is lost, plastic remodeling may cause the epiphyseal cartilage to gradually flatten and grow in a more lateral direction. The first radiographic sign of this may be broadening of the femoral neck and the presence of ossification lateral to a line projected up from the outer border of the femoral neck (see Fig. 12.16). The pressures that force the epiphyseal cartilage to grow laterally also broaden the underlying growth plate. This laterally extended growth plate then gradually increases the width of the femoral neck. In addition, this growth aberration may produce excess periosteal and perichondral growth, explaining the lamellar periosteal reaction occasionally seen along the femoral neck. Rarely, a bony protuberance forms and later resorbs. The acetabulum also enlarges to encompass this wide, flat femoral head, often with mild upsloping of the sourcil (the weight-bearing portion of the acetabulum).

Shortening of the femoral neck with relative trochanteric overgrowth is also seen, presumably due to interruption of the vascular supply to the cartilage cells of the growth plate, which inhibits linear growth of the femoral neck. The extent of trochanteric overgrowth and femoral neck shortening may be determined by assessing the articular-trochanteric distance. This is the length of a vertical line drawn perpendicular to horizontal tangents along the articular surface of the femoral head and the tip of the greater trochanter. In skeletally mature adolescents, this should measure 23 mm (standard deviation 5 mm) [52] (see Fig. 12.16). Increased femoral neck anteversion has been reported in LP disease, and the degree is associated with a worse prognosis.

When the unsupported cartilage of the femoral head is forced down around the neck, a characteristic metaphyseal line may be seen, the "sagging rope" sign (Fig. 12.18). This well-defined linear sclerosis is caused by either the cortical outline of the overhanging femoral head or reactive bone formed by the periosteum of the femoral neck adjacent to the cartilaginous epiphysis. If present, it is unlikely that femoral head contour will be restored to normal.

Late Stage

After the epiphysis ossifies into the pattern determined by the cartilage model, the newly deposited amorphous bone is gradually replaced by remodeled trabecular bone. The age at onset (with younger patients doing better), the magnitude of femoral head involvement, and the type of treatment influence the eventual size and shape of the bony epiphysis [53]. The final result ranges from complete restoration of normal size and contour to a large, flattened, misshapen femoral head with short femoral neck (i.e., coxa plana) [54] (see Figs. 12.17 and 12.18).

Nuclear Scintigraphy

Radionuclide imaging with Tc-99m MDP can help differentiate LP disease from other conditions. However, MRI has largely replaced this

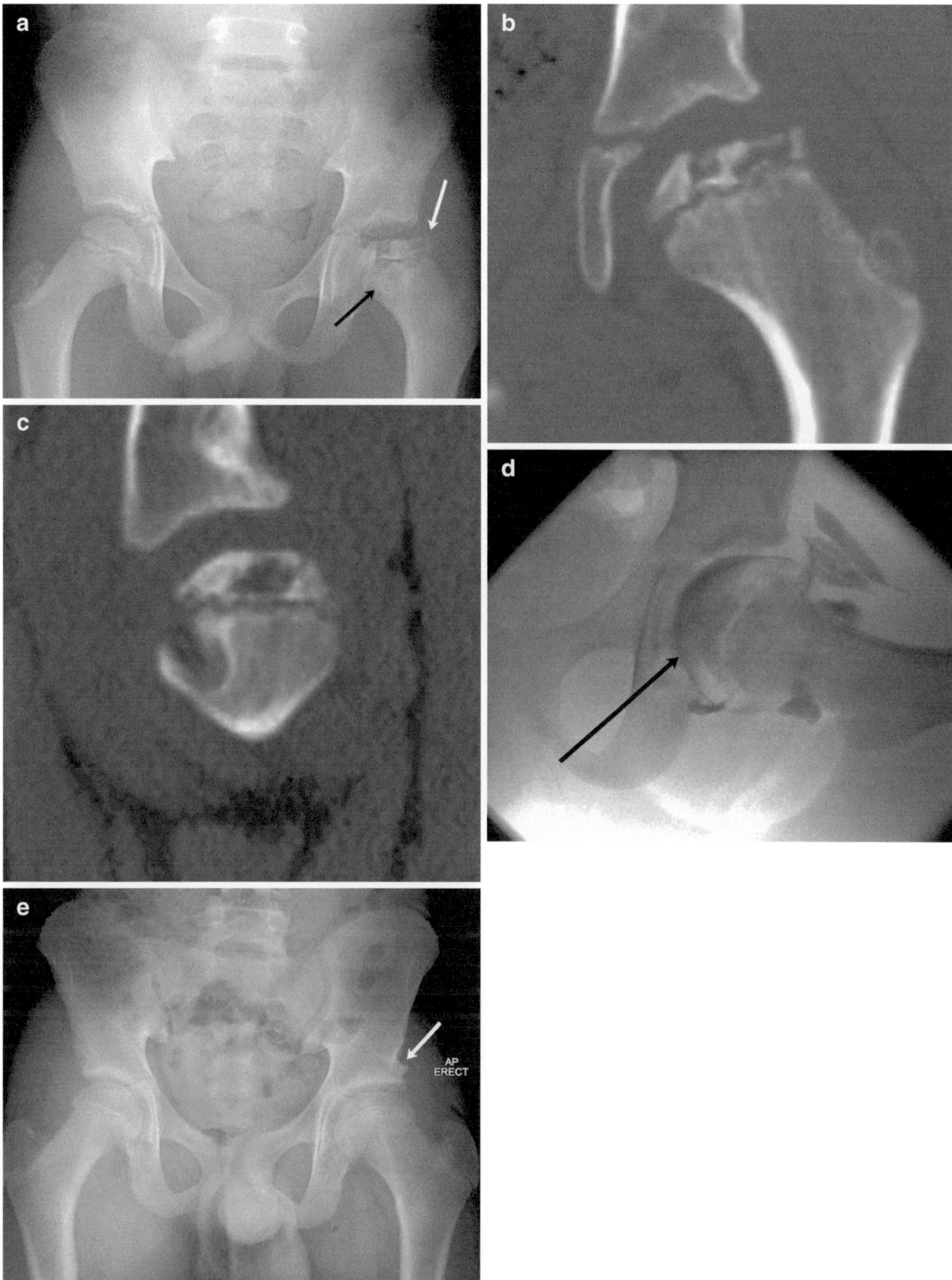

Fig. 12.17 Progressive LP disease in an 8-year-old boy with pain and limping. (**a**) At presentation, the left femoral epiphysis is already fragmented with mild lateral extrusion (*white arrow*), and there is cystic change (*black arrow*) in the broad femoral neck. Coronal (**b**) and sagittal (**c**) reformats from a CT 1 month later show similar findings. (**d**) An intraoperative arthrogram prior to shelf acetabuloplasty shows smooth, thick, spherical, unbroken articular cartilage (*arrow*) despite fragmentation of the ossific center. (**e**) Eight years later, the acetabuloplasty (*arrow*) has healed, and the joint is congruent despite mild broadening of the femoral head and neck. The patient is pain-free and able to engage fully in activities

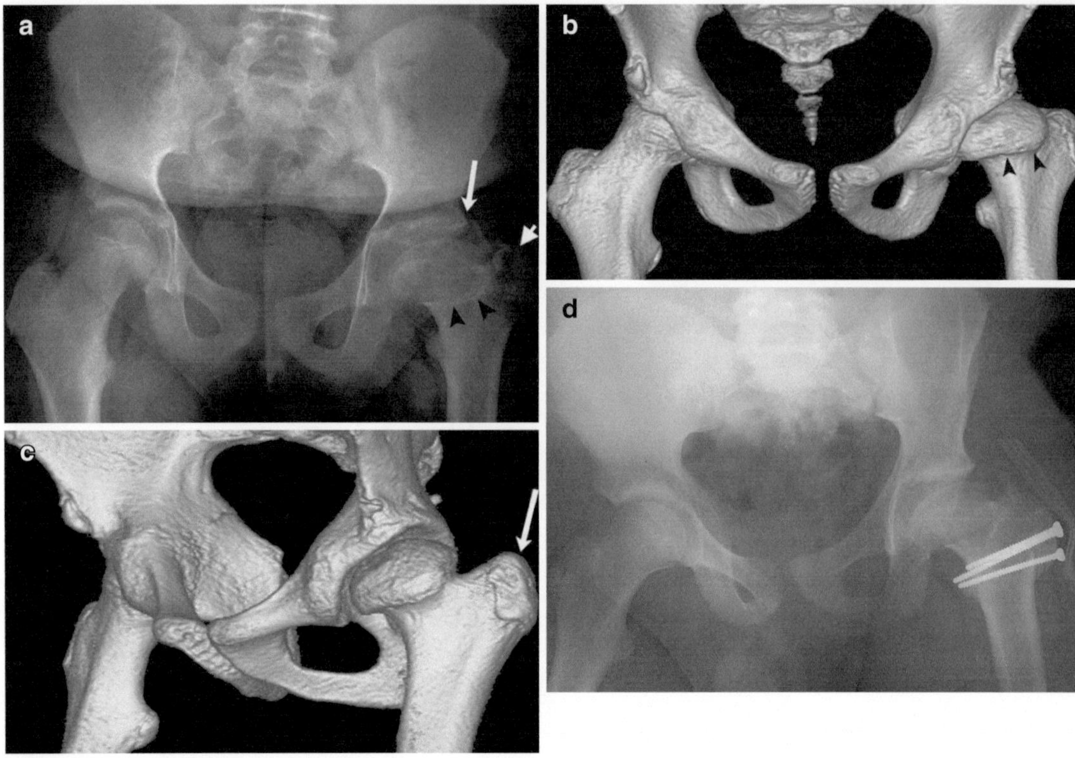

Fig. 12.18 Late LP disease in a 13-year-old boy complaining of pain, popping, and difficulty sitting. Preoperative radiograph (**a**) and 3D CT reconstructions (**b**, **c**) show typical broadening of the femoral head with marked shortening of the femoral neck. The greater trochanter is high riding and posteriorly positioned (*short white arrow*), and the acetabular-trochanteric distance is reduced. The sourcil of the acetabulum is laterally upsloped (*long arrow*). Note the "sagging rope" sign (*black arrowheads*). (**d**) Labral repair and femoral osteotomy for relative neck lengthening and advancement of the greater trochanter were performed, in order to alleviate impingement symptoms

modality for situations in which the radiographic findings are normal or equivocal, as MRI can reveal unexpected, clinically important causes of hip pain in one quarter of cases [55] (see subsequent section). Routine scintigraphic techniques are both sensitive (0.98) and specific (0.95) in demonstrating abnormal vascularity [56]; single-photon emission computed tomography (SPECT) imaging and quantitative segmental sampling techniques may be even more helpful.

Tc-99m MDP shows altered blood flow rather than actual bone formation. Focal decreased uptake is seen in the femoral head: in partial necrosis this generally involves only the anterolateral portion, whereas in complete epiphyseal involvement it extends across the entire width of the ossific nucleus (Fig. 12.19). This finding is visible as soon as symptoms occur and, in some cases of bilateral disease, precedes radiographic changes. The size of the defect correlates well with the length of the fracture fissure and the eventual area of necrosis [57, 58]. As regeneration occurs, sequential scanning shows that the areas of decreased uptake gradually develop increased or normal activity. This precedes radiographic evidence of healing by 3–6 months.

A scintigraphic classification system can predict prognosis earlier than can a radiograph [59, 60]. Categorization requires at least two bone scans, usually at presentation and 5 months later. This classification system is based on the location of radiotracer uptake within the femoral head. Pathway A hips demonstrate early appearance of uptake in the lateral column; they have a better prognosis, probably because of rapid recanalization of affected vessels. Pathway B hips show

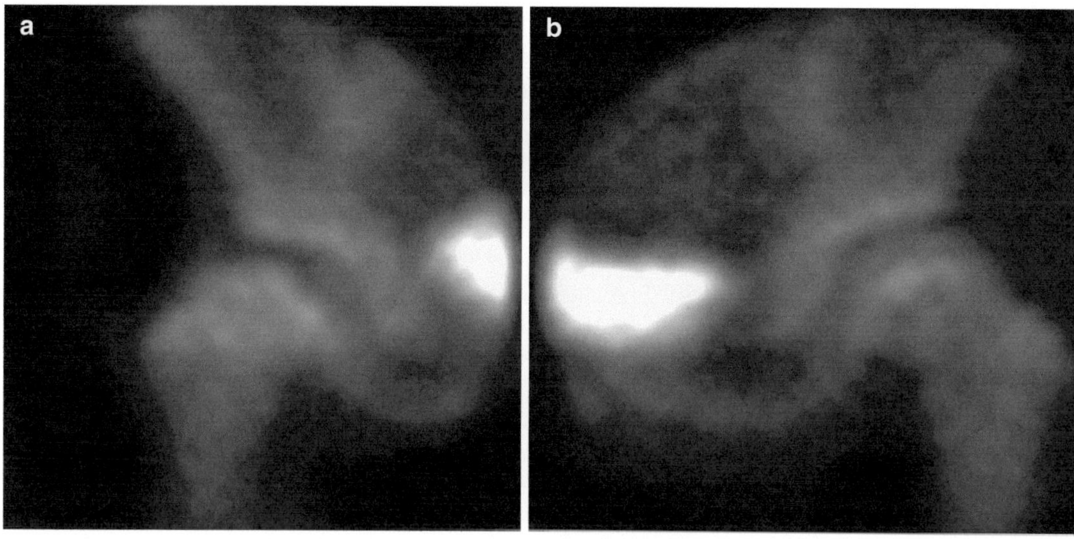

Fig. 12.19 AVN in a 5-year-old girl with hip pain. (**a**) Pinhole image from Tc-99m MDP bone scan shows photopenia in the right femoral head (**a**), consistent with avascular necrosis. Left hip (**b**) shows normal uptake, for comparison

uptake at the base and center of the epiphysis; this probably reflects transphyseal neovascular collateral vessel recruitment in response to persistent decreased vascularity. A subsequent scan may show diminished uptake in areas that were formerly well vascularized, presumably due to a second episode of infarction [61]. This scintigraphic classification system correlates well with the Herring and Catterall radiographic staging systems, providing prognostic information within 5 months of disease onset, several months or more before radiographic staging is possible [62]. Serial bone scans have a 97 % positive predictive value for a poor final outcome for pathway B hips and an 85 % positive predictive value for a good outcome for those in pathway A [63].

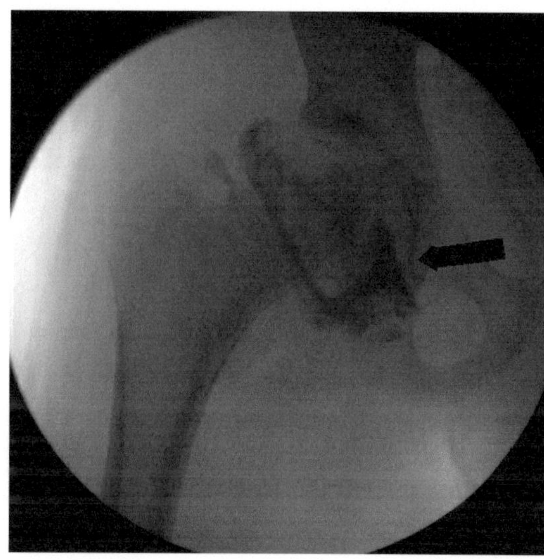

Fig. 12.20 LP disease in a 9-year-old boy. Intraoperative arthrogram shows medial contrast pooling (*arrow*) and lateral subluxation of the femoral head

Arthrography

Arthrography helps determine appropriate treatment, for although MRI demonstrates cartilage surfaces and para-articular structures, arthrography allows for direct observation of coverage and mobility during fluoroscopy [64, 65].

In early stages of LP disease, arthrography may be essentially normal, aside from subtle flattening of the cartilage over the fissure fracture (best shown with abduction views). The fissure does not penetrate the epiphyseal cartilage or otherwise communicate with the joint space, so it is not delineated by arthrography. The cartilaginous head outline is otherwise round and regular, and capsular laxity is unusual. The affected side does exhibit a measurable increase in width of both the femoral head and acetabular cartilage. Occasionally, true subluxation with medial contrast pooling occurs (Fig. 12.20). However, in general much of the epiphyseal center lateralization seen on radiographs results from cartilage overgrowth alone. The two can only be distinguished with arthrography or MRI.

In intermediate stages, it is difficult to ascertain cartilage shape and congruence with radiographs alone. However, arthrography usually shows that the surface outline is smoother than might be suspected based on the fragmented and nodular appearance of the ossification center (see Fig. 12.17). Although a normal femoral head should be perfectly spherical, an ovoid shape is often demonstrated. Furthermore, with severe collapse of the cartilage, the head becomes flattened around the femoral neck. Lateral extrusion of the head may result in a hump that can restrict motion or act as a fulcrum, opening up the medial joint space during abduction. This is termed "hinge abduction" and is generally a poor prognostic sign.

In late stages of remodeling, the shape of the cartilage determines the shape of the reconstituted ossification center. If there is an apparently non-united fragment of bone at the vertex of the femoral head, arthrography can help determine whether it is truly free or if it is covered by cartilage.

Computed Tomography

CT is reserved for later stages of healing. Although rarely essential, CT with multiplanar reformatting or three-dimensional (3D) reconstruction can contribute significantly to patient management (see Fig. 12.18) and may detect abnormalities in the contralateral ostensibly normal hip. CT is more sensitive to fractures in osteonecrosis than is radiography.

Magnetic Resonance Imaging

MRI best evaluates both early- and late-stage LP disease. However, MRI's extreme sensitivity results in false positive studies, and false negatives have also been documented. Some apparent false positives may in fact detect marrow edema that then resolves without frank necrosis [66].

During the early avascular stage, MRI may show focal or diffuse high signal intensity in the femoral head on fluid-sensitive sequences and low signal on T1-W images (see Fig. 12.16). T2-weighted (T2-W) images may show a bright anterosuperior subchondral "crescent" in the femoral head, representing a subchondral fracture. Gadolinium-enhanced MRI may show the early sign of asymmetric decreased enhancement on the affected side and more clearly delineates the area of involvement compared to non-contrast MR imaging [67]. Joint fluid and synovitis are also often evident. MRI excels at demonstrating ossific necrosis, joint effusion, and cartilage deformity, therefore replacing both nuclear scintigraphy and arthrography in the diagnosis of early disease [68].

During the reparative stage, MRI typically shows high signal intensity in the femoral head on fluid-sensitive sequences, delayed persistent enhancement after contrast administration, and possibly even increased early enhancement. Dynamic gadolinium-enhanced MRI with subtraction images can demonstrate the various revascularization patterns described in nuclear scintigraphy [69]. MRI is also unique in showing morphological changes in the femoral head as well in the epiphyseal cartilage, physis, femoral neck, and acetabular labrum. Late in the disease, MRI is useful in describing femoroacetabular incongruity and resultant impingement (Fig. 12.21).

Fig. 12.21 Severe deformity after LP disease that initially presented in an 8-year-old. (**a**, **b**) At presentation there is very mild decrease in height of the right femoral epiphysis (*arrow*, **a**) along with a subchondral fissure fracture (*arrow*, **b**) and slight sclerosis. (**c**) 1.5 years later, the femoral head is severely deformed and extensively resorbed. The pelvic crest and obturator foramen appear tilted, suggesting there may be a flexion contracture. (**d**, **e**) Arthrogram shows impingement on the labrum (*arrows*) in abduction. (**f**) Radial oblique proton density (PD) MRI shows increased signal and rounding of the anterosuperior labrum (*arrow*) with a large bony bump along the anterior aspect of femoral neck (*arrowhead*). There is severe femoroacetabular incongruity

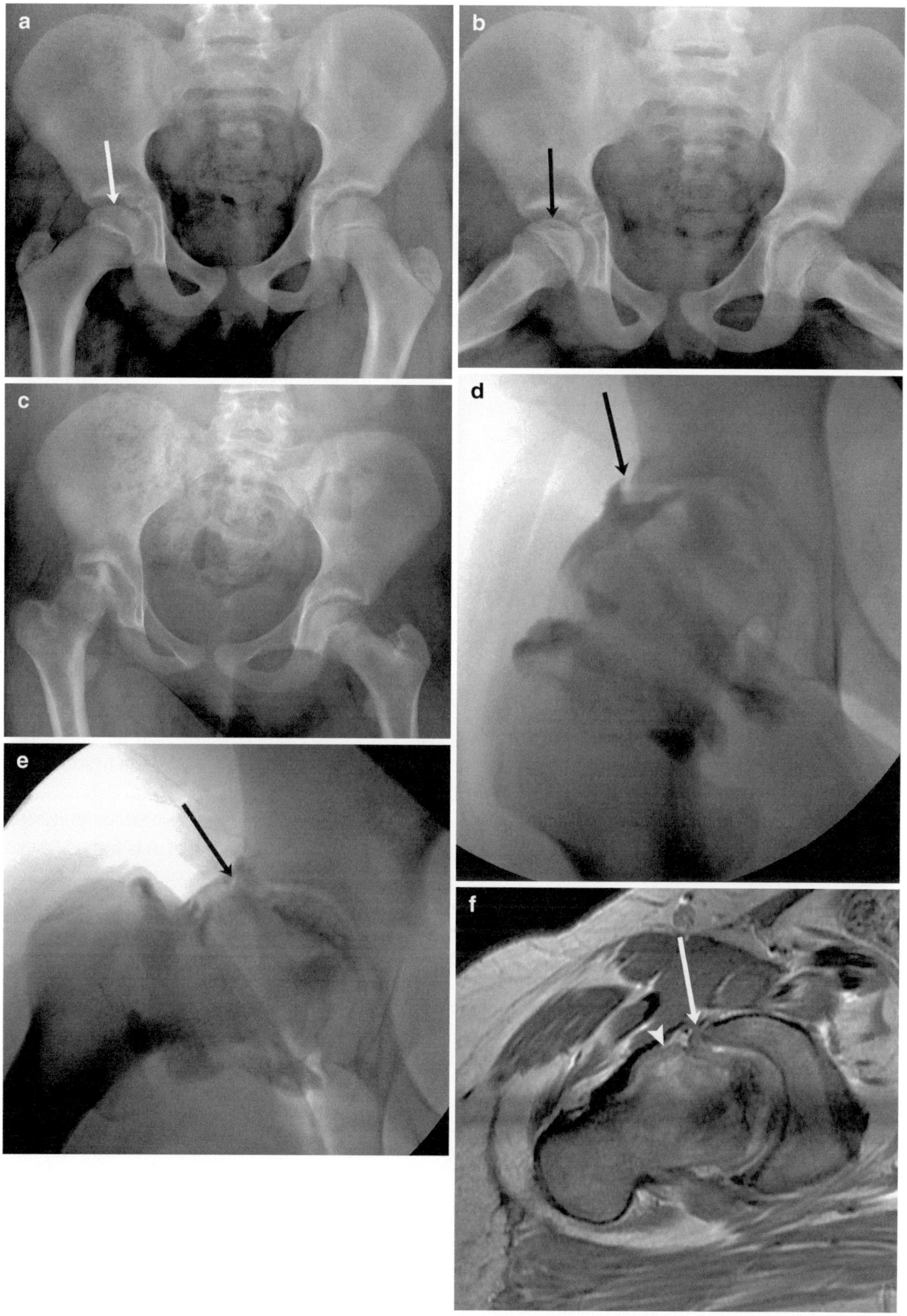
a
b
c
d
e
f

MRI techniques including diffusion-weighted imaging (DWI) and delayed gadolinium-enhanced MRI of cartilage (dGEMRIC) may provide additional information about perfusion as well as early cartilage damage. DWI shows increased diffusion in affected femoral heads in both early and reparative stages of disease [70]. The dGEMRIC technique may provide information about early cartilage damage that is not apparent on standard imaging. This technique exploits the fact that damaged cartilage has a smaller amount of negatively charged glycosaminoglycans, allowing greater accumulation of negatively charged gadolinium-diethylenetriamine pentaacetic acid (Gd-DTPA). Delayed imaging after contrast injection therefore shows T1 shortening in damaged cartilage [71].

Differential Diagnosis

LP disease is often mistaken clinically for transient synovitis. Pain and limp are similar in character but with transient synovitis symptoms have been present for days instead of weeks. Other types of AVN resemble LP disease radiographically, but clinical features help to differentiate these. Unilateral AVN in a white male in the appropriate age group is very likely to be due to LP disease. However, LP disease is rare in patients of African descent, so AVN in this population should initiate evaluation for possible sickle cell disease. Gaucher disease, steroid arthropathy, posttraumatic and post-osteomyelitic AVN, hypothyroid epiphyseal dysgenesis, hemophilia, Meyer dysplasia, and posttreatment necrosis in developmental dysplasia of the hip can also be considered in the differential diagnosis of pain and limp in the young child. Avascular changes identical to those of LP disease are seen in trichorhinophalangeal (Langer-Giedion) syndrome and familial dysautonomia. Some conditions encountered in adults, such as chronic alcoholism and caisson disease, do not apply to the pediatric age group.

Bilateral LP disease is unusual, occurring in only 13 % of patients. Bilateral disease should therefore raise concern for other etiology, especially if both hips appear to be in a similar stage of disease. Symmetric apparent AVN usually results from some type of multiple or femoral epiphyseal dysplasia.

Metaphyseal sclerosis in the early period helps exclude LP disease. Although it may be seen later (as metaphyseal cysts remodel), if encountered early, metaphyseal sclerosis is often related to medullary infarction, which may accompany non-idiopathic femoral head necrosis.

4.2 Femoral Head Necrosis of Known Etiology

Gaucher Disease

Gaucher disease is a rare autosomal recessive disorder caused by a mutation on chromosome 1q21, resulting in deficiency of glucocerebrosidase. Congenital deficiency of this enzyme prevents further metabolic degradation of the glucocerebrosides that result from normal breakdown of hematologic elements. The glucocerebroside-filled reticuloendothelial (Gaucher) cells, measuring 20–80 μm, infiltrate the bone marrow; resultant increased pressure causes atrophy of trabeculae as well as sludging and thrombosis in vessels supplying the femoral head and other bony structures. The subtypes of Gaucher disease are discussed in detail in Chap. 23. Type I, which has relatively late onset, is most common and very likely to manifest bone disease.

Significant orthopedic problems are common in children as well as adults. Skeletal manifestations progress more rapidly in children than in adults, but their course is unpredictable. Both intravascular thrombosis and medullary vascular compression lead to bone infarcts. AVN of the femoral head occurs in up to three-fourths of patients, and recurrent episodes of necrosis and healing are common. In addition, new bone production is decreased and osteoclast activity suppressed, leading to osteopenia, increased risk of pathologic fracture, and the classic "Erlenmeyer flask" remodeling defect in the distal femur (see Chap. 23). Other manifestations of the juvenile form include hepatosplenomegaly, anemia, thrombocytopenia, and osteomyelitis caused by unusual organisms.

The radiographic signs in the hip are similar to those of LP disease or any femoral head AVN [72]. Infarction usually begins in the latter half of the characteristic LP disease age range, and thus differential diagnosis may be difficult in an unrecognized case of Gaucher disease. However, bilaterality and femoral neck involvement are salient and common features of Gaucher disease. The latter, induced by marrow and medullary infarction, takes the form of metaphyseal sclerosis, ranging from a diffuse, smudged appearance to coarsening of the normal trabecular stress lines.

Radionuclide imaging can help distinguish between bone crisis and osteomyelitis. With MRI, marrow has abnormally low signal intensity due to replacement of fatty marrow with Gaucher cells (sparing the epiphysis). Quantitative chemical shift MRI helps assess disease status and response to therapy. Treatment options include enzyme replacement therapy, bone marrow transplant, or, in the future, possibly gene therapy with viral vectors.

Sickle Cell Disease and Other Hemoglobinopathies

AVN of the femoral head can occur in most sickle hemoglobin disorders. However, it is rare in the 7–9 % of the black population that carries the sickle trait [73]. Homozygous (SS) sickle cell anemia is more common than the SC dyscrasia, where the patient has two different abnormal hemoglobin genes, one "S," the other "C." The SC dyscrasia has by far the greatest incidence of femoral head necrosis: 20–60 % of all patients compared to about 10 % with the SS pattern. Silent osteonecrosis is much more common than symptomatic episodes, possibly raising the overall prevalence to 41 % in the SS disease group.

The femoral head often exhibits typical LP-like changes (Fig. 12.22), but there may also be metaphyseal sclerosis or trabecular thickening due to medullary infarction. Since marrow infarcts occur in areas of abnormal hyperplastic (red) marrow, these lesions are isointense on Tl-W MRI sequences but hyperintense on T2-W images. The vertex of the ossification center may show an osteochondritis dissecans-like contour defect. Since true LP disease is quite uncommon in people of African descent, hemoglobin electrophoresis is indicated in all such patients before diagnosing idiopathic femoral head necrosis. Managing osteonecrosis of the hip in children with sickle cell disease follows the same principles as with LP disease.

Corticosteroid-Induced Osteonecrosis

Systemic corticosteroid therapy is uncommonly but notoriously associated with femoral head collapse [74, 75] (Fig. 12.23). A variety of factors may contribute. Osteoporosis makes the bone vulnerable to microfracture. Ischemia may result from vasculitis, sludging, and fat emboli (the latter due to fatty degeneration in the liver and other organs). Steroid-induced osteocyte apoptosis may also play a role. Multiple genetic polymorphisms have been associated with increased susceptibility to steroid-induced osteonecrosis. Additionally, steroid-induced AVN is more likely in patients with renal insufficiency, graft versus host disease, inflammatory bowel disease, human immunodeficiency virus, and acute lymphoblastic leukemia and in those who have received organ transplants. These patients are often treated with steroids, and AVN may be secondary to either their underlying disease state or steroid intake.

On average, about 3 years elapse between initiation of corticosteroid therapy and onset of hip pain. Almost all patients have had more than 6 months of treatment, but femoral head necrosis may develop after as few as 7 days of therapy. No dose is considered safe but the risk of AVN increases with higher doses and prolonged treatment. After intraarticular administration of corticosteroids, Charcot-like osteocartilaginous collapse may also occur.

Avascular Necrosis in Treated Developmental Dysplasia of the Hip

AVN of the femoral ossification center is believed to occur only in patients whose developmental dysplasia has been treated. Untreated dislocation or subluxation is not predisposed to AVN (although myriad other problems ensue) [76]. Open surgical reduction appears to have higher risk for osteonecrosis than does successful closed reduction [77] (Fig. 12.24). Incidence decreased significantly after elimination of casting in extreme abduction. However, the condition remains a significant complication of treatment. AVN is very difficult to recognize, and accurate diagnosis relies on sequential observation. If the femoral head does not ossify within the first year after reduction or if an established center does not begin to grow, then AVN is strongly suggested.

Temporary irregular ossification, which may represent the mildest form of AVN, may be seen in about one-third of toddlers treated for developmental dysplasia of the hip (DDH) [78, 79]. In this condition, both the shape and the density of the ossifying femoral ahead appear irregular (Fig. 12.25). This phenomenon likely results

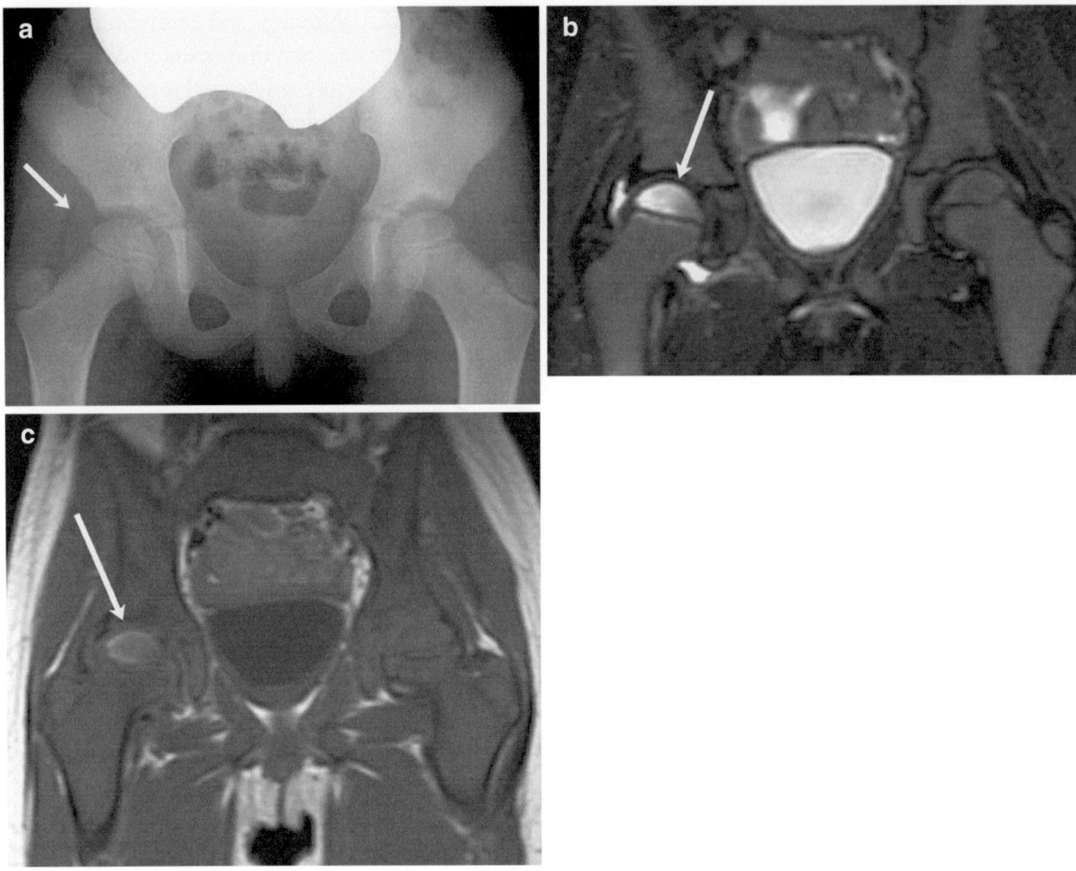

Fig. 12.22 AVN in a 7-year-old girl with sickle cell disease. (**a**) Bulging right hip fat plane (*arrow*) and increased medial joint width suggest a joint effusion. (**b**) Coronal T2-W FS image shows high signal throughout the femoral head (*arrow*) along with a joint effusion. (**c**) Coronal T1-W image shows a rim of high signal in the femoral head (*arrow*), possibly related to sludged blood products

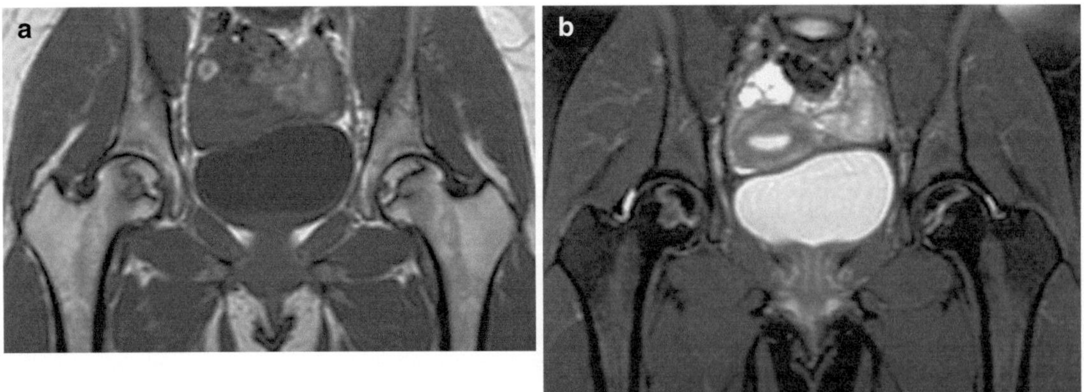

Fig. 12.23 AVN in a 17-year-old girl with lupus, treated with steroids. Coronal T1-W (**a**) and STIR (**b**) images of the pelvis show serpiginous signal alteration in both femoral heads, without articular surface collapse

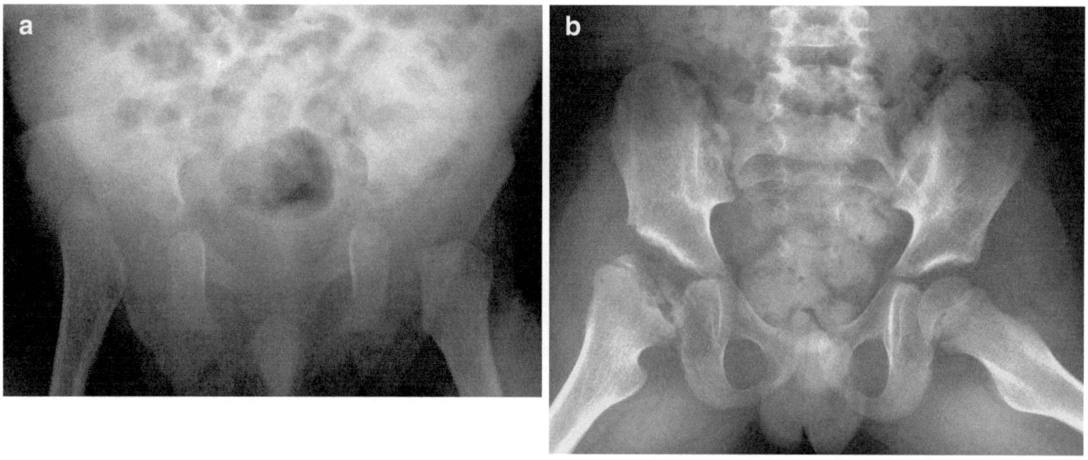

Fig. 12.24 AVN on the right in a 3-month-old with bilateral developmental hip dysplasia. (**a**) After unsuccessful harness treatment and closed reduction, the right hip is dislocated and the left hip is subluxated. (**b**) At age 6 years, following open surgical reduction on the right as well as prolonged casting, AVN has developed on the right. The left hip is normal

from a vascular insult but usually resolves with no significant long-term sequelae, except perhaps mild enlargement of the affected femoral head compared to the normal side.

Posttraumatic Femoral Head Necrosis

Femoral neck fractures are much less common in children than in adults and are nearly always due to high-energy trauma, mostly motor vehicle accidents and falls from a height. In an older series of 71 patients younger than 17 years of age, slightly over one-half of such fractures were transcervical and over one-third were basal; intertrochanteric and growth plate fractures were uncommon [1].

Older studies report a high incidence of AVN, encountered in about 40 % of patients with femoral neck fractures [1]. However, more recent series have found AVN in only about 20 % of cases [80]. AVN is more common in children younger than age 5 and is also more likely after transcervical fractures than after epiphyseal injury alone. Development of AVN depends on the severity of the original injury, associated regional fractures, and delay in reduction. Overall complications are lowest in those whose fractures are treated with open reduction and internal fixation, rather than conservative management [80].

Necrosis can involve the entire femoral head and neck, only the femoral head, or only the femoral neck. In the latter case, the epiphyseal ossification center retains a normal appearance while the femoral neck becomes sclerotic. Patients in this class are generally younger than 11 years, and premature growth plate fusion is common.

Avascular Necrosis in Osteomyelitis and Septic Arthritis

Many of the femoral head abnormalities that accompany metaphyseal osteomyelitis result from aseptic avascular necrosis rather than direct extension of the septic process into the joint or across the growth plate [81]. In young infants, this may result from septic thrombosis of vessels that terminate in the epiphysis after traversing an infected metaphysis, whereas in older children increased joint fluid may directly compress intraarticular vessels. The radiographic abnormalities are usually evident 6–8 weeks after infection, often when the condition has become clinically quiescent (see Chap. 19).

Femoral Head Dysplasia

Radiographs of older children with epiphyseal dysplasia affecting the femoral heads can closely resemble the appearance of old LP disease: bilateral, symmetric flattening of the epiphyseal ossification centers with short, wide femoral necks (see Chaps. 11 and 23). This pattern usually results from supervening AVN, which occurs in

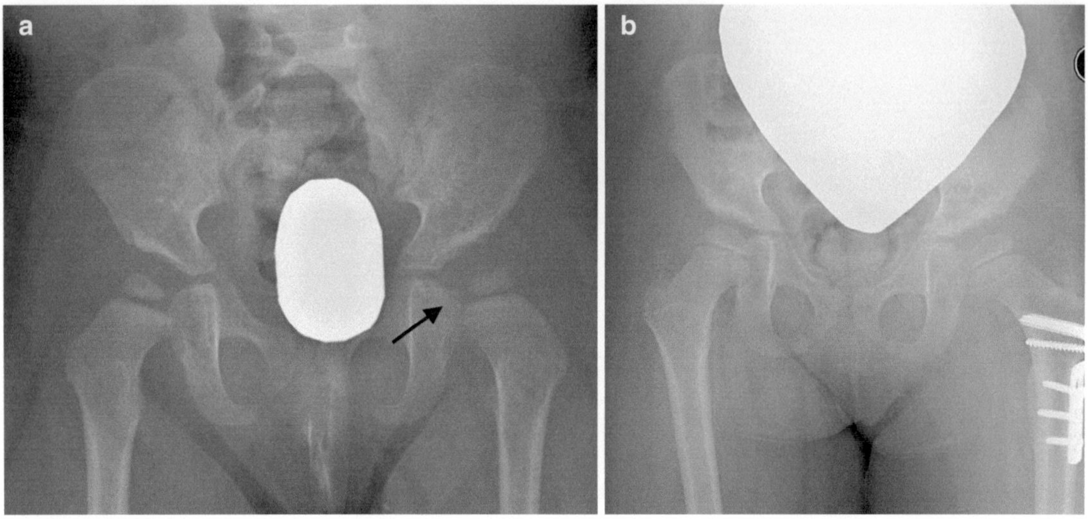

Fig. 12.25 Transient irregular ossification associated with treatment for DDH. (**a**) At age 2 years, after closed reduction, the left femoral head is small, irregular, and osteopenic (*arrow*). (**b**) Three years later, after proximal femoral osteotomy, both femoral heads are normal

some cases of isolated femoral head dysplasia or multiple epiphyseal dysplasia. Arthrography or MRI demonstrates striking mushrooming of the cartilage with the head extruded down over the neck; the inferior extent of the cartilage is marked by a metaphyseal sclerotic line. It is likely that most cases of bilaterally symmetric severe femoral head deformity are not LP disease but rather femoral head dysplasia.

5 Femoral Acetabular Impingement

Femoral acetabular impingement (FAI) is defined as pathological contact between the proximal end of the femur and the acetabulum during hip motion. This results in hip pain and limitation of motion—typically flexion and internal rotation—and may be a major cause of idiopathic osteoarthritis of the hip [82].

There are two categories of FAI: pincer impingement from the acetabular side of the joint and cam impingement from the femoral side of the joint (Fig. 12.26).[1] However, in up to 86 % of cases, a combination of the two is present [83]. FAI is usually encountered in teen and young adult athletes but can be evident at birth.

Pincer impingement arises from either over-coverage of the hip or unusual, supra-physiologic motion. The normal hip opening should be wider anteriorly than posteriorly, allowing for flexion of the leg. Generalized over-coverage can result from such entities as acetabular retroversion, coxa profunda, protrusio acetabuli, and os acetabuli. Alternatively, more limited over-coverage can result from focal acetabular retroversion or a prominent posterior wall. Ballet dancers and those with ligamentous laxity may develop pincer impingement due to supra-physiologic mobility. A more unusual cause of pincer impingement is extra-articular, resulting from a high riding greater or lesser trochanter, prominent anterior inferior iliac spine (Fig. 12.27), or osteochondromas (or less often other masses) in the proximal femur or near the anterior inferior iliac spine.

In these cases, contact between the femoral head-neck area and the acetabulum results in microtrauma to the anterior labrum, causing degeneration, cyst formation, and eventual ossification. Subtle subluxation causes "contrecoup" injury to the acetabular cartilage in the posteroinferior portion of the acetabulum [82]. With isolated pincer

[1] The term "cam" is derived from the Dutch word for "cog" and refers to an irregularly formed disk that articulates with a rocking motion.

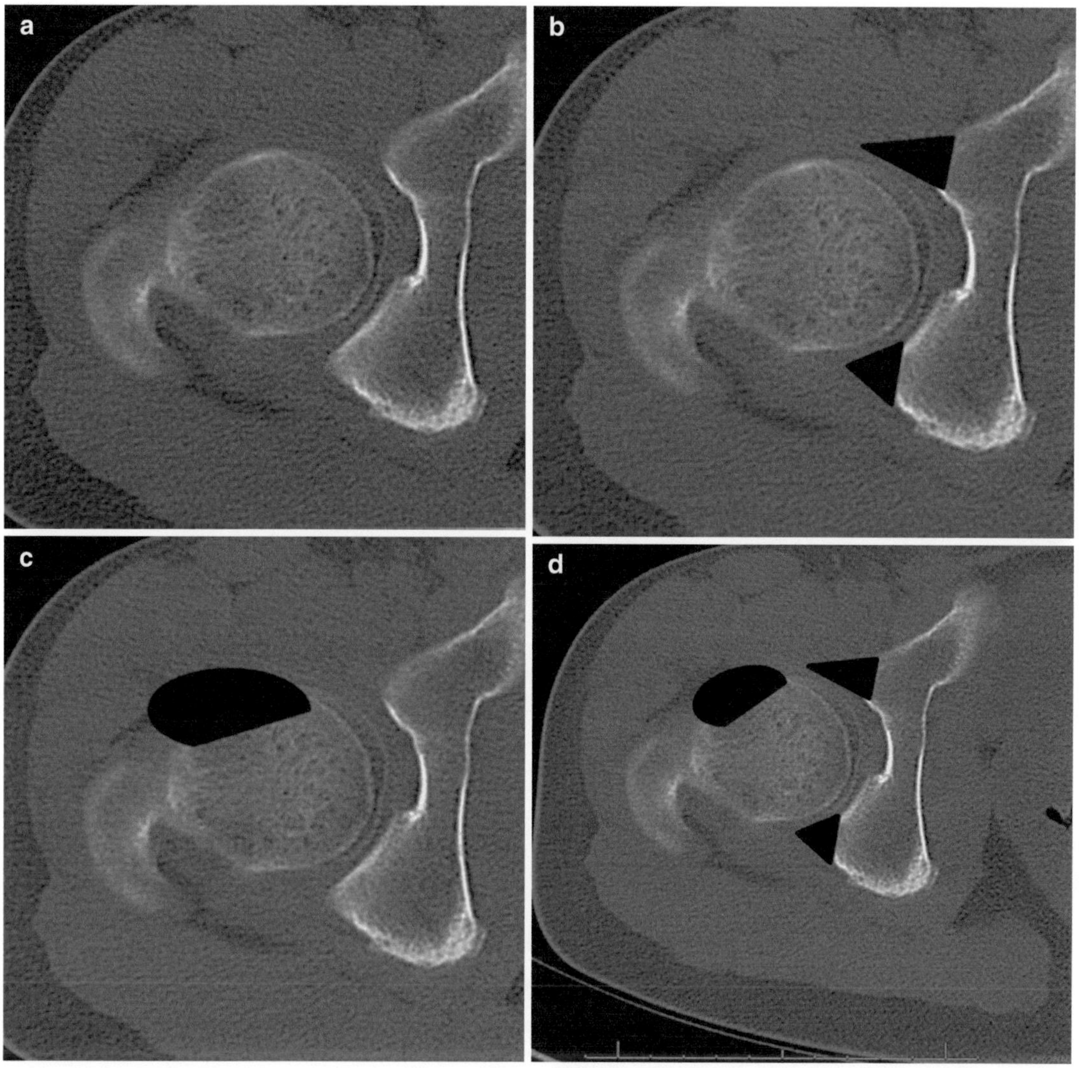

Fig. 12.26 The types of femoroacetabular impingement (FAI). (**a**) Normal: note that the anterior margin of the acetabulum is medial to the posterior margin. (**b**) *Black triangles* simulate excess bone in pincer impingement. (**c**) *Black bump* simulates asphericity of femoral head with cam impingement. (**d**) Combination of pincer and cam impingement, the most common configuration (Images modified from axial CT)

impingement, the area of chondral damage tends to be smaller than in isolated cam impingement.

Cam impingement results from an abnormal contour of the femoral neck or head (Fig. 12.28). The normal femoral neck is concave enough to accommodate the superolateral contour of the acetabulum. If the femoral neck is too thick, the femoral head too broad, or a focal bulge develops superiorly, the femur may collide with a normal acetabulum. When there is also pincer-type FAI, this problem is compounded. The chondro-osseous "bump" may be due to offset at the head-neck junction when the femoral head is no longer spherical. A common cause is the osseous bump that develops after slipped capital femoral epiphysis (SCFE) (discussed earlier in this chapter). Other causes include femoral retrotorsion, coxa vara, coxa magna, and any other condition that leads to abnormal growth of the proximal femur, such as septic arthritis and LP disease. It is also possible that abnormal contour of the femoral neck may develop if the continuous physis that initially extends from the proximal femoral physis to the greater trochanter fails to

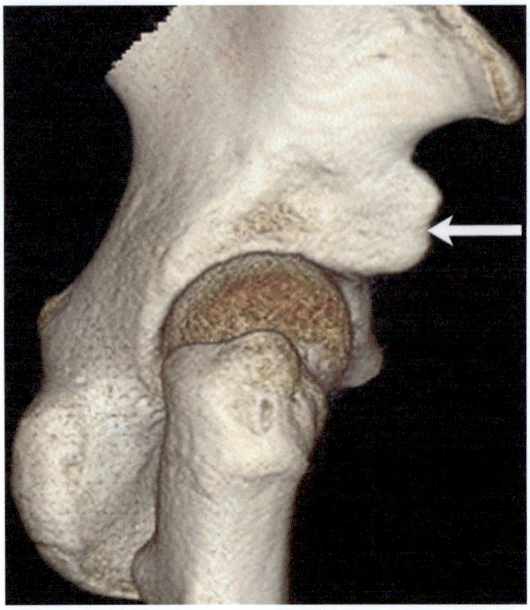

Fig. 12.27 Prominent anteroinferior iliac spine (*arrow*) causes extra-articular impingement (3D-CT reconstruction)

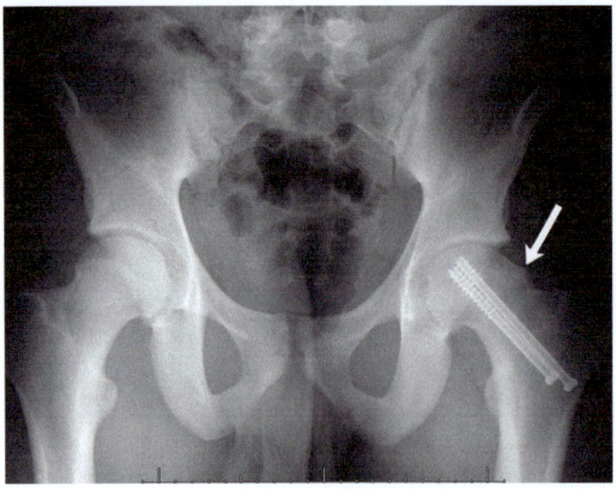

Fig. 12.28 Cam impingement attributed to slipped capitol femoral epiphysis (SCFE), with a bump (*arrow*) at the head-neck junction (Note that this view was obtained with the pelvis in extension (the sacrococcygeal junction overlaps the superior border of the symphysis) and should not therefore be used to evaluate acetabular configuration)

separate at age 5 or 6 years, leading to excessive growth in femoral neck width (see Chap. 11). In cases of cam impingement, the configuration of the femoral neck resembles that of a pistol grip.

The chondro-osseous bump can jam into the acetabulum, resulting in anterosuperior chondrolabral damage. The area of chondral damage tends to be larger than in pincer impingement, and delamination and fissuring of the acetabular cartilage may be extensive. This condition is usually seen in young men.

It is important to differentiate between focal and global acetabular retroversion, as treatment differs. A simple "rim trim" can be employed for focal retroversion. In this procedure, the overhanging portion of the cephalad part of the acetabulum is trimmed, either openly or arthroscopically, and the labrum is then reattached. However, global retroversion usually requires a more complex anteverting peri-acetabular osteotomy (also called a reverse PAO).

Untreated impingement leads to labral tears, chondral damage, and potential osteoarthritis of the hip. Imaging helps identify the cause of impingement and assess the extent of hip damage and thus facilitates appropriate treatment.

Radiographs help exclude other causes of hip pain such as avascular necrosis or inflammatory arthropathy and also evaluate the extent of damage. A variety of radiographic techniques allow assessment of acetabular and proximal femoral contour (Box 12.4). Proper technique and patient positioning are absolutely critical to diagnosing FAI correctly.

The anteroposterior (AP) view of the pelvis should be performed with the patient supine and the lower extremities internally rotated 15° (Fig. 12.29). This positioning helps eliminate the effect of femoral anteversion and also improves visualization of the femoral head-neck junction. The beam should be centered over the midpoint of a line that joins both anterior superior iliac spines and the center of the pubic symphysis. A beam centered over the hip instead may make a normal acetabulum appear abnormal [84]. It is therefore important that pelvis radiographs and not hip radiographs are used to assess for FAI.

A cross-table lateral view of the affected hip should be performed with the patient positioned as for the AP view but with the asymptomatic leg flexed. The beam is centered over the pelvis and directed cranially 45°, from the contralateral side.

A Dunn view is performed AP with hips in neutral rotation and flexed to 90° (Fig. 12.30) (for a modified Dunn, the hips are flexed to 45° and abducted 20°). This view helps identify abnormalities at the femoral head-neck junction.

Box 12.4: Radiographs for Assessing Femoroacetabular Impingement

View	Positioning	Beam
Anteroposterior (Fig. 12.29)	Supine Lower extremities internally rotated 15°	Centered over midpoint of a line joining both anterior superior iliac spines and the center of the pubic symphysis
Cross-table lateral	Supine Lower extremities internally rotated 15° Flexed contralateral leg	Centered over pelvis and directed cranially 45° from the contralateral side
Dunn (Fig. 12.30)	Anteroposterior (AP) Hips flexed to 90° Modified Dunn 45° flexion 20° abduction	
False profile of Lequesne and de Seze (Fig. 12.31)	Patient standing, pelvis rotated 65° away from cassette, affected hip against the cassette	Beam centered on the affected femoral head

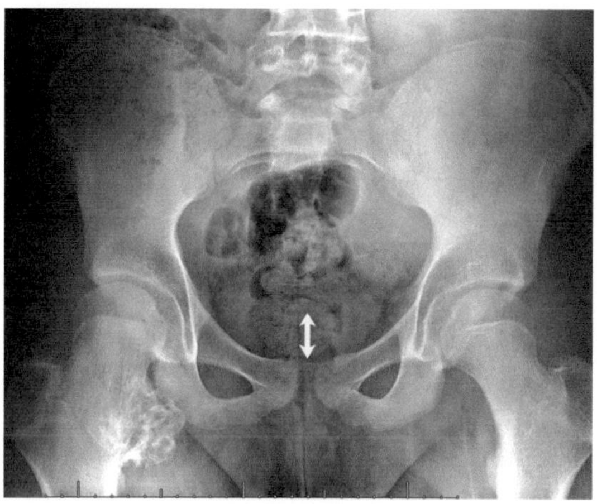

Fig. 12.29 Example of a satisfactory anteroposterior (AP) view of the pelvis that is centered over the pubic symphysis, with adequate distance between the pubic symphysis and the sacrococcygeal junction (*double arrow*). This child with multiple hereditary osteochondromatosis has extra-articular impingement along with cam impingement on the right and bilateral acetabular retroversion (pincer impingement) as evidenced by the bilateral crossover signs

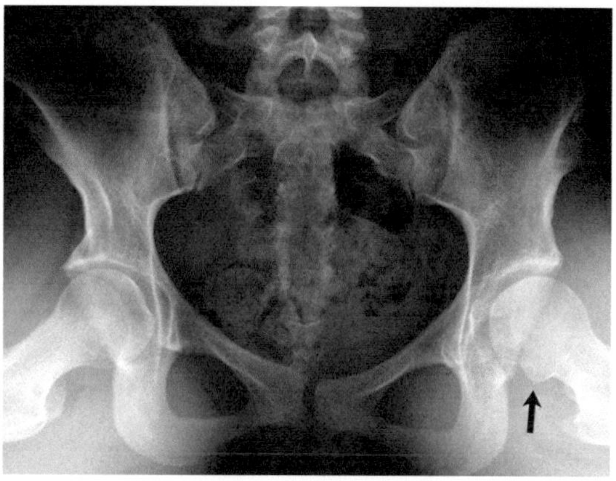

Fig. 12.30 Ninety degrees Dunn view demonstrates a "bump" (*arrow*) at the posterior portion of the left femoral head-neck junction

A false profile of Lequesne and de Seze is obtained with the pelvis rotated 65° with the affected hip against the X-ray cassette; the beam is centered on the more affected femoral head. This view helps determine the extent of anterior coverage by the acetabulum and may show that over-coverage has caused anterior impingement (Fig. 12.31).

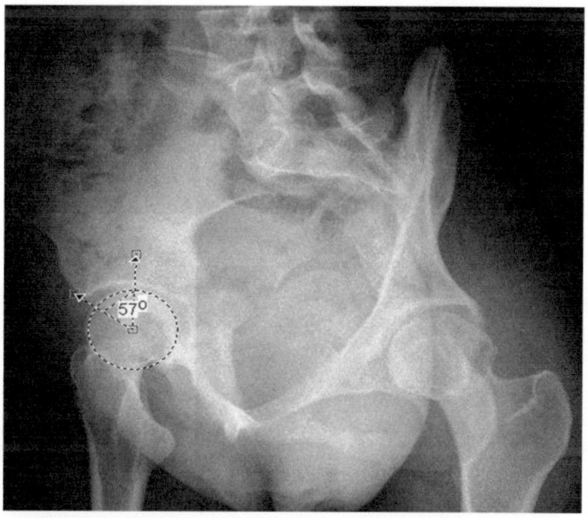

Fig. 12.31 False profile view demonstrates anterior over-coverage on the right with an anterior center edge angle of 57°

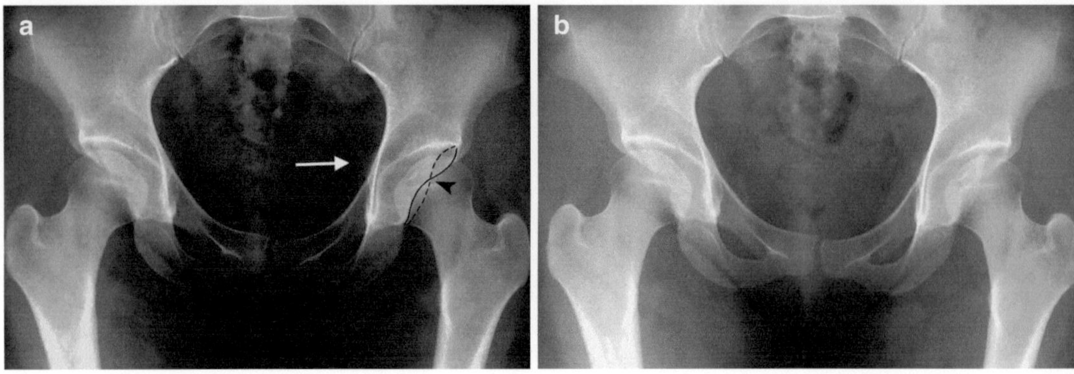

Fig. 12.32 Global retroversion. (**a**) AP view of the pelvis shows bilateral global acetabular retroversion with bilateral ischial spine sign (*white arrow*) and bilateral crossover signs. On the left, the anterior wall of the acetabulum is delineated with a solid line and the posterior wall with an interrupted line, with crossover (*arrowhead*) at the mid- to upper acetabulum. (**b**) Image provides bone detail without annotations

FAI can be properly assessed only if an image is obtained with the correct amount of pelvic tilt (or inclination) (see Fig. 12.29). Excessive anterior tilt gives the false impression of acetabular retroversion. This can be estimated on an AP view by comparing the position of the sacrococcygeal junction with the pubic symphysis. In a skeletally mature patient, the distance between these points is 1–3 cm if there is normal pelvic tilt. In addition, pelvic tilt can be assessed by correlating the AP view with a standing lateral view of the pelvis obtained without changing patient position. On the lateral, pelvic tilt is assessed by determining the angle formed between the horizontal and a line that joins the upper border of the symphysis pubis to the anterior edge of the sacral promontory. Normal pelvic inclination is about 60°. If the patient cannot be positioned with 60° of pelvic tilt, special software can be utilized to neutralize abnormal tilt (Hip2norm: University of Bern, Switzerland) [85].

A variety of radiographic findings suggest pincer impingement. These signs describe acetabular retroversion and overall configuration (which in general implies increased size). A prominent ischial spine on the AP view indicates global retroversion of the acetabulum (Fig. 12.32). In normal patients, the anterior, more horizontal wall of the acetabulum is medial to the more vertical posterior wall and may also be differentiated because the posterior wall ends at the ischium. Both can be identified on a well-positioned AP view of the pelvis, and either do not overlap at all or overlap very slightly at the upper outer corner of the acetabulum. If they cross lower down (such that a significant portion of the anterior acetabulum is lateral to the posterior), a "figure eight" or "crossover" sign is present, indicating acetabular retroversion (see Fig. 12.32). In the absence of an ischial spine sign, a crossover sign indicates focal or cephalic retroversion of the acetabulum, whereas if the ischial spine sign is also evident, there is global retroversion.

Anterior over-coverage is evident if the ventral or anterior center edge angle is more than 39° (see Fig. 12.31). On a false profile view, decreased joint space in the posteroinferior part of the joint may occur in cases with contrecoup injury from pincer impingement—this indicates increased likelihood of future arthritis and is a poor prognostic sign.

Excessive coverage of the femoral head can also result from an unusually large or deep acetabulum. Coxa profunda is seen when the medial wall of the acetabulum is at or medial to the ilio-ischial line, whereas acetabular protrusion is diagnosed if the medial wall of the femoral head is medial to the ilio-ischial line (see Chap. 11). An os acetabuli further deepens the acetabulum, predisposing the head to pincer impingement.

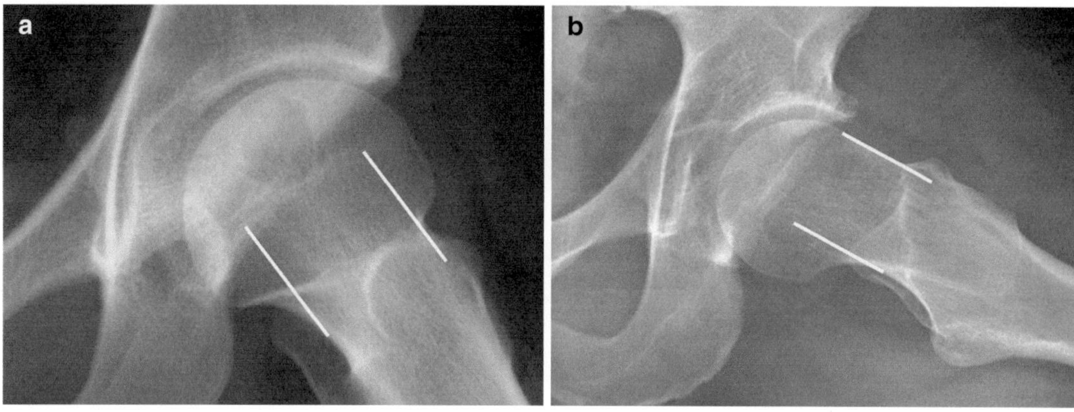

Fig. 12.33 Femoral head-neck offset on frog lateral views. (**a**) Normal anterior offset. (**b**) Lack of anterior offset in cam impingement

A Tönnis angle (the acetabular roof angle of the weight-bearing portion of the acetabular dome) of less than 0° also indicates over coverage of the femoral head.

Although less common, the posterior wall of the acetabulum can, like the anterior wall, project abnormally on an AP radiograph. The posterior wall normally projects at the center of the femoral head. If it projects lateral to this point, there is increased coverage, predisposing the patient to the less common posterior impingement and difficulty with extension. This is often associated with coxa profunda or acetabular protrusion but may be seen in isolation. Alternatively, if the posterior acetabular wall projects medial to the center of the femoral head, posterior coverage is deficient (often associated with excessive anterior coverage).

An abnormal contour of the femoral neck and head-neck junction can suggest cam impingement. A prominent superior bulge at the femoral neck may be seen after SCFE, or the upper femoral neck may be diffusely broad, resulting in the "pistol-grip" deformity (Fig. 12.33). The extent of deformity may be measured using the anterior offset, femoral head-neck offset ratio, or alpha angle. The anterior offset is defined as the difference between the radius of the anterior portion of the femoral head and the anterior femoral neck, determined on a cross-table view; normal is less than 10 mm. The femoral head-neck offset ratio is the ratio between the anterior offset and the diameter of the femoral head and if less than 0.15–0.18 predisposes to cam impingement [84].

The alpha angle is determined on either a radiograph or on an MRI (Fig. 12.34). It is formed by the intersection between a line drawn along the axis of the femoral neck and a line that connects the center of the femoral head to the point where the femoral head is no longer spherical (near the head-neck junction). Authorities disagree about the normal value for an alpha angle, but it is reasonable to consider the normal upper limit for this angle 55–60° [86]. Femoral head-neck offset may be more reliable.

If a cam lesion is advanced, there may be an accompanying small, lucent pit at the anterior femoral neck, presumably due to impact from the acetabulum. This is termed "fibrocystic change" or "impingement cyst" (Box 12.5).

The configuration of the acetabulum and femoral neck can also be assessed on CT. On axial images, the anterior acetabulum should be medial to the posterior acetabulum on every image. 3D CT can demonstrate deformity of the femoral neck in exquisite detail.

MRI is extremely useful for evaluating FAI, as it clearly identifies the cartilage, capsule, bone, surrounding soft-tissue anatomy, and extent of damage. Acetabular retroversion is best recognized on

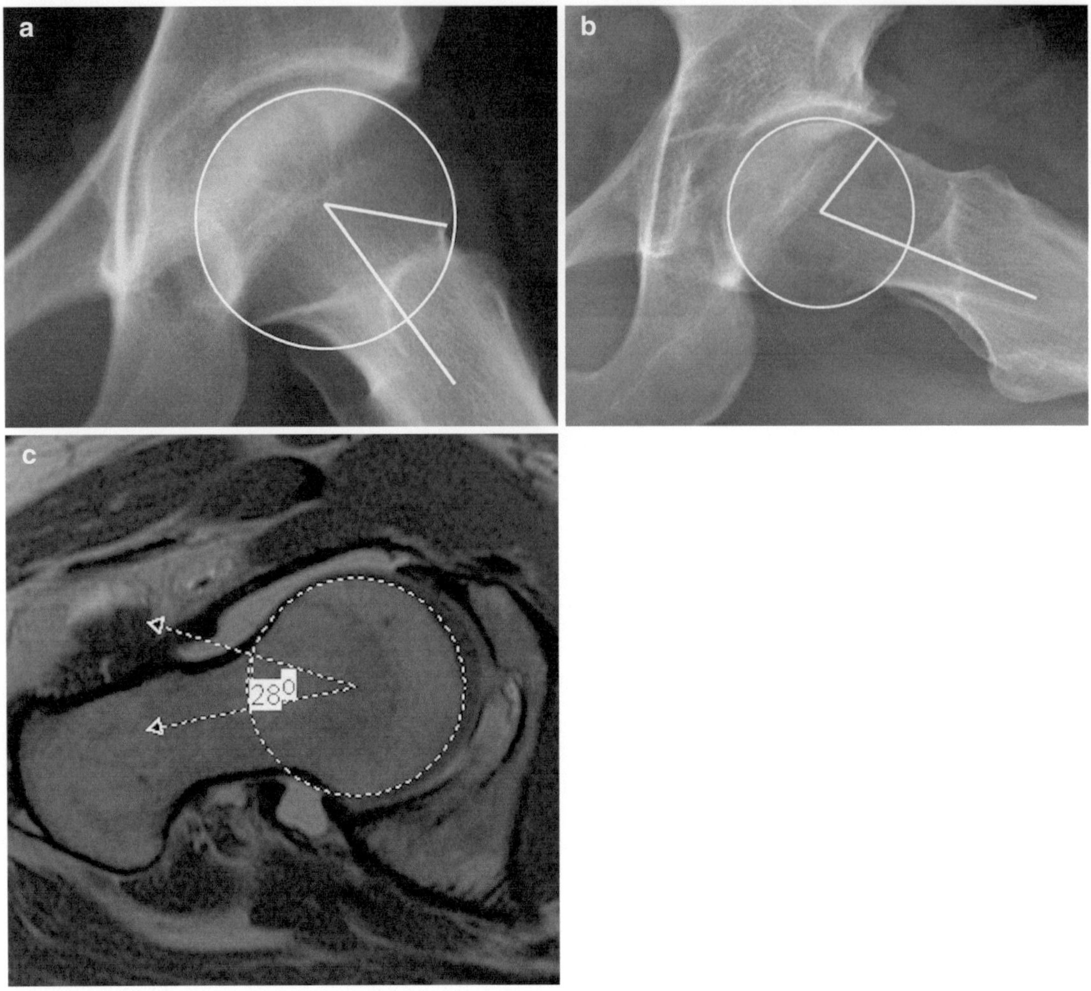

Fig. 12.34 Alpha angle on frog lateral views and MRI. (**a**) Normal angle of 42°. (**b**) Abnormal alpha angle of 67° in cam impingement. (**c**) Axial T1-W MRI shows normal angle of 28 degrees

axial images, especially the most cephalad image that includes a portion of the femoral head. Retroversion is present if the anterior acetabular margin projects lateral to the posterior acetabular margin on any image (Fig. 12.35a). Cam-type configuration of the femoral neck is recognized on axial or coronal images. The femoral neck should appear concave on all images, no matter the plane (Fig. 12.35b). True sagittal views and radial imaging play an important role in evaluating labral morphology. However, direct or magnetic resonance arthrography (MRA) is needed to adequately demonstrate conditions that predispose to eventual osteoarthritis, such as chondromalacia, loose bodies, and labral tears, degeneration, and hypertrophy.

Arthrography with either direct or indirect injection of contrast into the joint has been used to identify labral and chondral pathology. Noncontrast MRI, especially with fluid-sensitive sequences and higher field strength (e.g., 3.0 Tesla), may help identify labral tears. In general, routine MRI tends to underestimate the degree of chondral injury when compared to arthroscopy.

Box 12.5: Radiographic Findings in Femoroacetabular Impingement (FAI)

Adequate AP pelvic radiograph

Symmetric, open obturator foramina

Pelvic inclination about 60°

1–3 cm gap between sacrococcygeal junction and pubic symphysis

Pelvic inclination on lateral

Sacral promontory to top of symphysis (vs horizontal): 60°

Pincer impingement: acetabulum too large or abnormally angled

Prominent ischial spine	Global acetabular retroversion
Figure eight/ crossover	Focal (cephalic) retroversion
Posterior wall	
Too medial	Posterior wall sign: deficient posterior wall associated with anterior impingement
Too lateral	Posterior impingement (less common)
Coxa profunda	Medial contour of acetabulum medial to ilio-ischial line
Acetabular protrusion	Medial contour of femoral head medial to ilio-ischial line

Cam impingement

Femoral neck	Abnormally broad
	Focal bulge
Femoral head	Abnormally wide
Head-neck offset	Radius of femoral neck vs femoral head
	IIcad normally 10 mm larger than neck

5.1 Labral Tears

The normal labrum is uniformly hypointense, smooth, and triangular (Fig. 12.36). Labral tears are characterized by abnormal morphology, irregular contrast or fluid accumulation within the labral substance, or displaced fragments (Fig. 12.37). Tears are often associated with a superolateral paralabral cyst and are rarely found

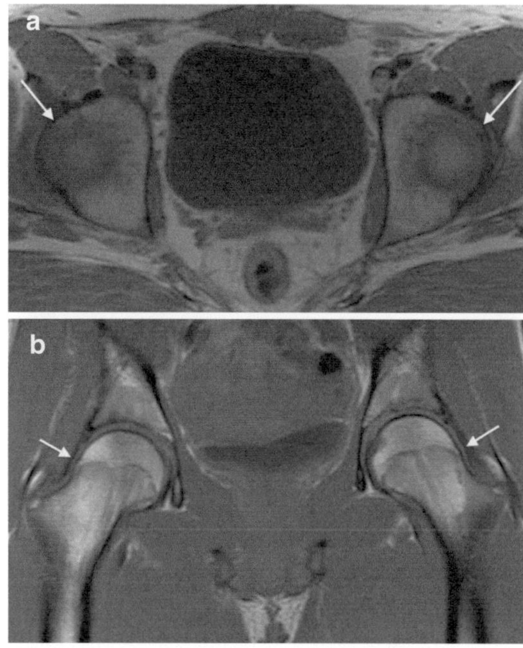

Fig. 12.35 FAI shown on MRI. (**a**) Axial T1-W MRI in a 15 y/o shows bilateral acetabular retroversion. The anterior margins (*arrows*) of the acetabula are lateral to the posterior margins. (**b**) Coronal T1-W MRI in a 17 y/o shows bilateral cam configuration of femoral necks, which lack normal concavity

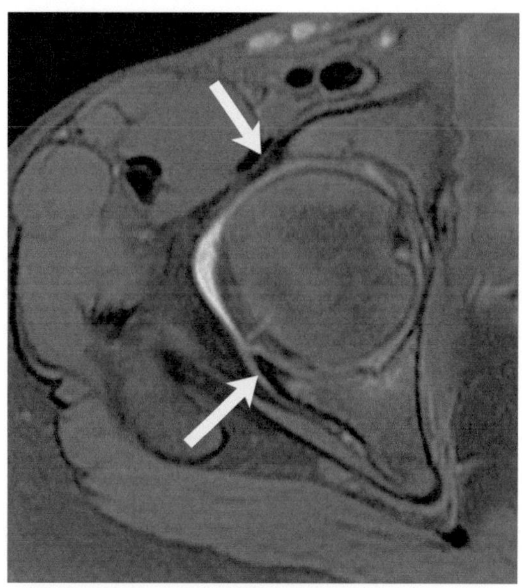

Fig. 12.36 Normal, triangular, uniformly hypointense labrum (*arrows*). Axial image from MR arthrogram (MRA)

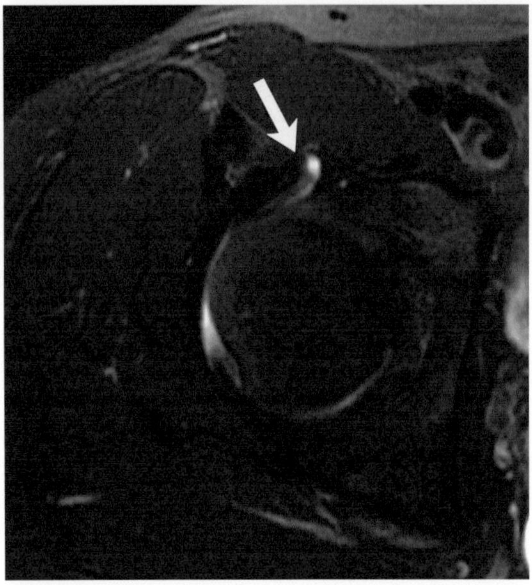

Fig. 12.37 Anterosuperior labral tear. Contrast extends beyond the base of the labrum (*arrow*) on this axial image from an MRA

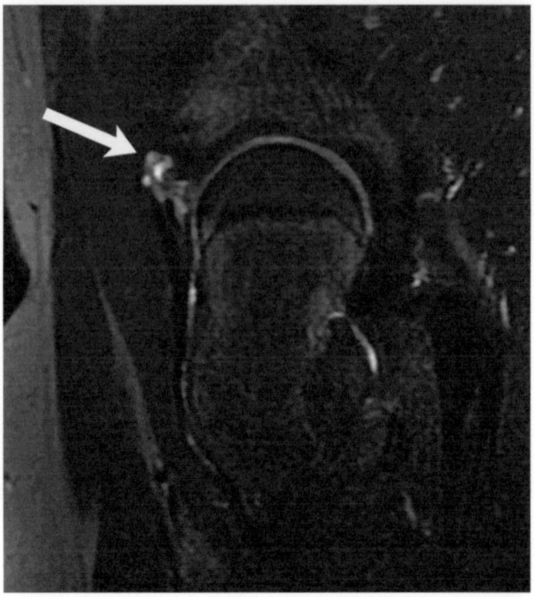

Fig. 12.38 Anterior labral detachment with paralabral cyst. Sagittal image from MRA shows fluid protruding through the labral separation and forming the paralabral cyst (*arrow*)

without an underlying osseous abnormality (Fig. 12.38) [87]. If a paralabral cyst is present, an accompanying labral tear is extremely likely. These tears may result from FAI or abnormal loading from hip dysplasia or instability.

Labral tears should be differentiated from a paralabral recess. This normal variant is usually positioned at the anteroinferior acetabulum near the 8-o'clock position. The recess is characterized by linear contrast interposition, only partial separation of the labrum, and absence of accompanying perilabral abnormalities [88, 89]. A labral tear can also be confused with a normal-variant cleft at the anteroinferior labral-transverse acetabular ligament junction; there may also be an associated recess.

5.2 Chondral Injury

Acetabular cartilage delamination occurs in almost half of all cases of cam impingement [83]. MRI—and especially MRA—can delineate the extent of cartilage damage. However, even MRA is relatively insensitive. The "inverted oreo cookie" sign is the most specific finding: hyperintense signal on either side of the delaminated, or hypointense, cartilage [90] (Fig. 12.39). However, this sign is insensitive, being seen in less than one-third of delamination cases [91]. The most useful sign of cartilage delamination is a hypointense area in the acetabular cartilage on intermediate weighted fat-suppressed (FS) or T1-W sequences [91]. dGEMRIC imaging can delineate abnormal cartilage in areas of delamination.

6 Chondrolysis of the Hip

Chondrolysis of the hip is a rare condition characterized by progressive loss of hip joint space along with pain, stiffness, and spasm [92]. It may be idiopathic or secondary to underlying conditions, such as SCFE, intraarticular penetration of SCFE pins, infection, inflammatory arthritis, prolonged immobilization, or severe trauma (Fig. 12.40).

Primary or idiopathic chondrolysis was initially described in adolescent African-American females but has since been reported in other populations as well as in males; it is now most frequently encountered in preadolescents [93]. The etiology is uncertain, but the process may involve a complement-mediated immunologic mechanism. Involvement may be unilateral or bilateral. On

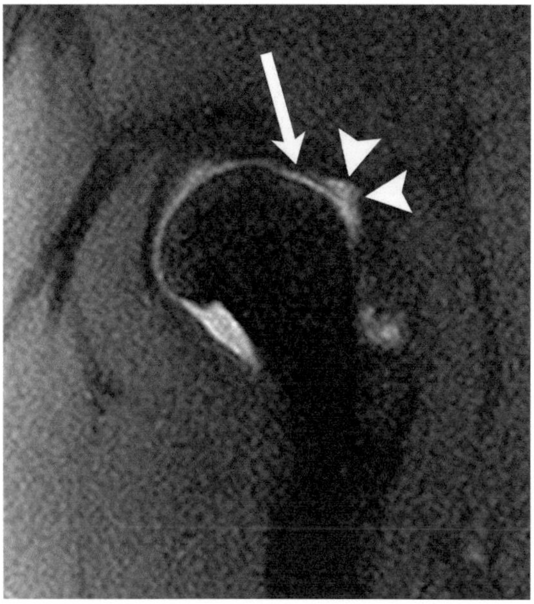

Fig. 12.39 Chondral injury showing "inverted oreo cookie" sign. Sagittal image from MRA shows delamination of the hypointense acetabular cartilage (*arrow*), which is surrounded by contrast (*arrowheads*) along the articular as well as deep (bony) surface

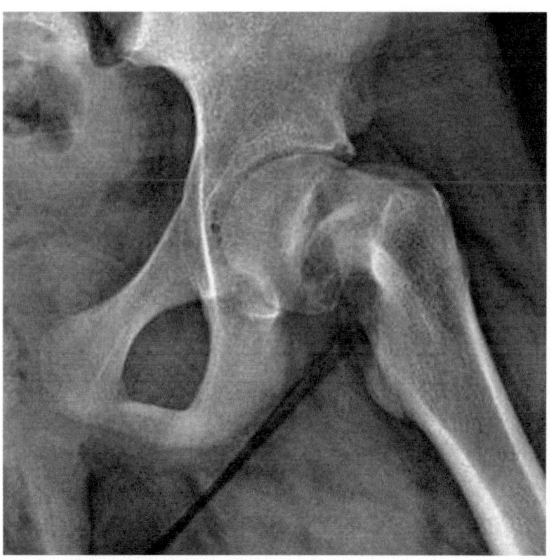

Fig. 12.40 Chondrolysis. Marked hip joint narrowing after remote, severe SCFE

physical examination there is typically a flexion, abduction, and external rotation contracture. Differential diagnosis includes infectious arthritis, juvenile idiopathic arthritis, pigmented villonodular synovitis, and rare tumors such as osteoid osteoma.

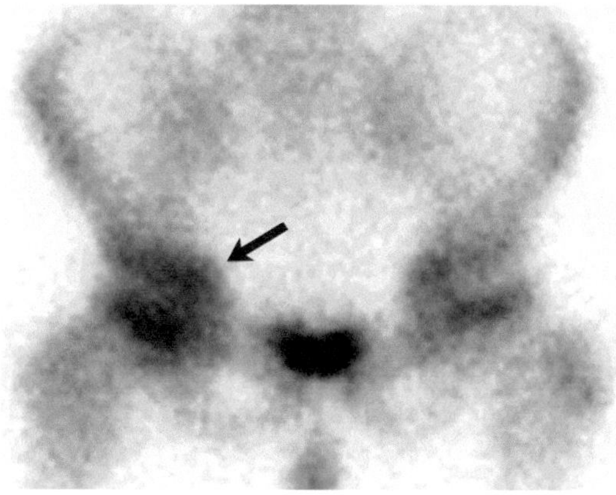

Fig. 12.41 Chondrolysis. Bone scan shows increased radiotracer uptake in the acetabulum (*arrow*) and adjacent femur

Imaging

Chondrolysis is defined as joint space narrowing to less than 3 mm [94]. Radiographs obtained early in the course of disease may reveal only mild diminution of joint space. However, serial imaging demonstrates progressive, asymmetric, and mainly central loss of joint space. On radiographs, there is usually abduction contracture with resultant pelvic tilt towards the affected side, along with asymmetry in the obturator foramina (reflecting flexion contracture). Bone scan demonstrates nonspecific increased radiotracer uptake in the femoral head and acetabulum (Fig. 12.41). MRI performed early in the course of the disease helps establish the diagnosis and also excludes other processes. Early findings include a small joint effusion, synovial enhancement, and segmental altered signal intensity within the middle third of the femoral head (best seen on coronal images) [95] (Fig. 12.42). As disease progresses, extensive edema develops in the femoral head and acetabulum, joint fluid increases, and the gluteal musculature atrophies [96].

Following examination under anesthesia to determine the degree of fixed contractures, treatment includes physical therapy and continuous use of a passive motion machine. Aggressive surgical release and hinged hip distraction are performed in recalcitrant cases [97]. The clinical course varies. Some hips will progress to end-stage arthritis or even spontaneous fusion (Fig. 12.43), whereas others may completely heal.

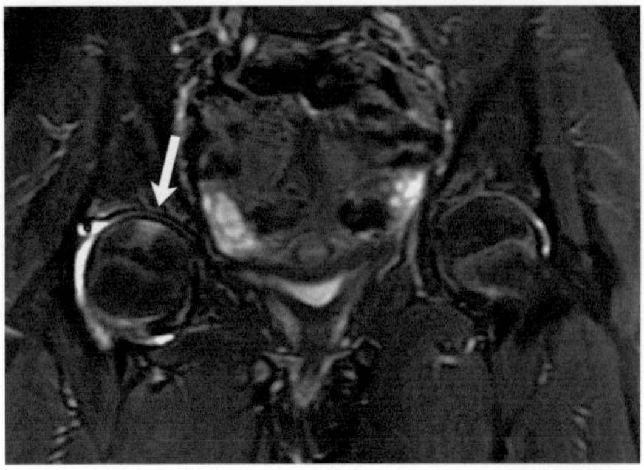

Fig. 12.42 Early chondrolysis. Coronal STIR MRI shows the characteristic geographic area of increased signal intensity in the central portion of the femoral head (*arrow*). There is also a small joint effusion

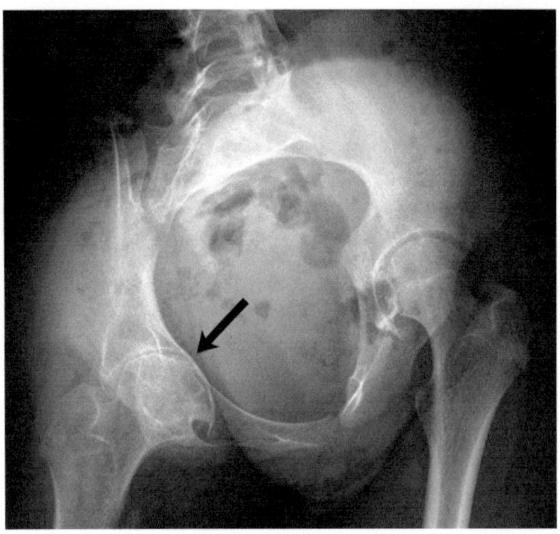

Fig. 12.43 Advanced chondrolysis with secondary arthritis and deformity (*arrow*)

7 Inflammatory/Infectious/Neoplastic Processes

7.1 Transient Synovitis

Transient synovitis (toxic synovitis, observation hip, irritable hip) presents with hip or knee pain, limp, and spasm, usually with acute onset. In contrast to patients with Legg-Perthes (LP) disease, children with transient synovitis tend to have had a shorter period of symptoms (6 days versus 6 weeks) and are less likely to have bilateral disease (1 % instead of 10 %). The typical age of onset differs: those with transient synovitis tend to be younger (3–5 years old, versus 4–8 for LP disease). The male to female ratio is 2:1 for toxic synovitis and 4:1 for LP disease [98]. Although the pathogenesis of transient synovitis is still not completely clear, evidence indicates a viral etiology [99].

Treatment consists of rest and pain management, since transient synovitis is a self-limited condition with no known long-term sequelae. Radiographic follow-up to exclude other diagnoses, like LP disease, is not necessary if symptoms resolve [100].

Imaging

While nonspecific, transient synovitis is characterized by joint effusion without associated findings (Fig. 12.44). Radiographs are most useful for excluding alternative diagnoses, as radiographic abnormalities are uncommon in transient synovitis. Asymmetry of the fat planes projected lateral to the femoral neck is misleading and probably a function of antalgic rotation and spasm, not joint capsule distension from the effusion. Widening of the medial joint space occurs with elevated intraarticular pressure but is usually minimal in simple transient synovitis.

The primary role of US is to document a joint effusion in children with hip pain and suspected transient synovitis. Hip US is performed in the anterior longitudinal plane parallel to the femoral neck. Bilateral imaging is performed for comparison as well as detection of unsuspected bilateral joint effusion. Gray scale and power Doppler cannot reliably differentiate transient synovitis from septic arthritis [101, 102].

There is considerable overlap in the MRI appearance of hips with transient synovitis and septic arthritis. Both show joint effusion and synovial thickening and enhancement. Transient synovitis is suggested by uniform normal signal in the proximal femoral bone marrow (see Fig. 12.44), and contralateral joint fluid is present in as many as 63 % [103]. Septic arthritis, on the other hand, is characterized by signal alternation in the bone marrow and surrounding soft tissues as well as decreased perfusion of the

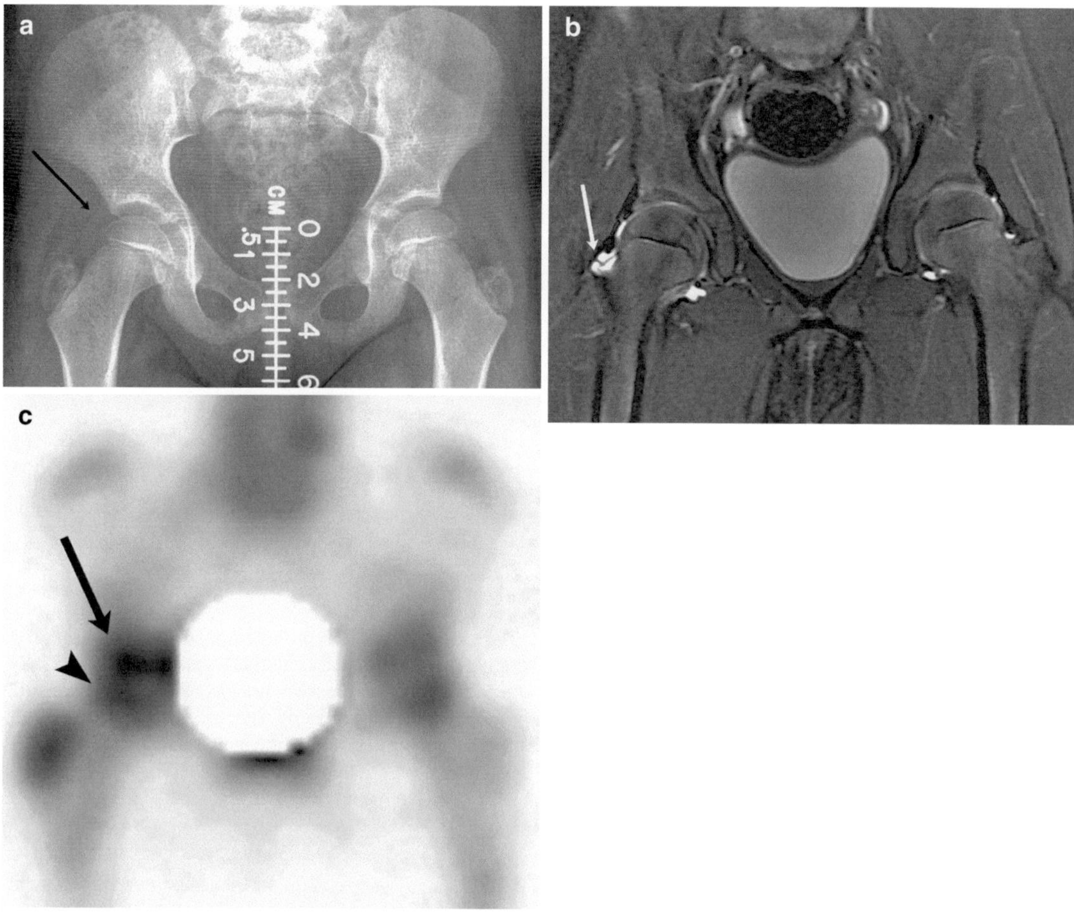

Fig. 12.44 Transient synovitis in a 5-year-old boy with hip pain. (**a**) Apparent bulging of the right hip fat plane (*arrow*) probably results from slight rotation of the femur. (**b**) Coronal T2-W FS MR image shows a joint effusion (but no significant bulging of the capsule) (*arrow*), without bone marrow edema or surrounding soft-tissue inflammation. (**c**) Corresponding coronal single photon emission computed tomography (SPECT) image from delayed phase of a triple-phase Tc-99 MDP bone scan shows increased activity at the right acetabulum (*arrow*) and growth plate of the right proximal femur (*arrowhead*). There was also mildly increased blood pool activity of the right hip (not shown). These mild periarticular findings favor toxic synovitis over septic arthritis

femoral head on contrast-enhanced images [103, 104]. MRI can also depict extra-articular causes of pain such as osteomyelitis and pyomyositis.

Radionuclide scintigraphy has been reported to be either normal or show periarticular increased uptake in transient synovitis (Figs. 12.44 and 12.45). If a bone scan is normal, radiographs obtained 6 months later should be normal as well.

The differential diagnosis of transient synovitis is extensive and includes bacterial and tuberculous infection, juvenile idiopathic arthritis, traumatic synovitis, LP disease, idiopathic chondrolysis, and leukemia. Clinical prediction algorithms for differentiating between septic arthritis and transient synovitis are inaccurate [105]. Transient synovitis is unlikely when marked deossification, soft-tissue swelling, and medial joint space widening are present.

7.2 Septic Arthritis

Children with septic arthritis often present with hip or knee pain and limp, usually with acute onset. Clinical features include fever, inability to

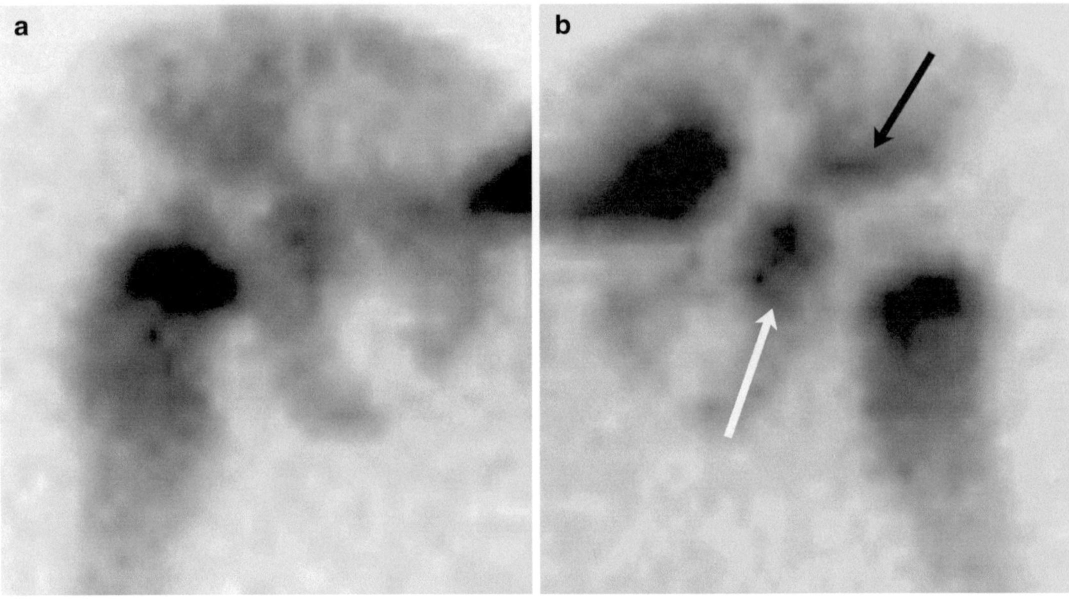

Fig. 12.45 Transient synovitis in an 11-month-old boy not bearing weight on his left leg. Pinhole images of the hips from delayed phase of a Tc-99 MDP bone scan (**a**, normal right hip (for comparison); **b**, symptomatic left hip). There is increased activity in the (**b**) left ischium (*white arrow*) and ilium (*black arrow*) compared to the normal right (**a**). Left femoral head activity is decreased, likely due to increased pressure from a joint effusion. Note that right and left pinhole images are acquired separately, and the intensity of uptake presented is not standardized between the two images. For this reason, the entire visualized pelvis in the image of the right hip appears to have greater uptake than the left. In fact, the left acetabulum has increased uptake, making the remainder of the pelvis in the left hip image appear to have decreased uptake

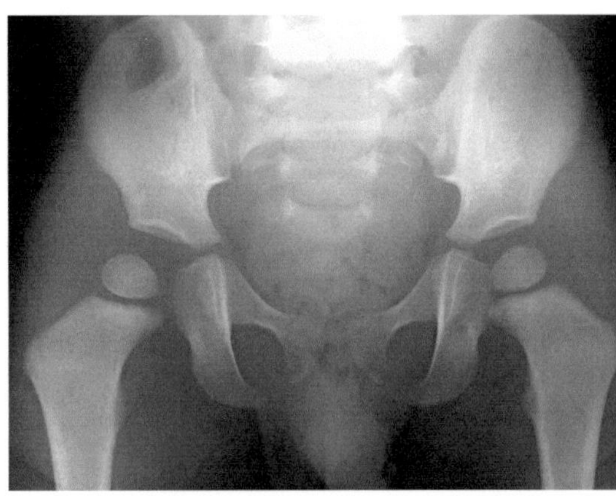

Fig. 12.46 Septic arthritis and osteomyelitis in a 2-year-old boy who refused to bear weight. The right femoral head is displaced laterally and the fat plane is effaced, a finding rarely seen in transient synovitis

bear weight, and elevated white blood cell count, C-reactive protein level, and erythrocyte sedimentation rate. Infants often lack classic signs of sepsis but instead present with irritability, lethargy, poor feeding, abdominal distention, and cyanosis. They may refuse to use the affected limb or have pseudoparalysis. The incidence of septic arthritis in children peaks between ages 1 and 3 years.

Septic arthritis may result from hematogenous seeding or as an extension of hip osteomyelitis. Severe osteocartilaginous changes may occur early due to bacterial enzymatic destruction of cartilage and to the compromised vascular supply incurred by increased joint pressures and arterial thrombosis; the latter may also cause AVN.

Radiographs are rarely helpful in the early stages of the disease, although if there is a large amount of joint fluid the femoral head may subluxate laterally (Fig. 12.46). US can demonstrate joint fluid (Fig. 12.47), but as with toxic synovitis the presence (or absence) of echogenic foci within the fluid does not help with diagnosis. A bone scan will be positive in all three phases. MRI is most helpful for delineating abscesses and the extent of

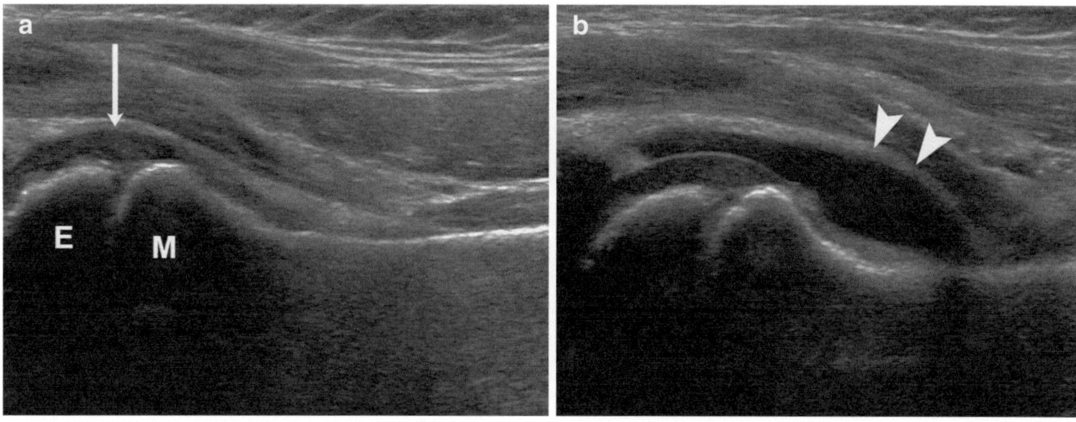

Fig. 12.47 A 2-year-old with pain and limp but no fever, diagnosed with septic arthritis after joint aspiration. (**a**) Anterior longitudinal ultrasound (US) image of the normal right hip (for comparison) shows hypoechoic articular cartilage (*arrow*), not to be confused with joint fluid. The bony epiphysis (E) and metaphysis (M) appear as echogenic lines. (**b**) On the left, there is a large anechoic joint effusion with bulging of the capsule (*arrowheads*)

osseous involvement. (See Chap. 19 for further discussion of septic arthritis.) Definitive diagnosis ultimately depends on joint aspiration.

7.3 Juvenile Idiopathic Arthritis

Juvenile idiopathic arthritis (JIA) is a chronic inflammatory disease with prominent joint involvement. At the time of diagnosis, the hip is affected in only 5 % of patients, but during the next few years, involvement increases to about 40 %. Hip involvement is more common in the systemic form of JIA, and it is usually bilateral. JIA is also characterized by developmental changes, such as femoral head overgrowth, premature growth plate fusion, and ultimately femoral head underdevelopment. Erosive changes lead to osteoarthritis (Fig. 12.48). Osteonecrosis can occur and resembles LP disease. Early recognition of hip involvement may help reduce disability. Therapy relies largely on antiinflammatory and immune modulating drugs, but hip joint replacement is ultimately required in 26–44 % of patients [106].

In addition to erosive bone and cartilage changes and synovial cysts, late sequelae include lateral subluxation, coxa valga, femoral head enlargement, premature growth plate fusion with femoral neck underdevelopment, and intrapelvic acetabular protrusion; many of these findings are probably secondary to femoral head and growth plate ischemia [107]. Those with hip symptoms often have severe involvement at MRI, but even asymptomatic patients may have abnormal findings [108]. MRI may demonstrate hip effusion, synovitis, bone marrow edema, erosions, cartilage loss, bone remodeling, and acetabular protrusion. Similar changes may be seen with other inflammatory arthritides as well (Fig. 12.49). (See Chap. 20 for additional discussion of JIA.)

7.4 Synovial Chondromatosis

The formation of intraarticular chondroid bodies characterizes this benign neoplastic condition. While the term osteochondromatosis is synonymous, synovial chondromatosis avoids confusion with multiple cartilaginous osteochondromas (MCE) syndrome. Synovial chondromatosis is uncommon and seen mostly in adults, but children may be affected. Pediatric disease is usually monoarticular and often involves the hip or, less commonly, the knee. Other synovial sites such as bursae and tendons are rarely involved [109, 110]. Males are affected two to four times more often than females [111]. Patients most commonly present with insidious development of nonspecific hip pain, swelling, and restricted range of motion. Physical examination may show

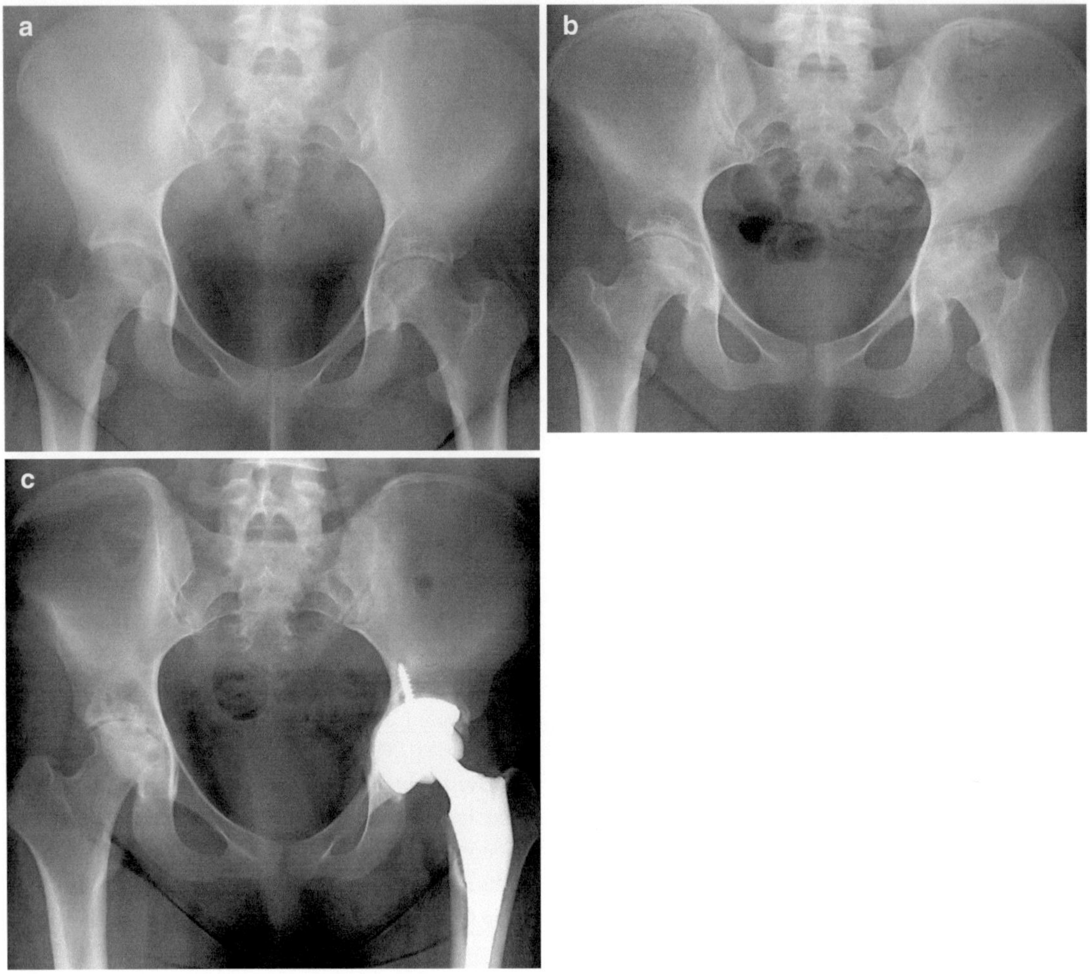

Fig. 12.48 Juvenile idiopathic arthritis in a teenage girl. (**a**) At age 16, there are bilateral erosions as well as hip joint space narrowing. (**b**) Three years later, there is complete loss of the left hip joint space, with extensive erosions and secondary osteoarthritis. Erosions on the right have progressed. (**c**) One year later, there had been further loss of cartilage on the right, and left hip arthroplasty has been performed

a swollen, enlarged hip joint with crepitus, locking, or, rarely, palpable nodules.

Since symptoms are nonspecific and progress slowly, several years often elapse between the onset of symptoms and diagnosis. The intraarticular bodies may cause extrinsic erosion of bone on both sides of the joint. In chronic cases, osteoarthritis and joint space narrowing may develop. Very rarely, synovial chondromatosis may undergo malignant transformation to chondrosarcoma.

Intraarticular chondroid bodies may remain cartilaginous, or they may calcify and ossify. When these subsynovial cartilaginous deposits grow large enough, they form sessile masses that may eventually become pedunculated. If detached from their pedicles, intraarticular free bodies result, nourished by the synovial fluid. Rare familial cases have been reported. Primary synovial chondromatosis should be distinguished from secondary disease, which is unusual in children and which follows previous injury to the joint cartilage.

On gross inspection, the intraarticular bodies consist of hyaline cartilage nodules covered by hyperplastic and attenuated synovium [112]. The number of bodies varies widely, but they are usually numerous and similar in size (Fig. 12.50);

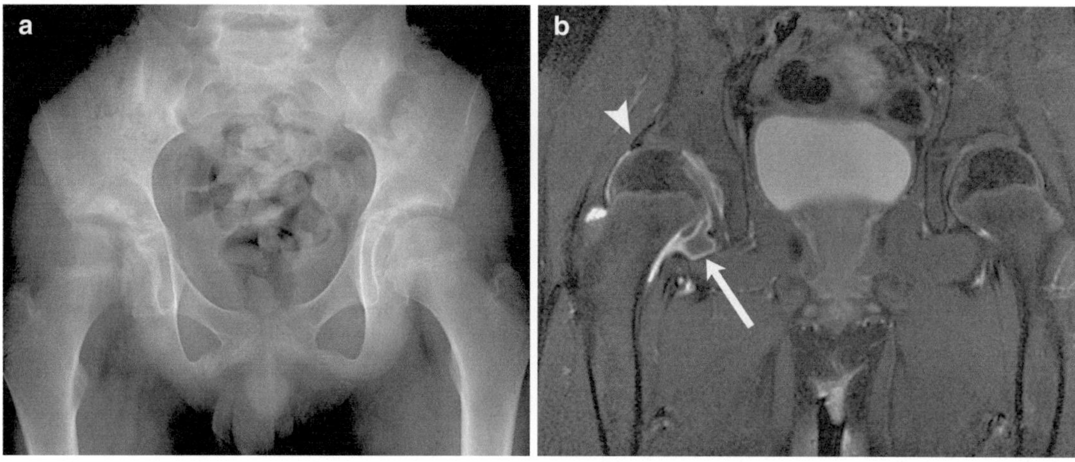

Fig. 12.49 A 12-year-old boy with spondyloarthropathy, who first presented with an abnormal gait. (**a**) The right hip is subluxated, the femoral head osteopenic, and there is irregular acetabular sclerosis with slight superolateral joint space narrowing. (**b**) Coronal T1-W FS gadolinium-enhanced image shows a right hip effusion with synovial thickening and enhancement (*arrow*), as well as subluxation. The labrum is uplifted (*arrowhead*)

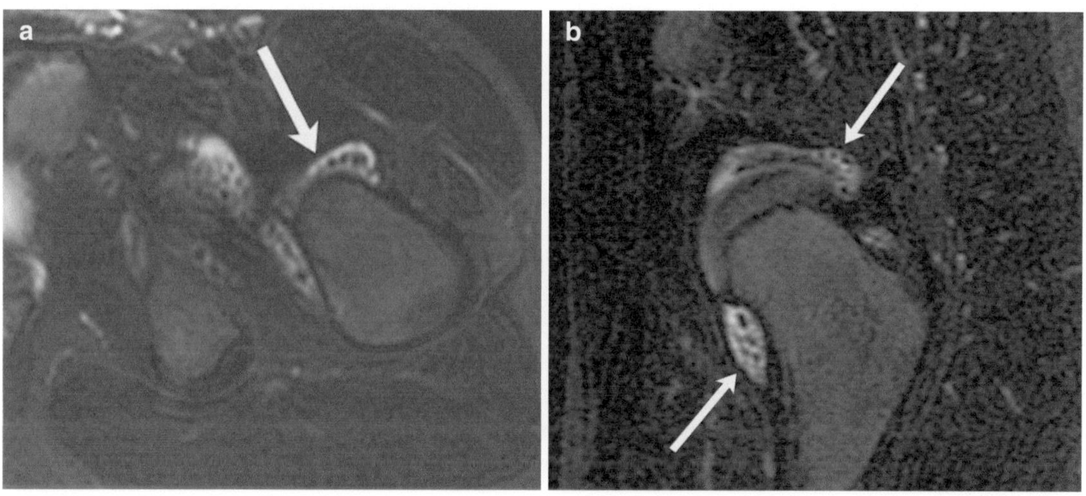

Fig. 12.50 Synovial chondromatosis in a 9-year-old boy. Axial (**a**) and sagittal (**b**) T2-W FS images of the left hip show numerous low signal intraarticular bodies of similar size distending the joint (*arrows*) (Courtesy of Tal Laor, Cincinnati Children's Hospital)

conglomerate bodies may form. Histologically, the chondromas have some malignant histologic features, but their behavior is benign. The nodules may undergo central dystrophic mineralization or peripheral enchondral ossification.

Surgical resection of the intraarticular bodies is the mainstay of treatment, often via arthroscopy. The role of synovectomy is controversial. Recurrence rate ranges from 3 to 23 %, often due to incomplete resection.

Imaging

About one-third of chondromas do not calcify or ossify, making it difficult to identify them on radiographs. However, these radiolucent cartilaginous bodies may be interposed within the joint space and displace the femoral head laterally. MRI or arthrography will better delineate cartilaginous chondromas. Those that calcify or ossify appear as clusters of stippled or mulberry-like calcifications. Extrinsic erosion of bone on both sides of the joint is more common in the hip joint than in the more capacious knee joint. If chondromas are located in the iliopectineal bursa (which communicates with the joint space in 15 % of persons), an intrapelvic mass may result, whereas chondromas within the iliopsoas bursa may present as a groin mass. The femoral head may enlarge due to chronic irritation and hyperemia.

US may show multiple heterogeneous echogenic foci in the joint with posterior shadowing, but extensive mineralization often obscures features. CT is best suited to document calcification within the chondromas, as it can identify calcification in most lesions—even those that appear lucent on radiographs. Erosions are also well imaged. Purely cartilaginous nodules appear as low attenuation, lobular areas of synovial thickening.

MRI appearance depends on the composition of the intraarticular bodies. The nodules most often demonstrate lobular, homogenous, intermediate signal similar to skeletal muscle on T1-W images and high signal on T2-W images. Areas of low signal on all pulse sequences indicate calcification. If nodules are truly ossified, central fatty marrow can be seen as high signal on T1-W images. MRI best shows possible extension of disease from the hip joint into the iliopsoas and obturator externus bursas; it is also useful to exclude true marrow invasion, which would suggest a more aggressive diagnosis.

References

1. Ratliff AH. Fractures of the neck of the femur in children. J Bone Joint Surg. 1962;44-B:528–42. PubMed PMID: 14038616.
2. Leung PC, Lam SF. Long-term follow-up of children with femoral neck fractures. J Bone Joint Surg. 1986;68(4):537–40. PubMed PMID: 3733826.
3. Bimmel R, Bakker A, Bosma B, Michielsen J. Paediatric hip fractures: a systematic review of incidence, treatment options and complications. Acta Orthop Belg. 2010;76(1):7–13. PubMed PMID: 20306957.
4. Herrera-Soto JA, Price CT. Traumatic hip dislocations in children and adolescents: pitfalls and complications. J Am Acad Orthop Surg. 2009;17(1):15–21. PubMed PMID: 19136423.
5. Speer KP, Spritzer CE, Harrelson JM, Nunley JA. Magnetic resonance imaging of the femoral head after acute intracapsular fracture of the femoral neck. J Bone Joint Surg Am. 1990;72(1):98–103. PubMed PMID: 2295679.
6. Rossi F, Dragoni S. Acute avulsion fractures of the pelvis in adolescent competitive athletes: prevalence, location and sports distribution of 203 cases collected. Skelet Radiol. 2001;30(3):127–31. PubMed PMID: 11357449.
7. Lehmann CL, Arons RR, Loder RT, Vitale MG. The epidemiology of slipped capital femoral epiphysis: an update. J Pediatr Orthop. 2006;26(3):286–90. PubMed PMID: 16670536.
8. Novais EN, Millis MB. Slipped capital femoral epiphysis: prevalence, pathogenesis, and natural history. Clin Orthop Relat Res. 2012;470(12):3432–8. PubMed PMID: 23054509, Pubmed Central PMCID: 3492592.
9. Benson EC, Miller M, Bosch P, Szalay EA. A new look at the incidence of slipped capital femoral epiphysis in new Mexico. J Pediatr Orthop. 2008;28(5):529–33. PubMed PMID: 18580367.
10. Rennie AM. The pathology of slipped upper femoral epiphysis. A new concept. J Bone Joint Surg. 1960;42-B:273–9. PubMed PMID: 13854494.
11. Carter JR, Leeson MC, Thompson GH, Kalamchi A, Kelly CM, Makley JT. Late-onset tibia vara: a histopathologic analysis. A comparative evaluation with infantile tibia vara and slipped capital femoral epiphysis. J Pediatr Orthop. 1988;8(2):187–95. PubMed PMID: 3350954.
12. Riad J, Bajelidze G, Gabos PG. Bilateral slipped capital femoral epiphysis: predictive factors for contralateral slip. J Pediatr Orthop. 2007;27(4):411–4. PubMed PMID: 17513962.
13. Popejoy D, Emara K, Birch J. Prediction of contralateral slipped capital femoral epiphysis using the modified Oxford bone age score. J Pediatr Orthop. 2012;32(3):290–4. PubMed PMID: 22411336.
14. Stasikelis PJ, Sullivan CM, Phillips WA, Polard JA. Slipped capital femoral epiphysis. Prediction of contralateral involvement. J Bone Joint Surg Am. 1996;78(8):1149–55. PubMed PMID: 8753706.
15. Nasreddine AY, Heyworth BE, Zurakowski D, Kocher MS. A reduction in body mass index lowers risk for bilateral slipped capital femoral epiphysis. Clin Orthop Relat Res. 2013;471(7):2137–44. PubMed PMID: 23378238, Pubmed Central PMCID: 3676625.
16. Loder RT, Richards BS, Shapiro PS, Reznick LR, Aronson DD. Acute slipped capital femoral epiphysis: the importance of physeal stability. J Bone Joint Surg Am. 1993;75(8):1134–40. PubMed PMID: 8354671. Epub 1993/08/01. eng.
17. Loder RT, Aronsson DD, Dobbs MB, Weinstein SL. Slipped capital femoral epiphysis. Instr Course Lect. 2001;50:555–70. PubMed PMID: 11372359. Epub 2001/05/25. eng.

18. Uglow MG, Clarke NM. The management of slipped capital femoral epiphysis. J Bone Joint Surg. 2004;86(5):631–5. PubMed PMID: 15274254.
19. Jarrett DY, Matheney T, Kleinman PK. Imaging SCFE: diagnosis, treatment and complications. Pediatr Radiol. 2013;43 Suppl 1:S71–82. PubMed PMID: 23478922.
20. Fragniere B, Chotel F, Vargas Barreto B, Berard J. The value of early postoperative bone scan in slipped capital femoral epiphysis. J Pediatr Orthop B. 2001;10(1):51–5. PubMed PMID: 11269811.
21. Monazzam S, Dwek JR, Hosalkar HS. Multiplanar CT assessment of femoral head displacement in slipped capital femoral epiphysis. Pediatr Radiol. 2013;43(12):1599–605. PubMed PMID: 23794055.
22. Lalaji A, Umans H, Schneider R, Mintz D, Liebling MS, Haramati N. MRI features of confirmed "pre-slip" capital femoral epiphysis: a report of two cases. Skelet Radiol. 2002;31(6):362–5. PubMed PMID: 12073122.
23. Umans H, Liebling MS, Moy L, Haramati N, Macy NJ, Pritzker HA. Slipped capital femoral epiphysis: a physeal lesion diagnosed by MRI, with radiographic and CT correlation. Skelet Radiol. 1998;27(3):139–44. PubMed PMID: 9554004.
24. Staatz G, Honnef D, Kochs A, Hohl C, Schmidt T, Rohrig H, et al. Evaluation of femoral head vascularization in slipped capital femoral epiphysis before and after cannulated screw fixation with use of contrast-enhanced MRI: initial results. Eur Radiol. 2007;17(1):163–8. PubMed PMID: 16625344.
25. Chung SM. The arterial supply of the developing proximal end of the human femur. J Bone Joint Surg Am. 1976;58(7):961–70. PubMed PMID: 977628.
26. Ogden JA. Changing patterns of proximal femoral vascularity. J Bone Joint Surg Am. 1974;56(5):941–50. PubMed PMID: 4847241.
27. Hulth A. Necrosis of the head of the femur. A roentgenological, microradiographic and histological study. Acta Chir Scand. 1961;122:75–84.
28. Perry DC, Green DJ, Bruce CE, Pope D, Dangerfield P, Platt MJ, et al. Abnormalities of vascular structure and function in children with Perthes disease. Pediatrics. 2012;130(1):e126–31. PubMed PMID: 22665417. Epub 2012/06/06. eng.
29. Legg AT. The cause of atrophy in joint disease. J Bone Joint Surg. 1908;6:84–90.
30. Waldenstrom H. Der obere tuberkulose cullumherd. Z Orthop Chir. 1909;24:487–512.
31. Calvé J. Sur une forme particuliere de pseudo-coxalgie greffee sur des deformations caracteristiques de l'extremite superieure du femur. Rev Chir. 1910;42: 54–84.
32. Perthes G. Uber arthritis deformans juvenilis. Deut Zietschrift Chir Leipzig. 1910;107:111–59.
33. Perry DC, Machin DM, Pope D, Bruce CE, Dangerfield P, Platt MJ, et al. Racial and geographic factors in the incidence of Legg-Calve-Perthes' disease: a systematic review. Am J Epidemiol. 2012; 175(3):159–66. PubMed PMID: 22223709.
34. Perry DC, Hall AJ. The epidemiology and etiology of Perthes disease. Orthop Clin North Am. 2011; 42(3):279–83, v. PubMed PMID: 21742139.
35. Girdany BR, Osman MZ. Longitudinal growth and skeletal maturation in Perthes' disease. Radiol Clin North Am. 1968;6(2):245–51. PubMed PMID: 5667500.
36. Harrison MH, Turner MH, Jacobs P. Skeletal immaturity in Perthes' disease. J Bone Joint Surg. 1976;58(1):37–40. PubMed PMID: 178665.
37. Fisher RL. An epidemiological study of Legg-Perthes disease. J Bone Joint Surg Am. 1972;54(4):769–78. PubMed PMID: 5055168.
38. Mattick A, Turner A, Ferguson J, Beattie T, Sharp J. Seven year follow up of children presenting to the accident and emergency department with irritable hip. J Accid Emerg Med. 1999;16(5):345–7. PubMed PMID: 10505915. Pubmed Central PMCID: 1347055. Epub 1999/10/03. eng.
39. Catterall A. The natural history of Perthes' disease. J Bone Joint Surg. 1971;53(1):37–53. PubMed PMID: 5578764.
40. Hardcastle PH, Ross R, Hamalainen M, Mata A. Catterall grouping of Perthes' disease. An assessment of observer error and prognosis using the Catterall classification. J Bone Joint Surg. 1980;62-B(4):428–31. PubMed PMID: 7430217.
41. Herring JA, Neustadt JB, Williams JJ, Early JS, Browne RH. The lateral pillar classification of Legg-Calve-Perthes disease. J Pediatr Orthop. 1992;12(2): 143–50. PubMed PMID: 1552014.
42. Cheng JC, Lam TP, Ng BK. Prognosis and prognostic factors of Legg-Calve-Perthes disease. J Pediatr Orthop. 2011;31(2 Suppl):S147–51. PubMed PMID: 21857429.
43. Herring JA, Kim HT, Browne R. Legg-Calve-Perthes disease. Part II: prospective multicenter study of the effect of treatment on outcome. J Bone Joint Surg Am. 2004;86-A(10):2121–34. PubMed PMID: 15466720.
44. Mose K. Methods of measuring in Legg-Calve-Perthes disease with special regard to the prognosis. Clin Orthop Relat Res. 1980 Jul–Aug(150):103–9. PubMed PMID: 7428206.
45. Joseph B, Varghese G, Mulpuri K, Narasimha Rao K, Nair NS. Natural evolution of Perthes disease: a study of 610 children under 12 years of age at disease onset. J Pediatr Orthop. 2003;23(5):590–600. PubMed PMID: 12960621.
46. Kamegaya M, Saisu T, Miura Y, Moriya H. A proposed prognostic formula for Perthes' disease. Clin Orthop Relat Res. 2005;440:205–8. PubMed PMID: 16239808.
47. Stulberg SD, Cooperman DR, Wallensten R. The natural history of Legg-Calve-Perthes disease. J Bone Joint Surg Am. 1981;63(7):1095–108. PubMed PMID: 7276045.

48. Jonsater S. Coxa plana; a histopathologic and arthrographic study. Acta Orthop Scand Suppl. 1953;12:5–98. PubMed PMID: 13065067.
49. Catterall A, Pringle J, Byers PD, Fulford GE, Kemp HB. Perthes' disease: is the epiphysial infarction complete? J Bone Joint Surg. 1982;64(3):276–81. PubMed PMID: 7096391.
50. Song HR, Dhar S, Na JB, Cho SH, Ahn BW, Ko SM, et al. Classification of metaphyseal change with magnetic resonance imaging in Legg-Calve-Perthes disease. J Pediatr Orthop. 2000;20(5):557–61. PubMed PMID: 11008730.
51. Johnson C, May DA, McCabe KM, Guse R, Resnick D. Non-cartilaginous metaphyseal cysts in Legg-Calve-Perthes disease: report of a case. Pediatr Radiol. 1997;27(10):824–6. PubMed PMID: 9323253.
52. Shah H, Siddesh ND, Joseph B, Nair SN. Effect of prophylactic trochanteric epiphyseodesis in older children with Perthes' disease. J Pediatr Orthop. 2009;29(8):889–95. PubMed PMID: 19934705.
53. Herring JA. Legg-Calve-Perthes disease at 100: a review of evidence-based treatment. J Pediatr Orthop. 2011;31(2 Suppl):S137–40. PubMed PMID: 21857427. Epub 2011/09/01. eng.
54. Catterall A, Pringle J, Byers PD, Fulford GE, Kemp HB, Dolman CL, et al. A review of the morphology of Perthes' disease. J Bone Joint Surg. 1982;64(3): 269–75. PubMed PMID: 6807991.
55. Lobert PF, Dillman JR, Strouse PJ, Hernandez RJ. Unexpected MRI findings in clinically suspected Legg-Calve-Perthes disease. Pediatr Radiol. 2011;41(3):369–73. PubMed PMID: 20865410.
56. Sutherland AD, Savage JP, Paterson DC, Foster BK. The nuclide bone-scan in the diagnosis and management of Perthes' disease. J Bone Joint Surg. 1980; 62(3):300–6. PubMed PMID: 7410461.
57. Danigelis JA. Pinhole imaging in Legg-Perthes disease: further observations. Semin Nucl Med. 1976;6(1):69–82. PubMed PMID: 1246636.
58. Fisher RL, Roderique JW, Brown DC, Danigelis JA, Ozonoff MB, Sziklas JJ. The relationship of isotopic bone imaging findings to prognosis in Legg-Perthes disease. Clin Orthop Relat Res. 1980 Jul–Aug(150):23–9. PubMed PMID: 7428227.
59. Conway JJ. A scintigraphic classification of Legg-Calve-Perthes disease. Semin Nucl Med. 1993; 23(4):274–95. PubMed PMID: 8256137.
60. Tsao AK, Dias LS, Conway JJ, Straka P. The prognostic value and significance of serial bone scintigraphy in Legg-Calve-Perthes disease. J Pediatr Orthop. 1997;17(2):230–9. PubMed PMID: 9075102.
61. Danigelis JA, Fisher RL, Ozonoff MB, Sziklas JJ. 99mTc-polyphosphate bone imaging in Legg-Perthes disease. Radiology. 1975;115(2):407–13. PubMed PMID: 1144759.
62. Van Campenhout A, Moens P, Fabry G. Serial bone scintigraphy in Legg-Calve-Perthes disease: correlation with the Catterall and Herring classification. J Pediatr Orthop B. 2006;15(1):6–10. PubMed PMID: 16280712.
63. Comte F, De Rosa V, Zekri H, Eberle MC, Dimeglio A, Rossi M, et al. Confirmation of the early prognostic value of bone scanning and pinhole imaging of the hip in Legg-Calve-Perthes disease. J Nucl Med. 2003;44(11):1761–6. PubMed PMID: 14602857.
64. Ozonoff MB. Controlled arthrography of the hip: a technic of fluoroscopic monitoring and recording. Clin Orthop Relat Res. 1973;93:260–4. PubMed PMID: 4722950.
65. Milani C, Dobashi ET. Arthrogram in Legg-Calve-Perthes disease. J Pediatr Orthop. 2011;31(2 Suppl):S156–62. PubMed PMID: 21857431.
66. Pay NT, Singer WS, Bartal E. Hip pain in three children accompanied by transient abnormal findings on MR images. Radiology. 1989;171(1):147–9. PubMed PMID: 2928519.
67. Kim HK, Kaste S, Dempsey M, Wilkes D. A comparison of non-contrast and contrast-enhanced MRI in the initial stage of Legg-Calve-Perthes disease. Pediatr Radiol. 2013;43(9):1166–73. PubMed PMID: 23478799.
68. Seiler 3rd JG, Christie MJ, Homra L. Correlation of the findings of magnetic resonance imaging with those of bone biopsy in patients who have stage-I or II ischemic necrosis of the femoral head. J Bone Joint Surg Am. 1989;71(1):28–32. PubMed PMID: 2912999.
69. Lamer S, Dorgeret S, Khairouni A, Mazda K, Brillet PY, Bacheville E, et al. Femoral head vascularisation in Legg-Calve-Perthes disease: comparison of dynamic gadolinium-enhanced subtraction MRI with bone scintigraphy. Pediatr Radiol. 2002;32(8): 580–5. PubMed PMID: 12136349.
70. Yoo WJ, Kim YJ, Menezes NM, Cheon JE, Jaramillo D. Diffusion-weighted MRI reveals epiphyseal and metaphyseal abnormalities in Legg-Calve-Perthes disease: a pilot study. Clin Orthop Relat Res. 2011;469(10):2881–8. PubMed PMID: 21660596. Pubmed Central PMCID: 3171554.
71. Holstein A, Zilkens C, Bittersohl B, Jager M, Haamberg T, Mamisch TC, et al. Delayed gadolinium-enhanced MRI of cartilage (dGEMRIC) and morphologic MRI of cartilage in the long-term follow-up after Legg-Calve-Perthes disease (LCPD). J Med Imaging Radiat Oncol. 2011;55(3):259–65. PubMed PMID: 21696558.
72. Lutsky KF, Tejwani NC. Orthopaedic manifestations of Gaucher disease. Bull NYU Hosp Jt Dis. 2007;65(1):37–42. PubMed PMID: 17539760.
73. Chung SM, Ralston EL. Necrosis of the femoral head associated with sickle-cell anemia and its genetic variants. A review of the literature and study of thirteen cases. J Bone Joint Surg Am. 1969;51(1):33–58. PubMed PMID: 4884827.
74. Fisher DE, Bickel WH. Corticosteroid-induced avascular necrosis. A clinical study of seventy-seven patients. J Bone Joint Surg Am. 1971;53(5):859–73. PubMed PMID: 4326745.
75. Weinstein RS. Glucocorticoid-induced osteonecrosis. Endocrine. 2012;41(2):183–90. PubMed PMID: 22169965. Pubmed Central PMCID: 3712793.

76. Salter RB, Kostuik J, Dallas S. Avascular necrosis of the femoral head as a complication of treatment for congenital dislocation of the hip in young children: a clinical and experimental investigation. Can J Surg J Can Chir. 1969;12(1):44–61. PubMed PMID: 5762671.
77. Firth GB, Robertson AJ, Schepers A, Fatti L. Developmental dysplasia of the hip: open reduction as a risk factor for substantial osteonecrosis. Clin Orthop Relat Res. 2010;468(9):2485–94. PubMed PMID: 20532719. Pubmed Central PMCID: 2919866.
78. Zionts LE, MacEwen GD. Treatment of congenital dislocation of the hip in children between the ages of one and three years. J Bone Joint Surg Am. 1986;68(6):829–46. PubMed PMID: 3733773.
79. Murray T, Cooperman DR, Thompson GH, Ballock RT. Closed reduction for treatment of developmental dysplasia of the hip in children. Am J Orthop. 2007;36(2):82–4. PubMed PMID: 17405637.
80. Bali K, Sudesh P, Patel S, Kumar V, Saini U, Dhillon MS. Pediatric femoral neck fractures: our 10 years of experience. Clin Orthop Surg. 2011;3(4):302–8. PubMed PMID: 22162793. Pubmed Central PMCID: 3232358.
81. Kemp HB, Lloyd-Roberts GC. Avascular necrosis of the capital epiphysis following osteomyelitis of the proximal femoral metaphysis. J Bone Joint Surg. 1974;56-B(4):688–97. PubMed PMID: 4452714.
82. Ganz R, Parvizi J, Beck M, Leunig M, Notzli H, Siebenrock KA. Femoroacetabular impingement: a cause for osteoarthritis of the hip. Clin Orthop Relat Res. 2003;417:112–20. PubMed PMID: 14646708.
83. Beck M, Kalhor M, Leunig M, Ganz R. Hip morphology influences the pattern of damage to the acetabular cartilage: femoroacetabular impingement as a cause of early osteoarthritis of the hip. J Bone Joint Surg. 2005;87(7):1012–8. PubMed PMID: 15972923.
84. Tannast M, Siebenrock KA, Anderson SE. Femoroacetabular impingement: radiographic diagnosis–what the radiologist should know. AJR Am J Roentgenol. 2007;188(6):1540–52. PubMed PMID: 17515374.
85. Tannast M, Mistry S, Steppacher SD, Reichenbach S, Langlotz F, Siebenrock KA, et al. Radiographic analysis of femoroacetabular impingement with Hip2Norm-reliable and validated. J Orthop Res. 2008;26(9):1199–205. PubMed PMID: 18404737.
86. Sutter R, Dietrich TJ, Zingg PO, Pfirrmann CW. How useful is the alpha angle for discriminating between symptomatic patients with cam-type femoroacetabular impingement and asymptomatic volunteers? Radiology. 2012;264(2):514–21. PubMed PMID: 22653190.
87. Wenger DE, Kendell KR, Miner MR, Trousdale RT. Acetabular labral tears rarely occur in the absence of bony abnormalities. Clin Orthop Relat Res. 2004;426:145–50. PubMed PMID: 15346066.
88. Dinauer PA, Murphy KP, Carroll JF. Sublabral sulcus at the posteroinferior acetabulum: a potential pitfall in MR arthrography diagnosis of acetabular labral tears. AJR Am J Roentgenol. 2004;183(6):1745–53. PubMed PMID: 15547222.
89. Studler U, Kalberer F, Leunig M, Zanetti M, Hodler J, Dora C, et al. MR arthrography of the hip: differentiation between an anterior sublabral recess as a normal variant and a labral tear. Radiology. 2008;249(3):947–54. PubMed PMID: 18840790.
90. Beaule PE, Zaragoza E, Copelan N. Magnetic resonance imaging with gadolinium arthrography to assess acetabular cartilage delamination. A report of four cases. J Bone Joint Surg Am. 2004;86-A(10):2294–8. PubMed PMID: 15466743.
91. Pfirrmann CW, Duc SR, Zanetti M, Dora C, Hodler J. MR arthrography of acetabular cartilage delamination in femoroacetabular cam impingement. Radiology. 2008;249(1):236–41. PubMed PMID: 18682585.
92. Jones BS. Adolescent chondrolysis of the hip joint. S Afr Med J. 1971;45(8):196–202.
93. Daluga DJ, Millar EA. Idiopathic chondrolysis of the hip. J Pediatr Orthop. 1989;9(4):405–11. PubMed PMID: 2732319.
94. Korula RJ, Jebaraj I, David KS. Idiopathic chondrolysis of the hip: medium- to long-term results. ANZ J Surg. 2005;75(9):750–3. PubMed PMID: 16173986.
95. Laor T, Crawford AH. Idiopathic chondrolysis of the hip in children: early MRI findings. AJR Am J Roentgenol. 2009;192(2):526–31. PubMed PMID: 19155420.
96. Johnson K, Haigh SF, Ehtisham S, Ryder C, Gardner-Medwin J. Childhood idiopathic chondrolysis of the hip: MRI features. Pediatr Radiol. 2003;33(3):194–9. PubMed PMID: 12612820.
97. Thacker MM, Feldman DS, Madan SS, Straight JJ, Scher DM. Hinged distraction of the adolescent arthritic hip. J Pediatr Orthop. 2005;25(2):178–82. PubMed PMID: 15718897.
98. Erken EH, Katz K. Irritable hip and Perthes' disease. J Pediatr Orthop. 1990;10(3):322–6. PubMed PMID: 2355074.
99. Kastrissianakis K, Beattie TF. Transient synovitis of the hip: more evidence for a viral aetiology. Eur J Emerg Med. 2010;17(5):270–3. PubMed PMID: 20523221.
100. Kallio P, Ryoppy S, Kunnamo I. Transient synovitis and Perthes' disease. Is there an aetiological connection? J Bone Joint Surg. 1986;68(5):808–11. PubMed PMID: 3782251.
101. Zamzam MM. The role of ultrasound in differentiating septic arthritis from transient synovitis of the hip in children. J Pediatr Orthop B. 2006;15(6):418–22. PubMed PMID: 17001248.
102. Strouse PJ, DiPietro MA, Adler RS. Pediatric hip effusions: evaluation with power Doppler sonography. Radiology. 1998;206(3):731–5. PubMed PMID: 9494493.
103. Yang WJ, Im SA, Lim GY, Chun HJ, Jung NY, Sung MS, et al. MR imaging of transient synovitis: differentiation from septic arthritis. Pediatr Radiol. 2006;36(11):1154–8. PubMed PMID: 17019590.

104. Kim EY, Kwack KS, Cho JH, Lee DH, Yoon SH. Usefulness of dynamic contrast-enhanced MRI in differentiating between septic arthritis and transient synovitis in the hip joint. AJR Am J Roentgenol. 2012;198(2):428–33. PubMed PMID: 22268189.
105. Sultan J, Hughes PJ. Septic arthritis or transient synovitis of the hip in children: the value of clinical prediction algorithms. J Bone Joint Surg. 2010;92(9):1289–93. PubMed PMID: 20798450.
106. Nistala K, Babar J, Johnson K, Campbell-Stokes P, Foster K, Ryder C, et al. Clinical assessment and core outcome variables are poor predictors of hip arthritis diagnosed by MRI in juvenile idiopathic arthritis. Rheumatology. 2007;46(4):699–702. PubMed PMID: 17158211.
107. Patriquin HB, Camerlain M, Trias A. Late sequelae of juvenile rheumatoid arthritis of the hip: a follow-up study into adulthood. Pediatr Radiol. 1984;14(3): 151–7. PubMed PMID: 6462810.
108. Argyropoulou MI, Fanis SL, Xenakis T, Efremidis SC, Siamopoulou A. The role of MRI in the evaluation of hip joint disease in clinical subtypes of juvenile idiopathic arthritis. Br J Radiol. 2002;75(891):229–33. PubMed PMID: 11932215.
109. Ginai AZ. Case report 607: Synovial (osteo) chondromatosis of left hip joint and ileopsoas bursa. Skelet Radiol. 1990;19(3):227–31. PubMed PMID: 2333566.
110. Pelker RR, Drennan JC, Ozonoff MB. Juvenile synovial chondromatosis of the hip. A case report. J Bone Joint Surg Am. 1983;65(4):552–4. PubMed PMID: 6833332.
111. Cahuzac JP, Lebarbier P, Germaneau J, Pasquie M. Synovial chondromatosis in children (author's transl). Chir Pediatr. 1979;20(2):89–93. PubMed PMID: 487502. La chrondromatose synoviale de l'enfant.
112. Murphey MD, Vidal JA, Fanburg-Smith JC, Gajewski DA. Imaging of synovial chondromatosis with radiologic-pathologic correlation. Radiographics. 2007; 27(5):1465–88. PubMed PMID: 17848703.

The Lower Extremity: Congenital and Developmental Conditions

13

Jeffrey S. Prince

Contents

J.S. Prince, MD
Department of Medical Imaging,
Primary Children's Hospital,
100 N. Mario Capecchi Drive,
Salt Lake City, UT 84113, USA
e-mail: jeffrey.prince@imail.org

Abstract

This chapter first discusses normal variants in the knee and lower leg, covering topics such as distal femoral epiphyseal ossification variants, benign cortical defects, cortical desmoids, tibial tuberosity development, and growth recovery lines. Variants of the fabella, patella, and patellofemoral articulation are discussed, as well as both congenital and developmental patellar instability. The chapter then presents congenital limb anomalies such as femoral bifurcation and duplication, longitudinal deficiency of the tibia, and longitudinal deficiency of the fibula. Bowing and alignment disorders follow, with sections on various forms of tibial and fibular bowing, and knee dislocation and hyperextension. Discussion of aberrant alignment includes physiological bowing, infantile tibia vara, rickets, genu valgum, and long bone rotational abnormalities. The chapter concludes with a discussion of leg-length discrepancy.

Variable osseous development leads to a changing appearance of the bones of the lower extremity during childhood. In order to recognize pathology, it is important to understand the ranges of normal. Developmental abnormalities of the lower extremity have a wide range of severity and can have significant impact on patient function.

R. Stein-Wexler et al. (eds.), *Pediatric Orthopedic Imaging*,
DOI 10.1007/978-3-642-45381-6_13, © Springer-Verlag Berlin Heidelberg 2015

1 Normal Development and Variants

1.1 Normal Development

Limb growth is stimulated by cells in the apical epidermal ridge, which first appears at the fifth week of development. The lower limb buds emerge from the fetal mesenchyme in the fourth or fifth fetal week, shortly after the upper limb buds appear. Preaxial and postaxial development of the limb then appears to be controlled by *Hox* genes, which are also influenced by a variety of growth-stimulating factors. Development of the limb primordium progresses in a proximal to distal fashion, with the proximal segments playing a role in inducing formation of the more distal structures. Growth and development occur in what have been termed developmental fields. Structures that arise in the same developmental field may all be affected by a single inciting event. For example, either mild femoral deficiency or proximal femoral focal deficiency (PFFD) is often associated with longitudinal deficiency of the fibula. This postaxial limb bud deficiency may include, from distal to proximal, lateral ray deficiency, tarsal coalition, ball-in-socket ankle, fibular deficiency, absence of the anterior cruciate ligament, and lateral femoral condylar hypoplasia.

Bone formation begins in the cartilage model of the femur at seven gestational weeks; this ossification process occurs second, following the clavicle. The tibial and fibular primary centers appear shortly afterward, in the seventh and eighth weeks. Differentiation of the ligaments and menisci is complete by the eighth gestational week. The distal femoral epiphyseal ossification center is visible at term in essentially all girls and in 95 % of boys. At the other extreme, the proximal fibular epiphysis rarely ossifies before age 4 years. As elsewhere in the body, girls mature earlier than boys.

In general, the centers that ossify first fuse last. For example, the progression in appearance of ossification centers in the femur is distal femur to femoral head to greater trochanter to lesser trochanter, whereas the pattern of fusion is the reverse, with the distal femur fusing last. Only in the fibula is this process reversed, with the distal fibular epiphysis appearing before and then fusing before the proximal fibular epiphysis. The proximal fibular epiphysis may begin to ossify as late as 4–6 years. (See Chap. 2 for further information about timing of ossification.)

The anlage of the patella can be identified as a condensation of cells in the future quadriceps femoris tendon as early as 8 weeks of fetal life, and the cartilaginous center develops shortly thereafter. Ossification does not become evident until a mean age of 2.5 years in girls and 4 years in boys (range 1.5–6 years). The patella is thus not amenable to radiographic investigation until this time, although its cartilaginous outline may sometimes be appreciated due to its contrast with surrounding fat. Ultrasound (US) and magnetic resonance imaging (MRI) can contribute important information, however. The patella matures during the late stages of skeletal maturation, when its cartilage assumes adult articular contours (age 10–12) [1].

As in the upper extremity, there is differential growth at the two ends of the long bones. The relative proportional contributions of the proximal and distal physes are, respectively: femur, 30/70; tibia, 55/45; and fibula, 60/40. The distal femoral physis is estimated to provide 37 % of the total length of the leg, and the proximal tibial physis provides 28 %.

1.2 Normal Variants of Ossification

Distal Femoral Epiphyseal Ossification Variants

Irregular ossification within the distal femoral epiphysis or along its posterior edge is extremely common during periods of rapid growth. Irregularities, often bilateral, are present in more than 80 % of subjects at age 4, but in only 10 % of subjects at age 12. The lateral femoral condyle is affected in 44 %, the medial condyle in 12 %, and both condyles in 44 %.

There may be ill-defined lucencies within the center of the distal femoral condyle, occasionally resulting in a stippled appearance (Fig. 13.1). Irregularity at the margins is more striking and can vary from a rough or knobby outline to deep

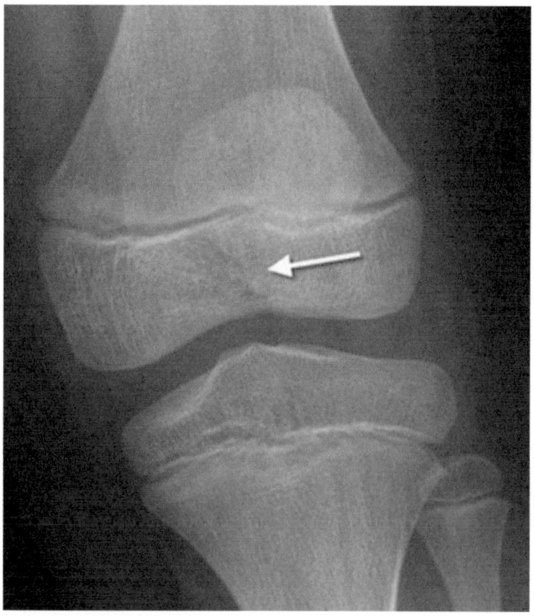

Fig. 13.1 Lucencies in the central portion of the distal femoral epiphysis (*white arrow*) of an 8-year-old boy

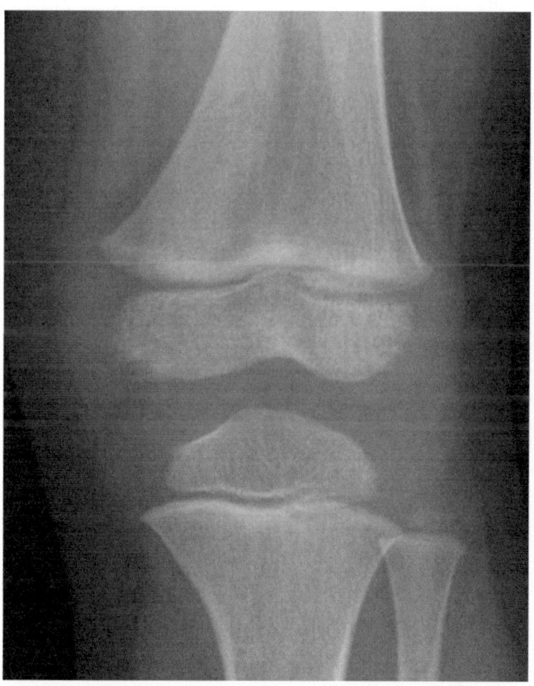

Fig. 13.2 Irregularities at the periphery of the medial (and, to a lesser extent, lateral) femoral condyle in a 3-year-old boy

fossa-like structures along the posteroinferior edge, although not on the weight-bearing surface (Figs. 13.2 and 13.3). One or more ossicles fre-

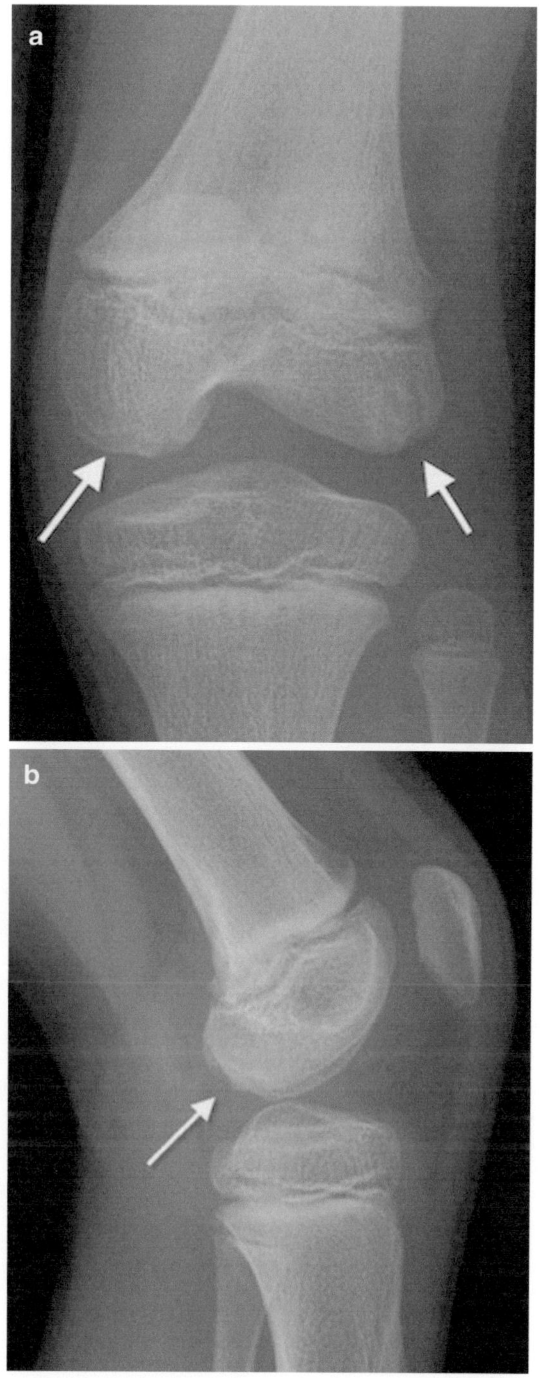

Fig. 13.3 Developmental irregular contours of the femoral condyles in an 8-year-old boy. (**a**) The irregularities are on the outer margin of the condyles (*white arrows*). (**b**) The defects in the contour project posteriorly and are not on the weight-bearing surface

quently project within these defects, and the defects fill in as the child matures.

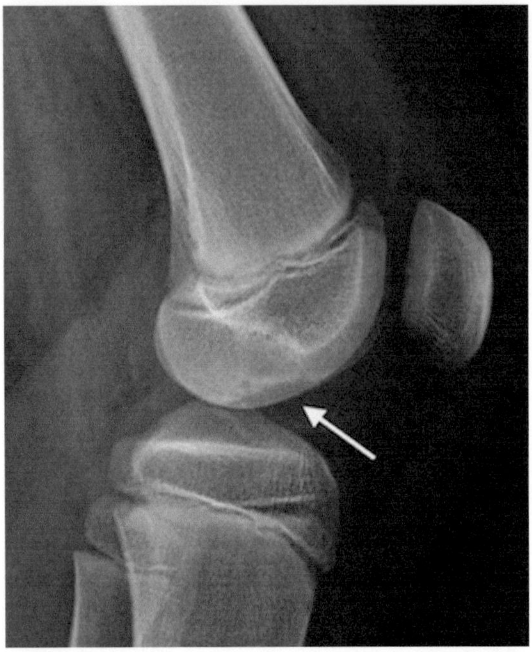

Fig. 13.4 Osteochondritis dissecans (OCD) in an 11-year-old boy. Unlike developmental irregularity of the femoral condyle, OCD is located on the weight-bearing surface (*arrow*)

The normal-variant depressions are often only evident on a tunnel radiograph that projects the posterior condyle in tangent and on a lateral view where they are clearly posterior. These irregularities resemble osteochondritis dissecans (OCD) but are differentiated by their position. OCD is located anteriorly or directly superior to the intercondyloid eminence inferior weight-bearing surface (Fig. 13.4), whereas the developmental variant is positioned posteriorly and does not affect the notch. These variants are present in almost one-third of young children. Note that it is occasionally impossible to distinguish variant ossification from OCD on radiographs. However, with the developmental variant, MRI demonstrates normal signal in the overlying cartilage and adjacent femoral condyle (Fig. 13.5). (See Chap. 14 for additional discussion of OCD.)

The appearance of the articular cartilage at the knee changes with maturation (Fig. 13.6). In infancy, signal intensity is homogeneous. As the child begins walking, signal decreases in the

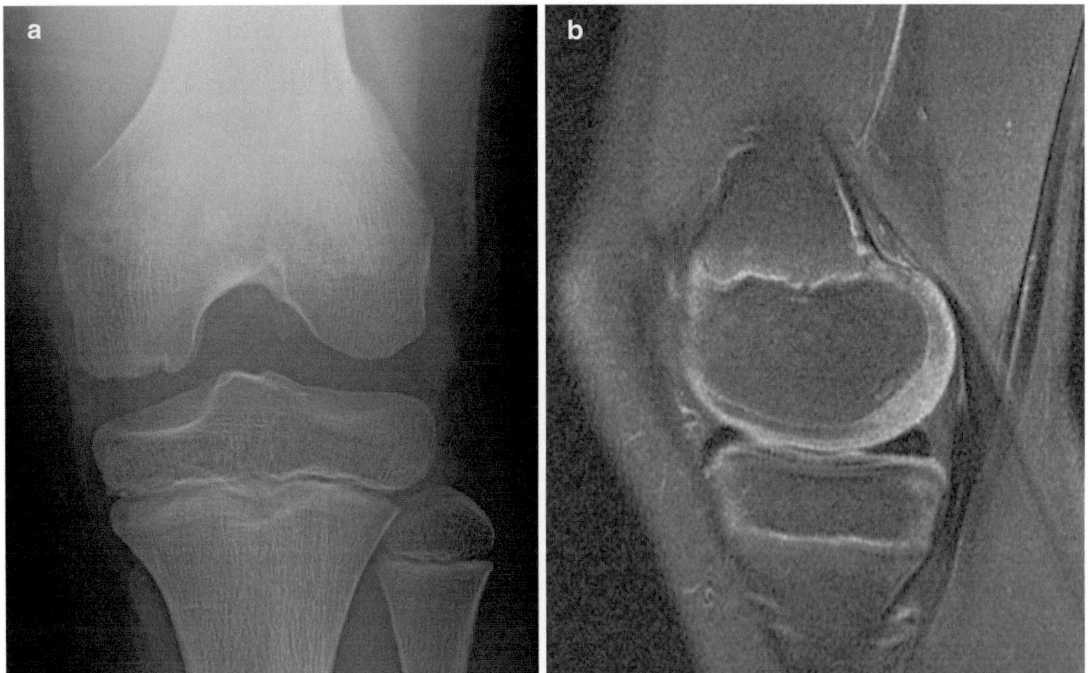

Fig. 13.5 Normal irregular ossification of medial femoral condyle in an 11-year-old. (**a**) Tunnel view shows irregular contour. (**b**) Sagittal proton density (PD) fat-suppressed (FS) image shows normal overlying cartilage and no marrow edema, differentiating this from OCD

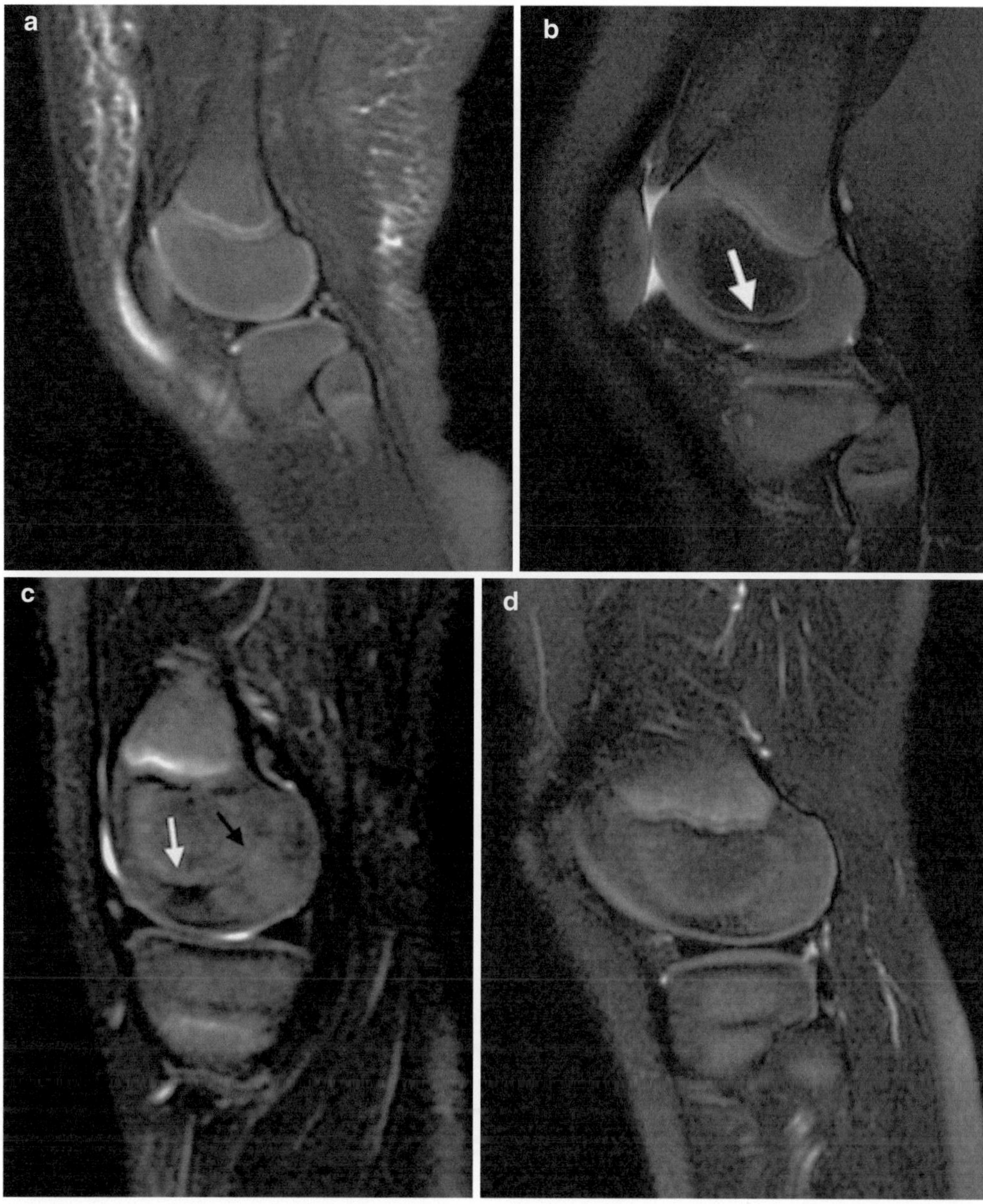

Fig. 13.6 Typical appearance of maturation of cartilage at the distal femoral epiphysis on T2-weighted (T2-W) magnetic resonance imaging (MRI). (**a**) At 9 months old, there is homogeneous high signal almost entirely throughout the epiphysis. (**b**) At 20 months old, the ossific nucleus is larger, and the weight-bearing portion is hypointense (*arrow*). (**c**) In a preschool-aged child, the posterior cartilage now appears heterogeneous and stippled, whereas the weight-bearing portion is even more hypointense (*arrow*). (**d**) With further maturation, the posterior cartilage becomes homogeneous

weight-bearing portion of the cartilage. By preschool age, the posterior portion of the condyle develops areas of stippled increased signal intensity, which eventually coalesce. These may be attributed to irregular ossification, as chondrocytes hypertrophy [2]. In the mature knee, the signal intensity of non-weight-bearing cartilage is relatively T2-hyperintense, whereas weight-bearing cartilage is hypointense. (See Chap. 2 for images and additional discussion of cartilage maturation.)

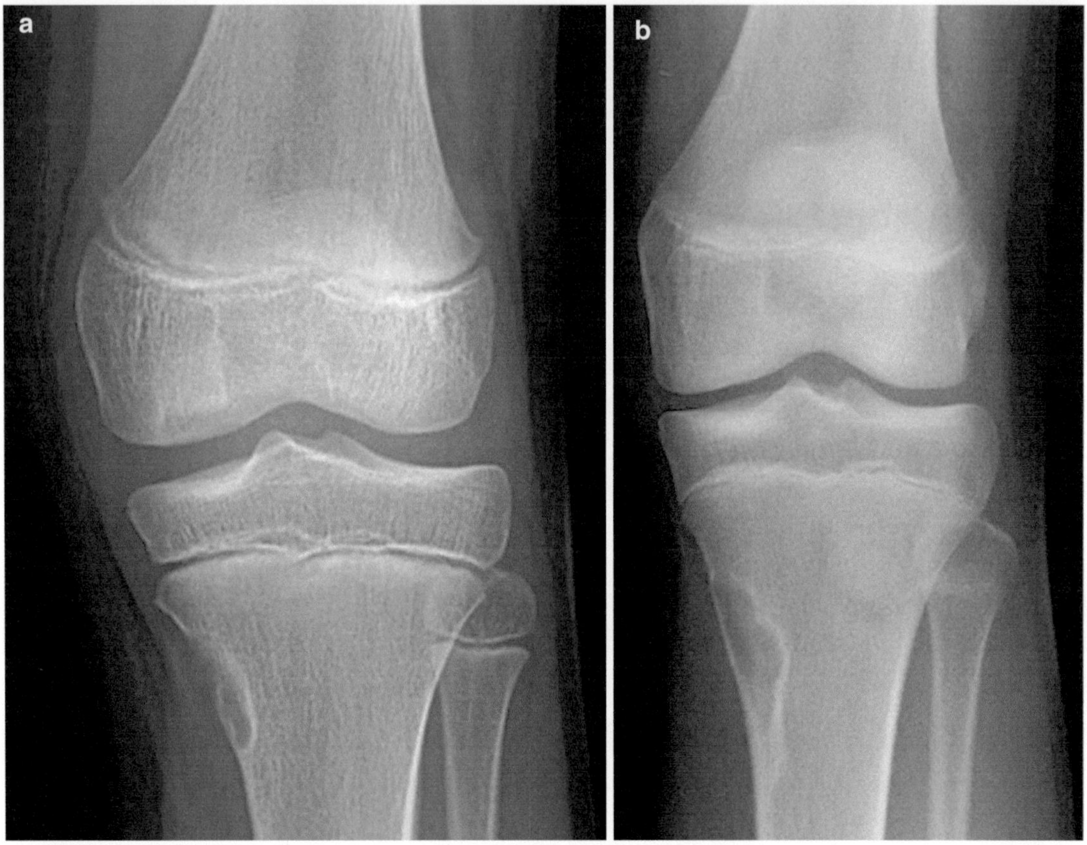

Fig. 13.7 Nonossifying fibroma. (**a**) Cortically based lesion with sclerotic margin and narrow zone of transition, without osseous matrix. (**b**) Four years later, the lesion is larger but retains benign characteristics. It is positioned further from the physis

Nonossifying Fibroma/Fibrous Cortical Defect

Nonossifying fibromas are very common benign, eccentric, cortically based lesions with an incidence as high as 40 % in boys and 20 % in girls. Most are asymptomatic. They belong to a continuum with fibrous cortical defects and are differentiated by size (fibrous cortical defects are smaller, less than 2 cm). These cortical lucencies are found close to the physis in younger children but appear to move toward the diaphysis with progressive bone growth (Fig. 13.7). Epiphyseal involvement has not been reported. They are not usually encountered before 18 months, peak at 5 or 6 years of age, and are rarely evident in adults. Lesions are commonly on the dorsal and medial aspect of the bone and may be bilateral. The vast majority occur in the lower extremity, and 82 % occur around the knee. They may be found simultaneously in the femur, tibia, and fibula.

These benign lesions probably originate at sites of tendinous or ligamentous insertion into the physeal perichondrium [3]. The traction force can be estimated by drawing a line toward the joint, along the long axis of the lucency. A defect in the dorsal medial femur thus results from traction by the adductor magnus muscle or medial gastrocnemius head; a defect in the dorsal medial tibia is due to pull from the semimembranosus muscle.

Imaging

When viewed en face, the defects appear as round, oval, multicystic, or irregularly marginated lucencies, often with sclerotic edges. When viewed tangentially on a lateral projection, they are almost invariably located in the posterior cortex, projecting either completely within the

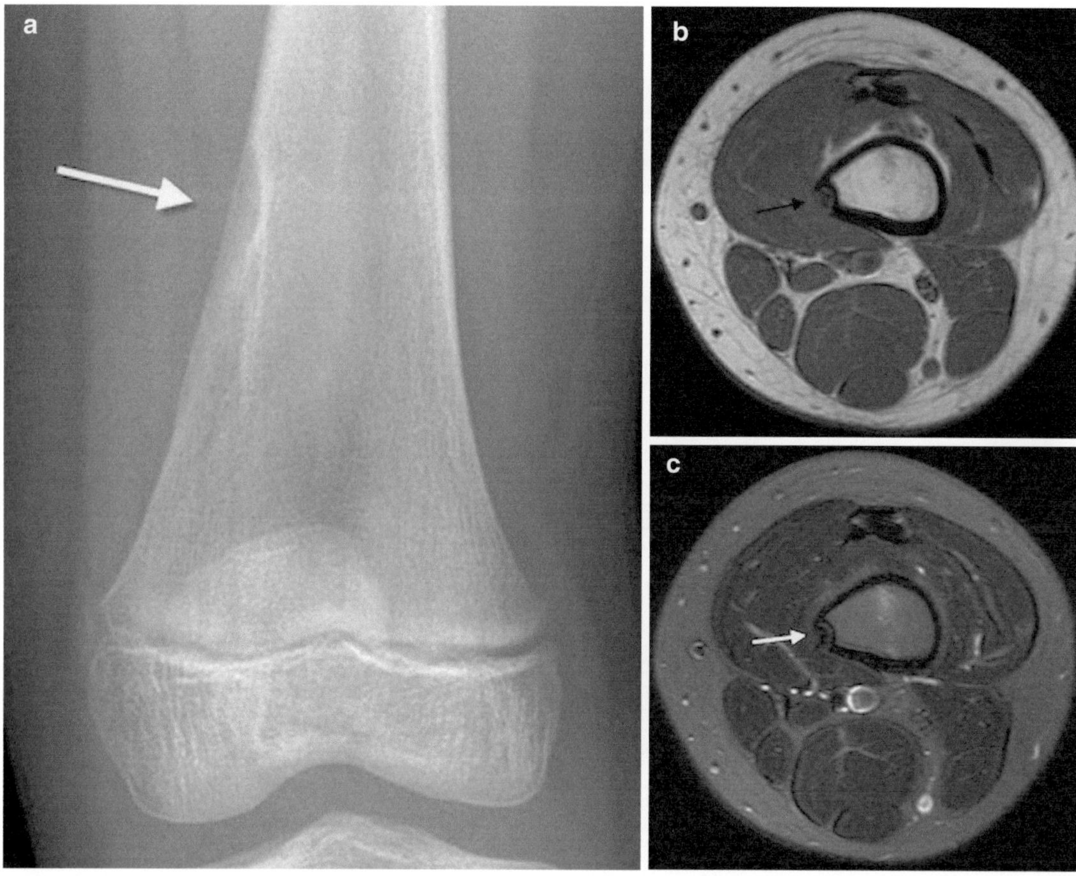

Fig. 13.8 Involuting nonossifying fibroma. (**a**) There is lucent scalloping within cortical sclerosis (*arrow*). Corresponding axial T1-weighted (T1-W) (**b**) and T2-W (**c**) images show focal subcortical hypointensity (*arrows*)

cortex or as shallow defect in its outer layer, and their greatest longitudinal axis parallels the long axis of the bone. They have a narrow zone of transition and lack aggressive features.

With longitudinal growth, the lesions appear to migrate away from the joint. Although initially ovoid and only faintly demarcated, they often become polycystic, with well-defined sclerotic margins and slight expansion of their thin cortical rim. During maturation the central lucency fills with sclerotic bone, beginning at the diaphyseal end. Once sclerosis is complete, the defect remodels to normal bone and usually disappears.

Radiographs are usually sufficient for diagnosis. Additional imaging should be performed only if the lesion is painful (in the absence of fracture). MRI shows lesions are initially low to intermediate on T1-weighted (T1-W) sequences and may initially demonstrate increased signal on T2-weighted (T2-W) images. As they involute, they become hypointense on all sequences (Fig. 13.8) [4]. The central tissue shows mild enhancement after gadolinium administration [3].

Stress fractures have been reported in association with nonossifying fibromas and fibrous cortical defects [5] (Figs. 13.9 and 13.10). Fractures are more likely with larger lesions that occupy more than half of the bone width, extending into the marrow cavity (Fig. 13.11).

Differential diagnoses include fibrous dysplasia, eosinophilic granuloma, and simple bone cysts. However, radiographic evaluation should show that benign cortical lesions are limited to the cortex, excluding these other diagnoses. In some cases, it may be difficult to completely exclude potentially intracortical lesions such as Brodie abscess or periosteal chondroma. Multiple nonossifying

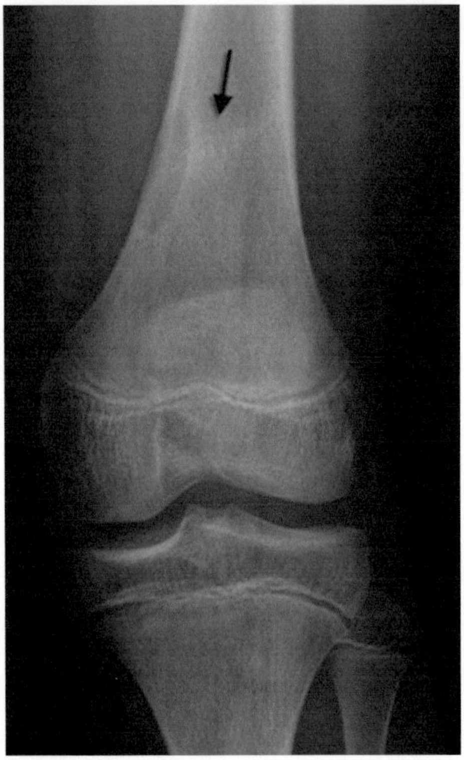

Fig. 13.9 Healing stress fracture through nonossifying fibroma. Linear sclerosis (*arrow*) extends laterally from the middle of the lesion

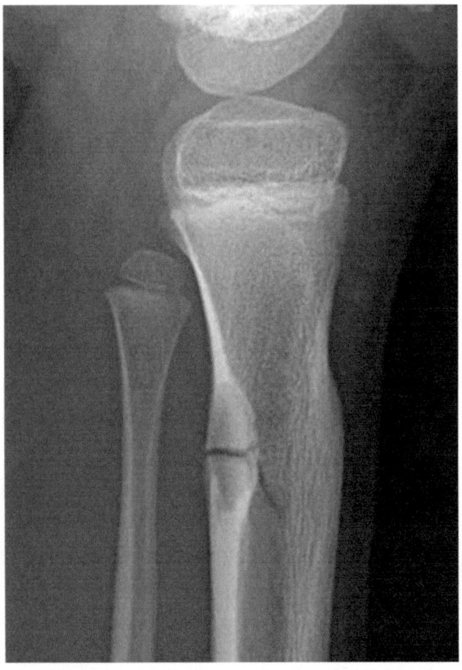

Fig. 13.10 Stress fracture through nonossifying fibroma in a 6-year-old boy. Stellate linear lucency traverses a cortically based lesion

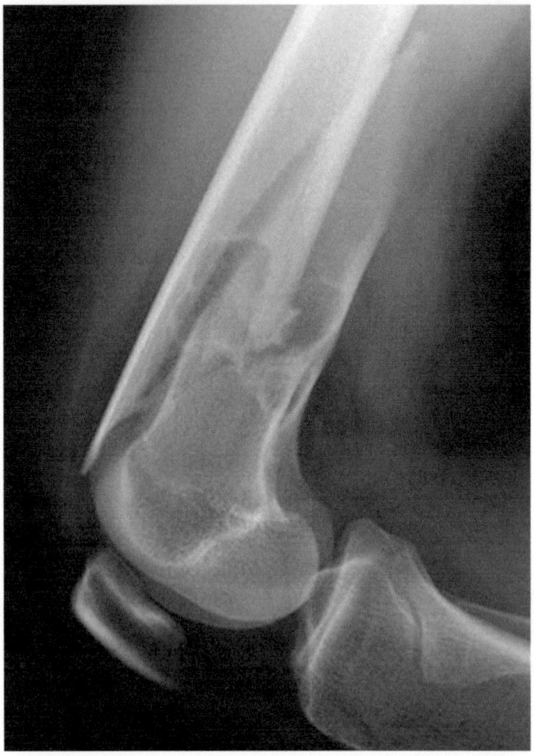

Fig. 13.11 Pathological fracture through a large nonossifying fibroma

fibromas/fibrous cortical defects occur in neurofibromatosis and Jaffe-Campanacci syndrome [6]. (See Chap. 21 for further discussion.)

Posterior Metaphyseal Stripe

A hyperintense band of tissue is common along the subperiostium at the posterior aspect of the distal femoral metaphysis as well as along the posterior aspect of the proximal tibial metaphysis. This band, composed of loose fibrovascular connective tissue, is more prominent on the femur than on the tibia. It is seen only in skeletally immature patients and on proton density (PD), T2-W, and inversion recovery (IR) sequences (Fig. 13.12); it is not evident on T1-W images. The tissue probably contributes to dynamic bone modeling that accompanies skeletal growth [7].

Cortical Desmoid

Cortical desmoids occur at the posteromedial metaphysis of the distal femur, at the insertion site of the medial head of the gastrocnemius muscle. This cortical roughening is common between ages 10 and 15, occurring in about 11 % of boys

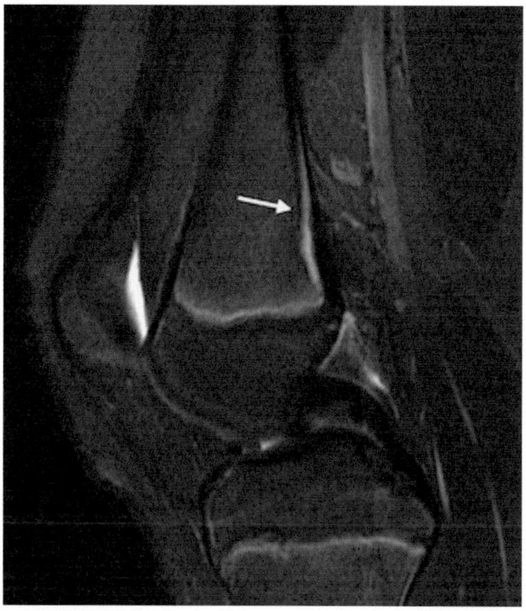

Fig. 13.12 Posterior metaphyseal stripe. Sagittal T2 FS sequence demonstrates linear subperiosteal hyperintensity along the posterior distal femoral metaphysis

and 3 % of girls [8]. The lesion is benign, self-limited, and usually asymptomatic, although there may be associated pain [9].

Etiology is uncertain. The lesion may represent a remodeling response to chronic or acute traction injury. It has also been theorized to result from chronic tension at the attachment of the medial head of the gastrocnemius or the adductor magnus aponeurosis, leading to the term "tug lesion." Very rapid growth may contribute as well. Subperiosteal connective tissue and osteoclasts within a cortical erosion have been identified at the attachment of the adductor magnus muscle [10]. Lesion shape may differ depending on the orientation of mechanical traction [9].

Imaging

Cortical desmoids are located in the posteromedial cortex, 1–2 cm proximal to the growth plate, and thus just above the adductor tubercle. Radiographic findings range from faint cortical fuzziness (Fig. 13.13) to irregular margination to

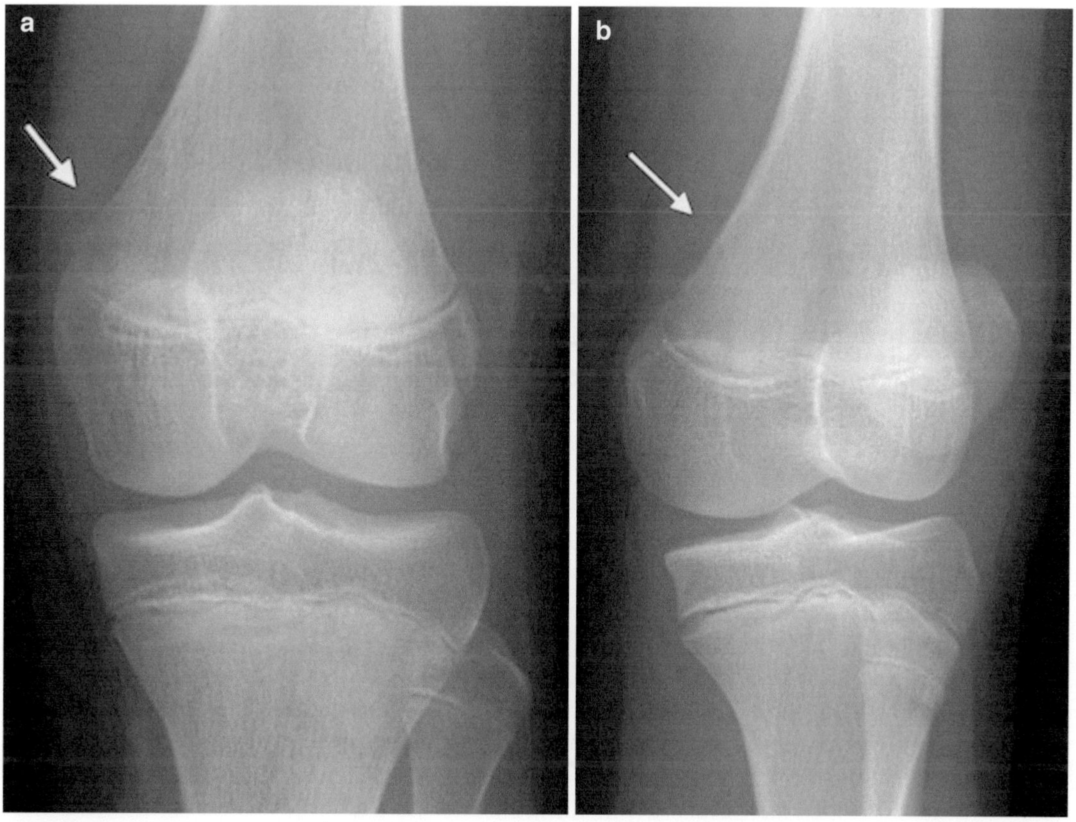

Fig. 13.13 Cortical desmoid. (**a**) Ill-defined lucency on frontal view. (**b**) Subtle cortical irregularity on projection obtained with slight external rotation

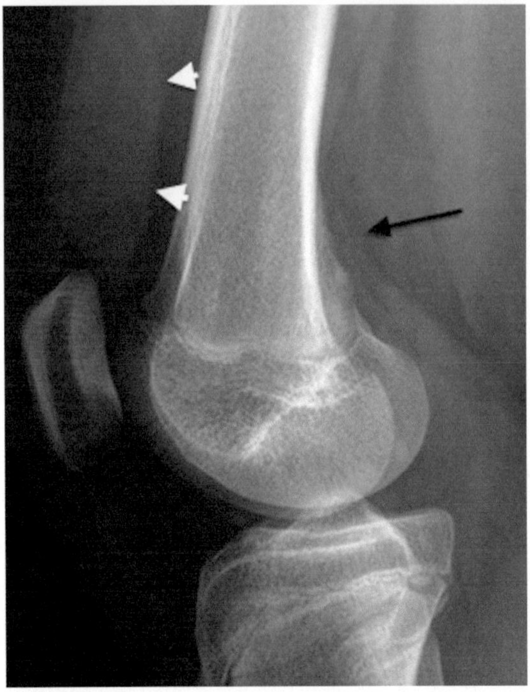

Fig. 13.14 Cortical desmoid in a 12-year-old girl. There is slight cortical irregularity (*arrow*) on the medial aspect of the posterior femur, at the site of the origin of the medial head of the gastrocnemius. Note unrelated joint effusion (*arrowheads*)

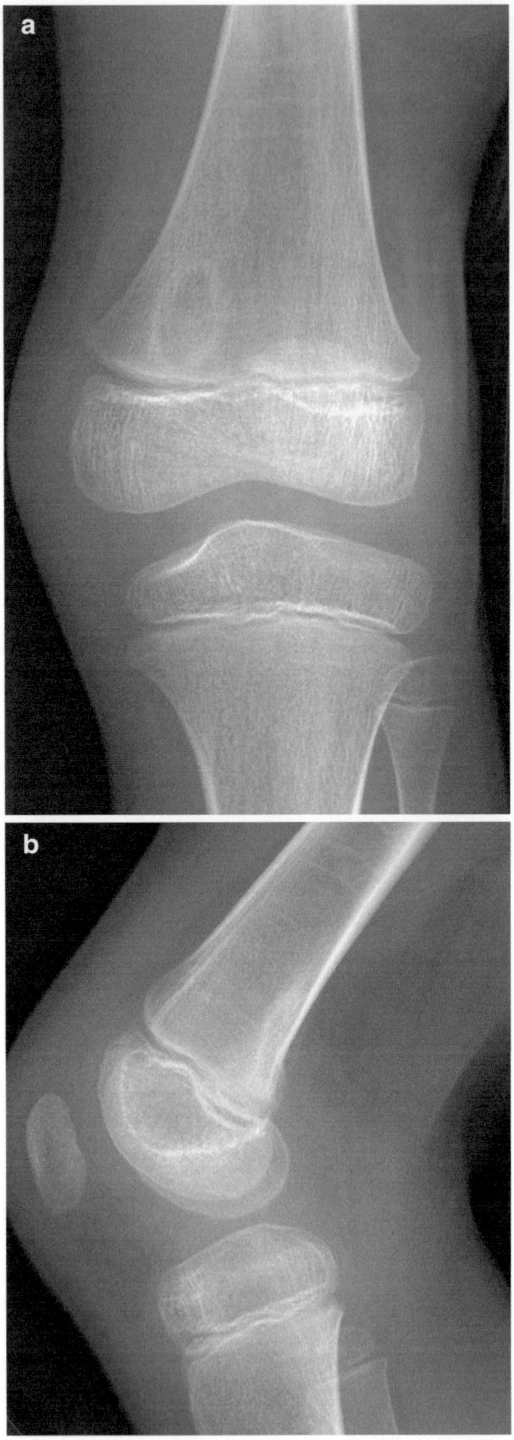

Fig. 13.15 Cortical desmoid in a 7-year-old boy. (**a**) Frontal projection demonstrates ovoid lucency with sclerotic margins. (**b**) Lateral shows posterior sclerosis with scalloped lucent defect (Courtesy of Tal Laor, Cincinnati Children's Hospital)

osseous spiculation perpendicular to the cortex, characteristic of rapid periosteal bone formation (Fig. 13.14). A scalloped cortical defect or bony prominence is often apparent (Fig. 13.15). Desmoids are most evident on a slightly externally rotated projection so that the posteromedial supracondylar area is projected in tangent (see Fig. 13.13).

At MRI, these lesions appear as T1-hypointense and T2-hyperintense cortical scalloping, with a dark rim of bony sclerosis along the attachment of the medial head of the gastrocnemius muscle (Fig. 13.16) [9]. If there has been acute trauma, marrow and intratendinous edema may be evident.

Although the appearance may resemble periosteal reaction with bony erosion, cortical desmoids should not be mistaken for a malignant or inflammatory process. If a pathological process is suspected, nuclear scintigraphy will not necessarily help differentiate, especially if the

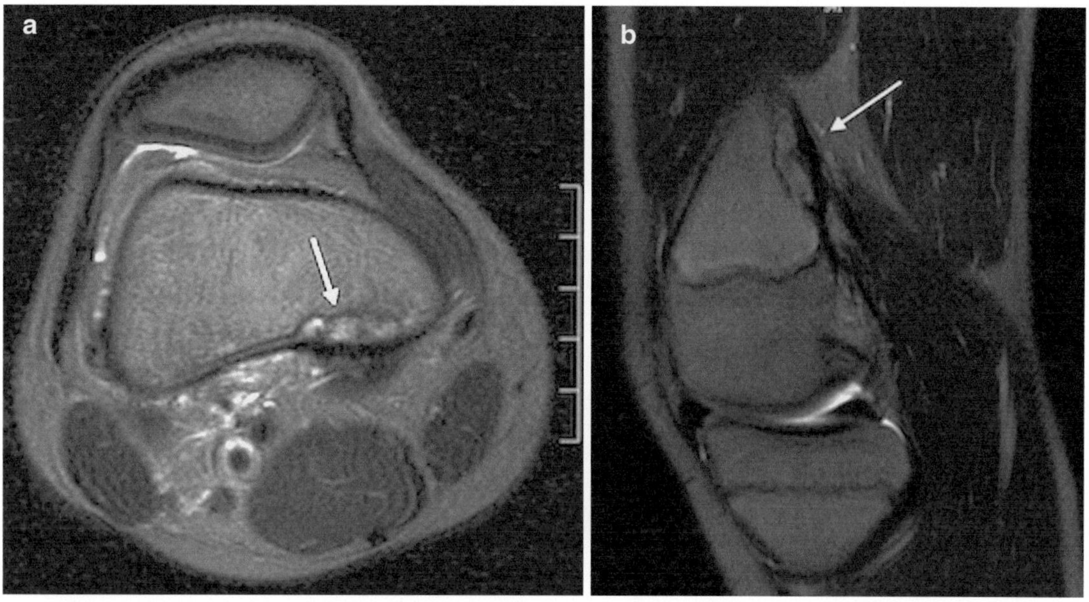

Fig. 13.16 Cortical desmoid. (**a**) Axial T2-W image shows heterogeneous signal along posteromedial distal femoral metaphysis, demarcated by hypointense cortex (*arrow*). (**b**) Sagittal T2-W image shows insertion of the medial head of the gastrocnemius muscle (*arrow*)

appearance is caused by a minor avulsion that might also generate increased radiotracer uptake. MRI may help confirm the benign nature of this lesion. Cortical desmoids are differentiated from nonossifying fibromas/fibrous cortical defects because the latter appear to migrate as the patient grows and also erode the cortex from within the bone, whereas cortical desmoids do not change position and do disrupt the outer surface [4].

Tibial Tuberosity

The tibial tuberosity forms from an anteroinferior cartilaginous extension of the tibial epiphysis. Before ossification of the tuberosity begins, it can appear as a large, abruptly scalloped defect, which can be smooth or show mild undulation (Fig. 13.17). It may mimic an erosive lesion or a buckle fracture (Fig. 13.18) [11]. Ossification begins as a distal extension of the primary epiphysis. However, a separate center occasionally develops and grows concentrically, eventually uniting with the more proximal portion of the epiphysis. The tuberosity fuses with the adjacent bone by age 15 in girls and age 19 in boys.

In most cases, the developing center is either multicentric or irregular. Lack of soft tissue swelling and clinical complaints help differentiate it from an avulsion fracture or Osgood-Schlatter disease (Fig. 13.19).

Growth Recovery Lines

Growth recovery lines appear as discrete horizontal lines of sclerosis parallel to the growth plate, developing after temporary growth cessation. They are quite common in both femoral and tibial metaphyses and are often present simultaneously at multiple metaphyses that significantly contribute to bone growth. They usually extend in a continuous line across the metaphysis and gradually remodel, apparently moving toward the diaphysis with continued growth (Fig. 13.20). While it seems logical that growth arrest lines would occur more often in children with frequent severe illnesses, in fact they are also common in healthy children or in those who have suffered the usual minor childhood illnesses. Persistence into early adulthood indicates a previous vigorous recovery response rather than chronic illness. Focal deformity of a growth arrest line can provide important information about adjacent growth arrest following physeal injury, before development of bony bridging or angular deformity.

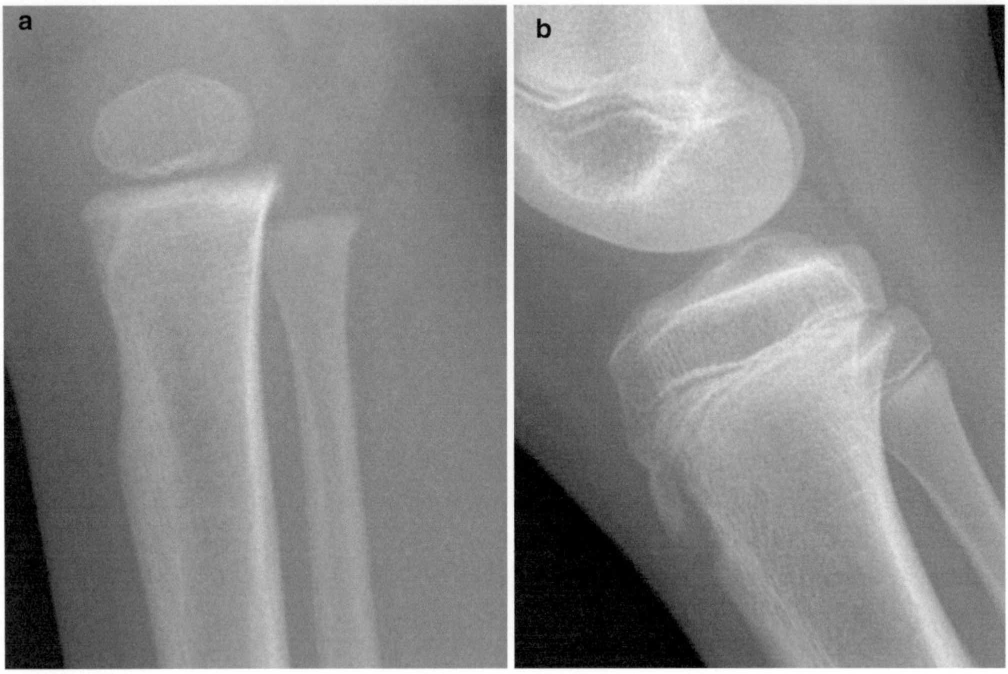

Fig. 13.17 Development of the tibial tuberosity. (**a**) In early childhood, the purely cartilaginous tibial tuberosity results in concavity of the anterior surface of the proximal tibia. (**b**) As the tuberosity ossifies, continuity with the proximal tibial metaphysis becomes apparent

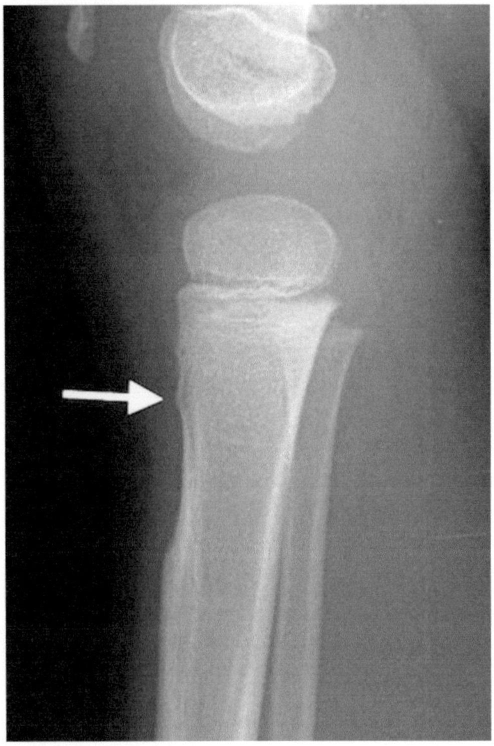

Fig. 13.18 Buckle fracture of the proximal tibia in a 3-year-old boy (*arrow*)

The Fabella

The fabella is an ovoid, occasionally multipartite, sesamoid bone in the lateral gastrocnemius muscle belly (the tendinous portion of this muscle is distal) (Figs. 13.21 and 13.22). It is found in about 12 % of the population and is bilateral in more than half [12]. Although the fabella is almost always of no clinical significance, teens occasionally complain of pain with full extension as well as local tenderness, and this may be relieved by excision of the fabella [13].

The Patella and Patellofemoral Articulation

The anterior surface of the bony patella has many vascular foramina and vertical striations. These appear on radiographs as lucencies or thin anterior fissures (Fig. 13.23) and on MRI as channels that parallel the long axis of the patella, generally with high signal on T2-W images (Fig. 13.24). The posterior surface of the patella has two facets, separated by a median ridge (Fig. 13.25). At birth the lateral facet is already larger than the medial, and it ultimately becomes 40 % longer.

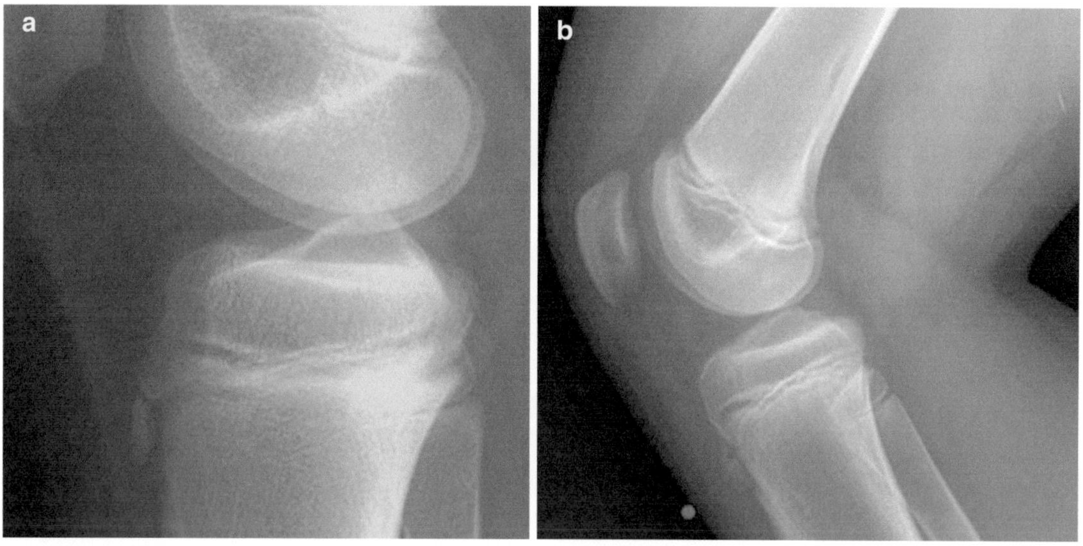

Fig. 13.19 Fragmentation of the tibial tuberosity. (**a**) Normal fragmentation of the tuberosity, with no overlying soft tissue swelling. (**b**) Osgood-Schlatter disease, with soft tissue swelling and thickened patellar tendon (metal marker indicates focal tenderness)

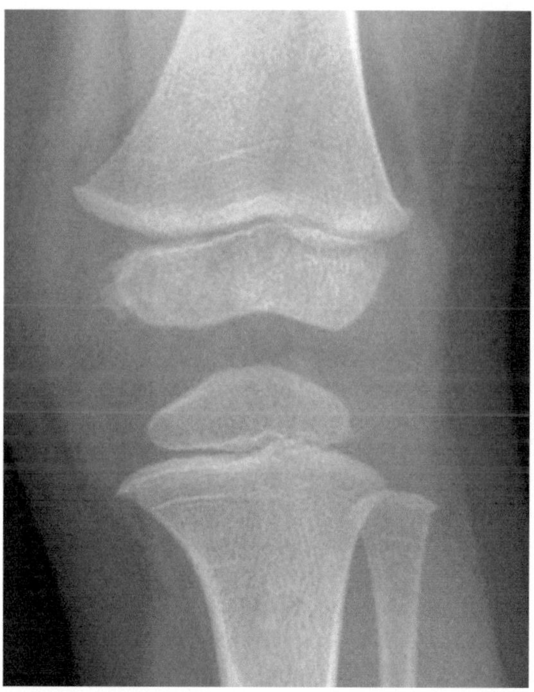

Fig. 13.20 Growth recovery lines appear as thin, sclerotic, horizontal lines traversing the metaphyses of all the bones about the knee

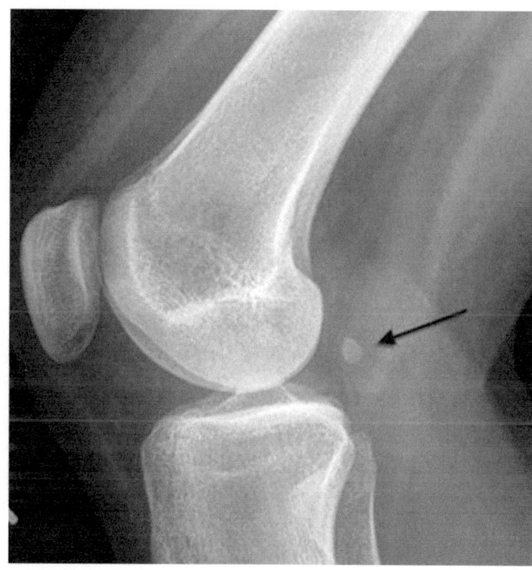

Fig. 13.21 Fabella. *Black arrow* indicates this sesamoid bone

The lateral facet is less steeply angled. The angle between the two facets averages 130°. The upper two-thirds of the posterior surface is covered with articular cartilage (Fig. 13.26), and—as the thickest cartilage in the mature body—it may be up to 5 mm deep in the adult.

The shape of the patella, the shape of the femoral condyles posterior to the patella, and the configuration of the proximal tibia affect the likelihood of developing patellar derangement. The

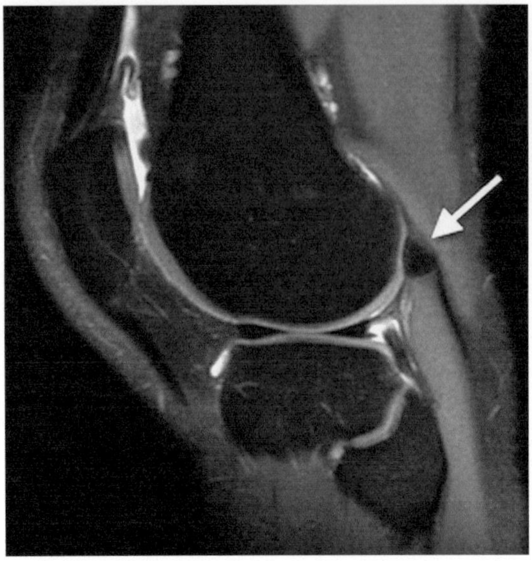

Fig. 13.22 Large fabella (*white arrow*) within the tendon of the lateral head of the gastrocnemius (sagittal T2-W fat-suppressed (FS) image)

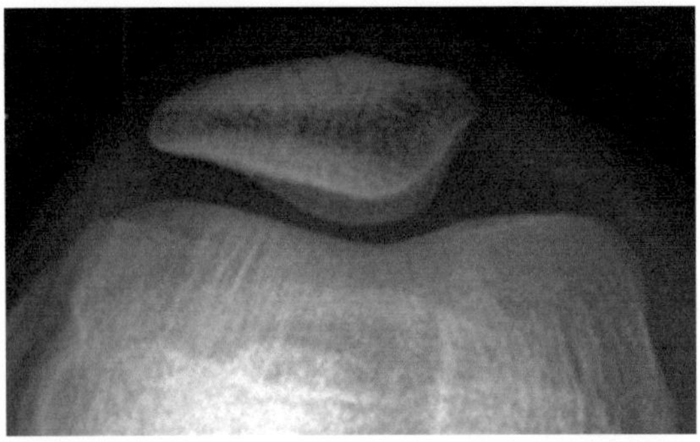

Fig. 13.23 Vascular grooves at the anterior patella. There are lucent striations at the anterior surface of the patella

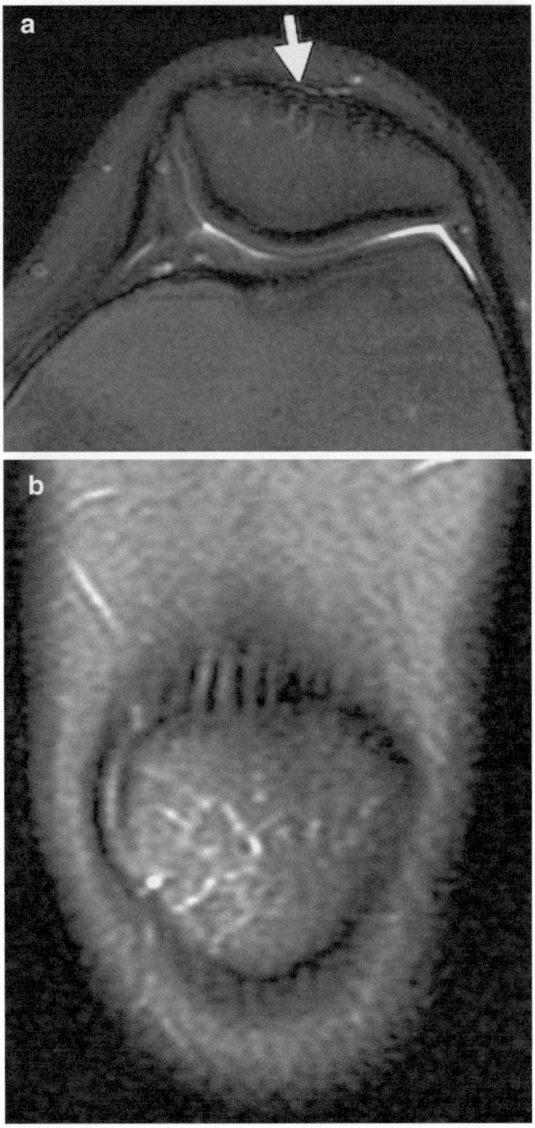

Fig. 13.24 Vascular grooves at the anterior patella. Axial (**a**) and coronal (**b**) T2-W images show hyperintense branching vessels (*arrow*)

patella lies in a sulcus that is a superior extension of the intercondylar notch. The sulcus is formed by the anterior contours of adjacent portions of the medial and lateral femoral condyles. The lateral surface of the sulcus projects more anteriorly than does the medial, restricting lateral patellar subluxation. (The force vectors of the quadriceps muscles apply both a major component of longitudinal force on the patella and a smaller component of lateral force: this lateral force may contribute to patellar subluxation.) Thus, the lateral facet of the femoral trochlea plays an important role in helping to stabilize the patellofemoral articulation. A shallow sulcus, as seen in children with longitudinal deficiency of the fibula, can contribute to instability.

Another important factor in evaluating patellar stability is alignment of the patella with respect to the tibial tuberosity. This can be assessed in several ways. The Q angle is calculated on MRI from the midline of the quadriceps as it inserts into the patella to the patellar tendon

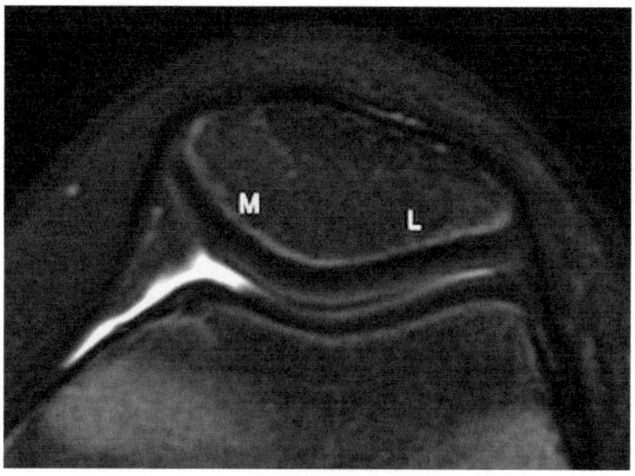

Fig. 13.25 Normal patella with a prominent ridge dividing the smaller medial (M) facet from the larger lateral (L) facet (axial T2-W image)

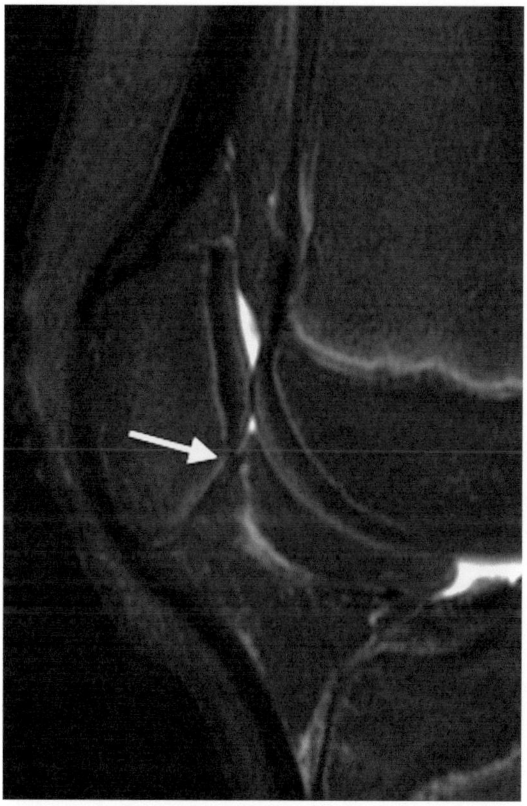

Fig. 13.26 Normal patella with articular cartilage covering only the upper two-thirds of the posterior surface (*arrow* denotes transition between cartilage and bone) (sagittal T2-W image)

as it aligns with the tibial tuberosity. Alternatively, the tibial tuberosity to trochlear groove (TT-TG) distance measures the space between the midpoint of the tibial tuberosity and the deepest part of the trochlear groove (described in detail in section below on developmental patellar instability and dislocation).

The suprapatellar pouch is usually an extension of the knee joint and very rarely a bursa that does not communicate with the joint. There is a small amount of fat anterior to this pouch, posterior and superior to the patella, and a larger amount of fat posterior to it, anterior to the femur. On a lateral knee radiograph, the pouch appears as soft tissue density outlined by fat. A joint effusion is present if the soft tissue between these two fat pads exceeds 10 mm in thickness (Fig. 13.27). If this distance is between 5 and 10 mm and the margins of the recess are fuzzy, an effusion is suggested.

The patella serves many functions: it decreases friction from the quadriceps around the femoral trochlea, transmits the vectors of the quadriceps system into one patellar tendon, protects against dislocation of the tendon from within the sulcus, and shields knee cartilage from injury.

Ossification variants are common. The ossified patella may be granular or nodular; it may have zones of sclerosis and lucency. Anterior lucencies as well as transverse and vertical anterior surface ridges are particularly common. Vertical fissures (larger than the thin branching fissures discussed above (see Figs. 13.23 and 13.24)) are most common (Fig. 13.28). Most variants are isolated, but they may mimic findings in multiple epiphyseal dysplasia or be confused with a patellar sleeve fracture.

A bipartite patella is the most common variation in patellar ossification, estimated to occur in 1–6 % of the population, and is slightly more likely to be unilateral than bilateral. The patella may form from multiple ossification centers, and if they fail to fuse a bi- (or tri-) partite patella results. The extra center is usually superolateral (Fig. 13.29), but in 20 % it is lateral and in 5 % at the lower pole (Fig. 13.30). There may be pain and increased mobility at the cartilaginous interspace adjacent to an accessory center.

It is possible that some bipartite patellae result from stress fracture rather than

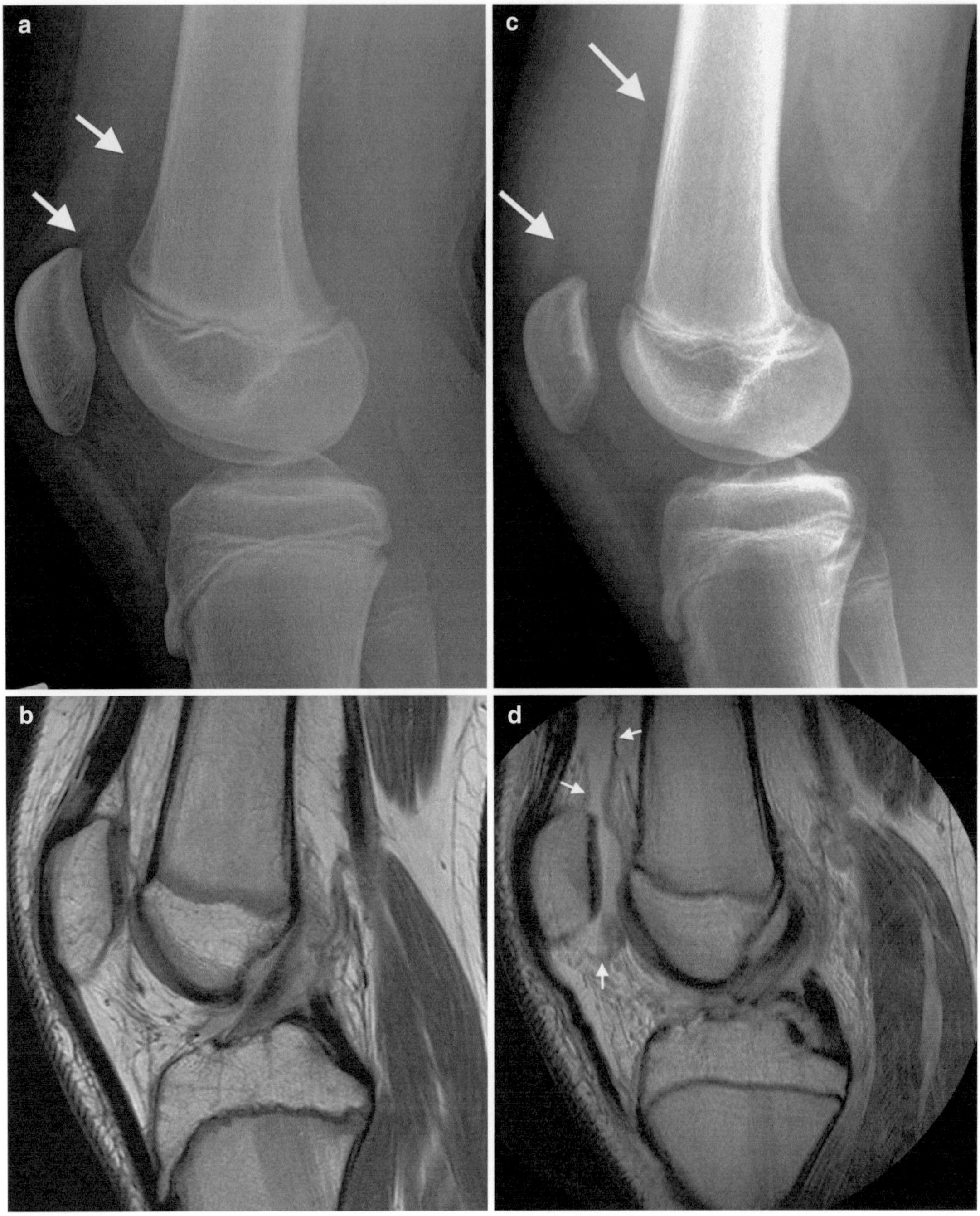

Fig. 13.27 Joint effusion. Cross-table lateral view (**a**) in a normal 12-year-old boy (for comparison) shows a normal, thin suprapatellar pouch, outlined by fatty tissue (*arrows*). (**b**) Accompanying sagittal PD MRI. (**c**) Hemarthrosis in a 14-year-old boy with tibial spine fracture and anterior cruciate ligament (ACL) tear shows the fat pads (*arrows*), along with thickening of the suprapatellar pouch. (**d**) PD MRI shows hemarthrosis (*short arrows*) with fluid-fluid level

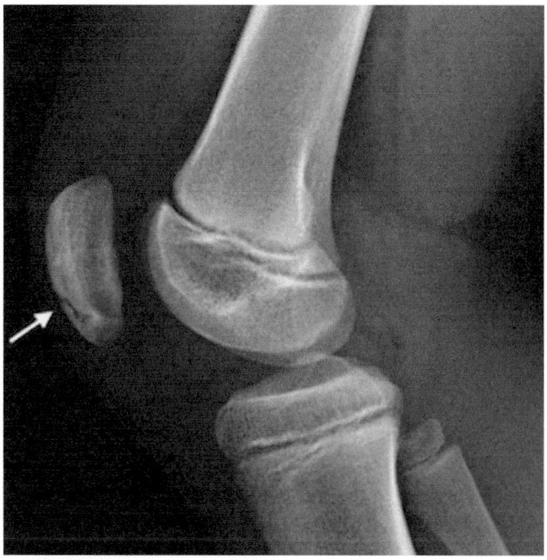

Fig. 13.28 Vertical patellar fissure (*white arrow*)

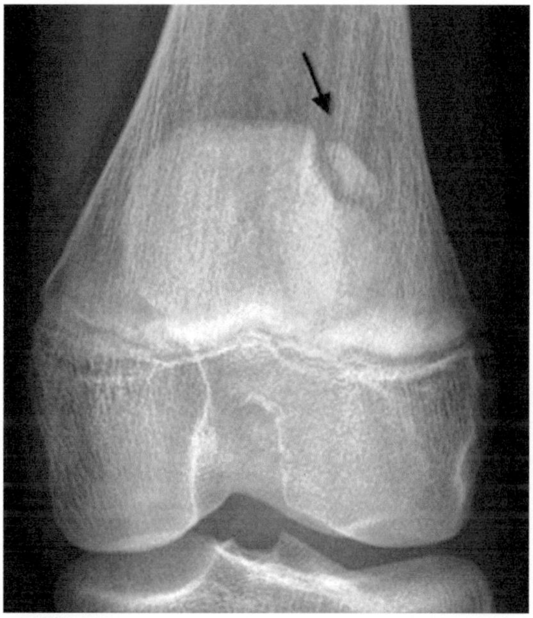

Fig. 13.29 Bipartite patella, most common at the supero-lateral patella (*arrow*)

developmental variation [14]. In addition, several pathological entities mimic the inferior accessory center at the lower pole. It may be confused with a traumatic patellar sleeve fracture (Figs. 13.31 and 13.32) a hyperflexion injury involving both cartilage and bone. If this fracture affects an incompletely ossified patella,

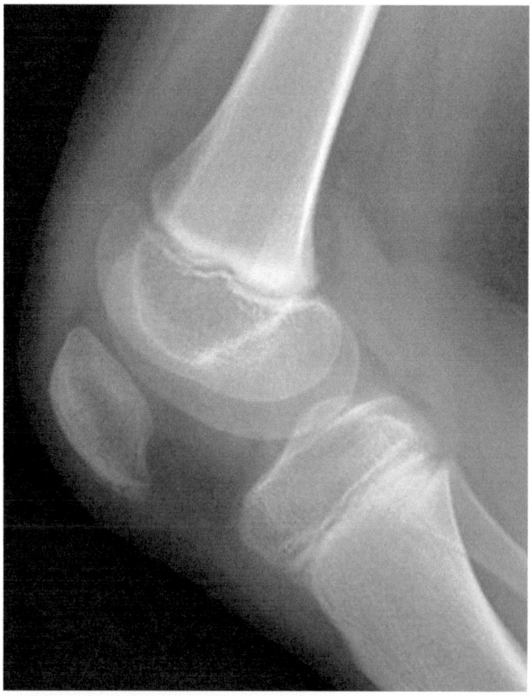

Fig. 13.30 Accessory ossification center at the lower pole of the patella in a 6-year-old boy

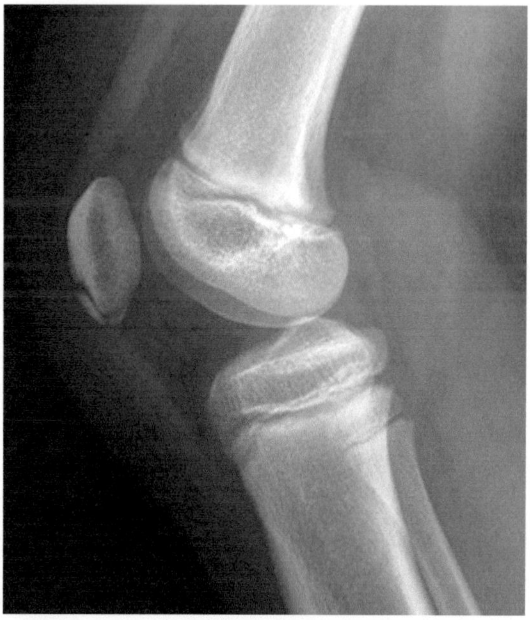

Fig. 13.31 Patellar sleeve avulsion fracture with two large fragments avulsed from the osseous lower pole. Note the associated soft tissue swelling in Hoffa's fat as well as thickening of the patellar tendon

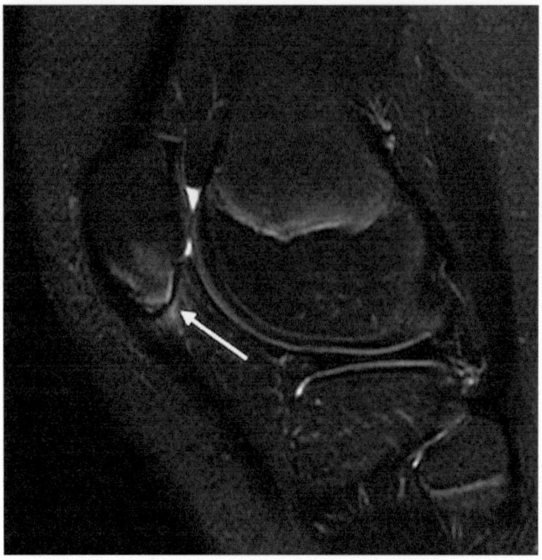

Fig. 13.32 Patellar sleeve avulsion fracture in a 12-year-old boy. Sagittal T2-W image shows transverse fracture through the lower pole of the patella with associated soft tissue edema. *Arrow* indicate avulsed fragment

it may be subtle, involving only the cartilaginous portion of the lower pole. In the setting of fracture, the patella is often high riding, with a small fragment avulsed from the inferior pole. Radiography underestimates the extent of cartilaginous involvement, and MRI is often necessary [15].

Another differential consideration is Sinding-Larsen-Johansson disease. This is most common in children between the ages of 10 and 14 and presents with restricted knee motion as well as localized tenderness and soft tissue swelling over the lower patella. As with Osgood-Schlatter avulsion, this is neither a "disease," osteochondritis, inflammation, nor avascular necrosis but is almost certainly traumatic. Radiographic findings of Sinding-Larsen-Johansson include an accessory ossification center or avulsed fragments at the lower border of the patella, with associated soft tissue swelling (Fig. 13.33). The

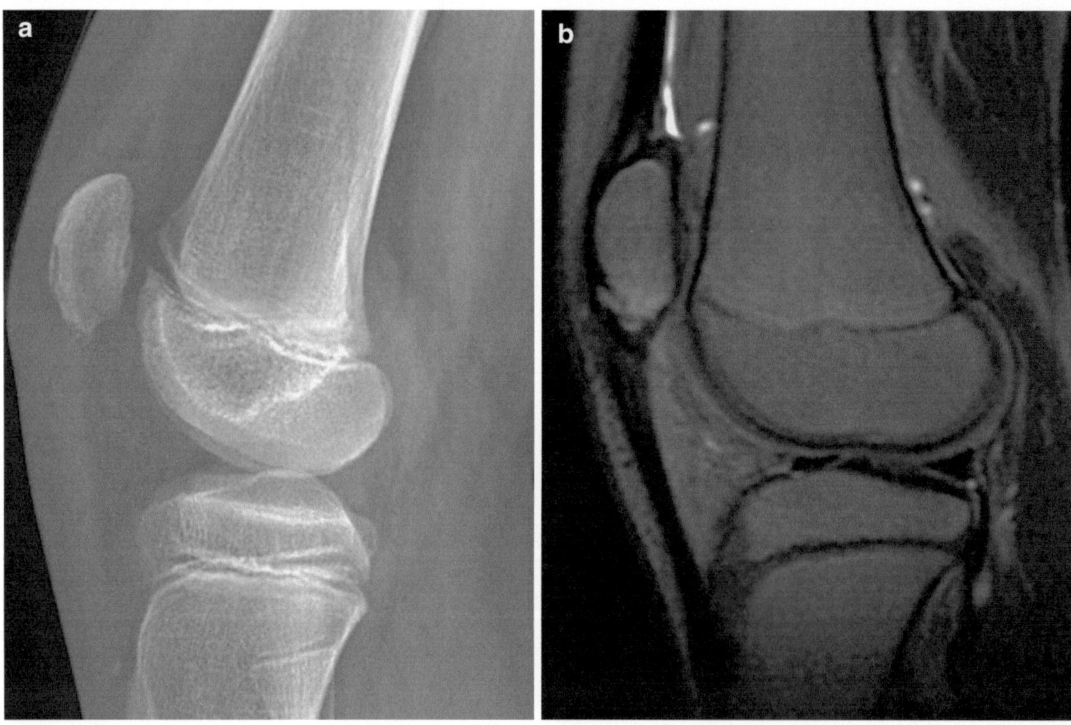

Fig. 13.33 Sinding-Larsen-Johansson disease in an 11-year-old boy with anterior knee pain. (**a**) The lower pole of the patella is slightly fragmented. (**b**) Sagittal T2-W FS image confirms fragmentation and shows mild bone marrow edema and patellar tendon thickening

appearance on both radiographs and MRI is essentially indistinguishable from patellar sleeve fracture, and differentiation relies on clinical history and examination.

Cerebral palsy is also associated with avulsion fractures of the lower pole of the patella, resembling an inferior patellar ossification center. There may be one or several fragments, separated from or adjacent to the patella. In spastic ambulatory children with cerebral palsy and flexion contractures, the patella may be high, elongated, and crescent shaped (see Chap. 24). The appearance probably reflects recurrent mechanical overload of the knee extensor mechanism with healed, subclinical avulsion fractures or ligamentous micro-tears. Ultrasound (US) can demonstrate patellar tendon thickening and local edema, probably due to contusion over (or avulsion of) an accessory center, a fracture-avulsion of the lower patella, or simply contusion of the patellar ligament with ligamentous ossification.

2 Patellar Abnormalities

2.1 Patellar Agenesis

A completely absent patella is rare as an isolated finding, generally running in families. Usually an absent patella indicates the patient has nail-patella (onycho-osteodysplasia, or Fong) syndrome, which consists of dysplasia of the fingernails, radial head and capitellar deformity with potential radial head dislocation, iliac horns, and renal disease. The patella has been found to be absent in approximately 15 % of patients with this disorder and to be small, angular, sclerotic, or otherwise dysplastic in about 85 % [16]. Femoral condylar dysplasia is often associated.

Patellar hypoplasia may also be encountered as an isolated variant, in families, or accompanying congenital dislocation of the patella or contracture of the quadriceps muscle. There are also many variations in facet size and orientation as well as median ridge development. Patellar and femoral cartilaginous and bony surfaces are not necessarily congruent, and radiographs may not portray the true anatomy. MRI may provide a more accurate assessment of contours. Patellar duplication is extremely rare.

2.2 Congenital Patellar Dislocation

Congenital patellar dislocation refers to lateral dislocation present at birth or shortly thereafter. It may be associated with arthrogryposis, Down syndrome, nail-patella syndrome, and other genetic syndromes. The association with Down syndrome suggests this disorder results from ligamentous laxity, but it may also be due to failed rotation of the quadriceps muscle myotome. Associated findings include anomalous insertions of fibrous bands into the lateral patella as well as tight lateral capsular structures and synovial fibrosis. Quadriceps fibrosis has also been found in many cases [17].

Infants with patellar dislocation may present with a fixed flexion contracture. However, the knee may have a normal range of motion, and the patella may dislocate only with flexion. Diagnosis is often made only after the patient begins walking. Surgery—generally release of the patella laterally and lengthening of the quadriceps tendon—should be performed promptly. Failure to recognize and treat this condition early may result in progressive flexion contracture at the knee, as well as genu valgum and torsional deformities.

Imaging

Patellar ossification does not begin until 1.5 years of age at the earliest, but its position may be deduced on radiographs by an ovoid increased soft tissue density. US can readily assess patellar position before ossification begins (Fig. 13.34). In extension, it may be normally positioned or dislocated (usually laterally). The dislocated patella may rotate 90° such that its articular surface abuts the lateral aspect of the relatively small

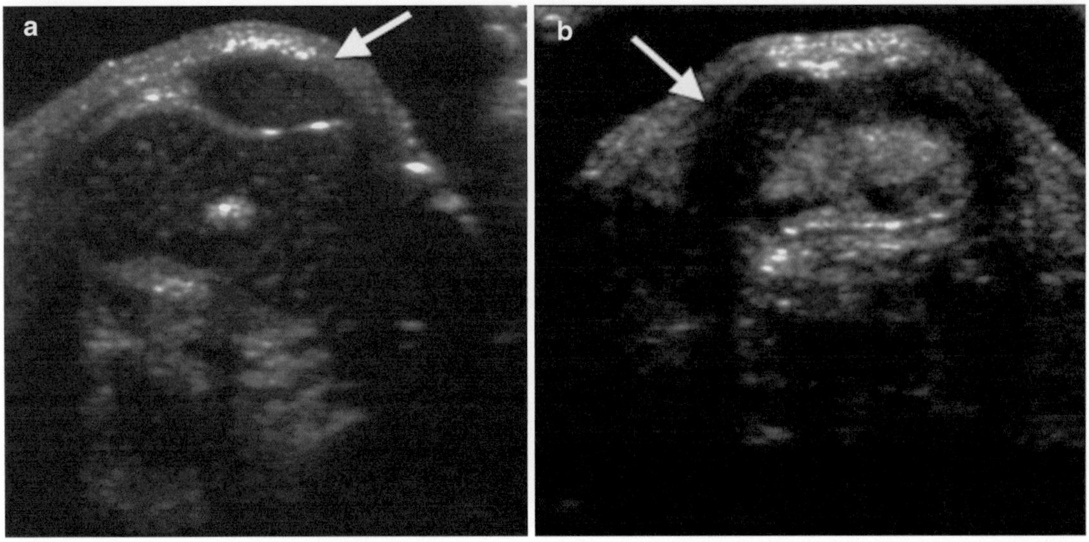

Fig. 13.34 Dislocated patella in an infant. (**a**) Normal side (for comparison) shows the hypoechoic patella (*arrow*) nestled in the intercondylar notch of the femur. (**b**) On the *right*, the distal femur is identified (*arrow*), but the intercondylar notch appears shallow, and the patella is not in its expected position (Courtesy of Rebecca Stein-Wexler)

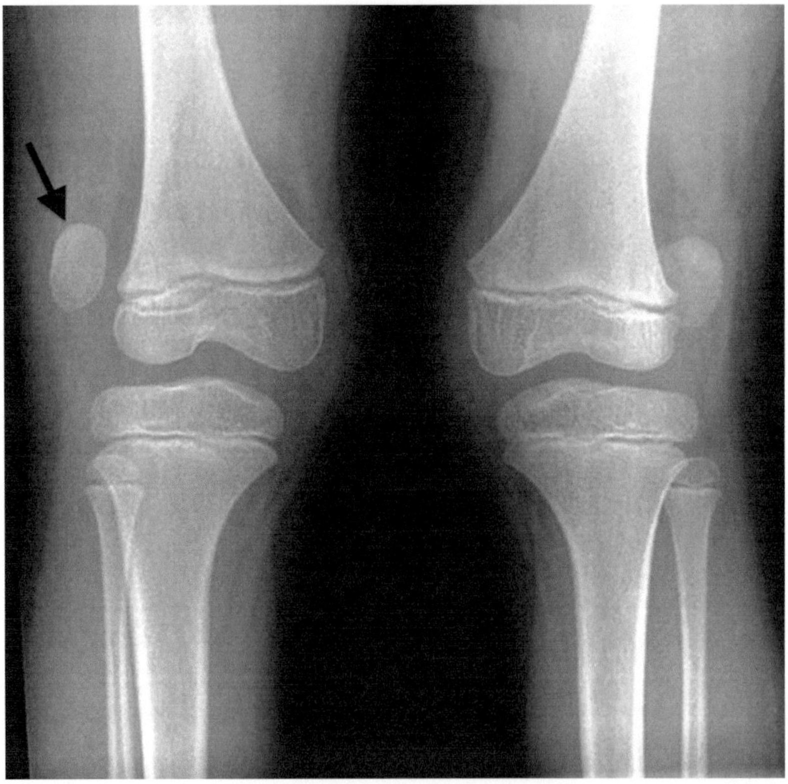

Fig. 13.35 Congenital patellar dislocation in a 6-year-old with bilateral lateral dislocation of the patella. The lateral femoral condyles are relatively small, and the right patella is rotated (*arrow*) (Courtesy of Hank Baskin)

lateral femoral condyle (Fig. 13.35). The axial projection shows a shallow sulcus, sometimes associated with hypoplasia of the femoral condyles [18]. MRI is also useful for assessing the position and configuration of a dislocated patella before it has ossified.

2.3 Developmental Patellar Instability and Dislocation

Patellar dislocation is common in young, active individuals, usually resulting from a twisting motion with the knee flexed. The annual incidence is approximately 43 per 100,000 children under age 16 years old [19]. The medial retinaculum, medial patellofemoral ligament, shape of the femoral trochlea, position of the tibial tuberosity, and the extensor muscles of the knee stabilize the patellofemoral articulation. Abnormal development of the femoral trochlea may lead to a shallow femoral trochlear sulcus, reducing the normal osseous barrier to lateral subluxation. This trochlear dysplasia thus leads to instability and recurrent patellar dislocations, and indeed 85 % of patients with patellar dislocation have imaging signs of trochlear dysplasia. In addition, an abnormally positioned tibial tuberosity may also contribute to patellofemoral instability by changing force vectors. If the medial stabilizing ligaments tear during an episode of dislocation, chronic instability results [20].

Surgery is frequently the definitive treatment. The type of surgery performed depends on imaging findings. Frequently, the stabilizing ligaments are repaired, specifically with medial patellofemoral ligament repair and medial capsular plication. A lateral capsular release is often performed as well. If lateralization of the tibial tuberosity contributes to instability, tibial tuberosity transfer can be performed after skeletal maturity (the tendon and an associated bone fragment are moved medially and reattached to the tibia). This decreases the lateral force vector of the quadriceps muscles, decreasing instability. In severe dysplasia, trochleoplasty may be performed, which involves deepening the trochlear sulcus by a curved osteotomy at the upper portion of the articular surface.

High-lying patella (patella alta) is associated with recurrent patellar subluxation, chondromalacia of the patella, Sinding-Larsen-Johansson lesion, recurrent effusion, and cerebral palsy. A low patella (patella baja or infera) occurs in achondroplasia, Osgood-Schlatter lesion, and poliomyelitis.

Imaging

Patellar position may be measured in several ways on a lateral radiograph or lateral MRI (Table 13.1). In a skeletally mature knee, the Insall-Salvati ratio and lateral trochlear inclination best predict both lateral patellar displacement and lateral tilt of the patella [21].

The *Koshino and Sugimoto method* is best used for children under 13 years of age, whose patella may not yet have ossified completely [22]. Lines are drawn along the distal femoral and proximal tibial growth plates. A line that connects them at their midpoints forms the femorotibial (FT) distance. The patello-tibial (PT) line is then drawn from the tibial midpoint to the center of the patellar axis (PT) (Fig. 13.36). A normal patello-tibial/femorotibial (PT/FT) ratio is 0.9–1.3.

The *Insall and Salvati method* should be used on radiographs only in patients over the age of 13, as a partially cartilaginous patella will yield misleading results [23]. The length of the patellar tendon is measured along its posterior edge—from the apex of the patella to its insertion into the tibial tuberosity (Figs. 13.37 and 13.38). The diagonal length of the patella is also measured. The patellar tendon and patellar lengths should be nearly equal. Patella alta is defined as a tendon/patella ratio greater than 1.3, and patella baja is defined as a ratio less than 0.7. This ratio is accurate on MRI's of younger children, while patellar ossification is still incomplete.

Patellar position may also be assessed with respect to the *Blumensaat line*, which is drawn along the roof of the intercondylar notch with the knee flexed to 30° (Fig. 13.39). The position of the patella is determined by measuring the distance from the lower pole of the patella to this line. Patella alta is present if the inferior pole of the patella is more than 29 mm above this line [24]. This technique is simple to perform but less accurate than either the Koshino and Sugimoto method or the Insall-Salvati ratio.

Table 13.1 Signs of trochlear dysplasia and patellar instability

	Normal value
Lateral trochlear inclination	>11°
Lateralization of tibial tuberosity	<15 mm
Patellar height ratio (Insall/Salvati)	<1.4
Patello-tibial/femorotibial ratio (PT/FT) (Koshino and Sugimoto)	>0.9, <1.3
Trochlear depth	>3 mm
Trochlear facet ratio	>0.4

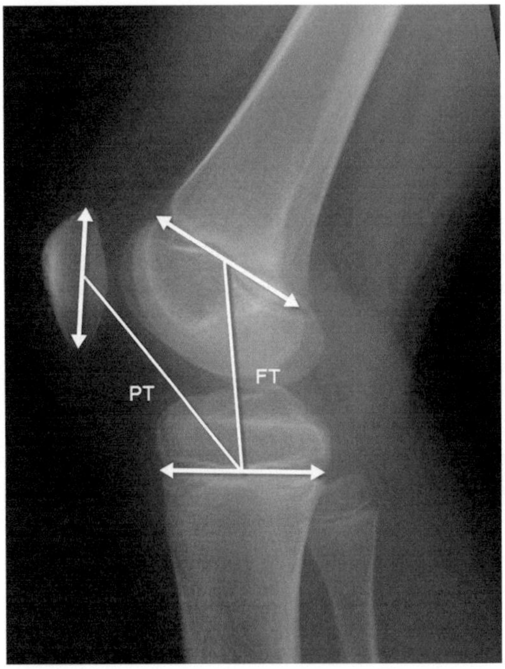

Fig. 13.36 Koshino-Sugimoto method for assessing patellar height ratio in a skeletally immature patient. The distance from the midpoint of the patella to the midpoint of the tibial physis (PT) is compared with the distance from the midpoint of the distal femoral physis to the midpoint of the proximal tibial physis (FT)

The axial projection helps evaluate patellar position and angulation, as well as the depth and configuration of the sulcus. MRI best evaluates articular cartilage, ligamentous structures, and the patellofemoral articulation [20]. Trochlear dysplasia can be evaluated on axial images.

Measurements of lateral trochlear inclination, sulcal depth, and facet ratio may be useful. The *lateral trochlear inclination* is measured on the first axial image that includes the trochlear

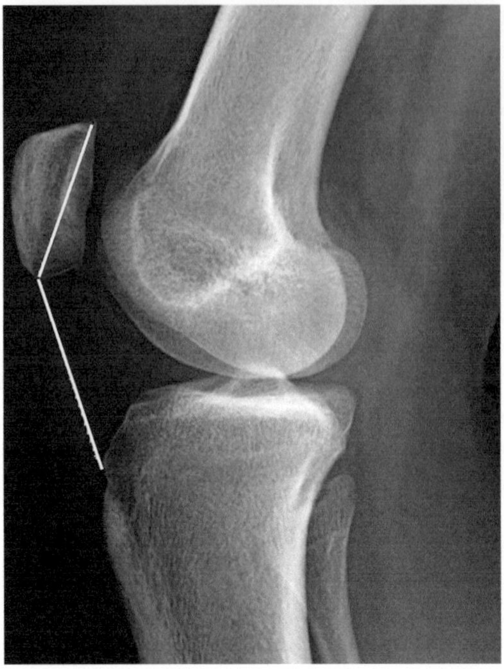

Fig. 13.37 Insall and Salvati method for assessing patellar height ratio in a skeletally mature 17-year-old girl: the diagonal length of the patellar tendon (measured from the apex of the patella to its insertion into the tibial tuberosity) is compared with the maximum diagonal length of the patella (Courtesy of Rebecca Stein-Wexler)

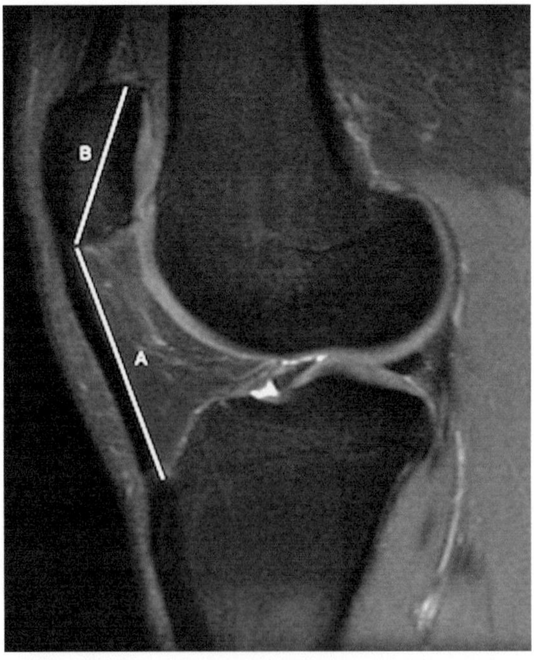

Fig. 13.38 Patella alta. Sagittal T2-W FS MRI shows the length of the patellar tendon (*A*) compared with the greatest height of the patella (*B*) is 1.55

cartilage by determining the angle formed by two lines. One line is tangent to the lateral trochlear facet, and the second is tangent to the posterior surface of the femoral condyles (Fig. 13.40). An abnormal angle is less than 11° [25].

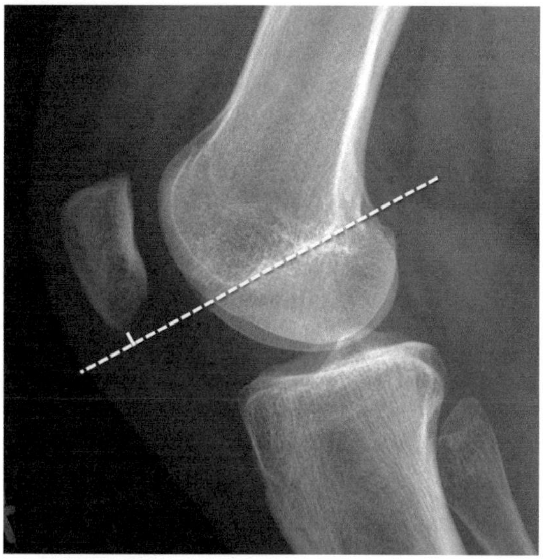

Fig. 13.39 Blumenstat method for assessing patellar position. Performed on a lateral radiograph with the knee in 30° of flexion, this technique determines the distance between the inferior tip of the patella and Blumenstat line (*long dashed line*). Blumenstat's line is tangent to the intercondylar roof

Trochlear depth is the maximum distance between a line connecting the highest points of the lateral and medial facets and the deepest point of the trochlear sulcus. This measurement is obtained 3 cm above the tibiofemoral joint cleft (Fig. 13.41). A sulcal depth less than 3 mm is abnormal [26].

The *trochlear facet ratio*, which is measured at the same level as the trochlear depth, compares the tangential length of the medial facet to that of the lateral facet (Fig. 13.42). A ratio of less than 0.4 is abnormal [27].

If the tibial tuberosity is too far lateral, the lateral force vector of the quadriceps femoris muscle at the patellofemoral articulation increases, contributing to patellar instability. The position of the tibial tuberosity in relation to the femoral trochlea is determined by measuring the horizontal distance between the midpoint of the anterior aspect of the tibial tuberosity and the deepest part of the trochlear groove (*tibial tuberosity to trochlear groove* (TT-TG) distance). The line through the trochlear groove is drawn perpendicular to a line drawn along the posterior femoral condyles. The line through

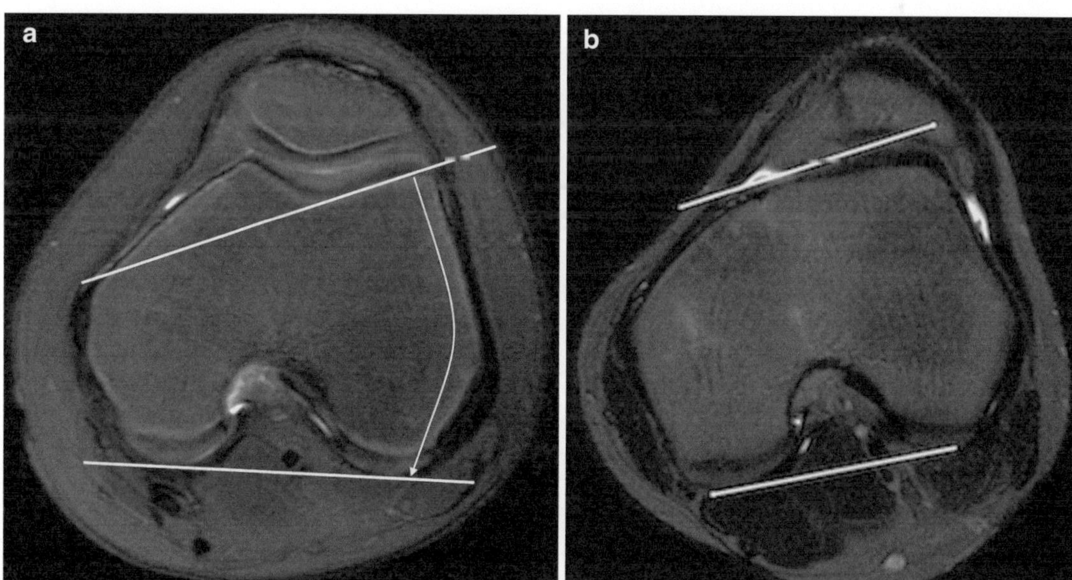

Fig. 13.40 Lateral trochlear inclination. The angle between a line tangent to the posterior aspect of the femoral condyles and a line tangent to the subchondral bone on the lateral trochlear facet. (**a**) Normal. (**b**) 10-year-old girl with abnormal trochlear inclination of 8° (axial T2-W FS MRI)

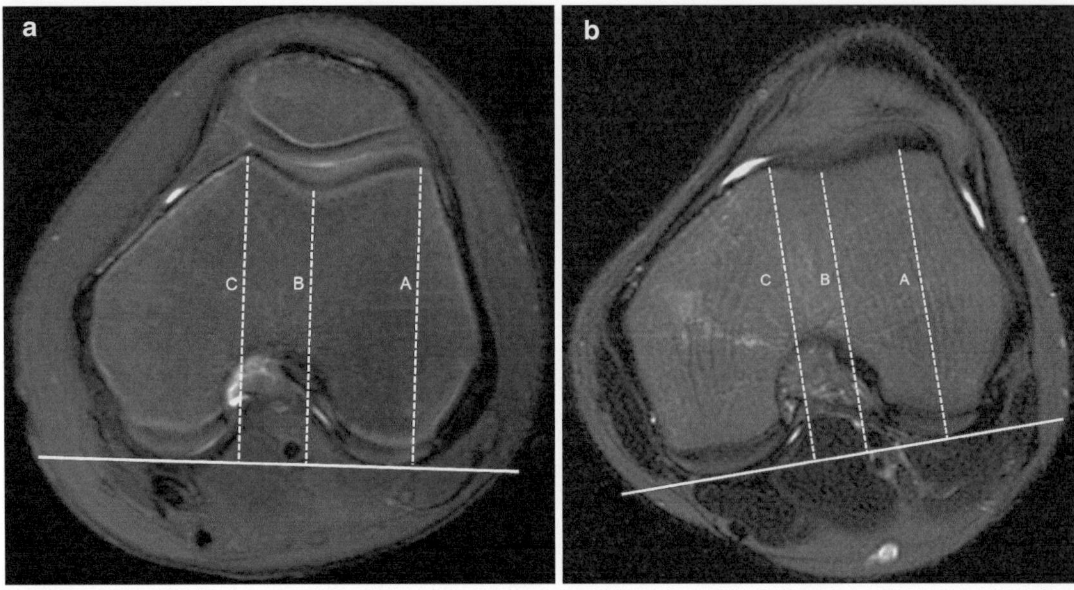

Fig. 13.41 Trochlear depth. An average of the difference between the highest point of the lateral (*A*) and medial (*B*) facets and the deepest point of the trochlear sulcus (*C*). (**a**) Normal. (**b**) Ten-year-old girl with very shallow trochlea, 1 mm deep (axial T2-W FS MRI)

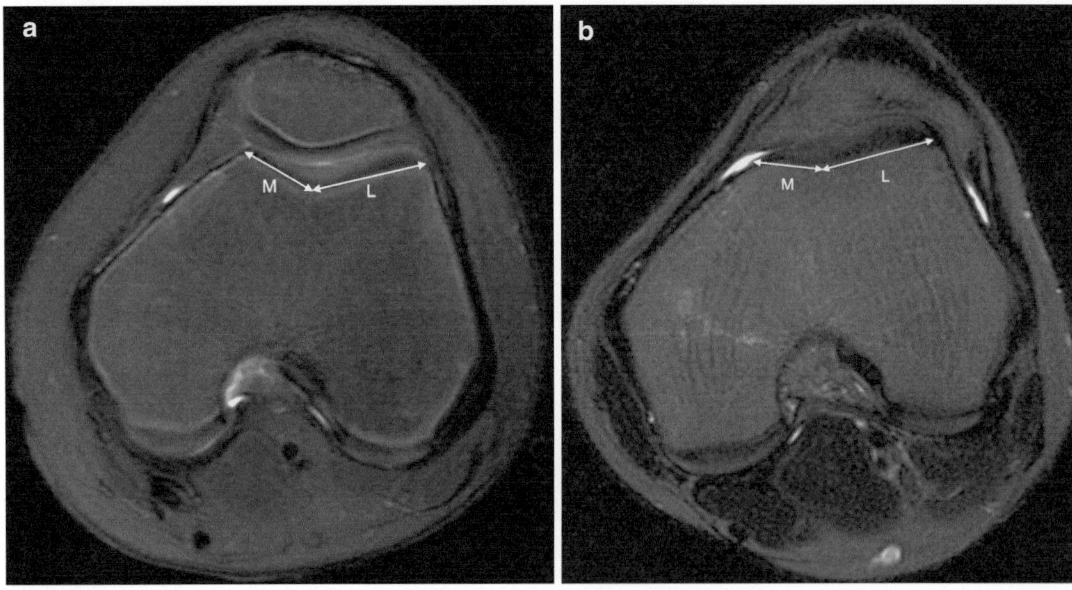

Fig. 13.42 Trochlear facet ratio. The transverse length of the medial trochlear facet compared to the lateral trochlear facet (M/L). (**a**) Normal. (**b**) Ten-year-old girl with abnormal facet ratio of 0.35 (axial T2-W FS MRI)

the tibial tubercle then parallels the trochlear groove line. If the distance between these lines is less than 15 mm, the value is normal, 15–20 mm is borderline, and over 20 mm is abnormal (Fig. 13.43).

If any of these measurements is abnormal, recurrent patellar dislocation is more likely (Fig. 13.44).

Patellar dislocation usually spontaneously reduces and is thus rarely encountered

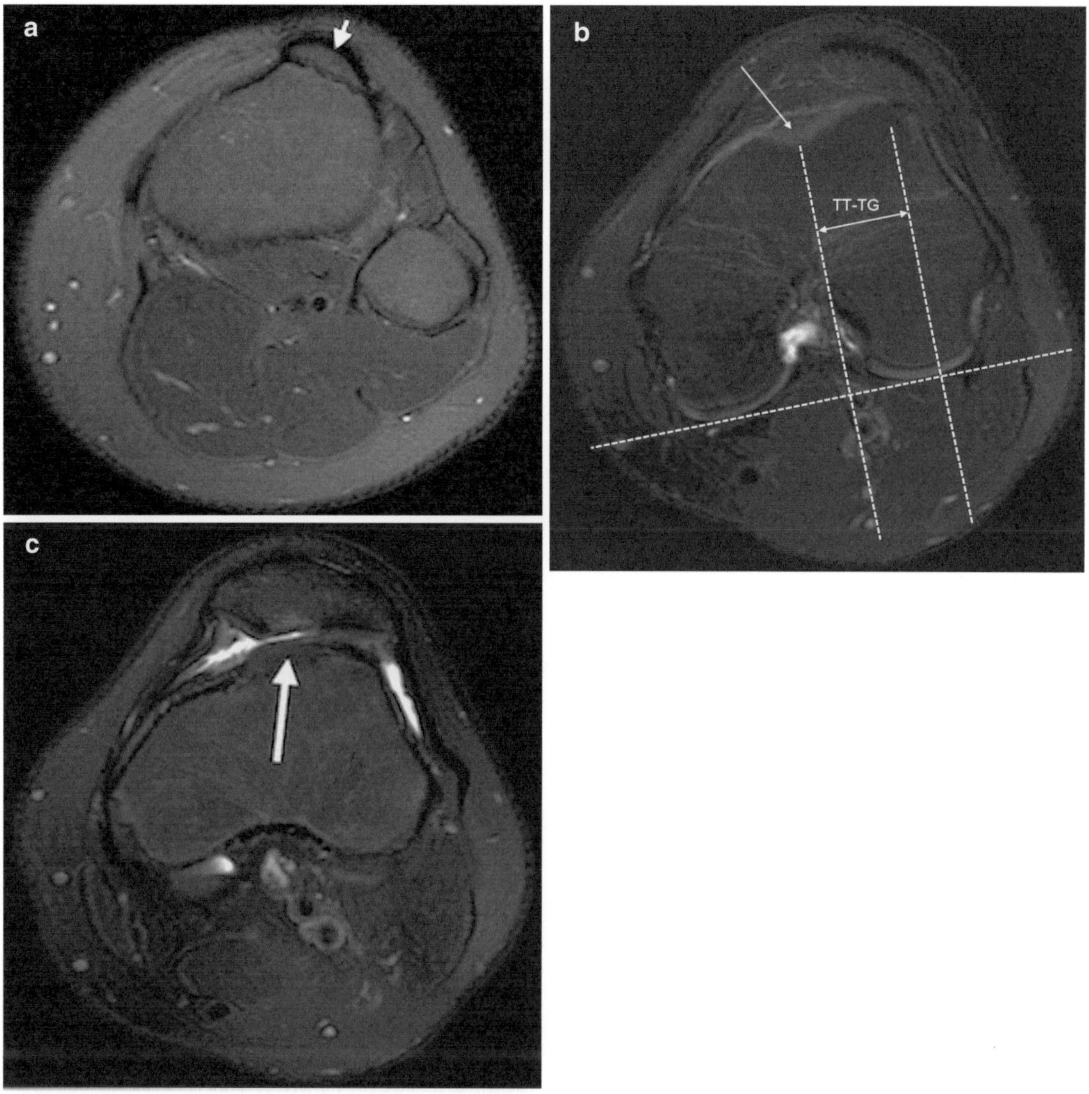

Fig. 13.43 Lateralization of the tibial tuberosity. The position of the tibial tuberosity relative to the femoral trochlea is assessed on axial images at two different levels: at the tibial tuberosity (**a**) and at the deepest point of the trochlea (**b**). The trochlear groove line is drawn through the deepest point of the trochlear groove (*long arrow*, **b**), perpendicular to a line tangent to the backs of the femoral condyle. The tibial tuberosity line is drawn through the midpoint of the tibial tuberosity (*short arrow*, **a**), parallel to the trochlear groove line. The distance between the *parallel lines* (*double arrow*, **b**) constitutes the tibial tuberosity-trochlear groove (TT-TG) distance. In this patient it measures 26 mm (normal less than 15 mm). (**c**) Axial T2-W FS image shows increased signal intensity in the patellar cartilage secondary to abnormal tracking, along with a small amount of joint fluid

radiographically. If present, it is more apparent on the frontal view than the sunrise view (Fig. 13.45), as the flexed position partially reduces dislocation. The patella is also rarely dislocated at MRI, but slightly abnormal alignment may suggest previous or recurrent dislocation. The patella may be slightly laterally subluxated, and the medial aspect of the articulation may open, causing the medial portion of the joint to be wider than the lateral. In addition, "kissing contusions" may be evident. This marrow edema results from impaction during

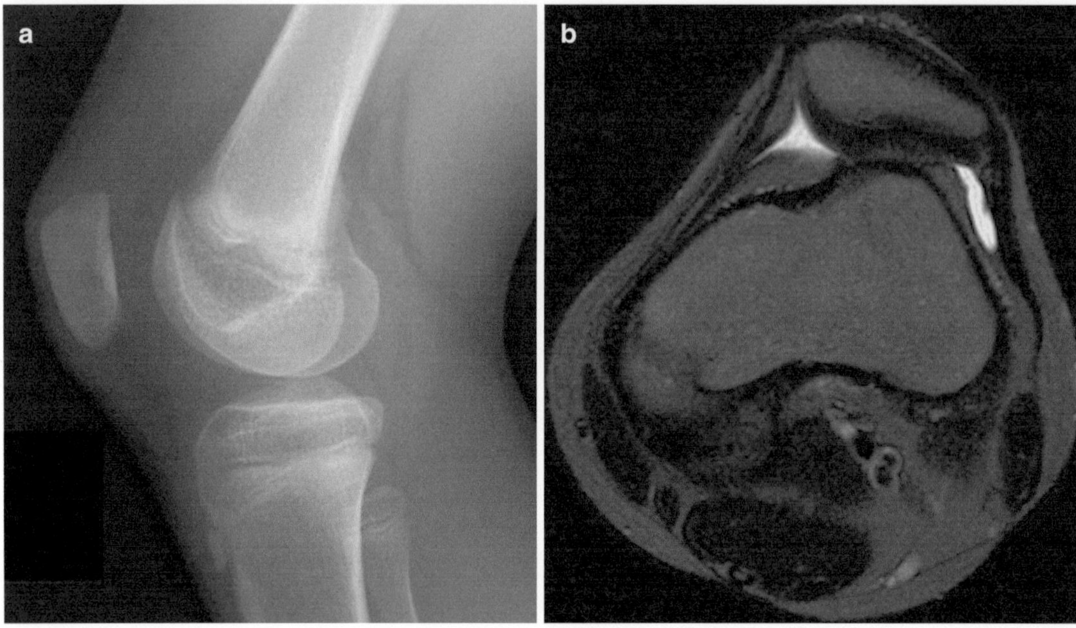

Fig. 13.44 Trochlear dysplasia in a 10-year-old girl. (**a**) Patella alta. (**b**) Axial T2-W FS MRI shows dysplastic trochlea with lateral subluxation of the patella (same patient as Figs. 13.40, 13.41, and 13.42b)

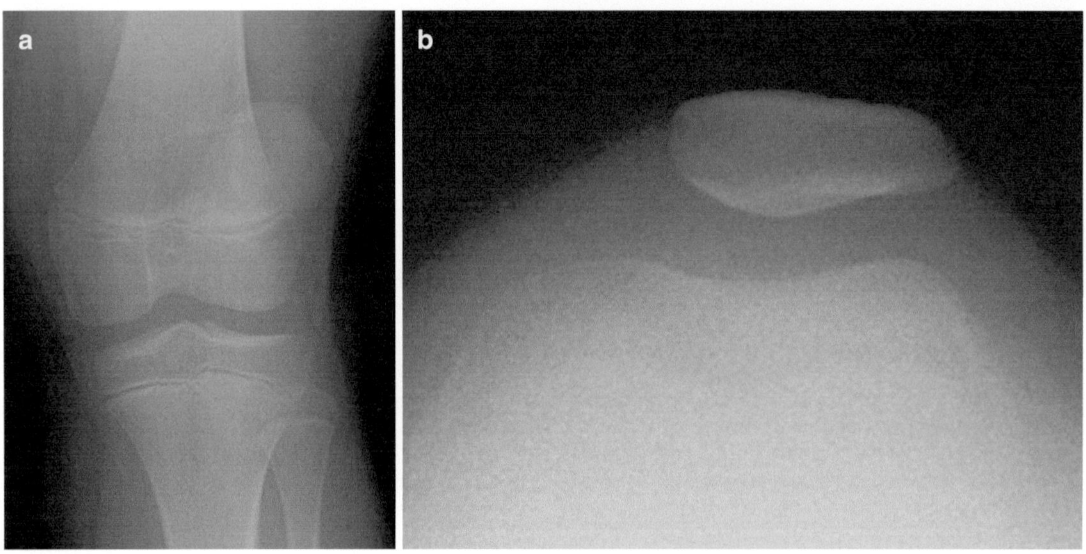

Fig. 13.45 Patellar dislocation in a 9-year-old girl with acute knee injury. (**a**) Frontal view of the right knee shows the patella is displaced laterally. (**b**) Sunrise view shows improved alignment with only mild lateral subluxation

dislocation and is evident on the lateral aspect of the lateral femoral condyle as well as the medial aspect of the patella (Fig. 13.46). Articular cartilage injury on the medial patellar facet may be associated as well.

The medial retinaculum may tear during dislocation and appear wavy or irregular (Fig. 13.47). This most frequently occurs at the patellar attachment in conjunction with an avulsion fracture of the patella's medial cortex.

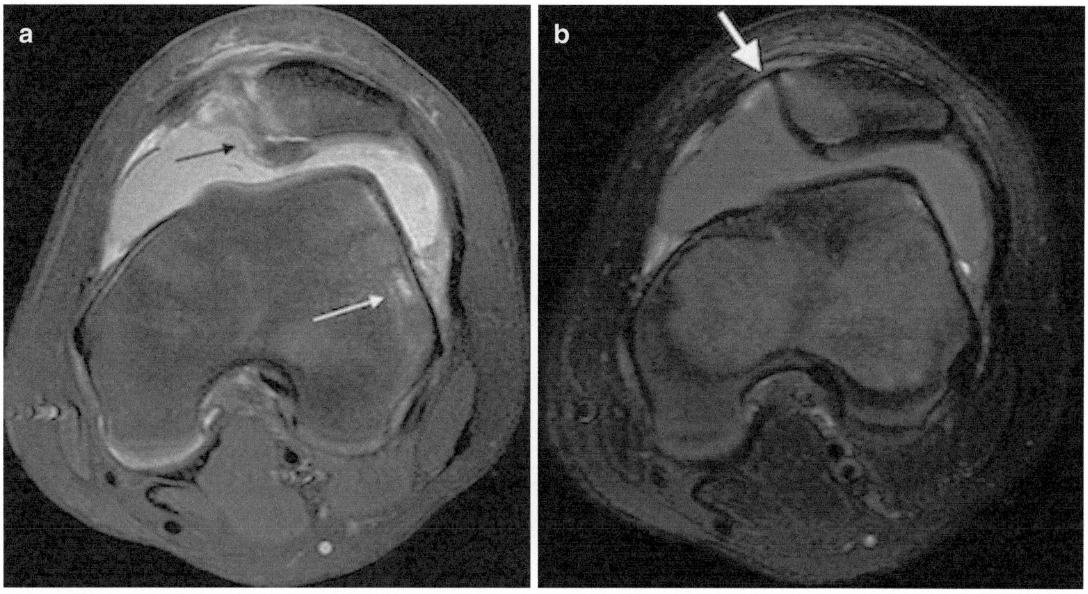

Fig. 13.46 Recent traumatic patellar dislocation in a 12-year-old boy. (**a**) Axial T2-W FS image shows kissing contusion, with cartilage injury at the medial aspect of the patella (*black arrow*) and marrow edema at the lateral aspect of the lateral femoral condyle (*white arrow*). (**b**) Axial T2-W FS image shows focal marrow edema and fluid where the medial retinaculum attaches to the patella (*white arrow*)

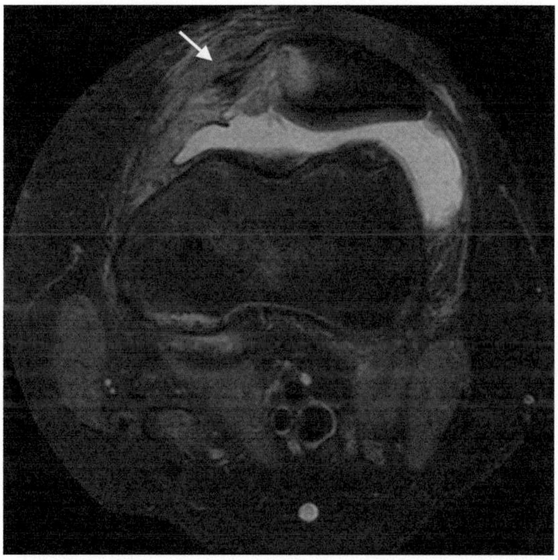

Fig. 13.47 Sequelae of recent traumatic transient patellar dislocation in a 15-year-old football player. Axial PD FS image shows tear of the medial retinaculum (*arrow*) as well as medial patellar marrow edema and cartilage injury (Courtesy of Sandra L. Wootton-Gorges)

However, tears can also occur in the mid-portion of the ligament or at the medial attachment of the retinaculum. With recurrent patellar dislocation, the retinaculum may be so attenuated that it cannot be identified.

3 Longitudinal Limb Deficiency (Hypoplasia and Aplasia)

3.1 General Considerations

Limb anomalies are encountered in the lower extremity about half as often as in the upper extremity [28]. Although patterns of malformation are generally similar in the upper and lower extremities, they differ in several interesting ways. In the upper extremity, if there is a significant abnormality in the proximal limb, the distal part of the extremity is almost certainly abnormal as well—for example, if the humerus is dysplastic, the radius and ulna are probably severely deformed. However, in the lower extremity, the femur may be markedly abnormal yet the tibia and fibula well formed or only slightly hypoplastic. In addition, the foot may be normal despite severe proximal anomalies—unlikely with the hand [29]. Another interesting difference is that although synostoses are relatively common in the forearm, they are very rare in the lower leg and in the lower extremity are essentially limited to the foot.

However, anomalies in some areas are often associated with nearby abnormalities, due to features of embryogenesis. For example, proximal focal femoral deficiency (PFFD) and fibular aplasia often occur together (i.e., postaxial limb bud deficiency). Some anomalies cluster as components of syndromes, whereas others are isolated. Proper limb development depends at least in part on sonic hedgehog gene clusters, and lack of these genes may contribute to severe truncation mutations [30].

As with the upper extremity, multiple classification systems have been devised (two are presented in detail in Chap. 7). These systems are generally either descriptive or based on treatment, and they can help guide therapeutic pathways as well as suggest prognosis.

The "International Standard" classification of limb deficiencies offers a practical system for describing limb deficiencies. It characterizes the deficiency as either transverse (if the limb developed normally to a specific level, beyond which there are no osseous elements) or longitudinal (if an element of the long axis is missing) [31]. Transverse deficiencies are designated by naming the segment beyond which there are no osseous structures. Longitudinal deficiencies are designated by naming the absent or deficient bone(s) and describing the extent of deformity (e.g., total or partial aplasia, or hypoplasia). With longitudinal deficiency, normal bones may be present distal to the deficient structures.

Other terminology may alternatively be used to describe anomalous limbs. For example, dysmelia is a broad term that denotes diminutive skeletal material and abnormal development, usually most severe distally [29]. It broadly encompasses hemimelia, defining absence of a large portion of a limb (partial longitudinal deficiency); amelia, defining complete absence of a limb (total longitudinal deficiency); and phocomelia, defining a flipper-like hand or foot attached directly to the trunk. Distal, proximal, and axial are used to describe the location of the abnormality. Terminal defects lack normal tissue distal to the level of the defect, whereas intercalary defects have some normal tissue beyond the level of the defect. Transverse defects extend across the entire limb, whereas longitudinal defects involve only the preaxial or postaxial portion of the limb.

Anomalies are also described according to the severity of involvement: hypoplasia, partial aplasia, and total aplasia. Dysmaturity refers to discordant maturation either in the area of the defect (where apparently absent segments ossify late) or in structures remote from the actual defect (as in delayed bone age in the hand accompanying more proximal abnormalities).

While usually easily recognizable at physical examination, imaging is often required to fully understand the abnormality. Radiography may be sufficient, but MRI determines the presence of cartilage anlage as well as anomalies of vasculature, muscles, and other soft tissue structures.

3.2 Proximal Femoral Focal Deficiency (PFFD)

Proximal femoral focal deficiency (PFFD) ranges from mild proximal hypoplasia with femoral neck varus to complete absence of both the femoral head and the proximal shaft. The femur below the defect may be practically normal, hypoplastic, or completely absent. A malpositioned or an absent femoral head induces secondary acetabular changes. One-fourth of patients have a contralateral lower limb abnormality, and up to one-half have ipsilateral fibular longitudinal deficiency (Fig. 13.48) (see Chap. 11 for further discussion).

3.3 Femoral Bifurcation and Duplication

Bifurcation of the distal portion of the femur is extremely rare. This anomaly probably results

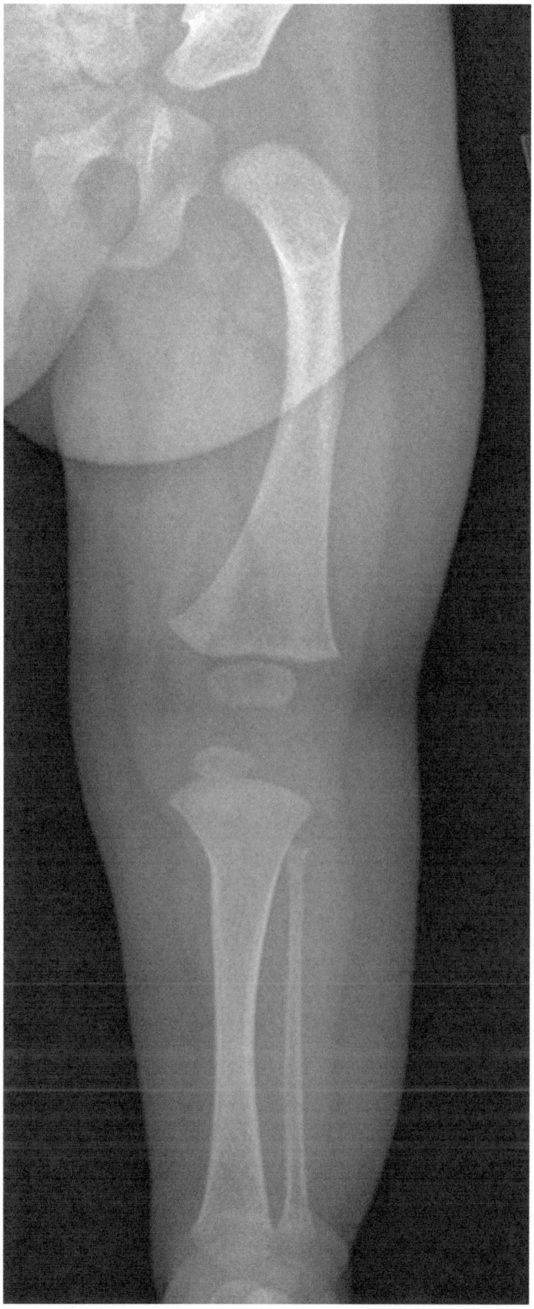

Fig. 13.48 Mild proximal femoral focal deficiency (PFFD) with fibular hypoplasia in a 7-month-old boy. The femur is short and slightly bowed, and ossification of the femoral head is delayed. The fibula is short and thin, indicating fibular longitudinal deficiency

from splitting of the mesenchymal or cartilaginous anlage with partial failure of proximal induction. Tibial longitudinal deficiency is always associated, and there is often ectrodactyly (congenital absence of all or part of a digit). The combination of femoral bifurcation and tibial longitudinal deficiency without ectrodactyly constitutes Gollop-Wolfgang complex [32].

In femoral bifurcation, the upper femur is relatively normal, with a single femoral head, acetabulum, and femoral neck. The extra, bifurcated segment extends anteriorly or medially, in a different plane than the normal axis of the extremity, and it usually has its own distal epiphysis. The less abnormal portion of the bifurcation may have an epiphysis as well, but although it may be near the fibula, the bones do not articulate.

Resection of the anteromedial limb treats femoral bifurcation. The accompanying tibial longitudinal deficiency must also be addressed.

3.4 Tibial Longitudinal Deficiency (Hemimelia)

Tibial longitudinal deficiency is a rare congenital abnormality that occurs in approximately one per one million live births, making it less common than fibular longitudinal deficiency. An autosomal dominant inheritance pattern is often present, and the condition is bilateral in about 30 %. The most severe cases, in which there is no ossified tibia, are termed complete longitudinal deficiency. In tibial dysplasia, a varying extent of the distal tibia is absent. If involvement is severe, the leg is short at birth, atrophic, flexed, and unstable at the knee. While the foot can be normal, aplasia or polydactyly is often present, and the foot is commonly in an equinovarus and adducted position. Claw hand and developmental dysplasia of the hip are often associated. Some cases also exhibit polydactyly in the hand or foot as well as tarsal coalition.

Older classification schemes are based on the presence of tibial aplasia/hypoplasia and on the status of the femoral epiphysis and ankle [33, 34]. A newer classification scheme considers the degree of abnormality of the tibia as well as presence of a cartilage anlage and the status of muscle function [35].

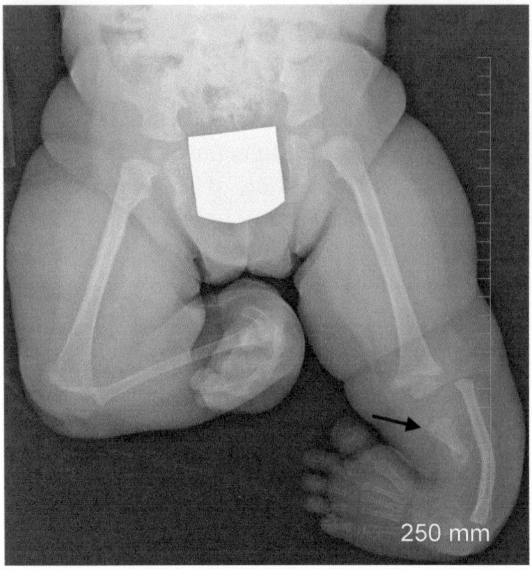

Fig. 13.49 Bilateral tibial longitudinal deficiency. There is complete right tibial longitudinal deficiency and partial left tibial longitudinal deficiency, with only a very small proximal left tibia present (*arrow*). The fibulas are flat and rib-like. Articulation at both knees, ankles, and feet is markedly abnormal (Courtesy of Rebecca Stein-Wexler)

Treatment aims to create a weight-bearing lower extremity. This is most often accomplished through amputation and prosthesis fitting. The nature of the surgical procedure depends heavily on how the deficiency is classified.

Imaging

With complete longitudinal deficiency, radiographs reveal an absent tibia (Fig. 13.49). The fibula is flat and resembles a rib. Alignment at the knee depends on the presence of the proximal portion of the tibia. Provided there is an ossified or cartilaginous proximal tibia, the fibula will initially be well aligned with respect to the femur, although varus deformity develops as the child grows. However, if the tibia is completely absent, the fibula will migrate proximal to the distal femur, and there will be no normal articulation at the knee. The distal femur is hypoplastic.

Possible variants include a hypoplastic tibia (Fig. 13.50), a proximal fragment articulating at the knee, bifocal aplasia with proximal and distal diminution, or the extremely rare distal fragment articulating at the ankle. Congenital distal diastasis is also considered a variant. The presence of a distal femoral condyle does not necessarily imply an extant cartilaginous tibial structure. MRI (US in infancy) best evaluates the cartilaginous elements. These modalities also depict anomalous arteries and muscles (most commonly an anomalous distal insertion of the quadriceps muscle).

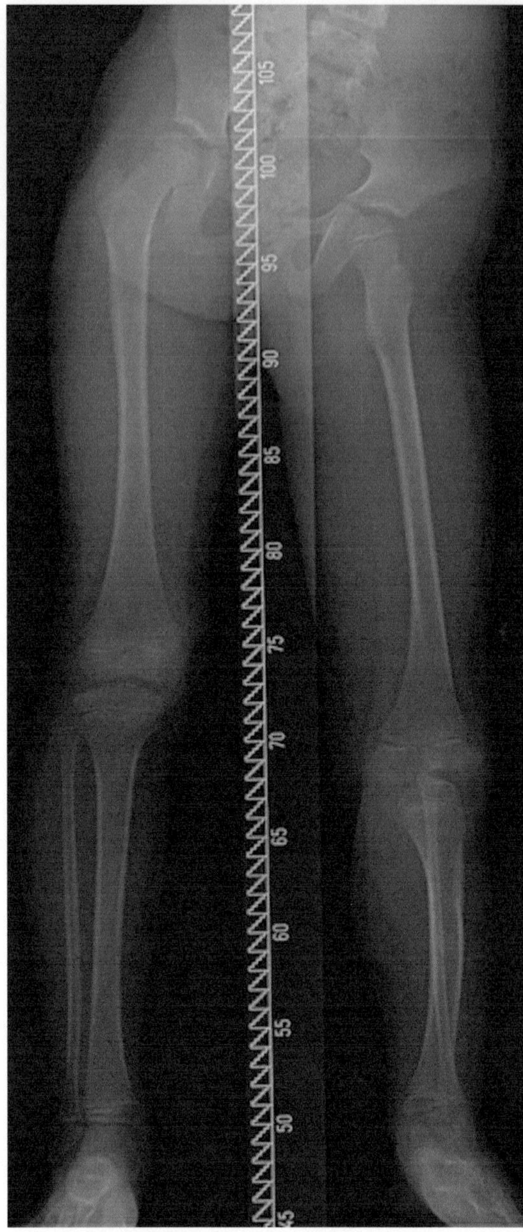

Fig. 13.50 Tibial longitudinal deficiency on the left in a 6-year-old boy with severe leg-length discrepancy. The left fibula is significantly longer than the tibia

3.5 Fibular Longitudinal Deficiency (Hemimelia) (Box 13.1)

Box 13.1: Fibular Longitudinal Deficiency

Much more common than tibial longitudinal deficiency

Normal levels	Superior proximal fibular epiphysis
	Normally at level of proximal tibial physis
	Distal fibular physis
	Normally at level of talar dome
Complete absence	Fibrous remnant may cause tibia to bow anterior/medial
	Tibia articulates with femur
	Absent lateral rays of foot
Partial absence	Thin, deformed fibula

Longitudinal deficiency of the fibula is the most common congenital longitudinal deficiency of the extremities, occurring in up to 20 per million live births [36]. It is caused by a defect in the fibular developmental field. The deformity usually occurs in isolation and ranges in severity from mild hypoplasia to complete absence of the fibula. It is strongly associated with other abnormalities of the fibular developmental field, most commonly PFFD (see Fig. 13.48). Other relatively common associated malformations include, coxa vara, clubfoot, and absent lateral foot structures [37]. The defect can be described as a postaxial or longitudinal fibular deficiency, either terminal (if there is an associated deficiency in the foot) or intercalary (if the foot is normal).

A completely absent fibula falls into the continuum of complete longitudinal deficiency of the limb. The incidence of femoral anomalies is greater with fibular hypoplasia than with complete aplasia.

If there is major deficiency below the knee, the diagnosis is obvious at birth. The femur may be slightly short as well, or there may be accompanying PFFD. Total initial leg-length discrepancy averages 19 %, with the tibia usually contributing 25 % and the femur 13 %; this discrepancy increases with growth [38]. Since the percent difference in length will be constant as the child grows, it is possible to predict the magnitude of eventual leg-length discrepancy, even in the young child.

In 60 % of patients with apparent complete absence of the fibula, a tight fibrous or sometimes cartilaginous band can be palpated, running from the posterior aspect of the proximal tibia to the calcaneus. This fibular anlage likely contributes to tibial bowing. Eighty percent of such bowing is apex-anterior, and one-third also bows with apex medial. The apex is at the junction of the medial and distal thirds of the tibia and usually exceeds 30°. In about 50 % of patients, a skin dimple overlies the apex. Normal weight-bearing during development usually rectifies bowing.

Foot abnormalities are common, especially severe equinovalgus. Between one and three of the lateral rays may be absent; the most lateral ray will have the muscle attachments of a normal fifth toe. The correlation between severity of abnormalities in the leg with those in the foot is uncertain. Some investigators have found that severe femoral shortening and leg-length discrepancy are often associated with a normal foot [39], whereas other have found a poor correlation between leg shortening, tibial bowing, and the condition of the foot [40].

Longitudinal deficiency of the fibula has been categorized according to the extent of radiographic preservation of the fibula [36], but categorization based on the magnitude of limb shortening and the condition of the foot assists with planning appropriate limb salvage treatment [41]. Accordingly, type 1 fibular longitudinal deficiency has a foot with at least three rays that can provide a stable base for ambulation; this is further subdivided according to the extent of limb-length discrepancy. With type 2 fibular longitudinal deficiency, the foot cannot be salvaged. Type 2 deficiency is then subcategorized according to whether there is an upper extremity deficiency as well, in which case the foot may be required to perform the functions of a hand.

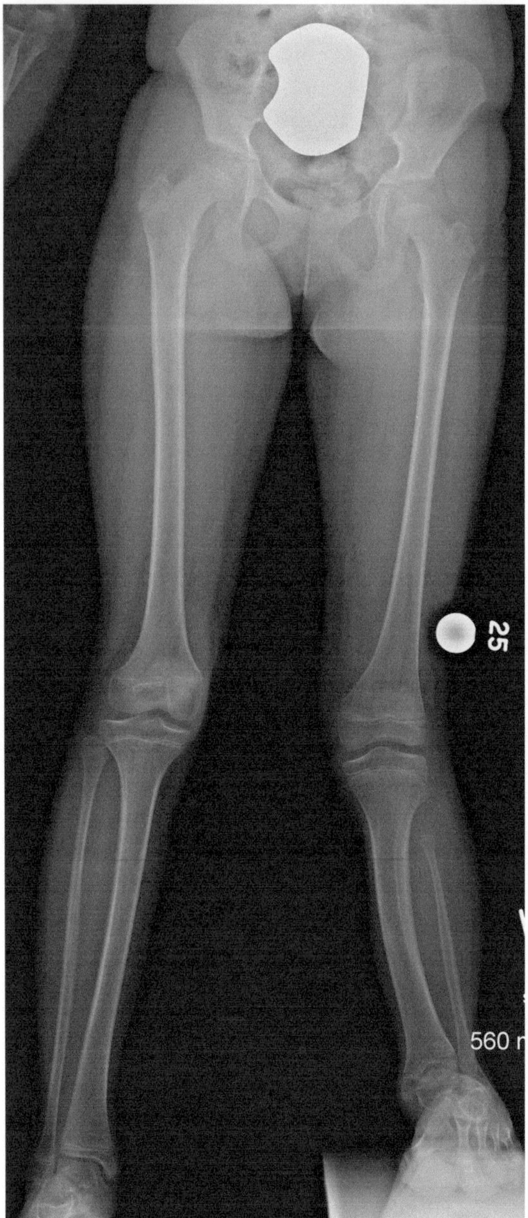

Fig. 13.51 Longitudinal deficiency of the fibula with hypoplastic tibia. The tibia is bowed medially, and there is sclerosis along the lateral concavity (Courtesy of Rebecca Stein-Wexler)

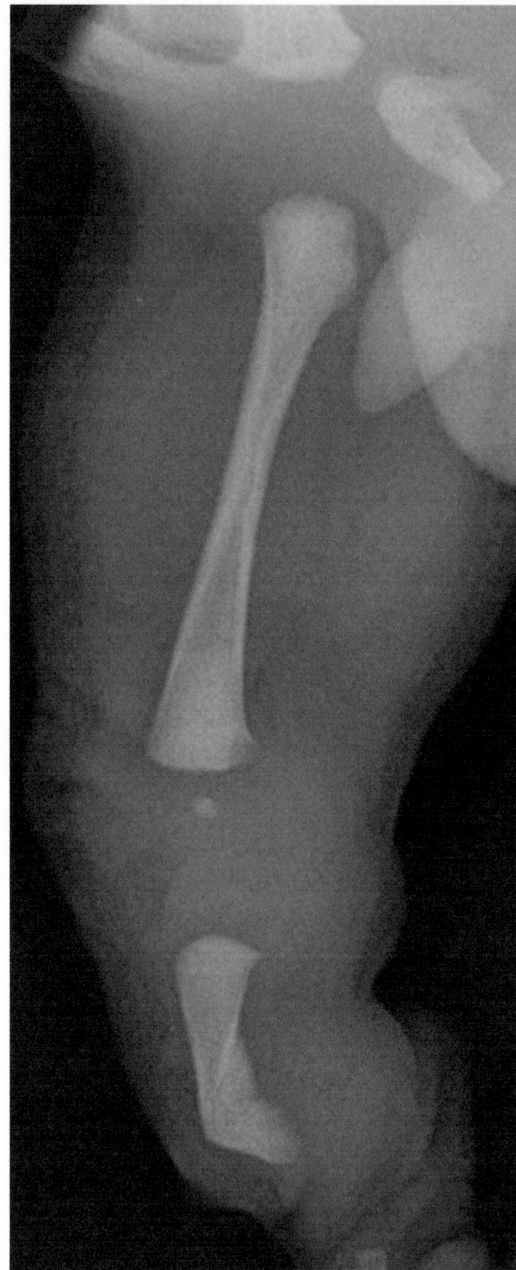

Fig. 13.52 Longitudinal deficiency of the fibula with aplastic fibula and a short, dysplastic tibia

Treatment attempts to establish a functional weight-bearing extremity without leg-length discrepancy, and the approach thus depends on the extent of disease. Procedures range from guided growth procedures to correct leg-length discrepancy to full amputation with prosthesis [37].

Imaging

Longitudinal deficiency of the fibula is characterized by a deficient (Fig. 13.51) or absent (Figs. 13.52 and 13.53) fibula. If there is no ossified fibula, the diagnosis is obvious. The tibia may be bowed anteriorly or medially, with

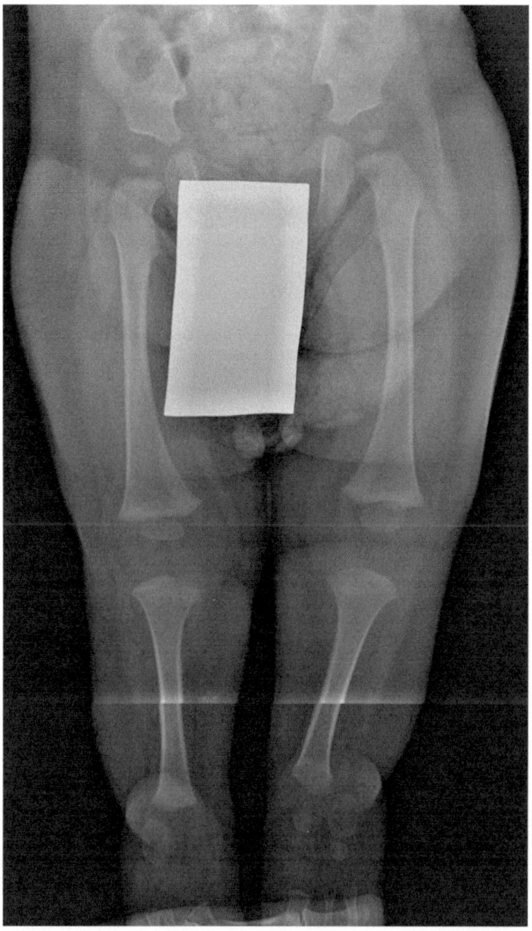

Fig. 13.53 Bilateral fibular hemimelia. The femurs are aplastic and the tibias hypoplastic. Each foot has only three rays, but tarsal development is asymmetric, more impaired on the right (Courtesy of Rebecca Stein-Wexler)

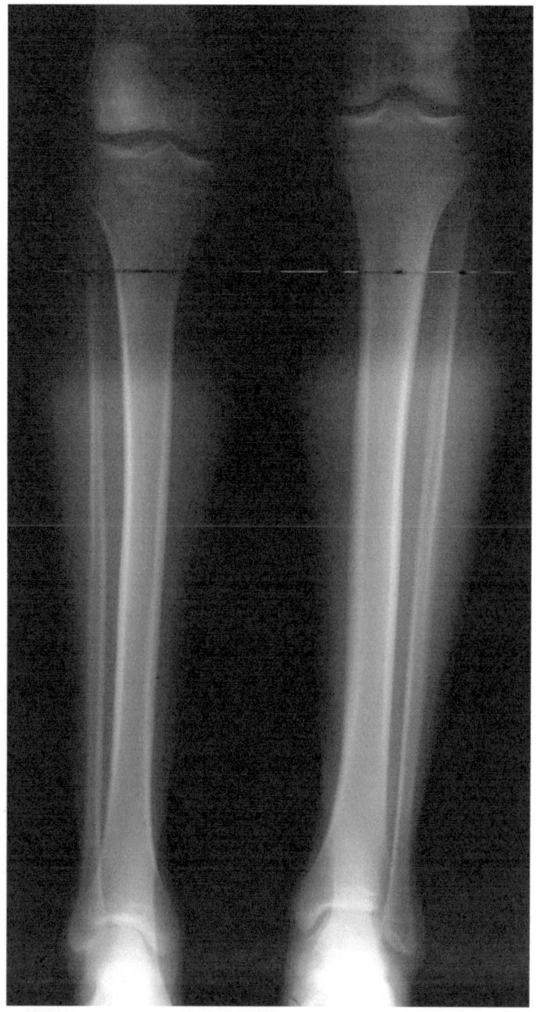

Fig. 13.54 Subtle fibular hemimelia in a 19-year-old male. The right fibula is slightly smaller than the left, and its distal fused physis is above the talar dome. Ball-and-socket ankle joint (Courtesy of Tal Laor, Cincinnati Children's Hospital)

cortical sclerosis along the concave side. The epiphyses may be small. The tibia articulates somewhat normally with the femur, but the cruciate ligaments are usually deficient, and the knee therefore potentially unstable. The tibial eminence may be flat, and the lateral condyle of the femur hypoplastic.

In some cases of fibular hypoplasia, the medullary canal is thin and the fibula obviously deformed. However, fibular hypoplasia may be clinically significant yet radiographically subtle (Fig. 13.54). It should be recognized if one is aware of and assesses the normal relationship of the fibula to surrounding structures. The superior edge of the proximal fibular epiphysis should be at the level of the proximal tibial growth plate, and the normal distal fibular growth plate should be at the level of the talar dome. Other anomalies such as aberrant vasculature, absent cruciate ligaments, or absent/malformed menisci will be recognized only on MRI, although flattening of the tibial eminence suggests deficiency of the cruciate ligaments. MRI may also identify a fibrous or cartilaginous anlage.

The lateral toes are commonly absent, but although this obvious deformity may lead to the diagnosis of fibular longitudinal deficiency, this finding alone has little clinical consequence. Ossification of rays may be delayed up to approximately age 5. Tarsal coalition is not uncommon, usually either talocalcaneal or talonavicular, although occasionally calcaneocuboid coalition occurs; it may be suggested by presence of a ball-and-socket ankle. The pelvis and hips should be assessed for PFFD and other hip abnormalities. MRI, or US in infancy, can help evaluate associated soft tissue deficiencies. Equinovalgus is common [42].

Fibular longitudinal deficiency and tibial longitudinal deficiency may be difficult to differentiate if a single abnormal-appearing bone is present. In tibial longitudinal deficiency, the fibula has normal curvature and does not articulate with the femur at the knee. In tibial longitudinal deficiency, the bone articulates with the femur at the knee. The foot is likely to show equinovarus alignment, whereas equinovalgus is common with fibular longitudinal deficiency.

4 Bowing and Other Malalignment

4.1 General Considerations

Bowing of the lower extremities is relatively common. This can represent a normal developmental phenomenon, and it is critical to differentiate physiological from pathological bowing. Bowing occurs at joints (e.g., genu varum) and within bones (e.g., tibial bowing). Proximal bowing can affect distal alignment, as in tibial torsion and intoeing. Convention dictates that bowing is described based on the direction of curve of the convex side of the bone, at the apex. Thus, a curved bone whose apex is convex posteriorly is described as "bowed posteriorly." Genu valgum (knock knees) and genu varum (bow legs) describe the angle the tibia makes in relation to the femur; these terms do not refer to intrinsic bowing of the individual bones.

4.2 Congenital Tibial and Fibular Bowing (Box 13.2)

Box 13.2: Congenital Tibial Bowing

Posteromedial	Often due to intrauterine position
	Spontaneous resolution with growth
	May be associated with limb-length discrepancy
Anterolateral	Likely to remodel if normal medullary canal (very rare)
	May lead to fracture/pseudarthrosis
	Narrow canal, cortical sclerosis
	Possible cystic changes with expansion
	Narrow diameter at angulation

Tibial bowing in the neonate may be unilateral or bilateral and is almost always associated with fibular bowing. It may be isolated or associated with other skeletal anomalies. Tibial bowing may follow a benign course with spontaneous resolution, result in significant leg-length discrepancy, or progress to fracture, often with subsequent pseudarthrosis.

Posteromedial bowing usually results from intrauterine positioning. However, the condition may alternatively be caused by localized skeletal dysplasia, fetal neurovascular insufficiency, or primordial cartilage abnormality. Anterolateral bowing may result from positional deformation as well, but it is often associated with such systemic conditions as neurofibromatosis, fibrous dysplasia, osteogenesis imperfecta, hypophosphatasia, thanatophoric dwarfism, and campomelic dwarfism. Furthermore, tibial bowing may accompany hypoplasia of the limb, soft tissue and bony hyperplasia, local gigantism, and syndactyly.

Isolated Tibial and Fibular Bowing

Posteromedial bowing due to intrauterine positioning (Fig. 13.55) is more common on the

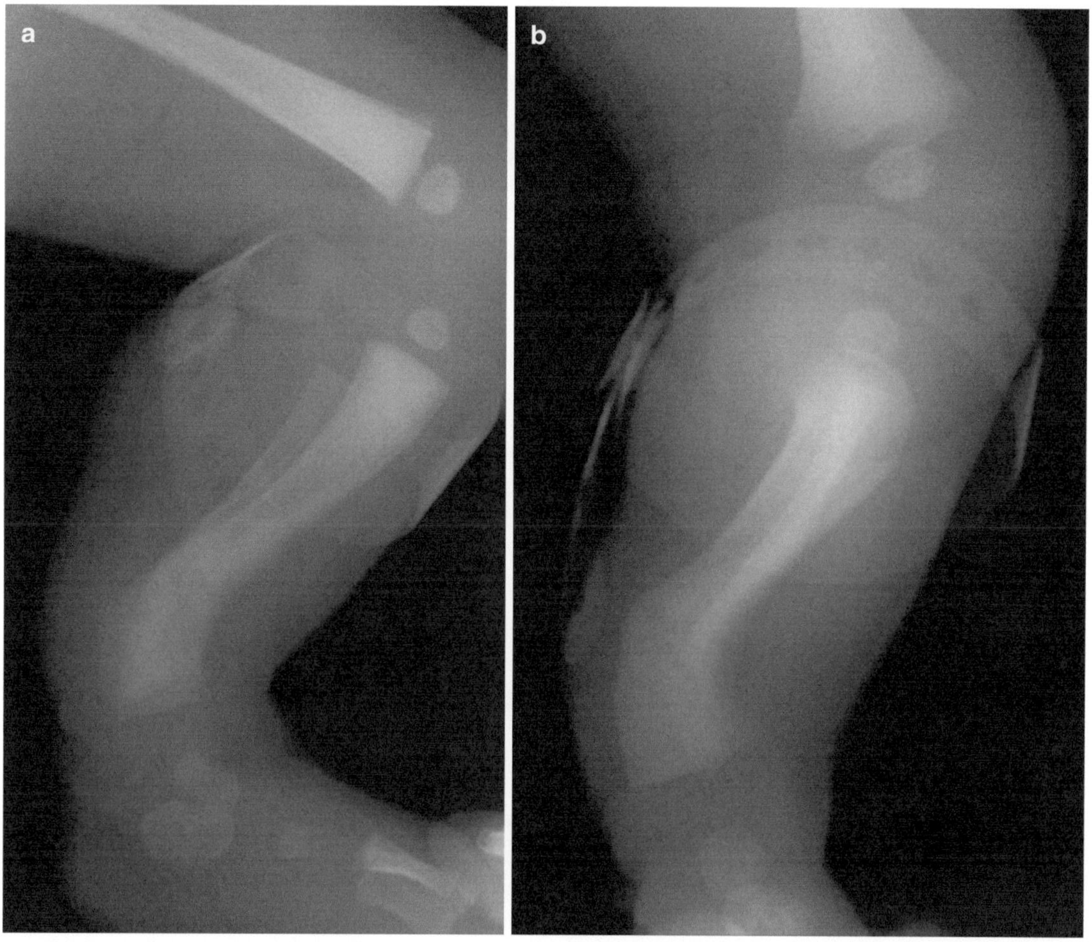

Fig. 13.55 Posteromedial bowing of the tibia and fibula in newborn secondary to intrauterine positioning (**a**, **b**)

right and in females. It is often unilateral but may occur bilaterally. Calcaneovalgus foot deformity is commonly associated. If the infant is examined shortly after birth while still folded in the fetal position, it is readily apparent how the extremities can press against and deform each other. Bone may respond by thickening on the concave side of the curve, and pressure from the uterine wall against the convex side of the limb may cause the skin to thin and dimple. Cortical thickening and sclerosis occur along the concavity, and the diaphysis may be broad.

Anterior tibial bowing may also have a medial or lateral component. If the width of the medullary canal is normal (Fig. 13.56), the prognosis for remodeling is good. However, if bowing is severe, residual deformity may persist into adulthood. Fracture of a bowed but otherwise normal bone is uncommon, and healing progresses normally.

The prognosis is worse when anterior tibial bowing is associated with a narrowed medullary canal, extensive cortical sclerosis, cystic change, or decreased tibial diameter at the point of maximum angulation (Fig. 13.57). Fractures are common and often unite incompletely, ultimately resulting in pseudarthrosis. Some of these cases may be the first indicator of the presence of underlying neurofibromatosis. Anterior tibial bowing is often seen with fibular longitudinal deficiency (see Fig. 13.52).

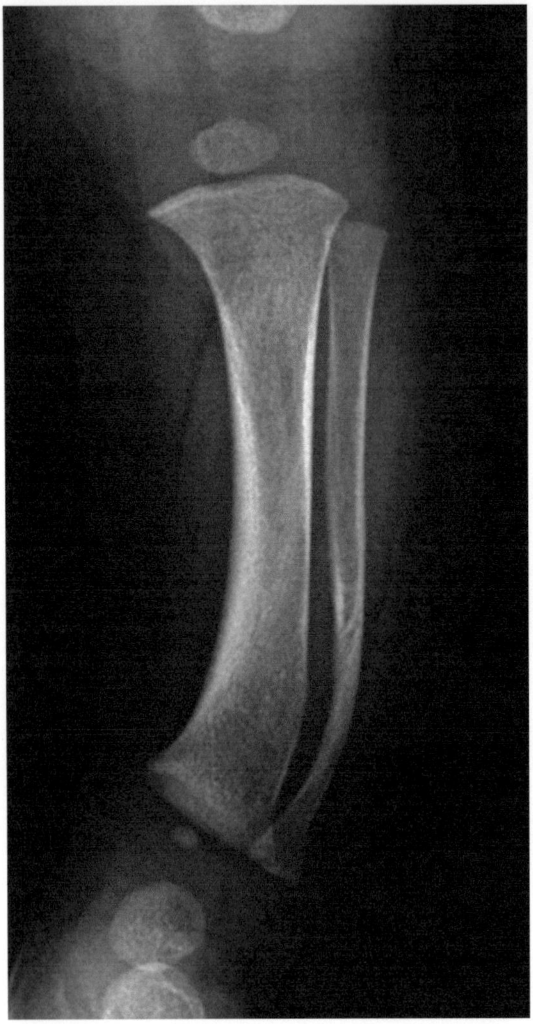

Fig. 13.56 Congenital anterolateral tibial bowing in a 5-month-old boy due to intrauterine packing abnormality. The cortex is thickened along the concave side, but the medullary canal of the tibia is not narrowed, and there is no bony lesion

Tibial Bowing Associated with Systemic Disorders

Tibial bowing is characteristic of several systemic diseases and congenital syndromes, of which neurofibromatosis type 1 (NF1) is the most common (Figs. 13.58 and 13.59) (see Chap. 23). Fracture and nonunion commonly (though not always) follow, and thus this form of bowing is usually considered in the spectrum of infantile pseudarthrosis. The tibial bowing is typically anterolateral, and the junction between the distal and middle thirds is most severely affected.

In osteogenesis imperfecta, the bowing results from intrauterine or postnatal bone softening, fracture, and subsequent deformity (Fig. 13.60). The diagnosis should be readily apparent, with healing or healed fractures elsewhere along with multiple cranial sutural bones (see Chap. 23).

In rickets, tibial bowing is associated with osteomalacia as well as characteristic metaphyseal flaring and fraying (see below). Secondary growth plate closure may exacerbate the deformity. Bowing is also seen in thanatophoric dysplasia and campomelic dysplasia (Fig. 13.61), both short-limbed dwarfisms.

Bowing may also result from local pathology in fibrous dysplasia, osteofibrous dysplasia (see Chap. 21), familial expansile osteolysis, and other conditions.

4.3 Congenital Pseudarthrosis of the Tibia (Tibial Dysplasia)

Congenital pseudarthrosis of the tibia generally develops from preexisting anterior tibial bowing and is not truly congenital. Fracture and pseudarthrosis may also occur in the fibula and are occasionally limited to that bone.

The deformity occurs in one per 140,000–190,000 neonates [43]. Approximately half of the patients with this disorder have NF1, and up to 11 % of patients with NF1 have tibial pseudarthrosis. Tibial pseudarthrosis may indeed be the initial manifestation of this condition. (See Chap. 23 for further discussion of NF1.) The pseudarthrosis is usually detected before age 2 years, with half of all cases becoming apparent before age 1. However, patients may present as late as age 12.

The cause of fracture and pseudarthrosis is uncertain. While the hamartomatous proliferation of fibrous tissue found in the pseudarthrosis is similar histologically to that of plexiform neurofibroma, schwannoma, and fibrous dysplasia, neurofibromas are not found at the point of fracture [44].

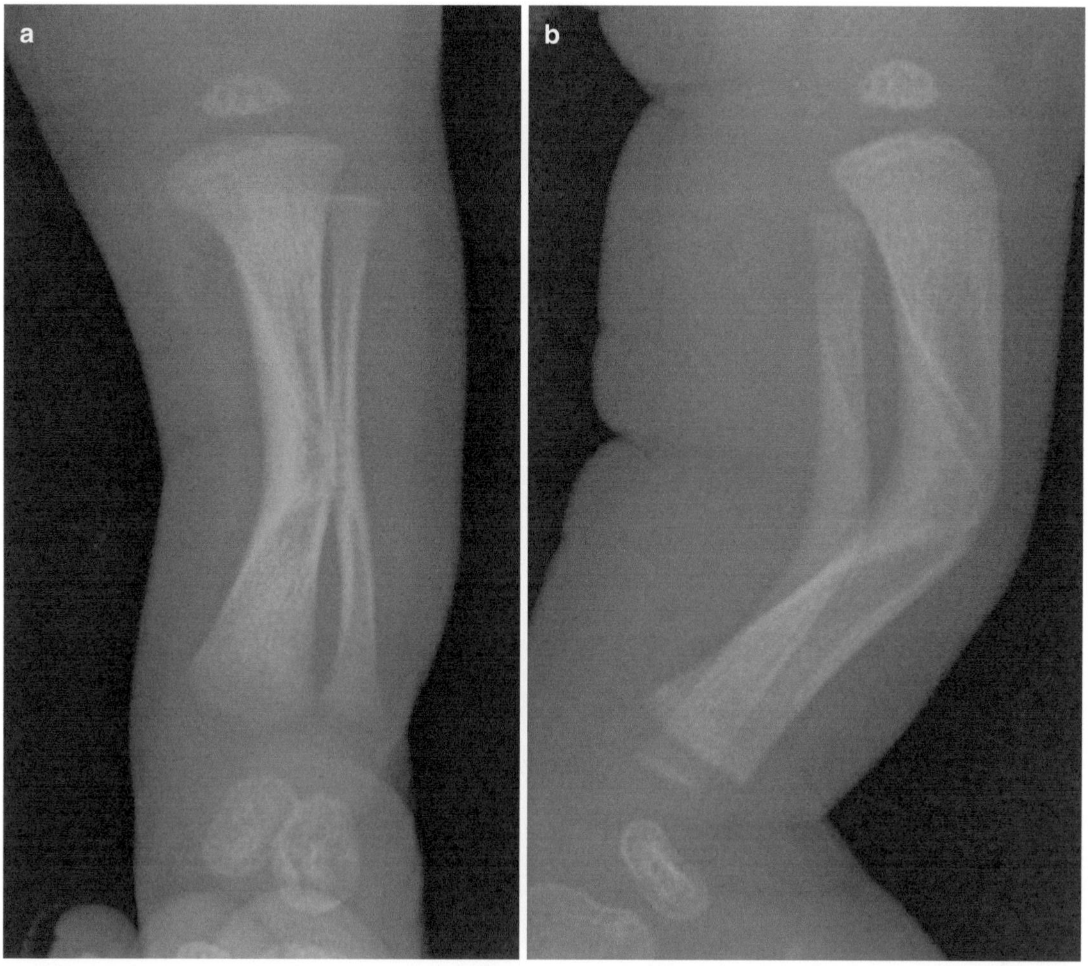

Fig. 13.57 Anterolateral bowing of the tibia and fibula in a 2-week-old boy. (**a**, **b**) There is striking sclerosis where angulation is most pronounced. The medullary canal is narrow, and there are subtle cortical lucencies, increasing the risk of fracture and pseudarthrosis

Treatment of tibial pseudarthrosis is challenging, especially if the goal is not just osseous union but a stable, weight-bearing extremity. Protective bracing is recommended at diagnosis. Treatment options include simple immobilization, internal fixation with intramedullary nails, external Ilizarov fixation, and vascularized free fibular bone grafting. None of these options is invariably successful and each has associated complications. The chance for union after grafting is independent of the presence of underlying neurofibromatosis. Using recombinant human bone morphogenic protein to aid healing at the bone graft site may help ameliorate some complications [45].

Surgery is more successful when the thick periostial cuff at the pseudarthrosis site is completely resected. Amputation is an option if multiple surgical attempts fail [44] and may be offered as primary treatment for severe cases (e.g., pseudarthrosis that develops before age two and that deforms the distal one-third of the tibia and fibula [46]). Significant numbers of patients whose radiographs demonstrate osseous union after surgical repair nevertheless require bracing in order to ambulate [46].

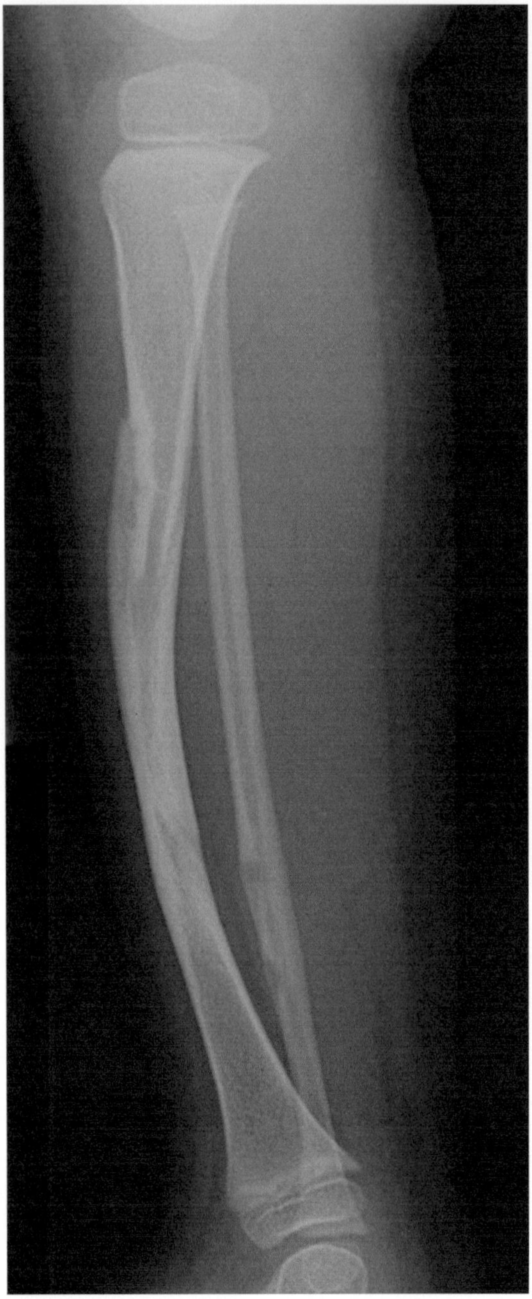

Fig. 13.58 Anterolateral tibial bowing in a 4-year-old boy with neurofibromatosis type 1 (NF1). The medullary canal is narrowed, and there is sclerosis and cortical thickening at the mid-tibia. Although the fibula is not bowed, there is focal lucency within its sclerotic cortex

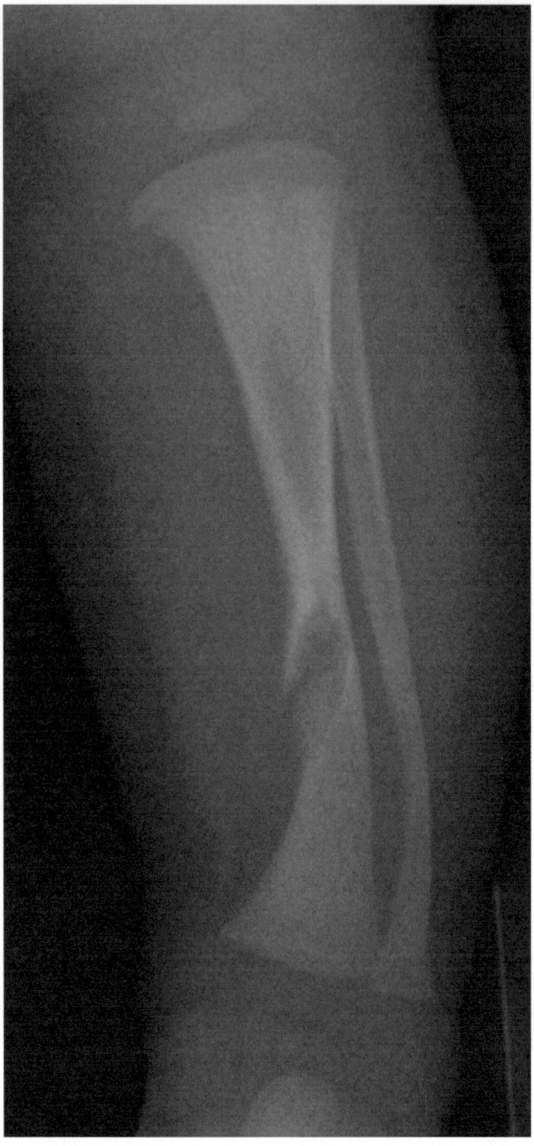

Fig. 13.59 Pathological fracture in a 3-week-old with NF1, which occurred during diaper change. The fracture traverses a lucent lesion that occupies most of the width of the tibia, and the medullary canal just above this area is tapered and sclerotic. Lateral tibial and fibular bowing

Imaging

Several radiographic findings suggest that a bowed tibia or fibula may fracture and eventually develop pseudarthrosis: regional sclerosis at the point of greatest angulation (Fig. 13.62), narrowing of the medullary canal (see Fig. 13.57), narrowing of the shaft into an hourglass shape, cystic change in the medulla or cortex of the bone (see Fig. 13.59), or clinical evidence of neurofibromatosis. However, bowed

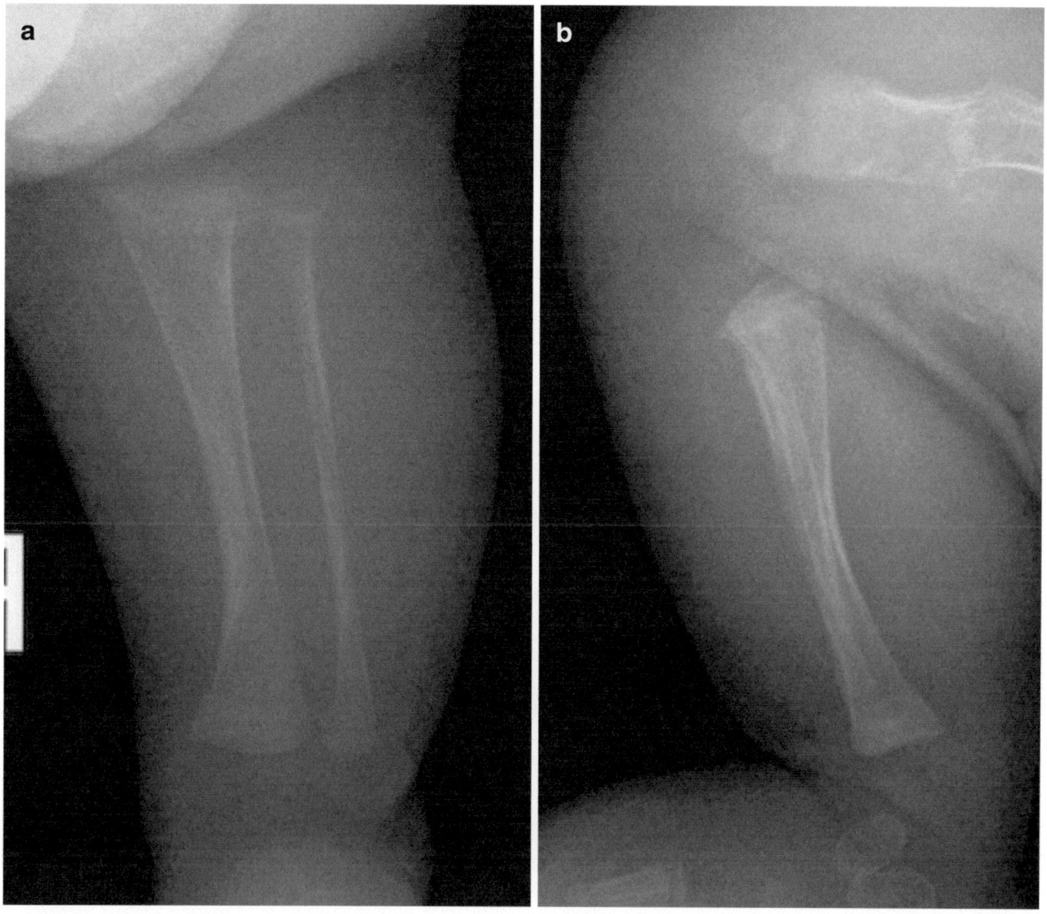

Fig. 13.60 Lateral tibial and fibular bowing in an infant with osteogenesis imperfecta. (**a**, **b**) The tibia and fibula are thin and osteopenic. There are fractures of the proximal and distal tibial metaphyses and of the distal femur

tibias that appear otherwise normal can fracture, and neurofibromatosis may affect a normal appearing bone.

The tibia generally demonstrates a chronic-appearing transverse defect with smooth, sclerotic margins, similar to chronic nonunion in a long bone fracture. Serial examination will demonstrate no callous formation or other evidence of healing. The fibula may also fracture.

MRI is generally unnecessary but demonstrates the pseudarthrosis as a linear area of decreased signal intensity at both T1- and T2-W sequences (Fig. 13.63). The dysplastic tibia may appear hypointense on T1- and hyperintense on T2-W sequences. Thickened periosteum may be intact across the pseudarthrosis.

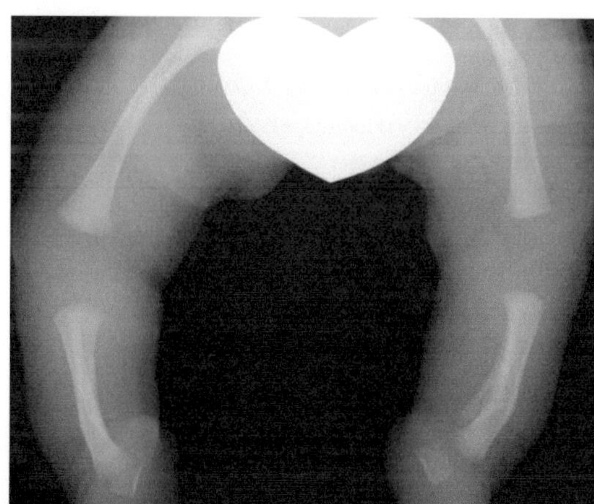

Fig. 13.61 Newborn with campomelic dysplasia. Apex anterior tibial bowing as well as femoral bowing. Delayed ossification of the epiphyses at the distal femurs and proximal tibias (Courtesy of Sandra L. Wootton-Gorges)

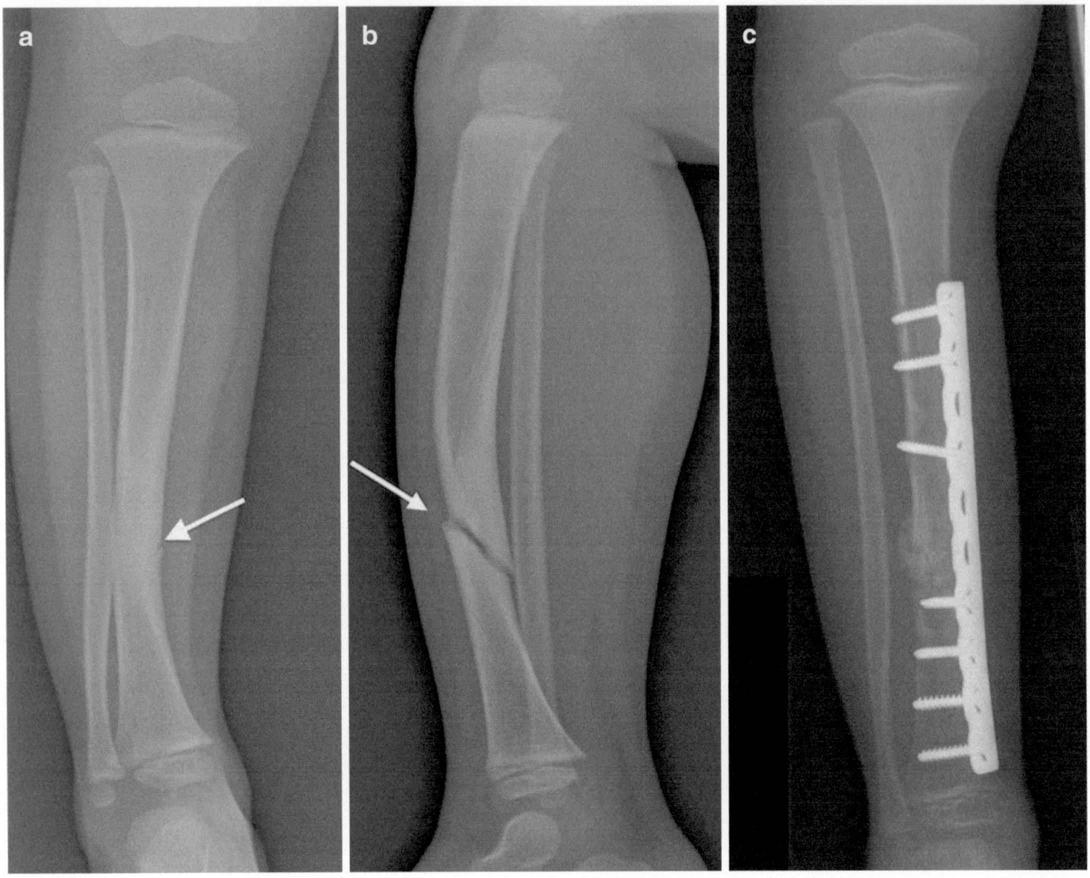

Fig. 13.62 Congenital tibial dysplasia with chronic pseudarthrosis in a 3-year-old boy with underlying anterolateral tibial bowing. (**a**, **b**) The tibial diaphysis is sclerotic, as are the margins of the pseudarthrosis (*arrows*). (**c**) After multiple attempts at casting failed, surgical fixation was required

4.4 Congenital Dislocation and Hyperextension of the Knee

Neonatal hyperextension at the knee may be associated with tibial dislocation, which is usually anterior. Segments may override, resulting in shortening of the affected extremity. Dislocation or hyperextension at the knee is much less common than developmental dysplasia of the hip, occurring in only approximately 1 in 100,000 live births. It is associated with female gender (girls affected three to four times more often than boys), breech presentation, oligohydramnios, and ligamentous laxity. Rarely occurring in isolation, its presence suggests Larsen syndrome, arthrogryposis (present in two-third), or another congenital abnormality. Etiology has not been established.

The knee is hyperextended at birth (genu recurvatum), with transverse skin folds anterior to the point of hyperextension. The femoral condyles are prominent posteriorly. Congenital snapping knee may be associated with recurrent anterior tibial subluxation. Approximately 50 % of patients also have hip dislocation, and 10 % have elbow dislocation. Calcaneovalgus or clubfoot deformity occurs in almost one-third.

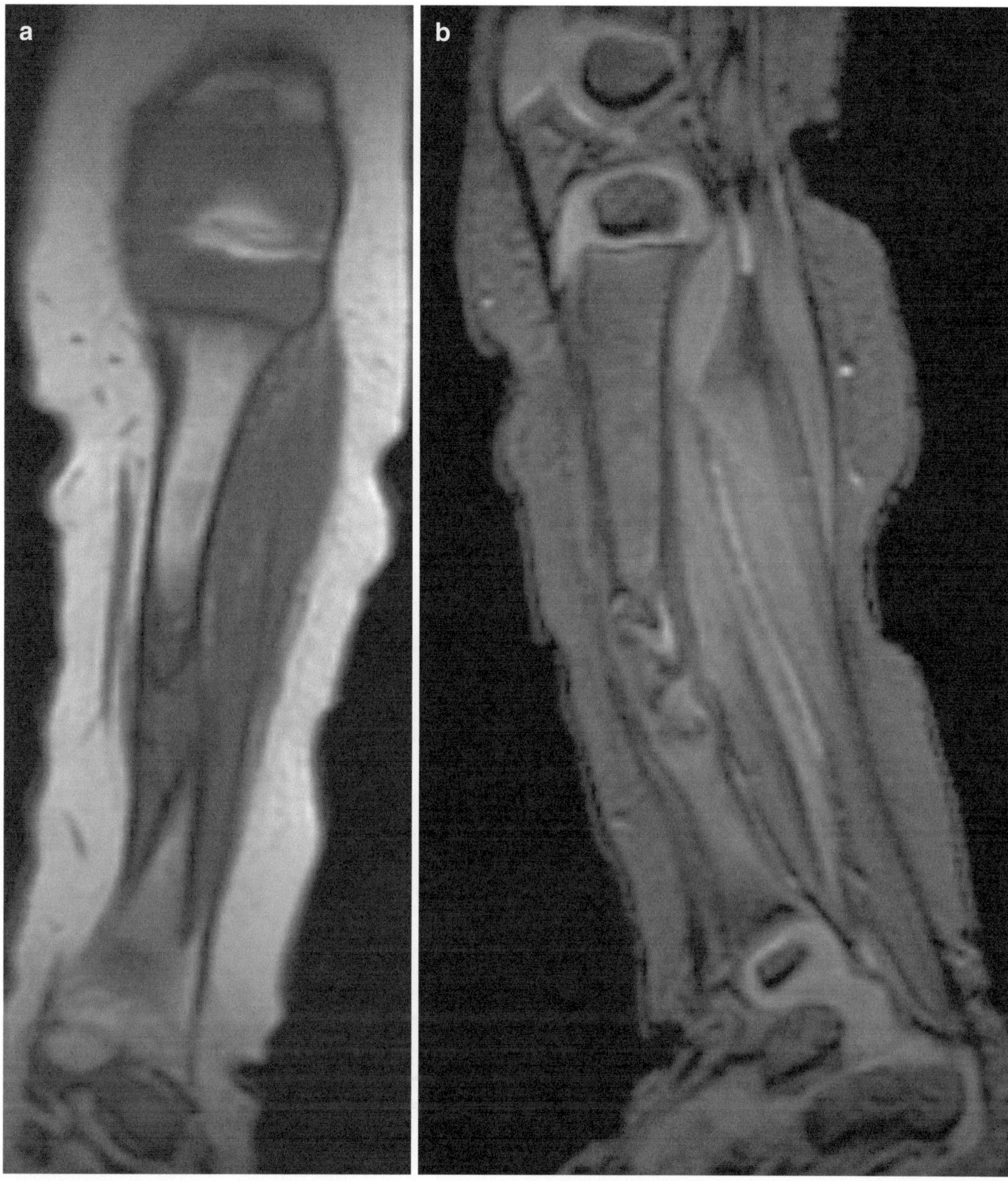

Fig. 13.63 Pseudarthrosis of the distal tibia in an 18-month-old girl. (**a**) T1-W coronal MRI shows the dysplastic portion of the tibia is isointense to muscle, and the pseudarthrosis appears as a linear area of more intense hypointensity. (**b**) Sagittal multiplanar gradient-recalled (MPGR) sequence shows the periosteum is intact and delineates the hypointense pseudarthrosis along with hyperintensity in the surrounding dysplastic bone (Courtesy of Tal Laor, Cincinnati Children's Hospital)

The quadriceps muscles are often short and fibrotic, especially laterally. A scarred suprapatellar pouch may bind these muscles to the femur. The hamstrings are positioned relatively anteriorly. The patella is usually laterally displaced, but it may be absent. The posterior capsule is redundant, and the cruciate ligaments may be absent, hypoplastic, or elongated [47].

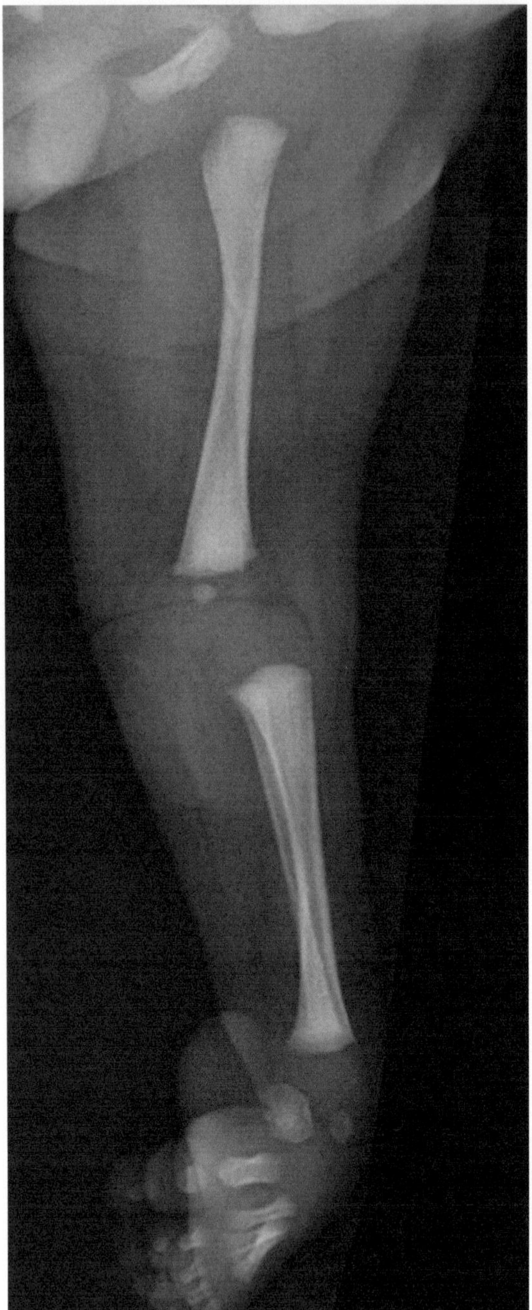

Fig. 13.64 Congenital dislocation of the knee in a newborn. The tibia is anterior and overlaps the fibula. Note clubfoot deformity

Treatment of congenital dislocation and hyperextension of the knee depends on its severity and ranges from stretching and bracing to closed reduction to more invasive surgery [48].

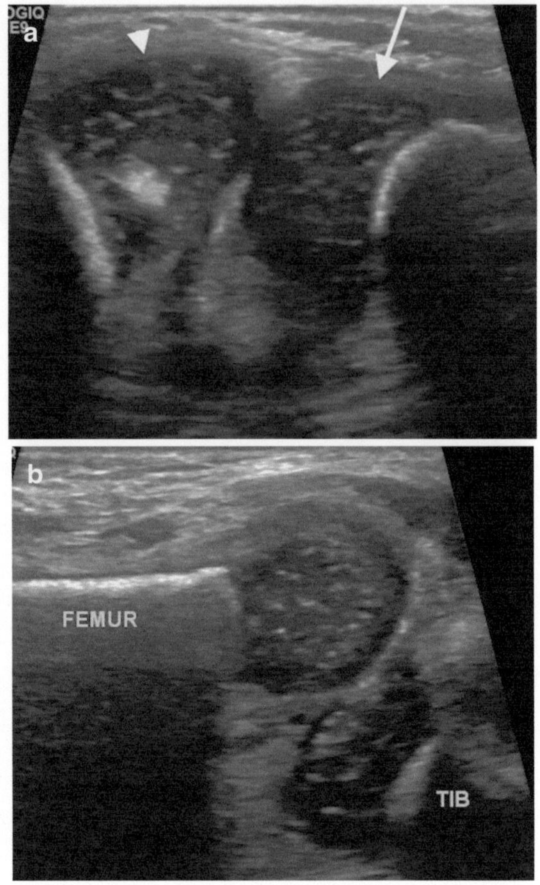

Fig. 13.65 Absent patella and anteriorly dislocated tibia in a newborn. Sagittal US images of both knees, scanned from posterior approach. (**a**) Normal left knee (for comparison) shows normal alignment of the femoral (*arrowhead*) and tibial (*arrow*) epiphyses. (**b**) On the right, the anteriorly dislocated tibia overlaps the distal femur. No patellar cartilage is evident on this image or elsewhere (Courtesy of Rebecca Stein-Wexler)

Imaging

In the infant, the tibia is usually hyperextended and either anteriorly subluxated or dislocated (Fig. 13.64). It may be in valgus alignment with respect to the femur. If the tibia is externally rotated, the fibula will appear superimposed over its lateral border. US readily delineates anatomy (Fig. 13.65). Arthrography or MRI may show flattening of cartilage, especially in the posterior tibial epiphysis, as well as obliteration of the suprapatellar pouch. During later childhood the posterior tibial plateau or anterior femur may become deformed (Fig. 13.66).

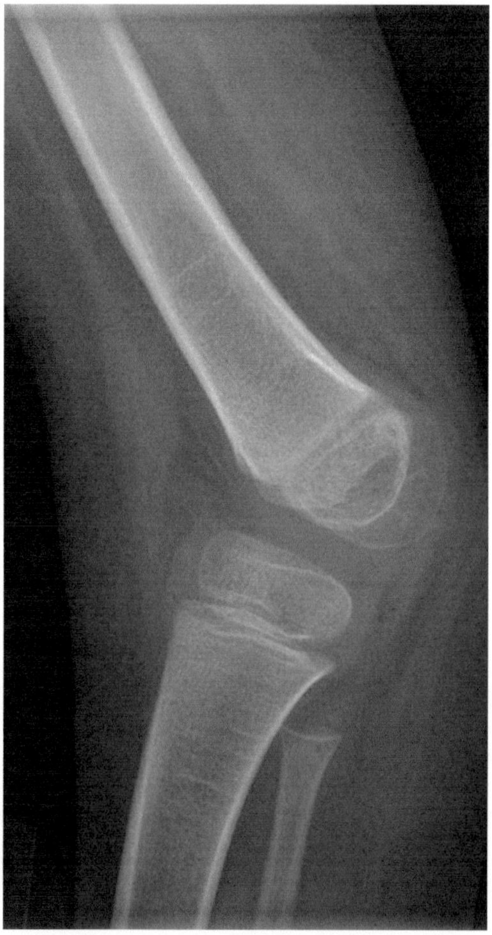

Fig. 13.66 Uncorrected congenital dislocation of the knee in a 5-year-old boy. The patella is absent, and there is genu recurvatum

4.5 Developmental Aberrant Alignment

Genu Varum

Physiological Bowing (Box 13.3)

Box 13.3: Physiological Bowing

Tibia/femur diaphyses: Bowed, apex lateral
  Tibia diaphysis: Medial cortical thickening
Distal femur/proximal tibia:
  Metaphyses: Prominent medial and posterior margins
    Beaks adjacent to growth plate
  Epiphyses: Wedge shaped
Distal tibial growth plate angled

During infancy, physiological bowing is the most common reason for lower extremity bowing. If patient age and physical examination are characteristic—and if nutritional or familial hypophosphatemic rickets, metaphyseal chondrodysplasia, osteogenesis imperfecta, neurofibromatosis, trauma, and congenital tibial bowing are excluded—extensive radiographic workup is unnecessary. Genetics appears to affect likelihood of tibiofemoral bowing, which is both more common and more pronounced in African-American children.

Prominent lateral bowing in very early childhood usually results either from molding deformity due to intrauterine position or from delayed transition to valgus. In the latter case, varus peaks at 18 months to 2 years. These patients are at increased risk of developing tibia vara, or Blount disease.

Imaging (Table 13.2, Box 13.4)

The tibiofemoral angle determines the angle of varus (or valgus) at the knee. This angle is calculated from the intersection of lines drawn longitudinally along the midshafts of the neutrally positioned femur and tibia. Normal varus angulation during infancy is approximately 15–20° (Fig. 13.67). With walking and weight-bearing, this angulation changes to approximately 10° valgus during the second to third year of life, and

Table 13.2 Tibial bowing and rotation

Tibial bowing		
	Metaphyseal diaphyseal angle	Comment
Normal (to 30 m/o)	5° (apex lateral)	Range 0–11°
Infantile tibia vara	16° (apex lateral)	Range 8–22°
Equivocal (get follow-up)	8–11° (apex lateral)	
Tibial rotation		
Newborn	4° external	
6 m/o	6° external	
1 y/o	10° external	
10 y/o	14° external	
Adult	14–20° external	20° external with knee flexed 40° external with knee extended

y/o year old

Box 13.4: Tibiofemoral Alignment (Genu Varus/Valgus)

Normal infant	15–20°	Varus
Normal 2–3 years old	10°	Valgus
Normal mature	6°	Valgus
Genu valgum	>15–20°	Valgus

any varus after age 2 years is abnormal. At skeletal maturity, normal alignment is approximately 6° valgus [49].

Typical features of developmental bowing include the following (Fig. 13.68):

1. The tibia is adducted relative to the femur. Both bones are bowed outward. External rotation of the upper tibia and internal rotation of the malleoli may be present, indicating internal tibial torsion.
2. The margins of the medial and posterior tibial and femoral metaphyses are accentuated, and prominent osseous beaks form adjacent to the growth plate. On the lateral projection, the beaks appear as discrete lines encircling the metaphysis as they project slightly away from the growth plate. There is no fragmentation.
3. The medial cortices of the femur and tibia are initially relatively thick. However, if the legs straighten during growth, thickening usually resolves.
4. The distal femoral and proximal tibial epiphyses appear wedge shaped due to increased medial pressure that inhibits ossification.
5. There is often an associated valgus deformity at the ankle, which may be unmasked by correction of the deformity at the knee.

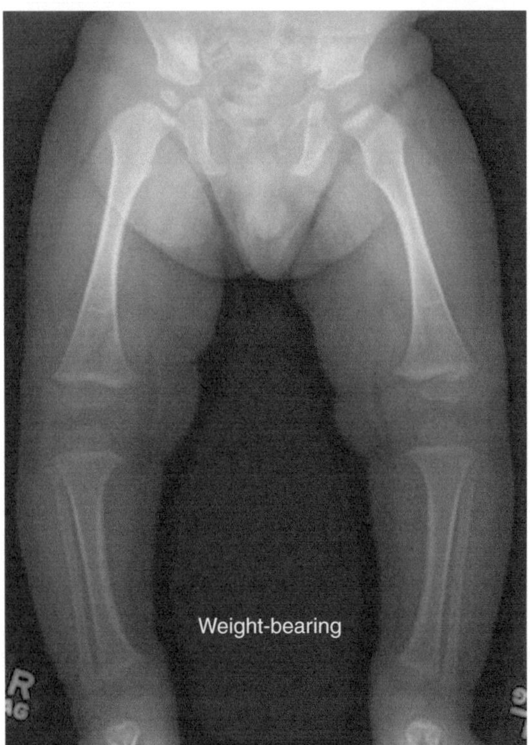

Fig. 13.67 Developmental bowing in a 1-year-old boy. Varus at the knee measures approximately 20°, well within normal range for this age

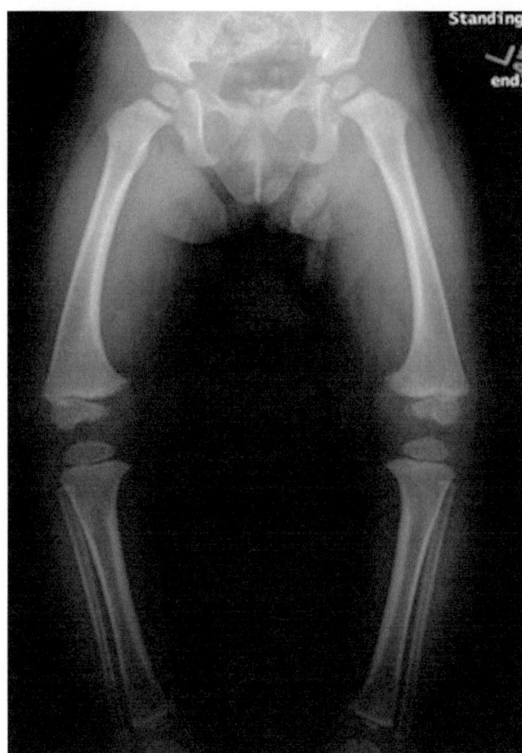

Fig. 13.68 Developmental physiologic bowing in an 18-month-old. The medial cortices of the femurs and tibias are thick, the tibias are adducted relative to the femurs, the epiphyses are *wedge shaped*, and there are prominent beaks at the medial aspect of the metaphyses

Pathological Bowing

Infantile Tibia Vara (Infantile Blount Disease) (Box 13.5)

Box 13.5: Infantile Tibia Vara (Infantile Blount Disease)

Abnormal	>8–11°
	Persists beyond age 3 years
Mild	Mild medial metaphyseal tibial beaking
Severe	Irregular, fragmented medial tibial metaphysis
	Wide tibial physis
	Lateral subluxation of tibia

Infantile tibia vara results from stress that early walking and/or obesity cause to the posteromedial aspect of the proximal tibial metaphysis. The child with tibia vara walks with hips abducted and externally rotated; the knees are flexed, and tibias show increased internal torsion. This places the body weight on the posterior and medial portions of the tibial plateau, resulting in continuous epiphyseal deformation and compression and progressive increased shear stress at the physis. Endochondral ossification at the corresponding region of the proximal tibial physis becomes disorganized. Growth of the tibial metaphysis is suppressed, causing excessive angulation of the knee.

This relatively common condition is—like developmental bowing more common in African-Americans. Incidence is also increased in those of Scandinavian descent. Infantile tibia vara and developmental bowing are closely related and may represent different points on a spectrum. Infantile tibia vara is differentiated from juvenile disease based on age of presentation before 4 years of age.

Mild cases of infantile tibia vara may be treated conservatively with orthoses and may normalize by age 3 or 4 but if untreated generally progress to marked varus deformity and internal torsion. Both juvenile and adolescent tibia vara may represent unrecognized infantile disease that has been allowed to progress (see Chap. 14).

Imaging (Table 13.2)

Alignment of tibia vara is best assessed on a standing frontal radiograph, although a supine view provides greater bony detail. The metaphyseal-diaphyseal angle is determined by measuring the angle between a line drawn perpendicular to the long axis of the tibia and a line drawn tangent to the proximal tibial metaphysis (Fig. 13.69). A normal angle is 5° (range 0–11°). Infantile Blount disease is defined by an angle of 16° (range 8–22°). In equivocal cases with a metaphyseal-diaphyseal angle between 8 and 11°, follow-up radiographs are suggested [50]. It may be very difficult to determine whether a clinically irretrievable situation has developed.

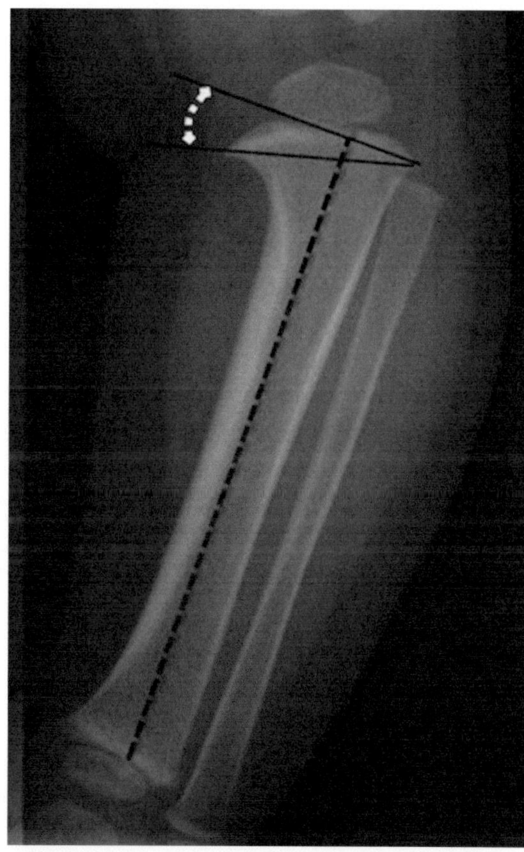

Fig. 13.69 Tibial metaphyseal-diaphyseal angle of 16° in a patient with infantile tibia vara. The angle is formed by a line drawn perpendicular to the long axis of the tibia and a line drawn tangent to the proximal tibial metaphysis. 0–8° is normal, and 8–11° is equivocal

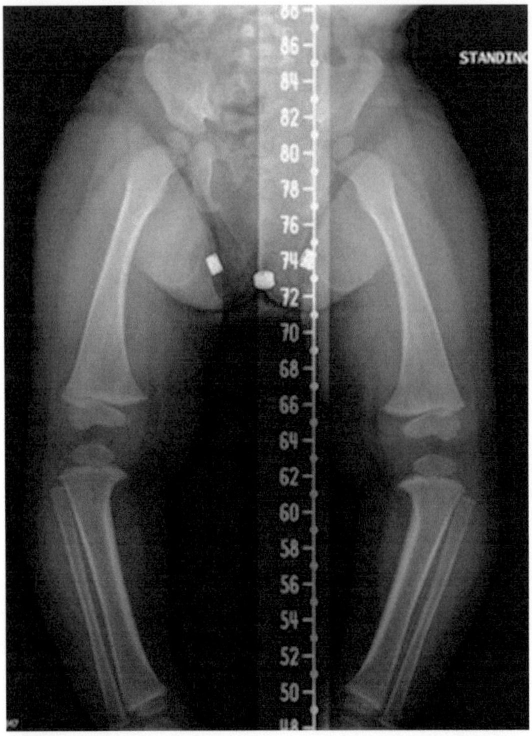

Fig. 13.70 Genu varum in a 1-year-old with infantile tibia vara. (**a**) There is genu varum, with 27° of angulation at the right knee and 35° at the left. In addition, the tibial metaphyseal-diaphyseal angle is abnormal, 14° on the right and 16° on the left, more severe than with developmental bowing (same patient as Fig. 13.69)

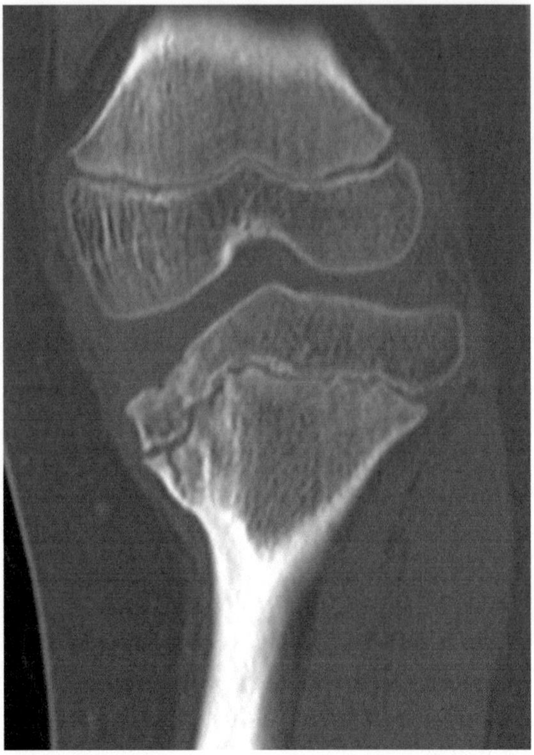

Fig. 13.71 Infantile tibia vara in a 5-year-old girl who presented with untreated disease. Coronally reformatted CT shows inferior tilt, sclerosis, and irregularity of the medial tibial metaphysis, along with thinning of the epiphysis

The extent of radiographic findings varies. Infantile tibia vara may simply demonstrate prominent beaking of the medial aspect of the proximal tibial metaphysis (Fig. 13.70). As the disorder becomes more advanced, the medial aspect of the metaphysis may become irregular and fragmented, and there may be widening of the proximal physis (Fig. 13.71). The medial portion of the tibial epiphysis is underdeveloped and wedge shaped, and the lateral physis may be unusually wide (perhaps as a result of persistent distraction or segmental cartilage hypertrophy). In severe cases the tibia may subluxate laterally, such that the medial plateau of the tibia is displaced into the intercondylar notch of the femur. The posteromedial cortex of the tibia is often thickened. The fibular head may appear prominent due to tibial varus and rotation. Unlike developmental bowing, infantile tibia vara is often unilateral or asymmetrical [51].

Orthopedic surgeons commonly use the Langenskiold classification to describe the appearance of the proximal tibia in Blount disease. The severity of metaphyseal depression and beaking, along with the extent of epiphyseal deformity, determines the Langenskiold stage from I to VI [52]. Surgical correction with osteotomy is generally used for stages III and above, which are characterized by progressively more severe metaphyseal beaking and depression [51].

MRI demonstrates angular deformity of the tibia (Fig. 13.72) [53, 54]. Ossification of the medial tibial epiphysis is delayed, and when ossified, its signal intensity is usually increased. In the medial compartment, decreased thickness of the cartilage at the mid-coronal epiphysis may be evident, along with focal joint space widening. The thickness of the unossified medial tibial epiphyseal cartilage is increased, and there may be both epiphyseal and metaphyseal edema. The

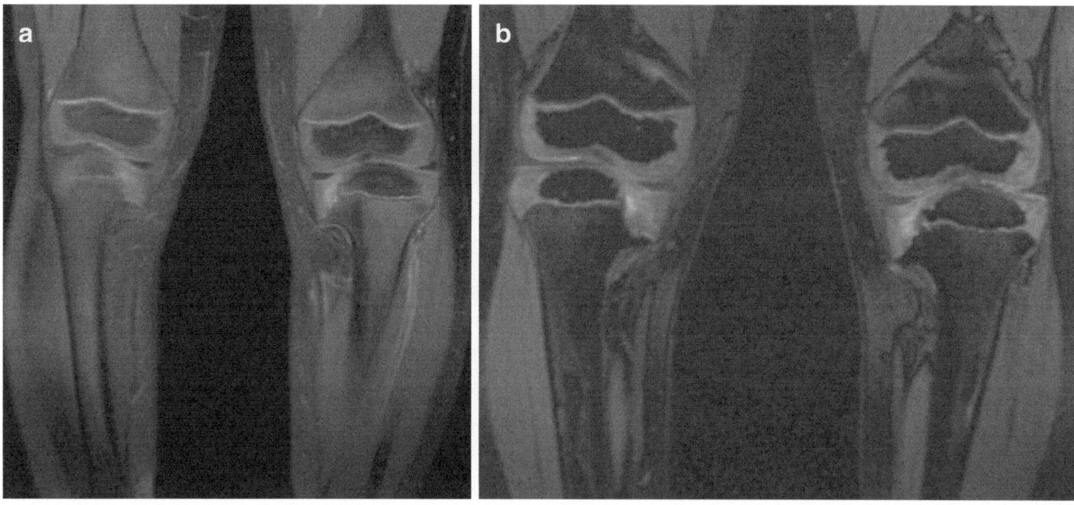

Fig. 13.72 Bilateral infantile tibia vara in a 4-year-old girl. Coronal FSE PD FS (**a**) and gradient echo (GRE) (**b**) images show medial proximal tibial metaphyseal depression and beaking with increased thickness of the medial cartilage. The mid-coronal cartilage appears thinned (Courtesy of Tal Laor, Cincinnati Children's Hospital)

medial portion of the physis is usually wide and depressed, and the lateral aspect of the tibial physis may also be widened [53]. Physeal cartilage may invaginate into the adjacent metaphysis, and the physis may close prematurely.

The distal femur is sometimes affected as well. Cyst-like T2 hyperintense foci may be seen in the distal femoral epiphysis of about half of patients. Irregularities of the medial and lateral metaphysis, along with widening of the physis may occur as well [53]. The medial meniscus is usually grossly enlarged, and it often demonstrates increased T2 signal, possibly representing hypertrophy and degeneration secondary to an increased compressive force. The anterior cruciate ligament may be lax.

The clinical utility of MRI is to determine the absence or presence of a medial physeal bar. If there is deformity but no bar, then realignment osteotomy will be successful. However, if there is a medial bar, realignment osteotomy alone will be followed by recurrent deformity with growth.

Differentiating developmental bowing from that associated with infantile Blount disease can be difficult. The two may represent parts of a continuum, with early walking and obesity leading to developmental bowing, which—if it does not resolve or is especially severe—eventually evolves into infantile Blount disease. Differentiating either phenomenon from bowing associated with skeletal dysplasia or metabolic abnormalities is usually more straightforward, as characteristic osseous findings typically distinguish these entities.

Metabolic Bowing (Rickets)

Rickets is a disorder of the growth plate characterized by deficient mineralization of cartilage and osteoid and retarded endochondral ossification, resulting in excessive accumulation of physeal cartilage, growth failure, and skeletal deformities [55].

Maintenance of normal circulating calcium and phosphate levels is crucial for a wide variety of physiological processes. Rickets may be classified by metabolic pathology: calcipenic (insufficient calcium absorption) and phosphopenic (excessive phosphate excretion) [56]. Calcipenic rickets usually results from vitamin D deficiency. Phosphopenic rickets results from renal tubular phosphate wasting, with X-linked hypophosphatemia being most common (Table 13.3).

Vitamin D is a prohormone that may be acquired from ingestion or by exposure to ultraviolet B light. It undergoes 25-hydroxylation in the liver and is then converted by renal tubular cells to active 1,25 dihydroxyvitamin D (calcitriol). Calcitriol acts on the intestine to increase calcium absorption.

Table 13.3 Etiologies of rickets

Calcipenic rickets		
Vitamin D deficiency	Nutritional	
	Malabsorption	GI disease
		Biliary disease
Vitamin D enzyme activation abnormalities	Vitamin D-dependent rickets	
Phosphopenic rickets		
X-linked hereditary hypophosphatemia	Tumor induced	
	Renal tubular disease	

GI gastrointestinal

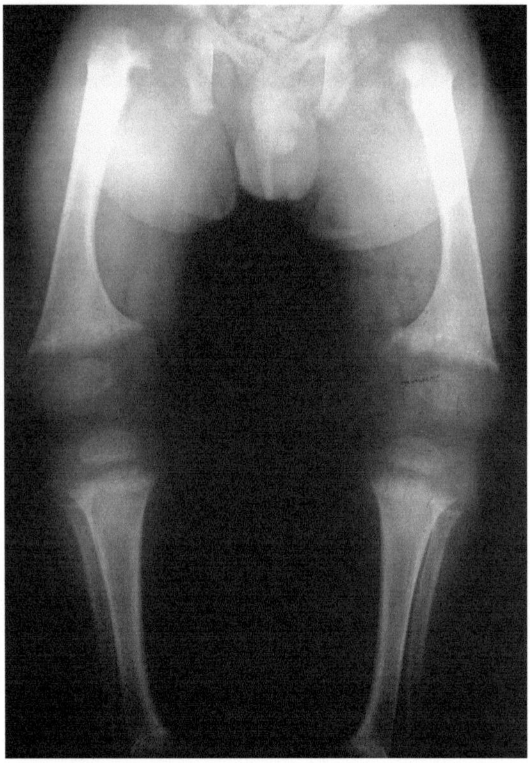

Fig. 13.73 Metaphyses are frayed and wide in this 3-year-old boy with vitamin D-dependent rickets (Courtesy of Rebecca Stein-Wexler)

The most common cause of rickets is nutritional vitamin D deficiency, which is most prevalent at 3–18 months of age. With low intake of vitamin D, intestinal calcium absorption is inadequate, and hypocalcemia results. This then causes release of parathyroid hormone (PTH), which mobilizes calcium and phosphate from the bone, also resulting in elevated alkaline phosphatase. In the kidney, PTH causes renal calcium reabsorption, phosphate wasting, and hypophosphatemia. At this point, the physeal manifestations of rickets become evident.

Hypophosphatemia is known to impair normal hypertrophic chondrocyte apoptosis [55, 56], leading to disorganized, excessive cartilage that widens the physis. In addition, the differentiated chondrocytes are unable to mineralize at the zone of provisional calcification, and metaphyseal fraying and cupping result. These findings are best seen in the metaphyses of the fastest growing bones, including the distal femur, proximal and distal tibia, and distal radius and ulna, as well as the anterior ends of the ribs (Figs. 13.73 and 13.74) [51, 56].

The findings in the diaphyses are less specific. They result from secondary hyperparathyroidism and osteomalacia and include insufficiency fractures, periosteal new bone formation, and bowing [56]. Both location and degree of bowing are age dependent, with lower extremity bowing most common after the child begins to stand. Genu varum is more common due to the lateral forces imparted in weight-bearing [56], but valgus or windswept deformity may be seen [57]. Interestingly, bone mineralization is often better preserved with X-linked hypophosphatemia than with vitamin D deficiency, as there is no secondary hyperparathyroidism in the former [56].

Imaging

Radiographic evaluation is sufficient for imaging rickets. Frontal views of the knees (Fig. 13.75), wrists, and ankles allow evaluation of the physes for widening and the metaphyses for fraying and cupping. Standing frontal views of the lower extremities define alignment abnormalities (Fig. 13.76). Changes of osteomalacia and hyperparathyroidism, with coarsening of the trabeculae, periosteal reaction, and insufficiency fractures, may be seen.

Genu Valgum (Knock Knees)

Often a physiological variant, mild valgus is normal from 2 to 12 years of age and usually resolves spontaneously. Genu valgum, however, describes

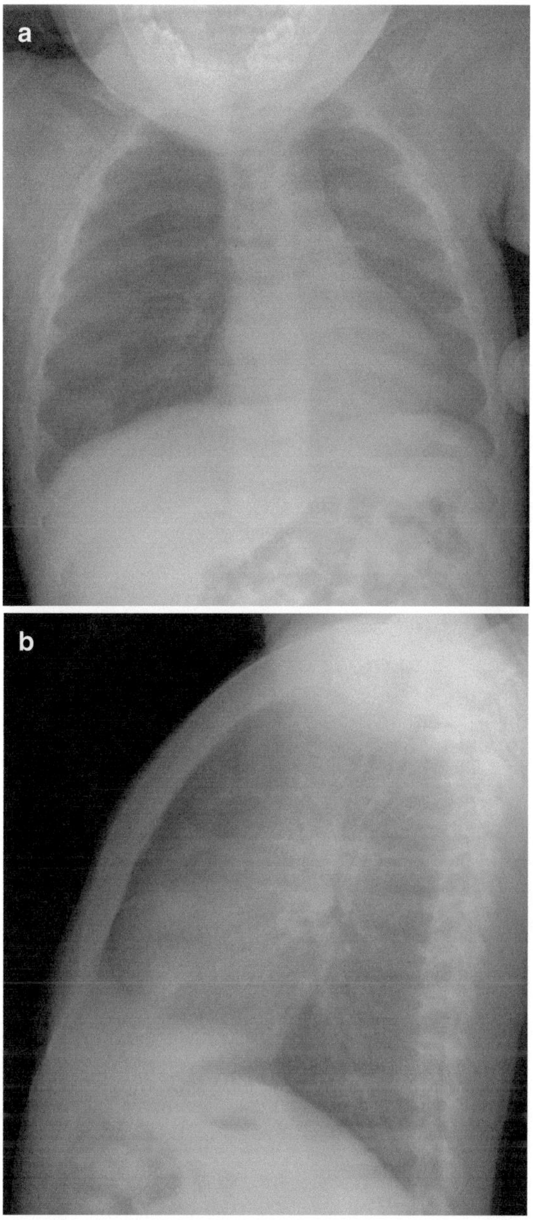

Fig. 13.74 Rachitic rosary in a 2-year-old with rickets. (**a**, **b**) The anterior rib ends are flared and irregular (Courtesy of Sandra L. Wootton-Gorges)

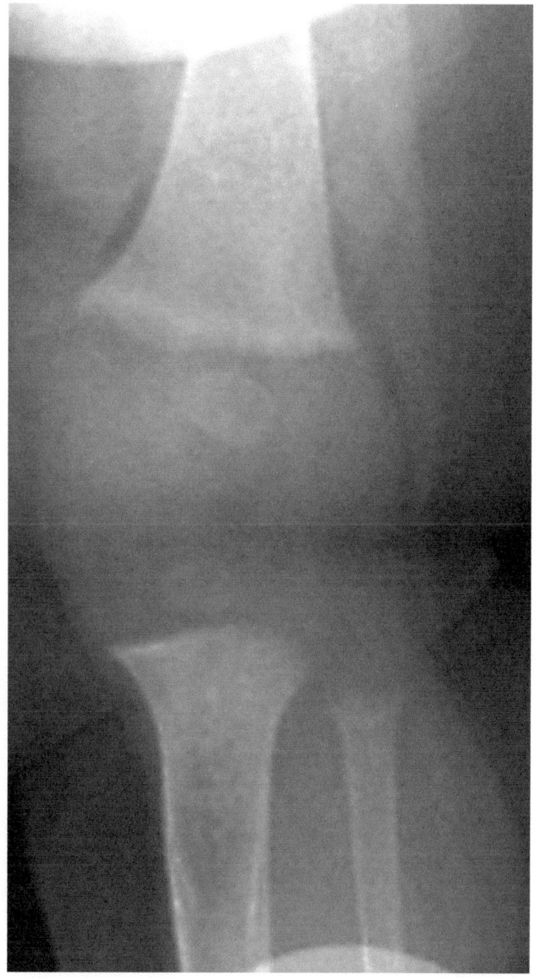

Fig. 13.75 Rickets in an African-American exclusively breast-fed 5-month-old girl who presented with hypocalcemic seizures due to nutritional vitamin D deficiency. There is physeal widening and metaphyseal fraying (Courtesy of Sandra L. Wootton-Gorges)

excessive (more than 6°) valgus alignment that persists. It is often associated with increased ligamentous laxity and external tibial torsion as well as pes planus and obesity.

Genu valgum may result from trauma or a variety of disease processes, such as renal osteodystrophy, rickets, cerebral palsy, and osteomyelitis involving the growth plate. Traumatic genu valgum usually results from injury to either the distal femoral or proximal tibial physis, although it can also follow tibial metaphyseal fracture (known as the Cozen phenomenon [58]). In this case, the fracture is remote from the growth plate, and gradual valgus orientation develops despite immediate postreduction satisfactory alignment (Fig. 13.77). Angulation continues to increase after the fracture line has united and then often corrects spontaneously, although some overgrowth may occur. Some of the many explanations for Cozen phenomenon include asymmetric

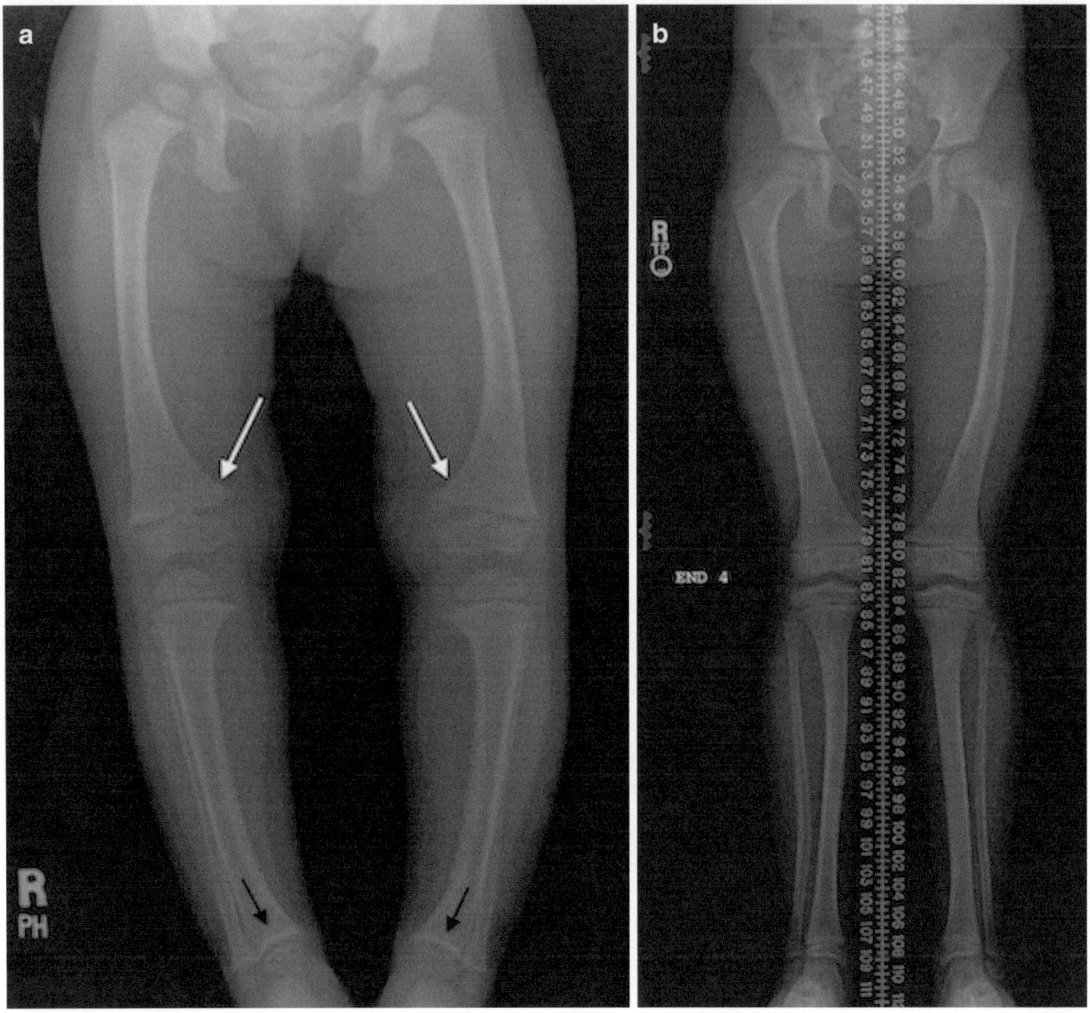

Fig. 13.76 Hypophosphatemic rickets in a 3-year-old girl with secondary lower extremity bowing. (**a**) The diaphyses of the tibias and the femurs are bowed, the distal femoral metaphyses are cupped and irregular (*white arrows*), and there are sclerotic bands in the distal tibial and distal fibular metaphyses (*black arrows*). (b) Five years after initial treatment, the metaphyses have improved. However, bowing in the femurs persists and results in mild genu valgum

medial growth plate stimulation, soft tissue imbalance or interposition, or growth plate damage with decreased lateral growth. Cozen phenomenon is most common between ages 3 and 6.

Physiological genu valgum generally does not require therapy and corrects over time. If angulation is severe, increased lateral pressure allows the medial condyle to grow more than the lateral, exacerbating the deformity; furthermore, differential growth may stretch the medial ligaments. If valgus is extreme or results from an underlying pathological process, medial hemiepiphysiodesis may be performed, limiting growth at the medial growth plate with staples or with a plate and screws [59]. Serial clinical and imaging follow-up allows guided growth and gradual correction of the deformity. Osteotomy is rarely required.

Imaging

On a standing view of the lower extremities with the patellae facing forward, the knees touch and the medial malleoli are separated (Fig. 13.78). The tibia is abducted relative to the femur, and

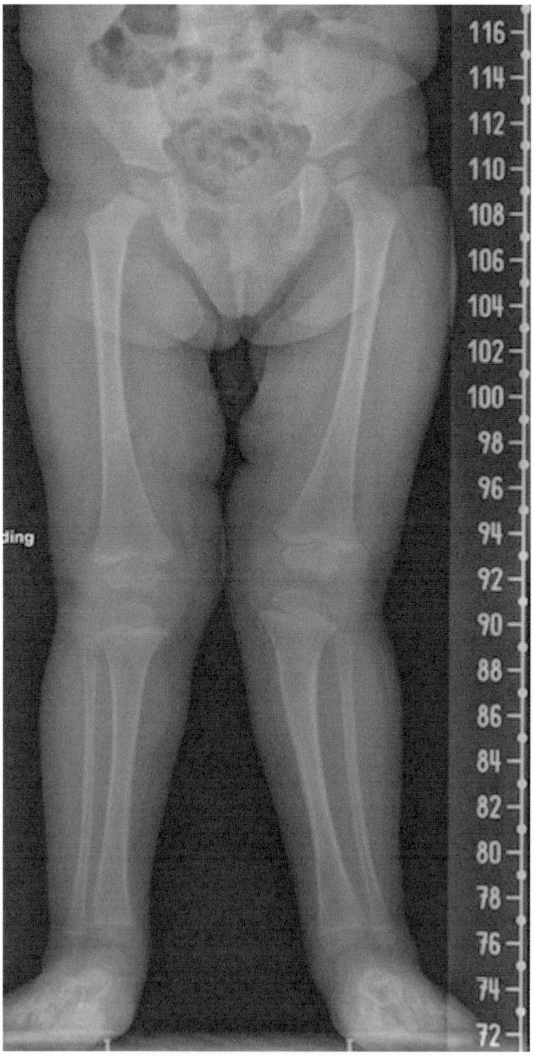

Fig. 13.77 Genu valgum secondary to proximal tibial metaphyseal fracture (Cozen phenomenon). This patient had a remote history of left proximal tibial metaphyseal fracture that resulted in overgrowth of the medial aspect of the proximal tibial metaphysis and genu valgum

the tibiofemoral angle measures greater than 15–20° (see section above on physiological bowing for measurement technique). The tibia may show apex-medial bowing, with increased thickness and sclerosis of the lateral cortex. The lateral aspect of the distal femoral ossification center may be underdeveloped due to increased stress. In some obese children the medial aspect of the growth plate may be abnormally wide, also due to stress.

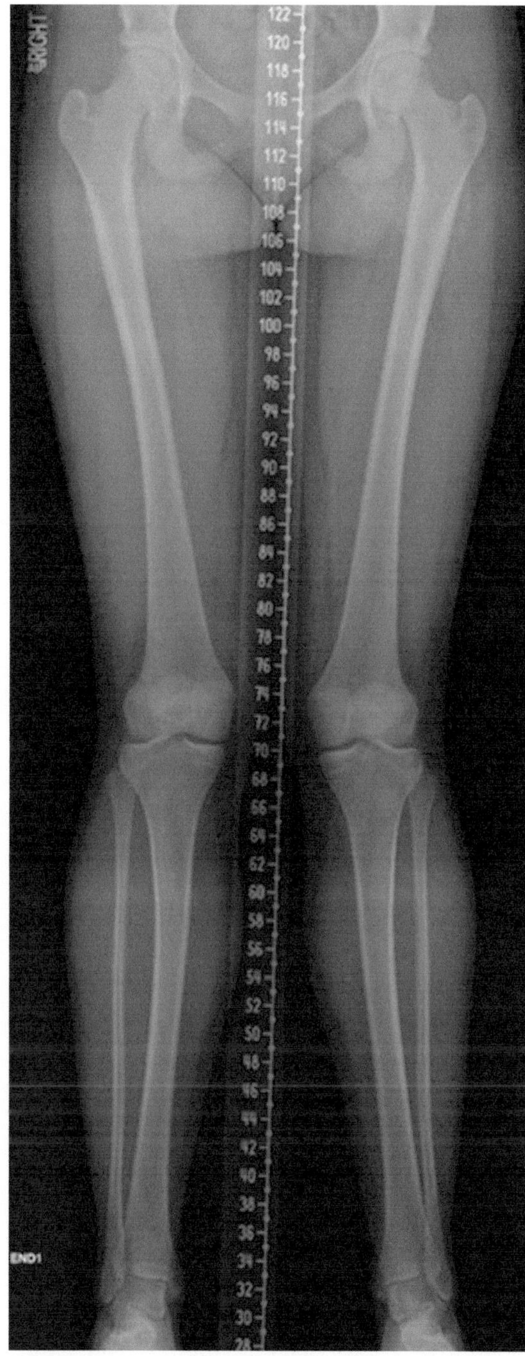

Fig. 13.78 Genu valgum in a 12-year-old girl. The tibiofemoral angle is 18° on the right and 16° on the left

Rotational Abnormalities of the Long Bones (Table 13.2)

Some rotation is normal in both the femur and the tibia: the femoral condyles are generally internally rotated in relation to the femoral neck, and the distal tibia is externally rotated in relation to the tibial plateau. The extent of rotation changes with development.

Compared to alignment in the adult, there is relative internal rotation of the lower tibia and fibula in the newborn, presumably due to intrauterine positioning. During normal development of the infant and child, the lower leg gradually rotates externally [60]. In the newborn, the bimalleolar axis averages 4° of external rotation in relation to the distal femur. By 6 months this external rotation increases to 6°, and by 1 year it averages 10°. By age 10, external rotation at the ankle averages 14°, and the lateral malleolus is posterior to the medial. By adulthood external rotation is 14–20° [61].

Tibial torsion refers to a twist in the longitudinal axis of the tibia resulting in internal or external malalignment. Persistent torsion in the newborn may lead to cosmetic and functional problems in adulthood. Abnormal internal tibial torsion occurs in about 5 % of children between the ages of 5 and 7 years and in 1 or 2 % of the adult population. Excessive femoral torsion has been seen in patients with intoeing gait, cerebral palsy, and myelomeningocele. Diminished femoral anteversion may be associated with slipped capital femoral epiphysis. Increased femoral anteversion and increased internal tibial torsion may affect patellofemoral alignment. The combination of increased femoral anteversion and increased external tibial torsion is known as miserable malalignment; this may cause knee pain with ambulation [62].

Aggressive therapy may be necessary if the rotational abnormality compromises function or puts the patient at risk for developing other pathological processes. During infancy and childhood, an external rotation splint may be applied, but this treatment is not necessarily either advised or efficacious. Severe rotation may be treated with rotational osteotomy.

Imaging

Physical examination is often sufficient for evaluation of tibial torsion. Radiographs may demonstrate thickening of the medial cortex of the tibia, as with the often-associated developmental bowing of the lower extremities. In severe cases, radiographs may demonstrate obvious rotational deformity of the femurs and tibias, and the knees may be directed medially (Fig. 13.79). If imaging assessment of the degree of torsion is required, cross-sectional imaging is usually considered necessary. Computed tomography (CT) or magnetic resonance (MR) images are obtained at the femoral neck, tibial plateau and ankle, and the angle formed by lines paralleling the tibial plateau and the malleoli is assessed (Figs. 13.80 and 13.81)

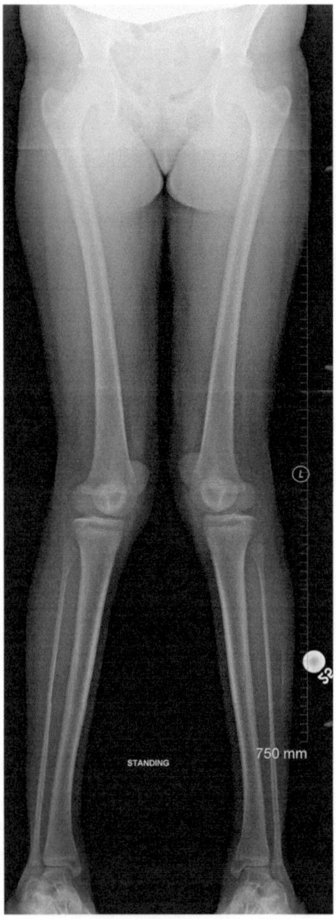

Fig. 13.79 Bilateral femoral anteversion and tibial torsion. Alignment at the hips and ankles is essentially normal, but the knees point medially so the patellae overlap the soft tissues on this frontal radiograph. There is also genu valgus (Courtesy of Rebecca Stein-Wexler)

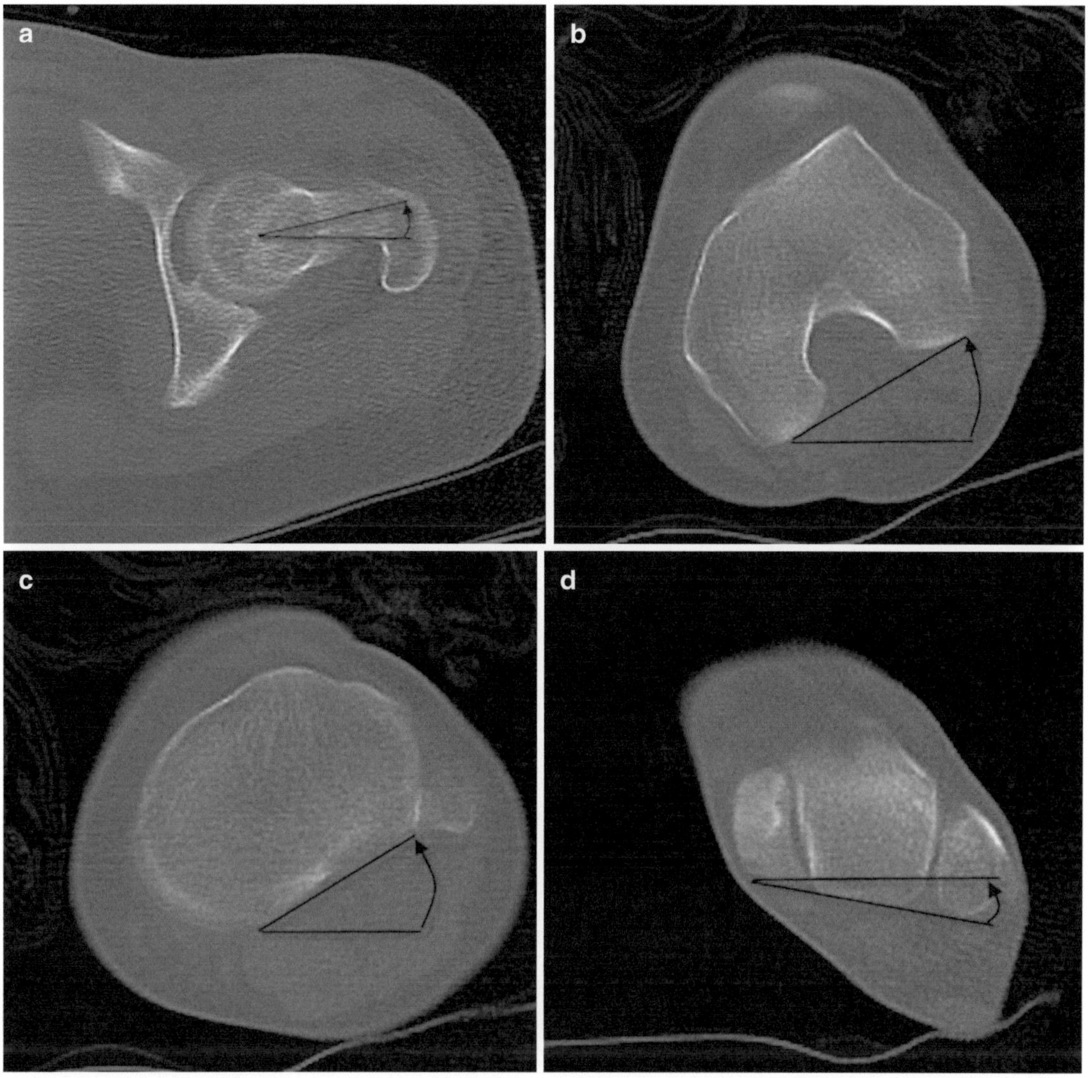

Fig. 13.80 Evaluation of femoral anteversion and tibial torsion with CT. Axial images at the femoral neck (**a**), femoral condyles (**b**), tibial plateau (**c**), and ankle (**d**) are obtained. The rotational angle of the femur (femoral anteversion) is assessed by determining the angle formed between two lines: one is parallel to the femoral neck and the other is tangent to the posterior femoral condyles. This can be done by measuring the angle that each of these lines forms against the horizontal and then subtracting or adding these values (depending on whether they are positioned above or below the horizontal). In this case, the two angles are added, and femoral anteversion measures 18°. The rotational angle of the tibia (tibial torsion) is then assessed by determining the angle formed between two lines that parallel the tibial plateau and that are tangent to the posterior portions of the peripheral aspects of the medial and lateral malleoli (the intermalleolar line). As with the femur, this can be done by measuring the angle that each of these lines forms against the horizontal and then subtracting or adding these values (depending on whether they are positioned above or below the horizontal). In this case, the values are added, and tibial torsion measures 41°. Measurement can also be performed on images that are superimposed

[63]. Alternatively, the EOS 2D/3D low-dose digital imaging device (EOS Imaging SA, Paris, France) provides images that can be manipulated in a variety of ways to allow both 2-dimensional and 3-dimensional evaluation of rotational abnormalities [64] (see Chap. 3).

5 Leg-Length Discrepancy (Anisomelia)

Asymmetry in size and contour of the skeleton and facial structures is common, but the lower extremities are usually remarkably symmetrical. Although a difference of 2 cm is considered normal, 60 % of legs measure within 1 mm of the other side. This is fortunate, since leg-length discrepancy may cause pelvic obliquity and compensatory scoliosis.

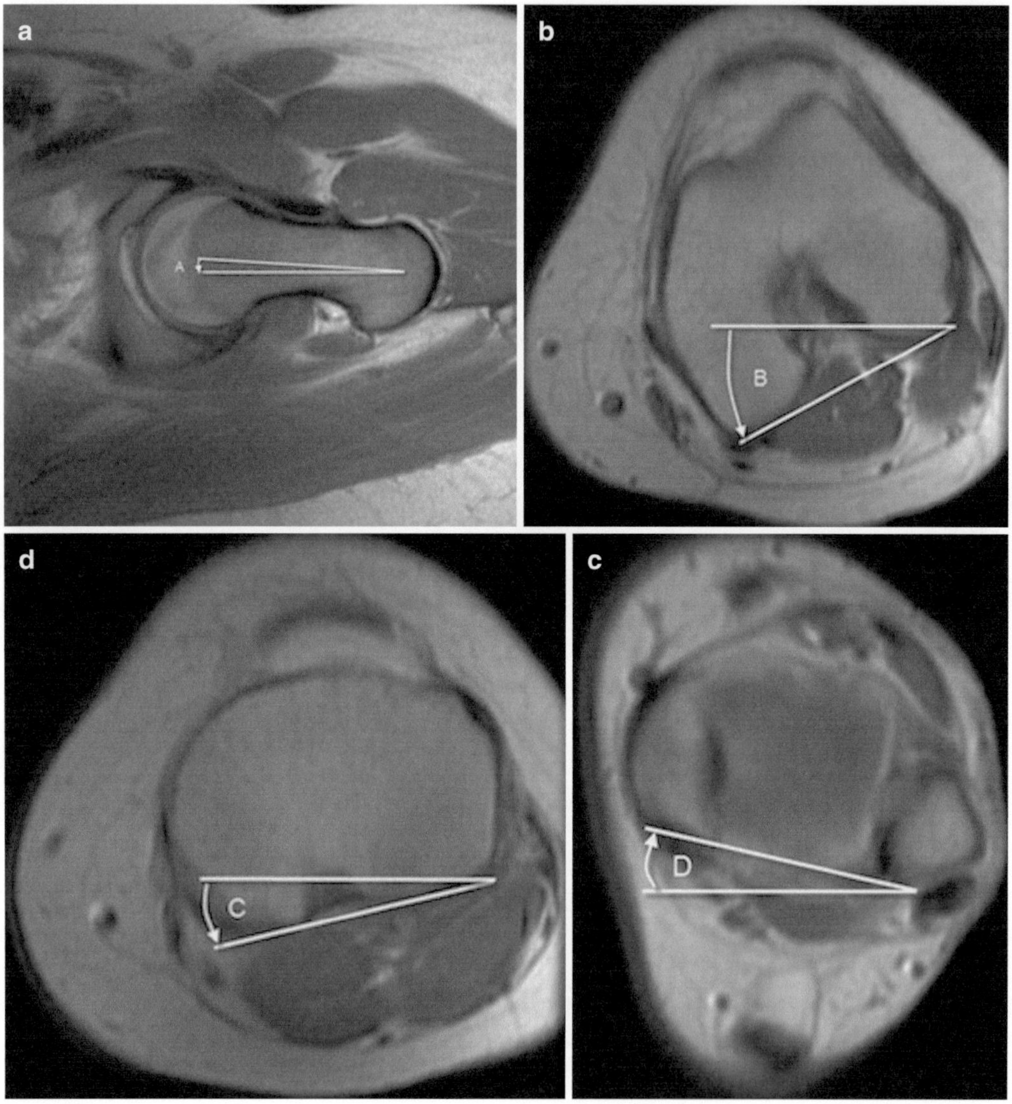

Fig. 13.81 Evaluation of femoral anteversion and tibial torsion with MRI. Axial images at the femoral neck (**a**), femoral condyles (**b**), tibial plateau (**c**), and ankle (**d**) are obtained. The femoral neck image can be acquired in a slightly oblique plane that parallels the true axis of the femoral neck. The rotational angle of the femur (femoral anteversion) is assessed by determining the angle formed between lines parallel to the femoral neck (**a**) and tangent to the posterior femoral condyles (**b**). In this case, femoral anteversion measures 35°. The rotational angle of the tibia (tibial torsion) is then assessed by determining the angle formed between two lines that parallel the tibial plateau (**c**) and the posterior portions of the peripheral aspects of the medial and lateral malleoli (the intermalleolar line) (**d**). In this case, tibial torsion measures 28°. Measurement can also be performed on images that are superimposed. (**e**) This patient's excessive femoral anteversion combines with tibial torsion to cause lateral subluxation of the patella

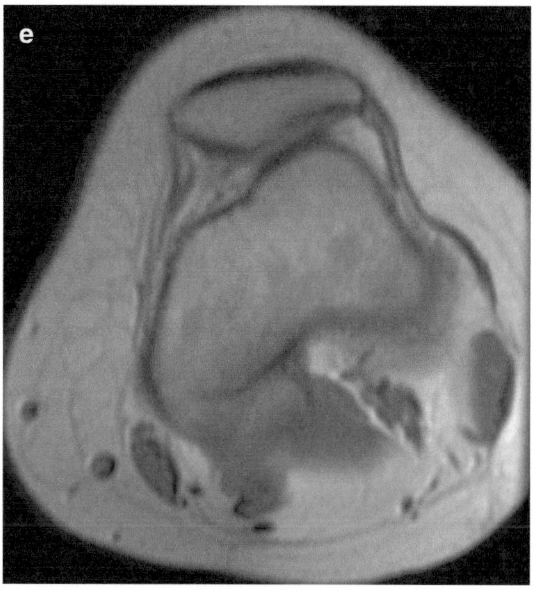

Fig. 13.81 (continued)

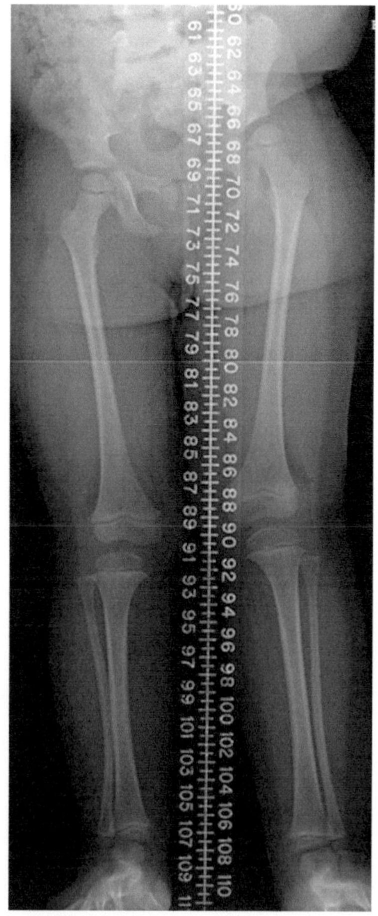

Fig. 13.82 Leg-length discrepancy secondary to hemihypertrophy in a 4-year-old girl. The bones of both legs appear grossly normal but when compared to the right side bones and soft tissues on the left are hypertrophied

Leg-length discrepancy may be due to either overgrowth of the long limb or reduced growth of the short limb (Figs. 13.82 and 13.83). Overgrowth may result from a generalized process, such as neurofibromatosis or hemihypertrophy, or it may be associated with such vascular anomalies as lymphangioma, hemangioma, and Klippel-Trenaunay-Weber syndrome (Fig. 13.84). Hyperemia and overstimulation may also cause overgrowth, as with long bone fractures (Fig. 13.85), chronic synovitis, or—infrequently—arteriovenous fistula. However, the cause of overgrowth is often unknown.

Reduced growth may be evident at birth, as a result of congenital hypoplasia or aplasia of a limb or segment. However, it is more common for growth impairment to develop postnatally, typically due to a growth plate disorder—either diminished growth or complete growth cessation and premature fusion. This can result from paralysis, long-term immobilization, vascular insufficiency, direct injury to the growth plate following thermal or radiation damage, osteomyelitis, fracture, or avascular necrosis (Fig. 13.86). Aortic or femoral artery thrombosis due to percutaneous or umbilical artery catheterization may result in vascular insufficiency. Developmental coxa vara also results in leg shortening.

Relatively small differences (between 2 and 4 cm) are addressed by inhibiting growth of the longer extremity. Permanent epiphysiodesis is often performed, ablating or interposing bone within the epiphysis in order to stop growth of the longer extremity. Results are predictable and complications uncommon. Alternatively, temporary epiphyseal stapling or bracketing may be performed, with the advantage that further growth may eventually be possible once the hardware is removed. However, with epiphyseal stapling, permanent fusion due to perichondrial or growth plate damage may cause unwanted angulation.

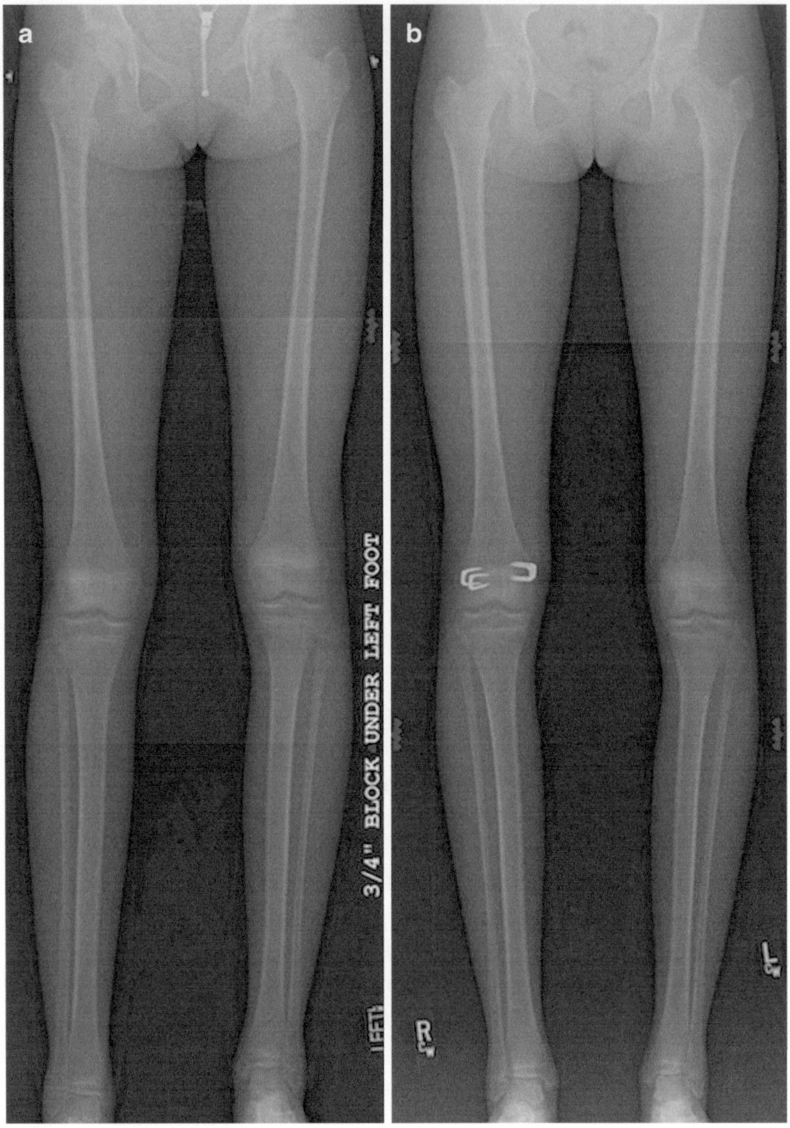

Fig. 13.83 Leg-length discrepancy in a 13-year-old girl. (**a**) Initial imaging with a ¾ inch block under the left foot shows the right femur is considerably longer than the left. (**b**) After 1 year of restricted growth at the distal right physis, the femurs appear symmetrical

If the patient is skeletally mature and growth can no longer be altered, a segment of the longer diaphysis may be removed.

Lengthening of the shorter limb is possible if shortening of the longer extremity is unacceptable, if discrepancy is too great to be equalized with epiphysiodesis (generally greater than 4 cm), or if a dwarf condition makes greater height appealing. As a general rule, a bone may be lengthened up to 15 % before significant soft tissue, neurovascular, and skeletal healing complications develop. Most limb-lengthening procedures involve diaphyseal transection and distraction with osteogenesis during gradual diastasis.

The most common methods of distraction involve pins or wires attached to either a cantilever device (e.g., uniplanar fixator technique) or encircling rings (such as the Ilizarov system). The latter method controls not only axial alignment but also angulation and rotation. Physeal distraction (or chondrodiatasis) lengthens the bone either by stimulating growth or by actual growth plate distraction. The latter is performed

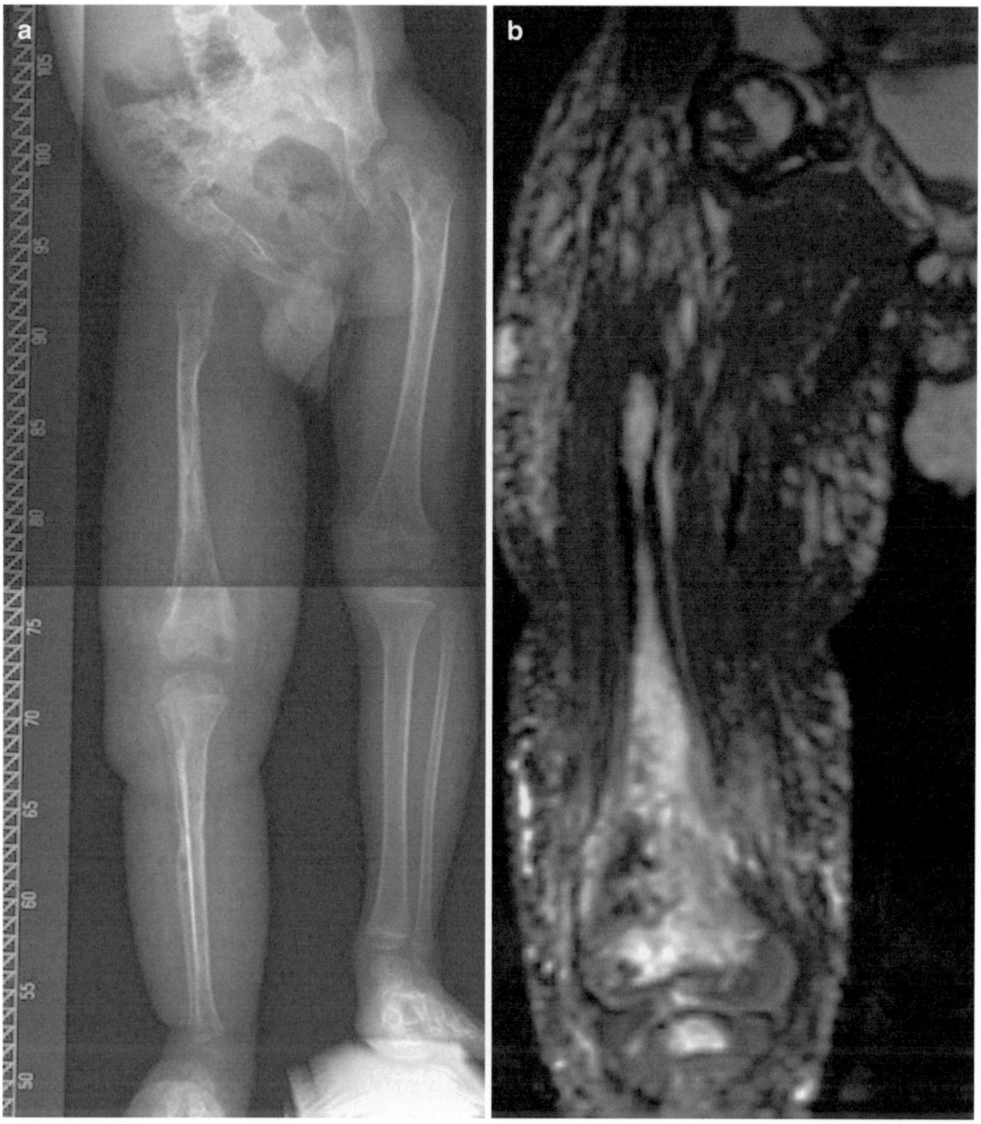

Fig. 13.84 Leg-length discrepancy secondary to vascular malformation in a 5-year-old boy. (**a**) Standing view with block under the left foot shows bony and soft tissue overgrowth of the right lower extremity. The vascular malformation also involves the bones, resulting in irregular lucencies. (**b**) Coronal T2-W MRI of the right upper leg shows extensive vascular malformation affecting bone and soft tissues

less frequently, usually just before skeletal maturity as the growth plate often closes after traction.

The rate of distraction is carefully controlled to allow for muscle, nerve, and vascular growth as well as osteogenesis, which may occur either at the periosteum, within the medulla, or as the result of stretching callus that has formed in the gap between the two pieces of bone (callotasis). Radiographs follow the progress of osteogenesis and realignment, and new bone formation is usually visible by 15 weeks. Bone grafting and plate fixation may be necessary after some procedures.

Complications are common, including pin-track infections, osteomyelitis, nonunion,

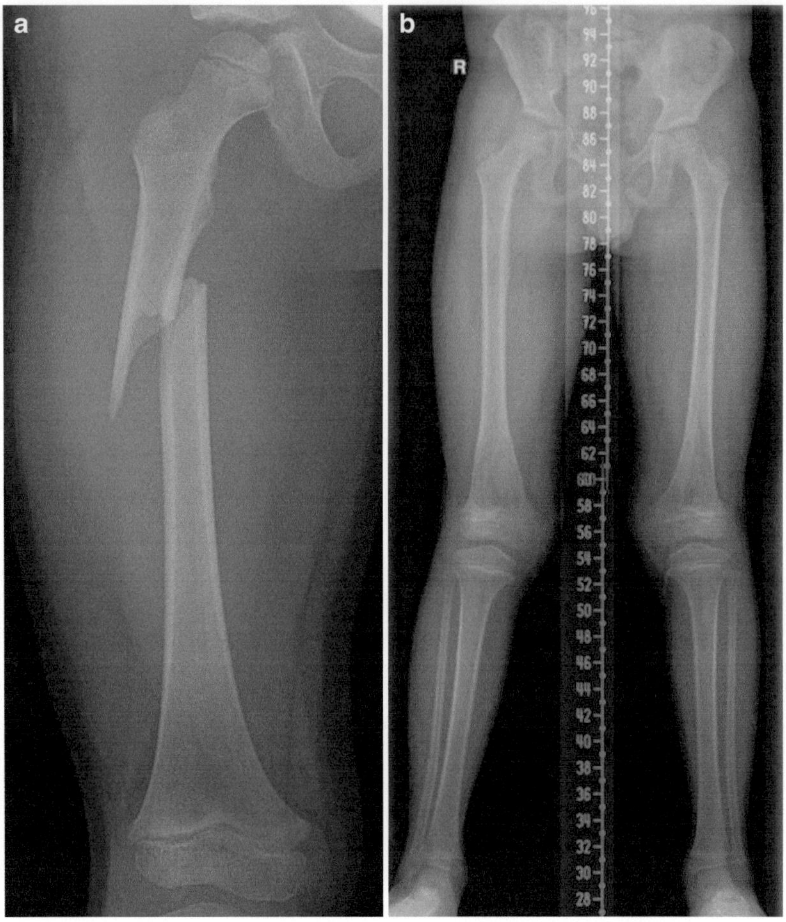

Fig. 13.85 Leg-length discrepancy in a 5-year-old boy due to overgrowth after right femoral fracture. (**a**) Acute femoral fracture with bayonet apposition. (**b**) Two years later (and after placement of an intramedullary rod), the fracture has healed, but the right femur is now 1 cm longer than the left

malunion, refracture, loss of motion, knee and ankle contractures, hypertension, peroneal nerve palsy, and angulation (usually varus in the femur and valgus in the tibia).

Imaging

There are several approaches to predicting limb-length discrepancy and thus determining timing and type of surgical intervention. The Paley multiplier method employs gender, age, and bone-specific values (or "multipliers") that are applied to one or preferably more measurements of the femur or tibia [65]. The Moseley straight-line graph method, on the other hand, calculates predicted limb-length discrepancy at skeletal maturity by correlating sequential radiographs of the lower extremities with sequential radiographs of the hand [66]. (See Chap. 2 for additional discussion of assessing skeletal maturity.) As a general guideline, the Moseley system requires three sequential studies performed 6–12 months apart to determine a trend, whereas the Paley method can if necessary be applied to a single radiograph.

When determining bone length and possible intervention, it is crucial to minimize the geometric magnification that results from using a single exposure for the entire extremity [67] (the "parallax" effect). Orthoroentgenography is the simplest method and requires no special equipment. Exposures at the hip, knee, and ankle are projected onto a single large cassette, along with an opaque ruler. The scanogram technique also employs separate exposures at the hip, knee, and ankle. They are collimated more tightly than for orthoroentgenography, so that all three exposures fit onto one standard size image (Fig. 13.87). Teloroentgenography uses a single exposure on a

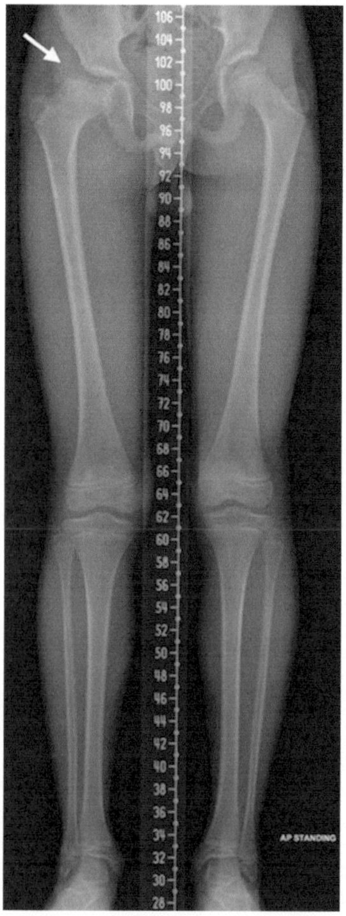

Fig. 13.86 Short right femur in a 12-year-old boy with Legg-Perthes disease. Resultant femoral head deformity (*arrow*), coxa vara, and impaired growth shorten the right femur. Pelvic tilt

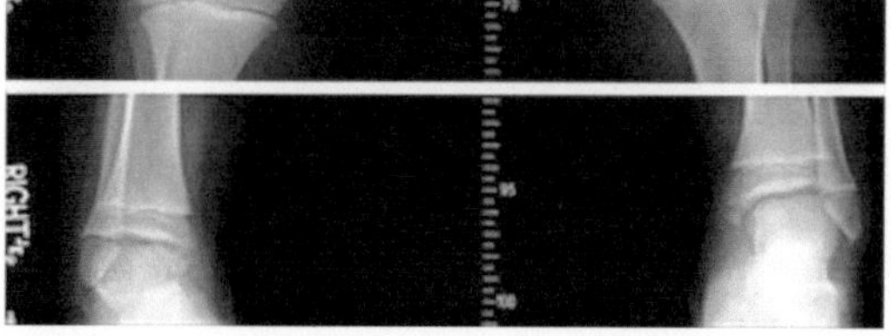

Fig. 13.87 Scanogram image capturing hips, knees, and ankles on a single cassette. Markings on the radiopaque ruler allow accurate determination of long bone length

long film with the tube detector 6 ft away. While this technique introduces magnification, it does accurately assess relative bone length (many images in this chapter employ this technique, e.g., Figs. 13.77, 13.78, 13.79, and 13.82).

Computed and digital radiography allow for full-length standing images with significantly lower doses (Fig. 13.83). Images are obtained on standard-sized digital cassettes and are digitally collated, allowing for manipulation on a picture archiving computer system (PACS). These techniques also image the entire bone with satisfactory detail and proportions. The scout view from a CT of the lower extremities also allows accurate measurement. The EOS 2D/3D low-dose digital imaging device may also be employed to determine leg length [64].

References

1. Ogden JA. Radiology of postnatal skeletal development. X. Patella and tibial tuberosity. Skeletal Radiol. 1984;11(4):246–57. PubMed PMID: 6729496. Epub 1984/01/01. eng.
2. Varich LJ, Laor T, Jaramillo D. Normal maturation of the distal femoral epiphyseal cartilage: age-related changes at MR imaging. Radiology. 2000; 214(3):705–9. PubMed PMID: 10715034. Epub 2000/03/14. eng.
3. Ritschl P, Hajek PC, Pechmann U. Fibrous metaphyseal defects. Magnetic resonance imaging appearances. Skeletal Radiol. 1989;18(4):253–9. PubMed PMID: 2781323. Epub 1989/01/01. eng.
4. Pai DR, Strouse PJ. MRI of the pediatric knee. AJR Am J Roentgenol. 2011;196(5):1019–27. PubMed PMID: 21512066. Epub 2011/04/23. eng.
5. Shimal A, Davies AM, James SL, Grimer RJ. Fatigue-type stress fractures of the lower limb associated with fibrous cortical defects/non-ossifying fibromas in the skeletally immature. Clin Radiol. 2010;65(5):382–6. PubMed PMID: 20380937. Epub 2010/04/13. eng.
6. Steinmetz JC, Pilon VA, Lee JK. Jaffe-Campanacci syndrome. J Pediatr Orthop. 1988;8(5):602–4. PubMed PMID: 3139710. Epub 1988/09/01.
7. Laor T, Chun GF, Dardzinski BJ, Bean JA, Witte DP. Posterior distal femoral and proximal tibial metaphyseal stripes at MR imaging in children and young adults. Radiology. 2002;224(3):669–74. PubMed PMID: 12202698. Epub 2002/08/31. eng.
8. Simon H. Medial distal metaphyseal femoral irregularity in children. Radiology. 1968;90(2):258–60.
9. Vieira RL, Bencardino JT, Rosenberg ZS, Nomikos G. MRI features of cortical desmoid in acute knee

trauma. AJR Am J Roentgenol. 2011;196(2):424–8. PubMed PMID: 21257896. Epub 2011/01/25. eng.
10. Resnick D, Greenway G. Distal femoral cortical defects, irregularities, and excavations. Radiology. 1982;143(2):345–54. PubMed PMID: 7041169. Epub 1982/05/01. eng.
11. Boyer RS, Jaffe RB, Nixon GW, Condon VR. Trampoline fracture of the proximal tibia in children. AJR Am J Roentgenol. 1986;146(1):83–5. PubMed PMID: 3484416. Epub 1986/01/01. eng.
12. Weiner D, Macnab I, Turner M. The Fabella syndrome. Clin Orthop Relat Res. 1977;126:213–5. PubMed PMID: 598120. Epub 1977/07/01. eng.
13. Weiner DS, Macnab I. The "fabella syndrome": an update. J Pediatr Orthop. 1982;2(4):405–8. PubMed PMID: 6815224. Epub 1982/10/01. eng.
14. Lawson JP. Symptomatic radiographic variants in extremities. Radiology. 1985;157(3):625–31. PubMed PMID: 4059550. Epub 1985/12/01. eng.
15. Bates DG, Hresko MT, Jaramillo D. Patellar sleeve fracture: demonstration with MR imaging. Radiology. 1994;193(3):825–7. PubMed PMID: 7972832. Epub 1994/12/01. eng.
16. Duncan JG, Souter WA. Hereditary onycho-osteodysplasia: the nail-patella syndrome. J Bone Joint Surg. 1963;45(2):242–58.
17. Wada A, Fujii T, Takamura K, Yanagida H, Surijamorn P. Congenital dislocation of the patella. J Child Orthop. 2008;2(2):119–23. PubMed PMID: 19308591. Pubmed Central PMCID: 2656798.
18. Koplewitz BZ, Babyn PS, Cole WG. Congenital dislocation of the patella. AJR Am J Roentgenol. 2005;184(5):1640–6. PubMed PMID: 15855131. Epub 2005/04/28. eng.
19. Nietosvaara Y, Aalto K, Kallio PE. Acute patellar dislocation in children: incidence and associated osteochondral fractures. J Pediatr Orthop. 1994;14(4):513–5. PubMed PMID: 8077438.
20. Diederichs G, Issever AS, Scheffler S. MR imaging of patellar instability: injury patterns and assessment of risk factors. Radiographics. 2010;30(4):961–81. PubMed PMID: 20631363.
21. Stefanik JJ, Zumwalt AC, Segal NA, Lynch JA, Powers CM. Association between measures of patella height, morphologic features of the trochlea, and patellofemoral joint alignment: the MOST study. Clin Orthop Relat Res. 2013;471(8):2641–8. PubMed PMID: 23546847. Pubmed Central PMCID: 3705075. Epub 2013/04/03. eng.
22. Koshino T, Sugimoto K. New measurement of patellar height in the knees of children using the epiphyseal line midpoint. J Pediatr Orthop. 1989;9(2):216–8. PubMed PMID: 2925858.
23. Insall J, Salvati E. Patella position in the normal knee joint. Radiology. 1971;101(1):101–4. PubMed PMID: 5111961.
24. Jacobsen K, Bertheussen K. The vertical location of the patella. Fundamental views on the concept patella alta, using a normal sample. Acta Orthop Scand. 1974;45(3):436–45.
25. Carrillon Y, Abidi H, Dejour D, Fantino O, Moyen B, Tran-Minh VA. Patellar instability: assessment on MR images by measuring the lateral trochlear inclination-initial experience. Radiology. 2000;216(2): 582–5. PubMed PMID: 10924589.
26. Ali SA, Helmer R, Terk MR. Analysis of the patellofemoral region on MRI: association of abnormal trochlear morphology with severe cartilage defects. AJR Am J Roentgenol. 2010;194(3):721–7. PubMed PMID: 20173151. Epub 2010/02/23. eng.
27. Pfirrmann CW, Zanetti M, Romero J, Hodler J. Femoral trochlear dysplasia: MR findings. Radiology. 2000;216(3):858–64. PubMed PMID: 10966723. Epub 2000/08/31. eng.
28. Dolk H, Loane M, Garne E. The prevalence of congenital anomalies in Europe. Adv Exp Med Biol. 2010;686:349–64. PubMed PMID: 20824455. Epub 2010/09/09. eng.
29. Henkel L, Willert HG. Dysmelia. A classification and a pattern of malformation in a group of congenital defects of the limbs. J Bone Joint Surg. 1969; 51(3):399–414. PubMed PMID: 5820783. Epub 1969/08/01. eng.
30. Kmita M, Tarchini B, Zakany J, Logan M, Tabin CJ, Duboule D. Early developmental arrest of mammalian limbs lacking HoxA/HoxD gene function. Nature. 2005;435(7045):1113–6. PubMed PMID: 15973411. Epub 2005/06/24. eng.
31. Day HJ. The ISO/ISPO classification of congenital limb deficiency. Prosthet Orthot Int. 1991;15(2):67–9. PubMed PMID: 1923724. Epub 1991/08/01. eng.
32. Wolfgang GL. Complex congenital anomalies of the lower extremities: femoral bifurcation, tibial hemimelia, and diastasis of the ankle. Case report and review of the literature. J Bone Joint Surg Am. 1984;66(3):453–8. PubMed PMID: 6699064.
33. Jones D, Barnes J, Lloyd-Roberts GC. Congenital aplasia and dysplasia of the tibia with intact fibula. Classification and management. J Bone Joint Surg. 1978;60(1):31–9. PubMed PMID: 627576.
34. Kalamchi A, Dawe RV. Congenital deficiency of the tibia. J Bone Joint Surg. 1985;67(4):581–4. PubMed PMID: 4030854.
35. Weber M. New classification and score for tibial hemimelia. J Child Orthop. 2008;2(3):169–75. PubMed PMID: 19308574. Pubmed Central PMCID: 2656800.
36. Stanitski DF, Stanitski CL. Fibular hemimelia: a new classification system. J Pediatr Orthop. 2003;23(1):30–4. PubMed PMID: 12499939. Epub 2002/12/25. eng.
37. Stevens PM, Arms D. Postaxial hypoplasia of the lower extremity. J Pediatr Orthop. 2000;20(2):166–72. PubMed PMID: 10739276. Epub 2000/03/30. eng.
38. Achterman C, Kalamchi A. Congenital deficiency of the fibula. J Bone Joint Surg. 1979;61-B(2):133–7. PubMed PMID: 438260.
39. Kruger LM, Talbott RD. Amputation and prosthesis as definitive treatment in congenital absence of the fibula. J Bone Joint Surg Am. 1961;43-A:625–42. PubMed PMID: 13831084.
40. Hootnick D, Boyd NA, Fixsen JA, Lloyd-Roberts GC. The natural history and management of congenital short tibia with dysplasia or absence of the fibula.

J Bone Joint Surg. 1977;59(3):267–71. PubMed PMID: 893503.
41. Birch JG, Lincoln TL, Mack PW, Birch CM. Congenital fibular deficiency: a review of thirty years' experience at one institution and a proposed classification system based on clinical deformity. J Bone Joint Surg Am. 2011;93(12):1144–51. PubMed PMID: 21776551. Epub 2011/07/22. eng.
42. Fordham LA, Applegate KE, Wilkes DC, Chung CJ. Fibular hemimelia: more than just an absent bone. Semin Musculoskelet Radiol. 1999;3(3):227–38. PubMed PMID: 11387140.
43. Johnston CE, Birch JG. A tale of two tibias: a review of treatment options for congenital pseudarthrosis of the tibia. J Child Orthop. 2008;2(2):133–49. PubMed PMID: 19308593. Pubmed Central PMCID: 2656794.
44. Vander Have KL, Hensinger RN, Caird M, Johnston C, Farley FA. Congenital pseudarthrosis of the tibia. J Am Acad Orthop Surg. 2008;16(4):228–36. PubMed PMID: 18390485.
45. Richards BS, Oetgen ME, Johnston CE. The use of rhBMP-2 for the treatment of congenital pseudarthrosis of the tibia: a case series. J Bone Joint Surg Am. 2010;92(1):177–85. PubMed PMID: 20048110. Epub 2010/01/06. eng.
46. Lehman WB, Abdelgawad AA, Sala DA. Congenital tibial dysplasia (congenital pseudoarthrosis of the tibia): an atypical variation. J Pediatr Orthop Part B. 2009;18(5):211–3. PubMed PMID: 19625879.
47. Ooishi T, Sugioka Y, Matsumoto S, Fujii T. Congenital dislocation of the knee. Its pathologic features and treatment. Clin Orthop Relat Res. 1993;287:187–92. PubMed PMID: 8448939.
48. Klingele KE, Stephens S. Management of ACL elongation in the surgical treatment of congenital knee dislocation. Orthopedics. 2012;35(7):e1094–8. PubMed PMID: 22784907.
49. Salenius P, Vankka E. The development of the tibiofemoral angle in children. J Bone Joint Surg Am. 1975;57(2):259–61. PubMed PMID: 1112851.
50. Levine AM, Drennan JC. Physiological bowing and tibia vara. The metaphyseal-diaphyseal angle in the measurement of bowleg deformities. J Bone Joint Surg Am. 1982;64(8):1158–63. PubMed PMID: 7130229. Epub 1982/10/01. eng.
51. Cheema JI, Grissom LE, Harcke HT. Radiographic characteristics of lower-extremity bowing in children. Radiographics. 2003;23(4):871–80. PubMed PMID: 12853662. Epub 2003/07/11. eng.
52. Langenskiold A. Tibia vara. A critical review. Clin Orthop Relat Res. 1989;246:195–207. PubMed PMID: 2670387. Epub 1989/09/01. eng.
53. Ho-Fung V, Jaimes C, Delgado J, Davidson RS, Jaramillo D. MRI evaluation of the knee in children with infantile Blount disease: tibial and extra-tibial findings. Pediatr Radiol. 2013;43(10):1316–26. PubMed PMID: 23615630. Epub 2013/04/26. eng.
54. Craig JG, van Holsbeeck M, Zaltz I. The utility of MR in assessing Blount disease. Skeletal Radiol. 2002;31(4):208–13. PubMed PMID: 11904688. Epub 2002/03/21. eng.
55. Shore RM, Chesney RW. Rickets: part I. Pediatr Radiol. 2013;43(2):140–51. PubMed PMID: 23208530. Epub 2012/12/05. eng.
56. Shore RM, Chesney RW. Rickets: part II. Pediatr Radiol. 2013;43(2):152–72. PubMed PMID: 23179485. Epub 2012/11/28. eng.
57. Al Kaissi A, Farr S, Ganger R, Klaushofer K, Grill F. Windswept lower limb deformities in patients with hypophosphataemic rickets. Swiss Med Wkly. 2013;143:w13904. PubMed PMID: 24318043. Epub 2013/12/10. eng.
58. Cozen L. Knock-knee deformity in children. Congenital and acquired. Clin Orthop Relat Res. 1990;258:191–203. PubMed PMID: 2203569.
59. Stevens PM. Guided growth for angular correction: a preliminary series using a tension band plate. J Pediatr Orthop. 2007;27(3):253–9. PubMed PMID: 17414005.
60. Staheli LT. Lower positional deformity in infants and children: a review. J Pediatr Orthop. 1990;10(4):559–63. PubMed PMID: 2193037.
61. Ritter MA, DeRosa GP, Babcock JL. Tibial torsion? Clin Orthop Relat Res. 1976;120:159–63. PubMed PMID: 975652.
62. Bruce WD, Stevens PM. Surgical correction of miserable malalignment syndrome. J Pediatr Orthop. 2004;24(4):392–6. PubMed PMID: 15205621. Epub 2004/06/19. eng.
63. Koenig JK, Pring ME, Dwek JR. MR evaluation of femoral neck version and tibial torsion. Pediatr Radiol. 2012;42(1):113–5. PubMed PMID: 21842328.
64. Wybier M, Bossard P. Musculoskeletal imaging in progress: the EOS imaging system. Joint Bone Spine Rev Rhum. 2013;80(3):238–43. PubMed PMID: 23177915.
65. Paley D, Bhave A, Herzenberg JE, Bowen JR. Multiplier method for predicting limb-length discrepancy. J Bone Joint Surg Am. 2000;82-A(10):1432–46. PubMed PMID: 11057472. Epub 2000/11/01. eng.
66. Moseley CF. A straight-line graph for leg-length discrepancies. J Bone Joint Surg Am. 1977;59(2):174–9. PubMed PMID: 845200.
67. Sabharwal S, Kumar A. Methods for assessing leg length discrepancy. Clin Orthop Relat Res. 2008;466(12):2910–22. PubMed PMID: 18836788. Pubmed Central PMCID: 2628227.

The Lower Extremity: Acquired Disorders

14

Ingrid Kjellin

Contents

Abstract

This chapter begins with a discussion of fractures that are encountered in the pediatric knee. Acute avulsion fractures are initially presented, such as intercondylar tibial eminence fractures, patellar sleeve fractures, and tibial tuberosity avulsion fractures. Chronic injuries of the extensor apparatus are then addressed, including Sinding-Larsen-Johansson disease, jumper's knee, and Osgood-Schlatter disease. The subsequent section presents a range of stress fractures from stress injuries in recreational and competitive sports to patellar stress fractures and toddler's fractures. Late-onset tibia vara is also discussed. Meniscal and ligamentous injuries are then addressed, as well as plica syndrome and popliteal cyst. The chapter concludes with a section on osteochondral lesions, covering acute chondral lesions, osteochondritis dissecans, and chondromalacia patella.

Many acquired disorders about the knee are unique to children, and those that occur in both children and adults typically have unique clinical and imaging characteristics in the pediatric age group. We present in detail disorders that are unique to children, whereas those that occur in both children and adults are discussed more briefly, highlighting the salient differentiating points. The maturing skeleton may respond

I. Kjellin, MD
Radsource, 400 S. Bridge View Drive,
Anaheim Hills, CA 92808, USA
e-mail: ingrid@drosenbergmd.com

R. Stein-Wexler et al. (eds.), *Pediatric Orthopedic Imaging*,
DOI 10.1007/978-3-642-45381-6_14, © Springer-Verlag Berlin Heidelberg 2015

to trauma with physeal fractures and avulsion fractures. Disorders such as Sinding-Larson-Johansson disease, jumper's knee, and Osgood-Schlatter disease are generally limited to the adolescent age group. The stress that occurs as a child begins to walk may result in the toddler's fracture, which is limited to very young children. Late-onset tibia vara, on the other hand, is unique to older children. Although meniscal and ligamentous injuries occur in both adults and children, some types of tears are more common in children, and developmental anomalies of the lateral meniscus may predispose it to injury.

1 Fractures

1.1 Acute Avulsion Fractures

Intercondylar Tibial Eminence Fracture (Box 14.1)

Box 14.1: Intercondylar Tibial Eminence Fracture

Forceful hyperextension or direct blow

Type	I	Minimal displacement of fragment
	II	Fragment elevated anteriorly
	III	Separation of fragment
	IV	Fragment separated and comminuted or rotated

Intercondylar tibial eminence avulsion fractures are one of the most common knee fractures in children and are typically caused by forceful knee hyperextension or a direct blow to the distal femur while the knee is in flexion. The traumatic tensile forces typically result in stretching or partial tearing of the anterior cruciate ligament (ACL) before the bone fractures at the tibial insertion of the ligament [1]. These fractures may be displaced and/or comminuted and are categorized into four types according to the Meyers and McKeever system (Fig. 14.1), which guides treatment [2]. In type I injury, the fragment is minimally displaced, and the fracture is treated conservatively with immobilization. The fragment is elevated anteriorly in type II injury, and closed reduction with immobilization usually suffices for this hinge-type fracture. In types III and IV, the fragment is separated from the tibia, but, in addition, in type IV, the fragment is comminuted or rotated. These displaced fractures were formerly treated with open reduction and internal fixation, but they are now managed arthroscopically. A partial ACL tear at the time of injury may result in postoperative joint laxity. This is a frequent finding on physical examination but rarely requires ligament reconstruction.

Imaging

Radiographs provide initial staging (the avulsed tibial eminence fragment should not be mistaken for an intra-articular osteochondral loose body) (Fig. 14.2). Cross-sectional imaging is often required for preoperative planning. Computed tomography (CT) shows the configuration and orientation of the displaced fragment, whereas magnetic resonance imaging (MRI) reveals concomitant meniscal and ligamentous tears, osteochondral lesions, and possible entrapment of tissue beneath the fragment (Fig. 14.3).

Patellar Sleeve Fracture (Box 14.2)

Box 14.2: Patellar Sleeve Fracture

Forceful contraction of quadriceps

Age: 8–12 years old (patellar ossification incomplete)

Radiographs	Subtle, small fragment distant from patellar lower pole
MRI	Important to define extent

A patellar sleeve fracture is an acute avulsion injury that affects the sleeve of the cartilaginous inferior pole of an incompletely ossified patella. The injury is seen in children between the ages of 8 and 12 years after forceful contraction of the quadriceps muscle against resistance. Clinical manifestations include a high-riding patella as well as limited ability to extend the knee.

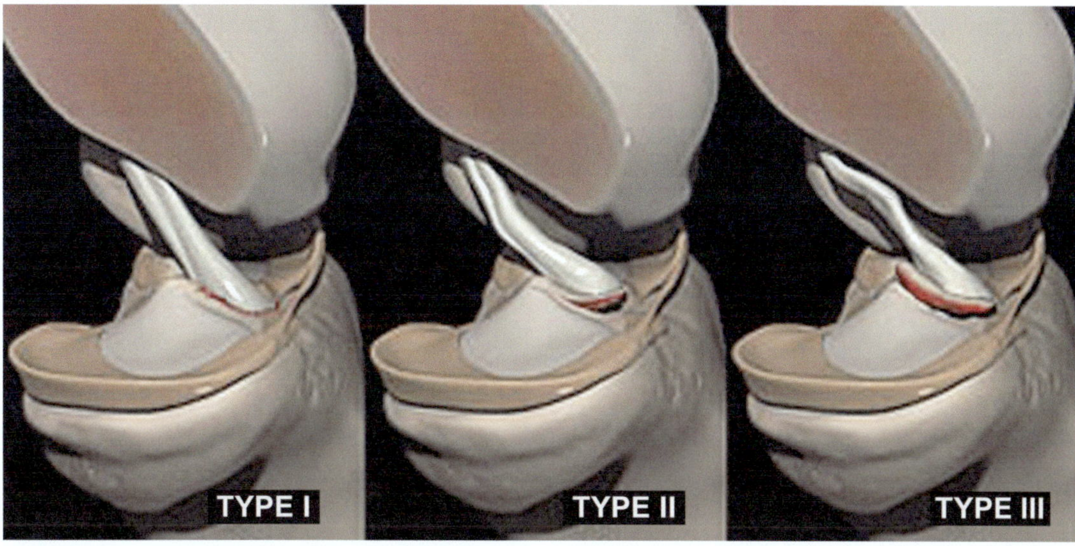

Fig. 14.1 Tibial intercondylar eminence fracture classification system (according to Meyers and McKeever). A type IV fracture, which is displaced and comminuted, was added to the original system (not shown here) (3D graphic representation courtesy of Michael Stadnick)

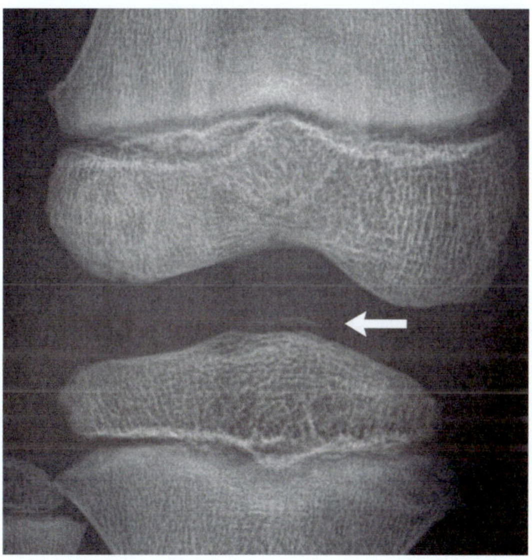

Fig. 14.2 Recent tibial intercondylar eminence fracture in a 7-year-old. There is a small avulsed fragment (*arrow*)

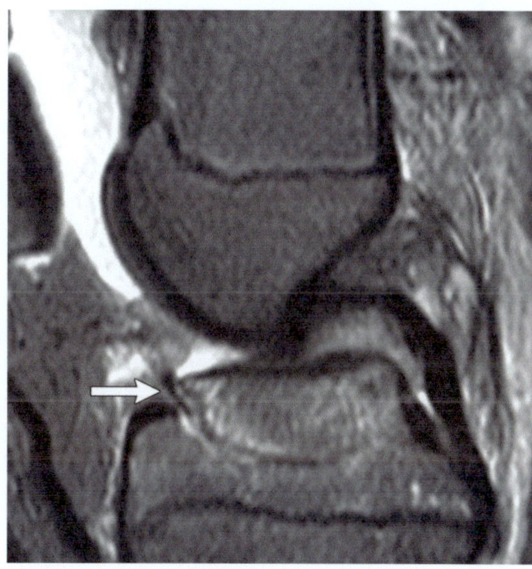

Fig. 14.3 Acute tibial intercondylar eminence fracture. T2-weighted (T2-W) fat-suppressed (FS) sagittal image shows elevation of the anterior aspect of the fragment, while the posterior aspect of the fragment is non-displaced (hinged, Type II). The transverse meniscal ligament (*arrow*) is trapped beneath the fragment

Imaging

Radiographic findings may be very subtle and are easily missed. A small avulsion fragment may be positioned a variable distance from the inferior pole of the patella. MRI may provide important information regarding the full extent of injury, such as the exact size and the full extent of displacement of the avulsed cartilage sleeve [3] (Fig. 14.4). MRI informs treatment and determines need for internal fixation.

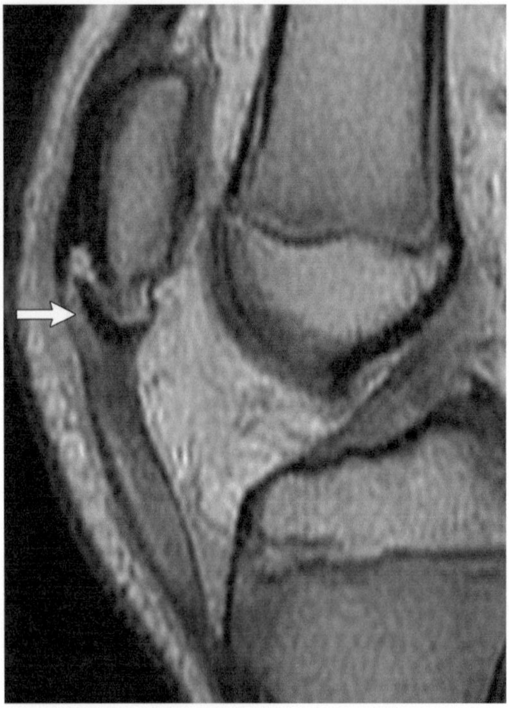

Fig. 14.4 Subacute non-displaced patellar sleeve fracture in an 11-year-old. T1-weighted (T1-W) sagittal image shows thickening and irregularity of the inferior aspect of the patellar growth cartilage (*arrow*)

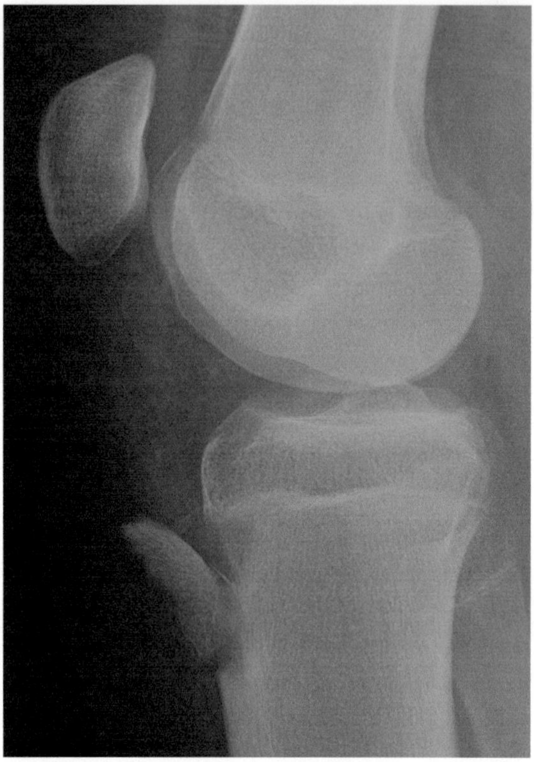

Fig. 14.5 Acute tibial tuberosity fracture in a 16-year-old male. The avulsed fragment is retracted and rotated almost 180°

Tibial Tuberosity Avulsion Fracture

The tibial tuberosity forms from an anteroinferior cartilaginous extension of the tibial epiphysis and fuses with the parent bone at age 13–15 in girls and age 15–19 in boys [4]. The physis of the tuberosity matures from fibrocartilage to columnar cartilage and ultimately to bone. During this maturation process the tibial tuberosity is relatively weak and especially susceptible to tensile forces. Acute avulsion of the tibial tuberosity is uncommon but may occur after active knee extension and vigorous contraction of the quadriceps muscle. Patients typically present with acute pain and swelling over the tibial tuberosity, usually preceded by jumping; the condition is most common in adolescent males involved in sports [5]. More severe fractures also involve hemarthrosis, loss of knee extension, and a high-riding patella. Osgood-Schlatter disease predisposes to the injury. The configuration of the proximal tibial epiphyseal cartilage explains the propensity for some tibial tuberosity fractures to involve the anterior aspect of the articular surface of the tibia.

Both degree of displacement and fragment size determine treatment. Small and minimally displaced fractures are treated with immobilization. Displaced fractures are managed surgically with open reduction and internal fixation. Significant complications after surgery are uncommon.

Imaging

Radiography shows fragment size and extent of displacement. The avulsed tuberosity is typically either hinged upward or proximally retracted (Fig. 14.5). MRI helps evaluate the articular surface and possible concomitant internal joint derangement (Fig. 14.6).

1.2 Chronic Avulsion Injuries of the Extensor Apparatus of the Knee

The extensor apparatus of the knee consists of several codependent structures. If chronically stressed by strong traction forces, this apparatus

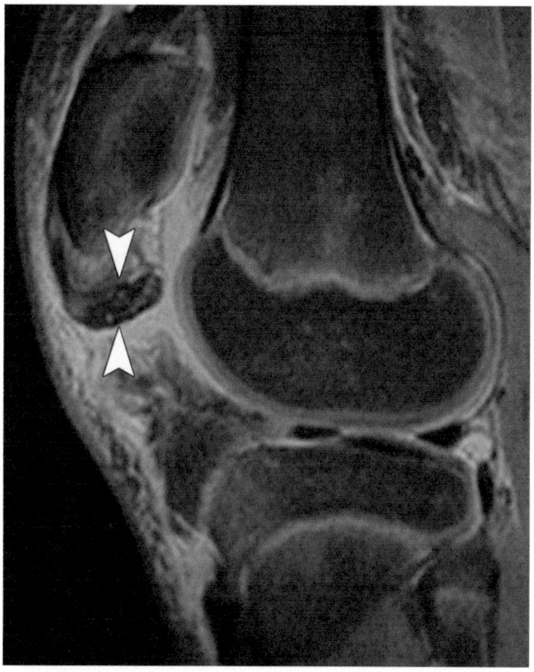

Fig. 14.6 Acute avulsion of the tibial tuberosity in a 14-year-old male. T2-W FS sagittal image shows severe retraction of the tuberosity fragment (*arrowheads*) and patella alta with diffuse edema of the anterior subcutaneous tissues and Hoffa's fat pad

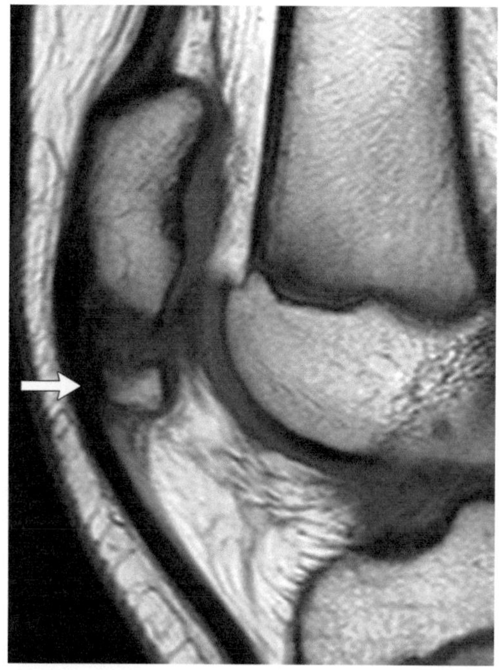

Fig. 14.7 Sinding-Larsen-Johansson disease. T1-W sagittal image shows chronic altered contour of the inferior pole of the patella with adjacent fragmentation. The proximal portion of the patellar tendon is mildly thickened, consistent with tendinosis (*arrow*)

can fail at the levels of the patella, patellar tendon, and tibial tuberosity. Although patients typically present with chronic anterior knee pain, chronic avulsion injury may be encountered as an incidental finding in a patient being imaged for other reasons.

Sinding-Larsen-Johansson Disease (Box 14.3)

Sinding-Larsen-Johansson disease is characterized by osseous avulsion injury at the inferior pole of the patella. It is most common in children between the ages of 10 and 14 years with a history of repetitive microtrauma. Patients present with limited knee motion as well as swelling and tenderness over the lower patella. Patella alta may be present. Successful nonoperative treatments include anti-inflammatory medication, quadriceps flexibility exercises, and activity modification. In most cases, as the lesion heals, fragments are gradually incorporated into the patella [6]. Symptoms generally resolve within 12–18 months; if they persist, surgical excision of non-united ossicles may be necessary [7].

Box 14.3: Sinding-Larsen-Johansson Disease (Inferior Patellar Pole Fracture)

Repetitive microtrauma

Age: 10–14 years

Radiographs	1 or more bone fragments near the inferior patella
MRI	Abnormal signal lower pole of the patella
	Thickened proximal patellar tendon
	Edematous Hoffa's fat pad

Imaging

Radiographs may demonstrate one or more osseous densities adjacent to the inferior patella. Ultrasound (US) can help with initial diagnosis and with monitoring of disease [8]. MRI shows abnormal signal within the inferior pole of the patella with adjacent fragmentation and changes in the osseous contour (Fig. 14.7). The proximal end of the patellar tendon is often thickened.

If there is superimposed acute injury, Hoffa's fat pad may be diffusely edematous [9].

Differential Diagnosis

Accessory ossification centers at the inferior patella may be confused with avulsion fragments, but these are rare. Fragmentation has been reported in patients with spastic lower extremities. After patellar dislocation, small fragments may be seen at the inferomedial patella, resembling findings of Sinding-Larsen-Johansson disease. However, other findings of patellar instability and dislocation should be apparent as well (see Chap. 13).

Jumper's Knee (Patellar Tendinosis) (Box 14.4)

Box 14.4: Jumper's Knee

Age: children approaching bone maturity

Usually affects proximal 1/3 of patellar tendon (occasionally distal 1/3)

Radiographs	Normal or soft tissue swelling
US	Thickened tendon with hypoechoic areas
MRI	Increased T1 and T2 signal
	Patellar marrow edema
	+/– Superimposed tendon tears

While Sinding-Larsen-Johansson disease results in osseous avulsion in children approaching osseous maturity, once the patella is fully developed and completely ossified, overuse and tensile forces injure the patellar tendon rather than the bone. Jumping and sports that involve repetitive jumping and landing tend to cause this injury. Usually, only the proximal third of the patellar tendon is affected, but occasionally the distal tendon is injured as well. Clinical manifestations are the same as in Sinding-Larsen-Johansson disease and are related to patellar tendinosis. Pathologic findings include mucoid degeneration, fibrinoid necrosis, and failure of tendon fibers. Accordingly, the preferred terminology is patellar "tendinosis" rather than "tendinitis." Patellar tracking abnormalities are associated with jumper's knee. Symptoms usually respond to conservative treatment, but a small number of patients require surgical tendon debridement [10]. The patellar tendon rarely ruptures.

Imaging

Radiographs are usually normal but occasionally demonstrate soft tissue swelling and patellar tendon thickening. US can assist with diagnosis and disease monitoring. The tendon appears enlarged and demonstrates hypoechoic regions [8]. MRI reveals anteroposterior thickening and increased signal within the tendon on T1-weighted (T1-W) and T2-weighted (T2-W) images (Fig. 14.8). The adjacent patella may exhibit marrow edema. Superimposed partial tendon tears typically affect the most proximal and posterior tendon fibers and appear hyperintense on T2-W images. However, caution must be exercised, as the normal tendon may demonstrate increased signal, especially on gradient-echo (GRE) sequences. Furthermore, the thickness of the normal patellar tendon varies, and this can lead to false-positive cases. Both ends of the tendon may normally appear slightly thickened.

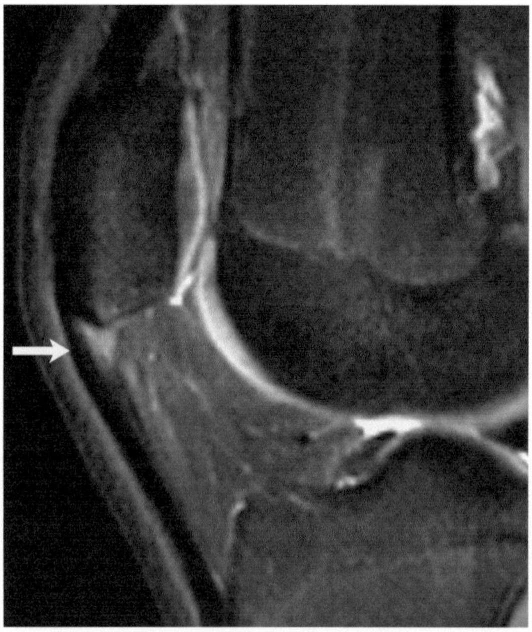

Fig. 14.8 Jumper's knee. T2-W FS sagittal image shows thickening and hyperintensity of the proximal portion of the tendon (*arrow*), indicating mild tendinosis

Osgood-Schlatter Disease (Box 14.5)

Box 14.5: Osgood-Schlatter Disease

Age: adolescent males during rapid growth

Radiographs	Soft tissue swelling, edema over tibial tuberosity
	Edema in Hoffa's fat pad
	Irregular bone densities at tibial tuberosity (if ossified)
	If cartilaginous, ossifications evident at 3–4 weeks
	Fragments normally fuse to tuberosity but may remain separate
MRI	Infrapatellar bursitis
	Thick distal patellar tendon
	Fragmentation of tibial tuberosity

Osgood-Schlatter disease has been described as traction "apophysitis" and affects the attachment of the extensor apparatus to the tibial tuberosity. This condition is typically encountered during periods of rapid growth in active adolescent males. Common clinical manifestations include activity-related recurrent pain as well as tenderness and swelling at the tibial tuberosity. Associated tibial tuberosity deformity may mimic a bone tumor. The pathogenesis of Osgood-Schlatter disease is similar to Sinding-Larsen-Johansson disease: repeated tensile forces lead to microfracture and avulsion of the unossified cartilage at the tibial tuberosity [11]. Bilateral involvement occurs in up to 50 % of cases. Patella alta, valgus alignment at the knee, and an internally rotated tibia or patella may predispose to the condition. The treatment and prognosis are also similar to Sinding-Larsen-Johansson disease. In most cases, the disorder is benign and self-limiting, resolving with skeletal maturity. Surgical treatment, specifically ossicle excision and tibial tubercleplasty, is reserved for patients who do not respond to conservative treatment and should only be performed after physeal closure [7].

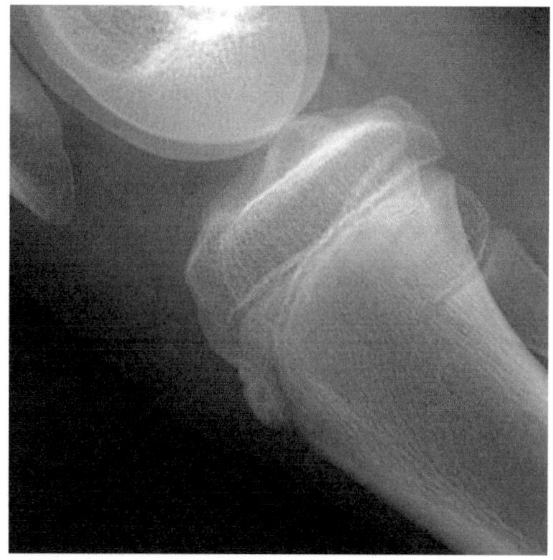

Fig. 14.9 Osgood-Schlatter disease in a 12-year-old boy. There is subcutaneous edema and swelling anterior to the tibial tuberosity without fragmentation. Diffuse edema in Hoffa's fat pad (Courtesy of Liliane Gibbs)

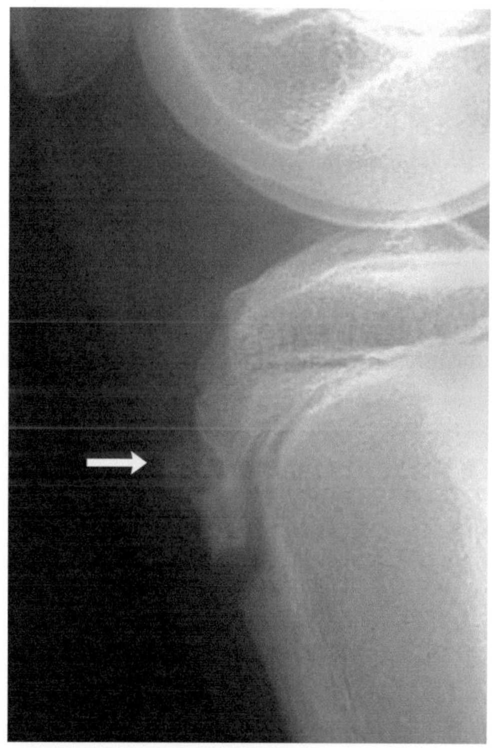

Fig. 14.10 Osgood-Schlatter disease. Fragmentation (*arrow*), subcutaneous edema, and swelling at the tibial tuberosity along with mild thickening of the deep infrapatellar bursa (Courtesy of Liliane Gibbs)

Imaging

Imaging findings depend on age as well as the duration and cyclic nature of disease. Radiographs help confirm the clinical diagnosis and exclude other entities that could cause pain. Typical radiographic findings include soft tissue swelling and edema over the tibial tuberosity, edema of Hoffa's fat pad, and one or more irregular osseous densities at the tibial tuberosity (Figs. 14.9 and 14.10). If the tuberosity is completely cartilaginous, there will initially be no direct evidence of avulsion; however, after 3–4 weeks, radiographs may show ossification of avulsed fragments. With time, soft tissue swelling and edema improve, but fragments continue to appear displaced. During the later phases of disease, findings vary. All fragments may unite, and the tibial tuberosity may resume its normal appearance. However, residual prominence and deformity of the tibial tuberosity related to malunion or nonunion of fragments may cause symptoms in adulthood. The normal irregular ossification of the cartilaginous extension of the proximal tibial epiphysis at the developing tibial tuberosity should not be mistaken for pathology [4].

US helps both in initial diagnosis and in monitoring disease course. It can document fragmentation and healing of the tibial tuberosity ossification center as well as the extent of inflammation at the deep infrapatellar bursa. MRI findings include infrapatellar bursitis, mild thickening of the distal patellar tendon, edema both within the subcutaneous fat and at Hoffa's fat pad at the tibial tuberosity, and fragmentation of the tibial tuberosity (Figs. 14.11 and 14.12).

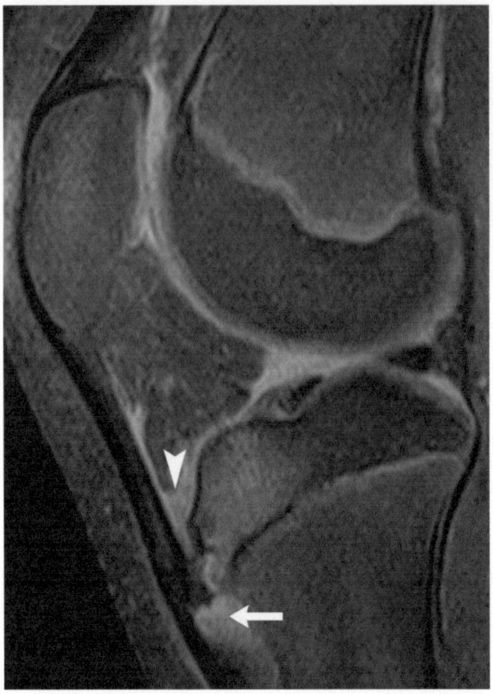

Fig. 14.11 Osgood-Schlatter disease. T2-W FS sagittal image shows mild diffuse edema within the subcutaneous fat at the tibial tuberosity, mild thickening of the deep infrapatellar bursa (*arrowhead*), and diffuse marrow edema of the anterior proximal tibia including the tibial tuberosity (*arrow*)

1.3 Stress Injuries

Osseous stress injury is a common cause of pain in the lower extremity in children and adolescents participating in competitive sports, especially running. The most common sites of involvement in the lower extremities are the tibia and fibula. The femur, tarsals, and metatarsals are less commonly affected [12, 13]. (See Chaps. 12 and 16 for discussion of stress fractures in the hip and foot.) Stress fractures have been divided into two types: fatigue fractures, occurring when normal bone is exposed to abnormal forces, and insufficiency fractures, resulting from demineralized bone exposed to normal loads.

Stress Injuries of the Tibia and Fibula (Box 14.6)

The tibia and fibula are common sites of stress injury. Clinical manifestations include pain, swelling, and limp. Pain often subsides with rest. Callus, swelling, and localized warmth may be palpable.

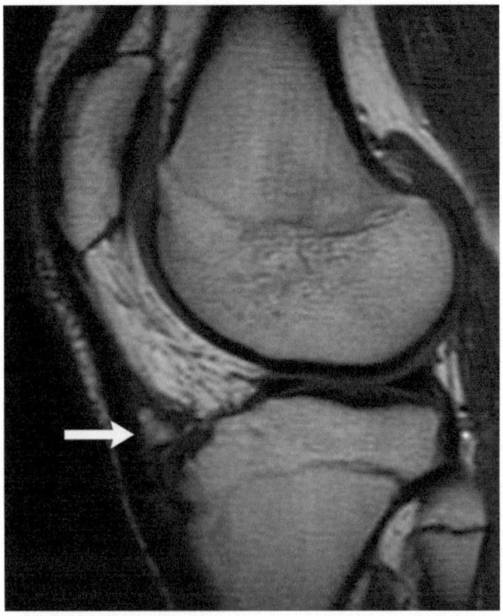

Fig. 14.12 Old avulsion of the tibial tuberosity secondary to Osgood-Schlatter disease in a 16-year-old boy. There is a well-corticated non-united fragment (*arrow*) in the distal patellar tendon. The distal patellar tendon is also slightly thickened, consistent with tendinosis

Box 14.6: Stress Injuries in the Tibia and Fibula

Fracture

Usually the *tibia*, transverse posteromedial proximal diaphysis

Occasionally longitudinal, anterior

Fibula: less common, isolated, or with tibia

Radiographs	Positive at 2 weeks in 50 %	
	Periosteal reaction	
	Focal lucency, transverse band of sclerosis	
NM	Early	Ill-defined increased uptake
	Late	Linear band-like uptake
MRI	Linear hypointense zone with surrounding edema	
	Grade I	Mild periosteal edema, normal marrow
	II	More periosteal edema
		Marrow edema only on T2
	III	Periosteal edema
		Marrow edema on T1 and T2
	IV	Fracture line
Shin splints		
NM	Increased uptake only on delayed sequence	
	Diffuse uptake at posteromedial cortex	

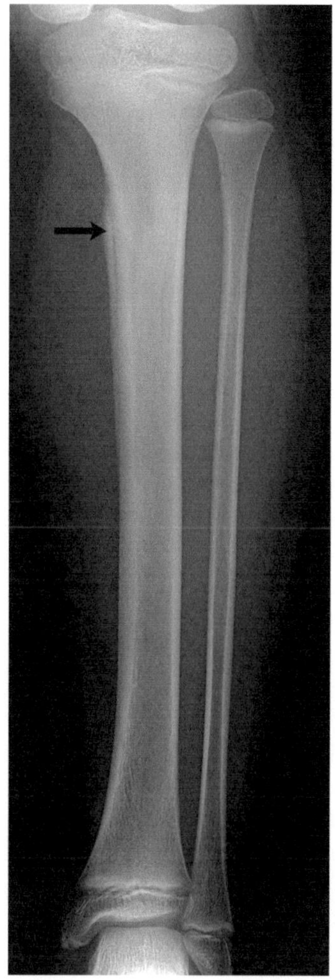

Fig. 14.13 Tibial stress fracture in an 8-year-old boy. There is periosteal reaction and a subtle linear lucency in the proximal tibial diaphysis (*arrow*) (Courtesy of Rebecca Stein-Wexler)

The term "shin splints" refers to activity-induced diffuse pain and tenderness at the posteromedial tibia caused by repetitive avulsion stress at tendinous insertions of the bone; shin splints are part of the spectrum of osseous stress injuries that fall under medial tibial stress syndrome.

Active patients suffer stress fractures when repetitive loads result in imbalanced cortical bone resorption and formation; microfractures then form in these regions. Excessive stress exerted by strong muscles at osseous insertion sites may be an additional cause of injury. The teenage "female athlete triad," a combination of eating disorder, amenorrhea, and osteoporosis, is among the many potential causes of bone stress injury.

Most tibial stress fractures are transverse and involve the posteromedial cortex of the proximal diaphysis. Tibial stress fractures occasionally have a longitudinal orientation or involve the anterior cortex. Fibular stress fractures present either in combination with tibial stress injuries or in isolation. Stress fractures of the tibia and fibula typically are treated with rest and heal 4–8 weeks after ceasing the offending activity. Patients can usually return to maximum exercise within 8–12 weeks [14].

Imaging

Radiographic findings are absent or minimal for the first few weeks, with a sensitivity of only 10–25 % for early fracture detection. Follow-up radiographs at 2 weeks or later are helpful in only 50 % of cases and may demonstrate periosteal reaction, focal cortical lucency, and a linear sclerotic band (Fig. 14.13).

Radionuclide bone scintigraphy is a useful imaging tool for confirming suspected stress fractures. In early stages of osseous stress injury, regions of radiotracer uptake are poorly defined; in more advanced stages, a band-like area of increased uptake corresponds to the fracture. Shin splints are diagnosed on bone scintigraphy when increased radionuclide activity is present only on the delayed phase of the study, with diffuse uptake along the posteromedial cortex of the tibia [15]. Scintigraphy should not be used to monitor stress fractures, because even after symptoms have resolved radionuclide uptake continues for up to 18 months due to ongoing healing and osseous remodeling.

MRI has similar sensitivity to bone scintigraphy but is much more specific. A stress fracture is characteristically incomplete and appears as a linear zone of decreased signal intensity on both T1- and T2-W images, with surrounding marrow edema. There are also varying degrees of endosteal sclerosis, cortical thickening, and periosteal edema. Extensive thickening of the anterior cortex of the tibial shaft is unusual and is difficult to treat. A grading system for medial tibial stress reaction using MRI is based on specific imaging sequences and increasing severity of osseous changes [16]. Grade 1 injuries have mild periosteal edema with normal-appearing marrow (Fig. 14.14). Grade 2 injuries have more advanced periosteal edema in combination with marrow edema evident on T2-W images only. Grade 3 injuries have periosteal edema in combination with marrow edema on both T1- and T2-W images. Grade 4 injuries are associated with a fracture line (Fig. 14.15). MRI is more accurate than radionuclide bone scan in correlating osseous involvement with symptoms; it also better evaluates healing.

Diagnostic difficulties may arise when radiographic findings show extensive periostitis and sclerosis, which can resemble infection, osteoid osteoma, and even a malignant neoplasm. MRI can aid in making the correct diagnosis. With infection, soft tissue involvement is generally more extensive than with osseous stress injury. An osteoid osteoma demonstrates a nidus within or near the cortex and is surrounded by extensive marrow edema. If there is a malignant osseous neoplasm, marrow edema is relatively mild, but there will be a mass with marrow infiltration. Normal vascular grooves within the bone should not be mistaken for stress fractures.

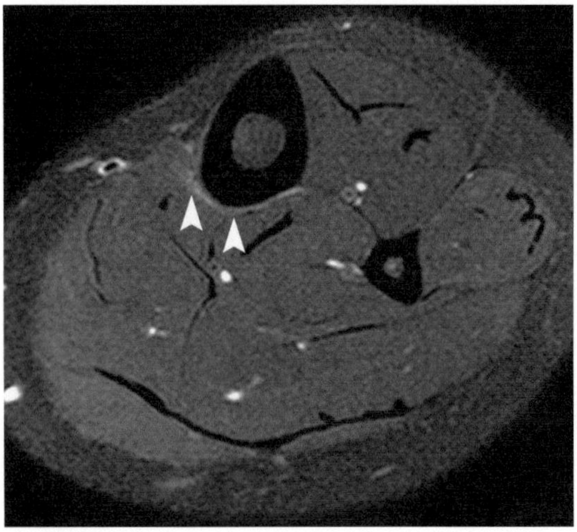

Fig. 14.14 Grade 1 medial tibial stress injury. T2-W FS axial image shows mild diffuse periosteal edema at the posteromedial tibia (*arrowheads*). Marrow signal is normal

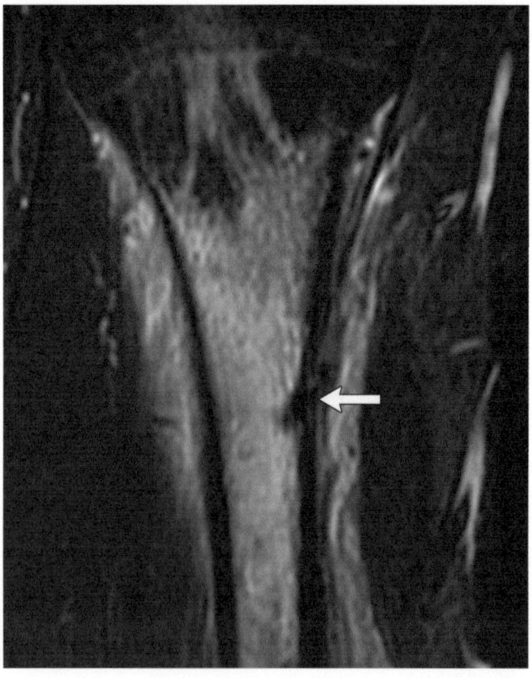

Fig. 14.15 Grade 4 medial tibial stress injury. T2-W FS coronal image of the proximal tibia shows an incomplete fracture (*arrow*) at the medial cortex with diffuse marrow edema. Soft tissue edema and mild diffuse periosteal reaction are also present

Adductor Insertion Avulsion Syndrome

Adductor insertion avulsion syndrome, also known as "thigh splints," presents with insidious onset of pain in the groin or thigh and is typically seen in young runners and ballet dancers. Repetitive avulsion stress at the insertions of the adductor muscle group can produce traction periostitis and even pseudotumors at the medial aspect of the proximal to mid femur [17]. These osseous changes can progress with continued stress and lead to a femoral shaft stress fracture. Treatment of adductor insertion avulsion syndrome consists of a short period of rest (1–4 weeks) followed by a gradual return to activity.

Imaging

Radiographs may be normal or there may be subtle periosteal reaction or cortical thickening at the medial aspect of the proximal to mid femoral diaphysis. Bone scintigraphy shows a distribution of uptake similar to that seen with shin splints (see discussion above). On MRI, the periosteum in the medial aspect of the femoral shaft is thickened and has abnormal signal on T2-W images (Fig. 14.16). Additional abnormalities include cortical thickening along with edema and endosteal sclerosis in the adjacent marrow cavity. The differential diagnosis is similar to that of other osseous stress injuries.

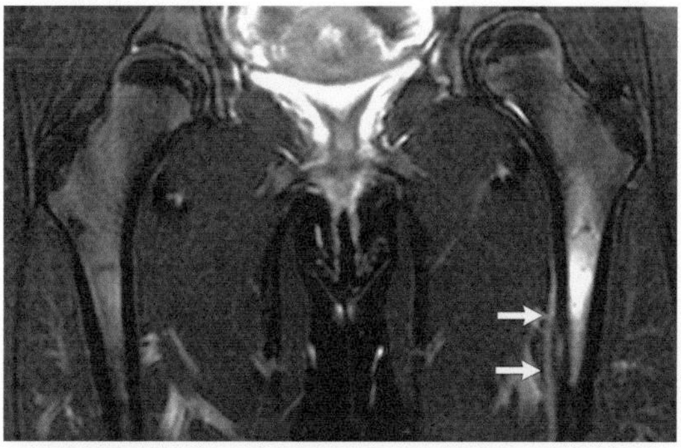

Fig. 14.16 Adductor insertion avulsion syndrome. Short tau inversion recovery (STIR) coronal image shows diffuse marrow hyperintensity with periosteal thickening and edema at the insertion site of the adductor muscles (*arrows*) on the left. The right femur is normal

Patellar Stress Fractures

Patellar stress fractures are rare in active children. However, if these fractures are not recognized and are then subjected to sudden quadriceps muscle contraction, they may propagate and become complete. Sports associated with this injury include basketball, tennis, soccer, high jumping, weight lifting, and hurdling. Patients present with anterior knee pain, aggravated by flexion. Bending forces across the patella, with tension on its superficial surface and compression on its deep surface, result in a transverse fracture, typically at the inferior pole [18]. Similar fractures have been reported in children with spastic cerebral palsy.

Imaging

Radiographic findings are absent or subtle if fractures are non-displaced. MRI shows transverse, linear hypointensity, usually in the anterior surface of the inferior pole of the patella (Fig. 14.17). A bipartite patella or an accessory ossification center should not be mistaken for a patellar stress fracture.

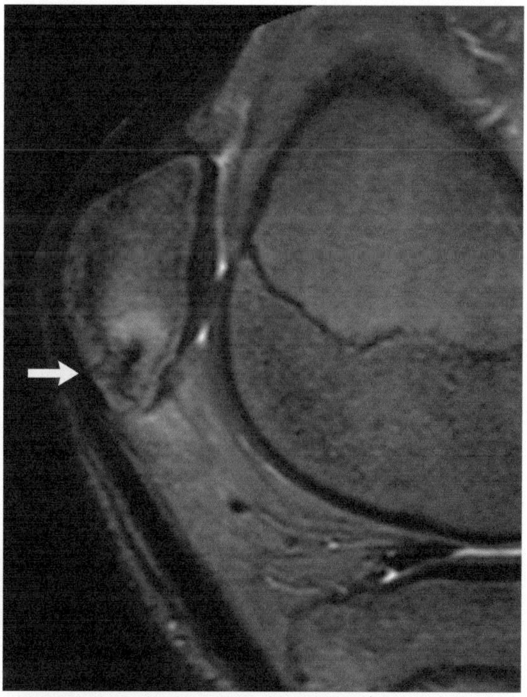

Fig. 14.17 Patellar stress fracture. T2-W FS sagittal image shows a non-displaced fracture (*arrow*) in the inferior pole of the patella with mild marrow edema

Chronic Physeal Stress Injury
(Box 14.7)

Box 14.7: Chronic Physeal Stress Injury

Age: 8–15-year-old high-level athletes

Radiographs	Physes of distal femur/proximal tibia wide
MRI	Wide physis, isointense to physeal cartilage
	Focal physeal irregularity

One of the many causes of chronic knee pain in high-level child athletes is physeal stress injury. Patients present between 8 and 15 years of age [19]. Chronic stress and repetitive microtrauma disrupt the microvascular blood supply to the physis, preventing normal endochondral bone formation. Failure to recognize this abnormality on imaging, or a patient's refusal to cease activity, may result in physeal bone bridging and permanent growth impairment or malalignment.

Imaging

Radiographs and MRI show broad physeal widening in the distal femur and proximal tibia (Fig. 14.18). The region of physeal widening is isointense to physeal cartilage on MRI due to metaphyseal extension of hypertrophic chondrocytes. Superimposed focal physeal irregularity correlates with localized tongue-like extensions of chondrocytes. No physeal or periphyseal fractures have been reported.

Other entities known to cause physeal widening include acute trauma, radiation therapy, infection, rickets, hypophosphatasia, and dysostosis multiplex. Periphyseal edema may be a normal MRI finding during the early stages of physeal closure and does not necessarily represent chronic physeal stress injury. Developmental marrow edema is located about the central portion of the physis (Fig. 14.19). Termed "focal periphyseal edema" (or "FOPE" zone), this marrow edema may be associated with pain but requires no further evaluation [20].

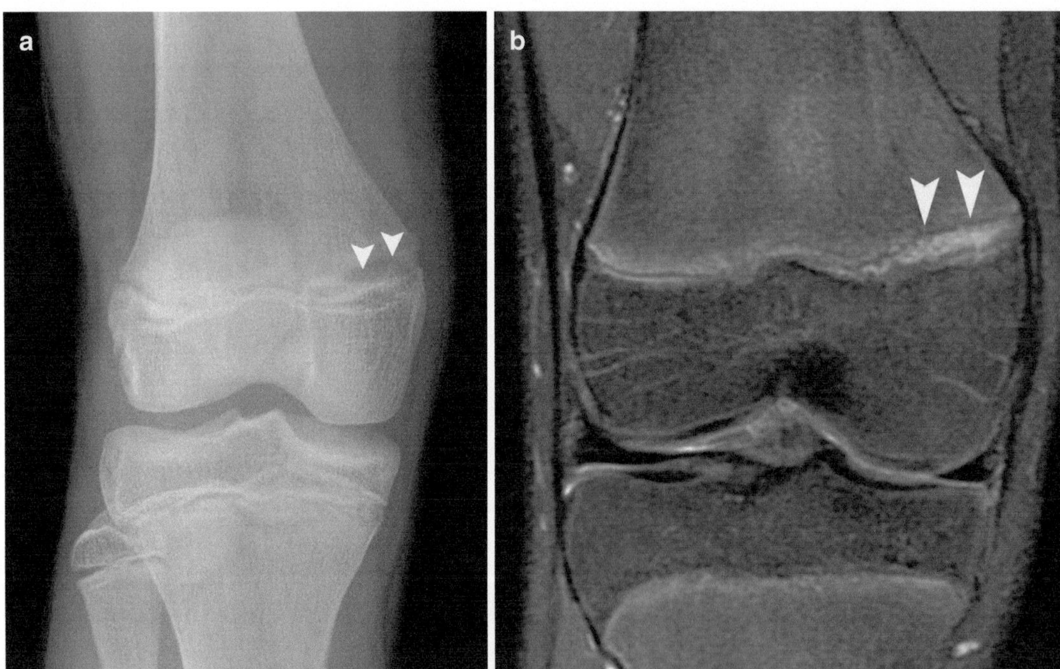

Fig. 14.18 Physeal stress injury in a 14-year-old girl who plays soccer. (**a**) The medial aspect of the distal femoral physis is slightly wide (*arrowheads*). (**b**) T2-W FS coronal image shows focal physeal widening (*arrowheads*) with mild edema of the adjacent marrow. Physeal irregularity results from metaphyseal extension of chondrocytes (Courtesy of Tal Laor, Cincinnati Children's Hospital)

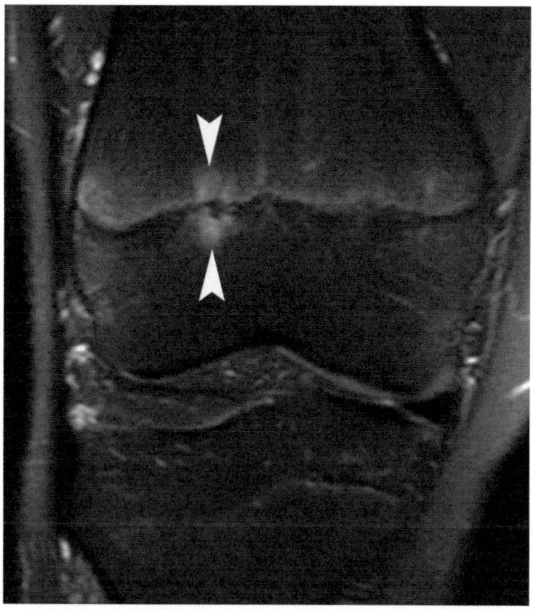

Fig. 14.19 Focal periphyseal edema ("FOPE" zone) in a 15-year-old. T2-W FS coronal image shows marrow edema in the central aspect of the distal femur adjacent to the physis (*arrowheads*)

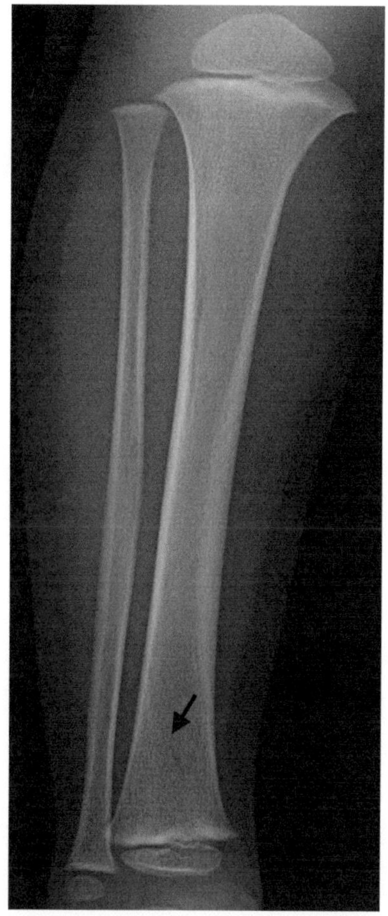

Fig. 14.20 Toddler's fracture in a 2-year-old girl. There is a minimal linear lucency (*arrow*) in the distal tibial diaphysis (Courtesy of Rebecca Stein-Wexler)

Toddler's Fracture

Around the time of early ambulation, young children are susceptible to fractures of the tibia, fibula, and bones of the foot and ankle. The presentation is often delayed because of nonexistent or vague history of injury, inability to localize symptoms, and relatively mild clinical symptoms. Torsional and hyperextension forces during stumbling and falling are plausible mechanisms. The classic toddler's fracture is a non-displaced oblique or spiral fracture of the distal tibial diaphysis [21]. Toddler's fracture also includes plastic bowing deformity of the fibula and transverse fractures of the proximal tibia [22].

Imaging

These fractures may be quite subtle (Fig. 14.20), and radiographs of the tibia and fibula are usually normal in patients with recent onset of symptoms. Oblique views may demonstrate a subtle lucency that is hidden on routine frontal and lateral views. Follow-up radiographs will demonstrate periosteal new bone and sclerosis in the healing phase of the fracture. Comparison to radiographs of the contralateral side may facilitate detection of the accompanying plastic bowing deformity of the fibula. However, follow-up radiographs are rarely useful for diagnosing plastic bowing deformity, as these injuries heal with minimal if any periosteal new bone.

Bone scintigraphy is highly sensitive and should be considered for the limping child younger than 5 years of age whose pathology does not localize. Disadvantages of scintigraphy include low specificity and high radiation exposure. MRI (Fig. 14.21) is highly sensitive to both osseous and soft tissue injury and lacks ionizing radiation but requires sedation in the young child, especially if symptoms are nonfocal and a large area must therefore be scanned.

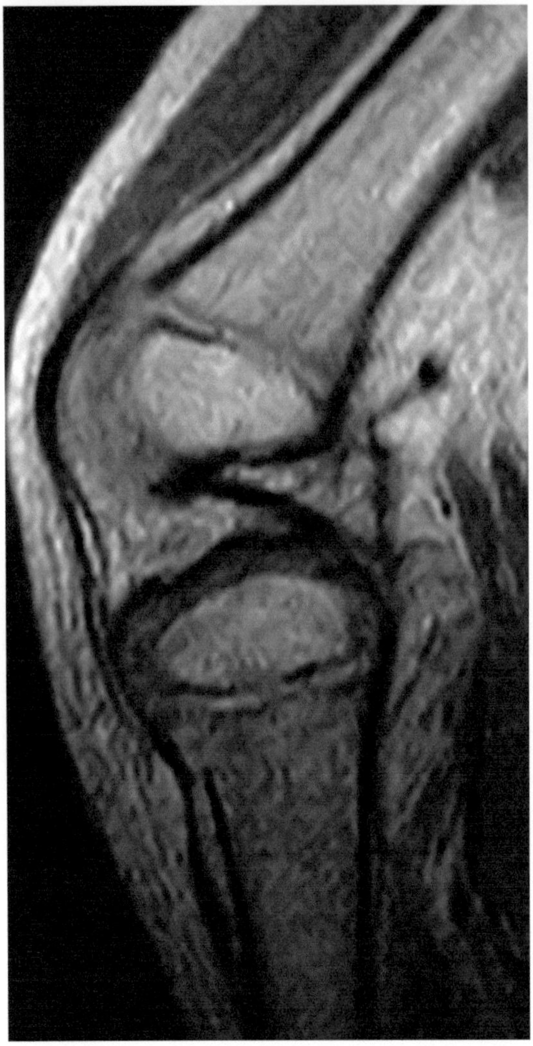

Fig. 14.21 Toddler's fracture in a 3-year-old boy unwilling to walk. T2-W FS sagittal image shows a non-displaced incomplete fracture of the proximal tibial metaphysis with elevation of the adjacent periosteum

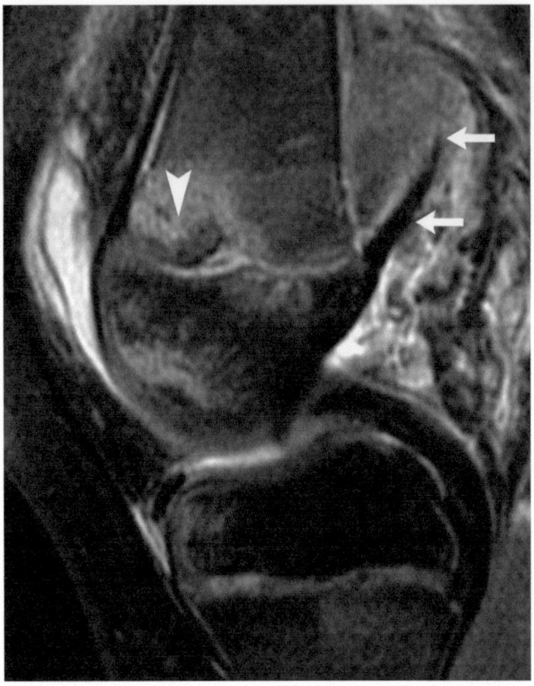

Fig. 14.22 Periosteal injury. T2-W FS sagittal image shows extensive stripping and disruption of the periosteum (*arrows*) of the posterior aspect of the femur, with a recent Salter-Harris II fracture (*arrowhead*)

1.4 Periosteal Injury

The periosteum in children is thicker than in adults, and it contributes to the child's relatively high rate of osteogenesis. This affects the types of pediatric fractures, how they heal, and complications that may arise. Thick periosteum reduces the negative effect of both shearing and tensile forces on the physis. If directly traumatized, the pediatric periosteum is frequently stripped from the bone, but it is less likely to be disrupted circumferentially than in adults. The severity of periosteal injury and the extent of the accompanying hematoma determine the amount of new bone formation. Ongoing osteogenesis of the periosteum contributes to the relative ease of fracture reduction in children and to an overall faster healing process.

The pattern and location of periosteal disruption shed light on the mechanism of injury. The periosteum is typically stripped from the bone surface on the distraction side, but remains intact on the compression side (Fig. 14.22). For example, posterior periosteal disruption at the distal femur suggests a hyperextension-varus-type injury [23]. The mechanism of injury should instigate a search for typical associated injuries, such as partial ACL tear after hyperextension.

In Salter-Harris fractures of the lower and upper limbs, disrupted periphyseal periosteum may be displaced into the physis, most commonly

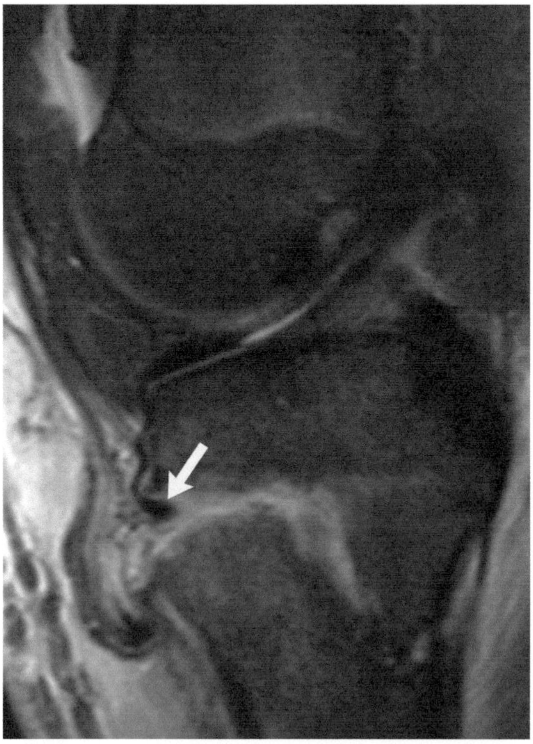

Fig. 14.23 Trapped periosteum with recent Salter II fracture. T2-W FS sagittal image shows hypointense periosteum (*arrow*) trapped in fractured physeal cartilage

at the distal femur or proximal and distal tibia. While these fractures may heal without complications, the trapped periosteum sometimes prevents satisfactory fracture reduction, in turn resulting in premature physeal closure. Open reduction and internal fixation best treat fractures that cannot be reduced due to periosteal entrapment.

Imaging

Damaged periosteum is initially radiographically occult, although eventually the cortical margin may appear slightly indistinct. The damaged periosteum appears hypointense on T2-W MRI. If disrupted periosteum has been displaced into the physis, radiographs performed after attempted reduction show a residual physeal gap. MRI can provide important information that affects clinical management, such as the extent of disruption and displacement of the periosteum [24] (Fig. 14.23).

2 Late-Onset Tibia Vara (Adolescent Blount Disease) (Box 14.8)

Box 14.8: Late-Onset Tibia Vara (Adolescent Blount Disease)

Segmental arrest of growth plate function

Age: 8–15 years old

Radiographs	Moderate	Fragmented proximal medial tibial metaphysis
		Depressed medial tibial plateau
	Advanced	Wide medial tibial physis
		Wedging proximal tibial epiphysis
		+/– Wide lateral tibial and distal femoral physis
MRI	Mild	Invagination of cartilage into metaphysis
		Wide and irregular proximal tibia physis
		T1 hypointensity at proximal medial tibial metaphysis
	Severe	Widening of the entire tibial physis
		Wide femoral physis (especially lateral)

Tibia vara is categorized according to age at onset. Late-onset or adolescent tibia vara affects children between the ages of 8 and 15 and is less common than either the infantile or juvenile forms (see Chap. 13 for discussion of early onset tibia vara). Unlike infantile or juvenile disease, adolescent tibia vara is usually unilateral (in as many as 90 % of patients). The pathologic process involves failure of endochondral ossification of the medial growth plate. This usually follows trauma, although it may follow osteomyelitis or occur without identifiable cause. The incidence of post-traumatic tibia vara is increased in obese males of African-American descent. Exaggerated medial stress likely causes aberrant ossification [25]. Angular deformity of the proximal tibia may be severe, although the diaphysis remains normal. Epiphysiodesis of the lateral tibial physis and proximal fibula prevents pro-

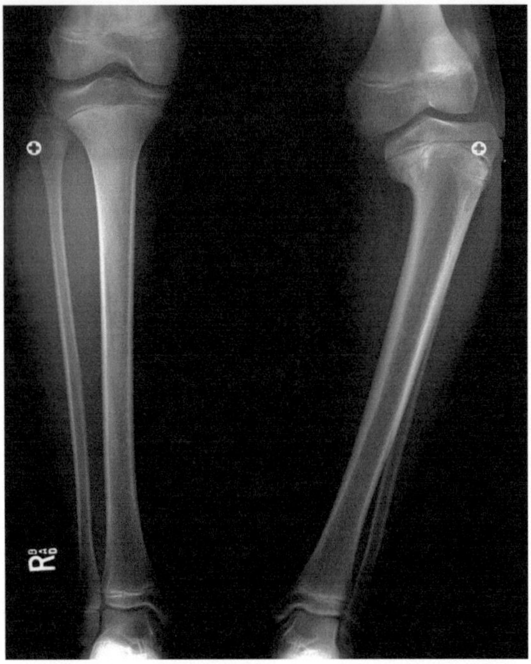

Fig. 14.24 Unilateral late-onset (adolescent) Blount disease in a 15 y/o. There is sclerosis, depression, and buttressing of the medial proximal tibial metaphysis. The adjacent epiphysis is narrow, resulting in depression of the medial tibial plateau (Courtesy of Leslie Grissom)

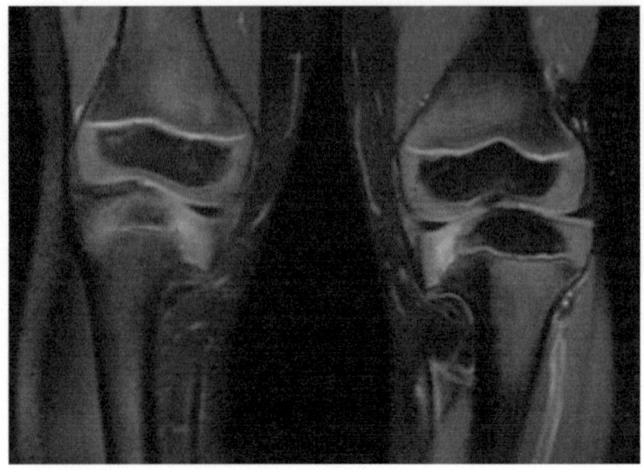

Fig. 14.25 Blount deformity. Coronal T2-W image of both knees shows decreased ossification of the medial tibial epiphysis with depression of the medial aspect of the physis. There is minimal lateral subluxation of the tibias (Courtesy of Tal Laor, Cincinnati Children's Hospital)

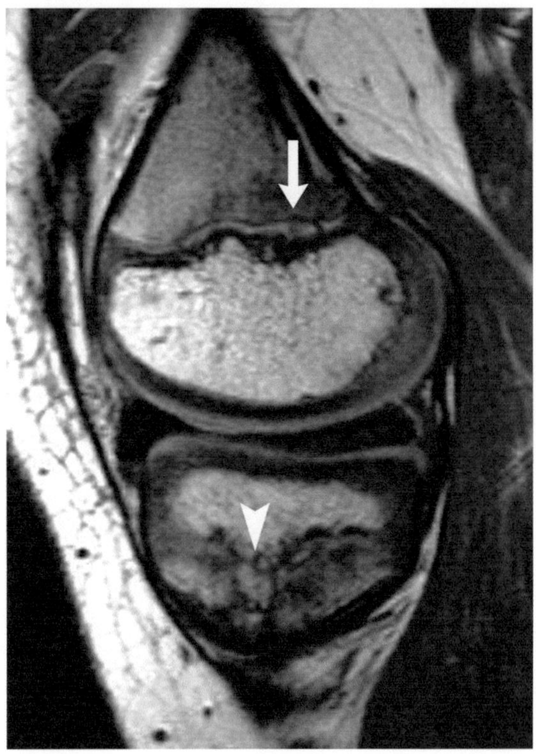

Fig. 14.26 Late-onset (adolescent) tibia vara. T1-W sagittal image shows focal physeal bone bridging (*arrowhead*). The distal femoral physis is mildly widened (*arrow*). Mild compensatory thickening of the posterior horn of the medial meniscus is also evident (Courtesy of Sjirk Westra)

gression, but tibial osteotomy may be necessary if deformity is severe.

Imaging

Radiographic findings vary with severity of disease. Moderate disease is characterized by fragmentation of the medial proximal tibial metaphysis and depression of the medial tibial plateau. With more advanced involvement, the growth plates appear abnormal. There is widening of the medial tibial growth plate and medial wedging of the proximal tibial epiphysis (Fig. 14.24). The lateral tibial and distal femoral physes may be widened as well. Sclerosis on either side of the growth plate probably represents stress-associated bone formation. Internal tibial torsion is a common component of the deformity. Femoral anteversion is also often increased; there is some evidence that this represents a response to therapeutic intervention [26].

In cases of mild late-onset tibia vara, MRI findings are limited to the medial aspect of the proximal tibial growth plate, which appears wide and irregular. There may be invagination of cartilage into the metaphysis. Decreased T1 signal intensity may be evident in the medial tibial metaphysis adjacent to the physis (Fig. 14.25). With severe disease, MRI shows widening of the entire proximal tibial physis as well as of the distal femoral physis (lateral more than medial). There is invagination of cartilage into the tibial and femoral metaphyses. Bone may bridge the physis [27] (Fig. 14.26).

3 Meniscal and Ligamentous Injury

3.1 Meniscal Tears

Meniscal injury in children is relatively rare. Diagnosis is often delayed, in part due to lack of a compelling clinical history and also because physical findings are often subtle. Children may present with pain and the sensation of snapping or locking; they may report a twisting injury. Joint line tenderness and a positive modified McMurray maneuver (provocative knee flexion to 30–40° with rotational varus and valgus) are moderately sensitive (about 55 %) but fairly specific (about 85 %) for detection of meniscal tears [28].

Meniscal tears often result from a single traumatic episode and are frequently encountered in patients with acute hemarthrosis. Up to 47 % of pediatric patients with acute hemarthrosis exhibit meniscal tears on arthroscopy [29]. Meniscal tears are frequently associated with ACL tears in the pediatric population and have been reported in as many as 79 % of patients [30]. As in adults, the medial meniscus is more commonly torn than the lateral, and the posterior horn is more frequently involved than the anterior horn [31]. (The exception to this is the discoid lateral meniscus, which is especially vulnerable to injury.) Isolated injury of the medial meniscus is more common than isolated injury of the ACL in children.

A discoid meniscus is an anatomic variant with a prevalence of 1.5–4.5 %. Thick and disc like, it typically involves the lateral meniscus, although medial discoid menisci have been reported. Symptoms, if present, include pain, clicking, snapping, and joint locking. In children with discoid lateral meniscus, this meniscus is more likely to tear than the medial, being especially vulnerable to injury.

Meniscal tears may be longitudinal horizontal, longitudinal vertical, bucket-handle, radial,

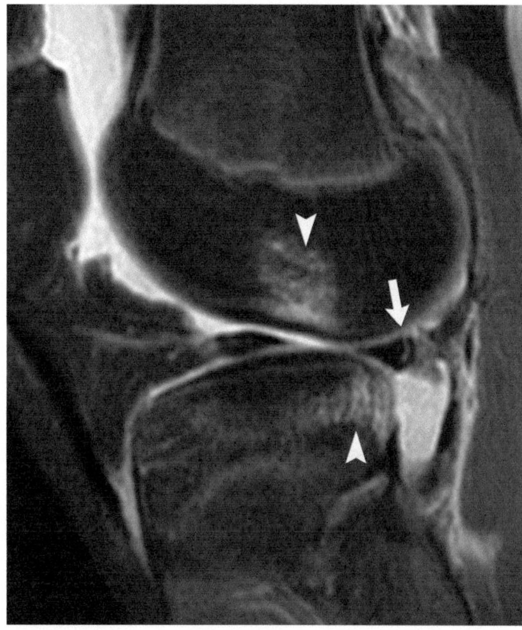

Fig. 14.27 Longitudinal vertical tear (*arrow*) of the posterior horn of the lateral meniscus. T2-W FS image shows contusions (*arrowheads*) of the femoral condyle and posterior tibia caused by rotatory subluxation and impaction at the time of injury. The patient also had an acute anterior cruciate ligament (ACL) tear (not included), suggested by this pattern of marrow edema and by the presence of anterior tibial translation

peripheral, flap, and root tears. The longitudinal vertical tear is most common in pediatrics (Fig. 14.27). This tear is located in the periphery of the meniscus and may progress to a bucket-handle tear if the inner portion of the meniscus is displaced centrally.

If surgically repaired, tears generally heal well due to the abundant blood supply of the developing meniscus [32], and surgical repair is recommended for most meniscal tears in skeletally immature patients [33] (longitudinal vertical tears in the vascular zone may heal spontaneously). Tears amenable to repair include most longitudinal vertical tears and bucket-handle tears in which the displaced portion of the meniscus is not significantly damaged. Short-term results from meniscal repair are encouraging, especially if the procedure is performed in conjunction with ACL reconstruction. Meniscal debridement or a limited partial meniscectomy is performed for longitudinal horizontal and radial tears. Likelihood of early osteoarthritis after meniscal repair is uncertain, but total meniscectomy commonly leads to premature osteoarthritis and chronic disability.

Imaging

When correlated with arthroscopic evaluation of meniscal tears, MRI is 83 % sensitive and 95 % specific [34]. However, artifacts and normal anatomic structures may simulate meniscal tears in patients of all ages. Young children may demonstrate intermediate signal predominantly within the posterior horn of the medial meniscus, likely a result of intrameniscal vascularity. This area develops a normal adult appearance by age 10. A common mistake in children and adults is diagnosing longitudinal vertical hyperintensity in the posterior medial meniscus at the meniscocapsular junction as an acute tear. In this setting, a tear is less likely if the hyperintensity extends to the superior but not to the inferior articular surface [35]. Small, peripheral tears of the posterior horn of the lateral meniscus are also commonly missed, particularly if the ACL is torn [36]. A thorough discussion of meniscal tears is beyond the scope of this text.

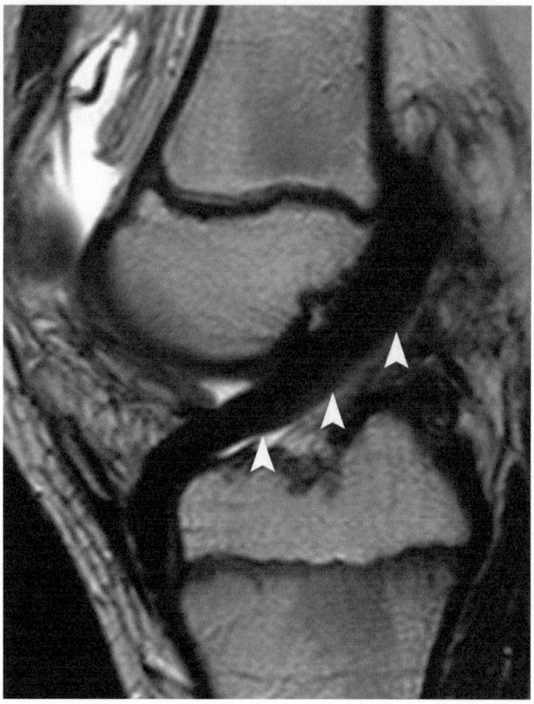

Fig. 14.28 Physeal-sparing ACL reconstruction using tendon autograft in a 12-year-old. T2-W FS image shows an intact graft (*arrowheads*) that does not bridge the physes of the distal femur and proximal tibia

3.2 Ligamentous Injuries of the Knee

Only 0.5–3 % of all Anterior cruciate ligament injuries occur in children [37]. However, with increased focus on single sports and with overall increase in training intensity, the incidence of intrasubstance ACL injury in children is increasing [38]. In those with a recent traumatic knee hemarthrosis who undergo arthroscopy, ACL tears are seen in 47 % of patients aged 7–12 years and in 65 % of patients aged 13–18 years [29]. Most skeletally immature patients with ACL injuries are boys, while most skeletally mature patients with ACL injuries are girls—especially those who engage in pivoting and jumping sports. This gender difference is due to anatomic, hormonal, and/or neuromuscular factors. Younger children with ACL injuries tend to have more partial ligament tears and avulsion fractures of the tibial intercondylar eminence than older children [39].

Traumatic traction forces cause the ACL to stretch and then partly tear. Eventually the incompletely ossified tibial intercondylar eminence, which is relatively weak, fractures. ACL injuries may be isolated or occur in combination with other ligament injuries and meniscal tears. Interestingly, in some Salter-Harris II fractures of the distal femur that result from hyperextension injury, the ACL remains intact, perhaps because the hyperextension force is absorbed by the osseous, cartilaginous, and supporting extra-articular soft tissue structures [23].

Nonsurgical management of ACL injuries leads to recurrent episodes of instability and progressive intra-articular damage; such management is not an option in patients with an active lifestyle. However, standard ACL reconstruction in skeletally immature patients is associated with physeal injury and growth disturbance. This can be avoided by delaying surgery until physeal closure or by applying newer techniques that have lower risk for growth arrest in prepubescent patients. Examples of these include physeal-sparing (Fig. 14.28), partial physeal-sparing, and complete transphyseal procedures [40].

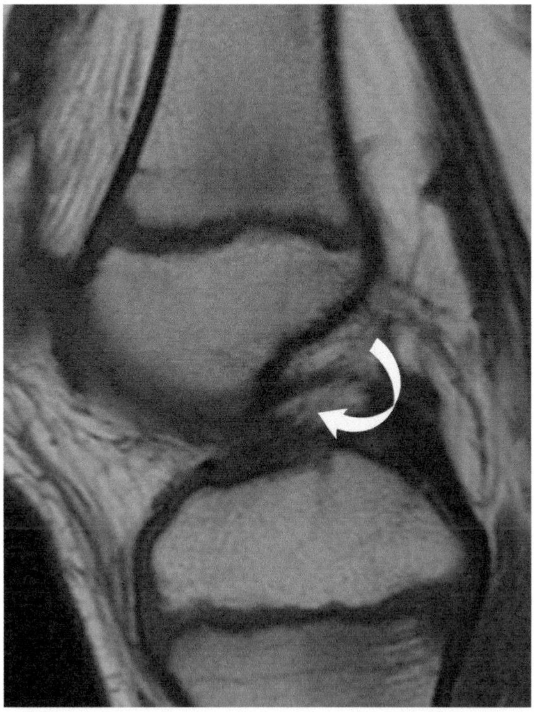

Fig. 14.29 Chronic ACL tear in a 10-year-old several months after injury, with near-complete absence of the ACL at arthroscopy. T1-W sagittal image shows fat (*curved arrow*) in the expected location of the ACL. The posterior cruciate ligament (PCL) was intact

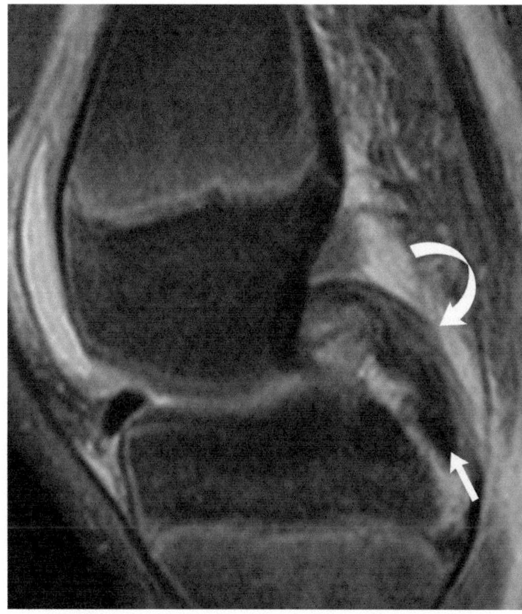

Fig. 14.30 Recent avulsion of the PCL. Sagittal T2-W FS image shows a cortical fragment (*arrow*) avulsed off the posterior margin of the tibial intercondylar eminence at the attachment of the PCL. The PCL is edematous and diffusely thickened (*curved arrow*)

Imaging

Radiographs cannot identify ACL tears but may demonstrate joint effusion, osteochondral fractures of the lateral femoral condyle, and, uncommonly, avulsion fractures of the intercondylar eminence of the tibia and lateral rim of the tibia (Segond fracture). However, MRI is highly sensitive and specific for diagnosing complete ACL tears in children [41]. It is unfortunately less accurate at diagnosing partial ACL tears, and these must be correlated with a physical examination performed by an experienced clinician. In interpreting knee MRIs, it is important to recognize that the angle the ACL makes with the proximal tibia normally increases as the child matures. In addition, patients with developmental anomalies of the lower extremity may have an abnormal ACL. However, in otherwise normal patients, an absent or small ACL is unlikely to be a developmental anomaly and probably results from resorption of ligament fibers related to remote injury (Fig. 14.29). The normal ACL may demonstrate linear increased signal within its substance, and this can be mistaken for a partial tear. It is important to recognize that secondary signs, such as femoral and tibial bone contusions that suggest ACL tears in adults, can be present in children in the absence of focal ACL disruption due to physiologic ligamentous laxity.

Posterior cruciate ligament (PCL) tears are uncommon but likely underreported because clinical and arthroscopic evaluation is difficult. Athletic injuries and motor vehicle accidents account for most PCL tears, which may be isolated or coexist with other ligamentous injures. Tears can be partial or complete. They are typically located in the mid-substance of the ligament, although the femoral or tibial attachment sites may be involved. Associated avulsion fractures at the posterior aspect of the tibial intercondylar eminence (Fig. 14.30) occur infrequently in children. In general, the injury patterns and MRI appearance of acute and chronic PCL tears in children and adults are similar [42].

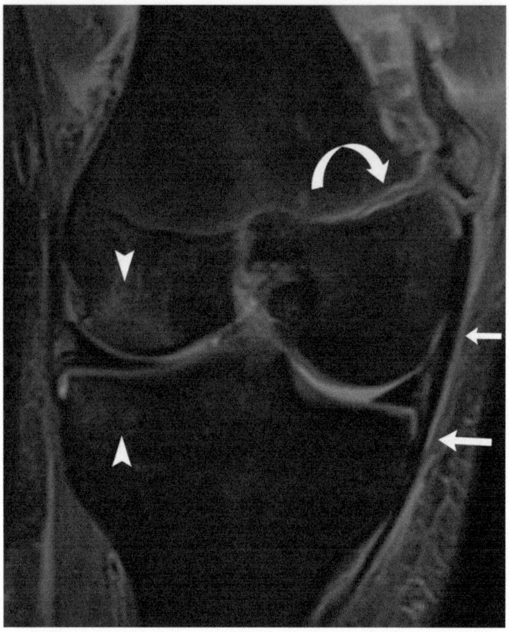

Fig. 14.31 Valgus injury of the knee in a 16-year-old football player. Coronal T2-W FS image shows contusions of the lateral femoral condyle and tibial plateau (*arrowheads*) from recent impaction injury. Tensile force at the medial knee has caused physeal injury (Salter-Harris III fracture), with mild medial physeal widening (*curved arrow*). Diffuse edema superficial to the medial collateral ligament (MCL) (*arrows*) reflects mild ligament sprain. Edema within the intercondylar notch results from ACL tear (not shown)

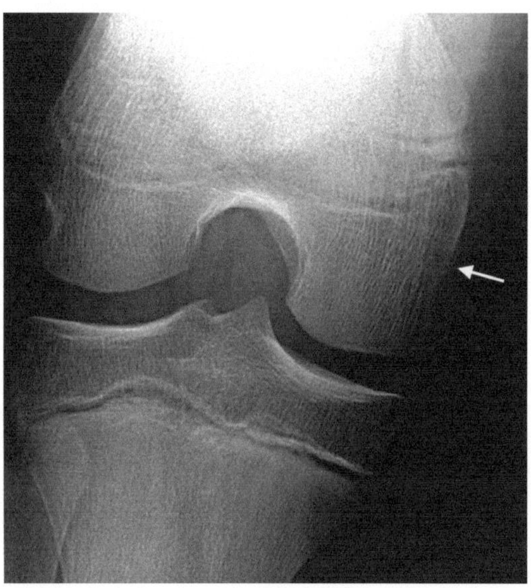

Fig. 14.32 Notch view of the knee shows a recent cortical avulsion (*arrow*) at the femoral attachment of the deep portion of the medial collateral ligament

Partial PCL tears and non-displaced avulsion injuries are treated nonoperatively with good outcome. PCL repair or reconstruction is a viable treatment for injuries involving more than one ligament and in patients who have failed conservative treatment [43]. In addition to MRI, CT is often used in preoperative evaluation of displaced and comminuted avulsion fractures of the tibial intercondylar eminence.

Collateral ligament injury in children is rare, as traumatic valgus and varus stress forces more likely result in physeal injury, rather than ligamentous failure, owing to the relatively weak physis (Fig. 14.31). Radiographs may show small, avulsed cortical fragments at the attachment sites of the collateral ligaments (Fig. 14.32). Collateral ligament injuries may be isolated or accompany cruciate ligament and meniscal injuries.

4 Plica Syndrome

Plica syndrome is characterized by thickening of the plica of the knee. It presents as a clicking, snapping sensation, with pain medial to the patella. The medial patellar plica is normally a delicate, 1–2 mm synovial band in the medial aspect of the knee joint, extending from the suprapatellar region to the synovial lining at Hoffa's fat pad [44]. The abnormal plica is more than 2 mm thick. Most patients with plica syndrome are active adolescents and young adults.

The exact etiology of plica thickening is uncertain. Proposed causes include trauma, overuse, synovitis, and intra-articular loose bodies. A thickened plica may be associated with chondromalacia of the patella and medial femoral condyle, presumably related to the plica constantly rubbing against these structures. Symptoms may respond to local cortisone injection, although arthroscopic resection may ultimately be necessary.

Imaging

Axial and sagittal MRI images best demonstrate the thickened plica and its relationship to the patella and medial femoral condyle (Fig. 14.33).

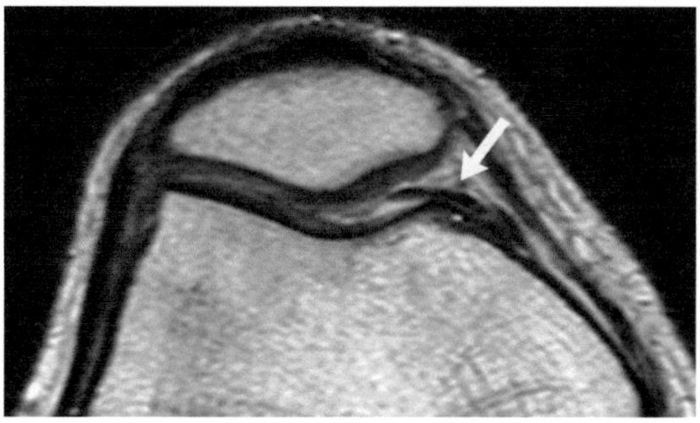

Fig. 14.33 Plica syndrome. Axial T2-W image shows a mildly thickened and irregular medial synovial plica (*arrow*). There is mild diffuse fraying of the adjacent cartilage of the medial facet of the patella

5 Popliteal Cyst

A popliteal cyst is a fluid-filled synovium-lined structure in the posterior aspect of the knee with its neck located between the tendons of the semimembranosus and medial head of the gastrocnemius muscles. Patients may present with a palpable mass or be entirely asymptomatic. Popliteal cysts are less common in children than in adults and are present in about 6 % of pediatric knee MRI studies. They are usually diagnosed at around age 8 [45]. Associated internal derangement is not as common in children as in adults. An accepted but not proven cause in the pediatric population includes irritation of the knee's posterior joint capsule due to repetitive trauma to the popliteal fossa. Most cysts disappear spontaneously.

Imaging

US is the best imaging method. However, if there is any suspicion of concomitant intra-articular pathology, MRI is preferred. Imaging usually demonstrates a well-defined fluid-filled structure in the posteromedial aspect of the knee adjacent to the semimembranosus muscle and the medial head of the gastrocnemius muscle (Fig. 14.34). It is important to identify a narrow neck that connects the cyst to the joint and confirms diagnosis. Cysts may extend into the calf or thigh. There may be intralesional septae, but debris and leakage are rare in children.

Differential diagnosis includes hematoma, parameniscal cyst, venous and lymphatic malformation, and malignant neoplasm such as synovial sarcoma. (See Chap. 22 for additional discussion of popliteal cysts.)

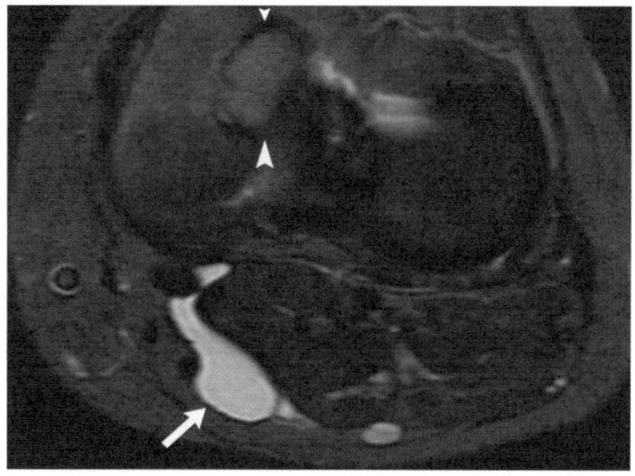

Fig. 14.34 Popliteal cyst. Axial T2-W FS image shows a popliteal cyst (*arrow*) with tail extending toward the joint between the semimembranosus and the medial head of the gastrocnemius muscle. There is also osteochondritis dissecans (OCD) (*arrowheads*) of the medial femoral condyle

6 Osteochondral Lesions of the Knee

6.1 Acute Chondral Lesions of the Knee

In children evaluated with MRI for internal derangement of the knee, chondral injuries are more common than meniscal or ligamentous injuries. This may be explained by the presence of a vulnerable interface between the articular cartilage and the subchondral bone in the developing juvenile joint. Shearing stress and direct impaction are the two basic mechanisms that result in chondral injuries; these forces also play a significant role in acute patellar dislocations. Osteochondral fractures are found in 25–50 % of patients after acute patellar dislocation. These fractures most often involve the medial patellar facet and the lateral femoral condyle (see Chap. 13). Chondral lesions of the distal femur are more likely to occur before physeal closure [46]. These injuries present with severe pain, swelling, difficulty bearing weight, and locking of the knee. The presence of intra-articular fragments may necessitate surgical intervention. Fixation of an osteochondral fragment is recommended if it is greater than 1 cm and involves a weight-bearing area.

Surgical techniques include microfracture, osteochondral autografting and allografting, and placement of resorbable synthetic scaffolds and autologous chondrocyte implants [47].

Imaging

MRI readily diagnoses partial-thickness and full-thickness chondral defects with acutely angulated margins, along with cartilage flaps and delamination in the setting of acute injury (Fig. 14.35). It is important to assess lesion size, location, depth, and containment, as well as associated marrow edema and subchondral cysts. It can be difficult to detect intra-articular chondral or osteochondral bodies; these may be more readily identified on CT. Except for the distribution, the MRI findings in children with acute chondral lesions do not differ significantly from those in adults.

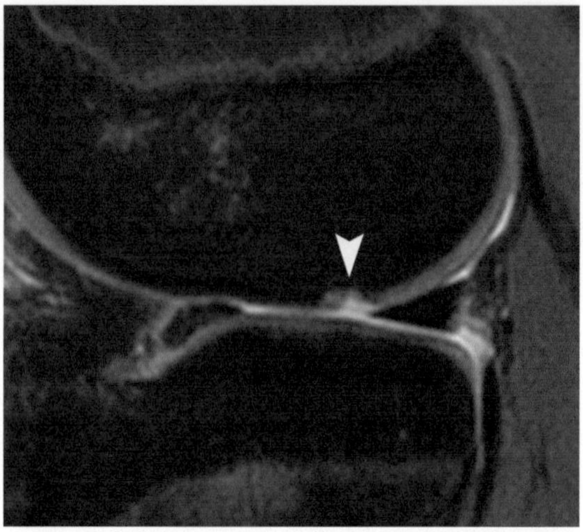

Fig. 14.35 Acute chondral fracture in a 15-year-old football player who dislocated the patella. T2-W FS image shows full-thickness chondral defect (*arrowhead*) in the weight-bearing portion of the lateral femoral condyle. A corresponding loose chondral fragment was identified adjacent to Hoffa's fat pad (not shown)

6.2 Osteochondritis Dissecans of the Knee (Box 14.9)

The term osteochondritis dissecans (OCD), which suggests "dissecting inflammation," is a misnomer [48], and some employ the more general term, osteochondral lesion. The lesion consists of a subchondral fracture and an osteochondral fragment, which may be attached at one edge or completely separated. Depending on which portion of the joint is affected, patients may be asymptomatic or present with knee pain, clicking, locking, and swelling. Younger patients present between the ages of 11 and 13 years, and older patients present after skeletal maturity, between age 17 and 35. OCD of the knee is slightly more common in males than in females. Opinions about etiology conflict, but experts presently believe that it relates to trauma, either a single event of significant magnitude or repetitive microtrauma [49]. Widening of the overlying epiphyseal cartilage suggests that OCD may be associated with disturbed endochondral ossification [50]. Familial cases have been reported, suggesting genetic factors probably also play a role. Bilateral knee involvement and multifocal unilateral involvement may occur.

Eighty-five percent of all OCD cases occur at the lateral aspect of the medial femoral condyle, and this location is even more common in children [51]. The proximity of this portion of the femur to the tibial intercondylar eminence suggests a tangential shearing stress against the condylar cartilage. Other

Box 14.9: Osteochondritis Dissecans

Subchondral fracture and osteochondral fragment
Age: 11–13 years old
Lateral aspect of medial femoral condyle in 85 %
Extends to intercondylar notch

Radiographs	Notch, tunnel, oblique views help
	Lucent crater with sclerotic margin
	+/– In situ fragment or loose body
MRI	*Unstable if* (best assessed on T2, STIR)
	Fluid signal rim (as bright as joint fluid)
	Hypointense rim
	Multiple disruptions in subchondral plate
	Cysts at margin, if multiple or >5 mm

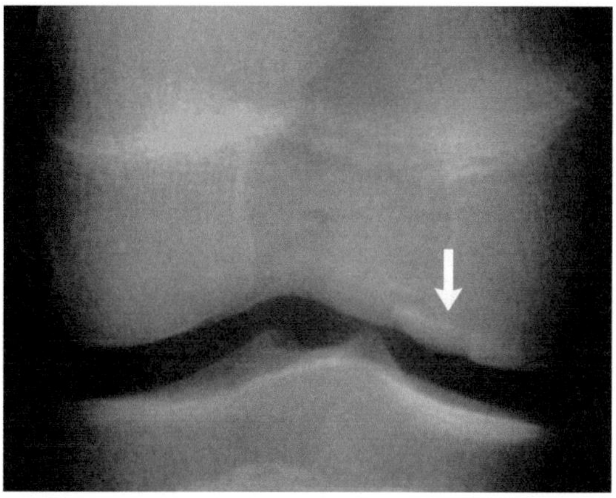

Fig. 14.36 Osteochondritis dissecans (OCD) of the medial femoral condyle in a 15-year-old boy with knee pain for 1 month. A defect with sclerotic margins (*arrow*) extends from the medial femoral condyle to the intercondylar notch

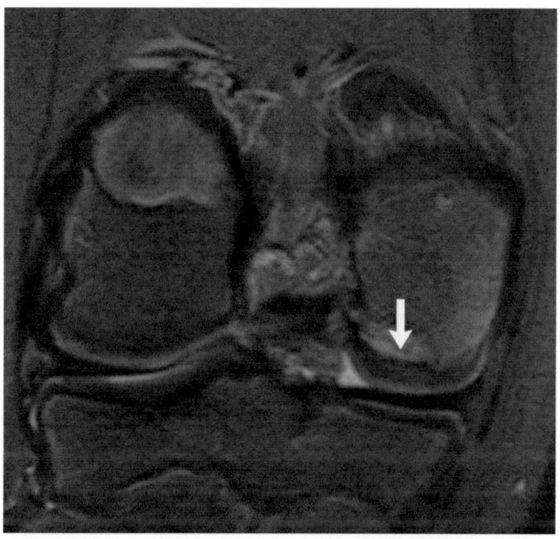

Fig. 14.37 Stable OCD of the medial femoral condyle. T2-W FS coronal image shows a rim of high T2 signal and mild marrow edema around the lesion (*arrow*). The signal intensity of the surrounding rim is lower than that of joint fluid. This lesion healed spontaneously 1.5 years later

sites of involvement include, in decreasing order of frequency, the lateral femoral condyle (anterior and inferior portions), the femoral trochlea, and the patella. OCD of the femoral trochlea is found at the anterior aspect of the lateral femoral condyle distal to the physis, while OCD of the patella is typically located at the medial facet [52].

OCD is much more likely to heal spontaneously in adolescents than in adults. Treatment depends on the stability of the osteochondral fragment, which can be assessed with MRI and arthroscopy. Surgical options include arthroscopic drilling, direct fixation by screw or pin, osteochondral plug fixation, and bone grafting [53]. The outcome is poor if large fragments must be excised.

Imaging

In addition to the standard frontal and lateral radiographic projections, notch, tunnel, and oblique views of the knee help evaluate the patellofemoral compartment and femoral OCD. The lesion typically extends into the intercondylar notch and is visualized as a lucent crater of variable depth, often with irregular or sclerotic margins (Fig. 14.36). In situ bone fragments or one or more displaced intra-articular osteochondral bodies may be present.

MRI helps diagnose OCD and assess lesion stability. Signs that indicate osteochondral lesion instability are best evaluated on T2-W or short tau inversion recovery (STIR) images and include a fluid signal rim surrounding the OCD, a low-signal rim (probably representing fibrous tissue or sclerotic bone) in the subchondral bone surrounding the OCD, and multiple disruptions in the subchondral bone plate. When the three signs are used together, the sensitivity and specificity have been reported to be 100 % [54]. It is important to note that if the T2 signal of the rim is less intense than that of joint fluid, the lesion is not necessarily unstable (Fig. 14.37). Cysts at the margins of the defect indicate instability in children only if they are multiple or measure at least 5 mm in diameter (Figs. 14.38 and 14.39), whereas in adults cysts of any size or number are associated with instability [54]. Computed tomographic arthrography (CTA) and direct and indirect MR arthrography (MRA) also evaluate OCD, and contrast agents potentially provide important information about the interface between the osteochondral fragment and underlying bone.

Differential diagnoses include osteonecrosis, subchondral stress fractures, epiphyseal dysplasia,

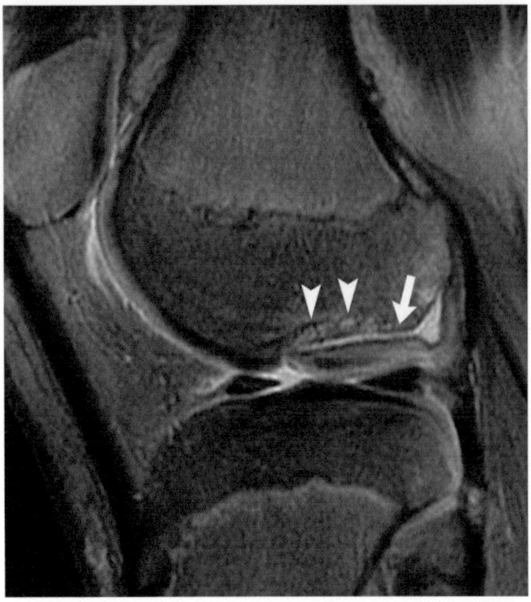

Fig. 14.38 OCD of the medial femoral condyle with an unstable osteochondral fragment. Sagittal T2-W FS image shows a fluid signal intensity rim (*arrow*) surrounding the fragment. There are also several cysts (*arrowheads*), and there is cartilage discontinuity at the margins

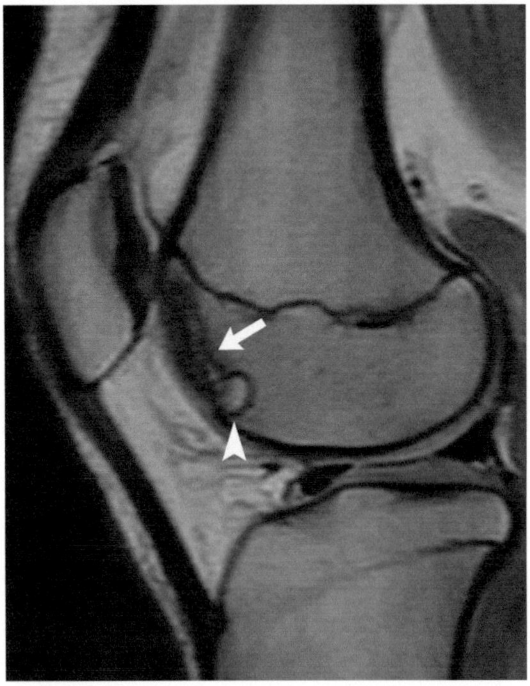

Fig. 14.39 OCD of the femoral trochlea with an unstable osteochondral fragment. Sagittal T2-W FS image shows a hypointense rim (*arrow*) representing fibrous tissue or sclerosis. A cyst (*arrowhead*) measuring >5 mm at the margin of the OCD is also associated with instability

and neuropathic arthropathy. Normal variant irregular ossification of the femoral condyles, commonly seen on radiographs and MRI, is located more posteriorly and laterally and does not involve the intercondylar notch. The configuration of normal variants may resemble a puzzle piece, or there may be irregular spiculated subchondral bone or multiple small, distinct ossification centers [55]. In addition, ossification variant tends to be deeper but extend over a smaller area of the condyle [56].

6.3 Chondromalacia Patella

Chondromalacia patella is a common cause of anterior knee pain in adults, and many have had related symptoms as adolescents. Clinical manifestations include retropatellar pain, crepitus with patellar motion, and locking of the knee. Although acute trauma may result in chondral fissures, fracture, and delamination, chondromalacia patella is generally thought to be caused by chronic repetitive compression and shear forces. Joint malalignment and chronic patellar tracking abnormalities predispose to the disorder. If the biomechanical forces that cross the joint exceed the strength of the tissue, femorotibial chondromalacia and osteoarthritis may develop. Valgus or varus malalignment results in an increased compressive load and a fivefold increased risk of osteoarthritis [57]. The lesions are classified according to their arthroscopic appearance and behavior when subjected to probing.

Imaging

Radiographs detect only advanced stages of chondromalacia. MRI best evaluates articular cartilage. Fast spin-echo (FSE) proton density (PD) and T2-W sequences with fat suppression (FS) can indicate cartilage fibrillation and partial-thickness chondral defects (Fig. 14.40), as well as progression to OCD (Fig. 14.41). MRI also shows knee malalignment, meniscal dysfunction, and osteochondral injury [58]. 3.0 tesla (T) MRI offers an advantage over 1.5 T MRI in cartilage imaging due to its higher spatial resolution and decreased slice thickness. However, even 3.0 T conventional MRI cannot detect the physiologic

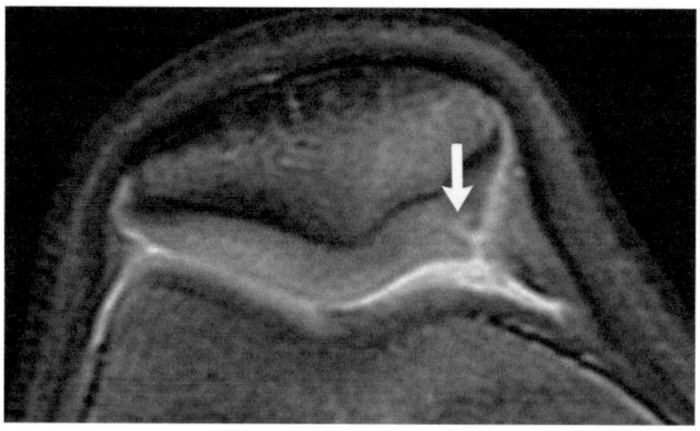

Fig. 14.40 Partial-thickness chondral defect of the medial facet of the patella. T2-W FS axial image shows a focal chondral fissure (*arrow*) involving about 50 % of the cartilage thickness

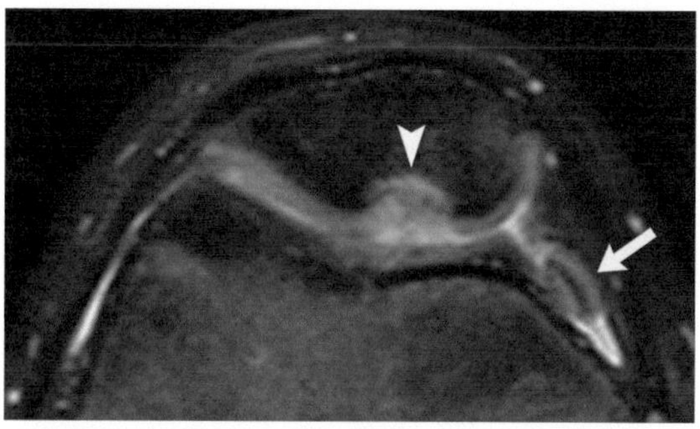

Fig. 14.41 OCD of the patella with an intra-articular loose body. T2-W FS axial image shows a well-demarcated osteochondral defect (*arrowhead*) in the central patella with minimal marrow edema. A corresponding loose body (*arrow*) is positioned within the medial aspect of the joint

and biochemical changes that occur with early cartilage degeneration. Special MRI techniques based on determination of proteoglycan content, collagen content and orientation, water mobility, and cartilage compressibility are available, but they heat tissues and require long imaging times, special coils, and intravenous contrast material [59].

References

1. Lafrance RM, Giordano B, Goldblatt J, Voloshin I, Maloney M. Pediatric tibial eminence fractures: evaluation and management. J Am Acad Orthop Surg. 2010;18(7):395–405. PubMed PMID: 20595132.
2. Meyers MH, McKeever FM. Fracture of the intercondylar eminence of the tibia. J Bone Joint Surg Am. 1970;52(8):1677–84. PubMed PMID: 5483091.
3. Bates DG, Hresko MT, Jaramillo D. Patellar sleeve fracture: demonstration with MR imaging. Radiology. 1994;193(3):825–7. PubMed PMID: 7972832.
4. Ogden JA. Radiology of postnatal skeletal development. X. Patella and tibial tuberosity. Skelet Radiol. 1984;11(4):246–57. PubMed PMID: 6729496.
5. Mirbey J, Besancenot J, Chambers RT, Durey A, Vichard P. Avulsion fractures of the tibial tuberosity in the adolescent athlete. Risk factors, mechanism of injury, and treatment. Am J Sports Med. 1988;16(4):336–40. PubMed PMID: 3189655.
6. Medlar RC, Lyne ED. Sinding-Larsen-Johansson disease. Its etiology and natural history. J Bone Joint Surg Am. 1978;60(8):1113–6. PubMed PMID: 721864.
7. Stanitski CL. Anterior knee pain syndromes in the adolescent. J Bone Joint Surg Am. 1993;75A(9):1407–16.
8. Carr JC, Hanly S, Griffin J, Gibney R. Sonography of the patellar tendon and adjacent structures in pediatric and adult patients. AJR Am J Roentgenol. 2001;176(6):1535–9. PubMed PMID: 11373229.
9. Dwek JR, Chung CB. The patellar extensor apparatus of the knee. Pediatr Radiol. 2008;38(9):925–35. PubMed PMID: 18265971.
10. Romeo AA, Larson RV. Arthroscopic treatment of infrapatellar tendonitis. Arthroscopy. 1999;15(3): 341–5. PubMed PMID: 10231119.
11. Ehrenborg G, Engfeldt B. Histologic changes in the Osgood-Schlatter lesion. Acta Chir Scand. 1961;121:328–37. PubMed PMID: 13725977.
12. Matheson GO, Clement DB, McKenzie DC, Taunton JE, Lloyd-Smith DR, MacIntyre JG. Stress fractures in athletes. A study of 320 cases. Am J Sports Med. 1987;15(1):46–58. PubMed PMID: 3812860.
13. Devas MB. Stress fractures in children. J Bone Joint Surg. 1963;45:528–41. PubMed PMID: 14058330.
14. Boden BP, Osbahr DC, Jimenez C. Low-risk stress fractures. Am J Sports Med. 2001;29(1):100–11. PubMed PMID: 11206247.
15. Rupani HD, Holder LE, Espinola DA, Engin SI. Three-phase radionuclide bone imaging in sports medicine. Radiology. 1985;156(1):187–96. PubMed PMID: 2860698.
16. Fredericson M, Bergman AG, Hoffman KL, Dillingham MS. Tibial stress reaction in runners. Correlation of clinical symptoms and scintigraphy with a new magnetic resonance imaging grading system. Am J Sports Med. 1995;23(4):472–81. PubMed PMID: 7573660.
17. Anderson SE, Johnston JO, O'Donnell R, Steinbach LS. MR imaging of sports-related pseudotumor in children: mid femoral diaphyseal periostitis at insertion site of adductor musculature. AJR Am J Roentgenol. 2001;176(5):1227–31. PubMed PMID: 11312186.
18. Garcia Mata S, Hidalgo Ovejero A, Martinez GM. Transverse stress fracture of the patella in a child. J Pediatr Orthop B. 1999;8(3):208–11. PubMed PMID: 10399126.
19. Laor T, Wall EJ, Vu LP. Physeal widening in the knee due to stress injury in child athletes. AJR Am J Roentgenol. 2006;186(5):1260–4. PubMed PMID: 16632716.
20. Zbojniewicz AM, Laor T. Focal Periphyseal Edema (FOPE) zone on MRI of the adolescent knee: a

potentially painful manifestation of physiologic physeal fusion? AJR Am J Roentgenol. 2011;197(4):998–1004. PubMed PMID: 21940591.
21. Dunbar JS, Owen HF, Nogrady MB, McLeese R. Obscure tibial fracture of infants–the toddler's fracture. J Can Assoc Radiol. 1964;15:136–44. PubMed PMID: 14212071.
22. John SD, Moorthy CS, Swischuk LE. Expanding the concept of the toddler's fracture. Radiographics. 1997;17(2):367–76. PubMed PMID: 9084078.
23. Kritsaneepaiboon S, Shah R, Murray MM, Kleinman PK. Posterior periosteal disruption in Salter-Harris Type II fractures of the distal femur: evidence for a hyperextension mechanism. AJR Am J Roentgenol. 2009;193(6):W540–5. PubMed PMID: 19933629.
24. Whan A, Breidahl W, Janes G. MRI of trapped periosteum in a proximal tibial physeal injury of a pediatric patient. AJR Am J Roentgenol. 2003;181(5):1397–9. PubMed PMID: 14573444.
25. Loder RT, Schaffer JJ, Bardenstein MB. Late-onset tibia vara. J Pediatr Orthop. 1991;11(2):162–7. PubMed PMID: 2010513.
26. Aird JJ, Hogg A, Rollinson P. Femoral torsion in patients with Blount's disease: a previously unrecognised component. J Bone Joint Surg. 2009;91(10):1388–93. PubMed PMID: 19794178.
27. Synder M, Vera J, Harcke HT, Bowen JR. Magnetic resonance imaging of the growth plate in late-onset tibia vara. Int Orthop. 2003;27(4):217–22. PubMed PMID: 12748828: Pubmed Central PMCID: 3458484.
28. Kocher MS, DiCanzio J, Zurakowski D, Micheli LJ. Diagnostic performance of clinical examination and selective magnetic resonance imaging in the evaluation of intraarticular knee disorders in children and adolescents. Am J Sports Med. 2001;29(3):292–6. PubMed PMID: 11394597.
29. Stanitski CL, Harvell JC, Fu F. Observations on acute knee hemarthrosis in children and adolescents. J Pediatr Orthop. 1993;13(4):506–10. PubMed PMID: 8370785.
30. Lee K, Siegel MJ, Lau DM, Hildebolt CF, Matava MJ. Anterior cruciate ligament tears: MR imaging-based diagnosis in a pediatric population. Radiology. 1999;213(3):697–704. PubMed PMID: 10580941.
31. Zobel MS, Borrello JA, Siegel MJ, Stewart NR. Pediatric knee MR imaging: pattern of injuries in the immature skeleton. Radiology. 1994;190(2): 397–401. PubMed PMID: 8284387.
32. Clark CR, Ogden JA. Development of the menisci of the human knee joint. Morphological changes and their potential role in childhood meniscal injury. J Bone Joint Surg Am. 1983;65(4):538–47. PubMed PMID: 6833331.
33. Kramer DE, Micheli LJ. Meniscal tears and discoid meniscus in children: diagnosis and treatment. J Am Acad Orthop Surg. 2009;17(11):698–707. PubMed PMID: 19880680.
34. Resnick D. Diagnosis of bone and joint disorders. 3rd ed. Philadelphia: W. B. Saunders; 1995.
35. De Smet AA, Nathan DH, Graf BK, Haaland BA, Fine JP. Clinical and MRI findings associated with false-positive knee MR diagnoses of medial meniscal tears. AJR Am J Roentgenol. 2008;191(1):93–9. PubMed PMID: 18562730.
36. De Smet AA, Graf BK. Meniscal tears missed on MR imaging: relationship to meniscal tear patterns and anterior cruciate ligament tears. AJR Am J Roentgenol. 1994;162(4):905–11. PubMed PMID: 8141016.
37. Andrish JT. Anterior cruciate ligament injuries in the skeletally immature patient. Am J Orthop. 2001;30(2):103–10. PubMed PMID: 11234936.
38. Frank JS, Gambacorta PL. Anterior cruciate ligament injuries in the skeletally immature athlete: diagnosis and management. J Am Acad Orthop Surg. 2013;21(2):78–87. PubMed PMID: 23378371.
39. Prince JS, Laor T, Bean JA. MRI of anterior cruciate ligament injuries and associated findings in the pediatric knee: changes with skeletal maturation. AJR Am J Roentgenol. 2005;185(3):756–62. PubMed PMID: 16120930.
40. McConkey MO, Bonasia DE, Amendola A. Pediatric anterior cruciate ligament reconstruction. Curr Rev Musculoskelet Med. 2011;4(2):37–44. PubMed PMID: 21594689: Pubmed Central PMCID: 3097323.
41. Ho-Fung VM, Jaimes C, Jaramillo D. MR imaging of ACL injuries in pediatric and adolescent patients. Clin Sports Med. 2011;30(4):707–26. PubMed PMID: 22018312.
42. Sonin AH, Fitzgerald SW, Hoff FL, Friedman H, Bresler ME. MR imaging of the posterior cruciate ligament: normal, abnormal, and associated injury patterns. Radiographics. 1995;15(3):551–61. PubMed PMID: 7624562.
43. Kocher MS, Shore B, Nasreddine AY, Heyworth BE. Treatment of posterior cruciate ligament injuries in pediatric and adolescent patients. J Pediatr Orthop. 2012;32(6):553–60. PubMed PMID: 22892615.
44. Garcia-Valtuille R, Abascal F, Cerezal L, Garcia-Valtuille A, Pereda T, Canga A, et al. Anatomy and MR imaging appearances of synovial plicae of the knee. Radiographics. 2002;22(4):775–84. PubMed PMID: 12110709.
45. De Maeseneer M, Debaere C, Desprechins B, Osteaux M. Popliteal cysts in children: prevalence, appearance and associated findings at MR imaging. Pediatr Radiol. 1999;29(8):605–9. PubMed PMID: 10415188.
46. Oeppen RS, Connolly SA, Bencardino JT, Jaramillo D. Acute injury of the articular cartilage and subchondral bone: a common but unrecognized lesion in the immature knee. AJR Am J Roentgenol. 2004;182(1):111–7. PubMed PMID: 14684522.
47. Mithofer K, Minas T, Peterson L, Yeon H, Micheli LJ. Functional outcome of knee articular cartilage repair in adolescent athletes. Am J Sports Med. 2005;33(8):1147–53. PubMed PMID: 16000659.
48. Barrie HJ. Osteochondritis dissecans 1887–1987. A centennial look at Konig's memorable phrase. J Bone Joint Surg Br. 1987;69(5):693–5. PubMed PMID: 3316236.

49. Flynn JM, Kocher MS, Ganley TJ. Osteochondritis dissecans of the knee. J Pediatr Orthop. 2004;24(4):434–43. PubMed PMID: 15205627.
50. Laor T, Zbojniewicz AM, Eismann EA, Wall EJ. Juvenile osteochondritis dissecans: is it a growth disturbance of the secondary physis of the epiphysis? AJR Am J Roentgenol. 2012;199(5):1121–8. PubMed PMID: 23096188.
51. Aichroth P. Osteochondritis dissecans of the knee. A clinical survey. The J Bone Joint Surg Br. 1971;53(3):440–7. PubMed PMID: 5562371.
52. Pfeiffer WH, Gross ML, Seeger LL. Osteochondritis dissecans of the patella. MRI evaluation and a case report. Clin Orthop Relat Res. 1991;271:207–11. PubMed PMID: 1914297.
53. Kocher MS, Tucker R, Ganley TJ, Flynn JM. Management of osteochondritis dissecans of the knee: current concepts review. Am J Sports Med. 2006;34(7):1181–91. PubMed PMID: 16794036.
54. Kijowski R, Blankenbaker DG, Shinki K, Fine JP, Graf BK, De Smet AA. Juvenile versus adult osteochondritis dissecans of the knee: appropriate MR imaging criteria for instability. Radiology. 2008;248(2):571–8. PubMed PMID: 18552309.
55. Jans L, Jaremko J, Ditchfield M, De Coninck T, Huysse W, Moon A, et al. Ossification variants of the femoral condyles are not associated with osteochondritis dissecans. Eur J Radiol. 2012;81(11):3384–9. PubMed PMID: 22297186.
56. Jans LB, Jaremko JL, Ditchfield M, Huysse WC, Verstraete KL. MRI differentiates femoral condylar ossification evolution from osteochondritis dissecans. A new sign. Eur Radiol. 2011;21(6):1170–9. PubMed PMID: 21267576.
57. Schouten JS, van den Ouweland FA, Valkenburg HA. A 12 year follow up study in the general population on prognostic factors of cartilage loss in osteoarthritis of the knee. Ann Rheum Dis. 1992;51(8):932–7. PubMed PMID: 1417116: Pubmed Central PMCID: 1004797.
58. Walker EA, Davis D, Mosher TJ. Rapidly progressive osteoarthritis: biomechanical considerations. Magn Reson Imaging Clin N Am. 2011;19(2):283–94. PubMed PMID: 21665091.
59. Choi JA, Gold GE. MR imaging of articular cartilage physiology. Magn Reson Imaging Clin N Am. 2011;19(2):249–82. PubMed PMID: 21665090: Pubmed Central PMCID: 3115556.

The Foot and Ankle: Congenital and Developmental Conditions

15

Matthew R. Hammer and Deepa R. Pai

Contents

Abstract

The radiographic evaluation of congenital and developmental abnormalities of the foot and ankle provides critical information to guide orthopedic treatment. This chapter begins by discussing the anatomy and normal variants of the ankle. Congenital and developmental abnormalities of the ankle are explored, including ball-and-socket ankle. The development and normal variants of the pediatric foot are then discussed. After describing radiographic techniques for imaging the foot, the chapter presents methods to evaluate and vocabulary to describe foot alignment. This is then applied to a broad spectrum of structural deformities of the foot, including clubfoot, cavus deformity, and multiple types of flatfoot (including tarsal coalition). A discussion of forefoot alignment follows, and the chapter concludes with a brief discussion of congenital foot malformations.

M.R. Hammer, MD
Department of Radiology,
University of Texas Southwestern Medical Center
and Children's Medical Center of Dallas,
1935 Medical District Drive, Dallas, TX 75235, USA
e-mail: MatthewRHammer@gmail.com

D.R. Pai, MD, MHSA (✉)
Department of Radiology,
C.S. Mott Children's Hospital,
1540 E. Hospital Drive, Ann Arbor,
MI 48109, USA
e-mail: dpai@med.umich.edu

In order to provide useful interpretations of foot and ankle radiographs, the radiologist must have a thorough knowledge of the many normal variants that affect this area, recognizing those that may mimic or obscure pathology. Analysis of alignment requires a careful, systematic approach, along with a clear understanding of normal alignment, the wide variety of possible deformities, and the many ways they may combine to create unique constellations of pathology.

R. Stein-Wexler et al. (eds.), *Pediatric Orthopedic Imaging*,
DOI 10.1007/978-3-642-45381-6_15, © Springer-Verlag Berlin Heidelberg 2015

This chapter first discusses the anatomy and normal variants of the ankle, providing essential background that makes accurate interpretation of pathology possible. It then analyzes normal alignment, presenting a useful vocabulary that can be applied to all foot and ankle malformations. It reviews a wide variety of common and unusual malalignments that affect the hindfoot, midfoot, and forefoot, such as clubfoot, cavus deformity, flatfoot (as well as tarsal coalition), rocker-bottom foot, congenital vertical talus, and metatarsus adductus.

1 The Ankle

1.1 Anatomy and Variants

The ankle is a complex joint comprised of the distal tibia, distal fibula, and talus and stabilized by multiple ligaments and tendons. These structures form a hinge joint that allows dorsiflexion and plantarflexion. The distal portions of the tibia and fibula form the medial malleolus and lateral malleolus, respectively. The ankle joint includes anterior and posterior recesses and sometimes communicates with the posterior subtalar and talocalcaneonavicular joints, including the pairs of anterior and middle subtalar facets [1].

The growth plates or physes of the distal tibia and fibula are often irregular and commonly appear fragmented [2]. Likely due to irregularity at the zone of provisional calcification, this is especially common at the distal fibula. The fragmentation may appear as discrete ossific densities, frequently adjacent to the physis. This appearance has been described as a *fibular ossicle* and should not be mistaken as a fracture in the absence of a radiographically apparent joint effusion (Fig. 15.1).

The distal tibial physis is also often irregular. A focal superiorly oriented notch at the medial aspect of the distal tibial physis is normal (*Kump bump*) (see Chap. 16).

Additional ossification centers are often encountered at the distal ends of the medial and lateral malleoli in children and are especially common medially. Many differentiate between these centers, labeling them either secondary or accessory centers of ossification. Accessory centers may be single or multiple and are visualized adjacent to or slightly separated from the main epiphyseal center (Fig. 15.2). They will not fuse with the adjacent bone and thus persist into adulthood. Examples at the ankle include the *os subtibiale* and *os subfibulare*. In contrast, secondary ossification centers will usually coalesce with other epiphyseal or apophyseal centers, eventually

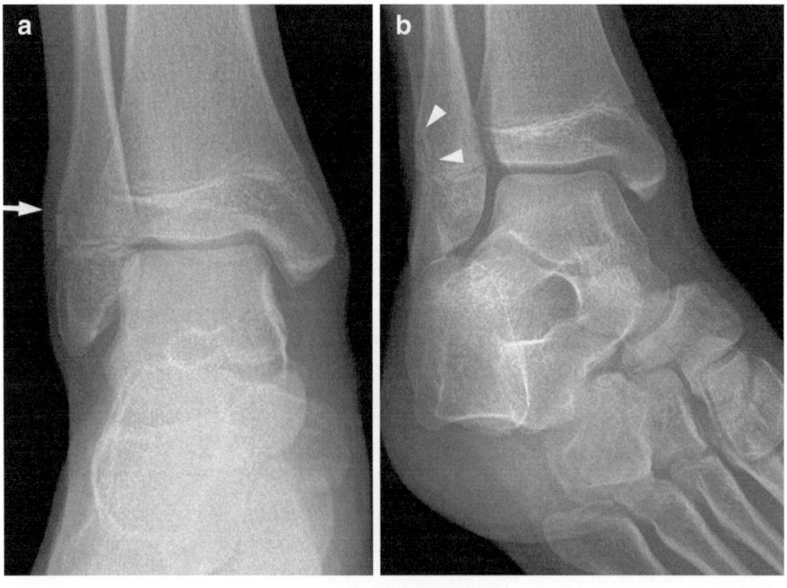

Fig. 15.1 Fibular ossicle in a 15-year-old boy. Apparent irregularity (*arrow*) along lateral fibular metaphysis on frontal view (**a**) has well-corticated margins (*arrowheads*) on oblique view (**b**). There is no soft tissue swelling

contributing to adult bone contours (Fig. 15.3). At the ankle, these are usually seen inferior to the tip of the medial malleolus. These secondary centers

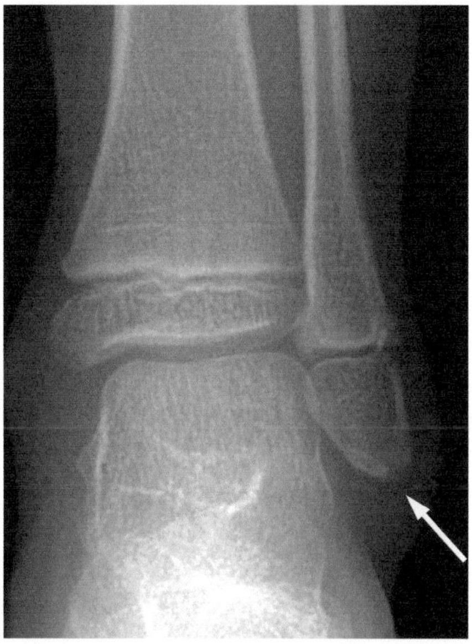

Fig. 15.2 Normal irregularity of the lateral malleolus in an asymptomatic 5-year-old girl. Oblique view shows small accessory ossification center adjacent to the distal fibula (*arrow*), without adjacent soft tissue swelling. This should not be mistaken for an avulsion injury

are encountered in 17–24 % of boys and in up to 47 % of girls. They are bilateral in more than two thirds of patients and more frequently so in girls. Generally appearing between ages 7 and 8, they usually unite with the main epiphysis 1–1.5 years after initial ossification [3]. By age 12, most will have fused with the main ossific epiphysis, but 1–2 % remain separate through adulthood—especially at the fibula [4]; these eventually become persistent ossification centers.

Old avulsion injuries, which appear as well-corticated, round ossific fragments in a similar location, are sometimes impossible to distinguish radiographically from an accessory or secondary ossification center. Indeed, some believe that these well-corticated fragments almost exclusively result from remote, unrecognized trauma [5]. Old injuries can usually be differentiated from acute fractures, in that acute fractures appear as curvilinear, irregular densities that lack corticated margins. It is possible, however, to injure the cartilaginous bridge between the accessory and main ossification centers. Clinically, there may be localized tenderness and swelling, but radiographs may not show an injury. This radiologically occult trauma will be evident on

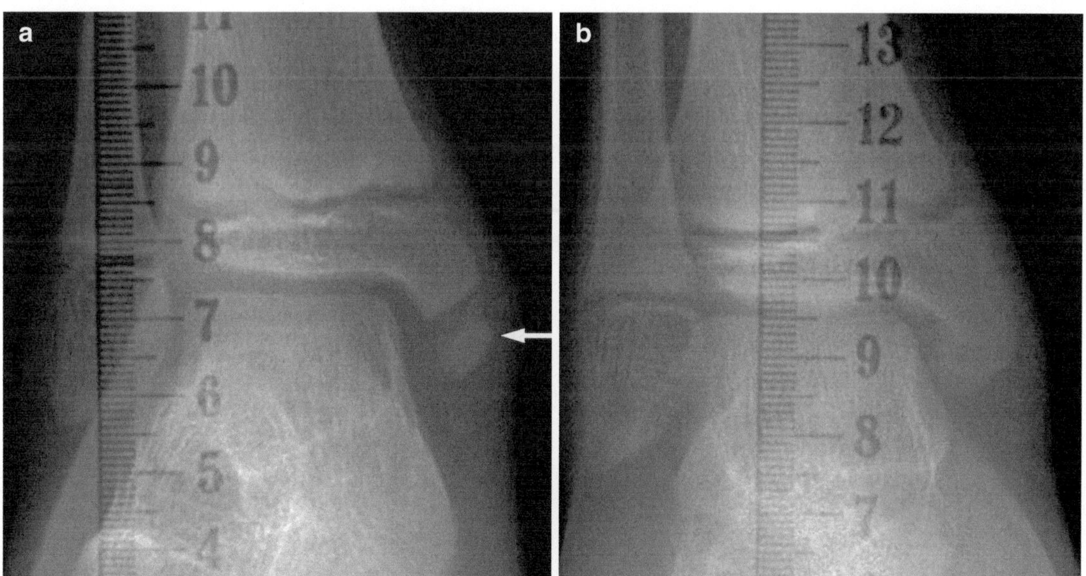

Fig. 15.3 Normal variant medial malleolar accessory ossification centers in a 12-year-old boy. (**a**) Frontal view shows a smoothly corticated osseous fragment (*arrow*) at the medial malleolus, consistent with an accessory ossification center. (**b**) Seven months later, the accessory ossification center has fused to the distal tibia. Both images were obtained as part of leg length studies

magnetic resonance imaging (MRI) as edema on T2-weighted (T2-W) sequences.

The tip of the lower fibular epiphysis is normally slightly inferior to that of the medial tibial epiphysis, with the physis of the fibula at the level of the ankle joint or slightly below it after age 4 years. The fibular growth plate should therefore be significantly more distal than the tibial growth plate. In infancy, the distal tibial and fibular growth plates initially provide most of the growth of the lower leg, but after 30 % of total bone length has been achieved, the proximal physes contribute the most longitudinal growth.

1.2 Imaging Examination and Analysis

The standard ankle series consists of anteroposterior (AP), lateral, and mortise views. Osseous detail is best evaluated on images obtained in the recumbent position. However, evaluation of ankle or hindfoot alignment requires weight-bearing views. These may be obtained with the child standing on radiolucent blocks or wood to accommodate the position of standard radiography equipment.

In order to obtain the best projection of the ankle mortise, the patient must be positioned supine with the foot in 15–20° of internal rotation. This oblique position compensates for normal external tibial rotation. For the lateral radiograph, the ankle should be parallel to the detector, with the fibula slightly posterior to the midline axis of the tibia. The standard oblique view requires medially rotating the ankle by 45°. Multiple other views have also been described but are less frequently utilized.

Radiography performed with stress applied to the ankle may be useful when chronic ligamentous injury or intrinsic malalignment is suspected. When there is an acute injury, stress views in children are quite painful and may require sedation. When stress is applied to the heel during eversion (whether by gravity or force), there should be no tilt of the talar dome in relation to the tibial plafond. With inversion the average obtainable tilt of the talar surface is 7°, with a normal range of up to 27°. With such marked change on inversion stress possible in normals, caution must be observed when using this to test for abnormal ligamentous laxity. Comparison views of both ankles can be obtained to look for asymmetry. Studies have shown that a 10° difference in inversion stress angulation between the two ankles is a specific but insensitive indicator of ligamentous injury [6]. Many consider stress radiography of the ankle unreliable and instead utilize clinical examination and dynamic imaging by ultrasound to directly evaluate the ligamentous structures.

In young children, there is normally a slight valgus angle of the distal tibial articular surface compared with the long axis of the tibia. This angle approaches 90° by age 10, when the articular surface becomes horizontal. This measurement may be altered in cases of marked developmental lower extremity bowing.

Slanting of the articular surface of the distal tibia with lateral side superior is termed "ankle valgus." This has been reported as a feature of paralysis, sickle cell anemia, juvenile idiopathic arthritis, multiple epiphyseal dysplasia, hemophilia, and many other entities. However, the appearance of distal tibial angulation may also result from improper positioning of the foot during imaging. A well-positioned, weight-bearing AP of the ankle is necessary to measure ankle valgus. If the knee is both flexed and externally rotated more than 20°, images may give a false impression of tibiotalar obliquity. Ankle varus usually follows trauma. "Calcaneus" and "equinus" deformities at the ankle are discussed below in the sections on radiographic analysis and deformities of the foot, since these dorsi- and plantar-flexion deformities are important in the evaluation of foot alignment.

MRI is useful for directly evaluating the soft tissue structures of the ankle, including ligaments and tendons. It also provides detailed anatomic information about cartilaginous, nonossified structures that can only be inferred from radiographs. Cartilage and soft tissues may also be evaluated by US.

1.3 Congenital Abnormalities

Congenital anomalies exclusively involving the ankle are uncommon. Aberrations of normal ankle relationships may accompany fibular or tibial longitudinal deficiency, as well as midfoot and

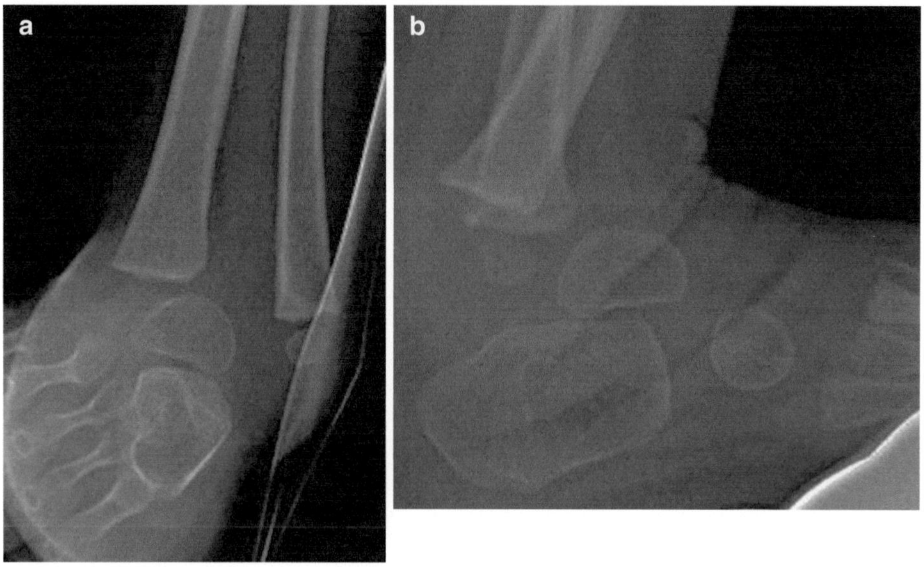

Fig. 15.4 Congenital diastasis of the inferior tibiofibular joint in a 2-year-old boy. Frontal (**a**) and simulated weight-bearing lateral views (**b**) show widening of the space between the distal tibia and fibula with superior migration of the talus, posteromedial displacement of the tibia, and dislocation of the distal fibula. This patient also had clubfoot, a commonly associated abnormality

hindfoot abnormalities such as congenital tarsal fusion. Congenital diastasis of the inferior tibiofibular joint is a very rare, severe deformity that may initially clinically resemble clubfoot [7] (Fig. 15.4). This entity has been considered part of a spectrum of distal tibial dysplasia with an intact fibula [8]. Diastasis of the distal tibia and fibula results in superior migration of the talus with resulting posteromedial displacement of the medial malleolus and dislocation of the distal fibula. Other congenital anomalies may be associated, including clubfoot and congenital heart disease. Treatment aims to preserve the foot, stabilize the ankle, and correct leg length discrepancies.

The ball-and-socket ankle is characterized by a hemispheric configuration of the articular surface of the talus on both frontal and lateral radiographs, with corresponding congruent concavity of the distal tibial articular surface (Fig. 15.5). Congenital and acquired etiologies of ball-and-socket ankle have been suggested (Table 15.1). Two major hypotheses have been proposed to explain the mechanical development: one postulates a secondary adaptation in shape to permit inversion and eversion in an ankle that has been limited by congenital tarsal fusions; the other states that the ball-and-socket ankle may be a characteristic component of a complex malformation with both deleted and fused foot bones. Regardless of etiology, this entity may not become symptomatic during childhood. However, its association with leg length discrepancy and other congenital abnormalities makes it important to recognize [9]. More recent studies have suggested that a surgical corrective approach to limb length discrepancies and malalignment in the setting of ball-and-socket ankle may prevent chronic osteoarthrosis and pain [10].

Congenital ball-and-socket ankle has been observed as early as 6 weeks of gestational age. During development, the abnormal talus ossifies more slowly than the normal side, and an abnormal shape of the talus may be detected on radiographs before 1 year of age [11]. Ball-and-socket ankle is associated with varying degrees of limb shortening. Anomalies of the forefoot rays are usually seen in conjunction with ball-and-socket ankle joint. Sixty percent of patients have some form of tarsal coalition, most commonly talonavicular or calcaneocuboid (see Fig. 15.5); occasionally all the hindfoot and midfoot structures are fused. By age 5 or 6, the ankle

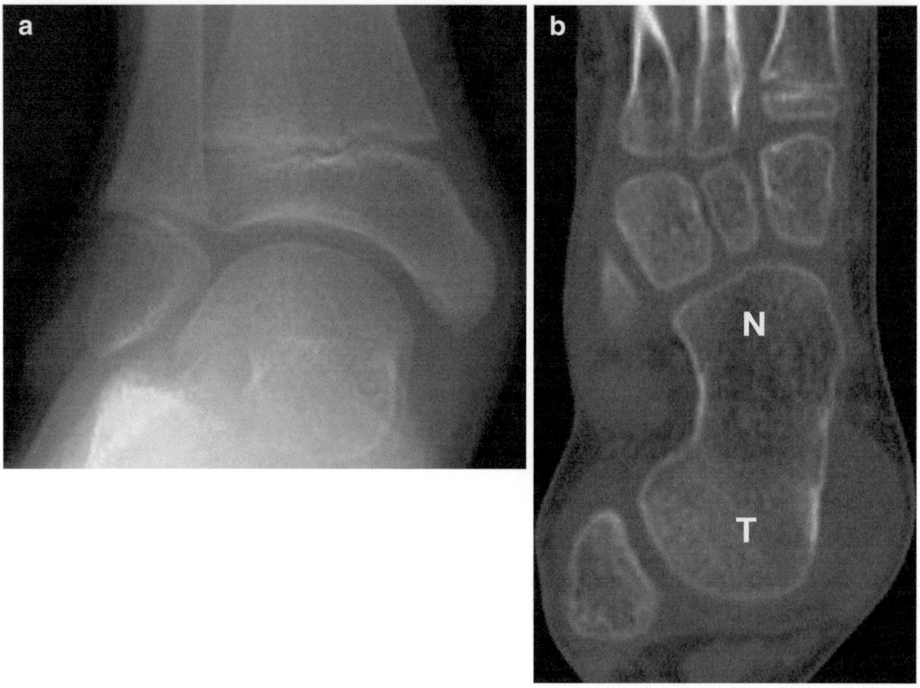

Fig. 15.5 Ball-and-socket ankle along with talonavicular coalition in a 12-year-old boy. (**a**) Frontal view shows hemispheric configuration of the talar dome, with concave distal tibial articular surface. (**b**) Axial-reformatted computed tomographic (CT) image from the same patient shows complete talonavicular osseous fusion and ray deletion. *T* talus, *N* navicular

Table 15.1 Associations and etiologies of ball-and-socket ankle

Congenital	Acquired
Short extremity	Tarsal coalitions
Tarsal coalition	Subtalar surgical arthrodesis at very young age
Absent or fused rays	Polio (after surgical arthrodesis at young age)
Hypoplastic fibula	Myelomeningocele
Skewfoot or clubfoot	Hyperlaxity
Acrocephalosyndactyly	Congenital insensitivity to pain

articulation has usually become a nearly perfectly congruent hemisphere.

Rounding of the talar dome may also be seen in older children without congenital fusions. For example, it may occur in patients with epiphyseal dysplasias or in the setting of ankle instability associated with chronic hyperlaxity from a young age, as seen in Larsen syndrome or myelomeningocele [12]. In these cases the talar trochlea is less rectangular than normal but usually does not have the near perfect rounding of congenital ball-and-socket ankle.

1.4 Developmental Abnormalities

In some situations, the plane of the ankle joint tilts into valgus. This may occur with paralytic conditions, such as myelomeningocele when growth of the distal fibula may be selectively impaired. Instead of the distal fibular physis sitting at the level of the ankle joint, undergrowth causes the distal fibular physis to be positioned above the level of the ankle joint (Fig. 15.6). Since ligaments tether the lateral edge of the distal tibial epiphysis to the fibula, poor development of the lateral malleolus may cause decreased growth and subsequent wedging of the lateral portion of the distal tibial epiphysis. Defective architecture of the ankle mortise may then lead to lateral instability of the ankle, with valgus tilt of

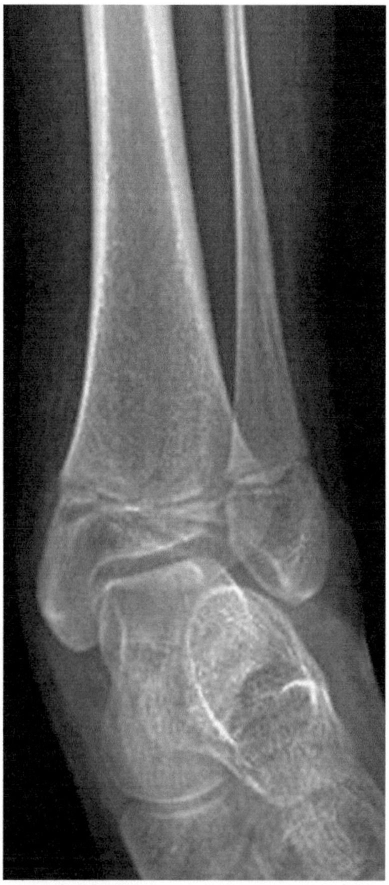

Fig. 15.6 Impaired growth of the fibula in a 9-year-old girl with myelomeningocele. Frontal view shows the fibula is relatively short compared with the tibia, since the distal fibular physis should be at or just below the level of the tibiotalar joint after age 4 years

the articular surface. Ankle valgus may occur in conjunction with genu valgum (Fig. 15.7), and in this setting the ossification of the fibular epiphysis may be delayed.

If the fibula is not intact, lack of weight-bearing forces on the fibula may cause growth inhibition and subsequent ankle valgus. This may occur in the setting of fibular resection or with fibular pseudarthrosis. Valgus ankle deformity also commonly occurs in the setting of multiple hereditary exostosis [13]. Relative fibular overgrowth with distal tibial or ankle varus may be seen in bone dysplasias such as achondroplasia, hypochondroplasia, and dyschondrosteosis [14, 15] and also after some fractures.

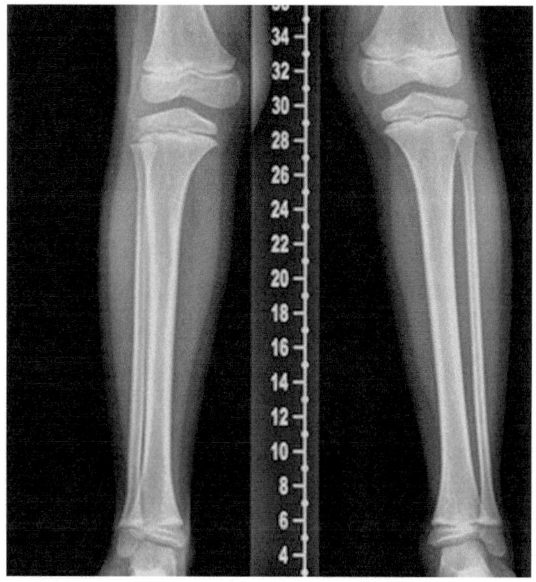

Fig. 15.7 Bilateral ankle valgus in a 7-year-old with genu valgum (Courtesy of Rebecca Stein-Wexler; Copyright Shriners Hospital for Children Northern California)

2 The Foot

2.1 Normal Anatomy and Variations

Anatomy and Development

The foot is a complex anatomical structure that performs a variety of biomechanical functions. These include weight bearing, shock absorption and propulsion during walking and running, and accommodating a variety of uneven surfaces. The foot is conventionally divided into three units: hindfoot, midfoot, and forefoot. These categories are useful to understand foot function, biomechanics, and pathophysiology. The hindfoot is composed of the talus and calcaneus, and the forefoot is composed of the metatarsals and phalanges. The midfoot includes the intervening tarsal bones: the cuneiforms, the navicular, and the cuboid. Although the last two are considered by some to be part of the hindfoot, from the viewpoint of radiologic analysis they are best considered midfoot structures. A variety of complex motions and deformities occur in all three regions, discussed below in the section on analysis of normal alignment.

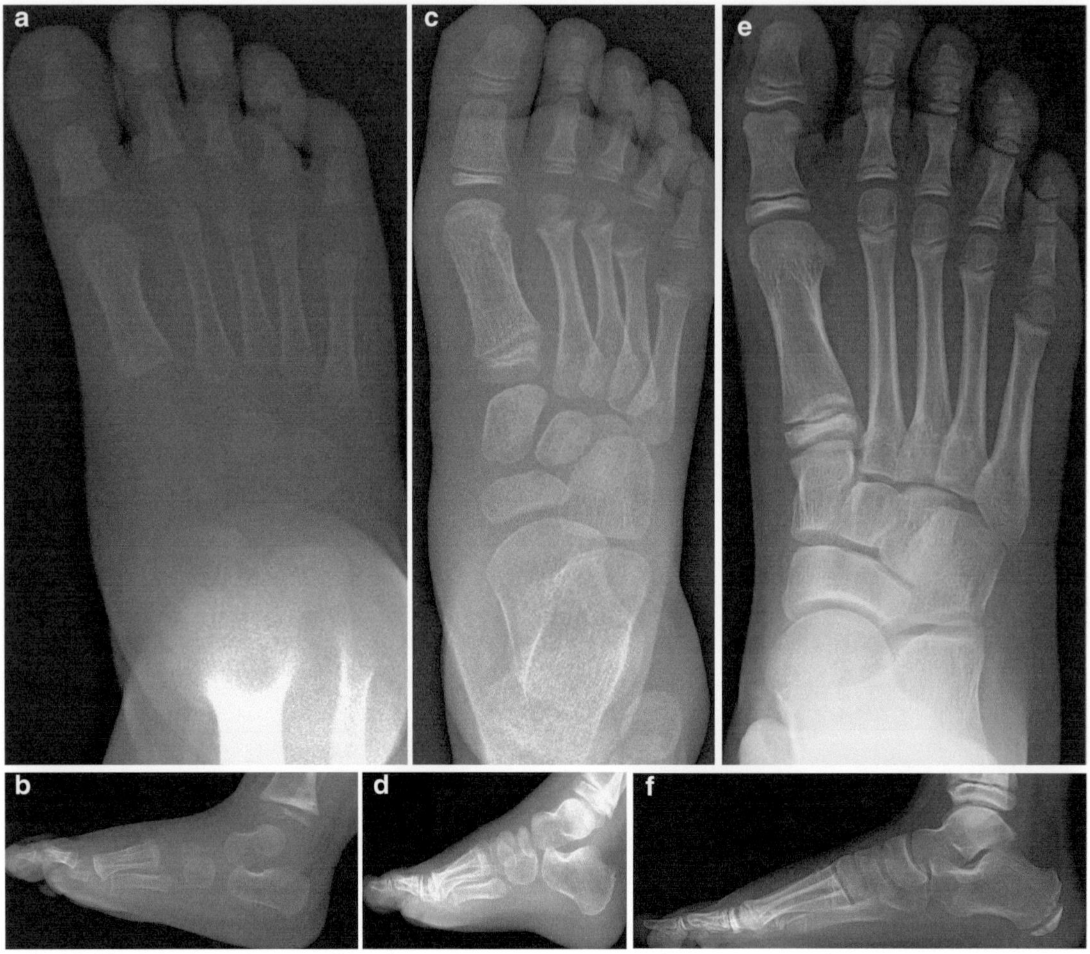

Fig. 15.8 Foot development. (**a**, **b**) At 1-year-old, the talus, calcaneus, cuboid, and lateral cuneiform have ossified. (**c**, **d**) At 5-year-old, all tarsal bones have ossified but their contours have not developed. (**e**, **f**) At 9-year-old, the foot has an adult configuration

The development of the cartilaginous structures that form the bones of the foot begins during approximately the 7th–9th week of gestation. Ossification typically follows a normal, sequential pattern within the foot, although congenital, infectious, and pregnancy-related abnormalities may alter the timeline. Ossification starts in the forefoot, beginning with the ends of metatarsals, with subsequent ossification of the metatarsals and then—sequentially—the proximal, middle, and distal phalanges. At birth all the metatarsals and phalanges are partially ossified. The tarsal bones ossify later, beginning at 24–28 weeks of gestation; only the talus and calcaneus are consistently partially ossified at birth. The sustentaculum tali do not begin to ossify until age 1–2 years and is not fully developed until age 5. The navicular is the last to ossify, usually between age 2 and 4 years [16] (Fig. 15.8).

Tarsal bone position is very important in evaluating foot deformities. However, limited tarsal ossification in the newborn and young child requires inference of their positions at radiography. Occasionally, US or MRI may be used to assess the developing tarsal bones before they ossify.

The foot grows rapidly from infancy to 5 years of age. It reaches one-half its adult size by age 5; growth slows and then usually ceases about age 12 years in girls and 14 years in boys, at which point the foot is considered mature. The anatomic relationship of the tarsal bones also changes during development. For example, the angle formed by the longitudinal axes of the talus and calcaneus gradually decreases with growth as the talus becomes less vertical, as indicated by a decrease in the lateral talocalcaneal angle from 45° on average in the newborn to 33° at age 4 years [17]. Similarly, the dorsiflexion-plantar flexion range of the foot decreases with age (76° at birth, 60° at age 1 year).

Normal Variants

Multipartite and Accessory Tarsal Centers

Ossification variants and accessory centers are common in the foot. Recognition of their characteristic appearance and location is important to avoid misdiagnosing a fracture or other injury. While some variants are common and readily recognized, others such as the striking vertical cleft of a bipartite talus are rare. A complete listing of the common accessory centers is provided in standard texts, but the most significant are discussed below.

It is unlikely that the presence of an ossification variant will lead to symptoms or later disability, since in most cases the multipartite or aberrantly ossifying nucleus is contained in a single normal cartilaginous anlage, with the centers fusing by maturity (Fig. 15.9).

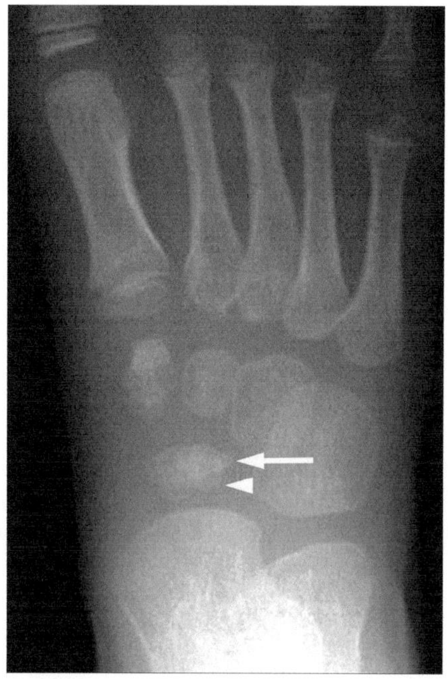

Fig. 15.9 Bipartite navicular in a 4-year-old girl. There are two separate ossification centers (*arrow* and *arrowhead*) for the navicular

The accessory navicular (*os naviculare*) is a common developmental variant that may be symptomatic, causing pain and peroneal spasm. This ossicle has been reported in 4–21 % of the population; 50–90 % are bilateral [18]. It ossifies around age 7–11 years [19] and is usually discovered incidentally when a child gets radiographs for foot pain or injury.

Three subtypes are generally recognized. The Type I accessory navicular accounts for about 30 % of cases. It appears as a 2–6 mm round or oval ossicle that represents a sesamoid bone within the posterior tibial tendon (Fig. 15.10). This ossicle is completely separate and is positioned about 2–5 mm proximal to the navicular body [20]. A Type 1 ossicle is also known as an *os tibiale externum* or *navicular secundarium*.

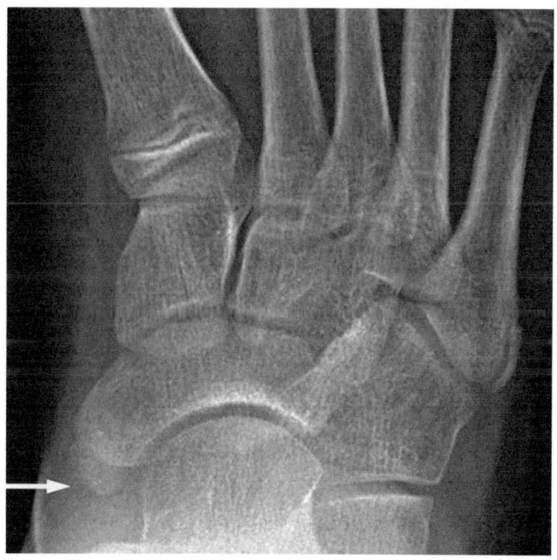

Fig. 15.10 Type 1 accessory navicular in an 11-year-old girl. There is a rounded ossicle (*arrow*) proximal to the navicular body

The Type 2 accessory navicular ossicle is also known as a *prehallux* or *bifurcated hallux*. It is more common than Type I, accounting for up to 70 % of accessory navicula. It is usually larger and has a flattened anterior surface that forms a facet with the medial proximal navicular tubercle, resulting in a triangular or heart-shaped ossicle (Fig. 15.11). The 1–2 mm interval separating this ossicle from the navicular represents a cartilaginous or fibrocartilaginous connection. Injury to

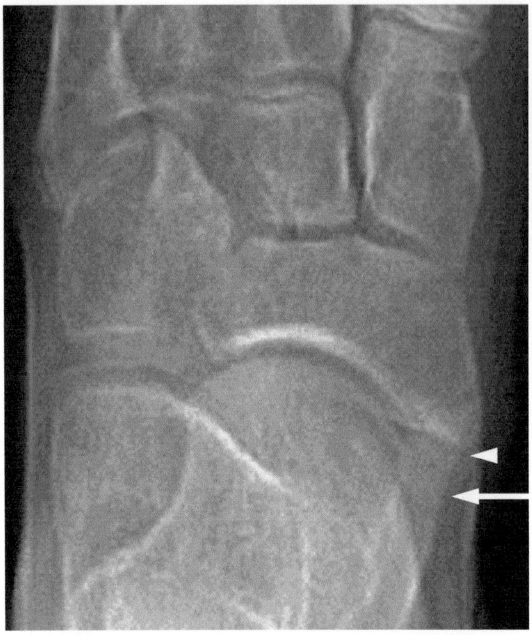

Fig. 15.11 Type 2 accessory navicular in a 12-year-old girl. There is characteristic flattening of the anterior surface (*arrow*), creating a facet with the medial proximal navicular tubercle (*arrowhead*)

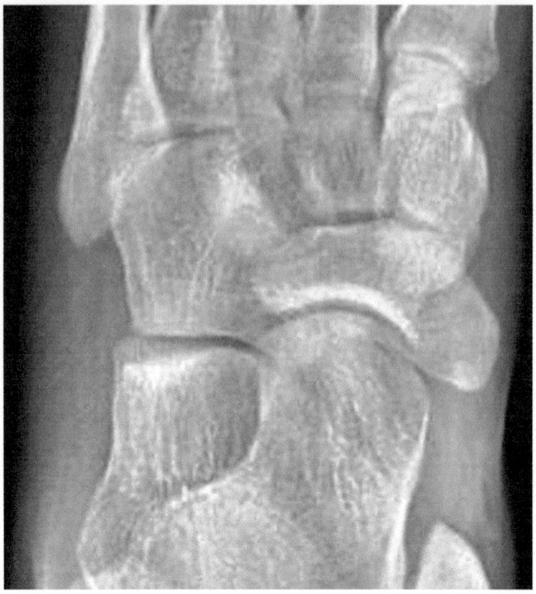

Fig. 15.12 Type 3 accessory navicular in a 16-year-old boy. The prominence of the medial margin of the navicular bone may be secondary to osseous bridging of previously separate ossification centers

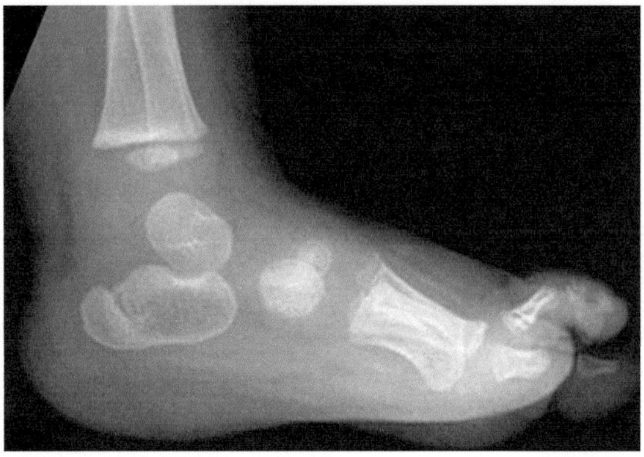

Fig. 15.13 Double ossification center of the calcaneus in a normal 17-month-old boy

this area may cause fracture and secondary pseudarthrosis of the synchondrosis or painful tendonosis or synovitis in some older children [21]. Fracture or pseudarthrosis of Type 2 accessory navicular ossicles is difficult to diagnose on radiographs. When symptomatic, an MRI is useful to evaluate for reactive bone marrow edema as well as secondary soft tissue findings, replacing technetium-99m bone scan [18] (see Chap. 16).

A Type 3 accessory navicular or *cornuate navicular* has been described as an especially prominent contiguous medial margin of the navicular, which may result from osseous bridging of a previously separate center. This causes a prominent, often symptomatic, protuberance (Fig. 15.12).

Bipartite or multiple ossification centers have also been reported at the cuboid and cuneiform bones, but these are generally asymptomatic. Double ossification centers within the calcaneus create a well-defined linear lucency through the central portion of this bone (Fig. 15.13), often associated with underlying conditions, such as trisomy 21 or Larsen syndrome. The formation of multiple ossification centers within a bone may also occasionally result in the appearance of an irregular-appearing central ossification site (Fig. 15.14). When this occurs in the navicular bone, it may be difficult if not impossible to distinguish the normal variant from Kohler osteonecrosis. This painful condition resembles variant ossification of the navicular, but flattening and sclerosis are more pronounced in Kohler osteochondrosis (see Chap. 16).

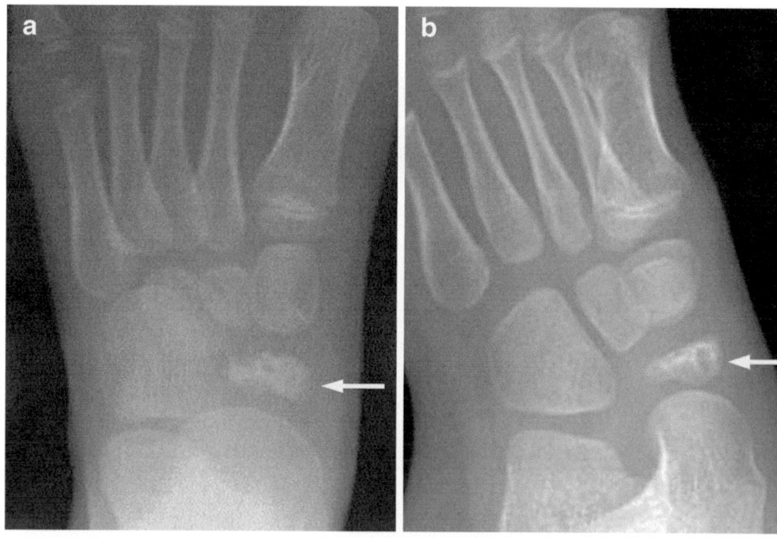

Fig. 15.14 Incidental irregular-appearing navicular in a 5-year-old boy, likely a normal variant given lack of focal symptoms. Frontal (**a**) and oblique (**b**) views show the margins of the navicular are sclerotic and irregular (*arrows*). Osteonecrosis may appear similar or the bone may appear flatter and more sclerotic; the patient will be symptomatic

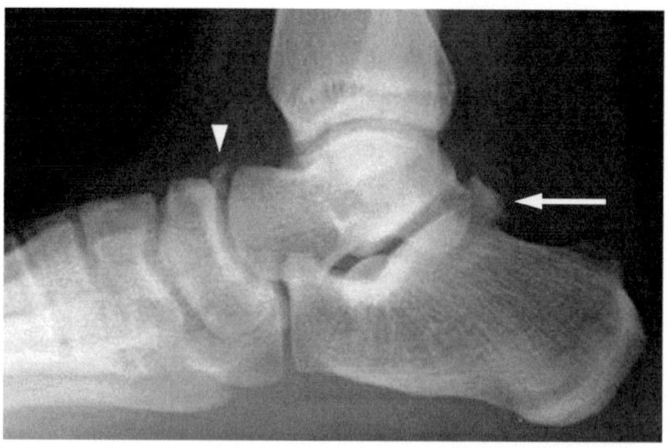

Fig. 15.15 Os trigonum and os supranaviculare in a 12-year-old girl. Well-corticated ossified fragment posterior to the talus is consistent with an os trigonum (*arrow*). Additional smooth fragment along the dorsal aspect of the talonavicular articulation is consistent with an os supranaviculare (*arrowhead*)

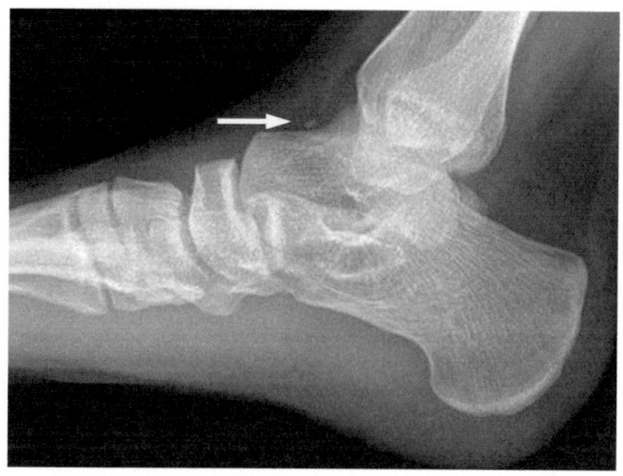

Fig. 15.16 Os supratalare in a 17-year-old boy. Small, oval ossific fragment (*arrow*) at the level of the talar neck is consistent with this accessory ossicle, particularly in the absence of focal symptoms or localized soft tissue swelling

A few of the many other accessory ossicles merit discussion. A normal accessory ossification center arises from the talus at the posterior ankle during normal development, ossifying around age 5 years and typically fusing with the talar body by age 20. Failure of fusion results in an ossicle called an *os trigonum* (Fig. 15.15). Posterior ankle impingement during plantar flexion may develop in dancers and other athletes. Chronic reactive changes from overuse or stress fracture may cause pain. MRI identifies edema, suggesting *os trigonum syndrome* [22] (see Chap. 16).

An *os supratalare* is a small, round ossicle along the dorsal aspect of the anterior talus on a lateral view; this may simulate a fracture (Fig. 15.16). An *os supranaviculare* is an irregular ossicle that typically fuses by about age 5 years; this too may look like a fracture or an accessory or bipartite navicular bone (see Fig. 15.15). Pain has been attributed to most ossicles, but aside from those highlighted above most are asymptomatic [23].

Calcaneal Apophysis

In the infant and young child, the posterior cortical margin of the calcaneus is smooth. An irregular, sawtooth outline often develops before the ossification centers for the apophysis appear. The

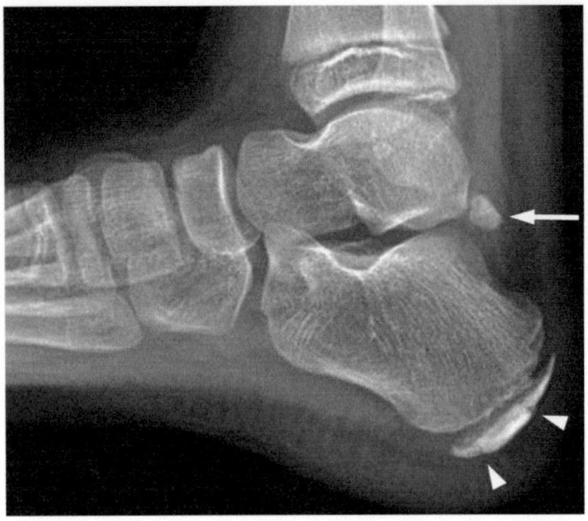

Fig. 15.17 Normal calcaneal apophysis in a 9-year-old boy. The apophysis is more sclerotic than the other bones, and it is traversed by several lucencies (*arrowheads*). An os trigonum (*arrow*) is also present

apophysis ossifies from several discrete centers, which then coalesce into one apophyseal center. The first of these appears between 4 and 7 years of age in girls and between 7 and 10 in boys. They usually demonstrate an extremely irregular outline, frequently traversed by several discrete linear lucencies. The normal ossification center(s) are often exceptionally dense, appearing more sclerotic than the calcaneal body on a lateral radiograph (Fig. 15.17).

A strikingly sclerotic, irregular calcaneal apophysis is often encountered in 8–10 year old girls and 9–12 year old boys who complain of heel pain during this period of rapid growth in length of the calcaneal tubercle. Perhaps best termed "calcaneal apophysitis," in the past this was considered diagnostic of "osteochondrosis" or Sever disease. The normal finding of increased density of the calcaneal apophysis may in part be a response to weight bearing. With bed rest (which is not recommended for this condition), the apophysis becomes osteopenic, eventually reaching the same density as the calcaneus. After 1 month of weight bearing, density is restored [24]. Eventually, as the apophysis fuses at age 12–15, the posterior margin of the calcaneus becomes isodense to the rest of the bone.

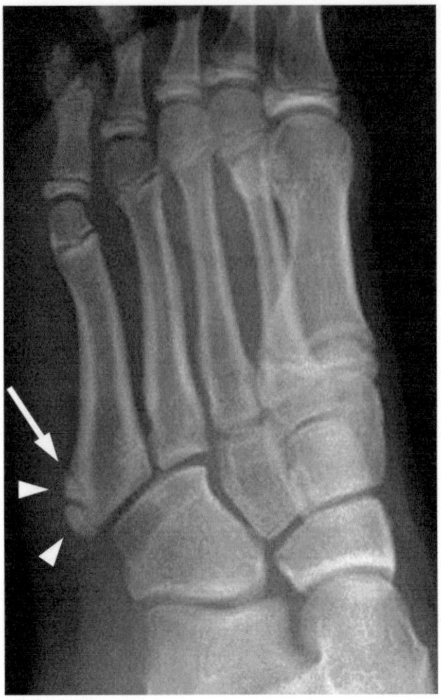

Fig. 15.18 Normal base of fifth metatarsal apophysis in a 12-year-old girl. Oblique view shows the normal apophysis paralleling the lateral cortex of the fifth metatarsal (*arrow*). Multiple ossification centers (*arrowheads*) may be present

Fifth Metatarsal Base Apophysis

This secondary ossification center parallels the lateral cortex of the fifth metatarsal. Multiple sliver-like centers may be present (Fig. 15.18). Fractures of the proximal fifth metatarsal, in contrast, are usually transverse to the metatarsal base, although oblique fractures may occur (see Chap. 16). The diagnosis of apophyseal separation should be made with caution, since the normal ossific portion of the apophysis may be quite lateral in the cartilaginous mass (Fig. 15.19). When in doubt, follow-up radiographs or images of the contralateral side may be helpful, as they may demonstrate evidence of healing or asymmetry. MRI may be performed but is usually not necessary.

Metatarsals and Phalanges

The fifth toe has only two phalanges in almost half the population, due to fusion of the distal interphalangeal joint. The epiphysis of the

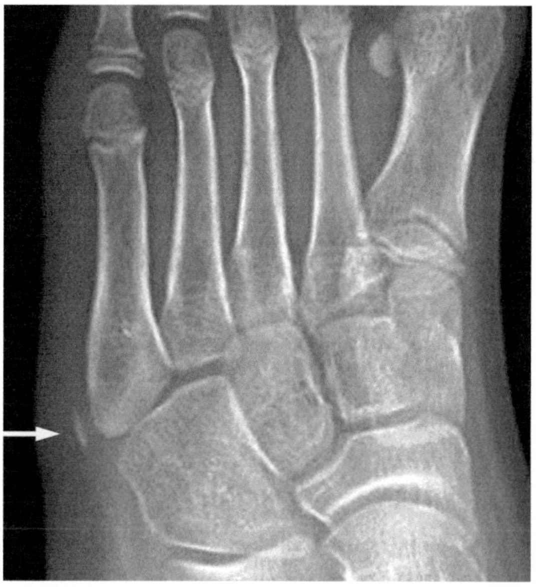

Fig. 15.19 Normal base of fifth metatarsal apophysis in a 10-year-old boy. Oblique view shows normal apparent separation of the ossific center from the adjacent metatarsal due to interposed cartilage (*arrow*). This should not be misinterpreted as an avulsion fracture

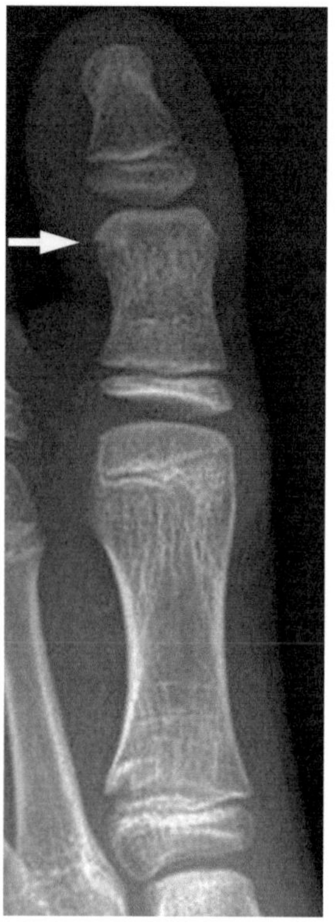

Fig. 15.21 Pseudoepiphysis of the first toe in a 10-year-old boy. There is an incomplete, transverse well-corticated lucency (*arrow*) at the distal aspect of the proximal phalanx

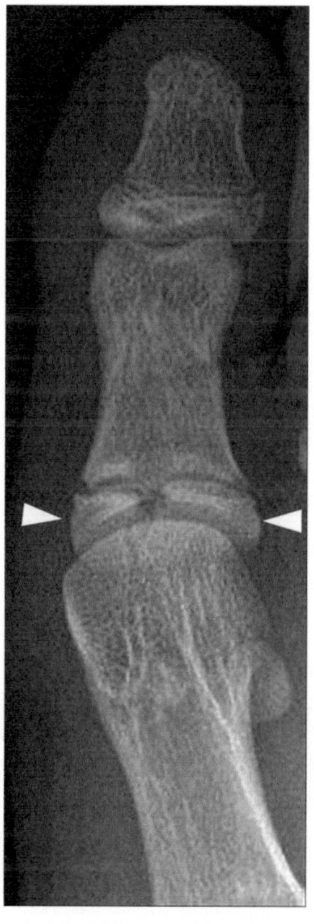

Fig. 15.20 Bifid epiphysis of the first toe in a 13-year-old boy. The epiphysis at the base of the proximal phalanx of the great toe is split and relatively sclerotic (*arrowheads*)

proximal phalanx of the first toe may have a central split (*bifid epiphysis*), due to incomplete ossification (Fig. 15.20). The bifid epiphysis may also appear sclerotic. Occasionally, the proximal epiphyses of other toes may be affected. Pseudoepiphyses may be seen at the base of the metatarsals and at the distal aspects of the phalanges (Figs. 15.21 and 15.22). The epiphyses of the proximal phalanges are frequently cone-shaped, perhaps due to premature closure of the central physis (see Fig. 15.22). Although often a normal variant, coned epiphyses are also found in a variety of syndromes.

A longitudinal epiphyseal bracket is rare, occurring in 2–14 % of congenital deformities of the hand and foot. Eleven percent of these cases involve the first toe [25]. In this entity, the normally transverse epiphysis is C-shaped and oriented along the longitudinal edge of the bone, causing abnormal transverse growth and shortening of the phalanx, as well as angular deformity (Fig. 15.23). This can be identified by radiographs or MRI and requires operative resection [26].

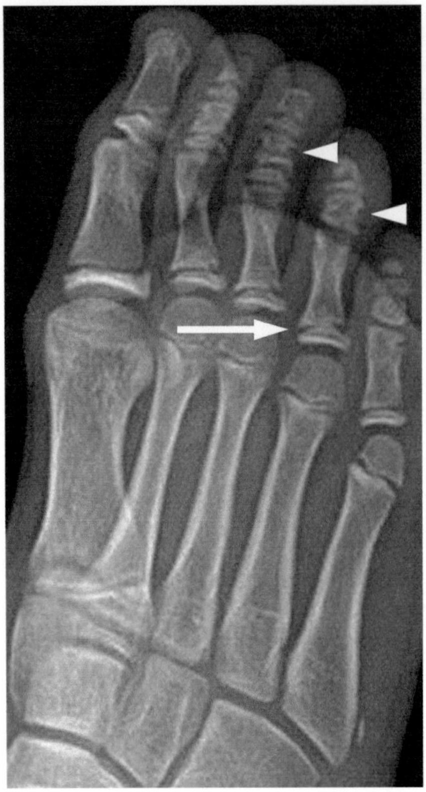

Fig. 15.22 Coned epiphysis in a 12-year-old girl. The epiphysis at the proximal phalanx of the fourth toe has a cone-like shape (*arrow*). There are also multiple pseudo-epiphyses (*arrowheads*)

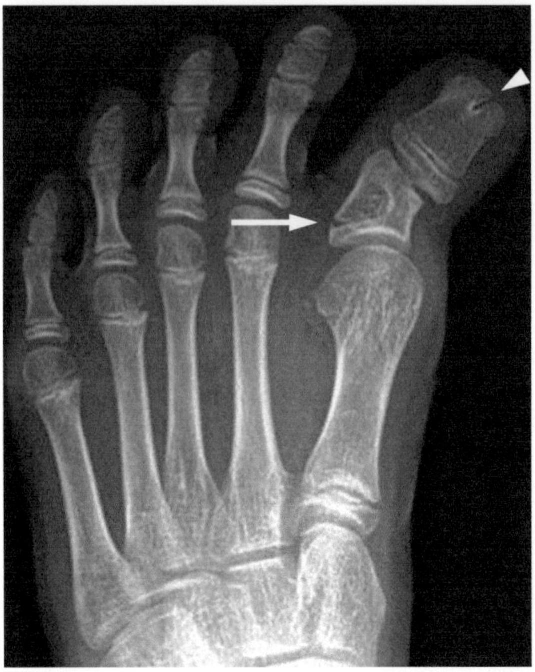

Fig. 15.23 Bracket epiphysis in a 10-year-old girl. Abnormal and fused proximal and distal epiphyses at the first toe proximal phalanx create a C-shape (*arrow*), widening, shortening, and tethering the phalanx. Note bifid appearance of the tuft of the great toe (*arrowhead*)

2.2 Imaging Examination and Analysis

Radiographs

The basic radiographic examination in the evaluation of foot deformities comprises a weight-bearing AP and a weight-bearing lateral projection of the foot. Weight bearing stresses the foot in a reproducible manner and shows the relationship of the bones in their functional state (Fig. 15.24). In an infant or non-ambulating older child, simulated weight-bearing radiographs may be acquired by using a wooden or plastic board to apply plantar pressure or an attendant may apply direct manipulation. Although every effort should be made to avoid radiation exposure of persons other than the patient, it is often impossible to achieve the correct plantar pressure and lateral positioning of the young infant's foot by any means other than a well-shielded assistant. Proper technique is essential.

An AP projection is obtained with the child standing, with tibias parallel to a sagittal plane perpendicular to the plane of imaging. Patients unable to stand may sit or lie supine with knees flexed and the feet plantigrade, pressed against the image receiver; the tibias should be aligned as for a standing radiograph. The central x-ray beam is angled about 15° toward the heel to eliminate overlap of the lower leg and posterior foot. Opinions vary about whether to attempt to correct alignment during imaging, as some surgeons prefer to have evidence of flexibility and the ability to correct deformity, while others prefer to view the uncorrected relationships.

A lateral projection is taken with the patient standing and leaning forward to show the foot in dorsiflexion (see Fig. 15.24). Similar positioning may be obtained in infants and non-ambulatory patients with directed plantar pressure with a radiolucent board. Care must be taken to ensure that the board used to produce plantar pressure is not tilted to produce a false impression of varus

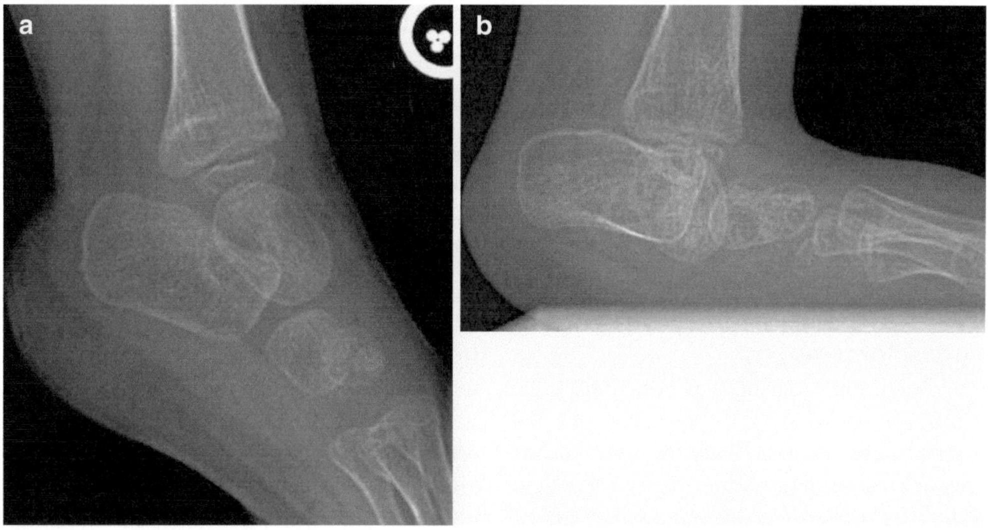

Fig. 15.24 The effect of weight bearing on hindfoot alignment. (**a**) Non-weight-bearing view shows markedly abnormal configuration of the hindfoot, including vertical talus in this 5-year-old with fibular longitudinal deficiency. (**b**) With simulated weight bearing, the configuration of the talus is even more abnormal, as it projects between the calcaneus and the cuboid. Rocker-bottom configuration becomes apparent, as well

or valgus. To avoid projectional distortion of the talar dome in a medially deviated foot, the ankle and hindfoot (not the forefoot) should be placed in a true lateral position.

Oblique projections of the foot are often useful in evaluation of trauma, surgical follow-up, or tarsal coalition. However, they are not necessary in the initial or serial evaluation of the structurally deformed foot.

Dedicated radiographic techniques for imaging the subtalar joints are useful in some circumstances, although definitive diagnosis of hindfoot pathology generally requires CT or MRI. In addition to the standard AP, lateral, and oblique views of the foot, several other views may be helpful in specific cases. Lateral foot radiographs in maximum plantar flexion and maximum dorsiflexion may help in assessing rigidity of foot deformity as well as subtalar motion. The 45° axially angulated Harris-Beath projection of the heel is the most commonly performed supplemental examination to see sustentaculum tali fracture or subtalar coalition. However, due to the wide variability in the orientation of the subtalar joint, 30–60° beam angulation may be necessary if the articular facets are not shown well at first. When successful, this projection will show the posterior subtalar joint laterally as well as the medial facet located medially, superiorly, and parallel. This view is not useful in young children, since the sustentaculum tali do not fully ossify until age 5 years.

Nuclear Medicine Imaging

Bone scans utilizing technetium-99m have relatively limited use in detecting occult trauma, infection, or areas of avascular necrosis, since MRI can provide similar information while also offering more anatomic detail without radiation exposure.

Ultrasound

The advantages of US are the same when imaging any part of the body—imaging is performed rapidly and without sedation, dynamic images can be obtained, and the modality is typically readily available and relatively inexpensive. US also provides the highest resolution of soft tissue detail. However, while US readily depicts the cartilaginous portions of bones, the limited depth of beam penetration precludes complete assessment of the complex articulations between the bones of the hindfoot and midfoot.

Directed US can provide measurements or depict relationships between specific structures [27]. In the setting of clubfoot, for example, defining the relationship between the talus and navicular is essential, and this can be directly visualized by observing the distance between the medial malleolus and the navicular [28]. Dynamic imaging can show reducibility of the navicular medially with respect to the talus during manipulation [29]. It can also evaluate the reducibility of the talonavicular joint in vertical talus [30] (see subsequent sections on clubfoot, pes planus, and congenital vertical talus).

Computed Tomography

With the ongoing development of multi-slice computed tomography (CT) systems and the ability to reduce radiation dose through various new image reconstruction algorithms, CT imaging of the foot is useful in many clinical settings, including tarsal coalition, fracture evaluation, postoperative imaging, and tumor evaluation (especially osteoid osteoma). Images can be acquired rapidly, typically without sedation, while minimizing radiation exposure and maintaining image quality [31]. CT can be performed with or without simulated weight bearing using similar techniques and with similar clinical applications, as described above for radiography. Multiplanar image reconstructions are now standard. Three-dimensional (3D)-reconstructed images are easily generated on most systems and are particularly useful for surgical planning.

CT has replaced conventional radiographic tomography in the investigation of the subtalar joint, as it provides a more definitive evaluation of the osseous structures while evaluating the soft tissue and cartilaginous structures as well. When evaluating for tarsal coalition, CT reformatted in the axial and coronal planes is often most useful [32].

Magnetic Resonance Imaging

Because of the superior soft tissue contrast available with MRI, this modality is best for delineating the relationship of the partially ossified cartilage templates of the tarsal bones during childhood. While other modalities such as US can also demonstrate the cartilaginous and soft tissue structures of the immature foot, MRI provides a complete, global assessment. MRI is also useful when evaluating tarsal coalition, as it characterizes non-osseous bridging and evaluates for reactive changes in the bones and adjacent tendons [33]. For routine evaluation, standard radiographs usually provide sufficient information, and additional imaging is limited to addressing specific clinical questions. The utility of MRI remains limited by long acquisition times and need for sedation in most young children.

Arthrography

Interventional direct contrast material injection to delineate the cartilage and joint surfaces has been replaced by US and MRI, but arthrography remains the modality of choice to establish joint continuity. The posterior subtalar (facet) joint, talocalcaneonavicular (anterior and middle facets), and ankle joints are all accessible to contrast material administration. Injection into the posterior subtalar joint may be useful for therapeutic and diagnostic purposes if there is a need to establish communication with the ankle joint.

Arteriography

An abnormal size and distribution of the small arterial vessels of the foot has been described in congenital deformities. However, conventional angiography is rarely performed for operative planning. If knowledge of arterial vascular anatomy is needed, CT angiography or MRI angiography of the lower extremities provides a noninvasive means to obtain this information.

2.3 Analysis of Alignment (Figs. 15.25 and 15.26)

The alignment of the ankle, hindfoot, midfoot, and forefoot is best evaluated separately, even though these structures are obviously intimately related both anatomically and functionally. The ankle, of course, consists of the distal tibia, distal fibula, and the talus. Two motions are possible: dorsiflexion and plantar flexion; the corresponding deformities consist of calcaneus and equinus. (Valgus and varus tilt are described above in the section on radiologic analysis of the ankle.)

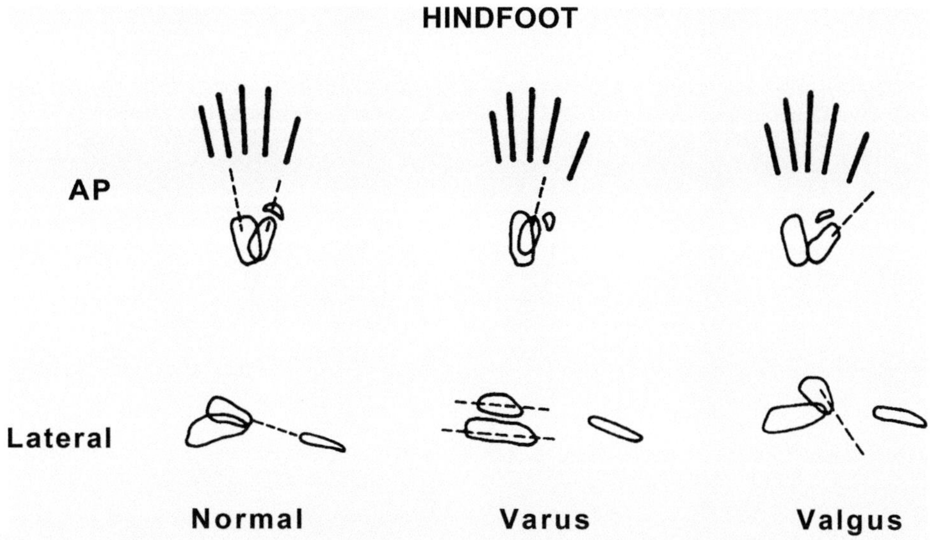

Fig. 15.25 Hindfoot relationships. In a *normally aligned foot*, the long axis of the calcaneus in an AP projection should pass through the base of the fourth metatarsal. A line drawn along the long axis of the talus should pass through or slightly medial to the base of the first metatarsal. In a normally aligned foot, a line drawn along the long axis of the talus on a lateral view should align with the long axis of the first metatarsal (the *Meary* angle). With *hindfoot varus*, the axis of the talus on the frontal view is laterally deviated from the midline. On a lateral view, the long axis of the talus is superior to that of the first metatarsal. The calcaneus and talus therefore appear more parallel on both views. With *hindfoot valgus*, the long axis of the talus is angled toward midline on the frontal view. On a lateral view, the long axis of the talus points inferior to the long axis of the first metatarsal. The calcaneus and talus therefore appear more divergent on both views

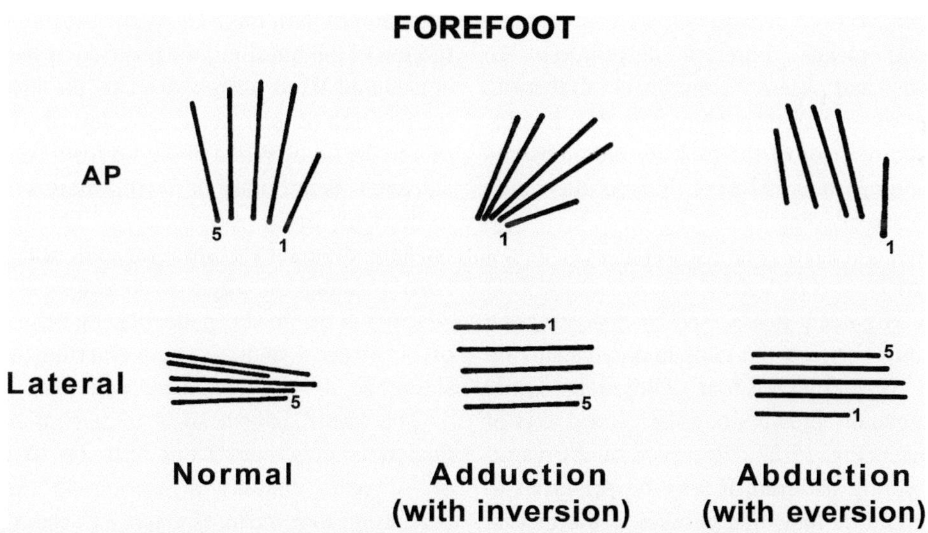

Fig. 15.26 Forefoot relationships: normal, adduction, and abduction. In the *normal forefoot*, the metatarsals are splayed, without significant overlap of the bases on an AP view. On a lateral view, the metatarsals converge distally. With *forefoot adduction*, the metatarsals are torqued so that the sole faces inward on an AP view. There is increased superimposition of the metatarsal bases, with the distal metatarsals swinging toward midline. On a lateral view, the metatarsals are generally configured in a ladder-like array due to concomitant *inversion*, with the fifth metatarsal being the most plantar. With *forefoot abduction*, the metatarsals are more parallel than normal on the frontal view, and there is less overlap at their bases, resulting in a broader forefoot. There may be a ladder-like array on a lateral view, with the first metatarsal most plantar (due to *eversion*), but this is rarely seen

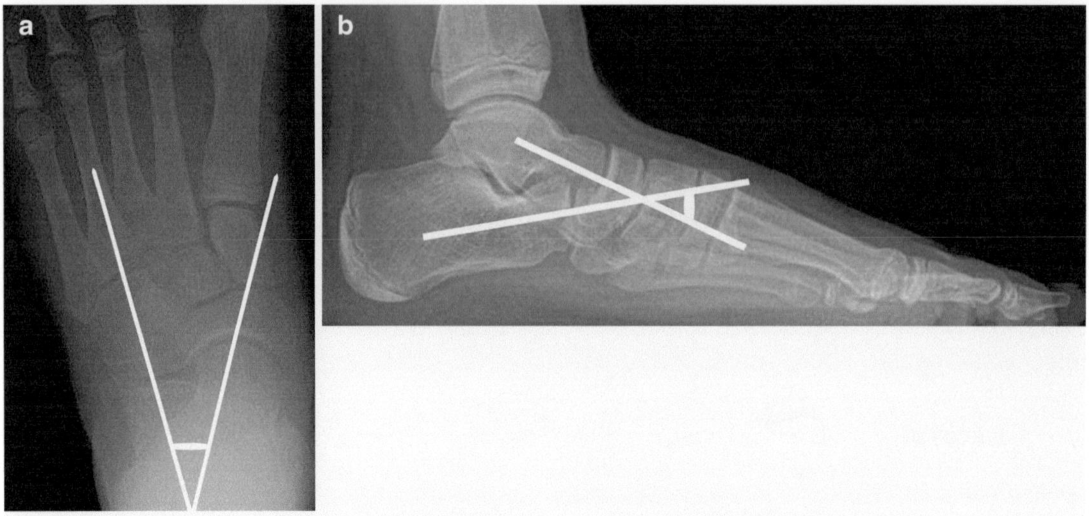

Fig. 15.27 Normal talocalcaneal relationships in a 13-year-old girl. Frontal (**a**) and lateral (**b**) views show *lines* drawn along the central axes of the talus and calcaneus. The intersection of these *lines* forms the talocalcaneal angle, which should be between 30 and 45° (weight-bearing views)

In radiologic practice, the hindfoot unit comprises the talus and calcaneus; the midfoot consists of the navicular, cuboid, and cuneiforms; and the forefoot, the metatarsals and phalanges. At the hindfoot, varus and valgus deformities may occur. Midfoot deformities are described as cavus and planus. Forefoot deformities are adduction and (less common) abduction. Inversion and eversion are more complex, involving motion of most of the foot around an essentially stationary talus. Most of this motion occurs at the intertarsal joints.

Hindfoot

Hindfoot alignment is assessed by analyzing the relationship between the talus and calcaneus on standard AP and lateral foot radiographs. Axial lines are usually drawn along the central axis of these bones (Fig. 15.27). However, on AP views of very young children, it may be preferred to draw the central talar line parallel to the medial cortex of the ossification center and the central calcaneal line parallel to the lateral cortex of the calcaneus. Similarly, on a lateral projection it may be preferred to draw central lines (see Figs. 15.25 and 15.27), although some suggest using the undersurface of the calcaneus [34]. The calculation of actual angles is often advocated, and some studies have shown excellent interobserver agreement when assessing standard measurements [34]. The placement of lines, however, remains somewhat arbitrary, and this limitation should always be considered.

During dorsiflexion and plantar flexion, the talus moves with the foot. With varus and valgus motion of the hindfoot, the position of the talus is considered fixed with respect to the ankle, and the position of the calcaneus is described in relation to the talus. When observed from behind, the calcaneus is normally in 5–10° valgus compared to the talus in the coronal plane. This translates on AP radiographs to midtalar and midcalcaneal lines forming an angle averaging 42° (range, 27–56°) in the newborn, decreasing to an average of 34° by age 4 years. As a general rule, this angle should be 30–45°, decreasing with age.

The lateral talocalcaneal alignment in dorsiflexion is maximum from birth up to the age of 2 years, initially measuring 45° and then decreasing to a mean of about 33°. As a general guideline, this angle should also be 30–45°. A similar evolution is seen in the range of the dorsiflexion and plantarflexion gliding motion of the talus: the average range of 76° in a child less than 1 year old decreases gradually as the child grows.

The calcaneus is mechanically linked to the midfoot and forefoot bones, and it is therefore

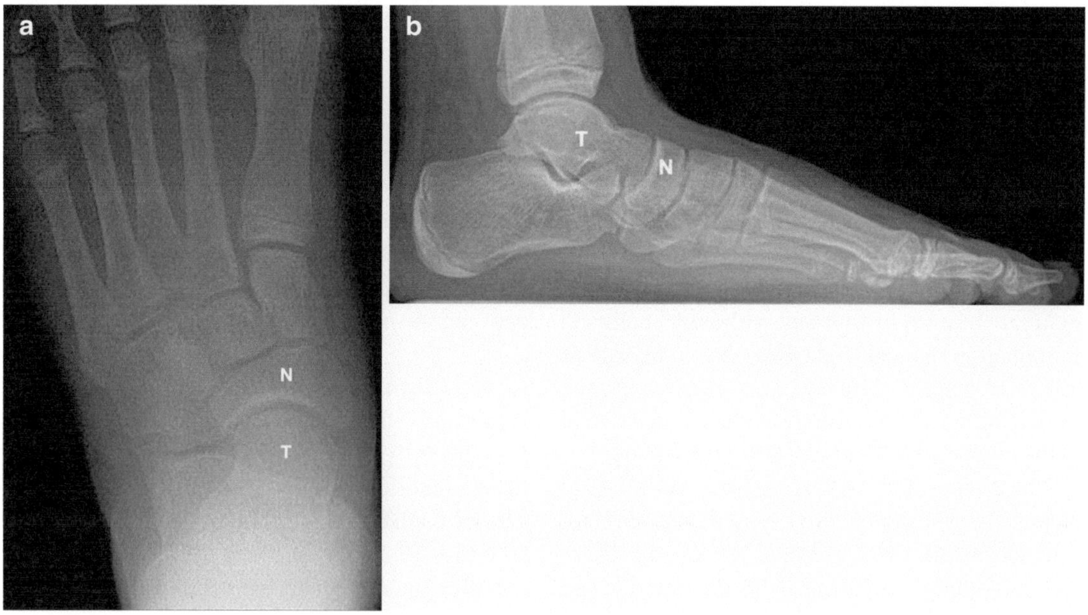

Fig. 15.28 Normal talonavicular relationship in a 13-year-old girl. The navicular is immediately distal to the middle of the talar head on frontal (**a**) and lateral (**b**) projections (weight-bearing views). *T* talus, *N* navicular

reasonable to consider the relation of the midtalar and midcalcaneal lines to the bases of the metatarsals. The midtalar line normally passes through or slightly medial to the base of the first metatarsal. The midcalcaneal line should pass through the base of the fourth metatarsal (see Figs. 15.25 and 15.27). When forefoot deformity is present, these lines do not necessarily pass down the shafts of the metatarsals.

The pitch of the calcaneus on a lateral view is measured with the tibiocalcaneal angle, which is the angle between the distal tibial shaft and the midcalcaneal line. This angle is about 77° at birth, decreasing to 67° by age 4 years. As a general rule, the tibiocalcaneal angle should be between 60 and 90°. The anterior calcaneus is therefore normally in slight dorsiflexion with respect to the tibia.

Midfoot

Ligaments link the midfoot bones to the calcaneus but not to the talus; therefore an abnormal position of the calcaneus relative to the talus should be made evident by a change in the relation of the midfoot bones to those of the hindfoot. Unfortunately, the navicular, which would be the key to this change, is the last to ossify. The navicular, when ossified, should be seen immediately distal to the middle portion of the talar head on both AP and lateral projections (Fig. 15.28); any shift in position indicates an abnormal relationship between the midfoot and the hindfoot. If the navicular is not yet ossified, assessment of alignment depends on the metatarsal bases, as discussed above. However, the lateral cuneiform, which begins to ossify between the newborn period and 19 months of age, may help indicate midfoot and hindfoot deformity.

Forefoot

This portion of the foot comprises the metatarsals and phalanges, but only the metatarsals are generally useful in the analysis of forefoot alignment. The forefoot is usually flexible, and thus metatarsal alignment may be altered during imaging by variable/inconsistent degrees of weight bearing, poor patient cooperation, and active attempts to straighten the foot. Analysis of the apparent metatarsal shaft alignment is therefore not necessarily reliable. However, the metatarsal bases should have a constant relationship to the distal tarsal row and through them to the remainder of the foot.

There is normally a slight overlap or convergence of the bases of the metatarsals on AP view (see Fig. 15.28). On a lateral projection, the central metatarsals should be superimposed, making it difficult to identify specific metatarsals—other than the short first and fifth metatarsals.

Plantar Arch

The longitudinal arch of the foot is identifiable on radiographs even in an infant, although at clinical examination the soft tissues and fat in the sole of the foot suggest flatness. The transverse arch causes the central metatarsals to be located dorsal to the more easily identified fifth metatarsal.

The plantar arch is best assessed on a lateral view by measuring the alignment of the hindfoot and metatarsals. On a lateral projection, the calcaneus is slightly dorsiflexed with the anterior end higher. The plantar angulation of the distal metatarsals completes the anterior portion of the arch.

The lateral talar-first metatarsal angle, also known as the angle of Meary, is used to measure the plantar arch in older children and adults. This is the angle formed between a line drawn along the central talus and a line drawn along the first metatarsal shaft. (The first metatarsal is easily distinguished because it is the shortest, widest metatarsal.) The Meary angle should be near zero (see Fig. 15.25). Normal values vary with age (see Table 15.3). As a general rule, an angle greater than 8° convex upward results in an exaggerated arch and *pes cavus*. An angle greater than 4° convex downward results in flattening of the plantar arch and *pes planus* or *flatfoot*.

2.4 Analysis of Foot Malalignment (Tables 15.2 and 15.3)

Several terms are traditionally employed to describe foot alignment, as presented in Table 15.2. The following discussion supplies specific details about each type of malalignment of the ankle, hindfoot, midfoot, and forefoot. Table 15.3 presents normative data for angular relationships between the hindfoot, forefoot, and distal tibia.

Ankle Alignment

Equinus (Talipes Equinus)

In a lateral projection, the calcaneus is plantar flexed, anterior end down, so that the angle of the axis of the calcaneus to that of the tibia exceeds 90° (Fig. 15.29), as opposed to the normal slight dorsiflexion of the anterior calcaneus (60–90°) (see Fig. 15.28).

Calcaneus Deformity

Calcaneus deformity of the hindfoot is determined on a lateral radiograph. For clarity, when discussing "calcaneus" deformity, it is helpful to refer to the bone as the *os calcis*. The os calcis is fixed in excessive dorsiflexion, with the anterior end higher than normal (Fig. 15.30); the tibiocalcaneal angle is less than 60°. The calcaneal position of the os calcis may contribute to the exaggerated plantar arch of pes cavus in a calcaneocavus deformity. This is commonly seen in S1 level myelomeningocele or polio patients who have paralysis of the gastrocsoleus muscle complex.

Table 15.2 Foot and ankle alignment terminology

Terminology	Meaning
Ankle valgus	Slanting of articular surface of distal tibia, lateral side superior
Ankle varus	Slanting of articular surface of distal tibia, lateral side inferior
Ankle calcaneus	Increased dorsiflexion of calcaneus, anterior end higher
Ankle equinus	Plantar flexion of calcaneus, anterior end lower
Hindfoot valgus	Axial reference line of calcaneus deviates away from body's midline on AP view of foot
Hindfoot varus	Axial reference line of calcaneus deviates toward body's midline on AP view of foot
Pes cavus	Increased depth of plantar arch
Pes planus	Flattening of plantar arch
Metatarsus abductus	Metatarsals move away from midline
Metatarsus adductus	Metatarsals move toward midline
Foot eversion	Plantar surface faces laterally: pronation, abduction, dorsiflexion
Foot inversion	Plantar surface faces midline: supination, adduction, plantar flexion

Table 15.3 Normal hindfoot-forefoot angular relationships

Angle	Newborn	2 years	4 years	6 years	9 years
AP view					
Talocalcaneal	42° (27–56°)	40° (27–50°)	34° (24–45°)	30° (20–40°)	18° (5–35°)
Calcaneal-fifth metatarsal	3° (−9 to +14°)	0° (−10 to +10°)	−1° (−10 to +8°	0° (−10 to +8°)	3°(−8 to +15°)
Talar-first metatarsal	20° (+12 to +31°)	15° (+2 to +27°)	10° (−4 to +23°)	7° (−7 to +20°)	4° (−9 to +17°)
Lateral view					
Talocalcaneal	39° (23–55°)	41° (27–56°)	44° (31–57°)	44° (33–56°)	40° (28–52°)
Talocalcaneal (maximum dorsiflexion)	45° (35–56°)	44° (33–54°)	43° (32–52°)	42° (31–51°)	41° (31–51°)
Tibiocalcaneal	77° (60–95°)	72° (57–87°)	68° (56–81°)	67° (58–76°)	68° (63–74°)
Tibiocalcaneal (maximum dorsiflexion)	42° (25–60°)	48° (27–68°)	50° (30–72°)	51° (33–71°)	50° (33–71°)
Tibiotalar	115° (86–145°)	114° (95–130°)	113° (100–122°)	111° (101–118°)	108° (89–123°)
Talar-first metatarsal (Meary angle)	18° (−2° to +44°)	12° (−4 to +28°)	8° (−5 to +22°)	7° (−5 to +18°)	7° (−7 to +20°)
Talar-horizontal	34° (14–55°)	32° (18–45°)	30° (20–40°)	26° (20–36°)	25° (13–35°)

Adapted from Vanderwilde et al. [17]
Mean values in degrees (ranges in parentheses)

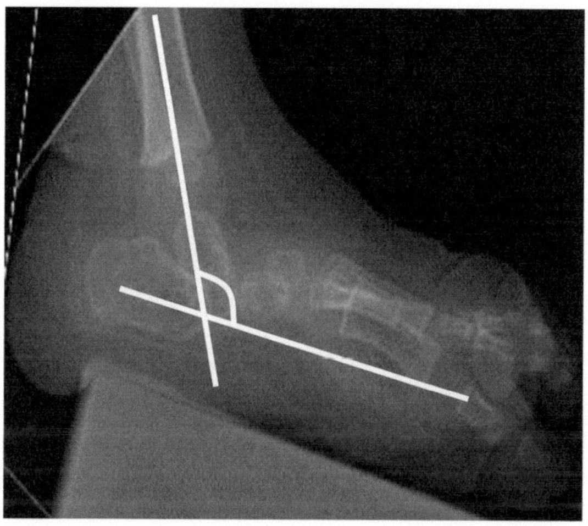

Fig. 15.29 Equinus foot. The angle between the long axes of the calcaneus and tibia exceeds 90° (normal ranges from 60 to 90°) (simulated weight bearing)

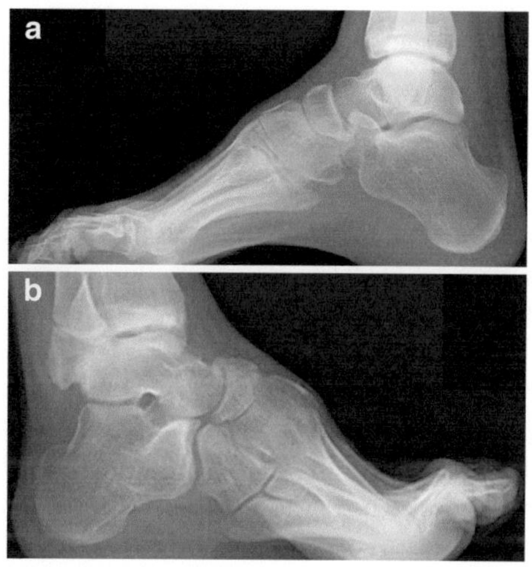

Fig. 15.30 Bilateral pes cavus. (**a**) (*right*), (**b**) (*left*). On both feet, the plantar arch is abnormally concave. The anterior margin of the calcaneus is directed superiorly (os calcis in "calcaneus"), and the metatarsals are abnormally plantar flexed. Note that this case illustrates the apparent flattening of the talus that is seen when the technologist "straightens" the foot, inadvertently causing obliquity of the ankle. On the right (**a**), a true lateral view of the ankle—with the fibula projecting over the middle of the tibia—the talar dome appears normally rounded, and the calcaneus is normally rectangular. On the left (**b**), performed with the ankle oblique as indicated by the dorsal position of the fibula, the talar dome appears to be flattened, as its convex contours are superimposed. The calcaneus appears square (weight-bearing views) (Courtesy of Rebecca Stein-Wexler; Copyright Shriners Hospital for Children Northern California)

Hindfoot

Hindfoot Valgus

The calcaneus rotates laterally under the talus so that its anterior part is lateral to the talus on AP radiograph. Its most posterior portion would be lateral to the center of the ankle when viewed from behind. Since it is difficult to get a true AP of the hindfoot, the following changes are conventionally identified on the standard weight-bearing AP and lateral foot views.

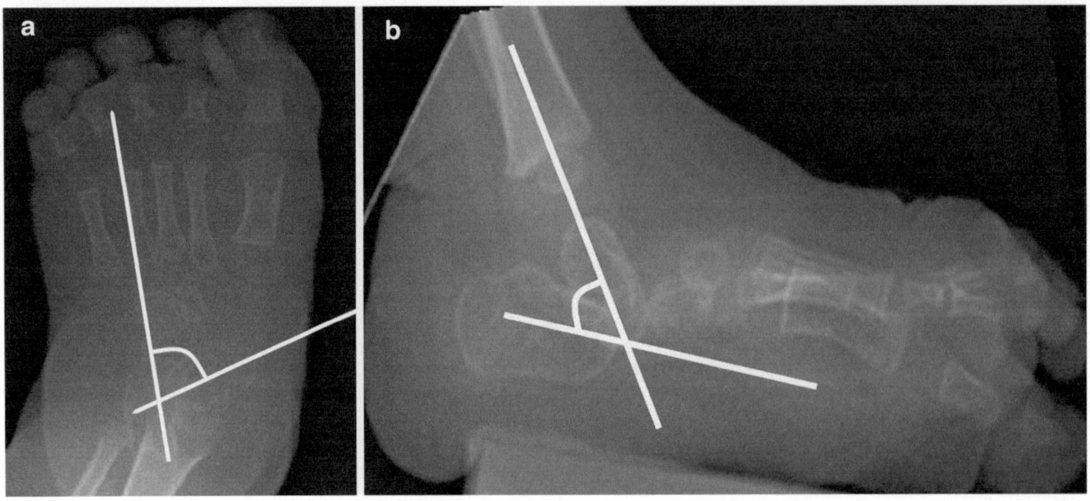

Fig. 15.31 Hindfoot valgus. (**a**) Frontal view shows medial deviation of the long axis of the talus, resulting in increased divergence of the calcaneus and talus and an abnormally large talocalcaneal angle. (**b**) Lateral view shows the long axis of the talus angled inferior to the long axis of the first metatarsal. The talocalcaneal angle is abnormally large due to increased divergence of the talus and calcaneus on this view as well (simulated weight-bearing views)

On an AP projection, the talocalcaneal angle is increased greater than 45°, since the calcaneus is laterally rotated from the midline. This gives the impression of medial deviation of the talus, so that a line through it points medial to the abducted first metatarsal base. However, the entire foot under and distal to the talus is abducted and everted (Figs. 15.25 and 15.31). The navicular moves with the calcaneus and if ossified appears displaced laterally from its normal position at the head of the talus.

On a lateral projection, the talus, having lost its medial support as a result of lateral displacement of the calcaneus, is more vertically oriented than normal, with a consequent increase in the talocalcaneal angle of greater than 45°. The navicular seems to be in an unusual plantar position, since it follows the calcaneus and the head of the talus downward.

Hindfoot valgus is present in many congenital and neurogenic deformities of the foot including flatfoot, skewfoot, congenital vertical talus, and cerebral palsy.

Hindfoot Varus

In hindfoot varus, the calcaneus is medially rotated under the talus, reducing the normal plantar angulation of the talus. On a lateral projection, a decreased talocalcaneal angle (less than 30°) and a more parallel orientation of the two bones are evident, as the calcaneus uplifts the anterior end of the talus. Axial lines through the two bones appear more horizontal and parallel than normal. On an AP projection, the calcaneal body is positioned under the talus, so that axes through the two bones are more parallel or even superimposed (Figs. 15.25 and 15.32). This decreases the normal talocalcaneal angle to less than 30°. Since the remainder of the foot also swings medially, a line through the talus points lateral to the first metatarsal base. The navicular is displaced medial to the talar head.

Varus deformity is seen in congenital clubfoot deformity (equinovarus) and in some neurological abnormalities, such as peripheral neuropathies.

Midfoot

Pes Planus

Pes planus is also known as flatfoot or flattening of the plantar arch. On a weight-bearing lateral projection, the calcaneus is more horizontal than usual (Fig. 15.33), and a line drawn along its plantar surface makes a flatter angle with one drawn along the shaft of the second or

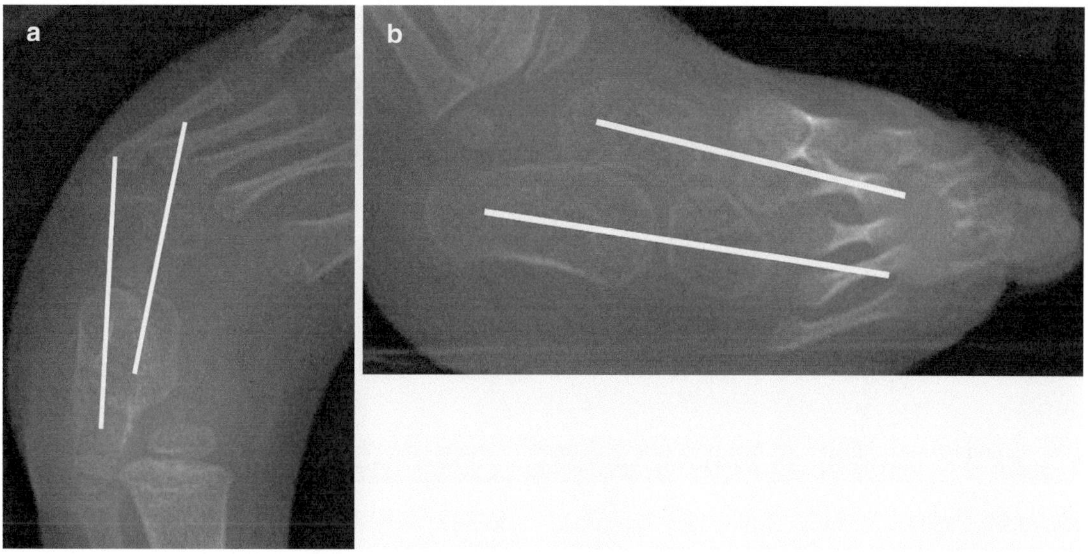

Fig. 15.32 Hindfoot varus in a 2-year-old. (**a**) Frontal view shows lateral deviation of the long axis of the talus relative to midline, resulting in a more parallel orientation of the talus relative to the calcaneus and an abnormally small talocalcaneal angle. (**b**) Lateral view also shows the parallel orientation of the talus relative to the calcaneus and a diminished talocalcaneal angle (simulated weight-bearing views)

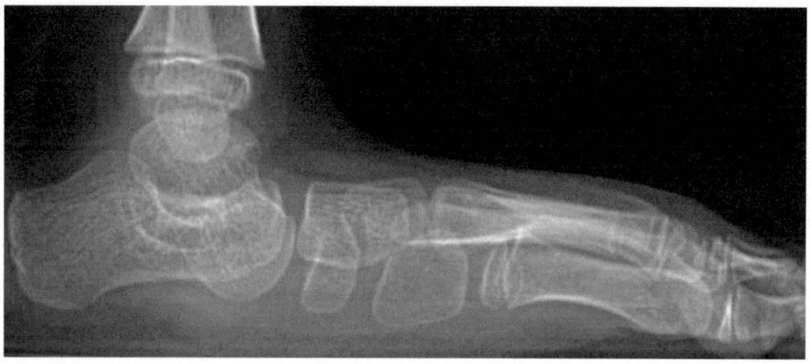

Fig. 15.33 Pes planus. Lateral view shows abnormal vertical orientation of the talus relative to the calcaneus and sagging midfoot compatible with pes planus. There are congenital and acquired causes of pes planus or "flat foot" deformity (weight-bearing view)

third metatarsal. The Meary angle is convex down. Lateral views in maximum dorsiflexion and plantar flexion can assess for hypermobility through the midfoot or stiffness at the hindfoot.

A flattened plantar arch is seen in conditions such as congenital or acquired flatfoot, including flexible planovalgus foot, tarsal coalition, peroneal spastic flatfoot, and cerebral palsy.

Rocker-Bottom Deformity

This entity represents a severe form of pes planus in which the plantar arch is convex, rather than concave. The calcaneus is in equinus position and the metatarsals are dorsiflexed, rounding the arch inferiorly.

This deformity may be seen in congenital vertical talus, severe cerebral palsy with hindfoot valgus, or clubfoot that has been overcorrected.

Pes Cavus

With cavus deformity, the height of the plantar arch is increased on a lateral projection. The os calcis may be tilted up in cases of calcaneus deformity, or it may be in equinus. From the apex of the arch in the midfoot, the metatarsals are then plantar flexed (see Fig. 15.30). Pes cavus may be seen as a primary congenital condition (as in clubfoot) or with neuromuscular disease, prolonged lack of weight bearing, and local trauma/irritation. The Hibbs angle quantifies the extent of cavus. This angle, formed by intersecting lines drawn along the

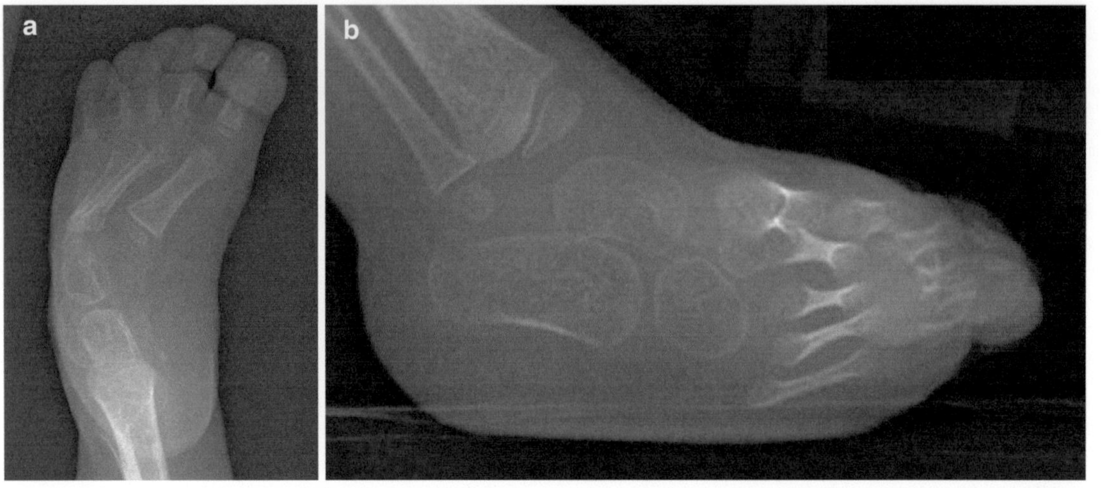

Fig. 15.34 Clubfoot in a 2-year-old boy. (**a**) Frontal view shows metatarsus adductus as well as inversion, with deviation of the metatarsals toward midline and increased overlap of the metatarsal bases. (**b**) Lateral shows the ladder-like array of metatarsus adductus with inversion, with the fifth metatarsal the most plantar. The talus and calcaneus are parallel on both projections, consistent with hindfoot varus (simulated weight-bearing views)

long axis of the calcaneus and the first metatarsal, should be at least 150° to be considered normal.

Forefoot: Adduction and Abduction

Adduction and abduction of the forefoot describes the position of the metatarsals solely in the plane of the foot, without inversion or eversion of the plantar surface. These alterations may be isolated, but they also occur in conjunction with complex foot deformities involving the hindfoot and midfoot. Significant forefoot abduction is not as common as forefoot adduction, although it may be severe in cases of cerebral palsy and congenital vertical talus.

On an AP projection, the metatarsals move essentially as a unit toward (adduction) or away from (abduction) the midline, pivoting at their bases. When viewed on a lateral projection, the normal superimposition of the central metatarsals is preserved, unless there is associated inversion or eversion.

Some use the term "varus" to describe adduction of the metatarsals and "valgus" to describe the far less common abduction. However, to avoid confusion with hindfoot varus and valgus, we use the terms "adduction" and "abduction" when describing forefoot malalignment. Inversion and eversion are often present concomitantly and are discussed more fully in the section below on complex foot deformities.

Complex Foot Deformity: Inversion and Eversion

Inversion and eversion are complex deformities of the entire foot. The talus moves only slightly, and the principal abnormality involves abnormal motion between tarsal joints. With inversion, the sole of the foot faces medially, whereas with eversion, it faces laterally. These two motions principally occur at the subtalar and transverse tarsal joints. Both these axes are oblique compared with standard anatomical planes. Inversion and eversion comprise three specific motions. Supination and pronation describe the medial and lateral rotation of the foot about an AP axis. Abduction and adduction describe motion of the anterior portion of the foot about a vertical axis. The third motion is dorsiflexion and plantar flexion. Inversion combines supination, adduction, and plantar flexion, whereas eversion combines pronation, abduction, and dorsiflexion. Inversion results from increased activity of the tibialis posterior and anterior muscles, whereas eversion results from the peroneal and extensor digitorum longus muscles.

On an AP view when the foot is supinated, the metatarsal bases are superimposed, and with adduction the distal metatarsals swing toward the midline (Figs. 15.26 and 15.34). This narrows the area of the forefoot on this projection. On a

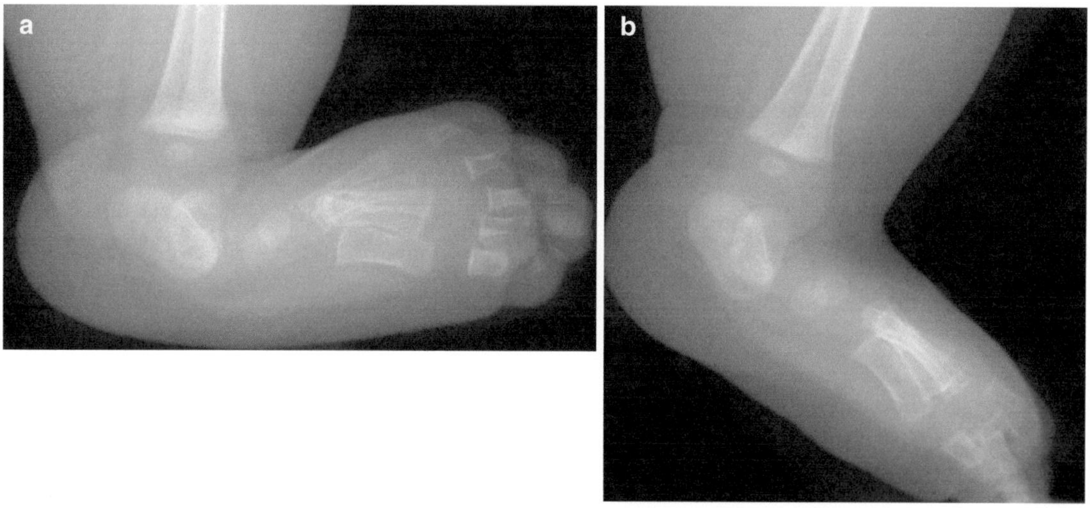

Fig. 15.35 Eversion in a 5-month-old with congenital vertical talus and teratologic dislocated hips. (**a**) Simulated weight-bearing lateral shows the talus is vertical and does not align with metatarsals, and the calcaneus is in equinus. In addition, the foot is everted, with the first metatarsal the most plantar. (**b**). With maximum plantar flexion, the heel/hindfoot alignment does not improve, but the eversion shows some flexibility. (Same patient as Fig. 15.50, which shows the other foot) (Courtesy of Sandra L. Wootton-Gorges; Copyright Shriners Hospital for Children Los Angeles)

lateral view, since the foot is now inverted, the fifth metatarsal is more plantar than the first, and a ladder-like array is seen, with the first metatarsal highest. The lateral radiograph may look almost like an AP view of the forefoot.

Forefoot inversion is most severe with congenital clubfoot, where there is over-pull of the tibialis anterior muscle. In contrast, inversion in cases of isolated metatarsus adductus is relatively mild, and associated hindfoot deformity is rare.

In eversion, the sole faces outward. This alignment may be more difficult to identify on radiographs compared to the usually obvious changes with inversion. On an AP view, there may be increased separation of the metatarsal bases, with less of the normal proximal convergence. The metatarsal shafts are more parallel and less divergent than normal. On a lateral view, a stepladder appearance may be seen, but with the orientation reversed from that with inversion (Fig. 15.35). With eversion, the first metatarsal is the most plantar, with the fifth metatarsal highest (see subsequent section on acquired pes planus). In general, however, the ladder-like distortion is rarely as striking as is seen in forefoot supination.

2.5 Structural Deformities (Figs. 15.36 and 15.37)

Congenital Clubfoot (Congenital Equinovarus) (Box 15.1)

Box 15.1: Congenital Clubfoot (Talipes Equinovarus)

Incidence 1:1,000 births, more common in males

Components	Ankle equinus (talus and calcaneus plantar flexed)
	Hindfoot varus (parallel talus and calcaneus)
	Forefoot adduction
	Foot inversion
Additional findings	Small talus and calcaneus
	Talar neck shows medial and plantar deviation
	Decreased convexity of talar dome
	Caveat: ankle radiograph must be true lateral
	Navicular shifted medially

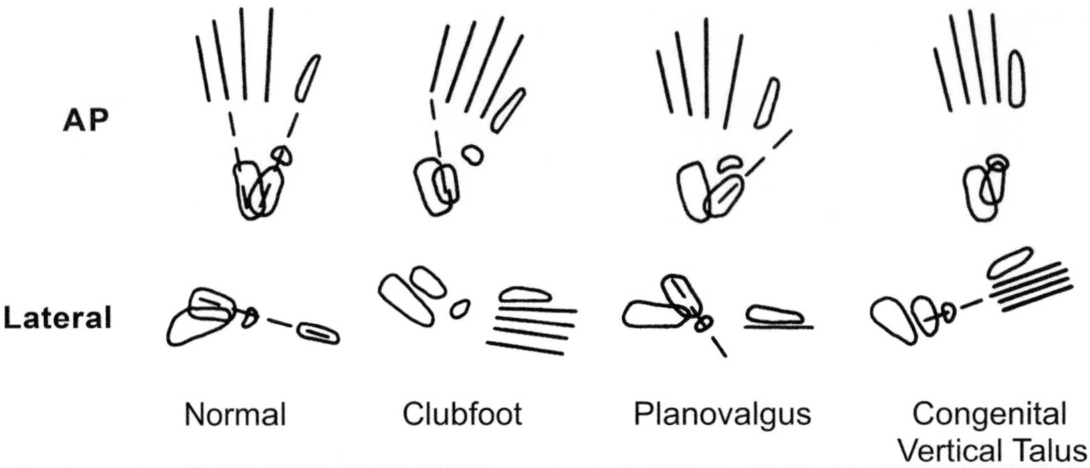

Fig. 15.36 Osseous relationships: normal, clubfoot, planovalgus, and congenital vertical talus. On the frontal view of the *normal foot*, the long axis of the talus intersects the base of the first metatarsal, and the long axis of the calcaneus intersects the base of the fourth metatarsal. On a lateral view, the long axis of the talus aligns with that of the first metatarsal. With *clubfoot*, there is hindfoot varus, and the long axis of the talus is thus laterally deviated from midline on the frontal view. The talus and calcaneus therefore appear more parallel on both views. The forefoot is also adducted and the foot inverted, so on a lateral view there is a ladder-like array of the metatarsals with the fifth metatarsal being the most plantar. With *planovalgus*, the talus is deviated toward midline on the frontal view, and the long axis of the talus is inferiorly oriented relative to the first metatarsal. The calcaneus and talus therefore appear more divergent on both views. In *congenital vertical talus*, the talus is abnormally vertically oriented on a lateral view, with fixed dorsal subluxation of the navicular relative to the talus. There may be hindfoot varus

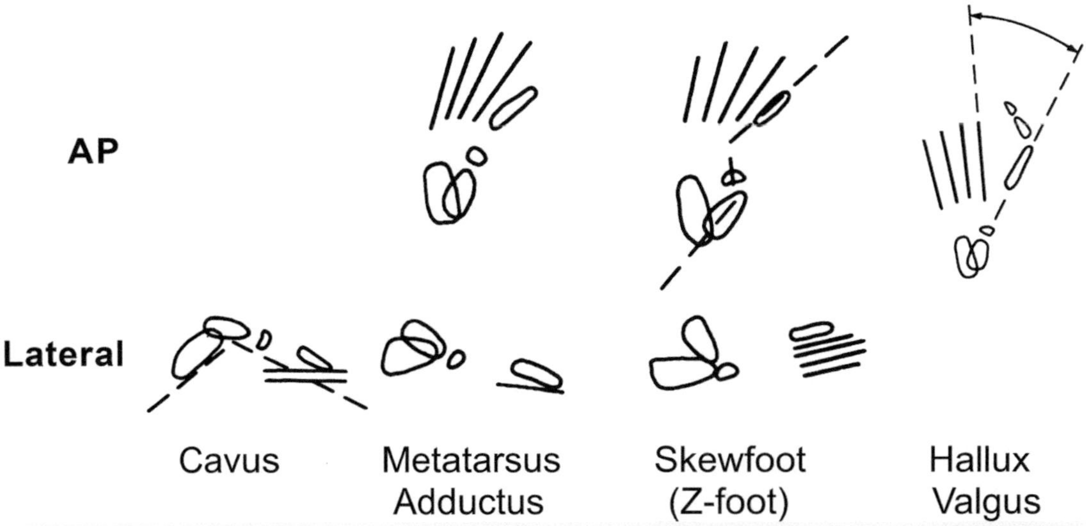

Fig. 15.37 Osseous relationships: pes cavus, metatarsus adductus, skewfoot, hallux valgus. In *pes cavus*, the anterior portion of the calcaneus is superiorly oriented ("calcaneus" hindfoot), and the metatarsals are plantar flexed. As a result, the depth of the plantar arch is abnormally increased. In *metatarsus adductus*, the metatarsals are abnormally medially deviated, whereas hindfoot alignment is normal. In *skewfoot*, there is severe metatarsus adductus as well as hindfoot valgus (increased talocalcaneal angle with divergent appearance of the talus and calcaneus on both frontal and lateral views). With *hallux valgus*, abnormal lateral deviation of the proximal phalanx of the first toe relative to the first metatarsal is associated with uncovering of the first metatarsal head

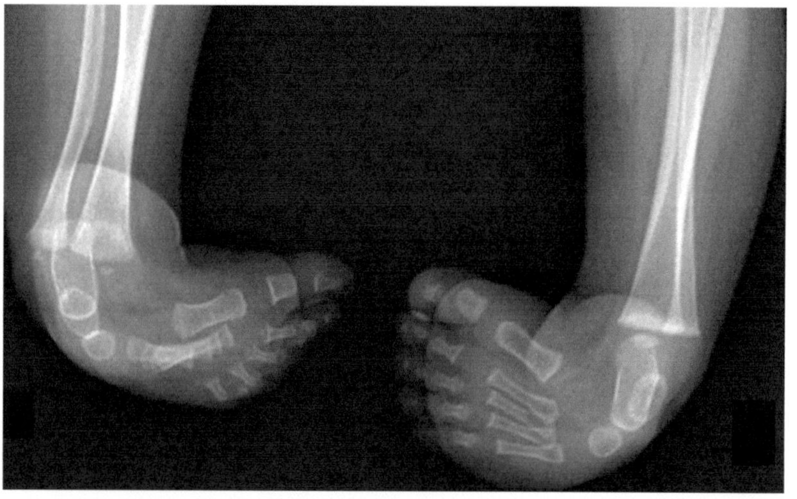

Fig. 15.38 Bilateral congenital equinovarus deformity in a neurologically impaired newborn. The feet are turned to face each other, and the lateral border of both feet is inferior. The talus and calcaneus are superimposed on each other, with loss of the normal angular relationships between them (Courtesy of Chirag V. Patel)

Idiopathic congenital clubfoot is relatively common, with an incidence of about 1:1,000 live births. It affects males more commonly than females and is bilateral in about half of cases. Its incidence is 30 times greater in those with an affected first-degree relative compared to the general population. Of children with clubfoot deformity, about 25 % have a known family history. Recent studies have suggested that clubfoot is a heterogeneous disorder with a polygenetic threshold model with specific transcription pathway mutations implicated [35]. Muscle imbalance, intrauterine positioning deformity, ligamentous laxity in the setting of defective connective tissues, and persistence of early normal fetal relationships have also been implicated as causes of clubfoot. To avoid confusion, the term *clubfoot* should be restricted to idiopathic congenital equinovarus deformity.

The non-idiopathic form of this disorder, preferably referred to by the descriptive term "equinovarus deformity," may result from mechanical factors in patients with such disorders as myelomeningocele, arthrogryposis, and tibial longitudinal deficiency (Fig. 15.38). Equinovarus deformity is common with a variety of syndromes as well.

Congenital clubfoot is also known as talipes equinovarus. However, the term *talipes*, a contraction of the words *talus* (ankle) and *pes* (foot), is archaic and best avoided. *Talipes* has also been applied to other congenital abnormalities of the foot, such as talipes varus, talipes calcaneovalgus, talipes equinovalgus, and talipes calcaneovarus. All of these conditions should instead be described with the alignment terminology introduced in earlier sections.

The clinical manifestations of clubfoot include plantar flexion at the ankle (equinus position) with varus of the hindfoot as well adduction of the forefoot and inversion of the foot. The exact mechanisms involved in embryologic development of the clubfoot are still not known.

Pathology investigations have revealed a fairly consistent pattern of deformity. The ossific nuclei of the talus and calcaneus are often small and immature, with poorly developed vascular channels [36]. The muscles, nerves, tendons, and blood vessels of the foot are typically normal except for shortening on the medial side of the foot and leg. The size and shape of the talus are often abnormal, contributing to the sometimes challenging radiographic evaluation [37]. The talus is usually small, with the dome less convex than normal and the neck demonstrating medial and plantar deviation. As a result, the articular surface for the navicular faces medially, and the subtalar surface is tilted into varus, equinus, and medial rotation. The calcaneus, which is also somewhat small, is also displaced into varus, equinus, and internal rotation so that the talonavicular and calcaneocuboid joints lie above each

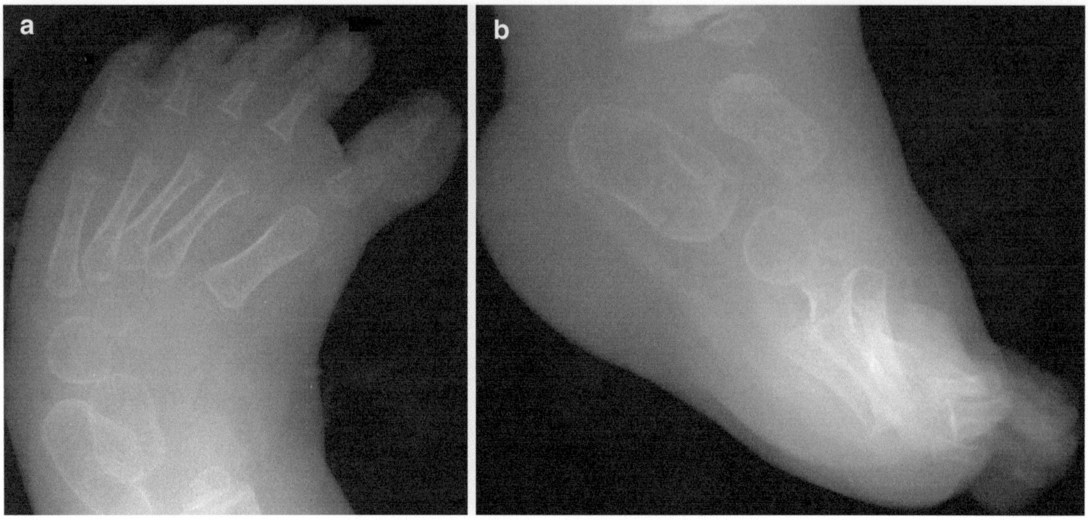

Fig. 15.39 Clubfoot in an infant. (**a**) (Frontal), (**b**) (lateral). There is ankle equinus and hindfoot valgus, with parallel talus and calcaneus. Metatarsus adductus with little inversion (simulated weight-bearing views)

other instead of side by side. The navicular shifts to a more medial position than normal.

Treatment of congenital clubfoot centers on the Ponseti method of serial casting, often weekly, until forefoot and midfoot alignment has been corrected [38]. This is often followed by Achilles tenotomy to correct the residual equinus position of the foot. Long-term foot bracing then prevents recurrent malalignment [39]. In some children, over-pull of the anterior tibialis after Ponseti treatment results in a condition termed "dynamic supination," which is almost always accompanied by flexible adduction.

Older children or refractory cases sometimes require more complex operations involving release of soft tissues, tendon transfers, and osteotomies to alter the mechanics of the medial, posterior, and/or lateral supporting structures [40]. Some centers perform surgeries without first attempting casting, generally performing posterior and medial soft tissue releases, along with transfer of the tibialis anterior tendon to a more lateral position. More invasive procedures, such as lateral column shortening, are performed if these measures fail (see Chap. 27).

Radiographic Technique

Radiographs have been used for clubfoot diagnosis since 1896. Imaging in multiple planes and measurement of angles have made it possible to standardize characterization of deformities [41]. AP (dorsoplantar) and lateral weight-bearing or simulated weight-bearing projections are sufficient for initial evaluation and routine follow-up. Oblique projections are rarely useful.

In order for the talus to be seen in a correct lateral projection, the ankle (rather than the foot) must be placed in a true lateral position. No attempt should be made to correct deformity of the forefoot, which may be flexible enough to change its relationship to the rest of the foot and leg. If instead the medially deviated foot is incorrectly placed in a true lateral position, the fibula will be displaced posteriorly, causing the talus to be seen obliquely (see Fig. 15.30). It is also important that the tibia must be parallel with the sagittal plane to avoid tilting the talus. Stressed dorsiflexion may be applied to determine the degree of uncorrectable equinus positioning.

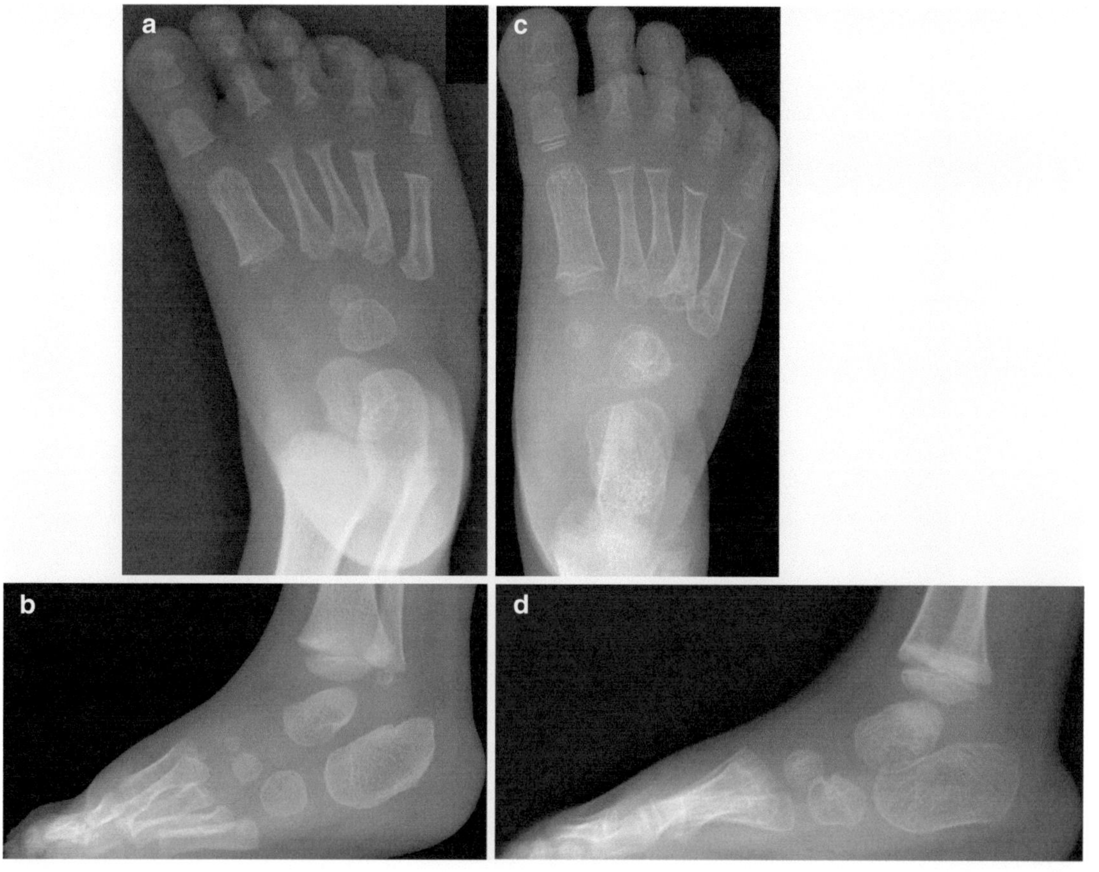

Fig. 15.40 Clubfoot in a 2-year-old girl, subsequently treated with Ponseti casting. (**a**, **b**) There is equinus deformity at the ankle, along with hindfoot valgus, metatarsus adductus, and inversion (with metatarsals in a ladder-like configuration, metatarsal plantar). (**c**, **d**) 1.5 years later, after serial casting, alignment is much improved. There is pes planus with residual mild equinus and hindfoot varus. The patient may later undergo additional surgery (Achilles lengthening and tibialis anterior tendon transfer) (weight-bearing views) (Courtesy of Ary Arauz; Copyright Shriners Hospital for Children Northern California)

Radiology Findings

Untreated Clubfoot

On an AP view of the hindfoot, the talus and calcaneus are parallel to each other or actually superimposed, with loss of the normal talocalcaneal angle (see Figs. 15.26, 15.34, 15.36, 15.39, 15.40, and 15.41). The cartilaginous navicular is not visible in the newborn; when ossified, it is displaced medially. A line drawn down the talus passes lateral to the base of the first metatarsal. The forefoot is adducted and the foot inverted, with increased superimposition of the metatarsal bases and apparent narrowing of the forefoot.

Increased parallelism of the talus and calcaneus is again evident on a lateral projection. The anterior portion of the calcaneus is less dorsiflexed than normal, and the calcaneus is usually in equinus position. Range of motion is decreased, with dorsiflexion limited. Foot inversion and forefoot adduction result in a ladder-like appearance of the metatarsals, which lose their normal superimposition. The first metatarsal is highest, since the foot rests laterally

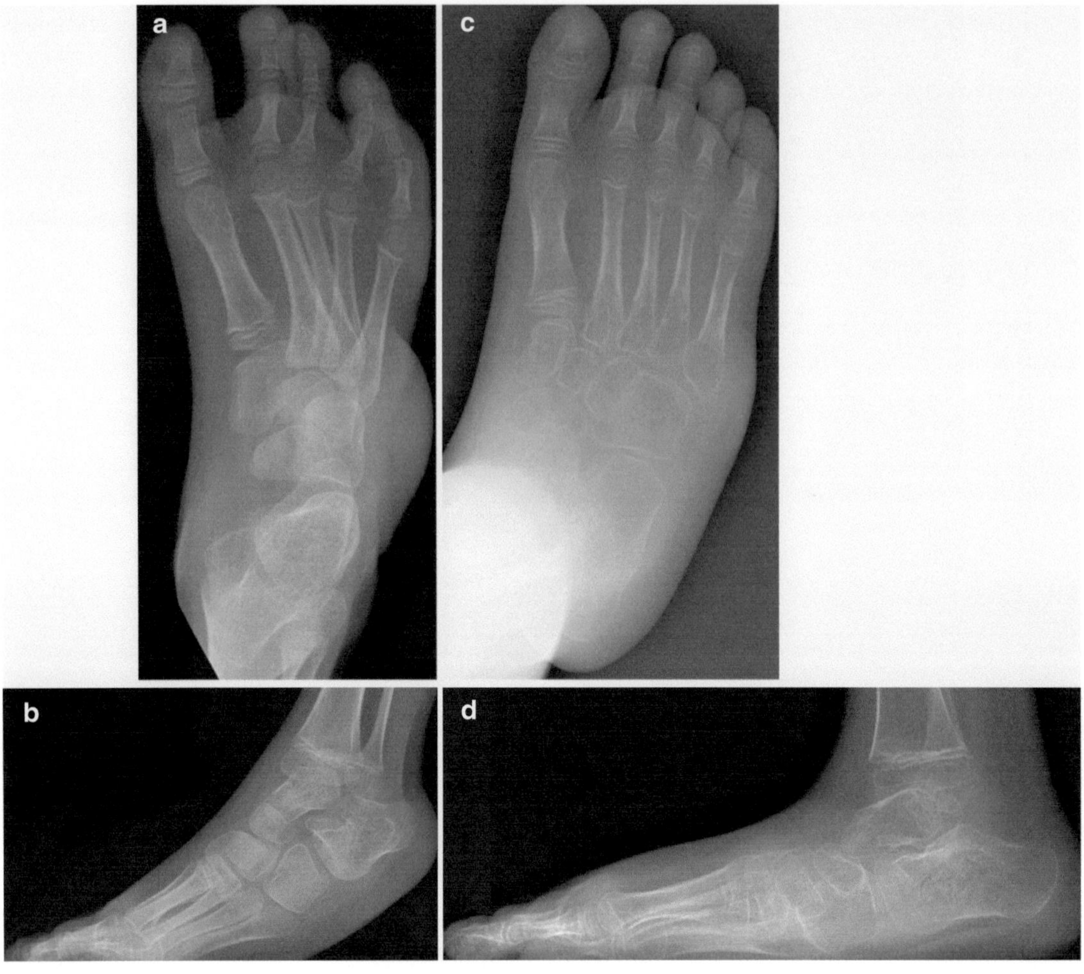

Fig. 15.41 Neglected clubfoot in a 7-year-old girl, subsequently treated with Ponseti casting. (**a**, **b**) At age 7 years, this untreated foot shows severe equinus and a small talus and calcaneus, as well as hindfoot valgus, metatarsus adductus, and inversion. (**c**, **d**) After 2 months of casting, typical residual deformities are present. There is mild equinus and hindfoot valgus as well as mild pes planus. Casting was halted before the os calcis achieved a "calcaneus" position to avoid overstretching the midfoot tissues and inducing subsequent rocker-bottom deformity. Planned Achilles lengthening will improve the position of the calcaneus (weight-bearing views) (Courtesy of Rebecca Stein-Wexler; Copyright Shriners Hospital for Children Northern California)

on the fifth metatarsal. In cases of longstanding severe untreated deformity, abnormal weight bearing on the lateral side of the foot may lead to periosteal reaction, sclerosis, and stress fractures at the lateral metatarsals (Fig. 15.42).

While many angles and measurements may be applied to clubfoot deformity, the talocalcaneal angle (see Figs. 15.32 and 15.36) is most often utilized on both AP and lateral views and has been shown to be reproducible [42].

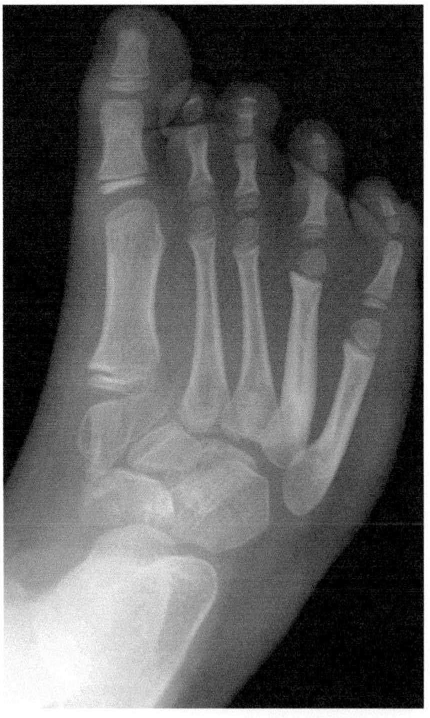

Fig. 15.42 Metatarsal sclerosis in a 4-year-old boy with an unclassified syndrome and equinovarus foot that was refractory to casting. Sclerosis at the fourth and fifth metatarsals results from stress induced by bearing weight on the lateral aspect of the foot (Courtesy of Rebecca Stein-Wexler; Copyright Shriners Hospital for Children Northern California)

Late Changes After Clubfoot Treatment

The incompletely treated or relapsed clubfoot demonstrates characteristic findings. Although the talocalcaneal angle may be restored to normal or actually converted to valgus on the AP radiograph, a lateral projection shows a more horizontal calcaneus than normal, indicating incomplete correction of calcaneal equinus (see Figs. 15.40 and 15.41). Increased parallelism of the talus and calcaneus on lateral view usually persists. Angle measurements do not always correlate with clinical findings after correction, as some feet with poor clinical outcomes show normal angle values [43]. Normalization of the tibial-calcaneal angle (correction of calcaneal equinus) has been shown to correlate with improved ankle dorsiflexion after treatment, specifically after Achilles tenotomy [44].

The plantar arch may remain abnormal after corrective measures (Fig. 15.43). If dorsiflexion is applied prematurely before the equinus and varus are corrected, a convex (rocker-bottom) arch may develop. In some cases, cavus deformity of the arch may result from incomplete correction of the midfoot deformity and/or overcorrection of the calcaneal position (Fig. 15.44). However, recurrence of cavus deformity suggests the presence of an underlying neurologic abnormality, such as tethered cord. As with neglected clubfoot, persistent inversion may result in stress-related changes involving the metatarsals.

Flattening of the talar dome has been noted in adults after clubfoot correction. This true flattening must be distinguished from the apparent flattening of the talar dome obtained when the foot, not ankle, is placed parallel with the cassette on a lateral projection, as discussed above. This results in a slightly oblique projection of the talus, in which the projected curvatures of the two sides of the talar dome give a false impression of flattening (see Fig. 15.30); this error in positioning can be recognized by the posterior position of the fibula.

In a late follow-up of some apparently completely corrected clubfeet, residual calcaneal supination and resulting hypoplasia of the sustentaculum may be evident.

Other Imaging Modalities

Ultrasound

Clubfoot deformity is readily recognized on prenatal US. Postnatal US is being increasingly employed to diagnose clubfoot and then evaluate its treatment. Although unable to provide global assessment of foot alignment, US

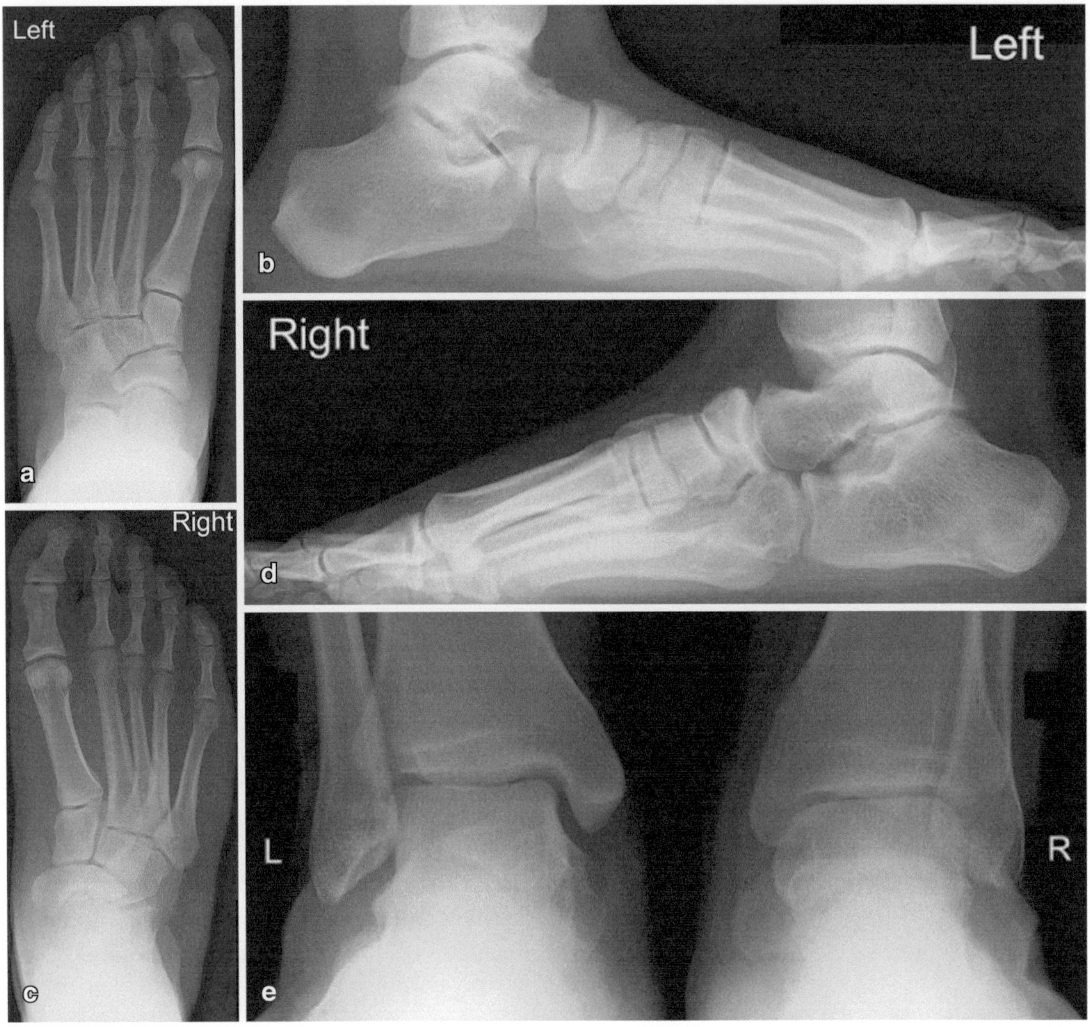

Fig. 15.43 Typical appearance of corrected clubfoot on the right in a 17-year-old male, treated surgically at age 1 year. (**a**, **b**) Normal left foot (for comparison). Note normal talar ridge. (**c**) On the *right*, an AP view shows mild hindfoot varus, medial subluxation of the navicular, and mild metatarsus adductus, resulting in mild skewfoot. (**d**) The *right* lateral also shows relatively parallel talus and calcaneus, small talus, boxy calcaneus, pes planus, and mild inversion. (**e**) The right ankle has a shallow ball-and-socket configuration (Courtesy of Rebecca Stein-Wexler)

demonstrates cartilaginous structures and their relationships [45]. For example, if the navicular bone is displaced medially, the distance between the cartilaginous medial malleolus and the navicular is decreased [46] (Fig. 15.45). The ability to assess the medial malleolar-navicular distance dynamically during simulated Ponseti maneuvers may aid in treatment planning [29].

MRI

MRI allows for visualization of cartilaginous structures of the foot while also providing a global assessment of alignment. Studies have characterized the complex malalignments of clubfoot as evaluated by MRI and associated them with disease severity [47]. However, in most practices sedation and relatively long scan times limit the use of MRI to unusually complex or refractory cases.

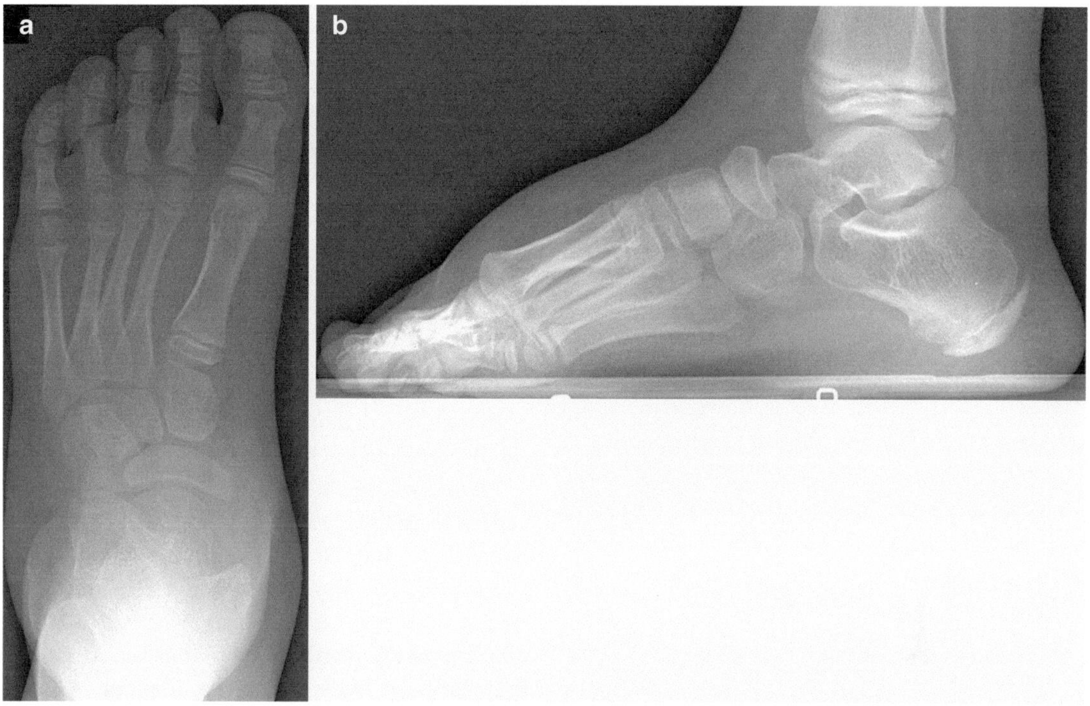

Fig. 15.44 Suboptimal result of posterior and medial soft tissue release (performed at age 7 months) in a 6-year-old girl with clubfoot (**a**, **b**). Excessive Achilles lengthening allows "calcaneus" position of the os calcis, which contributes to pes cavus. In addition, the navicular is dorsally and medially subluxated, and there is metatarsus adductus with a very mild skewfoot deformity (weight-bearing views) (Courtesy of Rebecca Stein-Wexler)

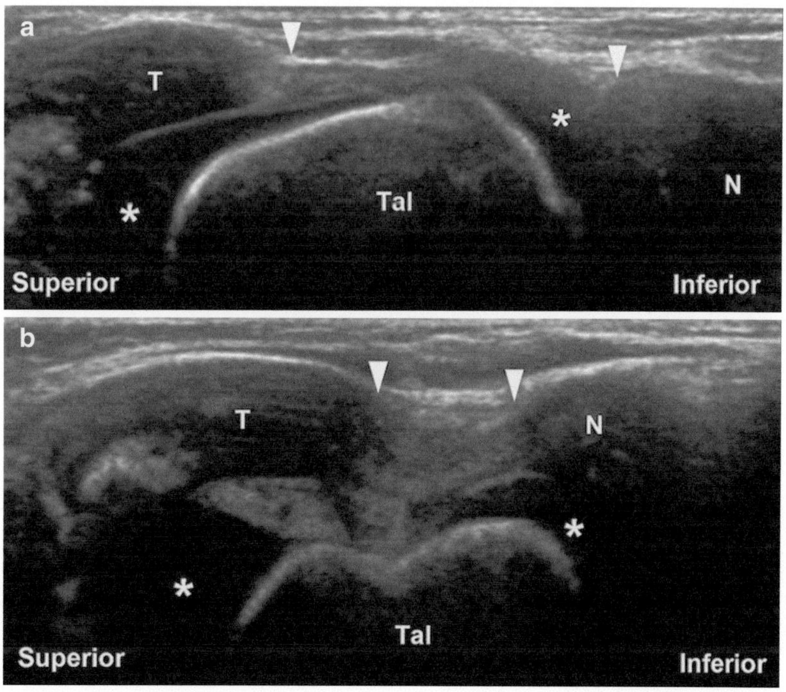

Fig. 15.45 Ultrasound of unilateral clubfoot in a 2-year-old girl. (**a**) Coronal US image of normal left foot (for comparison), obtained from a medial approach, shows the normal relatively large distance (*arrowheads*) between the medial malleolus and the navicular. (**b**) Corresponding image of the abnormal right foot shows an abnormally decreased distance (between *arrowheads*) between the navicular and medial malleolus due to metatarsus adductus and foot inversion. *Asterisks* denote normal hypoechoic cartilage. *T* tibia (medial malleolus), *Tal* talus, *N* navicular

Flatfoot (Pes Planus)
(Boxes 15.2, 15.3 and Table 15.4)

Box 15.2: Flatfoot (Pes Planus)

Components	Hindfoot valgus (talus is plantar flexed)
	Calcaneus and metatarsals more horizontal
	Possible foot eversion
Additional findings	Metatarsal adduction/abduction varies
	Navicular shifted laterally
	Talonavicular position usually normal

Box 15.3: Subtypes of Flatfoot

Congenital calcaneovalgus	Common in newborns, often bilateral
	Flexible, due to intrauterine position
Acquired planovalgus	Often asymptomatic, flexible
	Prevalence decreases with age
	Similar appearance with cerebral palsy
	Navicular usually normally aligned with talus
Congenital vertical talus	Talus near parallel to long axis of tibia
	Navicular dorsally dislocated
	Infer from 3rd cuneiform and 1st MT
	Calcaneus in equinus and valgus
	Rocker-bottom deformity
	Foot eversion
Congenital oblique talus	Resembles congenital vertical talus except:
	Talonavicular joint reduces on plantar flexion
Tarsal coalition	

Flatfoot (also termed pes planus and planovalgus) describes flattening of the plantar arch. The term is based on the clinical appearance of the foot. Flatfoot is seen in many different clinical settings, with dramatically different pathomechanics and ages of presentation. Knowledge of age of onset (congenital vs. acquired) and correctability (rigid and immobile vs. flexible and correctable by manipulation) helps determine etiology, as discussed below.

Table 15.4 Differential diagnosis of flatfoot

Onset	Flexible	Rigid
Congenital	Congenital calcaneovalgus	Rocker-bottom foot (CVT)
Acquired or late presenting	Common flatfoot/ planovalgus	Tarsal coalition/ peroneal spastic flatfoot

In general, ligamentous laxity permits the calcaneus to deviate into valgus angulation under the talus; there may also be forefoot abduction and eversion of the foot. These deformities decrease calcaneal support and cause increased load on relatively weak medial ligamentous structures. As the talar head loses its support, it becomes more vertical, and the arch flattens. The extent of hindfoot valgus, arch flattening, abduction, and eversion varies in different disorders. In addition, as the arch flattens, the Achilles tendon may become tight, causing the calcaneus to go into equinus.

Radiology Findings

In cases of pes planus, on an AP projection, the hindfoot is in valgus, with an increased talocalcaneal angle and the calcaneus abducted (see Fig. 15.36). The midtalar line passes medial to the first metatarsal base. The navicular is also displaced laterally from its usual position distal to the head of the talus, shifted because of the midfoot's connection to the calcaneus. The metatarsals' relationship to the midfoot and hindfoot depends on the specific cause and should be described according to the standard terminology of alignment. On a lateral projection, hindfoot valgus is evident, with the talus more vertical than normal (Fig. 15.46). Despite this, the close articulation between the talus and navicular is intact, except for in the relatively uncommon congenital vertical talus, where the navicular is dorsally displaced. The calcaneus and metatarsals are more horizontal than normal, which results in flattening of the plantar arch.

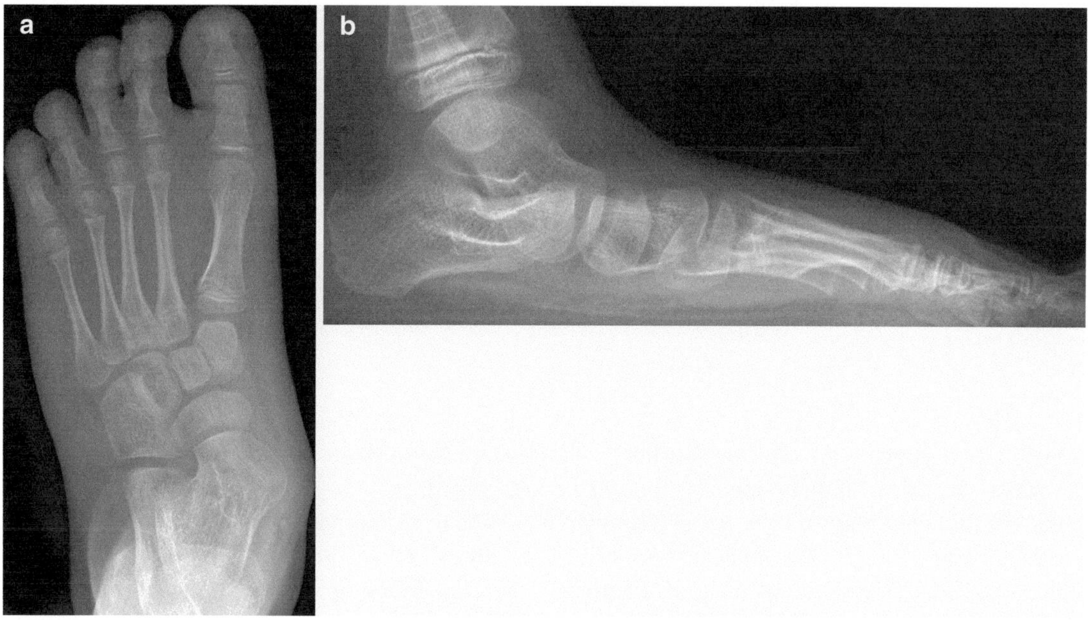

Fig. 15.46 Pes planus in an 8-year-old. (**a**) Hindfoot valgus, with medial deviation of the talus and lateral subluxation of the navicular. (**b**) Vertically oriented talus retains a normal relationship with the navicular. The arch is flattened (weight-bearing views) (Courtesy of Tal Laor, Cincinnati Children's Hospital)

Congenital Calcaneovalgus

This congenital, flexible foot deformity is seen in 30–50 % of newborns [48]. More than 90 % of cases of congenital calcaneovalgus are bilateral. Thought to result from intrauterine positioning, the foot is dorsiflexed against the lower leg and everted, with forefoot abduction (Fig. 15.47). The heel and hindfoot have a valgus configuration with a plantar-flexed talus, but the arch is only slightly flattened. This deformity is flexible and is usually almost fully correctable with passive manipulation. In contrast, other entities that clinically appear similar during infancy, such as congenital vertical talus, are rigid, and the heel is in equinus. Congenital calcaneovalgus foot usually resolves without treatment, rarely requiring corrective casting or operative management [49]. As the diagnosis is typically made clinically, imaging is usually unnecessary.

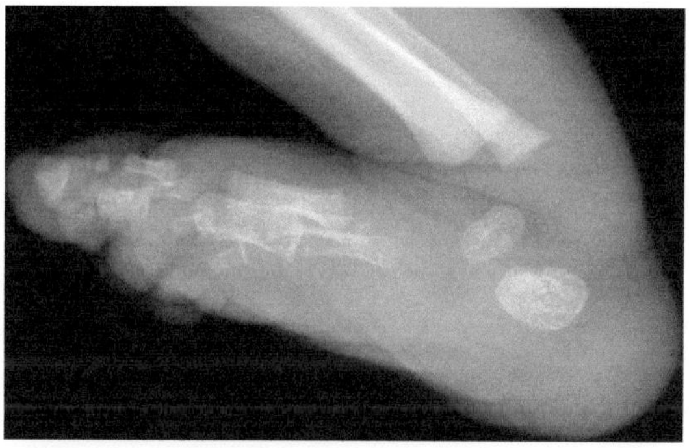

Fig. 15.47 Congenital calcaneovalgus deformity in a newborn, probably secondary to intrauterine positioning. Although the talus is vertical, the calcaneus is dorsiflexed (compare with congenital vertical talus, Fig. 15.50) (Courtesy of Jenny Boakes; Copyright Shriners Hospital for Children Northern California)

Acquired Planovalgus (Common Flatfoot)

An acquired, flexible foot deformity, flatfoot or planovalgus is the most common of the flatfoot deformities. Flattening of the plantar arch is considered normal in infants and very young children during the early walking years. From age 5 years onwards, the prevalence of flatfoot markedly decreases, and only 4 % of 10 year olds have flatfoot—near the percentage seen in adulthood [50]. Asymptomatic familial flatfoot is so common that it is considered a normal variant.

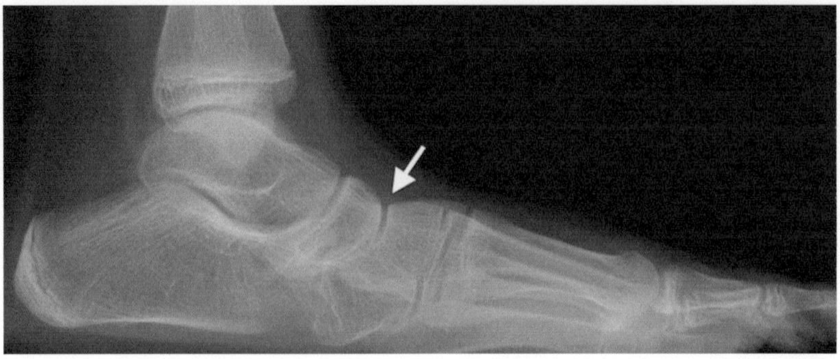

Fig. 15.48 Acquired flatfoot in a 12-year-old girl with spastic cerebral palsy. The calcaneus is in equinus, and the midfoot collapse is at the navicular-cuneiform joint (*arrow*) (weight-bearing view) (Courtesy of Jenny Boakes; Copyright Shriners Hospital for Children Northern California)

Indeed, pes planus has been noted in 6 % of predominantly asymptomatic military recruits.

While the cause of persistent pes planus is unknown, heredity plays a role. Some have suggested that abnormal ligamentous support structures contribute significantly to the disorder, particularly in children [51]. The usual mechanism of flatfoot follows, including a valgus shift of the calcaneus with resulting hindfoot valgus and foot eversion (see Fig. 15.33). Radiographic evaluation may be performed, and a variety of angles may be determined, including the Meary angle (see discussion of measurement technique, above). However, in many centers imaging is reserved for cases of painful flatfoot, predominantly to exclude other etiologies.

The abnormal position of the talus may cause synovitis or tendinosis, resulting in pain. Other lower extremity alignment abnormalities, such as genu valgum or increased femoral anteversion, can exacerbate symptoms, as can obesity [52]. Treatment usually involves supportive footwear, with surgical management reserved for very painful feet that have failed nonoperative measures.

Several entities resemble common flatfoot. For example, patients with cerebral palsy may develop hindfoot valgus with a pronated flatfoot (Fig. 15.48). In this case, the pathomechanics are similar to those for flexible flatfoot but probably result from muscular imbalance and spasticity. The foot is much stiffer, and there is often extreme forefoot abduction and hallux valgus. The talus may be almost completely vertical, as seen in congenital vertical talus, but the talonavicular relationship is normal. Although the planus deformity is most common at the talonavicular joint, it may occur elsewhere in the midfoot, such as at the navicular-cuboid articulation. This is especially common in patients with neuromuscular disorders.

The term "peroneal spastic flatfoot" describes a clinical, rather than imaging, diagnosis. In this case, the flatfoot is more rigid than with common flatfoot. This disorder is believed to result from peroneal muscle spasm, often secondary to tarsal coalition, trauma, or inflammatory arthropathy.

Congenital Vertical Talus

Congenital vertical talus is also known as congenital talipes convex pes valgus, reverse clubfoot, congenital rigid flatfoot, and congenital flatfoot with talonavicular dislocation. It is a rare condition, with an incidence of 1 in 10,000 births [53]. It may be slightly more common in males and is often bilateral [54]. While sometimes an isolated, idiopathic finding, at least 50 % of cases are syndromic. Congenital vertical talus occurs with craniocarpotarsal dysplasia (Freeman-Sheldon syndrome), trisomies [13, 18, 21], cerebral palsy, myelomeningocele, arthrogryposis, neurofibromatosis, congenital scoliosis, teratologic hip dislocation, and cardiopulmonary anomalies (Fig. 15.49).

The etiology of non-syndromic cases is unclear, but there may be a genetic predisposition. Proposed mechanisms include arrested normal rotational development of the foot during early fetal life as well as muscle imbalance. In the setting of myelomeningocele, congenital vertical talus is probably caused by overactive foot eversion and dorsiflexion muscles opposed by weak tibialis posterior muscles. A rare cause of congenital vertical talus is aplasia of the anterior calcaneus with loss of talar support.

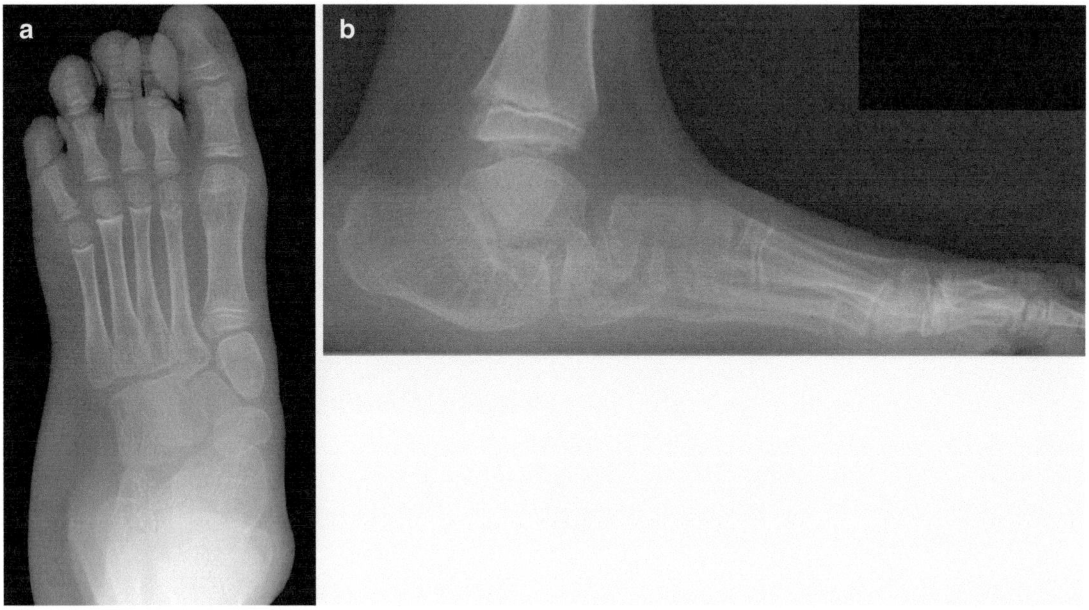

Fig. 15.49 Congenital vertical talus in a patient with Freeman-Sheldon syndrome. (**a**) There is hindfoot valgus, with the talus directed medial to the first metatarsal. (**b**) The talus is almost parallel to the long axis of the tibia, and the calcaneus is in equinus, resulting in rocker-bottom deformity. The other foot looked identical (weight-bearing views) (Courtesy of Rebecca Stein-Wexler; Copyright Shriners Hospital for Children Northern California)

Surgical and pathological analysis has shown that the tibialis posterior and peroneus longus tendons lie anterior to their usual positions and may function as dorsiflexors rather than plantar flexors. The talus is markedly plantar flexed and nearly parallel to the long axis of the tibia (Figs. 15.36, 15.49, and 15.50). Dislocation of the navicular distinguishes congenital vertical talus from other causes of flatfoot or planovalgus. With congenital vertical talus, the navicular is dorsally displaced so it lies on the neck of the talus. However, the navicular articulates normally with the bones of the midfoot. The calcaneus is in equinus, due to a short Achilles tendon. It is also laterally deviated into valgus, and the foot may be everted.

A pronated, rigid rocker-bottom foot (see section below) with marked medial prominence is evident at birth [55]. Current treatment consists of manipulation and casting, followed by talonavicular reduction and pinning, along with Achilles tenotomy [56]. Early treatment in infancy is preferred. If this fails, then more extensive soft tissue releases, tendon lengthening or transfer procedures, osteotomies, or arthrodesis are performed in the older walking-age child.

Imaging

Imaging is often employed to confirm the clinical diagnosis of congenital vertical talus. On an AP view of the foot, there is severe valgus deformity, with the calcaneus displaced laterally and the talus apparently pointing medially (see Figs. 15.24 and 15.49). The forefoot may be abducted, with decreased proximal convergence of the metatarsal bases due to eversion of the foot. On a lateral projection, the talus is in an abnormal vertical position, often aligned with the long axis of the tibia. The calcaneus is in severe equinus, and there is marked plantar flexion. The talus may indeed project into the interval between the calcaneus and cuboid. If the foot is everted, there will be a ladder-like configuration of the metatarsals, with the fifth metatarsal highest (see Fig. 15.35).

In the midfoot, the arch is convex, since the calcaneus is in marked equinus and the metatarsals are strikingly dorsiflexed, causing rocker-bottom deformity. The navicular is dorsally dislocated so that it is no longer adjacent to the head of the talus but rather dorsal to the talar neck. This relationship is only evident after the navicular ossifies. However, since the midfoot follows the displaced navicular,

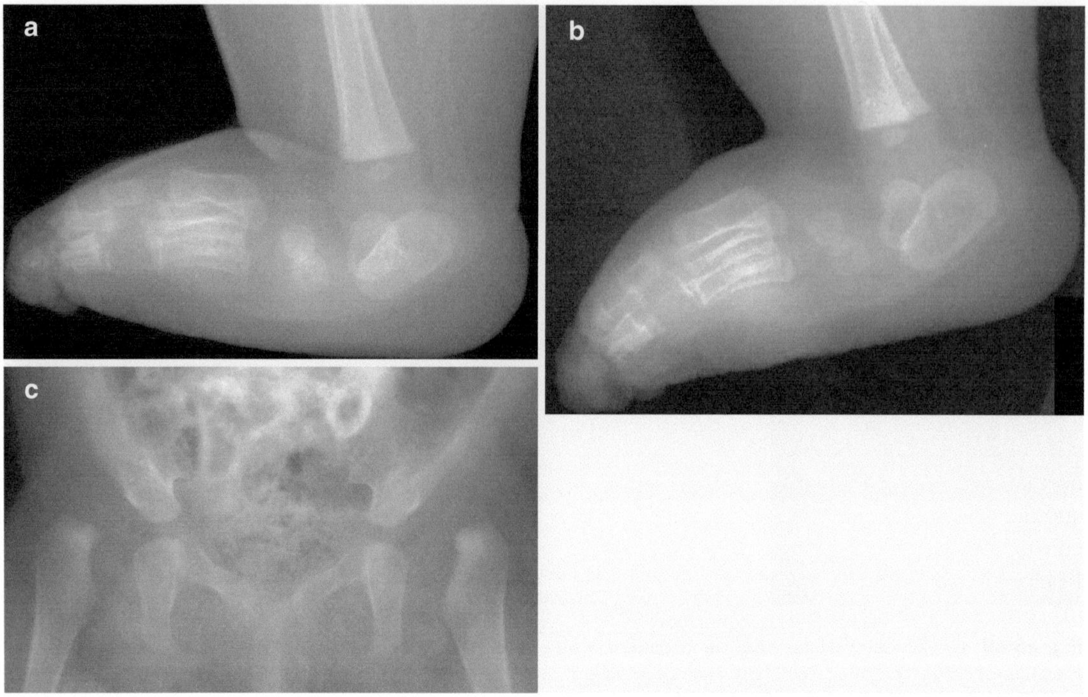

Fig. 15.50 Congenital vertical talus in a 5-month-old girl with teratologic dislocated hips. (**a**) There is a vertical talus that does not align with the metatarsals, calcaneus in equinus, and inversion (there was eversion on the other side, as shown in Fig. 15.35) (simulated weight-bearing view). (**b**) With maximum plantar flexion, there is no change. (**c**) Both acetabula are tiny, and the hips are widely dislocated (Courtesy of Sandra L. Wootton-Gorges; Copyright Shriners Hospital for Children Los Angeles)

shifting dorsally, the position of the navicular can be inferred from that of the ossified third cuneiform and base of the second metatarsal. If forced plantar flexion lateral images show that the navicular position does not correct, the diagnosis is confirmed (see Fig. 15.50). Late radiographic changes include hourglass deformity of the talus, wedging of the navicular, and secondary avascular necrosis or growth disturbance of the navicular.

US demonstrates talonavicular dislocation [57]. With dynamic plantar flexion, US also shows lack of reduction of the navicular, confirming the diagnosis of congenital vertical talus (Fig. 15.51). However, a lateral radiograph obtained with maximum plantar flexion would suggest the same abnormality and can be less expensive.

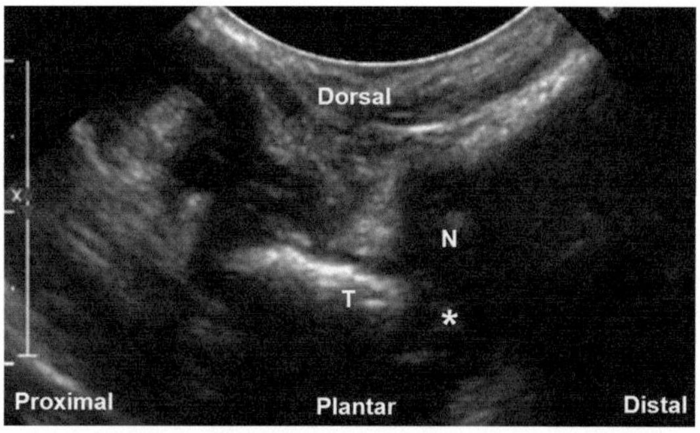

Fig. 15.51 Congenital vertical talus in a 1-month-old girl. Dorsal-plantar sagittal US readily demonstrates dorsal displacement of the cartilaginous navicular (*N*) with respect to the talus (*T*). In addition, dynamic plantar flexion maneuvers may be performed: lack of reduction of the navicular would confirm the diagnosis. *Asterisk* denotes the normal cartilaginous portion of the talus, which is expected at this age

The diagnosis of *oblique talus* may present with nearly identical clinical findings to congenital vertical talus, but the deformity is flexible (or reducible). While radiographs with forced plantar flexion may show correction of the malalignment, lack of ossification of the navicular remains a limitation. The ability of ultrasound to dynamically demonstrate reduction of talonavicular dislocation during plantar flexion confirms the presence of oblique, rather than vertical, talus. Since an oblique talus is often managed nonoperatively, it must be distinguished from congenital vertical talus [30].

The vertically aligned talus of severe planovalgus, especially as encountered in advanced cerebral palsy, is distinguished by a normal position of the navicular opposite the head of the talus and absence of calcaneal equinus (see Figs. 15.46 and 15.48). Valgus deformity of the hindfoot after clubfoot correction may resemble congenital vertical talus, but the clinical history and lack of talonavicular dislocation facilitate differentiation.

Congenital Rocker-Bottom Deformity

The "rocker-bottom" foot deformity is a nonspecific clinical descriptive term for reversal of the normal plantar arch. The calcaneus is in equinus and the metatarsals are dorsiflexed, resulting in a convex surface of the plantar aspect of the foot. Rocker-bottom deformity accompanies congenital vertical talus and congenital oblique talus, as discussed above. It may also be seen with hindfoot valgus in the setting of cerebral palsy and with overcorrected clubfoot.

Tarsal Coalition (Box 15.4)

Box 15.4: Tarsal Coalition

Classic presentation: peroneal spastic flatfoot (pes planus only in 50 %)

Fibrous coalition may progress to cartilaginous and then osseous

CT and MRI for definitive diagnosis

Talocalcaneal: most common, boys > girls

- Ossifies age 12–16 years, up to 50 % bilateral
- Usually middle facet
- Radiographs
  - Talus: beak; broad and round lateral process
  - Talar neck: undersurface short and concave
  - Apparent narrowing of posterior subtalar joint
  - C-sign on lateral

Calcaneonavicular: often asymptomatic, boys = girls

- Ossifies age 8–12 years
- Oblique radiographs
  - Elongated anterior dorsal calcaneus
  - Wide, flat anteromedial calcaneus
  - Talar head slightly small

Other coalitions: uncommon, likely syndromic

The abnormal fusion of tarsal bone centers is known as tarsal coalition, tarsal bar, or tarsal fusion. This entity is generally considered an acquired (or more precisely late-presenting) rigid flatfoot. The presentation varies depending on the specific type of fusion and which tarsal bones are involved, however, and the foot may be neither rigid nor flat. Talocalcaneal and calcaneonavicular coalitions are encountered most often.

The first widely reported series of tarsal coalitions was published in 1948 [58]. The classic clinical presentation is a constellation of signs and symptoms known as peroneal spastic flatfoot. Patients usually complain of vague midfoot pain that increases with activity, and they may have an increased incidence of ankle sprains. The foot may appear slightly everted. On physical examination, the hindfoot is stiff. Patients may find inversion stress painful, and they may guard against forced inversion [48]. There is no true spasm of the peroneal muscles, but rather shortening due to accompanying heel valgus.

This presentation, however, is nonspecific. Any process affecting the subtalar joint, including trauma, arthritis, infection, and tumor, can produce a similar clinical picture. Complicating the clinical diagnosis of coalition is the fact that up to half of patients do not present with flatfoot, and indeed some present with cavus deformity [59]. While most patients report symptoms beginning in the second decade, many present as adults. The less common talonavicular coalition, however, may present in the first decade.

The incidence of tarsal coalition is subject to debate, but most agree that it is present in about 1–3 % of the adult population. Most coalitions occur in isolation. However, there is sometimes a genetic component, with one study reporting coalitions in 39 % of first-degree relatives [60]. The osseous union is believed to begin with a fibrous (*syndesmosis*) or cartilaginous (*synchondrosis*) bridge, which in some cases eventually forms an ossified bridge (*synostosis*). The initial abnormal fusion may begin as failure of segmentation during early fetal life. The non-osseous bridge may initially be flexible, but with maturation joint

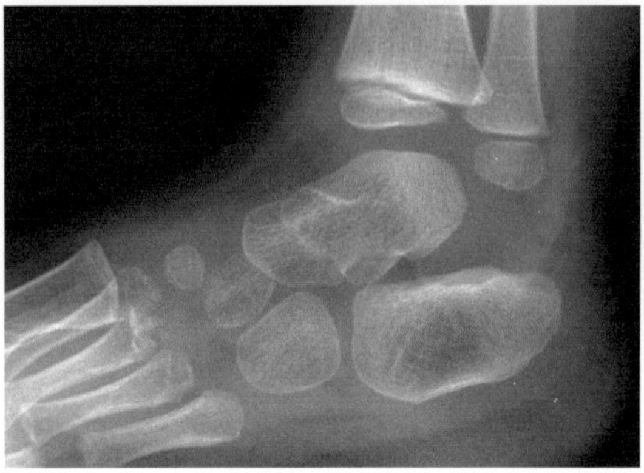

Fig. 15.52 Talonavicular coalition in a young child (Courtesy of Rebecca Stein-Wexler)

motion becomes more limited and the coalition often becomes symptomatic.

The talocalcaneal articulation is the most common site of symptomatic coalition, followed by the calcaneonavicular; together, these sites make up more than 90 % of symptomatic coalitions. Talonavicular (Fig. 15.52), calcaneocuboid, and cubonavicular coalitions are less commonly seen, perhaps because they are less often symptomatic. The presence of multiple or complex coalitions (especially involving the cuneiforms) suggests the possibility of an underlying syndrome or associated lower extremity anomalies such as fibular deficiency and the ball-and-socket ankle (see Fig. 15.5).

Most types of coalition are initially treated conservatively, beginning with a combination of anti-inflammatory medication, corticosteroid injections, orthotics or casting, and physical therapy. Surgical resection of the bone bridge or affected facet with interposition of the extensor digitorum brevis or adipose tissue may be necessary. In older patients with large coalitions not amenable to resection, subtalar fusion or triple arthrodesis may be necessary to alleviate pain [61].

Imaging

Imaging of suspected tarsal coalition begins with standard radiographs of the foot, including AP, lateral, and 45° oblique views. Some coalitions—especially talocalcaneal—are difficult to detect with standard radiographs. The axial Harris-Beath view may be helpful, as it demonstrates the orientation and patency of the medially located middle subtalar facet and its relationship to the posterior (lateral) subtalar joint (Fig. 15.53).

An understanding of the anatomy of the subtalar area is important in interpreting the Harris-Beath view and in both planning and interpreting more advanced imaging. The usually predominately fat-containing tarsal sinus with its enclosed ligamentous and vascular structures divides the plane between the talus and calcaneus into a posterior (and lateral) subtalar joint and an anteromedial talocalcaneonavicular joint. The subtalar joint posterior to the tarsal sinus contains the posterior calcaneal facet and communicates with the ankle joint in 14–20 % of patients [1]. The talocalcaneonavicular joint encompasses the anterior and medial calcaneal facets and is continuous through the talonavicular joint. A distinct anterior facet is variably present; this may be continuous with the medial facet. Another variant is the accessory anterolateral facet, which may cause pain in obese patients with rigid flatfoot [62].

CT and MRI have become essential to the workup of tarsal coalition. Both offer more definitive evaluation of known or radiographically occult coalitions and facilitate detection of additional coalitions.

CT provides information that is similar to but more detailed than radiographs, demonstrating osseous bridging as well as associated chronic reactive bone changes, such as sclerosis and subchondral cysts. It is often the preferred examination if clinical suspicion for coalition is high. CT of both feet is typically performed and reformatted in multiple planes. Coronal (short axis of foot, perpendicular to the ankle) and axial (long axis of foot, parallel to the ankle) reformats are important [63] as are sagittal reformats for evaluating calcaneonavicular coalition. Some advocate direct imaging in the plane of the subtalar articulations for talocalcaneal coalition [64].

Multiplanar MRI employing both T1-weighted (T1-W) and fluid-sensitive sequences demonstrates tarsal coalition and also depicts alternative diagnoses more readily than CT. Although

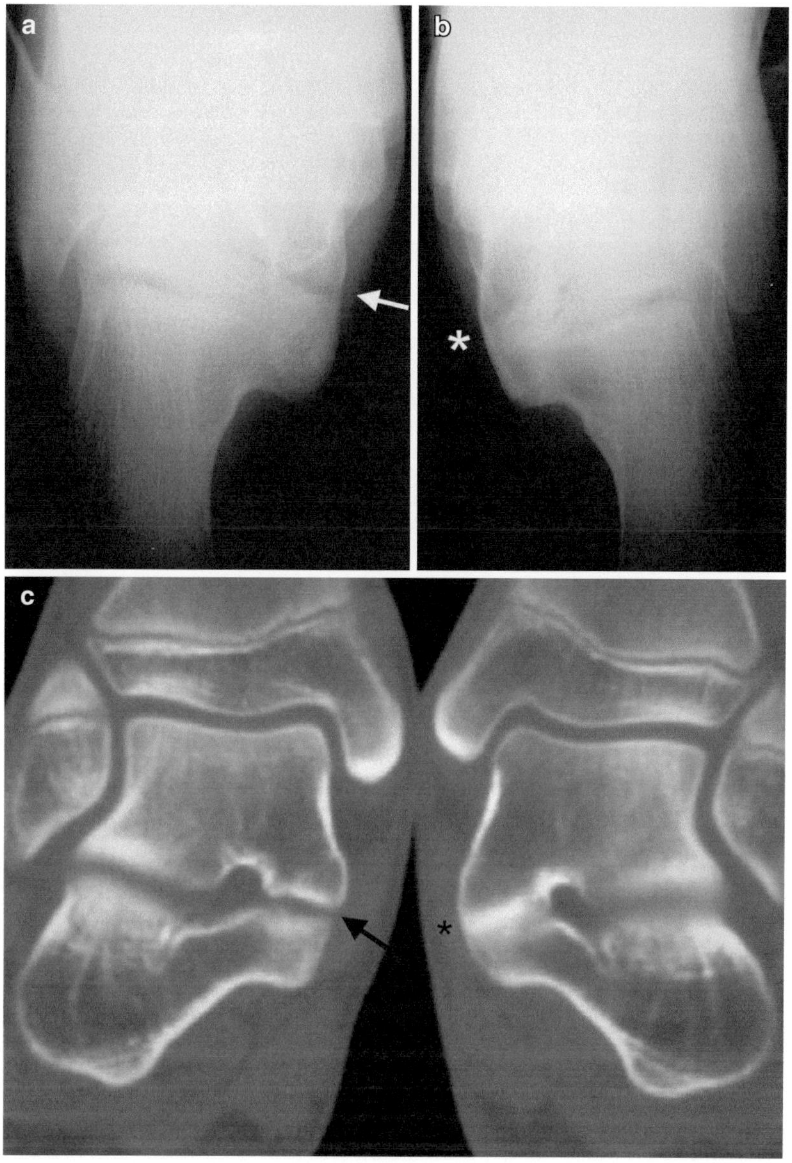

Fig. 15.53 Unilateral talocalcaneal coalition. (**a**) Harris-Beath view on normal side shows the talocalcaneal joint is intact (*arrow*). (**b**) On the affected side, the talocalcaneal joint is obliterated (*asterisk*). (**c**) CT correlation of radiographic findings (*arrow* denotes normal joint; *asterisk* denotes coalition) (Courtesy of Sandra L. Wootton-Gorges)

better shown on CT, osseous bridging is identified by bone signal crossing the fused articulation. Cartilaginous coalitions demonstrate T2-hyperintense interosseous signal, whereas fibrous coalitions show hypointense interosseous signal; mixed fibrocartilaginous coalitions demonstrate a combination of signal intensities. Reactive bone marrow edema is especially common with fibrous and/or cartilaginous coalitions; this is best evaluated on fluid-sensitive sequences. In addition, degenerative changes may be identified.

Skeletal scintigraphy may demonstrate abnormal radiotracer uptake, but this modality is not typically employed for diagnosis.

Talocalcaneal Coalition

Talocalcaneal coalition almost always involves the middle facet, including the talus and sustentaculum tali. Sometimes the fusion extends to the anterior facet or more posteriorly to involve the posterior facet [65]; isolated coalition of the posterior facet is rare. Talocalcaneal coalition

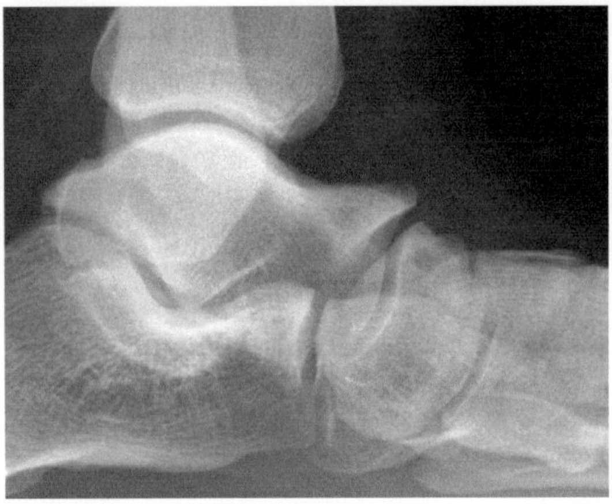

Fig. 15.54 Talar beak in a teen with talocalcaneal coalition extends from the anterosuperior margin of the talus (Courtesy of Sandra L. Wootton-Gorges; Copyright Shriners Hospital for Children Northern California)

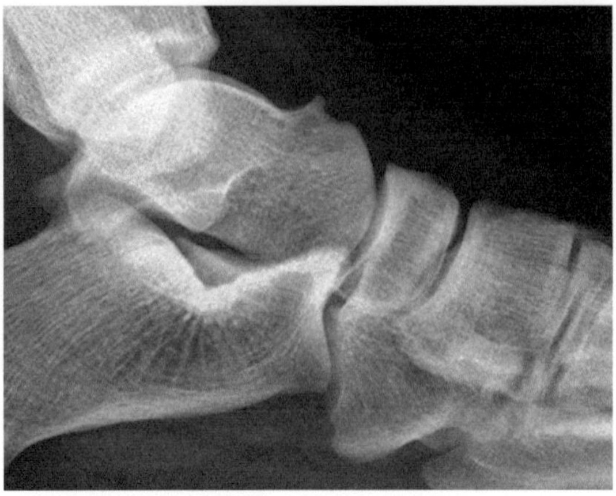

Fig. 15.55 Talar ridge in a 15-year-old girl without tarsal coalition is proximal to the distal talus (Courtesy of Tal Laor, Cincinnati Children's Hospital)

typically presents later than the other forms, with onset of symptoms usually between ages 12 and 16. It is three to four times more common in boys, and up to 50 % of cases are bilateral.

Although standard-view radiographs rarely demonstrate talocalcaneal coalition, several secondary signs have been described. These result from altered mechanics of the hindfoot. *Talar beaking* (Fig. 15.54) is the most common abnormality, appearing on lateral view as an osseous beak arising as a gradual slope from the talar ridge and ending as a steeply marginated dorsal projection at the talonavicular joint. This finding results from dorsal subluxation of the navicular caused by abnormal subtalar rigidity and subsequent elevation of the periosteum beneath the talonavicular ligament. A talar beak is seen in about 40–60 % of patients after age 10 but is rarely evident earlier. It is also seen with calcaneonavicular coalition. The talar beak must be distinguished from a more proximal talar ridge, located 7–14 mm anterior to the trochlear articular surface at the attachment sites of the tibiotalar joint capsule and talonavicular ligament (Fig. 15.55); this can be prominent in athletes [66]. This ridge has confusingly been called the *pseudobeak* or *talar beak* when not in the setting of coalition.

Other secondary signs of talocalcaneal coalition include broadening and rounding of the lateral process of the talus, seen in 60 % of patients, resulting from stress due to valgus position of the calcaneus. Apparent narrowing of the posterior subtalar joint as well as shortening and concavity of the undersurface of the talar neck may also be seen. A rounded, dysmorphic sustentaculum tali may be seen on lateral views.

The *C-sign* may be identified on lateral radiographs, and, while most often associated with talocalcaneal coalition, this may also be seen with other coalitions and indeed with flatfoot of any cause. The *C-sign* (Fig. 15.56) appears as an apparently continuous osseous structure outlining the medial talar dome and inferior sustentaculum tali; it may represent osseous or nonosseous bridging between these structures [67]. The sensitivity of the *C-sign* for talocalcaneal coalition is reported to be low, for example, 49 % in one study, and thus its absence does not exclude coalition [68].

The Harris-Beath view (see Fig. 15.53) may show osseous bridging or abnormal orientation of the subtalar facets, but this is better depicted on CT.

CT and MRI delineate the extent of fusion, including possible extension to the anterior sub-

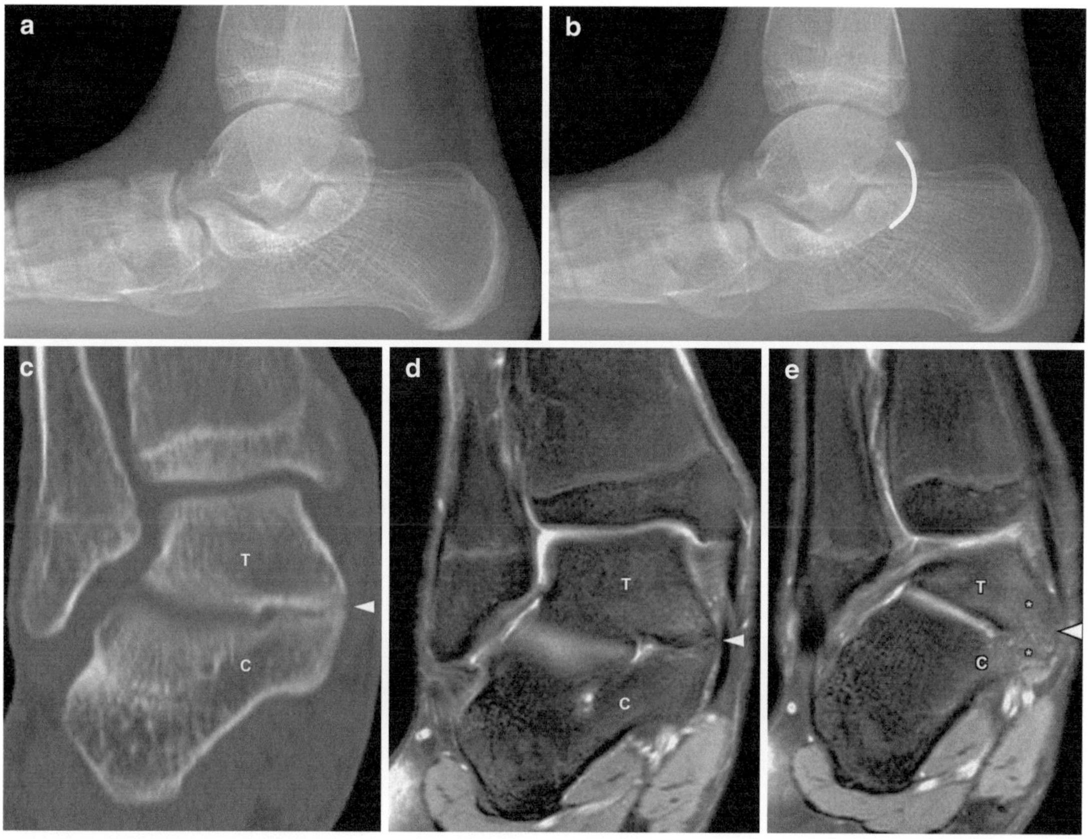

Fig. 15.56 Talocalcaneal coalition in a 15-year-old boy. (**a**, **b**) Apparent osseous continuity between the talus and calcaneus results in the "C-sign." (**c**) Coronally reformatted CT shows partial osseous continuity (*arrowhead*) of the talus and middle facet of the calcaneus. (**d**, **e**) Coronal T2-W fat suppressed (FS) MRI images show partially ossified coalition (*arrowhead*) with surrounding bone marrow edema (*asterisks*). *T* talus, *C* calcaneus

talar facet or posterolateral extension toward the tarsal tunnel. The orientation of the middle facet and sustentaculum tali is well evaluated. Instead of the normal slightly medial upward orientation, these structures may demonstrate a downward or horizontal orientation (see Fig. 15.56). Reactive bone sclerosis may be identified.

CT is useful for operative planning. Excellent results can be expected if the coalition involves up to one-third of the total joint surface area, but more extensive coalitions may not respond well to surgical intervention. Mapping the surface area of the coalition and comparing that to the entire surface area of the anteromedial and posterior facets determine the percentage of the articulations affected by the coalition [69].

Calcaneonavicular Coalition

Calcaneonavicular coalition is usually less painful than the other coalitions. It may indeed be entirely asymptomatic, or patients may complain of a rigid foot. This coalition has no gender preference and has shown autosomal dominant (with variable penetration) inheritance in many patients. The region may reossify after resection, without recurrence of symptoms.

Imaging

The calcaneus and navicular do not normally articulate directly, but the distance between these

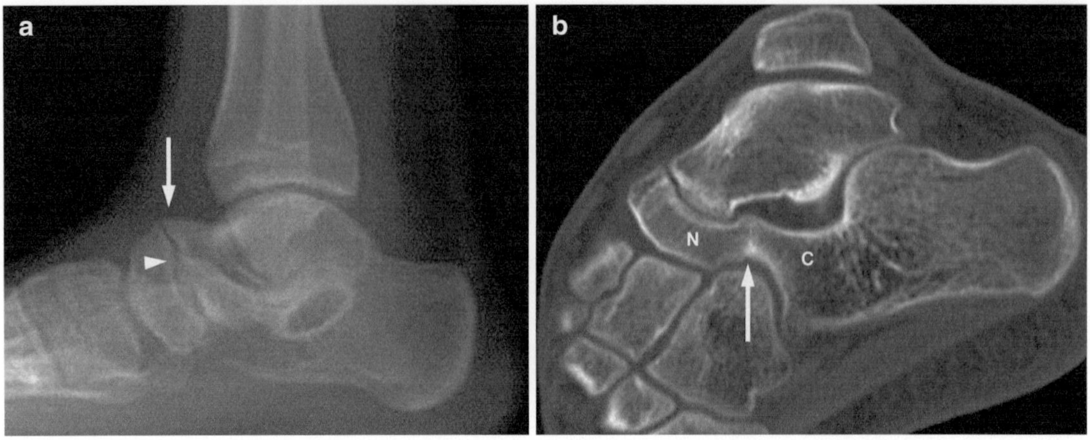

Fig. 15.57 Osseous calcaneonavicular coalition in a 15-year-old boy. (**a**) Secondary signs of coalition on a lateral view include the elongated appearance of the anterior process of the calcaneus (*arrowhead*) and beaking of the anterior talus (*arrow*) due to altered hindfoot mechanics. (**b**) Oblique sagittal reformatted CT shows osseous bridging (*arrow*) between the calcaneus and navicular. *N* navicular, *C* calcaneus

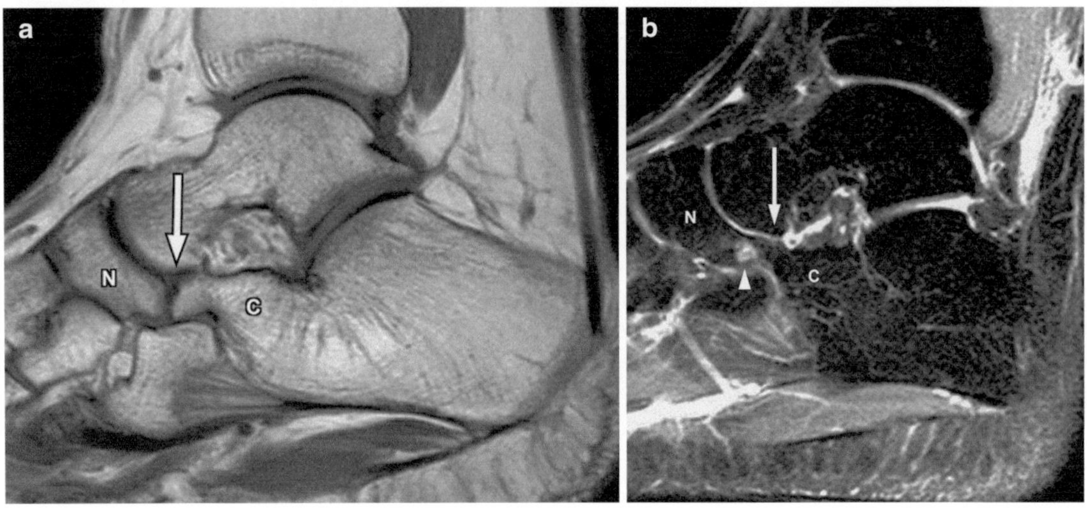

Fig. 15.58 Non-osseous calcaneonavicular coalition in an 18-year-old girl. (**a**) Sagittal T1-W image shows a non-osseous coalition (*arrow*) between the anterior process of the calcaneus and navicular. (**b**) Sagittal short tau inversion recovery (STIR) image shows cystic changes in the navicular (*arrowhead*) and edema at the level of the coalition (*arrow*). *N* navicular, *C* calcaneus

bones varies, and they may be quite close to each other in normal feet. Osseous coalition is frequently radiographically occult until age 8–12 years, although non-osseous abnormal connection is presumably present earlier.

The osseous bar of a calcaneonavicular coalition is best demonstrated on oblique foot radiographs. If there is a non-osseous coalition, there may be an abnormal articulation, with irregular, sclerotic surfaces and an abnormally wide and flat anteromedial calcaneus. On a lateral radiograph, there may be elongation of the anterior dorsal calcaneus, resulting in the *ant-eater nose* appearance (Fig. 15.57). The head of the talus is occasionally slightly smaller than normal.

CT and MRI findings resemble those on radiographs (Figs. 15.57 and 15.58). The abnormal anterior calcaneus at the site of coalition is usually best seen on sagittal reformats. However, the coalition may be quite small, so 0.625 or 1.25 mm thick images may be necessary to show the abnormality.

Cavus Foot (Box 15.5)

Box 15.5: Cavus Foot

Radiographs	Increased dorsiflexion of anterior calcaneus
	Calcaneus appears square
	Plantarflexion of metatarsals
Presentation	
With neuromuscular disorders (deformity more likely to be severe)	
Idiopathic congenital	
Cavoadductus	Hindfoot varus calcaneovalgus
	Midfoot plantar flexion
	Forefoot adduction
Simple cavus without adduction	
Cavovarus	

An abnormally high plantar arch results in pes cavus deformity. The cavus configuration forms part of several foot deformities. Cavovarus is most common, usually seen with neuromuscular disorders, such as Charcot-Marie-Tooth disease, cerebral palsy, and poliomyelitis when there is an imbalance between the weak peroneal muscles and the stronger inverter, posterior tibialis. Up to 78 % of children with bilateral cavovarus feet have Charcot-Marie-Tooth disease [70]. Cavovarus deformity may also follow incomplete clubfoot correction.

Calcaneocavus deformity, on the other hand, is usually associated with weak plantar flexors and strong toe extensors; this has been described in poliomyelitis when the gastrocsoleus complex is weak, Friedreich ataxia, S1 myelomeningocele, and peripheral neuropathy [71]. The historical practice of foot binding resulted in extreme cavus deformity [72]. In all these conditions, the deformity may initially be flexible, but it eventually becomes rigid. Given the likelihood of an underlying neuromuscular disorder, an MRI examination of the entire central nervous system should be considered.

There is also an idiopathic, congenital form of cavus deformity, which may be hereditary [73]. It is uncertain whether this is related to intrauterine positioning or an intrinsic anatomic defect. Several additional types of idiopathic pes cavus occur, the most common being cavoadductus foot. In this situation, the hindfoot is in calcaneovalgus, the midfoot in plantar flexion, and the forefoot in adduction, resulting in skewfoot deformity (see section below). The congenital forms may be milder and present later than those associated with underlying neuromuscular conditions.

Management of the cavus foot depends first on identifying a potential underlying cause. Nonoperative measures, including foot orthotics, may be successful in mild, nonprogressive deformities. However, many cases require soft tissue release, tendon transfers, and osteotomies to obtain good functional and anatomic results. Arthrodesis is performed only as a last resort. Correction of associated toe deformities is sometimes necessary.

Imaging

The anterior calcaneus looks foreshortened, often with a boxlike contour. This appearance results from radiographic projection and occurs when the foot is in varus and a lateral view of the foot is obtained instead of a true lateral view of the ankle. The actual shape of the calcaneus is normal. The plantar arch is deep, owing to simultaneous plantar flexion of the metatarsals (see Figs. 15.30 and 15.37). The angle formed by intersecting lines drawn along the long axis of the calcaneus and the first metatarsal, also known as the Hibbs angle, is less than the normal 150° and usually less than 140° [74]. Altered mechanics may lead to adventitious bursa formation along the plantar aspect of the foot; bursae may be demonstrated on US or MRI (Fig. 15.59).

Forefoot Adduction

In-toeing is a common concern among parents and primary care physicians, resulting in numerous referrals to orthopedic surgeons [75]. In-toeing is defined as internal rotation of the long

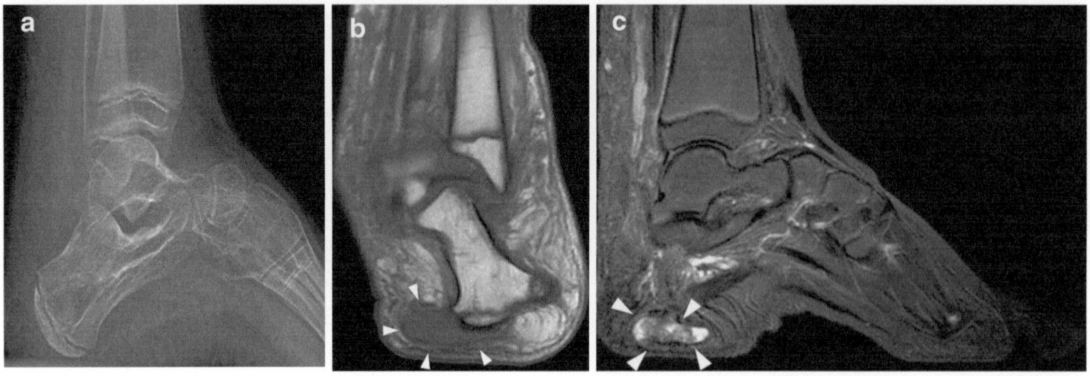

Fig. 15.59 Pes cavus with bursitis. (**a**) Severe pes cavus. Coronal T1-W (**b**) and sagittal T2-W FS (**c**) images show a well-defined T1 isointense (relative to muscle) and heterogeneously T2 hyperintense complex fluid collection (*arrowheads*) adjacent to the calcaneus, consistent with a bursa. This likely developed secondary to abnormal mechanics of the foot

axis of the foot in comparison to the direction of walking [76]. Increased femoral anteversion as well as internal tibial torsion are common causes. Clubfoot and cavus foot may cause in-toeing as well. In-toeing may also result from isolated forefoot adduction, due to abnormal insertion or forces on the abductor hallucis muscle, as well as from congenital abnormalities such as longitudinal epiphyseal bracket (discussed below).

The variable terminology used to denote forefoot adduction reflects the fact that a continuum exists, in which the deformity may be slight (forefoot adduction without foot inversion, with a relatively normal heel), moderate (forefoot adduction and foot inversion with mild heel valgus), or severe (serpentine or skewfoot with rigid forefoot adduction and foot inversion with marked heel valgus).

Metatarsus Adductus (Box 15.6)

> **Box 15.6: Metatarsus Adductus**
>
> Most common pediatric foot deformity
>
> Manifests by age 1 year
>
> Usually resolves, but up to 14 % progress to rigid deformity
>
> *Radiographs* Forefoot adduction
> Foot inversion (variable degree)
> Distal aspect of medial cuneiform may be wedged

Idiopathic metatarsus adductus is the most common pediatric foot deformity, occurring in 3 % of the population [77]. It is much more common than congenital clubfoot. Etiology is unknown, but muscle imbalance may play a role. In addition, the disorder may be inherited, since 25 % of affected children have a first-degree relative with a similar condition. Metatarsus adductus is recognizable at birth in two-thirds of patients and manifests during the first year of life in the other one-third. The forefoot is held in adduction. The degree of inversion varies. The medial border of the foot is concave, the lateral border convex, and the arch high. The distal aspect of the medial cuneiform may be wedged, resulting in malalignment of the tarsometatarsal articulations or medial deviation/adduction of the talar neck [78].

Pure forefoot adduction without foot inversion (true metatarsus adductus) is common and usually resolves without intervention, but 4–14 % of cases progress to a severe, rigid deformity. Serial casting may be sufficient, with more invasive interventions reserved for severe or late-presenting cases. Minimally invasive, percutaneous surgical techniques are effective in treating the adduction deformity refractory to casting [79].

After Ponseti treatment for clubfoot, the foot may resemble idiopathic metatarsus adductus. In this case, over-pull of the tibialis anterior results

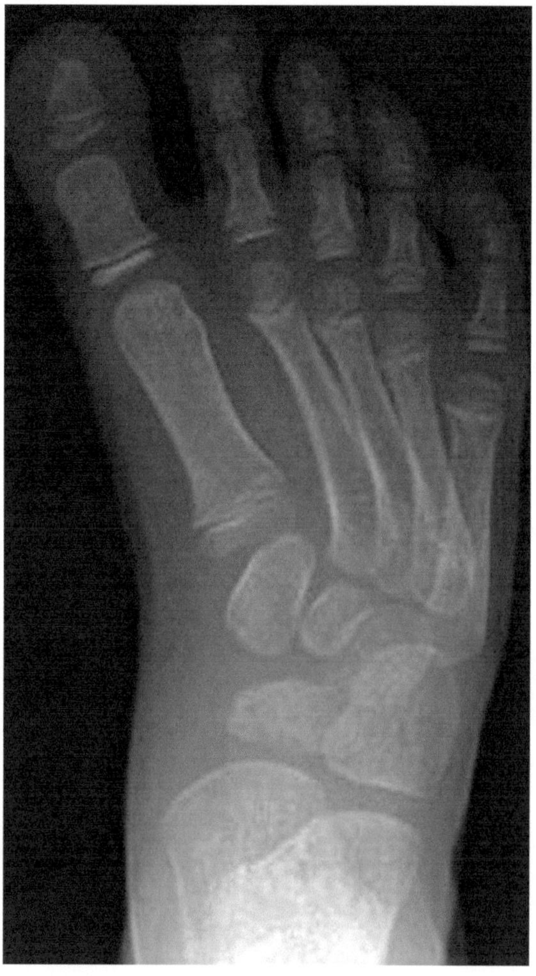

Fig. 15.60 Congenital metatarsus adductus in a 4-year-old boy. There is medial deviation of the metatarsals with normal hindfoot alignment (weight-bearing view)

in a condition termed "dynamic supination." The resulting supination is almost always accompanied by a degree of adduction.

Imaging

On radiographs, the forefoot is adducted relative to the midfoot on an AP view (Figs. 15.37 and 15.60). Mild inversion may be corrected with plantar pressure. In true metatarsus adductus, the hindfoot is normal. Varying amounts of inversion may be assessed on a lateral view by examining the alignment of the metatarsals and looking for the "stepladder" deformity with the first metatarsal highest.

Skewfoot

Skewfoot, or serpentine metatarsus adductus, is sometimes considered to be a severe form of metatarsus adductus but is actually a distinct entity. This deformity is quite rare, and it should not be mistaken for common metatarsus adductus. In skewfoot, forefoot adduction is associated with hindfoot valgus. In a sense, the hindfoot and forefoot deformities balance each other so that the foot has a Z or zigzag appearance (see Fig. 15.37). This deformity is most often encountered in otherwise normal children. Patients with severe cerebral palsy may develop a similar deformity, sometimes accompanied with hallux valgus. Incompletely treated clubfoot and syndromes such as Larsen, Proteus, and Ehlers-Danlos may also have a similar appearance [80] (see Fig. 15.44). Because the foot is usually flexible and the hindfoot valgus is balanced by forefoot adduction and cavus, operative management is generally unnecessary.

Imaging

The hindfoot is in valgus, with an increased talocalcaneal angle and medial deviation of the talus. There is midfoot angulation, with the navicular shifted lateral to the talar head (Fig. 15.61). The metatarsals are adducted. Axial lines drawn along the talus and metatarsals are roughly parallel, and a line connecting the center of the talar head and base of the first metatarsal completes a Z-figure with the axial lines (see Fig. 15.37).

Hallux Valgus

Increased valgus angulation of the first metatarsophalangeal joint is usually considered a disorder of adults, but up to 40 % of adult patients report the deformity being present before age 10 [81]. Pain, deformity, and difficulty fitting shoes may occur as early as age 7, and in this setting the entity is called *juvenile hallux valgus*. The deformity is ten times more common in girls and is bilateral in more than 75 % of patients. A positive family history is present in up to 83 % [82].

The etiology of isolated hallux valgus is not clearly understood. It may result from a primary change in the first metatarsophalangeal joint or be secondary to abnormal angulation of the first

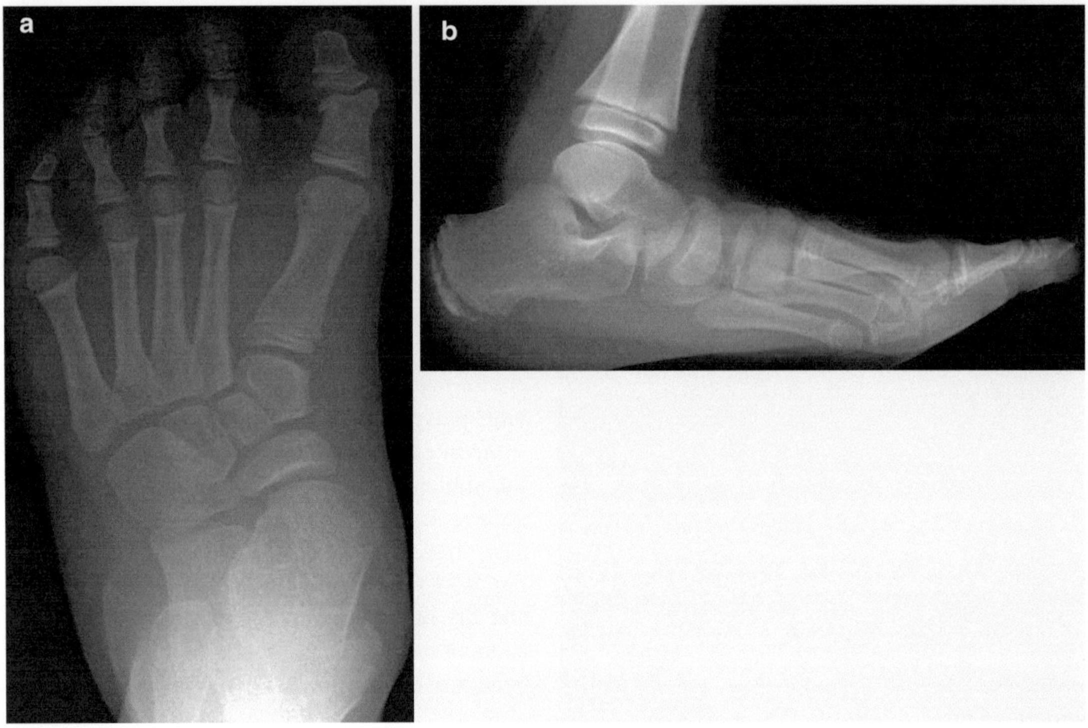

Fig. 15.61 (**a**, **b**) Skewfoot in a 9-year-old boy. There is hindfoot valgus and forefoot adduction (weight-bearing views)

and second metatarsals. This angulation, termed *metatarsus primus varus*, is defined as an abnormally increased angle between the first and second metatarsals [83]. Hallux valgus may also be seen in patients with cerebral palsy. In the setting of cerebral palsy, it is likely due to muscle imbalance and increased spasticity of the adductor hallucis.

Imaging

Radiographs typically reveal an adducted first metatarsal that is shorter than the second metatarsal (Figs. 15.37 and 15.62). The angle between the first metatarsal and first proximal phalanx (metatarsophalangeal angle) exceeds 15° in adolescents. Splaying of the first and second metatarsals is also seen, assessed by the intermetatarsal angle on a weight-bearing AP radiograph. This angle is formed by the intersection between a line drawn along the first metatarsal, connecting the centers of the proximal articular surface and base, and a similar line drawn along the second metatarsal. A normal angle is less than 10° (normal range, 6–9°).

In addition to these increased angles, there should also be medial uncovering of the first metatarsal head. Tilt of the articular surface of the first metatarsal without medial uncovering may be considered a normal variant and usually does not progress. An increased metatarsophalangeal angle associated with uncovering of the medial portion of the first metatarsal head, however, is considered abnormal and may progress to frank subluxation. In addition, the hallux sesamoids are usually laterally displaced.

During adolescence, the joint capsule may contract, limiting flexibility and causing inflammation of the bursa over the metatarsal head. However, an osseous protuberance at the medial first metatarsal head is not usually seen until adulthood. Other measurements (interphalangeal angles and first metatarsal-cuneiform angles,

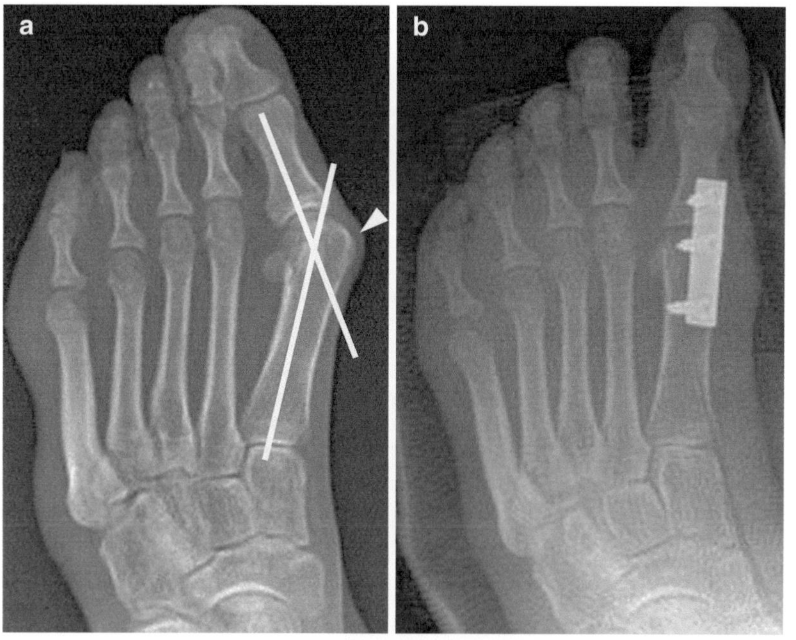

Fig. 15.62 Hallux valgus in a 13-year-old girl. (**a**) The angle between the shafts of the first metatarsal and proximal phalanx is abnormally increased, and the medial aspect of the head of the first metatarsal is uncovered (*arrowhead*). (**b**) After plate and screw fixation across the first metatarsophalangeal joint, the angle is normal, and the proximal phalanx is centered on the first metatarsal head

metatarsal lengths, sesamoid position, and others) may be used for operative planning [84].

2.6 Structural Malformations

Abnormalities of individual or multiple foot bones are encountered in many congenital syndromes. Foot pathology may occur in isolation or be associated with other elements of a syndrome. Rarely does a specific anomaly suggest a particular syndrome, with diagnosis of a syndrome resting on a combination of physical examination, radiographs, and often genetic evaluation.

Abnormalities of the Digits

Polydactyly involves supernumerary digits that may be preaxial (anatomically medial to the first toe), postaxial (lateral to the small toe), or central/intercalary (Fig. 15.63). Factors such as the presence of syndactyly, axis deviation and metatarsal extension are important for treatment planning and outcome [85]. Polydactyly occurs in isolation and is also seen in skeletal dysplasias, such as chondroectodermal dysplasia and trisomies 13 and 21.

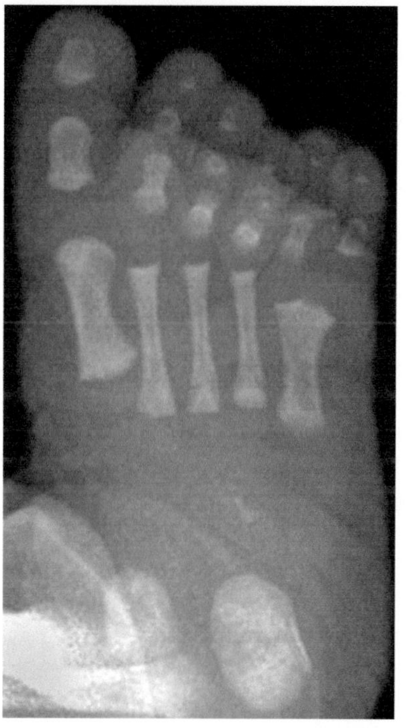

Fig. 15.63 Polydactyly in a newborn. Oblique view shows postaxial polydactyly. The two proximal phalanges articulate with an unusually broad fifth metatarsal

Syndactyly—fusion of adjacent digits—involves soft tissue (simple) or bone (complex). A portion of the digit (incomplete) or an entire digit (complete) may be affected. Like polydactyly, syndactyly may be isolated or syndromic; it is a feature of both Poland and Apert syndromes.

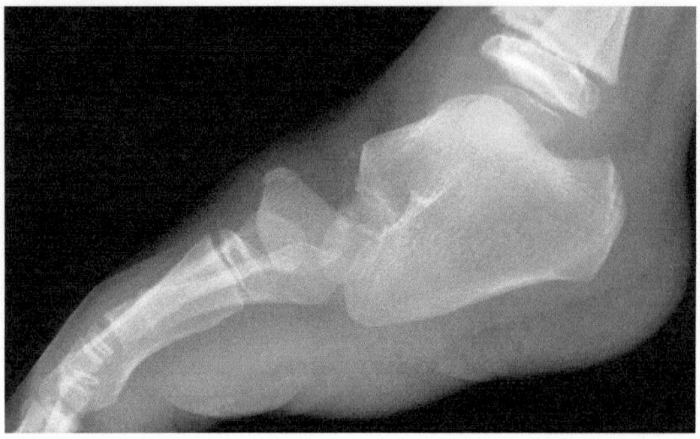

Fig. 15.64 Calcaneocuboid, talocalcaneal, and partial navicular-cuneiform fusion, along with ray deletion (lateral with forced flexion) (Courtesy of Rebecca Stein-Wexler) Shriners permission

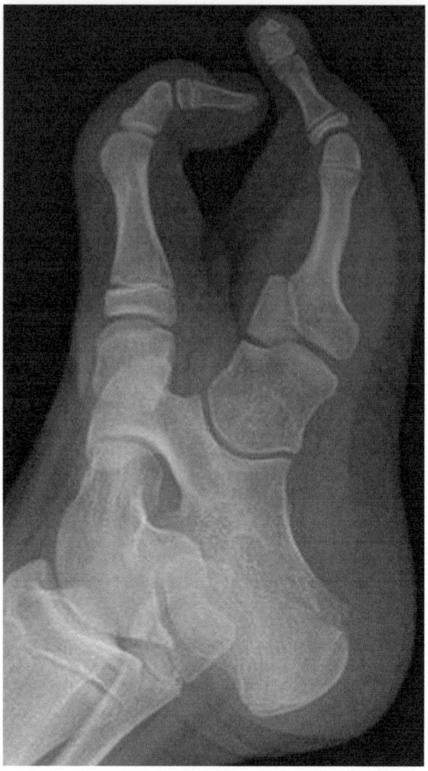

Fig. 15.65 Split foot deformity in an 18-year-old girl. Oblique view shows essentially two rays, with a remnant of the base of the fourth metatarsal. The midfoot is incomplete, and there is calcaneonavicular coalition

Symphalangism is a rare, autosomal dominant abnormality characterized by joint fusion. It affects the foot or hand, most often the proximal interphalangeal joints; this disorder may be associated with other digit abnormalities along with hip and spine problems. Other foot anomalies, such as short metatarsals, short digits (brachydactyly), and cone-shaped epiphyses, are seen in many syndromes.

Specific abnormalities of the great toe are characteristic of—and indeed suggest the diagnosis of—Rubinstein-Taybi syndrome and myositis ossificans progressiva congenita [86]. Great toe abnormalities are also seen in trisomy 18, Apert syndrome, and Cornelia de Lange syndrome, among others.

Tarsal Fusions

Congenital tarsal fusion associated with underlying syndromes often involves the cuneiforms, although this may not be apparent radiographically in early childhood due to the lack of ossification. The more common tarsal coalitions (discussed above) rarely involve the cuneiforms. Fusion may be distal, fusing the midfoot to the metatarsal, or along the same midfoot row. Massive fusion of multiple bones (Fig. 15.64) may be associated with symphalangism, arthrogryposis, and acrocephalosyndactyly. Tarsal fusions are integral to Nievergelt and Fuhrmann syndromes. Talonavicular and calcaneocuboid coalitions are common with ball-and-socket ankle joints (see Fig. 15.5).

Split Foot

This characteristic malformation involves a variable number of digits missing from the central foot (or hand), resulting in a central V- or U-shaped cleft (Fig. 15.65). The term "split foot" is preferred over older terminology (ectrodactyly, cleft foot, and lobster-claw malformation) [87]. The malformation is rare, occurring in 1 in 8,500–25,000 newborns. It is associated with various genetic abnormalities [88]. Although it may occur in isolation, split foot is also seen with more than 75 different syndromes. The most common of these is ectrodactyly-ectodermal dysplasia-cleft lip/palate syndrome (or EEC). The degree and type of deformity guide surgical management.

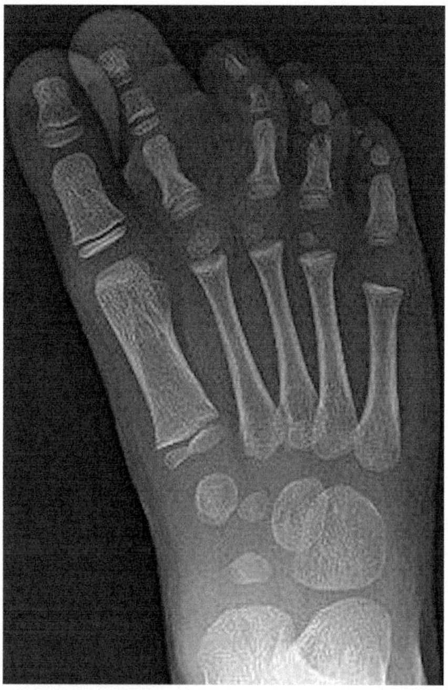

Fig. 15.66 Macrodystrophia lipomatosa in a 6-year-old girl. There is osseous and soft tissue overgrowth of the second toe with secondary deformity of the third toe

Structural Abnormalities Associated with Syndromes

Clubfoot deformity is seen in diverse syndromes, such as diastrophic dwarfism and arthrogryposis. Congenital vertical talus is associated with teratologic hip dislocation and with microstomia in craniocarpotarsal dysplasia (Freeman-Sheldon or whistling face syndrome).

Localized Gigantism

Soft tissue and osseous overgrowth may be associated with local hemangiomatosis, lymphangiomatosis, macrodystrophia lipomatosa (Fig. 15.66), and neurofibromatosis (see Chaps. 9, 22, and 23).

References

1. Carmont MR, Tomlinson JE, Blundell C, Davies MB, Moore DJ. Variability of joint communications in the foot and ankle demonstrated by contrast-enhanced diagnostic injections. Foot Ankle Int Am Orthop Foot Ankle Soc Swiss Foot Ankle Soc. 2009;30(5):439–42. PubMed PMID: 19439145.
2. Love SM, Ganey T, Ogden JA. Postnatal epiphyseal development: the distal tibia and fibula. J Pediatr Orthop. 1990;10(3):298–305. PubMed PMID: 2355072.
3. Selby S. Separate centers of ossification of the tip of the internal malleolus. Am J Roentgenol Radium Ther Nucl Med. 1961;86:496–501. PubMed PMID: 13749864.
4. Mellado JM, Ramos A, Salvado E, Camins A, Danus M, Sauri A. Accessory ossicles and sesamoid bones of the ankle and foot: imaging findings, clinical significance and differential diagnosis. Eur Radiol. 2003;13 Suppl 6:L164–77. PubMed PMID: 16440220.
5. Carty H. Accessory ossicles at the lateral malleolus: a review of the incidence. Eur J Radiol. 1992;14(3):181–4. PubMed PMID: 1563424.
6. Sauser DD, Nelson RC, Lavine MH, Wu CW. Acute injuries of the lateral ligaments of the ankle: comparison of stress radiography and arthrography. Radiology. 1983;148(3):653–7. PubMed PMID: 6878679.
7. Skolan V, Smigovec I, Ethapic T, Anticevic D. Long-term follow-up of congenital distal tibiofibular diastasis: a report of two female patients. J Pediatr Orthop B. 2013;22(5):464–9. PubMed PMID: 23337613.
8. Jones D, Barnes J, Lloyd-Roberts GC. Congenital aplasia and dysplasia of the tibia with intact fibula. Classification and management. J Bone Joint Surg. 1978;60(1):31–9. PubMed PMID: 627576.
9. Pistoia F, Ozonoff MB, Wintz P. Ball-and-socket ankle joint. Skelet Radiol. 1987;16(6):447–51. PubMed PMID: 3659990.
10. Stevens PM, Aoki S, Olson P. Ball-and-socket ankle. J Pediatr Orthop. 2006;26(4):427–31. PubMed PMID: 16791056.
11. Takakura Y, Tanaka Y, Kumai T, Sugimoto K. Development of the ball-and-socket ankle as assessed by radiography and arthrography. A long-term follow-up report. J Bone Joint Surg. 1999;81(6):1001–4. PubMed PMID: 10615975.
12. Ilyas I, Wade WJ, Al Barrag M, Al Hussainan TS, Lotaibi LA, Alssayad M. A rare pentad of foot and ankle deformities in hyperlax children. J Child Orthop. 2009;3(2):115–20. PubMed PMID: 19308622. Pubmed Central PMCID: 2656954.
13. Takikawa K, Haga N, Tanaka H, Okada K. Characteristic factors of ankle valgus with multiple cartilaginous exostoses. J Pediatr Orthop. 2008;28(7):761–5. PubMed PMID: 18812904.
14. Dawe C, Wynne-Davies R, Fulford GE. Clinical variation in dyschondrosteosis. A report on 13 individuals in 8 families. J Bone Joint Surg. 1982;64(3):377–81.
15. Kaissi AA, Farr S, Ganger R, Hofstaetter JG, Klaushofer K, Grill F. Treatment of varus deformities of the lower limbs in patients with achondroplasia and hypochondroplasia. Open Orthop J. 2013;7:33–9. PubMed PMID: 23459260. Pubmed Central PMCID: 3580759. Epub 2013/03/06. eng.
16. Vallejo JM, Jaramillo D. Normal MR imaging anatomy of the ankle and foot in the pediatric population. Magn Reson Imaging Clin N Am. 2001;9(3):435–46.

17. Vanderwilde R, Staheli LT, Chew DE, Malagon V. Measurements on radiographs of the foot in normal infants and children. J Bone Joint Surg Am. 1988;70(3):407–15. PubMed PMID: 3346265.
18. Miller TT, Staron RB, Feldman F, Parisien M, Glucksman WJ, Gandolfo LH. The symptomatic accessory tarsal navicular bone: assessment with MR imaging. Radiology. 1995;195(3):849–53. PubMed PMID: 7754020.
19. Lawson JP. International Skeletal Society Lecture in honor of Howard D. Dorfman. Clinically significant radiologic anatomic variants of the skeleton. AJR Am J Roentgenol. 1994;163(2):249–55. PubMed PMID: 8037009. Epub 1994/08/01. eng.
20. Lawson JP, Ogden JA, Sella E, Barwick KW. The painful accessory navicular. Skelet Radiol. 1984; 12(4):250–62. PubMed PMID: 6239377.
21. Bennett GL, Weiner DS, Leighley B. Surgical treatment of symptomatic accessory tarsal navicular. J Pediatr Orthop. 1990;10(4):445–9. PubMed PMID: 2358479.
22. Bureau NJ, Cardinal E, Hobden R, Aubin B. Posterior ankle impingement syndrome: MR imaging findings in seven patients. Radiology. 2000;215(2):497–503. PubMed PMID: 10796931.
23. Miller TT. Painful accessory bones of the foot. Semin Musculoskelet Radiol. 2002;6(2):153–61. PubMed PMID: 12077704.
24. Shopfner CE, Coin CG. Effect of weight-bearing on the appearance and development of the secondary calcaneal epiphysis. Radiology. 1966;86(2):201–6. PubMed PMID: 5902461.
25. Schreck MA. Pediatric longitudinal epiphyseal bracket: review and case presentation. J Foot Ankle Surg Am Coll Foot Ankle Surg. 2006;45(5):342–5. PubMed PMID: 16949533.
26. Mahboubi S, Davidson R. MR imaging in longitudinal epiphyseal bracket in children. Pediatr Radiol. 1999;29(4):259–61. PubMed PMID: 10199903.
27. Aurell Y, Johansson A, Hansson G, Wallander H, Jonsson K. Ultrasound anatomy in the normal neonatal and infant foot: an anatomic introduction to ultrasound assessment of foot deformities. Eur Radiol. 2002;12(9):2306–12. PubMed PMID: 12195486.
28. Agrawal S, Srivastava D, Gangwar HS, Agrawal S, Agrawal PK. Sonography as an objective tool for monitoring serial corrections and detecting spurious corrections in clubfoot: a review. Foot. 2012;22(4):315–8. PubMed PMID: 22985728.
29. Kuhns LR, Koujok K, Hall JM, Craig C. Ultrasound of the navicular during the simulated Ponseti maneuver. J Pediatr Orthop. 2003;23(2):243–5. PubMed PMID: 12604958.
30. Supakul N, Loder RT, Karmazyn B. Dynamic US study in the evaluation of infants with vertical or oblique talus deformities. Pediatr Radiol. 2013;43(3):376–80. PubMed PMID: 23184066.
31. Smith EA, Dillman JR, Goodsitt MM, Christodoulou EG, Keshavarzi N, Strouse PJ. Model-based iterative reconstruction: effect on patient radiation dose and image quality in pediatric body CT. Radiology. 2014;270(2):526–34. PubMed PMID: 24091359.
32. Harty MP. Imaging of pediatric foot disorders. Radiol Clin N Am. 2001;39(4):733–48. PubMed PMID: 11549168.
33. Patel CV. The foot and ankle: MR imaging of uniquely pediatric disorders. Magn Reson Imaging Clin N Am. 2009;17(3):539–47. PubMed PMID: 19524201.
34. Davids JR, Gibson TW, Pugh LI. Quantitative segmental analysis of weight-bearing radiographs of the foot and ankle for children: normal alignment. J Pediatr Orthop. 2005;25(6):769–76. PubMed PMID: 16294134.
35. Dobbs MB, Gurnett CA. Genetics of clubfoot. J Pediatr Orthop B. 2012;21(1):7–9. PubMed PMID: 21817922. Pubmed Central PMCID: 3229717.
36. Waisbrod H. Congenital club foot. An anatomical study. J Bone Joint Surg. 1973;55(4):796–801. PubMed PMID: 4766184.
37. Settle GW. The anatomy of congenital talipes equinovarus: sixteen dissected specimens. J Bone Joint Surg Am. 1963;45:1341–54. PubMed PMID: 14069774.
38. Ponseti IV. Treatment of congenital club foot. J Bone Joint Surg Am. 1992;74(3):448–54. PubMed PMID: 1548277.
39. Dobbs MB, Rudzki JR, Purcell DB, Walton T, Porter KR, Gurnett CA. Factors predictive of outcome after use of the Ponseti method for the treatment of idiopathic clubfeet. J Bone Joint Surg Am. 2004; 86-A(1):22–7. PubMed PMID: 14711941.
40. Park SS, Kim SW, Jung BS, Lee HS, Kim JS. Selective soft-tissue release for recurrent or residual deformity after conservative treatment of idiopathic clubfoot. J Bone Joint Surg. 2009;91(11):1526–30. PubMed PMID: 19880901.
41. Simons GW. A standardized method for the radiographic evaluation of clubfeet. Clin Orthop Relat Res. 1978;135:107–18. PubMed PMID: 709918.
42. Thometz J, Manz R, Liu XC, Klein J, Manz-Friesth B. Reproducibility of radiographic measurements in assessment of congenital talipes equinovarus. Am J Orthop. 2009;38(12):617–20. PubMed PMID: 20145787.
43. Herbsthofer B, Eckardt A, Rompe JD, Kullmer K. Significance of radiographic angle measurements in evaluation of congenital clubfoot. Arch Orthop Trauma Surg. 1998;117(6–7):324–9. PubMed PMID: 9709844.
44. Radler C, Manner HM, Suda R, Burghardt R, Herzenberg JE, Ganger R, et al. Radiographic evaluation of idiopathic clubfeet undergoing Ponseti treatment. J Bone Joint Surg Am. 2007;89(6):1177–83. PubMed PMID: 17545419.
45. Aurell Y, Johansson A, Hansson G, Jonsson K. Ultrasound anatomy in the neonatal clubfoot. Eur Radiol. 2002;12(10):2509–17. PubMed PMID: 12271392.

46. Desai S, Aroojis A, Mehta R. Ultrasound evaluation of clubfoot correction during Ponseti treatment: a preliminary report. J Pediatr Orthop. 2008;28(1):53–9. PubMed PMID: 18157047.
47. Kamegaya M, Shinohara Y, Kokuji Y, Moriya H. Evaluation of pathologic abnormalities of clubfoot by magnetic resonance imaging. Clin Orthop Relat Res. 2000;379:218–23. PubMed PMID: 11039809.
48. Sullivan JA. Pediatric flatfoot: evaluation and management. J Am Acad Orthop Surg. 1999;7(1):44–53. PubMed PMID: 9916191.
49. Yu GV, Hladik J. Residual calcaneovalgus deformity: review of the literature and case study. J Foot Ankle Surg Am Coll Foot Ankle Surg. 1994;33(3):228–38. PubMed PMID: 8081328.
50. Rao UB, Joseph B. The influence of footwear on the prevalence of flat foot. A survey of 2300 children. J Bone Joint Surg. 1992;74(4):525–7. PubMed PMID: 1624509.
51. Basmajian JV, Stecko G. The role of muscles in arch support of the foot. J Bone Joint Surg Am. 1963;45:1184–90. PubMed PMID: 14077983.
52. Villarroya MA, Esquivel JM, Tomas C, Moreno LA, Buenafe A, Bueno G. Assessment of the medial longitudinal arch in children and adolescents with obesity: footprints and radiographic study. Eur J Pediatr. 2009;168(5):559–67. PubMed PMID: 18751725.
53. Aslani H, Sadigi A, Tabrizi A, Bazavar M, Mousavi M. Primary outcomes of the congenital vertical talus correction using the Dobbs method of serial casting and limited surgery. J Child Orthop. 2012;6(4):307–11. PubMed PMID: 23904897. Pubmed Central PMCID: 3425696.
54. Bosker BH, Goosen JH, Castelein RM, Mostert AK. Congenital convex pes valgus (congenital vertical talus). The condition and its treatment: a review of the literature. Acta Orthop Belg. 2007;73(3):366–72. PubMed PMID: 17715728.
55. Becker-Andersen H, Reimann I. Congenital vertical talus. Reevaluation of early manipulative treatment. Acta Orthop Scand. 1974;45(1):130–44. PubMed PMID: 4451046.
56. Dobbs MB, Purcell DB, Nunley R, Morcuende JA. Early results of a new method of treatment for idiopathic congenital vertical talus. J Bone Joint Surg Am. 2006;88(6):1192–200. PubMed PMID: 16757750.
57. Violas P, Chapuis M, Treguier C, Darnault P, Bracq H. Ultrasound: a helpful technique in the analysis of congenital vertical talus. A case report. J Pediatr Orthop B. 2006;15(1):70–2. PubMed PMID: 16280725.
58. Harris RI, Beath T. Etiology of peroneal spastic flat foot. J Bone Joint Surg. 1948;30B(4):624–34. PubMed PMID: 18894612.
59. Crim J. Imaging of tarsal coalition. Radiol Clin N Am. 2008;46(6):1017–26. PubMed PMID: 19038610.
60. Leonard MA. The inheritance of tarsal coalition and its relationship to spastic flat foot. J Bone Joint Surg. 1974;56B(3):520–6. PubMed PMID: 4421359.
61. Cass AD, Camasta CA. A review of tarsal coalition and pes planovalgus: clinical examination, diagnostic imaging, and surgical planning. J Foot Ankle Surg Am Coll Foot Ankle Surg. 2010;49(3):274–93. PubMed PMID: 20356770.
62. Martus JE, Femino JE, Caird MS, Kuhns LR, Craig CL, Farley FA. Accessory anterolateral talar facet as an etiology of painful talocalcaneal impingement in the rigid flatfoot: a new diagnosis. Iowa Orthop J. 2008;28:1–8. PubMed PMID: 19223941. Pubmed Central PMCID: 2603342.
63. Newman JS, Newberg AH. Congenital tarsal coalition: multimodality evaluation with emphasis on CT and MR imaging. Radiogr Radiol Soc N Am. 2000;20(2):321–32; quiz 526–7, 32. PubMed PMID: 10715334.
64. Wechsler RJ, Karasick D, Schweitzer ME. Computed tomography of talocalcaneal coalition: imaging techniques. Skelet Radiol. 1992;21(6):353–8. PubMed PMID: 1523429.
65. Lee MS, Harcke HT, Kumar SJ, Bassett GS. Subtalar joint coalition in children: new observations. Radiology. 1989;172(3):635–9. PubMed PMID: 2772169.
66. Resnick D. Talar ridges, osteophytes, and beaks: a radiologic commentary. Radiology. 1984;151(2):329–32. PubMed PMID: 6709899.
67. Lateur LM, Van Hoe LR, Van Ghillewe KV, Gryspeerdt SS, Baert AL, Dereymaeker GE. Subtalar coalition: diagnosis with the C sign on lateral radiographs of the ankle. Radiology. 1994;193(3):847–51. PubMed PMID: 7972836.
68. Taniguchi A, Tanaka Y, Kadono K, Takakura Y, Kurumatani N. C sign for diagnosis of talocalcaneal coalition. Radiology. 2003;228(2):501–5. PubMed PMID: 12819337.
69. Comfort TK, Johnson LO. Resection for symptomatic talocalcaneal coalition. J Pediatr Orthop. 1998;18(3):283–8. PubMed PMID: 9600549.
70. Nagai MK, Chan G, Guille JT, Kumar SJ, Scavina M, Mackenzie WG. Prevalence of Charcot-Marie-tooth disease in patients who have bilateral cavovarus feet. J Pediatr Orthop. 2006;26(4):438–43. PubMed PMID: 16791058.
71. Schwend RM, Drennan JC. Cavus foot deformity in children. J Am Acad Orthop Surg. 2003;11(3):201–11. PubMed PMID: 12828450.
72. Mottram ME, Pyle IR. Mandarin feet. Am J Roentgenol Ther Nucl Med. 1973;118(2):318–9. PubMed PMID: 4576452.
73. Barenfeld PA, Weseley MS, Shea JM. The congenital cavus foot. Clin Orthop Relat Res. 1971;79:119–26. PubMed PMID: 5097456.
74. Weseley MS, Barenfeld PA, Shea JM, Eisenstein AL. The congenital cavus foot. A follow-up report. Bull Hosp Jt Orthop Inst. 1982;42(2):217–29. PubMed PMID: 6309296.
75. Blackmur JP, Murray AW. Do children who in-toe need to be referred to an orthopaedic clinic? J Pediatr Orthop B. 2010;19(5):415–7. PubMed PMID: 20520580.

76. Harris E. The intoeing child: etiology, prognosis, and current treatment options. Clin Podiatr Med Surg. 2013;30(4):531–65. PubMed PMID: 24075135.
77. Widhe T. Foot deformities at birth: a longitudinal prospective study over a 16-year period. J Pediatr Orthop. 1997;17(1):20–4. PubMed PMID: 8989696.
78. Bleck EE. Developmental orthopaedics. III: toddlers. Dev Med Child Neurol. 1982;24(4):533–55. PubMed PMID: 7117713.
79. Knorr J, Soldado F, Pham TT, Torres A, Cahuzac JP, de Gauzy JS. Percutaneous correction of persistent severe metatarsus adductus in children. J Pediatr Orthop. 2014;34(4):447–52. PubMed PMID: 24276227.
80. Hagmann S, Dreher T, Wenz W. Skewfoot. Foot Ankle Clin. 2009;14(3):409–34. PubMed PMID: 19712883.
81. Coughlin MJ, Mann Award RA. Juvenile hallux valgus: etiology and treatment. Foot Ankle Int Am Orthop Foot Ankle Soc Swiss Foot Ankle Soc. 1995;16(11):682–97. PubMed PMID: 8589807.
82. Coughlin MJ, Jones CP. Hallux valgus: demographics, etiology, and radiographic assessment. Foot Ankle Int Am Orthop Foot Ankle Soc Swiss Foot Ankle Soc. 2007;28(7):759–77. PubMed PMID: 17666168.
83. Davids JR, McBrayer D, Blackhurst DW. Juvenile hallux valgus deformity: surgical management by lateral hemiepiphyseodesis of the great toe metatarsa. J Pediatr Orthop. 2007;27(7):826–30. PubMed PMID: 17878793.
84. Karasick D, Wapner KL. Hallux valgus deformity: preoperative radiologic assessment. AJR Am J Roentgenol. 1990;155(1):119–23. PubMed PMID: 2112832.
85. Seok HH, Park JU, Kwon ST. New classification of polydactyly of the foot on the basis of syndactylism, axis deviation, and metatarsal extent of extra digit. Arch Plast Surg. 2013;40(3):232–7. PubMed PMID: 23730599. Pubmed Central PMCID: 3665867.
86. Poznansk A. Foot manifestations of congenital malformation syndromes. Semin Roentgenol. 1970;5(4):354. PubMed PMID: WOS:A1970H660200003. English.
87. Elliott AM, Evans JA, Chudley AE. Split hand foot malformation (SHFM). Clin Genet. 2005;68(6): 501–5. PubMed PMID: WOS:000233169500006. English.
88. Gurrieri F, Everman DB. Clinical, genetic, and molecular aspects of split-hand/foot malformation: an update. Am J Med Genet A. 2013;161A(11):2860–72. PubMed PMID: 24115638.

The Foot and Ankle: Acquired Disorders

16

J. Herman Kan

Contents

Abstract

Injuries to the pediatric ankle and foot are common and increasing due to the popularity of organized youth sports. Fracture and dislocation patterns vary based on skeletal maturity, position of the ankle and foot at the time of injury, and direction of force. Ankle fractures unique to children, such as triplane and juvenile Tillaux, are addressed initially. Fractures of the foot are then presented based on their position within the hindfoot, midfoot, and forefoot. Discussions of osteochondritis dissecans of the talar dome and the various osteochondroses of the mid- and forefoot follow, and the chapter concludes with a brief review of ankle impingement syndromes.

Injuries to the pediatric ankle and foot are common and increasing due to the popularity of organized youth sports. Fracture and dislocation patterns vary based on skeletal maturity, position of the ankle and foot at the time of injury, and direction of force. Ankle fractures have unique patterns in children, such as triplane and juvenile Tillaux fractures. Fractures of the foot are addressed based on their position within the hindfoot (talus and calcaneus), midfoot (cuneiforms, cuboid, navicular), and forefoot (metatarsals and phalanges). Osteochondritis dissecans of the talar dome and the various osteochondroses of the mid- and forefoot may cause chronic pain

J.H. Kan, MD
Department of Radiology,
Texas Children's Hospital, 6701 Fannin Street,
Suite 470, Houston, TX 77005, USA

Department of Radiology,
Baylor College of Medicine, Houston, TX, USA
e-mail: jhkan@texaschildrens.org

R. Stein-Wexler et al. (eds.), *Pediatric Orthopedic Imaging*,
DOI 10.1007/978-3-642-45381-6_16, © Springer-Verlag Berlin Heidelberg 2015

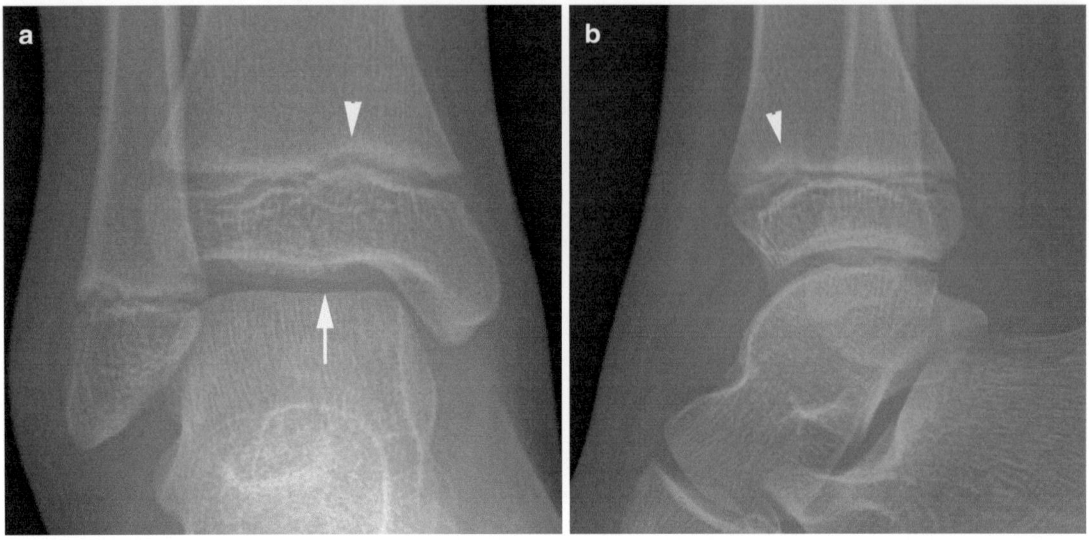

Fig. 16.1 Juvenile Tillaux fracture in an 11-year-old boy. (**a**, **b**) There is a nondisplaced Salter-Harris III fracture, with the vertical epiphyseal fracture line (*arrow*) lateral to Kump bump (*arrowhead*). The physis anterolateral to Kump bump is widened

in children. Anterior and posterior impingement syndromes are encountered less often in the pediatric age group.

1 Fractures

1.1 Fractures About the Ankle

The ankle joint includes the tibiotalar, tibiofibular, and talofibular articulations, and injury to the ankle may cause a variety of fractures as well as damage ligaments and other soft tissues in these areas. However, the physis is the weakest component of the pediatric ankle in the skeletally immature child [1]. Therefore, when the musculoskeletal unit is subjected to acute or chronic stress, the physis often fails before ligaments, tendons, or trabecular/cortical bone. In circumstances where an adult would suffer an ankle sprain, a child may suffer a physeal fracture instead.

The configuration of the distal tibial physis changes with age, affecting the type of fracture that occurs at this location. The physis of the young child is smooth, but it becomes progressively more irregular until it eventually fuses. The most prominent distal tibial physeal undulation is located anteromedially and is known as Kump bump (Fig. 16.1). The anteromedial aspect of the distal tibial physis fuses first, and fusion then progresses posteriorly and laterally [2]. Fusion begins at approximately age 11 in girls and age 12 in boys and is usually complete by age 14 in girls and age 16 in boys. The distal fibular physis closes at approximately the same time as the distal tibial physis [3].

Salter-Harris I fractures are limited to young children, whose physes are still smooth; these fractures, along with Salter-Harris II fractures, are the most common distal tibia fractures in children (see Chap. 17 for further discussion of the Salter-Harris and Ogden classification systems). Salter-Harris II fractures tend to occur after age 10. Older children, who have an undulating or partly fused physis, are prone to more complex Salter-Harris fractures. Focal physeal fusion or undulation may alter fracture force propagation. Fractures propagate along the path of least resistance; therefore, the open physis is usually first to fail, rather than the metaphyseal or epiphyseal bone. Similarly, fractures are more likely to propagate along an open, smooth physis than along an undulating physis. Physeal fracture propagation will usually terminate at sites of undulation, such as Kump bump, or at sites where there is already bony physeal fusion. These areas resist transmission of force more than the open, smooth physis.

The juvenile Tillaux and triplane fractures are affected by the contour of the distal tibial physis (Box 16.1). Both of these fractures usually occur when the foot is in supination and subject to external rotational forces [4], usually during a fall. They are most common between ages 12 and 15, especially during the approximately 18-month transitional period when the distal tibial physis begins closure [5, 6].

Box 16.1: Tibial Fractures

Accompany about 25 % of fibular fractures

Juvenile Tillaux and triplane fractures

- Twelve to fifteen years old, especially as distal tibial physeal closure begins
- Operative reduction if >2 mm displaced

Juvenile Tillaux fracture (Salter-Harris III)

- Fracture through the anterolateral smooth distal tibial physis to Kump bump
- Vertical fracture line in the epiphysis anterolateral to Kump bump
- Distal tibial fragment may rotate

Triplane fracture (Salter-Harris IV)

- At least three orthogonal planes; two-, three-, or four-part fractures (two-part most common)
- Classic two-part: sagittal in epiphysis, axial in physis, coronal in metaphysis
- Distal fibula also fractured in about 50 %

The Salter-Harris III juvenile Tillaux fracture occurs in early adolescence and is most common in girls. The force initially propagates along the anterolateral smooth distal tibial physis. However, physeal fracture propagation stops at Kump bump, where the force deviates vertically into the epiphyseal bone anterolateral to Kump bump [6]. The older the child, the more lateral the epiphyseal fracture line, since more of the physis is fused. The anterior tibiofibular ligament inserts into the epiphyseal fragment, and therefore some degree of separation of the fracture fragments is common.

Triplane fractures are Salter-Harris IV fractures; the degree of physeal undulation and fusion affects propagation of this fracture and the resultant number of bone fragments. As a general rule, there is a sagittal component in the epiphysis, an axial component through the physis, and a coronal component in the metaphysis [5]. The distal fibula is fractured in about 50 % of cases.

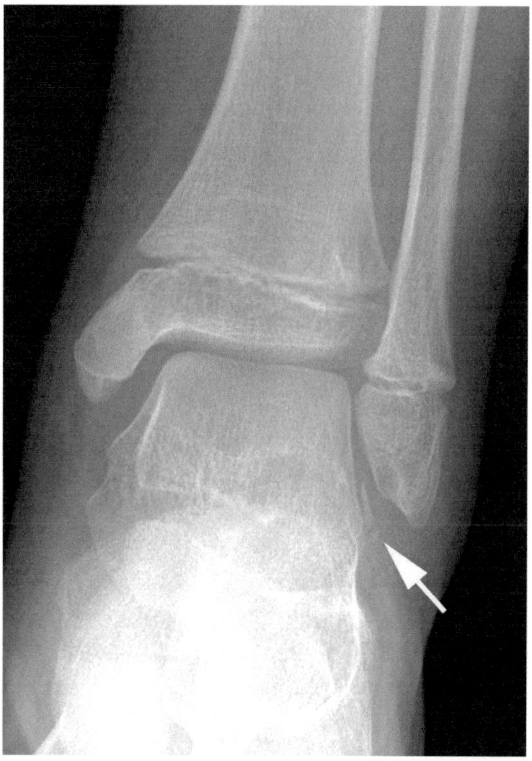

Fig. 16.2 Avulsion fracture at attachment site of anterior talofibular ligament in a 12-year-old girl. A thin, linear bone fragment (*arrow*) is separated from the talus

Distal fibular physeal fractures have been described with any mechanism of injury. Tibial fractures accompany approximately 25 % of fibular fractures [7], so if there is a fibular fracture the tibia should be closely examined.

Periosteal avulsion fractures about the ankle may occur at the medial or lateral collateral ligament insertion sites (Fig. 16.2). These are frequently seen in skeletally immature children, in whom the periosteum where ligaments attach is less resilient than are ligaments and tendons [8]. Maisonneuve fractures result from pronation/external rotation of the ankle and consist of the combination of proximal tibial/tibiofibular injury and ligamentous injury at the medial ankle.

The objective of treatment of ankle physeal fractures is to avoid premature physeal fusion by minimizing the degree of physeal injury and displacement. If the epiphysis is involved, incongruity at the articular surface may lead to early osteoarthritis if left untreated. Therefore, the threshold for operative intervention is relatively low for epiphyseal fractures. In addition, Salter-Harris fractures may lead to physeal bars, especially those that are higher grade. When physeal bars are eccentrically located in the tibia, varus or valgus deformity of the ankle may result, whereas central physeal bars may lead to restricted growth without angular deformity [7].

Operative reduction is indicated for juvenile Tillaux and triplane fractures when the gap between fragments exceeds 2 mm [4]. If the gap is less than or equal to 2 mm, the fracture may be treated conservatively with 4 weeks of non-weight bearing with a long leg cast followed by 4 weeks of relative non-weight bearing in a boot [9]. Maisonneuve fractures are considered unstable and require operative reduction.

Imaging

Radiography is the first-line imaging in children with suspected ankle fractures. The Ottawa ankle rules have been validated in children over 5 years of age and are useful in limiting the number of unnecessary radiographic exams [10] (see Chap. 1). The Ottawa ankle rules recommend that radiographs should be ordered if the child complains of pain over the malleoli and if there is either bony tenderness along the distal 6 cm of the posterior edge of either malleolus or if the child cannot bear weight for four steps both immediately after the injury and at the time of clinical examination. The standard views for the ankle include frontal, mortise, and lateral views, preferably with weight bearing if the child is capable since this stresses the ankle and foot and may make subtle fractures more obvious.

Computed tomography (CT) is helpful for comprehensive delineation of the fracture pattern, particularly if operative reduction is planned. CT allows more accurate measurement of fracture displacement, assessment of articular surface congruity as well as location and extent of physeal involvement, and determination of the number and location of fracture fragments.

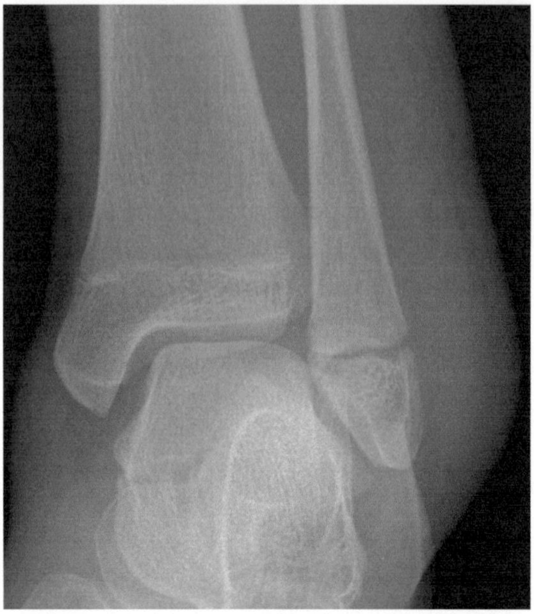

Fig. 16.3 Salter-Harris I fracture of the distal fibula in a 13-year-old girl. There is extensive soft tissue swelling centered at the level of the widened fibular physis

Salter-Harris I and II distal tibial and fibular fractures are the most common ankle fractures. It is important to search for a metaphyseal fragment or small flake (the so-called *Thurston Holland* fragment) in order to differentiate between a Salter-Harris I and a subtle Salter-Harris II. The degree of displacement and extent of physeal widening determine operative versus nonoperative management. Isolated Salter-Harris I and II fractures at the level of the distal fibular physis are not uncommon (Fig. 16.3).

It can be difficult to identify Salter-Harris I fractures of the distal fibula (or elsewhere). Isolated soft tissue swelling centered at the level of the open physis should be considered a Salter-Harris I fracture until proven otherwise (Fig. 16.3). However, in children younger than 10, the cartilaginous epiphysis of the medial or lateral malleolus may be confused with soft tissue swelling. If there is any question, comparison views of the asymptomatic distal fibula may help assess for physeal widening on the affected side.

The juvenile Tillaux fracture subgroup of distal tibial Salter-Harris III fractures has a vertical

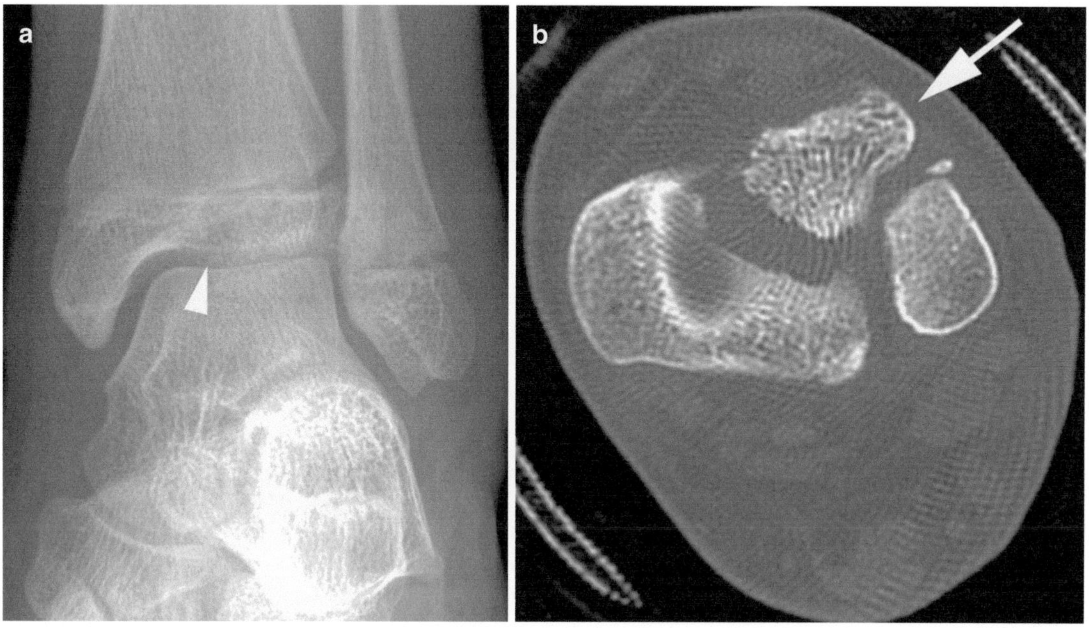

Fig. 16.4 Juvenile Tillaux fracture in a 12-year-old girl. (**a**) There is a minimally displaced vertical epiphyseal fracture (*arrowhead*), and the lateral tibial physis is widened. (**b**) Axial computed tomography (CT) shows an avulsion injury with lateral rotation of the anterolateral tibial epiphyseal fracture fragment (*arrow*) due to traction from the anterior syndesmosis

epiphyseal fracture line that is usually anterolateral to Kump bump (see Fig. 16.1) [9]. The older the child, the more lateral this vertical epiphyseal fracture line tends to be. The distal tibial epiphyseal fragment may rotate anterolaterally due to traction from the anterior syndesmosis (or tibiofibular ligament) at the level of the tibial plafond (Fig. 16.4). Although the anterolateral physis is fractured, it does not always appear widened.

The triplane subgroup of Salter-Harris IV fractures of the distal tibia must have at least three orthogonal fracture planes. These fractures can be divided into two-, three-, and even four-part fractures. Each category has several subtypes, which creates a confusing classification system [5]. Rather than trying to label these fractures according to their type and subtype, it is useful to define and describe the fracture components and extent of displacement. The two-part fracture is most common, followed by the three-part [11]. The classic two-part triplane fracture consists of a sagittal fracture plane through the tibial epiphysis, an axial fracture plane through the physis, and a coronal fracture plane through the metaphysis (Fig. 16.5). The posterolateral epiphyseal fracture fragment usually moves with the distal fibula, whereas the distal tibial epiphysis between the medial malleolus and Kump bump (or the anteromedially fused physis) follows the rest of the tibia. In younger patients, a three-part medial triplane fracture may have an axial fracture plane that extends through the anteromedial physis where Kump bump will develop. Once Kump bump appears, the medial fracture fragment in a three-part triplane fracture may include the medial epiphysis as well as Kump bump (Fig. 16.6).

Additional fractures about the ankle include avulsion fractures related to the lateral collateral ligament, syndesmosis (anterior or posterior tibiofibular ligament) (see Fig. 16.4), and peroneal sheath. Lateral and medial avulsion fractures usually appear as sharply defined flecks of bone along the tibia or talus (see Fig. 16.2); these should not be confused with the normal fragmentary ossification pattern of the malleoli or accessory ossicles such as the os subfibulare, which are corticated and round or ovoid in shape.

The Maisonneuve fracture has several components (Box 16.2). There is a medial malleolar fracture or deltoid ligament injury (Fig. 16.7), along

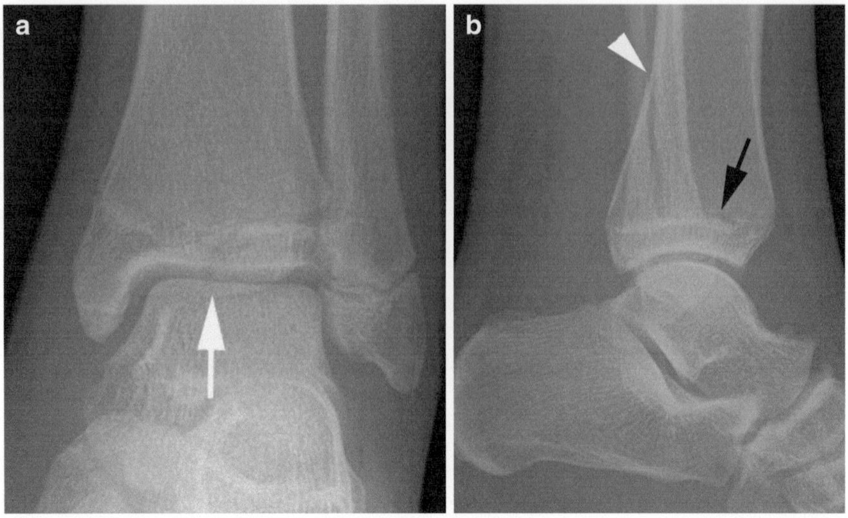

Fig. 16.5 Two-part triplane fracture in a 14-year-old boy. (**a**, **b**) There is a vertical epiphyseal component (*white arrow*), an axial component extending through the plane of the physis (*black arrow*), and a metaphyseal oblique component (*arrowhead*). This is a Salter-Harris IV fracture

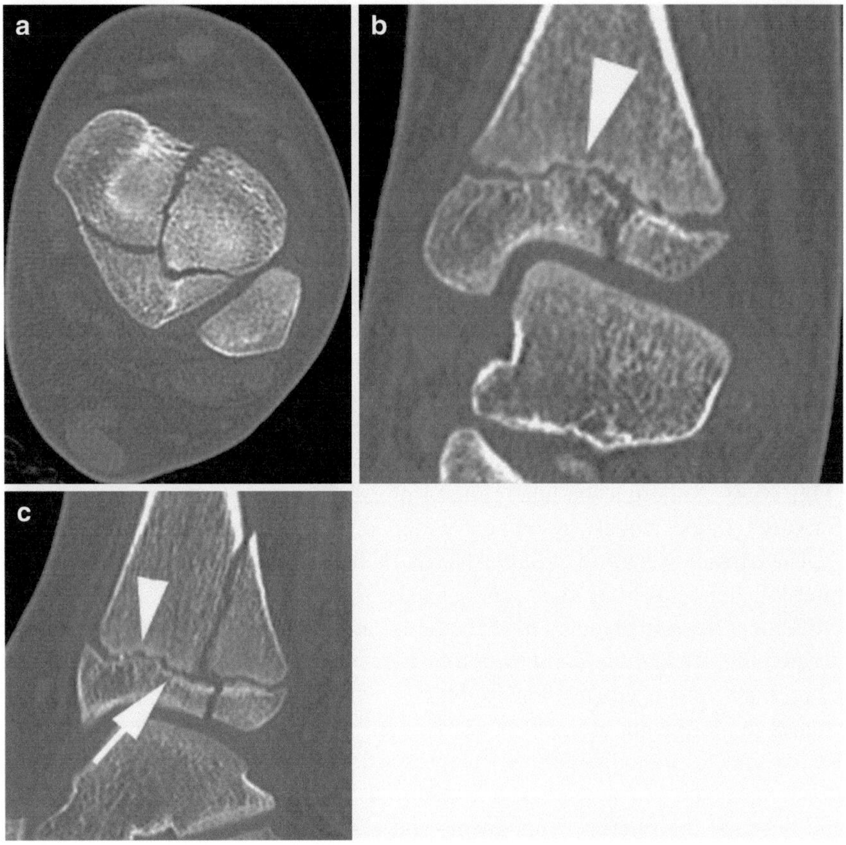

Fig. 16.6 Classic three-part triplane fracture in a 10-year-old girl. Axial (**a**), coronal (**b**), and sagittal (**c**) reformatted CT shows that the medial main fracture fragment includes the anteromedial epiphysis and Kump bump (*arrowhead*). The lateral physeal fracture (*arrow*) stops at Kump bump (*arrowhead*)

with injury to the syndesmosis and interosseous tibiofibular ligament, which results in widening of the medial tibiotalar joint. In addition, there is a proximal fibular fracture or proximal tibiofibular dislocation. Therefore, if the medial tibiotalar joint is widened or there is a medial malleolar fracture on ankle radiographs, radiographs of the upper tibia and fibula near the knee are recommended to

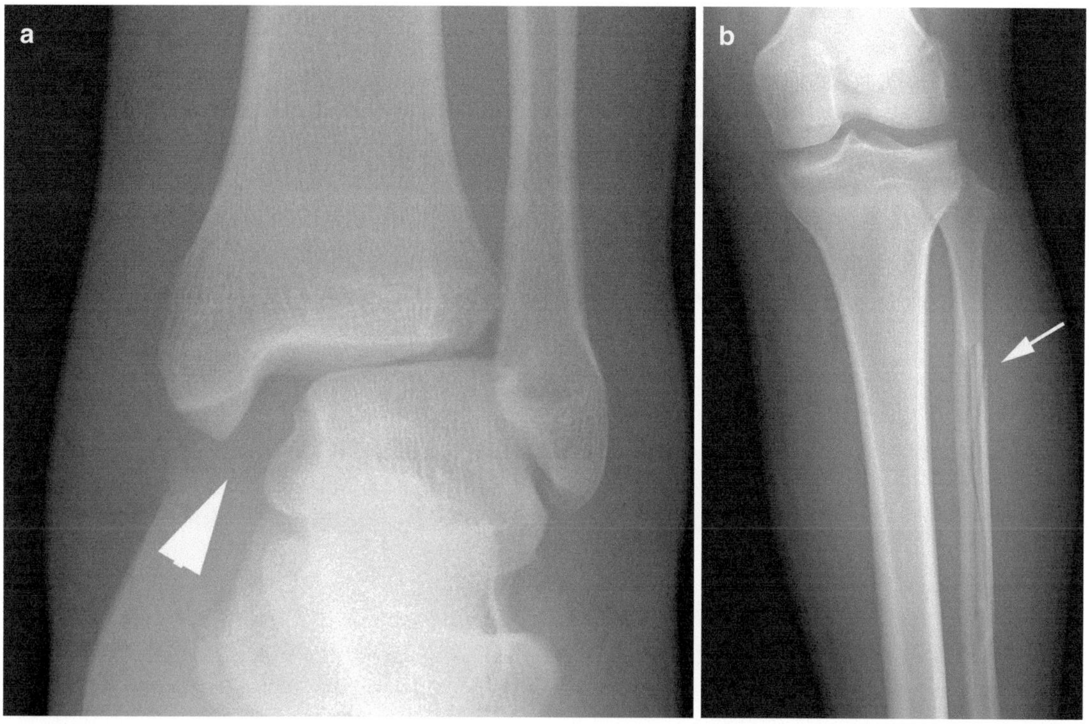

Fig. 16.7 Maisonneuve fracture in a 14-year-old boy. (**a**) Ankle radiograph shows medial tibiotalar joint space widening (*arrowhead*) consistent with a deltoid ligament injury. (**b**) Leg radiograph in the same patient demonstrates an oblique longitudinal fracture of the proximal fibular diaphysis (*arrow*)

evaluate for a concomitant proximal fibular fracture or proximal tibiofibular dislocation.

Box 16.2: Maisonneuve Fracture

Mechanism: pronation/external rotation

Associated with medial malleolar fracture or deltoid ligament injury

Injury to syndesmosis and interosseous tibiofibular ligament

Proximal fibular fracture or proximal tibiofibular dislocation

Key: if there is medial malleolar fracture/deltoid ligament injury, evaluate the proximal fibula

1.2 Midfoot and Hindfoot Fractures

The toddler spectrum of fractures may affect the bones of the midfoot and hindfoot, especially the cuboid (Fig. 16.8) [12]. The most likely mechanism is forced plantar flexion of the foot resulting in compression force at the cuboid.

Fractures of the talus most often affect the neck [13] (Box 16.3). The usual mechanism is forced dorsiflexion of the foot, resulting in abutment of the anterior lip of the tibial plafond and the talar neck. Since most of the arteries to the talus (which include branches from the posterior tibial, dorsalis pedis, and peroneal) enter the talus at the level of the neck, there is a relatively high incidence of osteonecrosis after this type of fracture. The likelihood of post-traumatic osteonecrosis increases with the degree of talar neck displacement and increasing patient age [14, 15].

Calcaneal fractures usually result from falls from a height or direct injury (such as from a lawn mower) [13, 16]. Fractures that result from falls are usually less severe in skeletally immature patients because cartilage is plastic compared with adult bone. Stress fractures are fairly common in the calcaneus [17].

Box 16.3: Talar Fracture

Mechanism: forced dorsiflexion of the foot

Usually affects the neck

High incidence of osteonecrosis (tenuous blood supply)

- More likely with greater talar neck displacement and increasing patient age
- Follow for 18 months

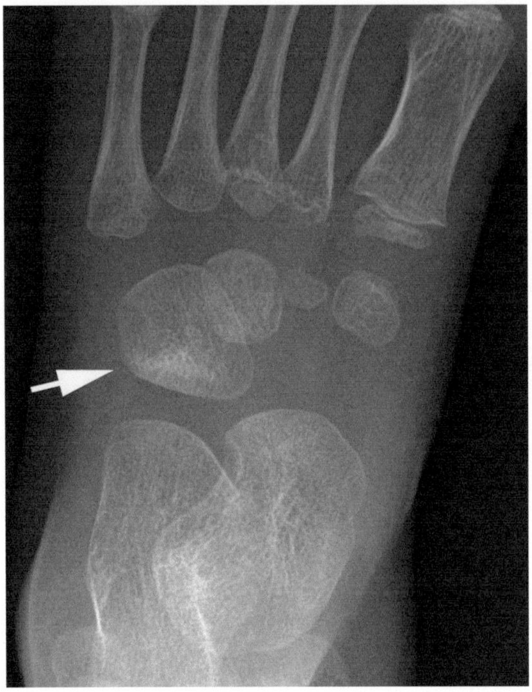

Fig. 16.8 Toddler's fracture of the cuboid in a 3-year-old boy. There is a transverse band of sclerosis at the proximal cuboid (*arrow*)

The navicular bone is affected by stress fractures [18] as well as avulsion injuries. Avulsion injuries generally occur at the insertion of the tibialis posterior tendon along the medial pole of the navicular. This is also the location of accessory ossicles, which are relatively mobile, leading to avulsion and/or symptomatic stress reaction. Accessory navicular ossicles are categorized according to the position of the ossicle with respect to the tendon. The type 1 ossicle is embedded in the tibialis posterior tendon, whereas the tendon fibers insert on the type 2 ossicle, which has a synchondrosis with the navicular [18].

Displaced talar neck fractures should be reduced to anatomic alignment. Nondisplaced fractures should be followed for at least 18 months to monitor for talar dome osteonecrosis [13]. Calcaneal fractures in children carry a better prognosis compared with adults and are likely to remodel without operative fixation. Symptomatic accessory navicular ossicles may be resected if conservative management fails to alleviate symptoms [19].

Imaging

Frontal, lateral, and oblique radiographs should be performed, preferably with weight bearing. The stress placed on the bones with weight bearing may help reveal subtle nondisplaced fractures, assess for longitudinal alignment of the foot, and—if there is a calcaneal fracture—provide a more accurate estimate of Bohler angle. Ankle radiographs should include the base of the metatarsals to assess the tarsometatarsal joints.

Calcaneal fractures are more likely to be extra-articular in children than in adults [18]. A Harris-Beath view may help evaluate fracture displacement in the mediolateral direction as well as intra-articular extension to the middle and posterior facets of the subtalar joint (Fig. 16.9). CT complements radiography and facilitates preoperative planning by quantifying the extent of displacement and intra-articular extension.

Follow-up of talar neck fractures should include evaluation for talar dome osteonecrosis, which appears as subchondral sclerosis, collapse, and fragmentation. Hawkins sign, which is first seen from 6 to 8 weeks after injury, indicates that there is adequate blood supply to the talar dome and low probability of osteonecrosis [20]. This sign appears as subchondral lucency that parallels the talar dome, and it results from imbalanced bone resorption relative to bone formation in the setting of hyperemia [21]. Determining the presence of Hawkins sign is probably less important in the era of MRI (magnetic resonance imaging).

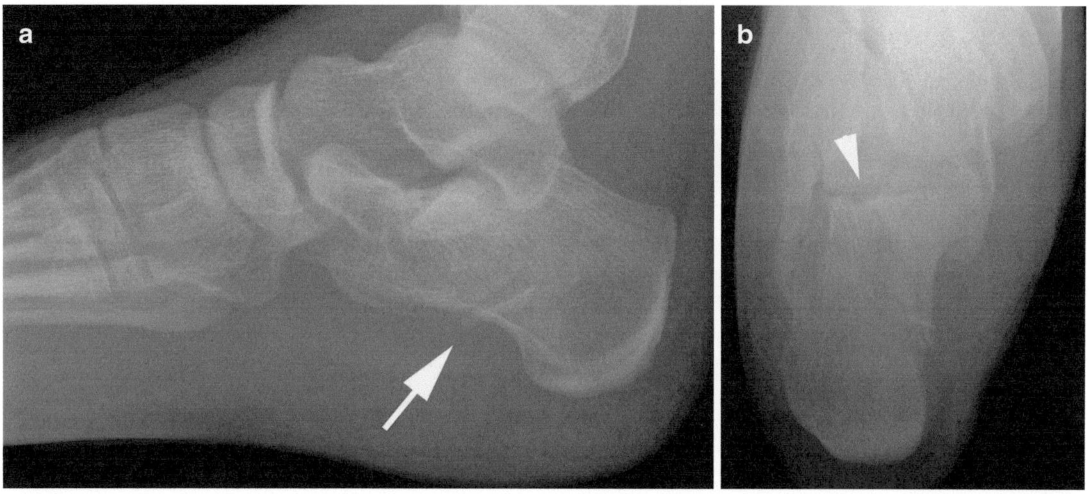

Fig. 16.9 Intra-articular calcaneal body fracture in a 15-year-old boy. (**a**) Lateral view shows a nondisplaced calcaneal body fracture (*arrow*). (**b**) Subtalar involvement is often apparent on the Harris-Beath view (*arrowhead*)

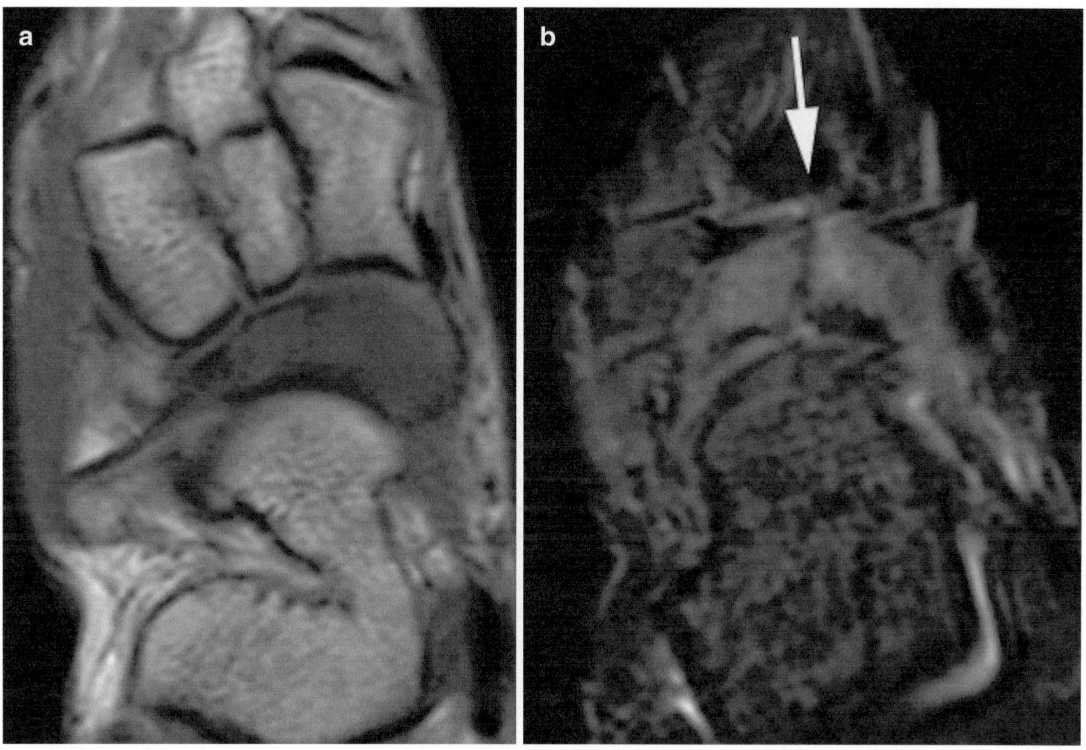

Fig. 16.10 Nondisplaced navicular stress fracture in a 14-year-old boy. (**a**) Axial T1-weighted (T1-W) image shows diffuse decreased signal throughout the navicular. (**b**) Axial short tau inversion recovery (STIR) image shows diffuse navicular marrow edema and a nondisplaced longitudinal fracture (*arrow*)

MRI is helpful when radiographic findings are normal and an occult fracture or stress reaction is suspected (Fig. 16.10). MRI is also helpful in the evaluation of a symptomatic accessory navicular to assess for associated marrow edema and juxtacortical soft tissue edema (Fig. 16.11) [22].

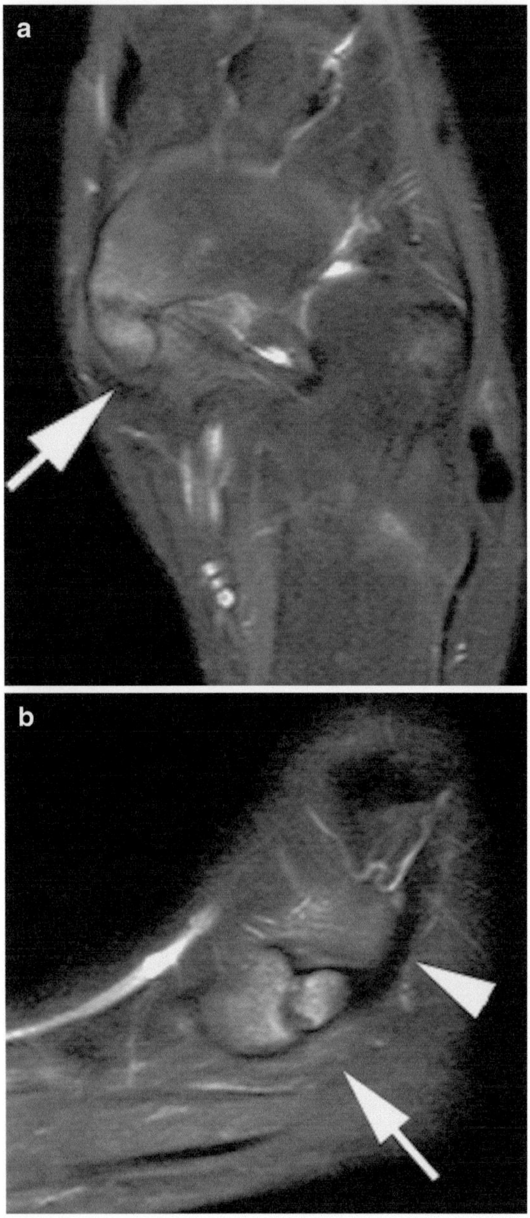

Fig. 16.11 Symptomatic type 2 accessory navicular in an 11-year-old girl. Axial T2-weighted (T2-W) fat-suppressed (FS) (**a**) and sagittal proton density (PD) FS (**b**) views show marrow edema at the navicular and accessory navicular as well as juxtacortical soft tissues (*arrows*). Tibialis posterior tendon (*arrowhead*)

1.3 Metatarsal Fractures (Box 16.4)

Toddler-type fractures can affect the metatarsals due to either impaction or twisting forces [12]. Stress fractures of the foot are especially common in athletes and dancers, most often affecting the metatarsals [23]. The pediatric bunk bed fracture is thought to be the pediatric equivalent of an adult Lisfranc fracture-dislocation injury [24]. This injury occurs when a child jumps or falls from a height, landing with the foot plantar flexed. The vertical impaction force is transmitted to the proximal first metatarsal, possibly causing ligamentous injury along with fracture.

Three types of fractures affect the proximal fifth metatarsal. Avulsion fractures of the tubercle at the peroneus brevis tendon insertion are the most common type of metatarsal fracture in children over age 5 [25]. These fractures occur when the ankle twists with a fixed forefoot. The other common type of proximal fifth metatarsal fracture affects the diaphysis and is usually an overuse stress injury in adolescent athletes. The Jones fracture, which is a transverse fracture distal to the peroneus brevis tendon insertion into the tubercle, is relatively uncommon in children, although it does occur in adolescents. Differentiating a Jones fracture from a proximal fifth metatarsal diaphyseal stress-type fracture can be challenging because the boundaries overlap and descriptions in the literature conflict [25]. Therefore, fifth metatarsal metadiaphyseal

Box 16.4: Metatarsal Fractures

First metatarsal
- Pediatric bunk bed fracture, common in young children
- Flexion force wedges oblique first cuneiform-first MT epiphysis into first MT-second MR interspace
- Salter-Harris type II or buckle fracture at metatarsal base
- Pathogenesis similar to adult-type Lisfranc injury to ligaments

Fifth metatarsal
- Fifth metatarsal tuberosity avulsion fracture: tubercle at the peroneus brevis tendon insertion
  - Most common metatarsal fracture in children >5 years old
  - Mechanism: ankle rotation with fixed forefoot
- Proximal fifth metatarsal diaphyseal fracture
  - Overuse stress injury in adolescent athletes
  - In vascular watershed, so heals poorly without screw fixation
  - Jones fracture is more proximal

fractures should be described including distance from the tubercle rather than labeling them as either a Jones fracture or diaphyseal stress-type fracture.

Even minimally displaced fifth metatarsal tubercle avulsion fractures respond well to casting, but comminution or displacement more than 2 mm usually mandates operative intervention. Unlike fifth metatarsal tuberosity avulsion fractures, proximal fifth metatarsal diaphyseal fractures heal poorly and are at risk for fracture-nonunion. This is because a vascular watershed zone is present at the level of the proximal fifth metatarsal diaphysis. Therefore, screw fixation is often recommended-especially if the fracture is displaced [25, 26].

Imaging

Frontal, lateral, and oblique foot radiographs with weight bearing are usually sufficient to evaluate metatarsal fractures, and advanced imaging is seldom necessary. Weight bearing in the frontal plane helps assess for Lisfranc injuries, since this stresses the Lisfranc joint and opens the joint space if the Lisfranc ligament complex is disrupted (Fig. 16.12). Non-weight-bearing views may spuriously show reduction of the Lisfranc joint and thus result in a false-negative study. The pediatric bunk bed fracture is usually a Salter-Harris type II fracture or buckle fracture at the base of the first metatarsal (Fig. 16.13).

The fifth metatarsal apophysis should not be confused with peroneus brevis tubercle avulsion fractures. The normal fifth metatarsal apophysis is longitudinally oriented with respect to the shaft and has well-formed ossicles (Fig. 16.14). Avulsion fractures of the fifth metatarsal tuberosity are usually transversely oriented (Fig. 16.15). These fractures should be distinguished from stress fractures, which, being diaphyseal, are more distal (Fig. 16.16).

1.4 Phalangeal Fractures

Phalangeal fractures usually result from a heavy object falling on the toes. Turf toe is a hyperextension injury at the level of the metatarsophalangeal joint that results in capsular injury and disruption of the plantar plate [27]. A Seymour fracture is a Salter-Harris-type fracture of the terminal phalanx, usually resulting from a plantar flexion injury at the level of the interphalangeal joint [28] (Box 16.5). These relatively benign appearing fractures are at high risk of developing osteomyelitis because the nail bed and physis are intimately associated. Along the dorsum of the terminal phalanx, the dermis attaches directly to the bony periosteum near the physis with no intervening subcutaneous tissue [28]. Therefore, any physeal injury of the terminal phalanx that also involves the nail bed is presumed to be an open fracture. Because Seymour fractures are considered open,

Box 16.5: Seymour Fracture

Physeal fracture of distal phalanx

Dermis of nail bed attaches to the periosteum near the physis

Considered open fracture until proven otherwise

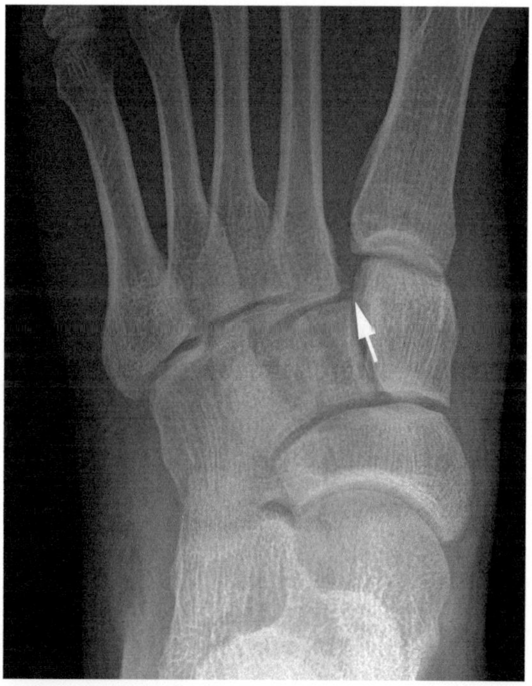

Fig. 16.12 Lisfranc avulsion fracture in a 16-year-old boy. Standing anteroposterior (AP) view shows punctate avulsion fragments (*arrow*) arising from the medial base of the second metatarsal bone and widening of the Lisfranc joint

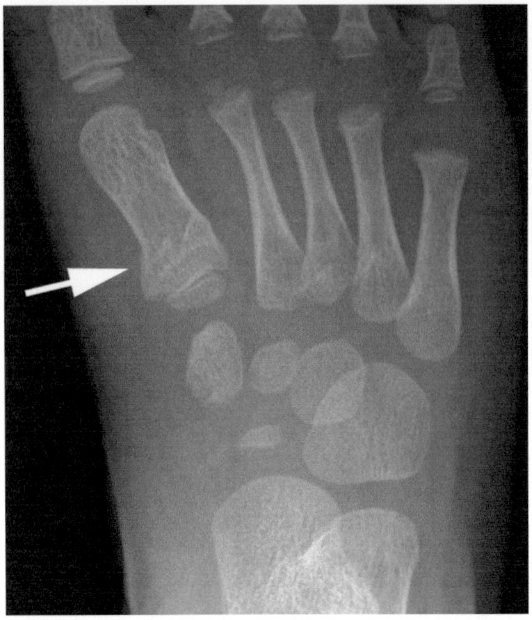

Fig. 16.13 Bunk bed fracture in a 3-year-old girl. There is a Salter-Harris II fracture (*arrow*) at the base of the first metatarsal

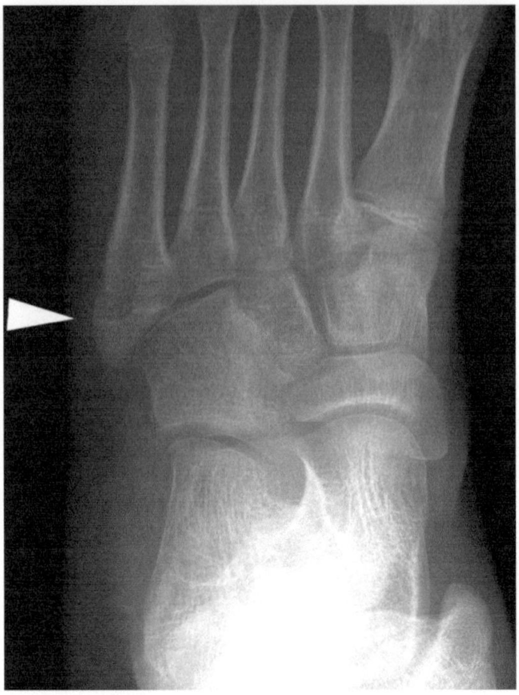

Fig. 16.15 Nondisplaced avulsion fracture of the fifth metatarsal tubercle in a 13-year-old boy. This transversely oriented lucency (*arrowhead*) extends to the articular surface

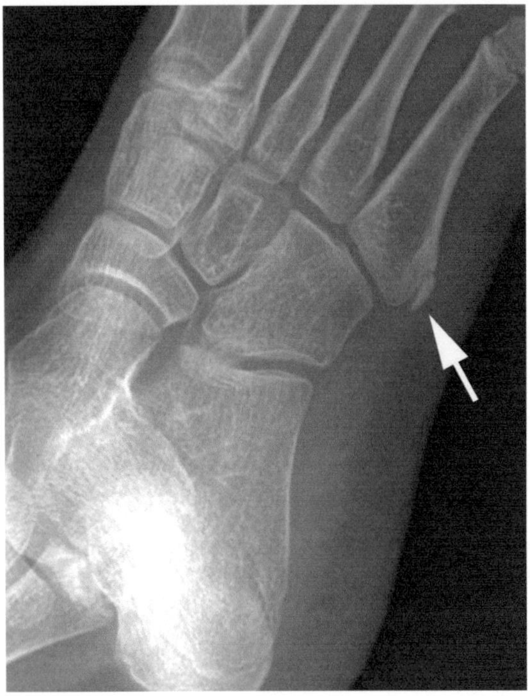

Fig. 16.14 Normal fifth metatarsal apophysis in an 11-year-old girl. Oblique view shows a normal longitudinally oriented apophysis (*arrow*)

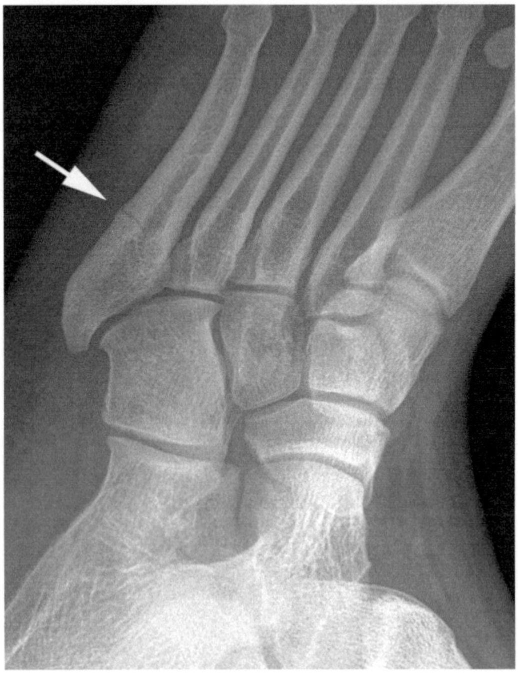

Fig. 16.16 Fifth metatarsal proximal diaphyseal stress fracture in a 17-year-old boy. Subtle lucency (*arrow*) is limited to the lateral one-third of the bone

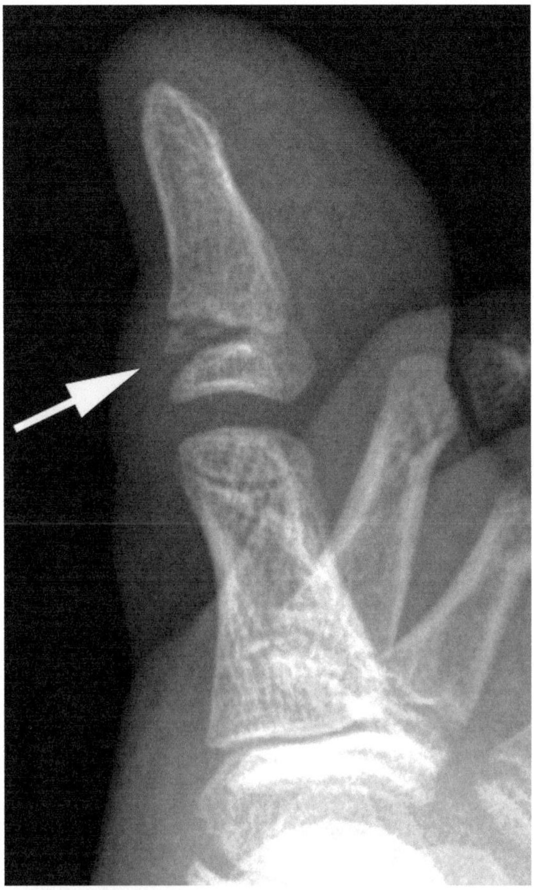

Fig. 16.17 Seymour fracture in a 9-year-old boy. Salter-Harris II fracture of the terminal phalanx of the great toe (*arrow*)

treatment includes immobilization and, particularly if there is skin or nail bed violation, antibiotic therapy and even irrigation and debridement to treat osteomyelitis [29]. Other phalangeal fractures are usually taped to the adjacent digit.

Imaging

Dedicated radiography of the affected toe in frontal, oblique, and lateral views minimizes radiation to the entire foot. A Salter-Harris type fracture of the terminal phalanx should suggest the diagnosis of a Seymour fracture, and the radiology report should indicate that the injury is considered to be an open fracture (Fig. 16.17). On follow-up radiography, if there are increased physeal widening and juxtaphyseal osteopenia, osteomyelitis should be suggested.

2 Osteochondritis Dissecans of the Talus (Box 16.6)

> **Box 16.6: Talar Osteochondritis Dissecans (OCD)**
>
> Frequency: anteromedial > posterolateral > mid-talar dome
>
> Radiographs: focal subchondral bone fragmentation, osteolysis, cyst formation, loose bodies
>
> MRI: unstable if
>
> - Fluid signal between OCD and parent bone
> - Subchondral bone plate disrupted
> - Junctional cysts
> - Loose bodies

Osteochondritis dissecans (OCD) is most common along the anteromedial talar dome, followed by the posterolateral and mid-talar dome. OCD of the talar head is very rare [30]. Lateral talar dome lesions are thought to be post-traumatic. It is controversial whether the etiology of medial lesions is developmental or traumatic [31]. Talar OCD is more common in boys than in girls.

Patients usually complain of pain and restricted tibiotalar movement; locking and instability are less common. There is usually no specific antecedent acute injury. Etiology is thought to be chronic repetitive microtrauma. Lateral OCDs may result from repetitive inversion and dorsiflexion with impingement at the tibiotalar joint; they are usually symptomatic. Because medial OCDs may be developmental, these lesions may be asymptomatic and discovered incidentally; they are more likely to be stable compared with lateral OCDs.

OCD of the talar dome may lead to deformity, probably as a result of trauma-related damage to the spherical growth plate and secondary growth disturbance [32]. (The spherical growth plate is responsible for primary ossification of the epiphyses and short bones of the hands and feet (see Chap. 2).) Post-traumatic ischemia to subchondral bone may also lead to deformity in the setting of OCD [31].

Treatment

Stable lesions are usually treated nonoperatively, whereas unstable lesions require operative fixation.

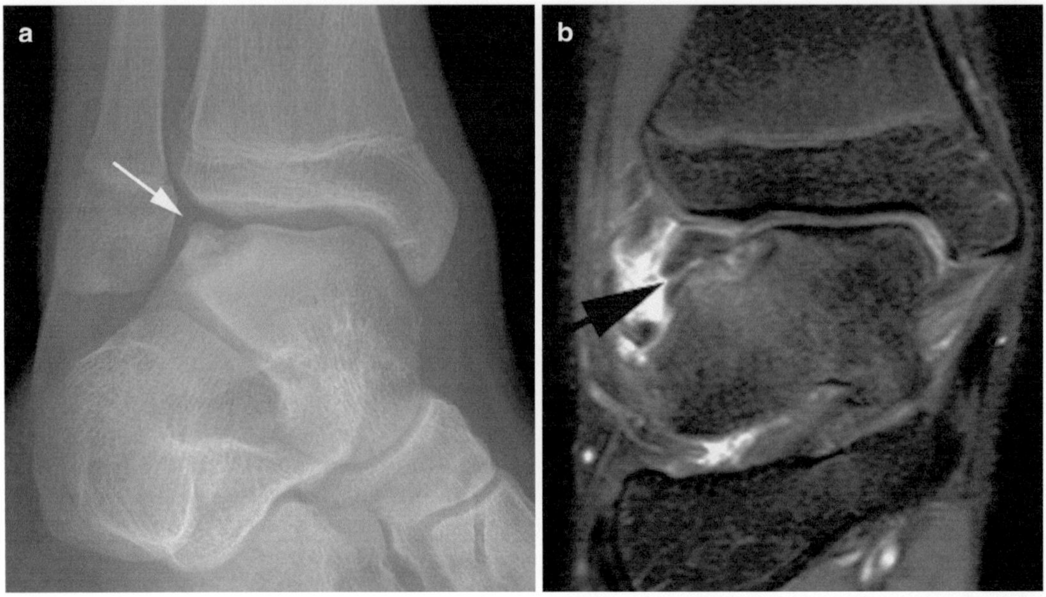

Fig. 16.18 Unstable lateral talar dome osteochondritis dissecans (OCD) fragment in a 15-year-old boy. (**a**) Oblique radiograph shows a subchondral fragment (*arrow*). (**b**) Coronal T2-weighted (T2-W) fat-suppressed (FS) image shows extensive marrow edema, discongruity of the articular joint surface, and subtle fluid insinuating (*arrow*) between the OCD lesion and parent bone

In addition, some authors advocate operative intervention if there is persistent pain after 6 months of conservative treatment [33]. The threshold to treat lateral lesions is usually lower compared with medial lesions, since medial lesions have a propensity to heal spontaneously. Patient age also influences the decision to treat, since younger children with OCD tend to heal spontaneously, whereas adolescents, like adults, often require operative stabilization. The open spherical growth plate in the skeletally immature child may facilitate more rapid remodeling and healing.

Surgical treatment includes debridement, internal fixation of the fragment, excision and curettage, drilling, microfracture, cancellous bone grafting, osteochondral transplantation, and autologous chondrocyte transplantation [34].

Imaging

Radiography is useful for screening for OCD. Radiographic features include focal subchondral bone fragmentation (Fig. 16.18) and/or osteolysis (Fig. 16.19), cyst formation, loose bodies, and (rarely) secondary osteoarthritis with tibiotalar joint space loss. It is important to comment on the size of the OCD and whether the lesion is in situ or displaced.

MRI is the optimal study to evaluate OCD because it can help determine if lesions are stable or unstable. A talar dome OCD fragment is considered unstable if fluid signal insinuates between the OCD and parent bone, if the subchondral bone plate is disrupted, if there are junctional cysts, or if loose bodies are present (see Figs. 16.18 and 16.19) [35]. However, balancing sensitivity and specificity can be difficult with this diagnosis, and, depending on how these criteria are applied, the correlation between MRI and arthroscopy may be as low as 30 %. In the pediatric age group, if only one criterion for instability is applied, most lesions will be overcalled, with a specificity of only 15 % (although the sensitivity will be 100 %). If two criteria are applied, diagnosis will be much more specific (about 90 %), but instability will be missed half the time [36]. Overcalling high-signal fluid between the fragment and parent bone may contribute to low specificity.

Both the fragment and the parent bone may demonstrate marrow edema, although this does not necessarily correlate with symptoms. Indeed, marrow edema often persists for months although the child is symptom-free.

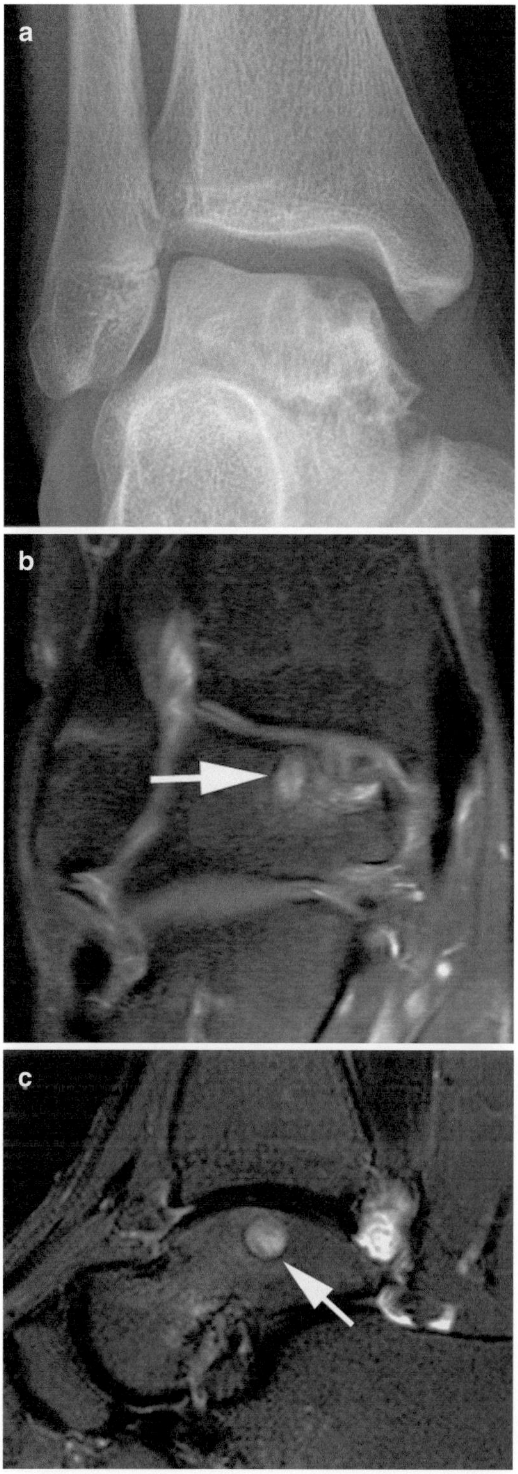

Fig. 16.19 Unstable medial talar dome OCD lesion in a 12-year-old girl. (**a**) Oblique radiograph shows subchondral osteolysis. Coronal proton density (PD) FS (**b**) and sagittal T2-W FS (**c**) images show junctional cyst formation (*arrows*) as well as perilesional marrow edema

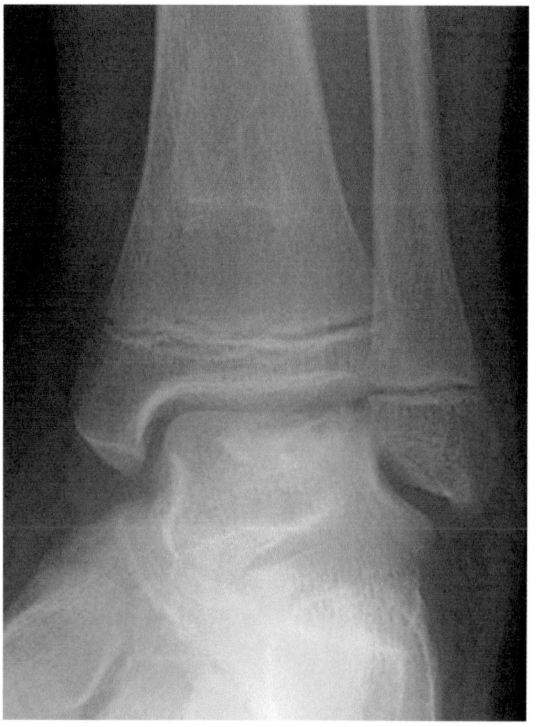

Fig. 16.20 Talar subchondral osteonecrosis in a 15-year-old boy who had received chemotherapy for lymphoma. There are patchy sclerosis and lucency in the subchondral region of the lateral talar dome. Also note tibial metadiaphyseal bone infarct

Magnetic resonance arthrography (MRA) is rarely necessary. However, if there is question of instability, it may contribute additional information, since insinuation of intra-articular gadolinium between the OCD fragment and the parent bone indicates instability. CT provides superior delineation of OCD bone fragments and complements MRI findings, but is not routinely performed in the initial workup and preoperative evaluation of OCD.

Differential diagnosis

Subchondral osteonecrosis and acute osteochondral fractures may mimic OCD. However, the principal abnormality in talar subchondral osteonecrosis involves the marrow rather than the spherical growth plate, and although chondral injury may eventually develop, this results from subchondral bone collapse. Furthermore, lesions of subchondral osteonecrosis tend to be larger and occur in at-risk patients (Fig. 16.20). Acute osteochondral fractures have well-defined sharp margins and usually appear as flecks of bone, whereas OCD fragments, being chronic, have undergone remodeling and therefore have a round or ovoid configuration. In addition, the articular surface of OCD is usually partly reconstituted.

3 Osteochondroses of the Foot

Osteochondroses are a group of poorly defined conditions that probably result from repetitive microtrauma and/or ischemia in the skeletally immature patient [37]. Three osteochondroses occur in the feet: Freiberg infraction (second or third metatarsal head), Kohler disease (navicular), and Sever disease (calcaneal apophyses).

Freiberg infraction usually presents in adolescent female dancers who complain of pain during activity, tenderness to palpation over the affected metatarsal, and swelling. The disorder is bilateral in less than 10 % of patients. Kohler disease is most common in boys, especially between ages 3 and 10 [38]; about 25 % of patients have bilateral involvement. An antecedent history of trauma is rare. The most common presentation is midfoot pain and limping with point tenderness over the navicular. Sever disease occurs in children and adolescents during athletic activity and manifests as focal tenderness over the calcaneal apophysis.

Freiberg infraction, Kohler disease, and Sever disease all respond favorably to conservative management, including activity restriction, foot padding, and shoe modification [37].

Imaging

The diagnosis of Freiberg infraction and Kohler disease is based on both clinical and imaging findings. Radiographic findings of Freiberg infraction (Box 16.7) include sclerosis, fragmentation, and asphericity of either the second or third metatarsal head (Fig. 16.21). MRI may show marrow edema, metatarsophalangeal (MTP) joint effusion, and juxtacortical soft tissue edema. Depending on the extent of osteonecrosis, there may be focal hypointensity in the metatarsal head on both T1-weighted (T1-W) and T2-weighted (T2-W) sequences [38].

Box 16.7: Freiberg Infraction (Second or Third Metatarsal Head)

Adolescent female dancers, bilateral in <10 %

Radiographs: sclerosis, fragmentation, asphericity of second or third metatarsal head

MRI	Marrow edema, MTP joint effusion, juxtacortical soft tissue edema
	T1 and T2 focal hypointensity in the metatarsal head if osteonecrosis is extensive

Kohler disease appears as sclerosis, fragmentation, and diminished height and width of the navicular (Box 16.8). Since the navicular may demonstrate similar findings in the course of normal development, comparison with the asymptomatic foot and/or previous radiographs may be helpful (Fig. 16.22). MRI features include

Box 16.8: Kohler Disease (Navicular)

Boys 3–10 years old, bilateral in 25 %

Rarely history of trauma

Radiographs	Sclerosis, fragmentation, diminished height/width of navicular
	Comparison with asymptomatic foot and/or previous radiographs may help
	Similar appearance to normal ossification variant
MRI	Marrow edema, midfoot joint effusions, soft tissue edema near navicular

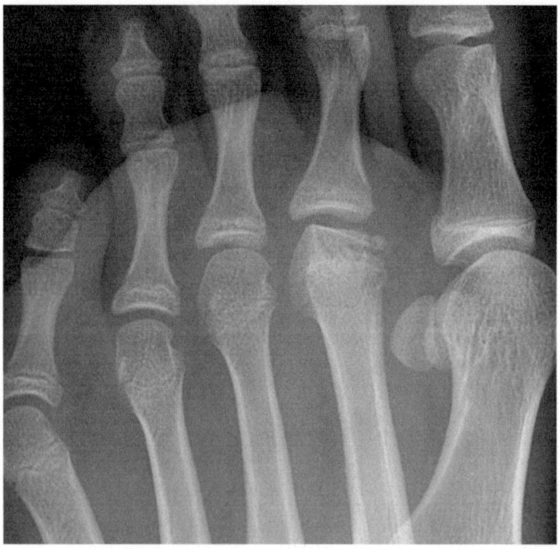

Fig. 16.21 Freiberg infraction in an 11-year-old girl. There are flattening, sclerosis, and resultant asphericity of the second metatarsal head

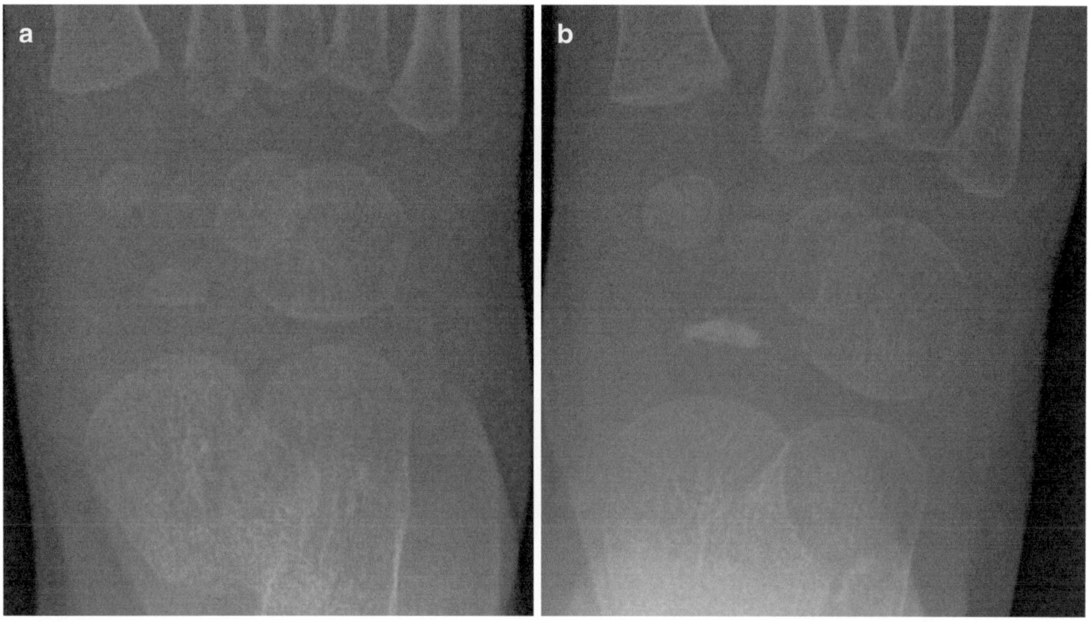

Fig. 16.22 Kohler disease in a 2-year-old boy. (**a**) Normal forefoot obtained 9 months earlier shows a normal navicular ossification center. (**b**) Nine months later, the navicular is flat and sclerotic

marrow edema, midfoot joint effusions, and soft tissue edema about the navicular.

The diagnosis of Sever disease is purely clinical. Historically, Sever disease was radiographically defined as sclerosis and fragmentation of the calcaneal apophyses, but this is now understood to be a normal developmental phenomenon [39]. However, radiographs are useful to exclude alternative etiologies for focal pain over the calcaneal tuberosity. In one study, 5.1 % of radiographs obtained in children with focal pain over the calcaneal tuberosity demonstrated an abnormality that affected treatment, such as unicameral bone cysts and calcaneal stress fractures [40].

Box 16.9: Ankle Impingement

Proliferation of soft tissues (hypertrophied synovium) or bone (bone spurs, bone protrusion, ossicle)

Symptoms must correlate with imaging findings

Anterior: talar neck and tibial plafond bone spurs

MRI	Marrow edema helps identify symptomatic spurs
	Synovial hypertrophy, capsular thickening, ganglion cysts

Posterior: prominent posterolateral process, os trigonum

Os trigonum common in children 8–13 years old

MRI	Marrow edema near prominent posterolateral process or os trigonum
	Cystic degeneration at os trigonum and talus, soft tissue edema

4 Ankle Impingement Disorders (Box 16.9)

Ankle impingement can be either anterior or posterior. Anterior impingement may be caused by mechanical inhibition of end-range motion related to abnormal proliferation of either soft tissues (usually hypertrophied synovium) or bone (bone spurs and bone protrusion) [41]. Anterior impingement is associated with a history of ankle sprains in some patients and may be due to proliferation of the anterior-inferior tibiofibular ligament. Posterior ankle impingement is caused by an os trigonum, which may become symptomatic in athletes who frequently plantarflex their ankles. The diagnosis of both types of impingement is based on clinical symptomatology, since many patients have the same anatomical deformities seen with ankle impingement but are asymptomatic. Therefore, when imaging features of ankle impingement are present, the diagnosis should be suggested only if symptoms correlate.

Patients with ankle impingement complain of pain or restricted motion at end-range movement of the joint. Impingement disorders may result from repetitive supraphysiologic ankle dorsiflexion or plantar flexion; this may therefore be seen in ballet dancers. Ankle impingement may also result from bone remodeling or synovial reaction after an acute traumatic event or repetitive direct microtrauma.

Patients are usually treated conservatively, with rest and nonsteroidal anti-inflammatory drugs [23]. For symptomatic anterior impingement, arthroscopic resection of bone spur(s) and debridement of hypertrophic soft tissues may be performed. For posterior impingement, resection of osseous protrusion or a symptomatic os trigonum accessory ossicle may be performed.

Imaging

Radiographic findings of anterior impingement include talar neck and tibial plafond bone spurs (Fig. 16.23). However, MRI best identifies symptomatic spurs by demonstrating associated marrow edema. It also helps define soft tissue causes for ankle impingement, such as synovial hypertrophy, capsular thickening, and ganglion cyst formation. Meniscoid fibrous tissue in the anterolateral gutter may contribute to anterolateral impingement as well (the anterolateral gutter is defined by the tibia posteromedially, fibula posterolaterally, and the anterior talofibular ligament anterolaterally). In order to diagnose anterior impingement, it is essential that MRI findings are correlated with clinical manifestations, as MRI findings alone have a sensitivity and specificity of only 39 and 50 %, respectively [42].

With posterior impingement, radiographs may demonstrate a prominent posterolateral process. This is defined as bone that extends abnormally from the talus, beyond the posterior talar dome arc. An os trigonum may also cause posterior impingement. The os trigonum is a normal secondary ossification center of the posterior aspect of the talus, which appears between ages 8 and 13 and fuses to the talus within 1 year of initial ossification [41]. In 7 % of the population, this secondary ossification center fails to fuse.

MRI features of posterior impingement include marrow edema related to the prominent posterolateral process of the talus or the os trigonum (Fig. 16.24). Cystic degeneration at the os trigonum and talus may be seen, as well as adjacent soft tissue edema. Additional imaging features of posterior impingement include ganglion cyst formation, synovial thickening, posterior talofibular ligament tears, and flexor hallucis longus tenosynovitis. Because the flexor hallucis

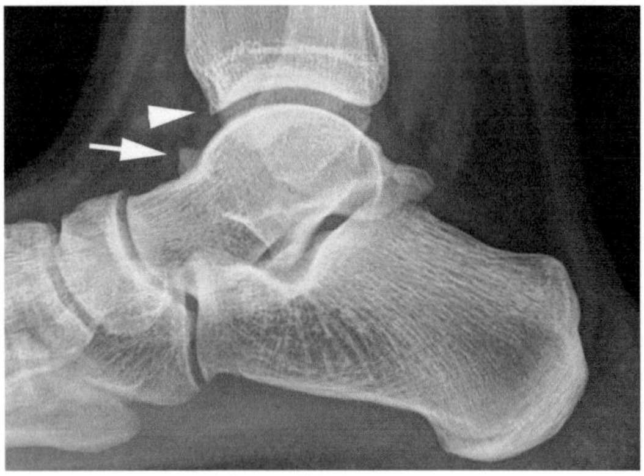

Fig. 16.23 Anterior impingement in a 15-year-old girl. There are spurs at the talar neck (*arrow*) and anterior tibial plafond (*arrowhead*)

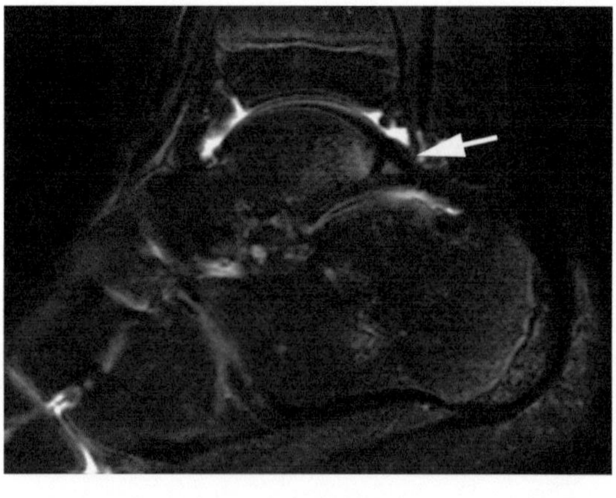

Fig. 16.24 Posterior impingement in an 8-year-old girl. Sagittal short tau inversion recovery (STIR) image shows edema of the os trigonum (*arrow*) and adjacent posterior process of the talus

longus tendon communicates with the tibiotalar joint in approximately 20 % of patients, fluid surrounding the tendon should not be the sole determinant of tenosynovitis [43]. Additional features such as tendon thickening or longitudinal tears should be present to diagnose flexor hallucis longus tendon pathology.

Differential Diagnosis

Talar neck spurs associated with anterior impingement should not be confused with talar beaking that occurs with calcaneonavicular coalitions. Talar beaking occurs at the dorsal aspect of the talar head, not the neck. An os trigonum is usually a normal finding, present in many children between 8 and 13 years of age. As a general rule, it should be mentioned in the radiography report only in the context of symptoms related to posterior impingement.

References

1. Ecklund K. Magnetic resonance imaging of pediatric musculoskeletal trauma. Top Magn Reson Imaging. 2002;13(4):203–17.
2. Ecklund K, Jaramillo D. Patterns of premature physeal arrest: MR imaging of 111 children. AJR Am J Roentgenol. 2002;178:967–72.
3. Chung T, Jaramillo. Normal maturing distal tibia and fibula: changes with age at MR imaging. Radiology. 1995;194:227–32.
4. Crawford AH. Triplane and Tillaux fractures: is a 2 mm residual gap acceptable? J Pediatr Orthop. 2012;32:S69–73.
5. Schnetzler KA, Hoernschemeyer D. The pediatric triplane ankle fracture. J Am Acad Orthop Surg. 2007; 15(12):738–47.
6. Horn BD, Crisci K, Krug M, Pizutillo PD, MacEwen GD. Radiologic evaluation of juvenile Tillaux fractures of the distal tibia. J Pediatr Orthop. 2001;21:162–4.
7. Podeszwa DA, Mubarak SJ. Physeal fractures of the distal tibia and fibula (Salter-Harris Type 1, II, III, and IV fractures). J Pediatr Orthop. 2012;32:S62–8.
8. Stevens MA, El-Khoury GY, Kathol MH, Brandser EA, Chow S. Imaging features of avulsion injuries. Radiographics. 1999;19:655–72.
9. Wuerz TH, Gurd DP. Pediatric physeal ankle fracture. J Am Acad Orthop Surg. 2013;21:234–44.
10. Dowling S, Spooner CH, Liang Y, Dryden DM, Friesen C, Klassen TP, Wright RB. Accuracy of Ottawa ankle rules to exclude fractures of the ankle and midfoot in children: a meta-analysis. Acad Emerg Med. 2009;16:277–87.
11. Brown SD, Kasser JR, Zurakowski D, Jaramillo D. Analysis of 51 tibial triplane fractures using CT with multiplanar reconstruction. AJR Am J Roentgenol. 2004;183:1489–95.
12. John SD, Moorthy CS, Swischuk LE. Expanding the concept of the Toddler's fracture. Radiographics. 1997;17:367–76.
13. Ribbans WJ, Natarajan R, Alavala S. Pediatric foot fractures. Clin Orthop Relat Res. 2005;432:107–15.
14. Eberl R, Singer G, Schalamon J, Hausbrandt P, Hoellwarth ME. Fractures of the talus- differences between children and adolescents. J Trauma. 2010; 68(1):126–30.
15. Smith JT, Curtis TA, Spencer S, Kasser JR, Mahan ST. Complications of talus fractures in children. J Pediatr Orthop. 2010;30(8):779–84.
16. Laing TA, O'Sullivan JB, Nugent N, O'Shaughnessy M, O'Sullivan ST. Paediatric ride-on mower related injuries and plastic surgical management. J Plast Reconstr Aesthet Surg. 2011;64(5):638–42.
17. Oestreich AE, Bhojwani N. Stress fractures of ankle and wrist in childhood: nature and frequency. Pediatr Radiol. 2010;40(8):1387–9.
18. Davis KW. Imaging pediatric sports injuries: lower extremity. Radiol Clin North Am. 2010;48: 1213–35.
19. Leonard ZC, Fortin PT. Adolescent accessory navicular. Foot Ankle Clin. 2010;15(2):337–47.
20. Pearce DH, Mongiardi CN, Fornasier VL, Daniels TR. Avascular necrosis of the talus: a pictorial essay. Radiographics. 2005;25(2):399–410.
21. Donnelly EF. The Hawkins sign. Radiology. 1999; 210:195–6.
22. Miller TT, Staron RB, Feldman F, Parisien M, Glucksman WJ, Gandolfo LH. The symptomatic accessory tarsal navicular bone: assessment with MR imaging. Radiology. 1995;195:849–53.
23. Chambers HG. Ankle and foot disorders in skeletally immature athletes. Orthop Clin North Am. 2003;34: 445–59.
24. Johnson GF. Pediatric Lisfranc injury: "bunk bed" fracture. AJR Am J Roentgenol. 1981;137:1041–4.
25. Zwitser EW, Breederveld RS. Fractures of the fifth metatarsal; diagnosis and treatment. Injury. 2010;41: 555–62.
26. Polzer H, Polzer S, Mutschler W, Prall WC. Acute fractures to the proximal fifth metatarsal bone: developing of classification and treatment recommendations based on current evidence. Injury. 2012; 43:1626–32.
27. Tewes DP, Fischer DA, Fritts HM, Guanche CA. MRI findings of acute turf toe. A case report and review of anatomy. Clin Orthop Relat Res. 1994;304:200–3.
28. Pinckney LE, Currarino G, Kennedy LA. The stubbed great toe: a cause of occult compound fracture and infection. Radiology. 1981;138:375–7.
29. Kensinger DR, Guille JT, Horn BD, Herman MJ. The stubbed great toe: importance of early recognition and treatment of open fractures of the distal phalanx. J Pediatr Orthop. 2001;21:31–4.

30. Thacker MM, Dabney KW, MacKenzie WG. Osteochondritis dissecans of the talar head: natural history and review of the literature. J Pediatr Orthop B. 2012;21(4):373–6.
31. Letts M, Davidson D, Ahmer A. Osteochondritis dissecans of the talus in children. J Pediatr Orthop. 2003; 23:617–25.
32. Laor T, Zbojniewicz, Eismann EA, Wall EJ. Juvenile osteochondritis dissecans: is it a growth disturbance of the secondary physis of the epiphysis? AJR Am J Roentgenol. 2012;199(5):1121–8.
33. Perumal V, Wall E, Babekir N. Juvenile osteochondritis dissecans of the talus. J Pediatr Orthop. 2007;27(7): 821–5.
34. Zwingmann J, Sudkamp NP, Schmal H, Niemeyer P. Surgical treatment of osteochondritis dissecans of the talus: a systematic review. Arch Orthop Trauma Surg. 2012;132:1241–50.
35. De Smet AA, Fisher DR, Burnstein MI, Graf BK, Lange RH. Value of MR imaging in staging osteochondral lesions of the talus (osteochondritis dissecans): results in 14 patients. AJR Am J Roentgenol. 1990;154(3):555–8.
36. Heywood CS, Benke MT, Brindle K, Fine KM. Correlation of magnetic resonance imaging to arthroscopic findings of stability in juvenile osteochondritis dissecans. Arthroscopy. 2011;27(2):194–9.
37. Atanda A, Shah SA, O'brien K. Osteochondrosis: common causes of pain in growing bones. Am Fam Physician. 2011;83(3):285–91.
38. Patel CV. The foot and ankle: MR imaging of uniquely pediatric disorders. Magn Reson Imaging Clin N Am. 2009;17:539–47.
39. Volpon JB, de FilhoCarvalho G. Calcaneal apophysitis: a quantitative radiographic evaluation of the secondary ossification center. Arch Orthop Trauma Surg. 2002;122:338–41.
40. Rachel JN, Williams JB, Sawyer JR, Warner WC, Kelly DM. Is radiographic evaluation necessary in children with a clinical diagnosis of calcaneal apophysitis (Sever disease)? J Pediatr Orthop. 2011;31: 548–50.
41. Dimmick S, Linklater J. Ankle impingement syndromes. Radiol Clin N Am. 2013;51:479–510.
42. Liu SH, Nuccion SL, Finerman G. Diagnosis of anterolateral ankle impingement comparison between magnetic resonance imaging and clinical exam. Am J Sports Med. 1997;25(3):394–401.
43. Na J, Bergman AG, Oloff LM, Beaulieu CF. The flexor hallucis longus: tenographic technique correlation of imaging findings with surgery in 39 ankles. Radiology. 2005;236:974–82.

Part III

Generalized and Systemic Diseases

Skeletal Trauma: General and Unique Considerations in Children

17

Marilyn Ranson

Contents

M. Ranson, BSc, MD, FRCPC
Radiology Department,
The Hospital for Sick Children,
University of Toronto,
555 University Avenue,
Toronto, ON M5G 1X8, Canada
e-mail: marilyn.ranson@sickkids.ca

Abstract

This chapter presents common and unusual pediatric fracture patterns and mechanisms of injury. A detailed discussion of growth cartilage injury follows a brief presentation on cartilage development, reviewing the Salter-Harris classification and the Ogden extended classification. Other unique pediatric injuries including apophyseal avulsion fractures and pediatric stress fractures are also discussed. Pediatric fracture healing and remodeling and potential complications are presented. Finally, there is a brief discussion of pediatric articular trauma.

The dynamic state of the developing skeleton makes children susceptible to unique mechanisms of injury, resulting in specific fracture patterns. Pediatric fractures may result from acute or chronic/repetitive trauma; typical mechanisms of injury include a fall, motor vehicle collision, or sporting injury. The type of fracture that occurs depends on the child's age. Fractures in infants are often diaphyseal, whereas older children commonly sustain fractures involving the metaphysis or metadiaphysis (Fig. 17.1) [1]. Since pediatric bone is relatively elastic, several fractures—such as greenstick, buckle, and bowing injuries—are essentially limited to children. Growth plate fractures represent up to 25 % of all pediatric fractures, and additional growth cartilage injuries include osteochondral and apophyseal fractures [2, 3].

R. Stein-Wexler et al. (eds.), *Pediatric Orthopedic Imaging*,
DOI 10.1007/978-3-642-45381-6_17, © Springer-Verlag Berlin Heidelberg 2015

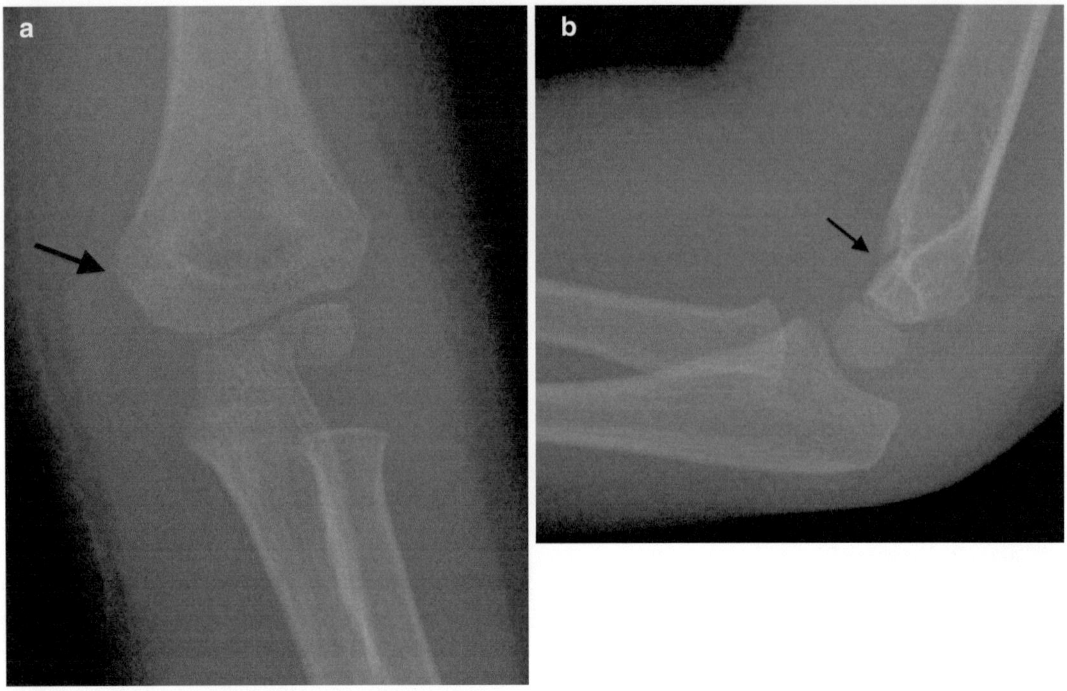

Fig. 17.1 Supracondylar fracture involving the metaphysis of the distal humerus. (**a**, **b**) This is the most common fracture (*arrows*) in the pediatric elbow. Note joint effusion

1 Pediatric Fracture Patterns and Mechanisms of Injury

The pediatric bone is mainly composed of woven bone, which has less mechanical strength than mature trabeculated adult bone [4]. The woven bone is highly cellular and porous and contains a large amount of collagen. This results in decreased tensile and compressive strength and predisposes children to fractures rather than ligament injuries [3].

Buckle (torus) fractures result from compressive forces and constitute one of the most common pediatric fractures. They consist of cortical buckling, typically at the metadiaphysis, usually extending only partway around the bone circumference. Buckle fractures most frequently occur in the distal radius, typically after a fall on an outstretched hand. Displacement and angulation are usually minimal (Fig. 17.2) [4]. These stable fractures require only symptomatic treatment with a splint [5]. Greenstick fractures occur when a bone bends before beginning to break, and the fracture does not extend through the entire bone [6]. The cortical break is seen on the convex or tension side, and the fracture line propagates vertically within the medulla without breaking the cortex on the concave or compression side. Greenstick fractures most commonly involve the diaphysis of the radius or ulna, and radiographs typically show an incomplete fracture with angulation deformity (Fig. 17.3). Bowing injury is a plastic deformation, with the bone bent just short of the fracture or failure point [4, 7]. This may result from low-energy bending forces, and the adjacent bone often fractures [5]. Bowing injury most frequently occurs in the ulnar diaphysis and sometimes in the radial or fibular diaphysis. Radiographs show excessive bowing without cortical disruption (Fig. 17.4) [4, 6].

Abundant growth cartilage in the physes, epiphyses, and apophyses makes these areas vulnerable to specific injuries. The physis, the major contributor to longitudinal bone growth, is usually injured due to a shearing or avulsive force (Fig. 17.5). The epiphysis, responsible for spherical

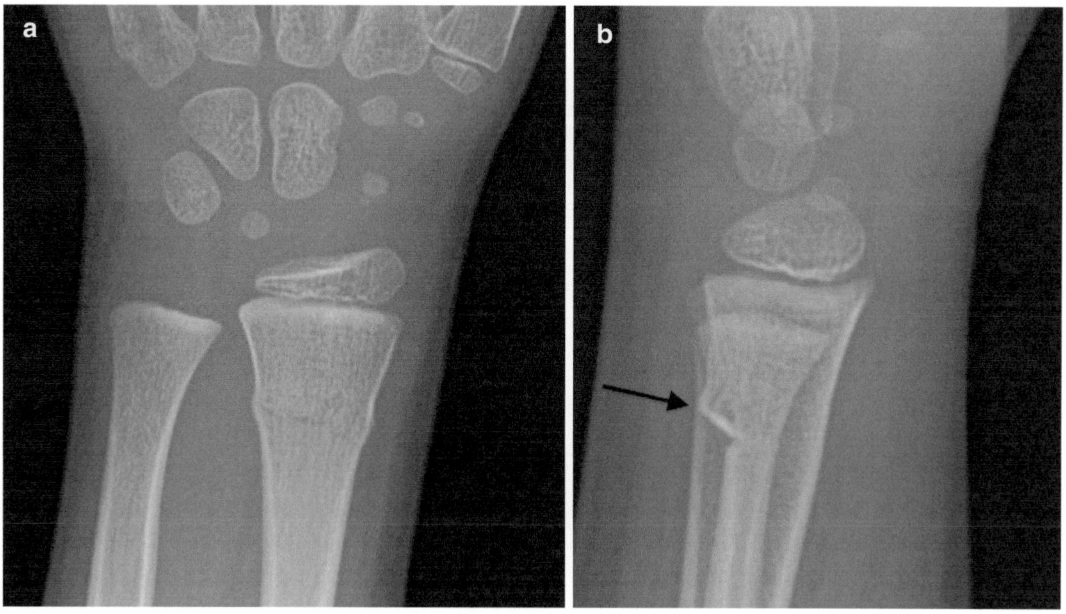

Fig. 17.2 Buckle fracture (*arrow*) of the distal radial metadiaphysis (**a**, **b**)

growth at the ends of the long bones, is primarily subject to compressive forces, which may cause osteochondral injuries (Fig. 17.6). The apophyses, secondary ossification centers at the attachment sites of major tendons, contribute to bone shape and may be injured by tensile forces (Fig. 17.7) [4]. The incidence of growth cartilage injury is highest during periods of maximal growth, such as the pubertal growth spurt. This may be because mineralization lags behind linear growth in rapidly growing bone, resulting in a thicker and more fragile physis. In addition, the increased rate of longitudinal bone growth may cause a temporary disparity with muscle-tendon elongation, resulting in decreased flexibility and increased susceptibility to growth cartilage injury [4].

2 Imaging of Pediatric Fractures

Orthogonal radiographs are usually sufficient to diagnose pediatric fractures. Oblique views may provide further information about subtle fractures, particularly at the elbow, knee, and ankle. For example, internal oblique and external oblique views of the pediatric elbow are essential for accurate diagnosis of lateral condyle and medial condyle or epicondyle fractures. Tunnel views of the knee are important for imaging osteochondral fractures of the condyles, and mortise views of the ankle assist in characterizing the extent of ligamentous injury in ankle fractures. Axillary views of the shoulder are essential for evaluating glenohumeral dislocation.

Cross-sectional imaging is sometimes indicated to evaluate equivocal fractures and growth cartilage injuries or to distinguish trauma from other pathology such as infection or tumor. Ultrasound (US) is currently underutilized but can delineate cartilaginous structures and further assess osseous and physeal fractures. It is particularly helpful in evaluating radiographically occult epiphyseal avulsion fractures in infants. Sonographic findings include cortical discontinuity and growth plate widening; subperiosteal fluid or hematoma may be evident as well (Fig. 17.8) [8].

The high-resolution cortical detail of computed tomography (CT) makes this modality excellent for delineating and confirming subtle fractures [6]. However, CT is most often used for presurgical assessment of complex intra-articular

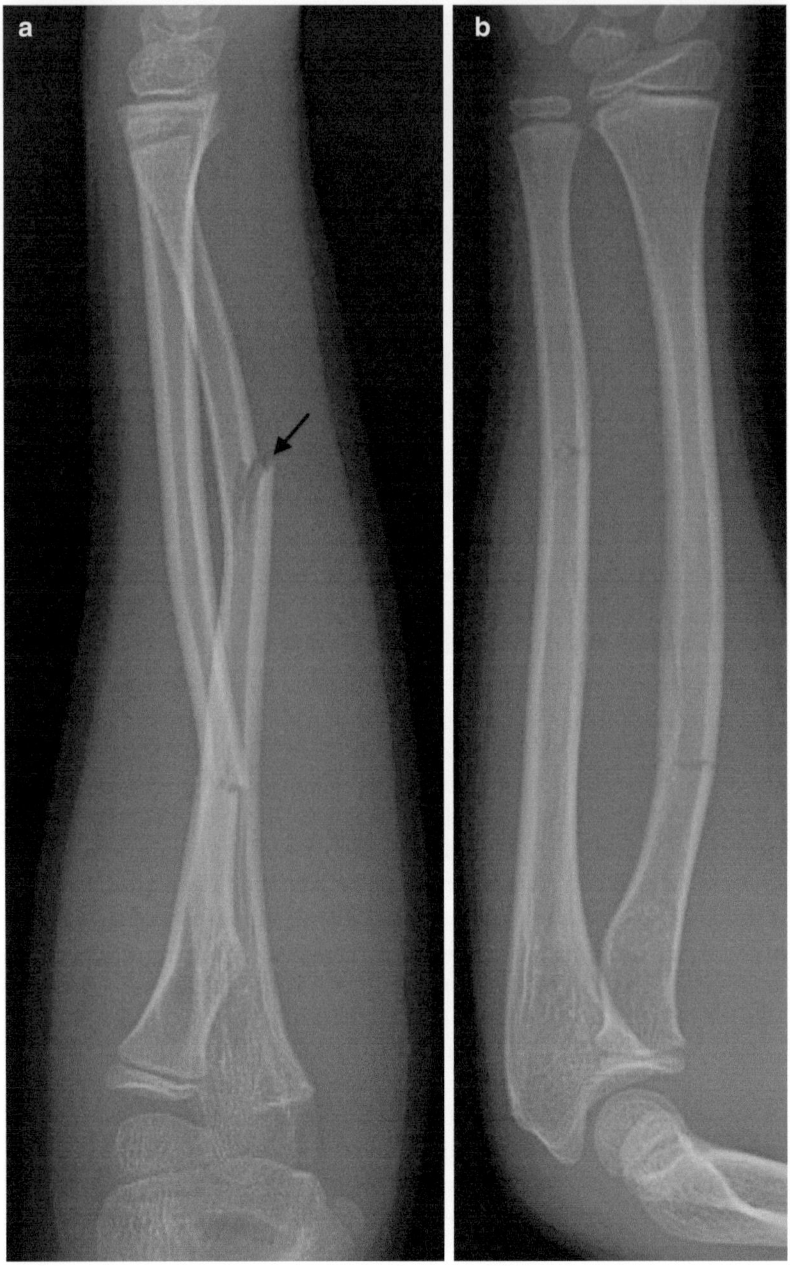

Fig. 17.3 Greenstick fracture of the ulnar diaphysis with vertical extension in the medullary space (*arrow*). There is also an incomplete transverse fracture of the radial shaft (**a**, **b**)

and growth plate fractures. CT can be performed in a cast with a single acquisition. The isotropic volume data of 64-detector technology can then be manipulated into multiplanar high-resolution two-dimensional (2D) and three-dimensional (3D) images (Fig. 17.9). Rapid acquisition speed nearly eliminates motion artifact, greatly decreasing the need for sedation [9].

Magnetic resonance imaging (MRI) depicts occult osseous fractures, which are usually hypointense on T1-weighted (T1-W) images and hyperintense on fluid-sensitive sequences, including T2-weighted (T2-W) and short tau inversion recovery (STIR) (Fig. 17.10). MRI is particularly useful for assessing epiphyseal and physeal injuries, due to its multiplanar capability and superb soft tissue con-

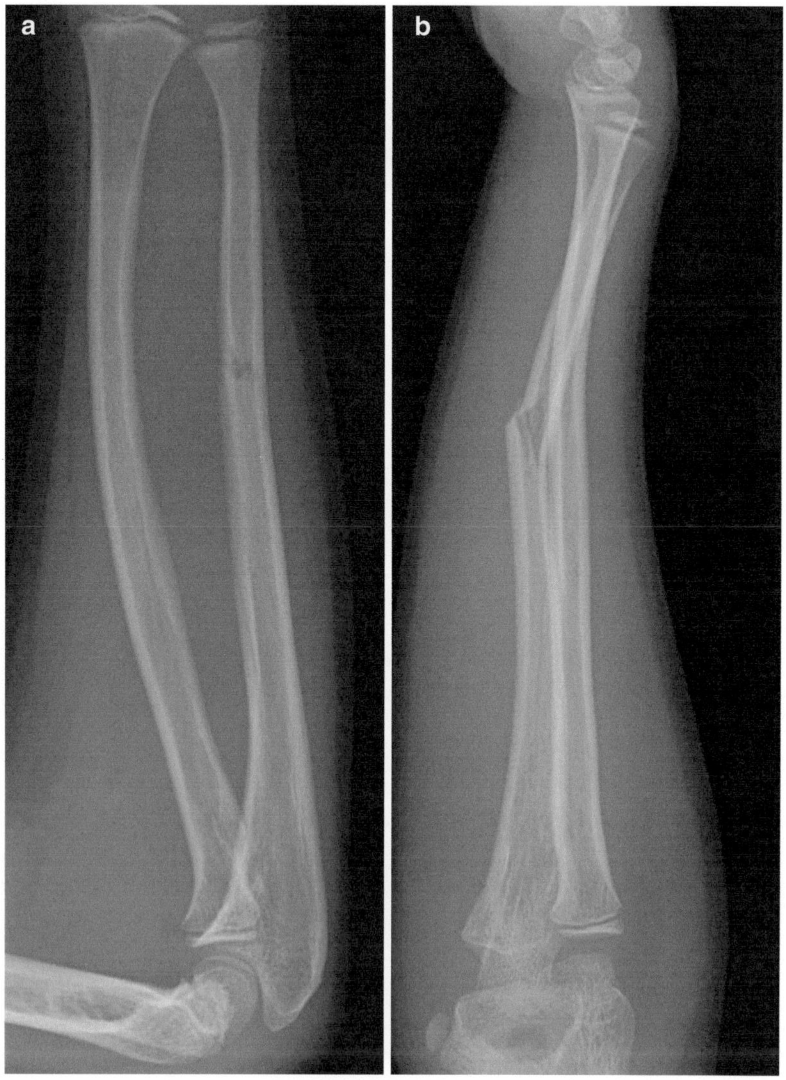

Fig. 17.4 Bowing injury of the radius and greenstick fracture of the ulnar diaphysis (**a**, **b**)

trast [10]. MRI findings that suggest growth plate fracture include increased physeal thickness and T2 hyperintensity as well as disruption of the perichondrium. Gas within a physeal fracture cleft may be visible as a hypointensity, contrasted with the hyperintense physis on water-sensitive and multiplanar gradient echo (MPGR) images [6]. Fluid within a fracture cleft is hyperintense on water-sensitive sequences; it may be obscured, since the growth plate is also hyperintense. However, on gadolinium-enhanced 3D spoiled gradient-recalled echo (SPGR) images, growth plate fracture clefts that contain fluid are hypointense, compared to the enhancing physeal cartilage [11].

3 Normal Development and Imaging of Growth Cartilage

Knowledge of bone growth facilitates understanding and imaging interpretation of fractures and other osseous injuries. However, growth plate architecture and cartilage imaging are addressed only briefly here, as they are discussed in depth in Chap. 2.

Of the four distinct zones of the growth plate, the zone of provisional calcification (ZPC) is most vulnerable to trauma. This zone, adjacent to the metaphysis and the site of mineralization

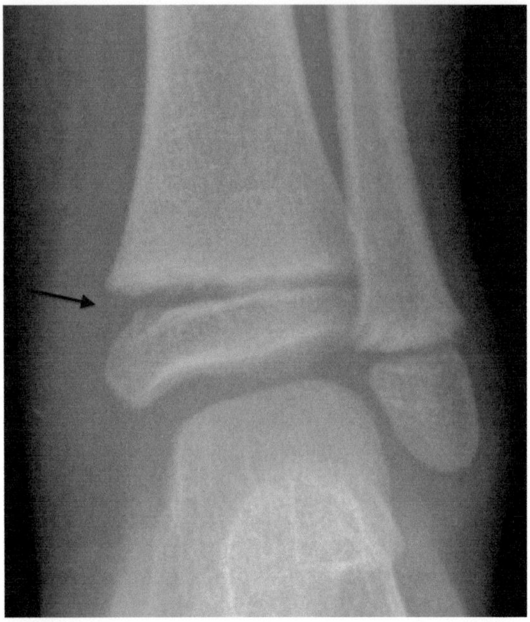

Fig. 17.5 Type I fracture of the distal tibial growth plate with widening of the physis (*arrow*) and adjacent soft tissue swelling

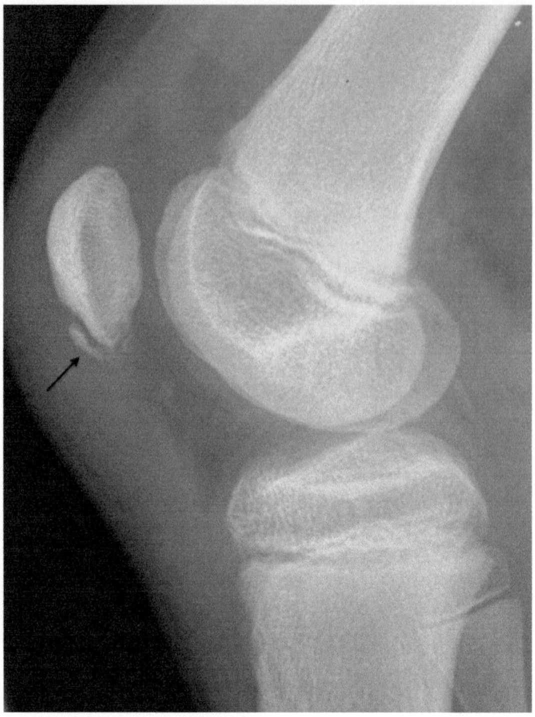

Fig. 17.7 Acute avulsion fracture of the inferior pole of the patella (*arrow*) at the origin of the patellar tendon

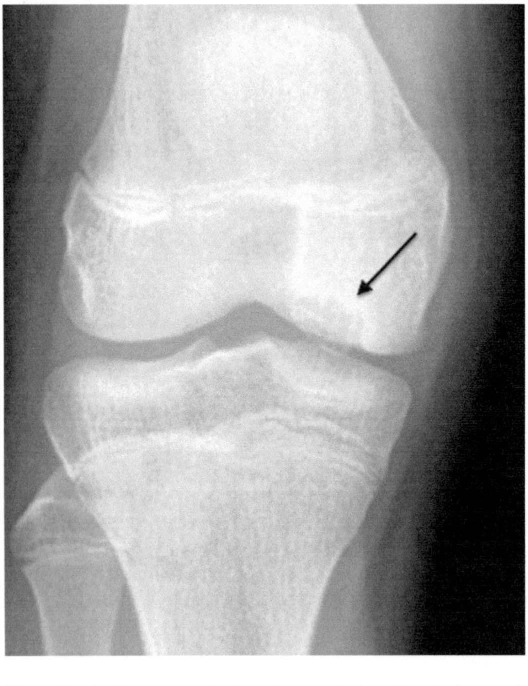

Fig. 17.6 Osteochondral injury of the distal femoral epiphysis (*arrow*)

from cartilage to bone, is the weakest part of the growth plate. The thickness of the physis is relatively constant throughout growth due to a balance between the rate of cartilage production in the proliferative zone and cartilage removal and mineralization in the hypertrophic zone [12]. Although the physis is initially smooth and flat, differential growth rates lead to an undulating contour. Circumferential growth of the epiphyses, apophyses, and small bones proceeds by a similar mechanism. There is a fibrocartilaginous perichondrial ring, at the periphery of the physis, which provides structural support to the chondro-osseous junction [6, 13].

Unique characteristics of blood supply to the epiphysis and metaphysis affect the likelihood of complications after fracture or chronic repetitive cartilage injury. The epiphyseal cartilage is initially perfused by vessels within cartilage canals, which decrease in number and size during childhood. Cartilage canals also traverse the growth plate during infancy, but these disappear after

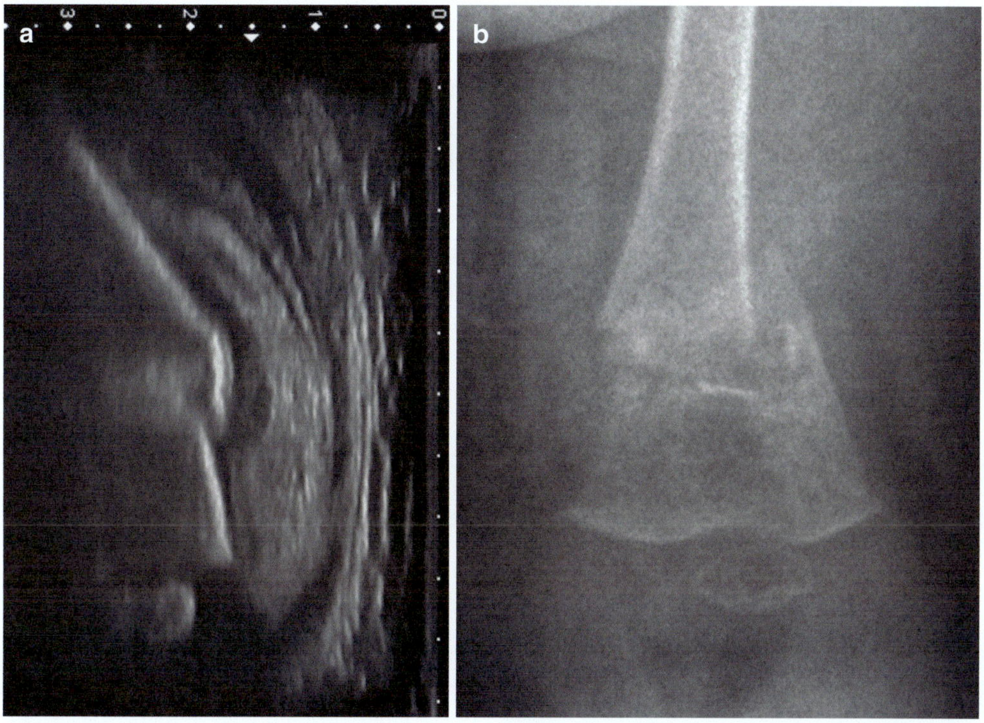

Fig. 17.8 Pathologic fracture in a 6-month-old boy with congenital renal insufficiency, who developed pain and swelling after routine vaccinations. (**a**) Ultrasound (US) shows a displaced fracture, with overlying hematoma (the US was performed to evaluate for deep venous thrombosis and has been rotated to correspond to the radiograph). (**b**) Osteopenia and displaced fracture (Courtesy of Willemijn M. Klein, MD, PhD, radiologist, Radboud University Medical Center, Nijmegen, the Netherlands)

about 18 months [14]. The physis thus has a dual vascular supply, with the epiphyseal artery supporting cartilage growth and the metaphyseal nutrient arteries supporting ossification (Fig. 17.11) [6]. The epiphyseal artery supplies the germinal and proliferative zones of the physis. The metaphyseal arteries supply the hypertrophic zone and zone of provisional calcification, but these nutrient arteries loop within the metaphysis before reaching the growth plate, and the hypertrophic zone is therefore relatively avascular. The tenuous nature of this blood supply makes the primary physis and epiphysis particularly prone to ischemic injury. Focal physeal ischemia may cause bone bridge formation, whereas epiphyseal ischemia may cause fragmentation and decreased size of the epiphyseal ossification center [13]. Fractures involving the germinal and proliferative zones have a higher incidence of complications than those involving the hypertrophic zone [10].

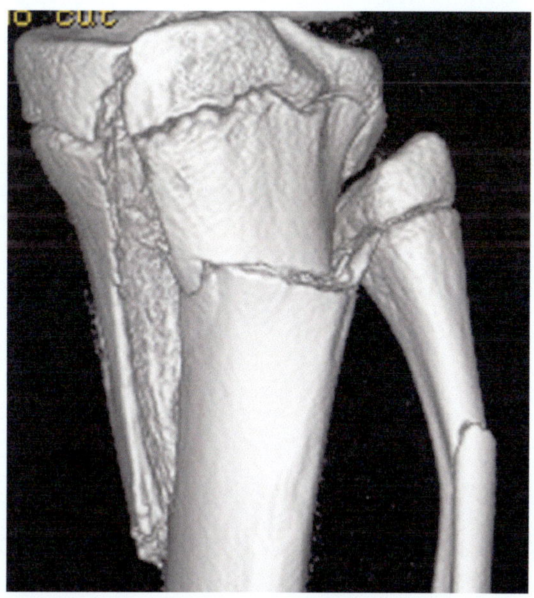

Fig. 17.9 Intra-articular Type IV proximal tibial fracture shown on reconstructed three-dimensional (3D) CT. There is also a fracture of the proximal fibular diaphysis

Several normal growth-related findings may mimic pathology. For example, although in infants and young children the growth plate is smooth and flat, uneven growth leads to physeal undulation. The thickness of the normal physis remains uniform. However, the wavy contour of the growth plate (Fig. 17.12) makes it difficult to obtain images perpendicular to the entire physis, and multiple planes and 3D sequences help evaluate this area [15]. As skeletal maturation approaches, the physis thins, and after it closes there is a residual very thin low signal physeal scar that could be misinterpreted as a fracture. This often persists into adulthood but eventually disappears [15]. The epiphyseal ossification center may develop from several ossification centers (Fig. 17.13) or may have an irregular contour in younger children (Fig. 17.14). However, the overlying cartilage is intact, which helps differentiate this appearance from pathology [16].

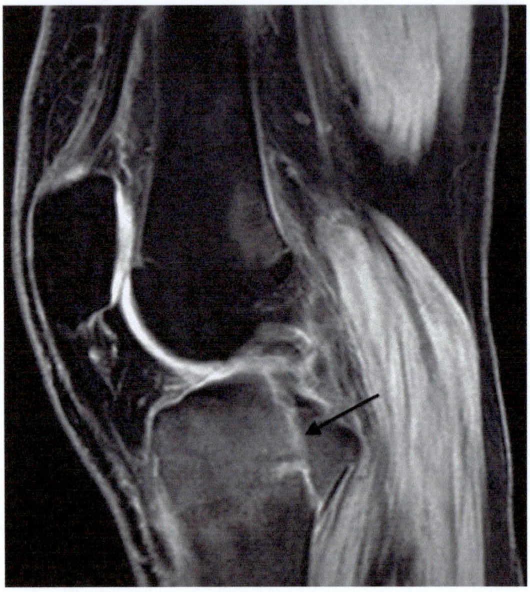

Fig. 17.10 Intra-articular proximal tibial fracture. Sagittal T2-weighted (T2-W) fat-suppressed (FS) image shows the vertical linear hyperintense fracture (*arrow*) with diffuse surrounding ill-defined hyperintense marrow edema (Courtesy of J. Herman Kan)

4 Classification of Growth Plate Injury

Several classification schemes have been developed since Poland's systematic description of epiphyseal injuries in 1898. Salter and Harris (1963) devised the simplest and most widely used classification system, which describes five types of growth plate injury, according to radiographic findings in the epiphysis, physis, and metaphysis (Table 17.1) [17]. Ogden subsequently extended this system to include nine

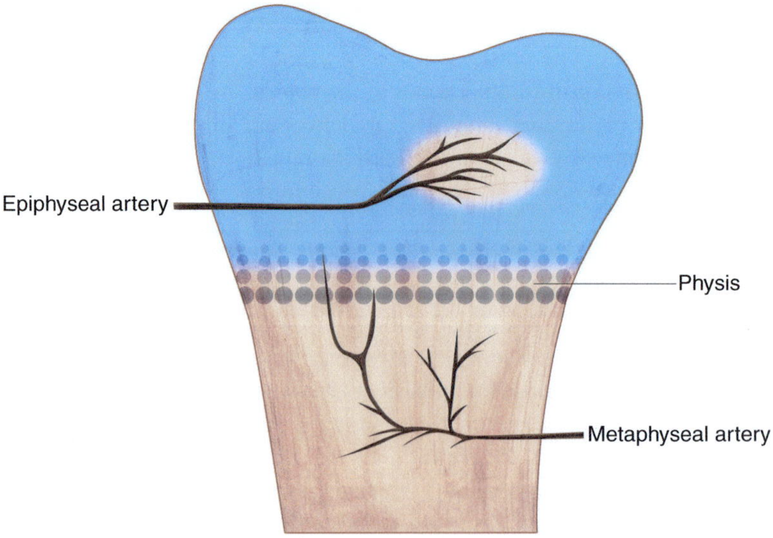

Fig. 17.11 After 18 months of age, the transphyseal vessels disappear, and the arterial supply of the metaphysis and epiphysis is separated by the growth plate

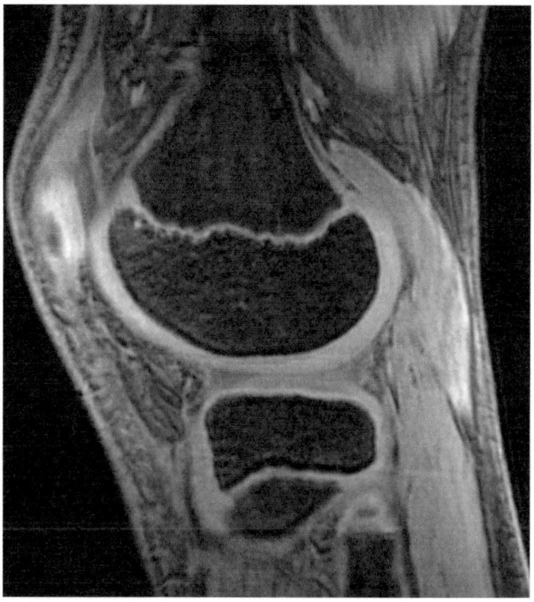

Fig. 17.12 Normal undulation of the distal femoral growth plate related to differential growth in a 12-year-old (sagittal fast spoiled gradient-recalled echo [FSPR])

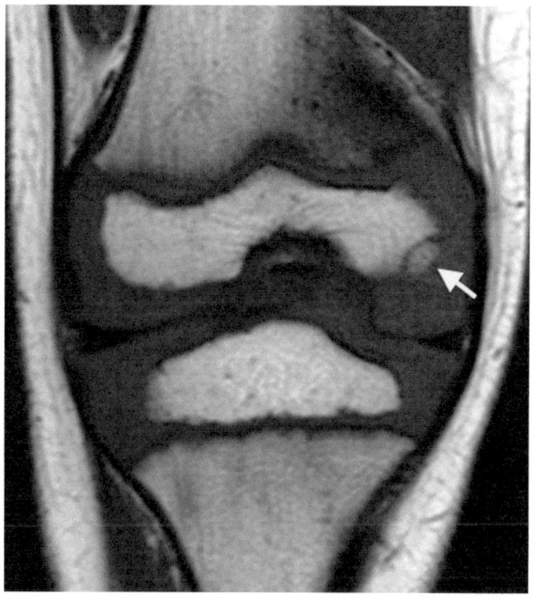

Fig. 17.13 Secondary ossification center (*arrow*) at distal femoral epiphysis has hyperintense signal due to marrow fat in this young child (coronal T1-weighted (T1-W) image)

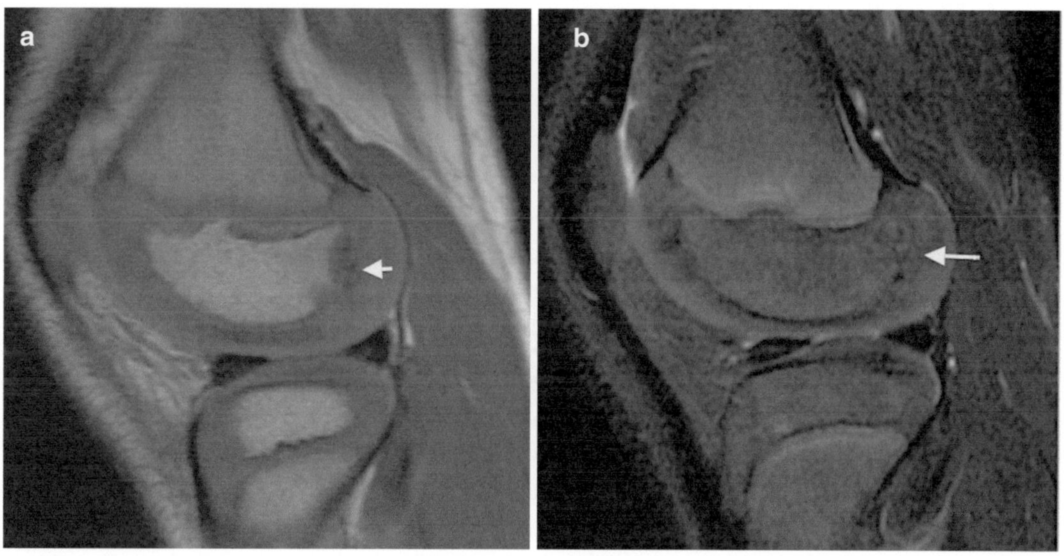

Fig. 17.14 Normal cortical irregularity in a 7-year-old. Sagittal proton density (PD) (**a**) and T2-W FS (**b**) images show irregularity of the posterior aspect of the lateral femoral condylar ossification center without edema or cartilage defect (*arrows*)

fracture types that affect bone growth at any site, including appositional growth of the diaphysis (Fig. 17.15) [18]. However, with the exception of Type VII, isolated epiphyseal fractures, the additional types only account for a small percentage of injuries [6].

Table 17.1 Salter-Harris growth plate fractures

Incidence	Age/common location	Radiographic findings	Cross-sectional imaging
Type I 6 %	Usually <5 y/o Proximal/distal humerus Proximal femur Older child Distal radius Proximal humerus Proximal femur	Soft tissue swelling Fracture often unapparent Growth plate widening Epiphyseal displacement Blurring of distal metaphysis Tiny fragments within physis	MRI: physeal widening T2 hyperintense
Type II 75 %	Usually >10 y/o Distal radius Distal tibia Distal fibula Phalanges	Triangular metaphyseal fragment adjacent to physis May extend into diaphysis Growth plate widening Epiphyseal displacement	Infrequently performed Exceptions Distal femur Proximal tibia
Type III 8 %	Usually adolescent Distal tibia Proximal tibia Distal femur Phalanges	Intra-articular sagittal or oblique fracture through epiphysis Growth plate widening	CT or MRI to assess alignment Low T1, low or high T2 fracture line through epiphysis Wide high T2 physis
Type IV 10 %	5–10 y/o Distal humerus (lateral condyle) Older child Distal radius Adolescent Distal tibia	Intra-articular fracture Through physis, epiphysis, and metaphysis	CT or MRI to assess alignment Low T1, low or high T2 fracture line through epiphysis and metaphysis Wide high T2 physis
Type V 1 %	Severe trauma	May see physeal narrowing Usually diagnosed retrospectively Present with complications of growth arrest	MRI may show hemorrhage or hematoma within growth plate immediately after injury

y/o year(s) old

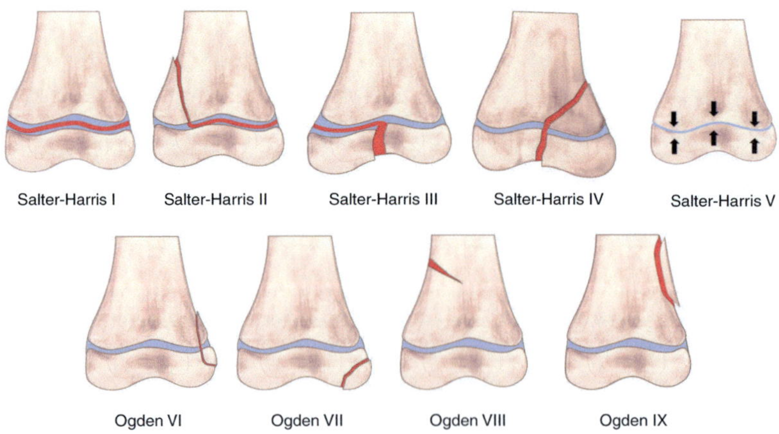

Fig. 17.15 The Salter-Harris I–V and extended Ogden VI–IX classification of fractures at or near the growth plate

4.1 Salter-Harris Fractures

Type I Fractures

These fractures are confined to the physis and usually result from a shearing or avulsion force that parallels the growth plate. Type I fractures occur most often in children less than 5 years old but are relatively uncommon, representing around 6 % of all growth plate injuries. In infancy, they usually occur in the proximal humerus, distal humerus, and proximal femur, resulting from birth trauma or non-accidental trauma [6]. In older children, Type I fractures are most common in the distal radius, proximal humerus, and proximal femur. "Little Leaguer's shoulder," a Type I fracture of the proximal humerus, occurs around age 10–12 in throwing athletes. Slipped capital femoral epiphysis (SCFE), also a Type I fracture, occurs around puberty, usually without specific antecedent trauma. Most Type I injuries have an excellent prognosis [6], but SCFE may be complicated by avascular necrosis of the femoral head, since the artery supplying the epiphysis courses along the physis and may be injured at epiphyseal separation.

The classic but relatively uncommon radiographic finding is displacement of the epiphysis without an osseous fracture. This may be seen in infants with traumatic separation of the distal humerus, which usually results in posteromedial displacement of the distal fragment [19] (Fig. 17.16) (see Chap. 8). However, in many cases the fracture reduces spontaneously after the initial slip, and radiological diagnosis may be difficult. Findings that suggest a Type I fracture include slight widening of the growth plate or poor definition of the metaphyseal margin adjacent to the growth plate, due to slight angulation. Very small, thin bone fragments may be seen along the physis, due to fracture propagation from the hypertrophic zone into the zone of provisional calcification [6] (Fig. 17.17). In infants whose epiphysis has not yet ossified, a slipped epiphysis may mimic a dislocation. Ultrasound may confirm a Type I fracture by showing malalignment between the metaphysis and cartilaginous

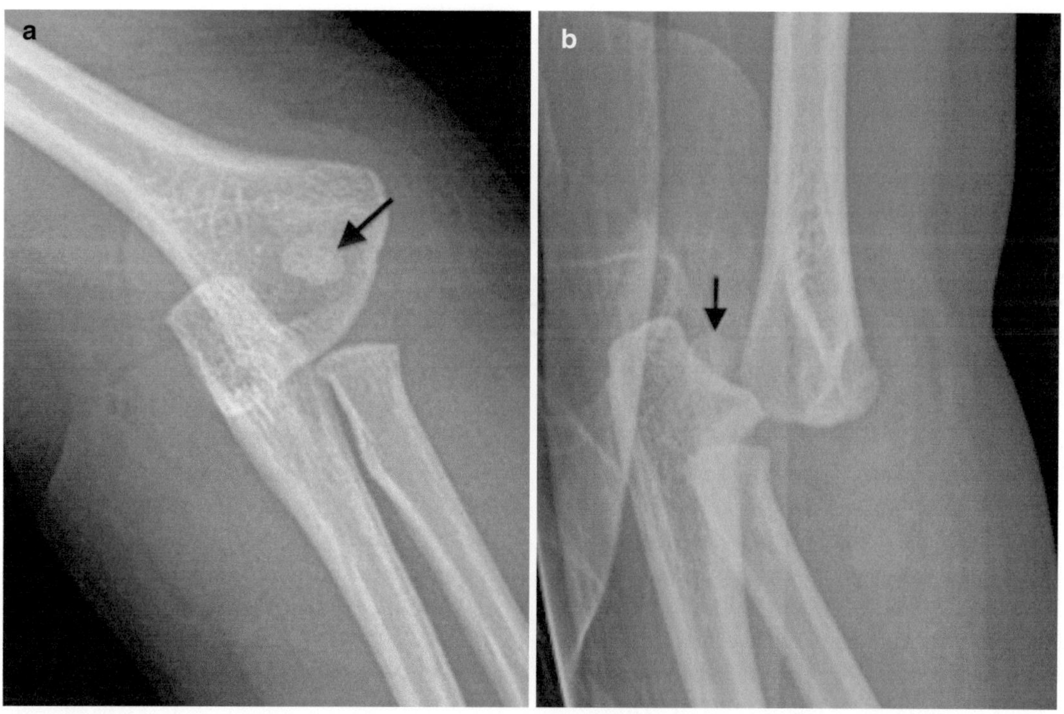

Fig. 17.16 Type I distal humeral fracture in a young child. (**a**, **b**) The capitellum (*arrow*) is displaced posteromedially with respect to the distal humeral metaphysis but maintains alignment with the radius and ulna

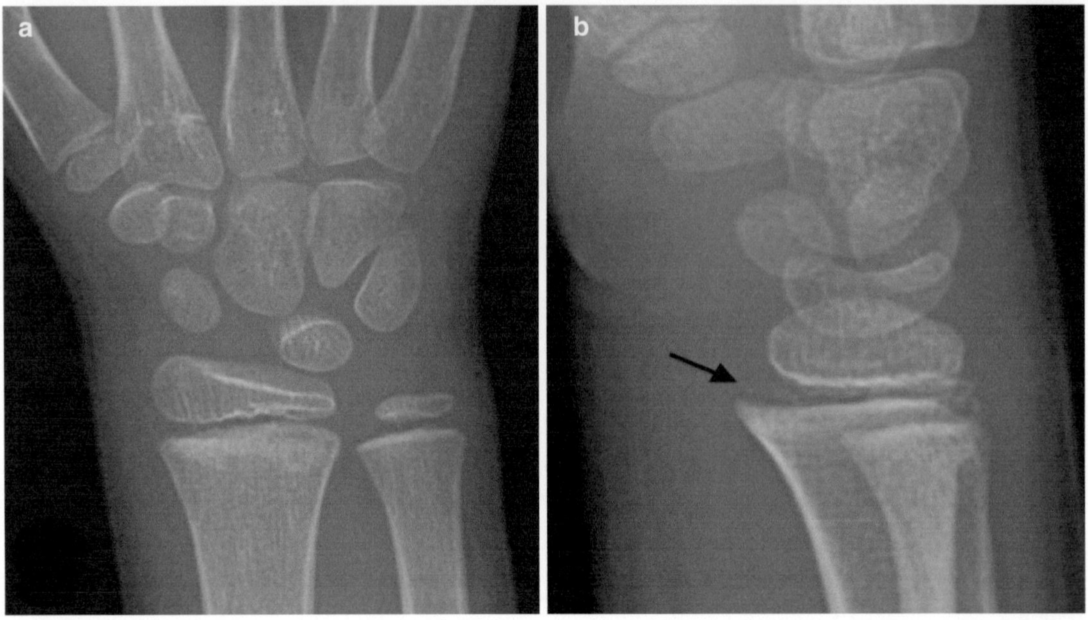

Fig. 17.17 Type I fracture with mild posterior displacement of the distal radial epiphysis. (**a**, **b**) Note tiny fragments along the physis (*arrow*)

epiphysis (Fig. 17.18). MRI may be used to assess for occult Type I injury, particularly in regions where growth plate damage could cause significant growth arrest, such as the knee. Water-sensitive sequences typically show a wide, hyperintense physis, with adjacent marrow and soft tissue edema (Fig. 17.19). Follow-up radiographs in 7–10 days may show periosteal new bone formation in the adjacent metaphysis, due to healing.

Type II Fractures

Type II fractures extend along the growth plate into the metaphysis and usually result from a shearing or avulsive force. They are the most common physeal injury, representing 75 % of growth plate fractures. Type II injuries are rare in infancy and usually occur in children older than age 10. The distal radius is most often affected, accounting for up to 50 % of Type II fractures [6]. Other common sites include the distal tibia, distal fibula, and phalanges. Growth usually continues undisturbed or with minimal shortening, as the germinal matrix is often preserved. However, Type II fractures at the knee, especially at the distal femur, have a guarded prognosis, as the force required to produce these injuries may crush the germinal cells [6]. Distal femoral growth plate fractures are usually caused by severe force, such as high-speed motor vehicle collisions, but these fractures also have an increased incidence in adolescents playing contact sports.

Imaging

The classic radiographic finding of a Type II fracture is a triangular metaphyseal fragment adjacent to the growth plate (the Thurston-Holland sign) (Fig. 17.20). Variations include a metaphyseal fracture parallel to the growth plate or extending into the diaphysis. The metaphyseal fragment is usually visible on radiographs, and there is often epiphyseal displacement and growth plate widening (Fig. 17.21). The periosteum is intact along the metaphyseal fracture but torn at the site of growth plate separation.

Type III Fractures

Type III fractures extend both vertically and obliquely through the epiphysis to the articular

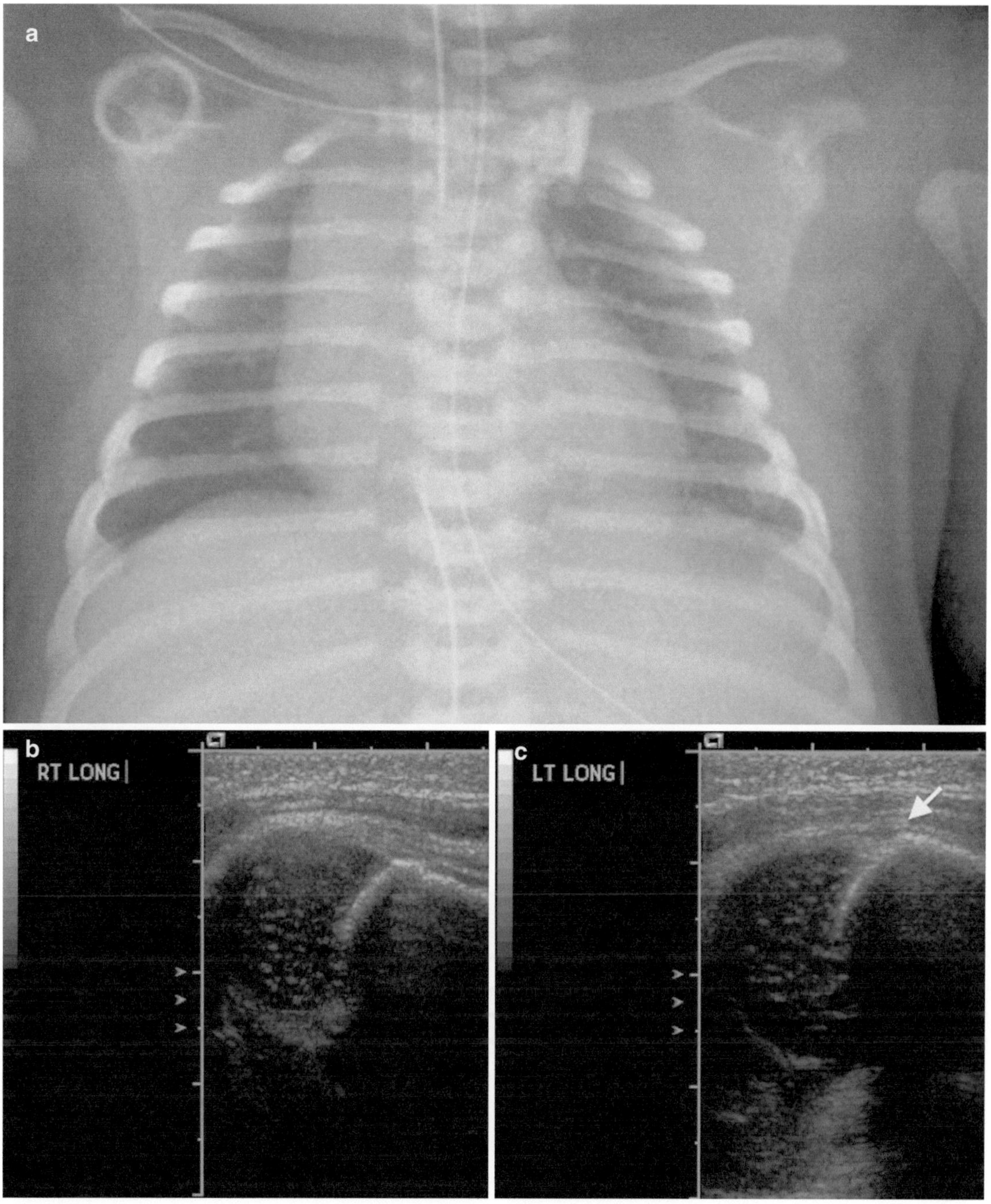

Fig. 17.18 Type I fracture in a newborn who did not move the left arm after a difficult delivery. (**a**) The distance between the left glenoid and proximal humeral metaphysis may be slightly wide, perhaps suggesting dislocation or Type I fracture. (**b**) Sagittal US on right side (for comparison) shows normal alignment. (**c**) Sagittal US on left shows malalignment of the hypoechoic cartilaginous epiphysis and echogenic cortical bone

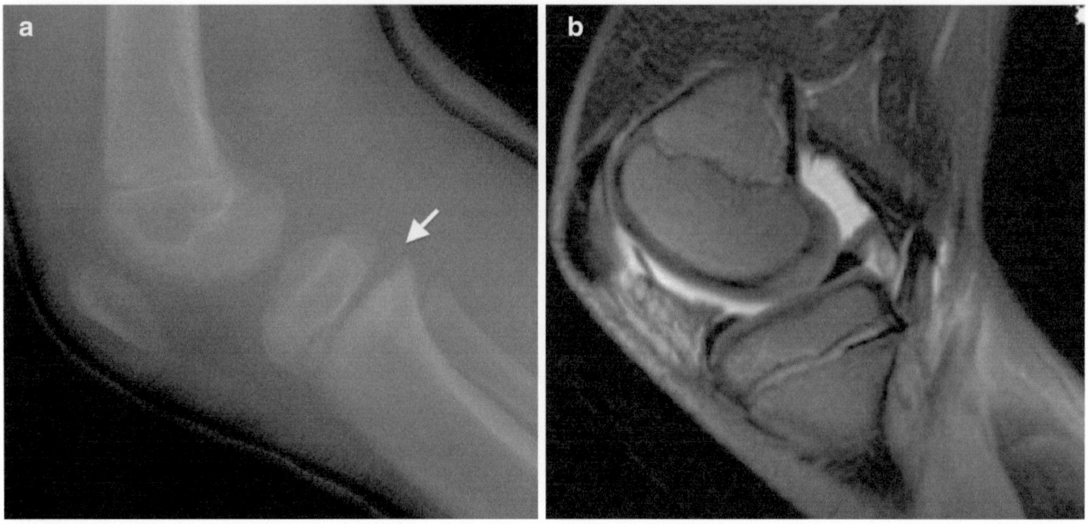

Fig. 17.19 Type I fracture of proximal tibial physis. (**a**) Widening of the posterior portion of proximal tibial physis (*arrow*). (**b**) Sagittal T2-W FS image shows increased signal and widening of the proximal tibial physis with adjacent marrow edema and a joint effusion

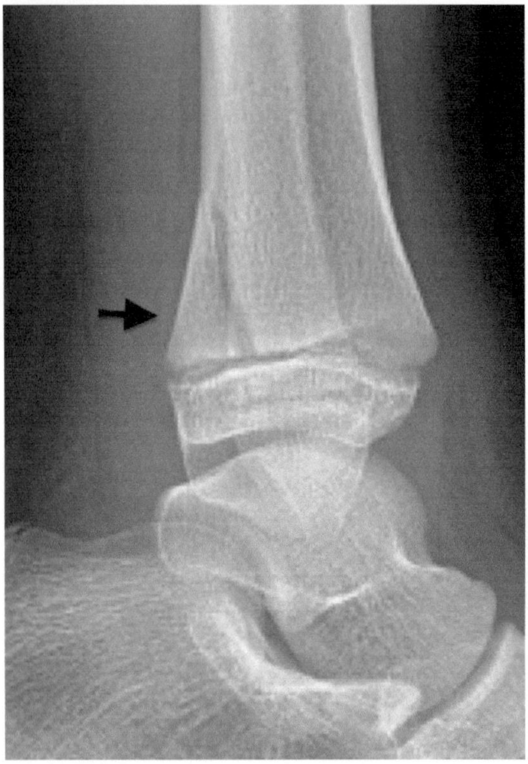

Fig. 17.20 Type II fracture of the distal tibia. Growth plate widening and a posterior triangular metaphyseal fragment (*arrow*)

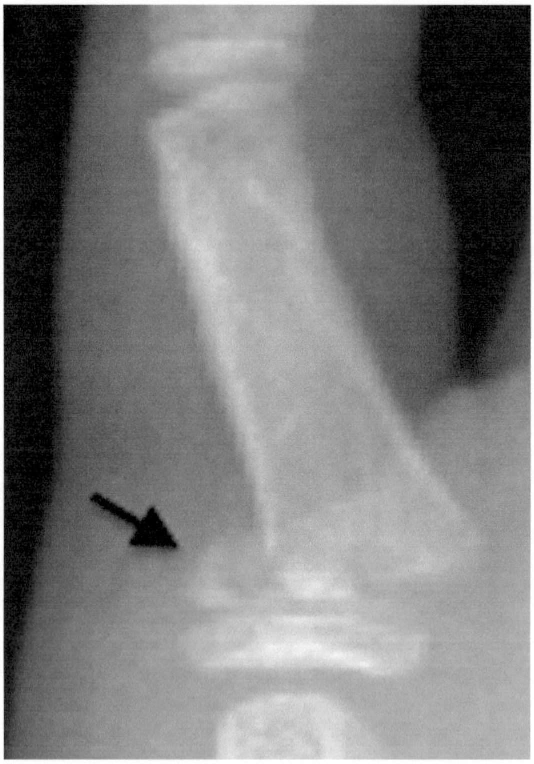

Fig. 17.21 Type II fracture with small metaphyseal fragment (*arrow*)

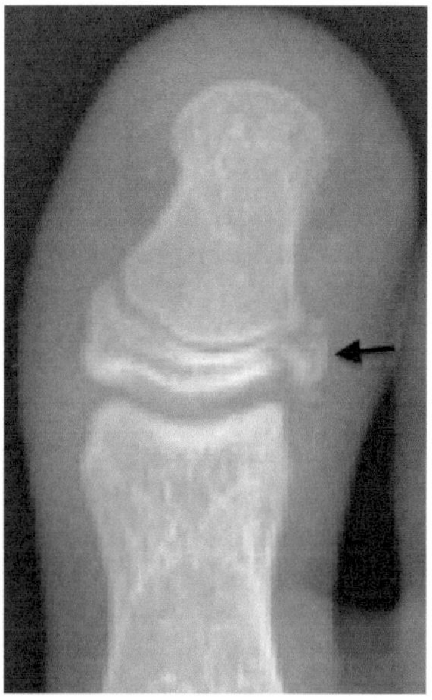

Fig. 17.22 Type III fracture. The epiphyseal fragment is rotated (*arrow*)

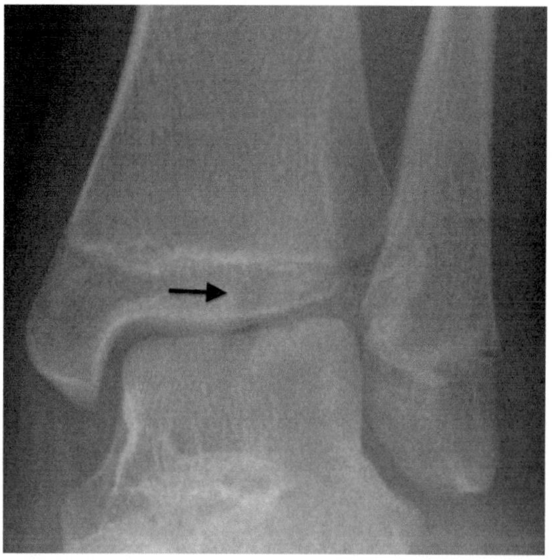

Fig. 17.24 Type II fracture (Tillaux) in a 13-year-old who fell while Rollerblading. Vertical fracture (*arrow*) through epiphysis

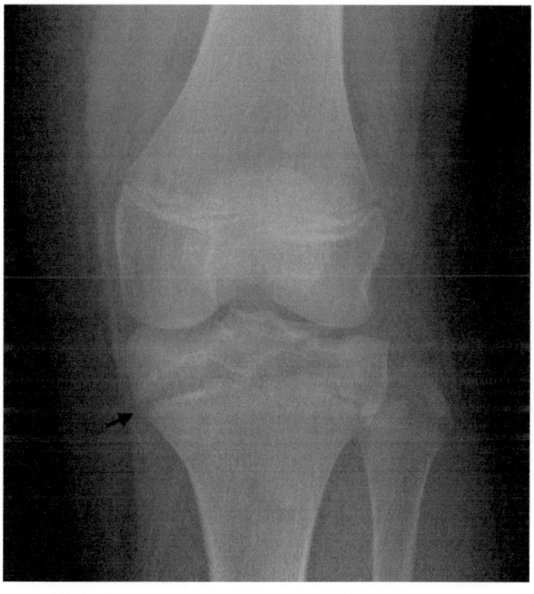

Fig. 17.23 Type III fracture of the proximal tibia. An oblique fracture line traverses the epiphysis, and the medial physis is widened (*arrow*)

surface, and horizontally through the physis, resulting in separation of a portion of the epiphysis. They represent 8 % of growth plate fractures and most commonly occur during adolescence. These fractures usually result from vertical shearing force, and fragments are typically at most minimally displaced [6]. The prognosis is generally good, provided the fracture is not significantly displaced and the epiphyseal blood supply is intact. However, if a displaced fracture is incompletely reduced, bone bridging and/or articular incongruity may result. The most common locations for these fractures are the distal tibia, proximal tibia, distal femur, and phalanges [6].

Imaging

Type III fractures are usually visible on radiographs (Figs. 17.22 and 17.23), but additional oblique views may be needed for diagnosis. The juvenile Tillaux fracture, which affects the distal tibial epiphysis, occurs when physeal fusion is incomplete (see Chap. 16). Forced supination and external rotation of the ankle cause stress on the anterior tibiofibular ligament, with resultant avulsion of a small fragment of the bone from the anterolateral corner of the distal tibial epiphysis (Figs. 17.24 and 17.25). Type III fractures of the distal femur usually result from severe valgus stress, sometimes due to direct force against the lateral portion of the knee (as in a football "clip"

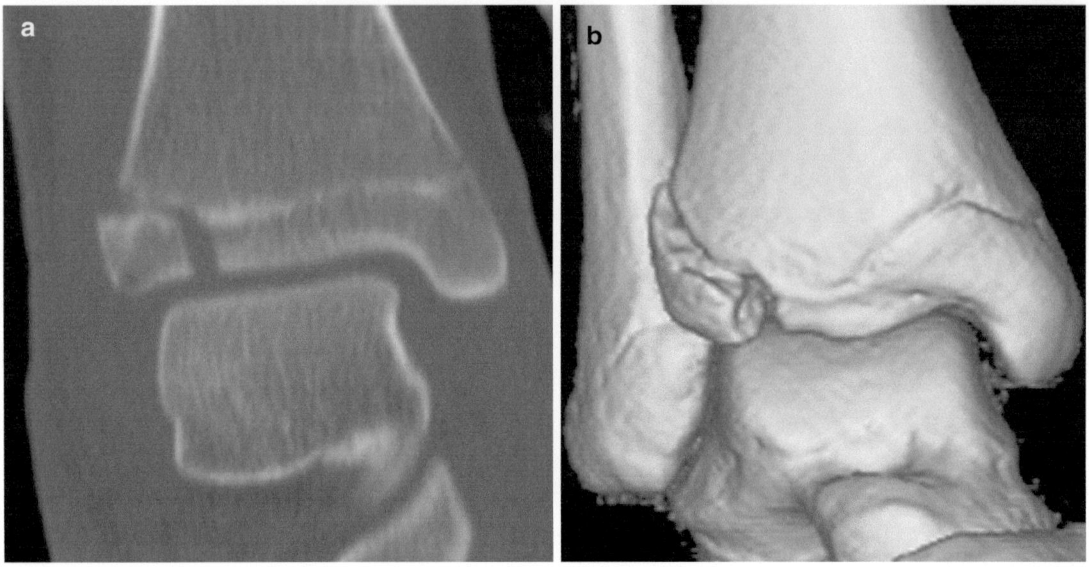

Fig. 17.25 Type III fracture (Tillaux). Coronal two-dimensional (2D) (**a**) and three-dimensional (3D) (**b**) computed tomography (CT) reformatted images

or wrestling). CT or MRI may help delineate these fractures and assess alignment, particularly at the distal femur, proximal tibia, and distal tibia (Fig. 17.26).

Type IV Fractures

These fractures usually result from a vertical compression or shearing force that extends through the metaphysis, epiphysis, and intervening physis. They represent 10 % of growth plate fractures and most commonly occur at the distal humerus (lateral condyle), distal tibia, and distal radius [20]. Because these fractures are intra-articular, they must be reduced to near-anatomic alignment to prevent long-term complications such as joint deformity, accelerated osteoarthritis, or bone bridge formation. Such complications are most likely at the elbow, knee, and ankle.

Imaging

Radiologic findings of Type IV fractures include a fracture line extending through the epiphysis, growth plate, and metaphysis (Fig. 17.27). Lateral condylar fractures of the distal humerus, which represent about 20 % of pediatric elbow fractures and which usually occur in children age 4–10 years, are often Type IV fractures (Figs. 17.28 and 17.29) [21] (see Chap. 8). Internal oblique views may demonstrate a subtle, minimally displaced lateral condylar fracture [22]. CT more accurately evaluates the degree of fracture displacement and can determine if the articular cartilage is intact [23, 24]. However, MRI, with its superior cartilage detail, is the best method for distinguishing between Type II and IV lateral condylar fractures (Fig. 17.30). Lateral condylar fractures have the highest incidence of nonunion of all pediatric fractures [22].

The triplane fracture is a Type IV injury of the distal tibia, occurring at the end of puberty, as the physis is fusing (see Chap. 16). Usually a result of eversion injury, it may result from a fall [25]. This fracture consists of a coronal fracture through the posterior metaphysis, a transverse fracture along the lateral physis and a sagittal fracture through the anterior epiphysis. This complex pattern is related to asymmetric fusion of the distal tibial growth plate, which begins medially at a physeal undulation, “Kump’s bump” [26]. Radiographs typically show widening of the lateral physis, with the epiphyseal fracture evident on the frontal or oblique view and the metaphyseal fracture evident on the lateral view (Fig. 17.31). CT with multiplanar reformats is indicated for presurgical assessment (Fig. 17.32). Since these fractures occur near skeletal maturity, limb shortening is

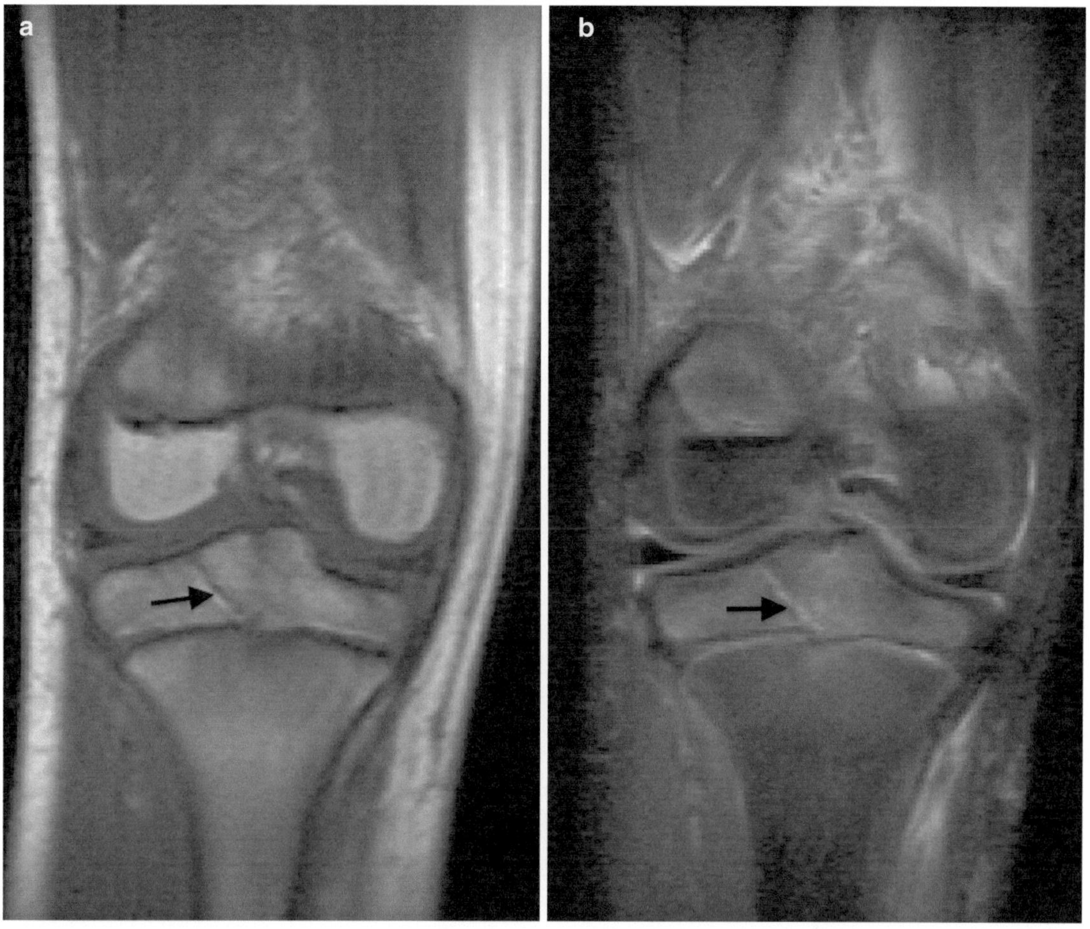

Fig. 17.26 Type III fracture of the proximal tibial epiphysis. Coronal T1-W (**a**) and T2-W FS (**b**) images show an oblique non-displaced fracture line extending to the growth plate, which is T1 hypointense and T2 hyperintense (*arrows*)

uncommon; the prognosis is largely determined by the integrity of the tibial plafond [12, 20].

Type V Fractures

These injuries represent only 1 % of growth plate fractures and result from severe axial loading with physeal compression or crush injury. This damages the vascular supply and germinal cells of the physis, and subsequent growth arrest is therefore common and the prognosis poor [6]. Type V fractures are most common in the distal femur, proximal tibia, and distal tibia and may also coexist with other types of complex growth plate injuries [12]. Radiographic diagnosis is difficult and often made retrospectively, when premature physeal fusion is observed. Type V injuries may be suspected after significant axial loading injury of the knee or ankle, especially if associated with adjacent fractures. MRI can establish the diagnosis immediately after injury, if hemorrhage or hematoma is identified within the growth plate [6].

4.2 Ogden Extension of Salter-Harris Fractures

Type VI Fractures

This injury is very rare and damages the perichondrial ring. It frequently involves a lawn mower or farm machinery and is often associated with a compound or open fracture. With healing, a bone bridge forms, connecting the epiphysis to the metaphysis and leading to angular deformity. The distal femur and distal tibia are common locations. Radiographs may demonstrate a small, sliver-like fragment at the lateral margin of the epiphysis [6].

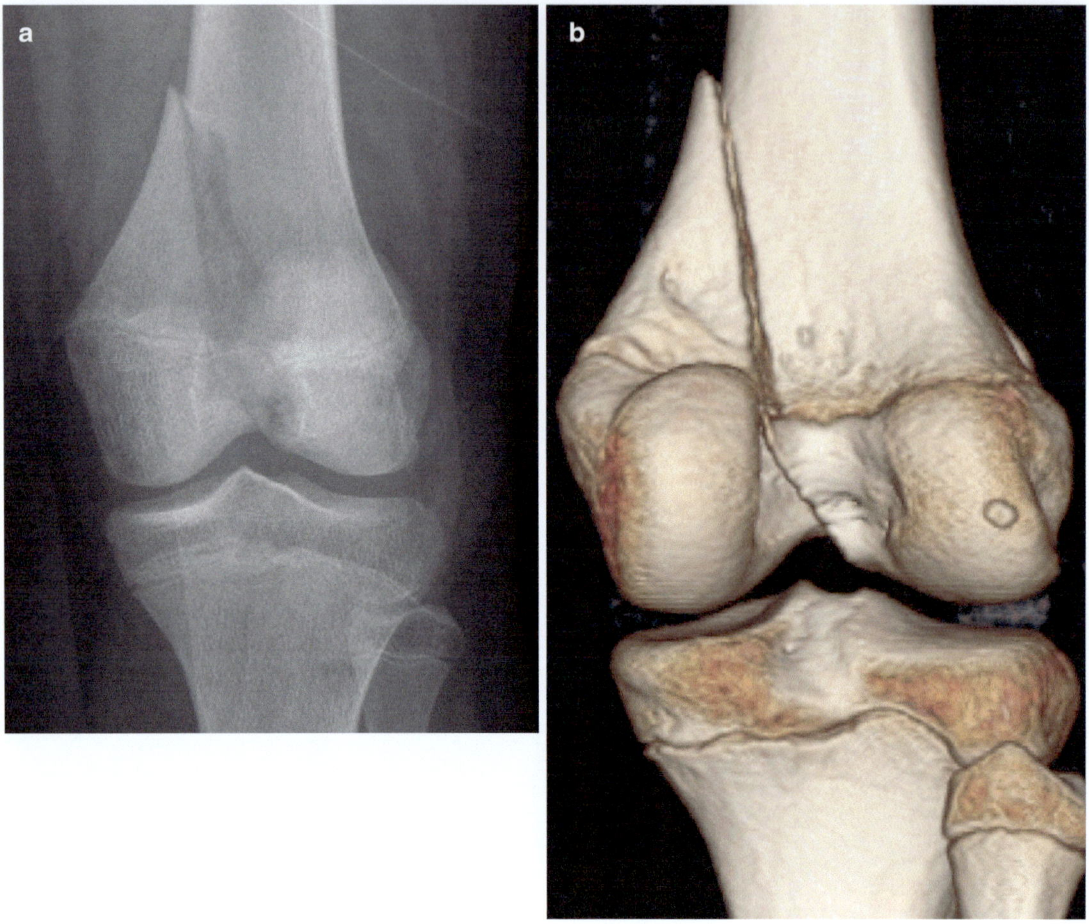

Fig. 17.27 Type IV fracture of the distal femur. (**a**) There is a vertical fracture of the distal femur, extending from the metadiaphysis, across the physis, and through the intercondylar region of the epiphysis. (**b**) 3D CT reconstruction

Type VII Fractures

These purely epiphyseal fractures do not involve the primary physis (see section below on osteochondral injuries and tendon/ligament injuries).

Type VIII Fractures

These purely metaphyseal fractures disrupt the blood supply of the primary spongiosa, leading to temporary disruption of normal ossification. Normal remodeling of the metaphysis into a normal funnel shape may be affected [6, 27].

Type IX Fractures

This injury strips the periosteum and interferes with appositional bone growth of the metadiaphysis [6].

5 Osteochondral Injuries (Box 17.1)

Box 17.1: Sites of Osteochondral Fracture/ Osteochondritis Dissecans (Type VII)

Most common	Medial femoral condyle
	Talus
	Capitellum
Other sites	Lateral femoral condyle
	Femoral head
	Trochlea
	Radial head
	Patella

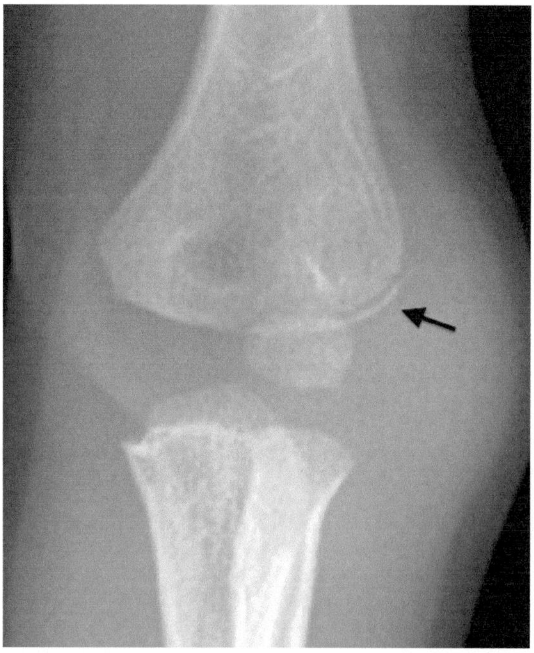

Fig. 17.28 Lateral condylar fracture. There is a thin, non-displaced metaphyseal fragment (*arrow*). Distinction between a Type II and IV fracture cannot be made radiographically as the epiphysis is largely cartilaginous

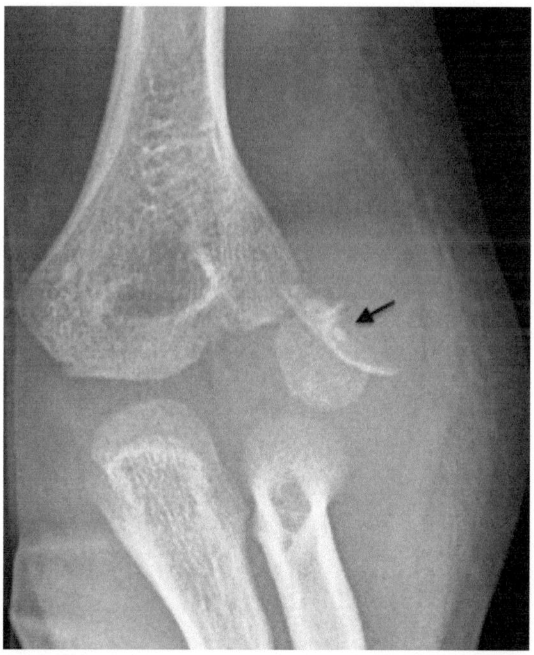

Fig. 17.29 Type IV lateral condylar fracture in a 5-year-old who fell from a play structure. There is striking displacement and rotation of the capitellum and metaphyseal fragment (*arrow*)

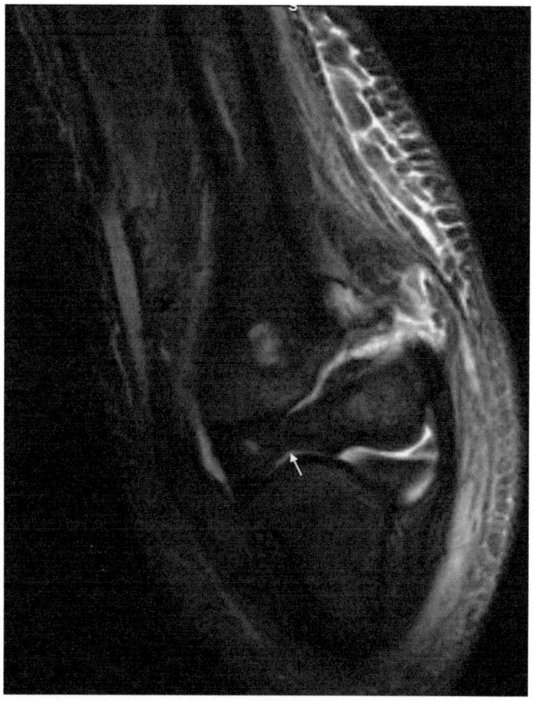

Fig. 17.30 Type IV fracture. Coronal T2-W FS image shows high T2 signal in the fracture, extending from the lateral metaphysis into the cartilaginous epiphysis, with an intact cartilage flap (*arrow*) (Courtesy of J. Herman Kan)

Osteochondral fractures of the articular surface usually result from shearing and rotatory forces that cause dissection of a fragment of epiphyseal articular cartilage and subchondral bone. A single episode of trauma may result in an acute fracture. Alternatively, repetitive microtrauma may lead to osteochondritis dissecans (OCD). The latter is encountered most often in adolescent boys, especially in very active children and high-level athletes. Like chronic metaphyseal stress injuries that impair endochondral ossification at the primary physis (see discussion of stress fractures, below), OCD may result from damage to the secondary subchondral physis [16]. If the vascular supply to the secondary physis is disrupted, cartilage may extend deep into the epiphyseal ossification center.

The most common locations of osteochondral injury are the medial femoral condyle, talus, and capitellum (Figs. 17.33 and 17.34). Other less common sites include the lateral femoral condyle, femoral head, trochlea, radial head, and patella. Prognosis is better in younger children. The lesion may heal

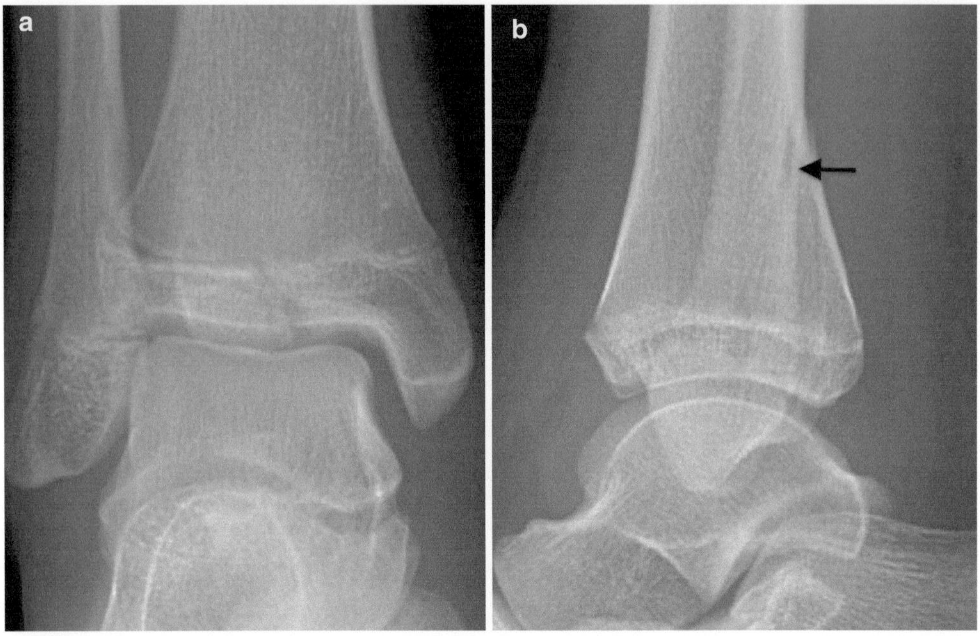

Fig. 17.31 Type IV triplane fracture. (**a**) Vertical fracture through the distal tibial epiphysis with widening of the lateral aspect of the growth plate. (**b**) Oblique fracture component through the posterior aspect of the distal tibial metaphysis (*arrow*)

with conservative treatment, if the fragment is not displaced. However, after skeletal maturity, the secondary physis no longer forms endochondral new bone, and healing is limited (Fig. 17.35). Osteochondral lesions in adults may represent residual non-healed lesions that developed in childhood [16]. Similar pathophysiology applies to the bony epiphysis or its equivalent, such as with Kohler disease of the tarsal navicular or Panner disease of the capitellum (Fig. 17.36) (see Chaps. 8, 14, and 16).

Imaging

Acute and chronic osteochondral injuries have similar clinical symptoms and radiographic appearance. When accompanied with standard views, tunnel views of the knee and mortise views of the ankle are helpful in accurately diagnosing OCD lesions in the knee and talus, respectively. While radiographs are often diagnostic, MRI is helpful in demonstrating occult osteochondral injuries and isolated cartilage injuries (Fig. 17.37). MRI can also better assess fragment size and the degree of instability because it highlights fluid extending around an in situ fragment and shows subchondral cysts (Figs. 17.38 and 17.39). Such findings direct the most appropriate surgical treatment, such as drilling, debridement, in situ fixation, or cartilage replacement. MRI or CT may also demonstrate free intra-articular osteochondral fragments, which require arthroscopic removal (Figs. 17.40 and 17.41).

6 Apophyseal Avulsion Fractures (Box 17.2)

The apophysis is a secondary ossification center at the attachment site of a major muscle-tendon unit to bone. The apophyseal growth plate is suscepti-

Box 17.2: Apophyseal Avulsion Fractures

Pelvis		
	Most common	Ischial tuberosity (hamstring)
		Anterior-superior iliac spine (sartorius)
		Anterior-inferior iliac spine (rectus femoris)
	Less common	Lesser trochanter (iliopsoas)
		Pubis (adductor)
		Iliac crest apophysis (abdominal muscles)
Knee		Inferior patellar pole (patellar sleeve injury)
		Tibial tuberosity
Elbow		Medial epicondyle

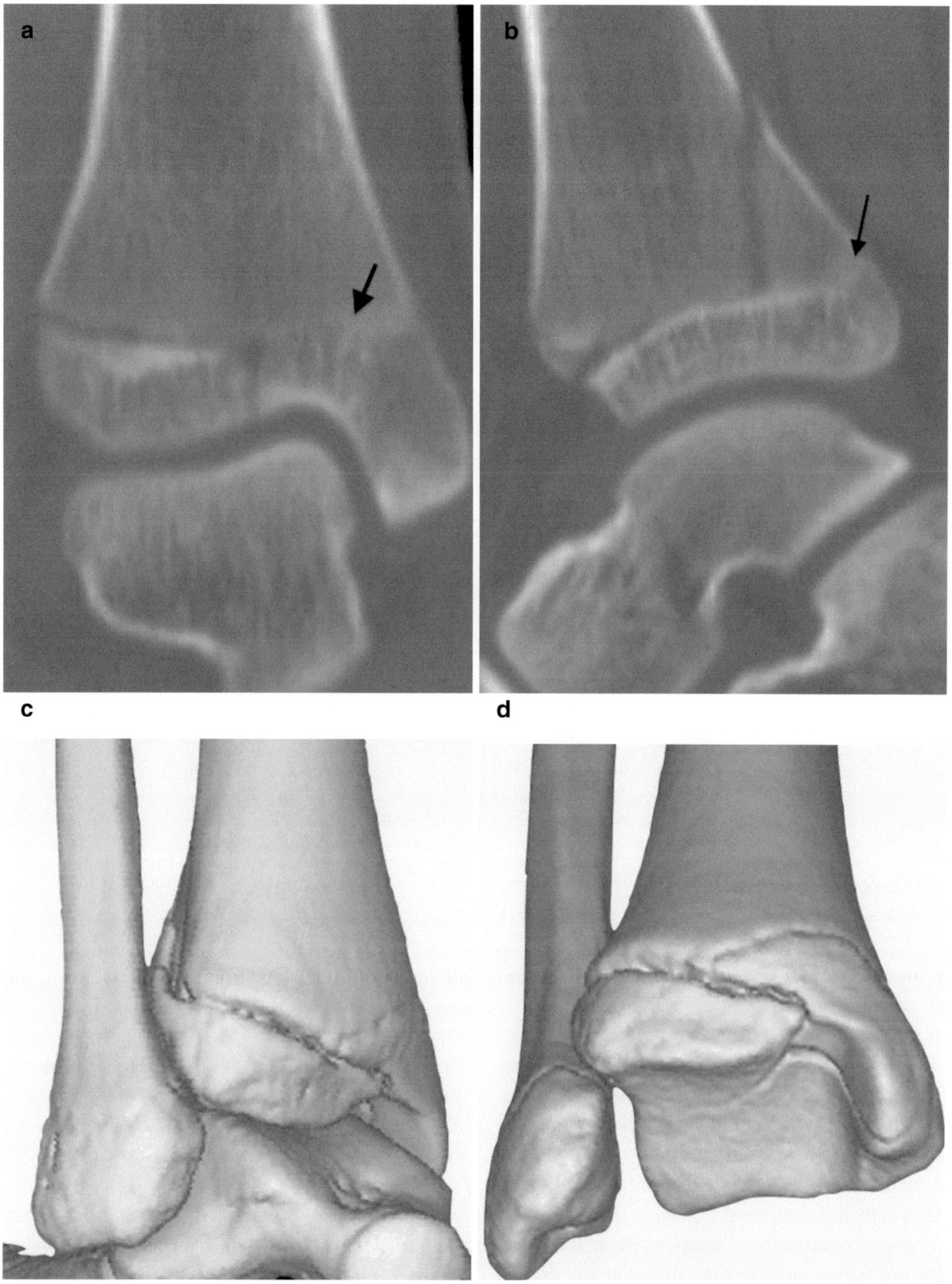

Fig. 17.32 Type IV triplane fracture. Coronal (**a**) and sagittal (**b**) CT reformats show partial fusion at the medial and posterior distal tibial growth plate (*arrows*). 3D CT reformats (**c**, **d**) show all three fracture planes

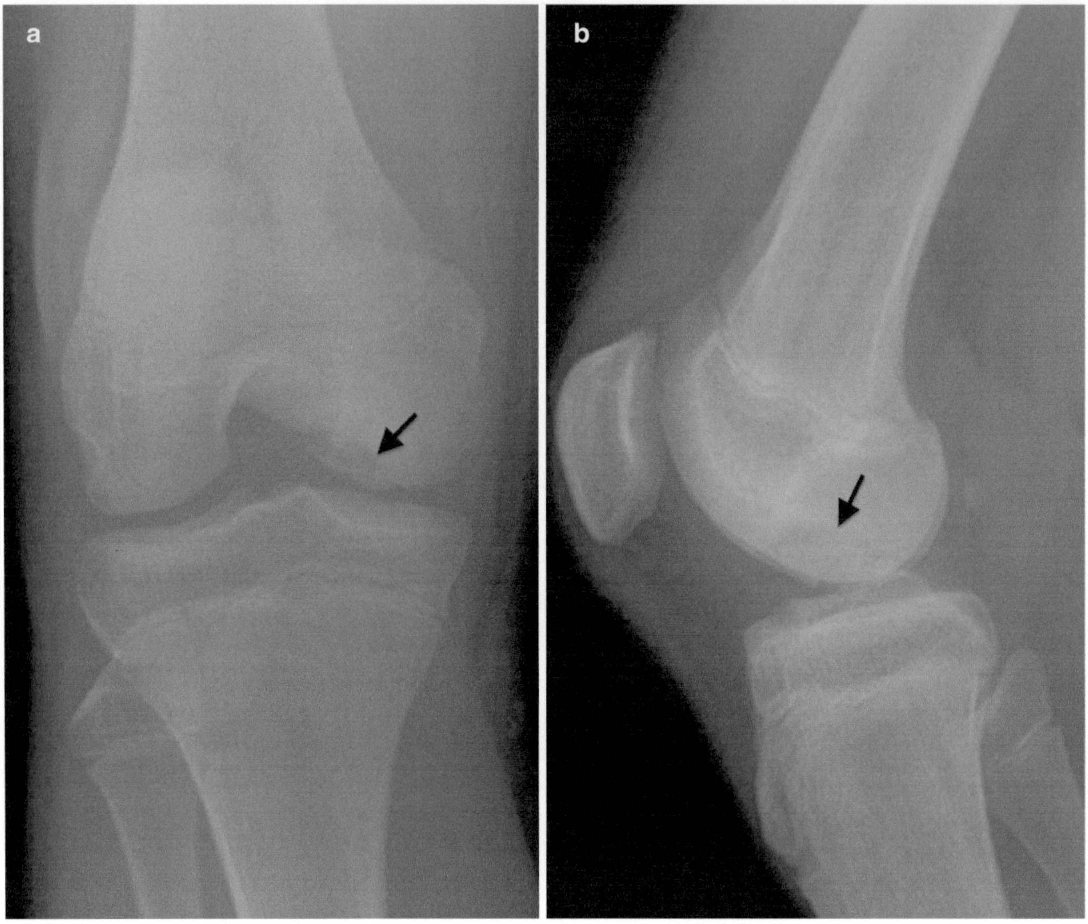

Fig. 17.33 Osteochondritis dissecans (OCD) of the distal femur. (**a**, **b**) There is a subchondral fragment along the medial femoral condyle (*arrows*)

ble to injury from tensile forces, which may result in avulsion fractures (in adults, comparable injury will damage the musculotendinous junction). Although apophyses develop at various times during childhood, they are usually injured during the adolescent growth spurt, due to relative weakening of the apophyseal growth plate and increased tension on the apophysis at this time. Acute apophyseal avulsion fractures are often associated with sudden pain and a popping sensation during forceful muscle contraction. They most commonly affect the pelvis but can also occur at the major tendon insertion sites in the knee and elbow.

Imaging

Apophyseal avulsion fractures of the pelvis generally occur in sports with running, kicking, or jumping. A frontal radiograph of the pelvis is usually sufficient for diagnosis and typically shows a crescent-shaped bone fragment displaced from the apophysis. The most common sites are the ischial tuberosity (hamstring) (Fig. 17.42), anterior-superior iliac spine (sartorius) (Fig. 17.43), and anterior-inferior iliac spine (rectus femoris) (Fig. 17.44). Other sites include the lesser trochanter (iliopsoas) (Fig. 17.45), pubis (adductor), and iliac crest apophysis (abdominal muscles) (Fig. 17.46). Occasionally, there may be no history of trauma, and exuberant callus related to healing may mimic an aggressive bone lesion (see Fig. 17.42). However, short-term follow-up radiographs usually establish the diagnosis. MRI may be helpful in certain cases, to confirm equivocal or occult apophyseal avulsion fractures. (See Chap. 12 for further discussion.)

Acute avulsion fractures at the knee may occur at either end of the patellar tendon, at the

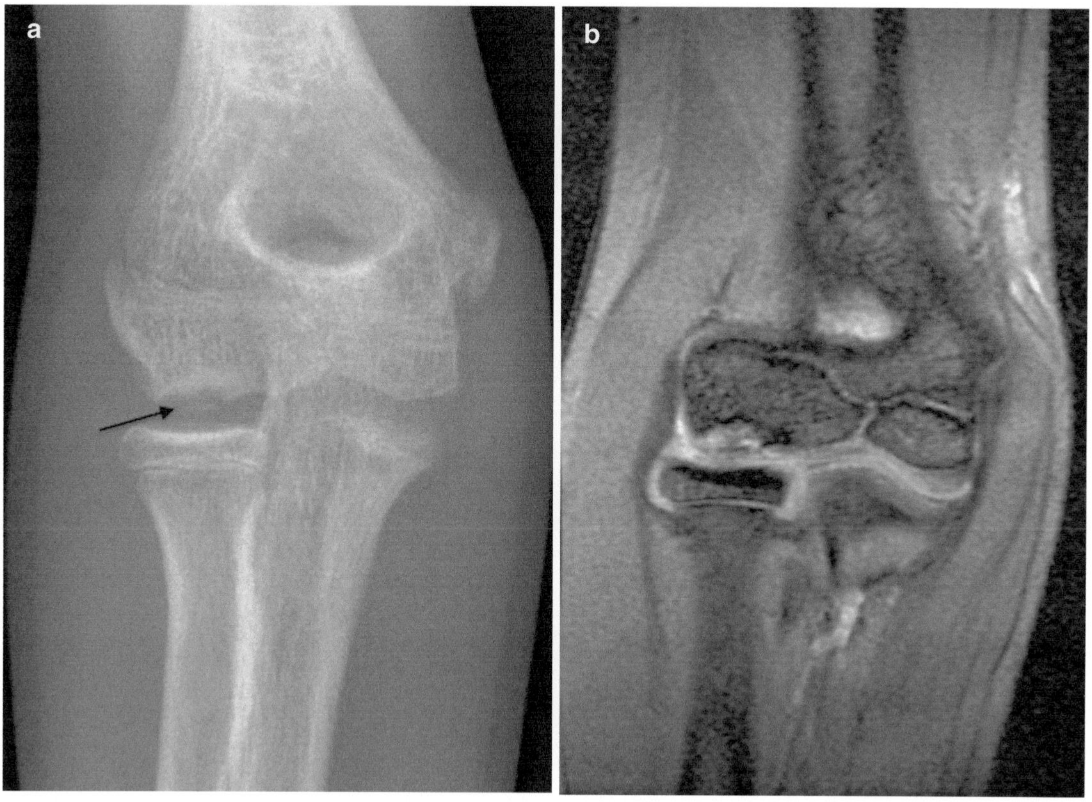

Fig. 17.34 OCD of the capitellum. (**a**) There is a subchondral defect with sclerotic margin and small in situ fragment (*arrow*). (**b**) Coronal MPGR image shows hyperintense subchondral defect with hypointense fragment

tibial tuberosity, or at the inferior pole of the patella (patellar sleeve injury). As injuries of the extensor mechanism, these fractures typically occur during sports activities associated with jumping. Tibial tuberosity avulsion fractures are usually seen in boys, age 12–17 years, and may be confined to the apophysis (Fig. 17.47) or extend superiorly through the proximal tibial epiphysis into the knee joint [28] (Fig. 17.48). Lateral radiographs are usually diagnostic, but oblique views help assess for intra-articular extension [29]. Patellar sleeve fractures occur in slightly younger children, age 8–12 years. They consist of avulsion of a sleeve of periosteum, cartilage, and bone from the inferior patellar pole [29]. Radiographs may show patella alta, related to disruption of the extensor mechanism, along with an osseous fragment inferior to the patella. However, the diagnosis may be missed if the bone fragment is so small that it is imperceptible on radiography. MRI may then show a small osteocartilaginous fragment and also more accurately demonstrate the extent of patellar sleeve injury [28, 30] (Fig. 17.49). (See Chap. 14 for additional discussion of avulsion injuries at the knee.)

Medial epicondyle avulsion fractures are most common in children 7–15 years of age [3]. The forearm flexors insert into the medial epicondyle, and significant valgus stress may result in an acute avulsion fracture. Patients classically present with an acute episode of pain during throwing, often related to baseball pitching (a variant of Little Leaguer's elbow) [24]. Medial epicondyle fractures may also follow direct trauma, fall on an outstretched hand, or elbow dislocation. They are usually Type I growth plate fractures, but occasionally Type II or III injuries occur if the fracture extends through the adjacent metaphysis or apophyseal ossification center (Fig. 17.50). Medial epicondyle fractures with more than 15 mm of displacement generally require reduction and internal fixation.

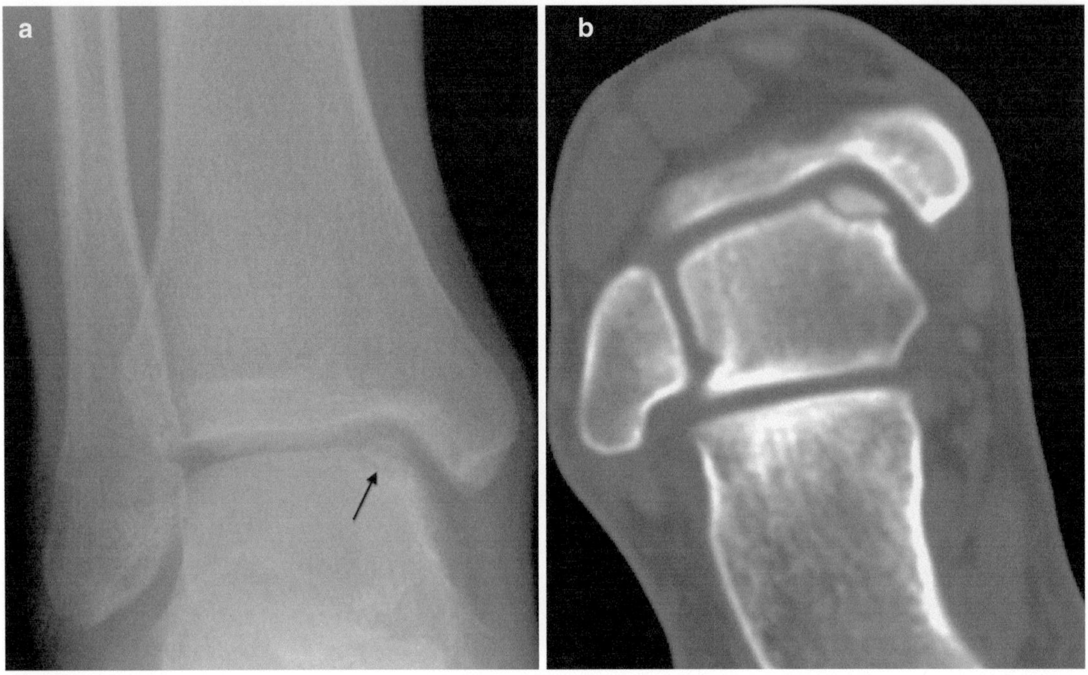

Fig. 17.35 OCD of the talar dome in a skeletally mature adolescent. (**a**) In situ osteochondral fragment at medial talar dome (*arrow*). (**b**) 2D coronally reformatted CT shows sclerosis in the talus but no evidence that the fragment is fusing to adjacent bone

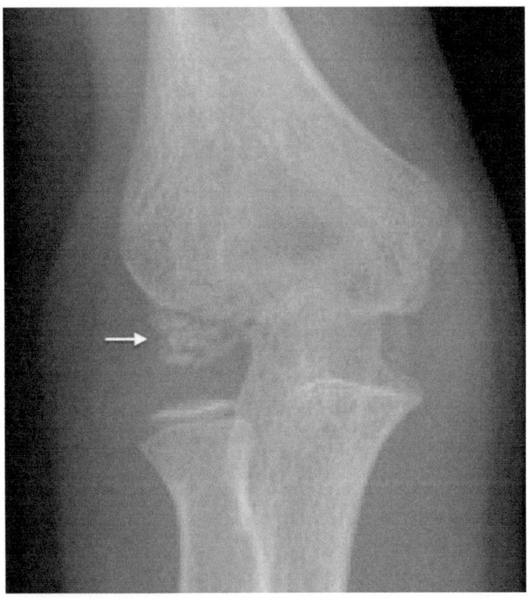

Fig. 17.36 Panner disease. The capitellum is small and fragmented (*arrow*)

7 Stress Fractures (Box 17.3)

Box 17.3: Pediatric Stress Fractures

Osseous stress fracture	
Toddler's fracture—9 months to 3 years	Tibial diaphysis Fibular diaphysis Calcaneus Cuboid Talus
Stress fracture in older child	Tibial diaphysis Fibular diaphysis Femoral diaphysis Tarsal Metatarsal
Growth cartilage stress fracture	
Older child/adolescent	Proximal tibia Distal radius and ulna Proximal humerus Distal femur

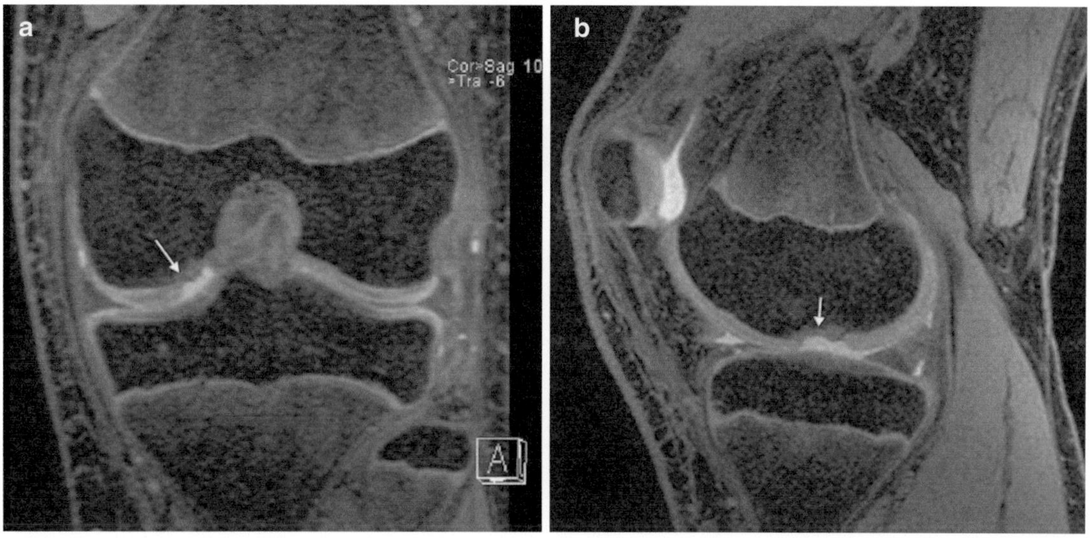

Fig. 17.37 OCD of the medial femoral condyle. Coronal (**a**) and sagittal (**b**) gadolinium-enhanced images show a largely cartilaginous defect (*arrows*), delineated by the adjacent hyperintense joint fluid

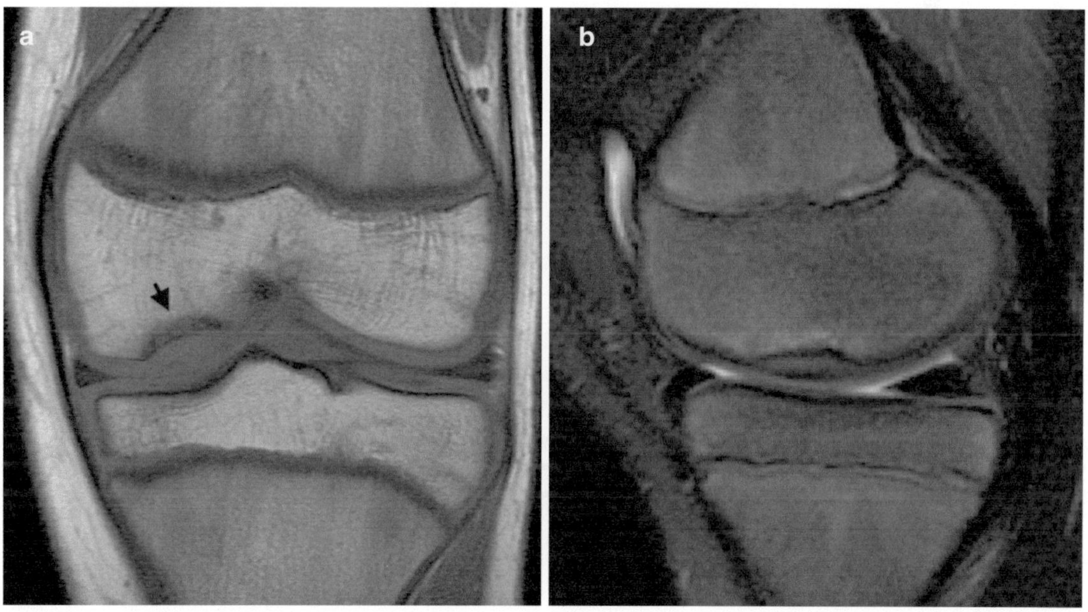

Fig. 17.38 OCD with stable in situ fragment. (**a**) Coronal T1-W image shows lenticular osseous defect along the medial femoral condyle (*arrow*). (**b**) Sagittal T2-W FS image shows in situ fragment with adjacent ill-defined hyperintense edema and intact overlying cartilage

Stress fractures in young children that are associated with the onset of ambulation are termed "*toddler's fracture*" and most commonly involve the tibia [31]. Less common locations include the fibula, calcaneus, cuboid, and talus. Toddler's fractures usually occur between 1 and 4 years of age, with history of at most minor trauma, such as a fall. Radiographs typically

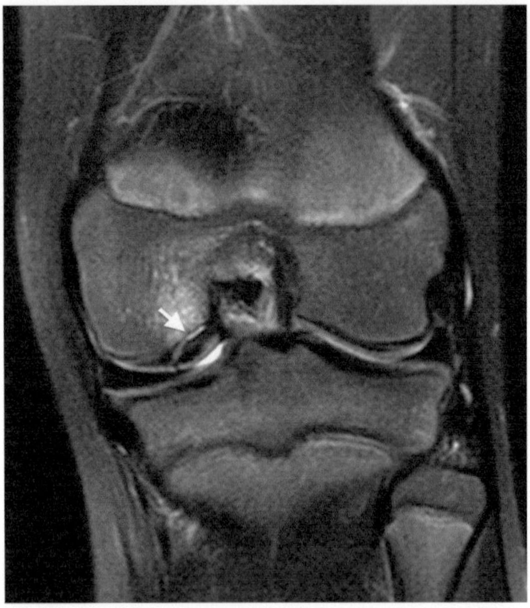

Fig. 17.39 OCD with unstable in situ fragment. Coronal T2-W FS image shows hyperintense rim of fluid (*arrow*) around the medial condylar fragment, compatible with loosening

show a non-displaced oblique fracture of the distal tibial diaphysis, but the fracture may be occult and become evident only on follow-up radiographs that show healing (Fig. 17.51).

Stress fractures in older children usually result from sports injuries but may be precipitated by abnormal weight bearing or extremity malalignment. They most commonly involve the lower limbs, including the proximal tibia, distal fibula, proximal femur, tarsal bones, and metatarsals [31]. They are most common between 10 and 15 years of age, especially in adolescent girls. This may be related to the female athlete triad, which includes disordered eating leading to decreased body mass and fat, prolonged amenorrhea resulting in decreased ovarian hormones, and osteoporosis causing increased susceptibility to stress fractures. Early diagnosis of stress injury is important to avoid progression to a complete fracture [32]. Initial radiographs have low sensitivity for stress fractures, and follow-up imaging is helpful in only 50 % of patients.

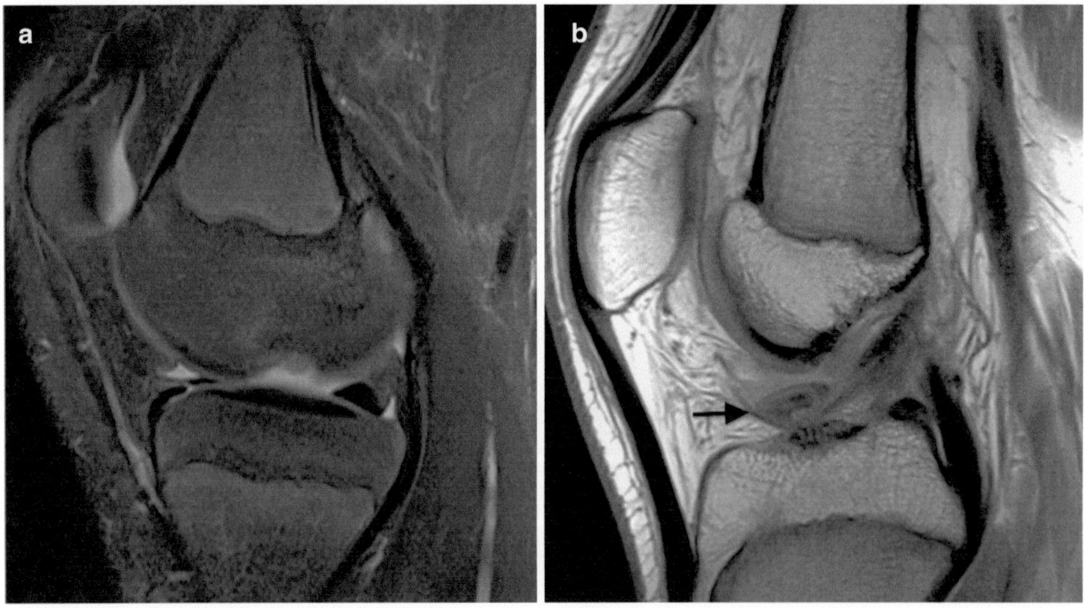

Fig. 17.40 OCD with free fragment. (**a**) Sagittal T2-W FS image shows an osteochondral defect at the medial femoral condyle. (**b**) Sagittal PD image shows the donor free fragment (*arrow*) in the intercondylar notch, anterior to the anterior cruciate ligament

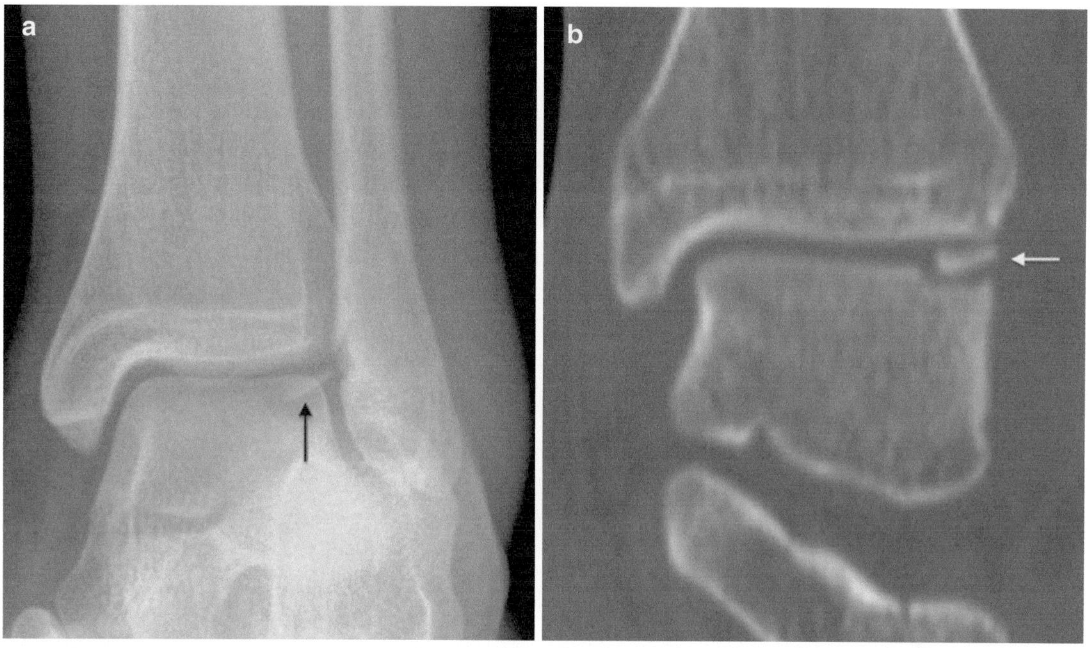

Fig. 17.41 Osteochondral lesion of talar dome. (**a**) Osteochondral fracture (*arrow*) at lateral talar dome. (**b**) 2D coronally reformatted CT shows displaced, flipped fragment (*arrow*)

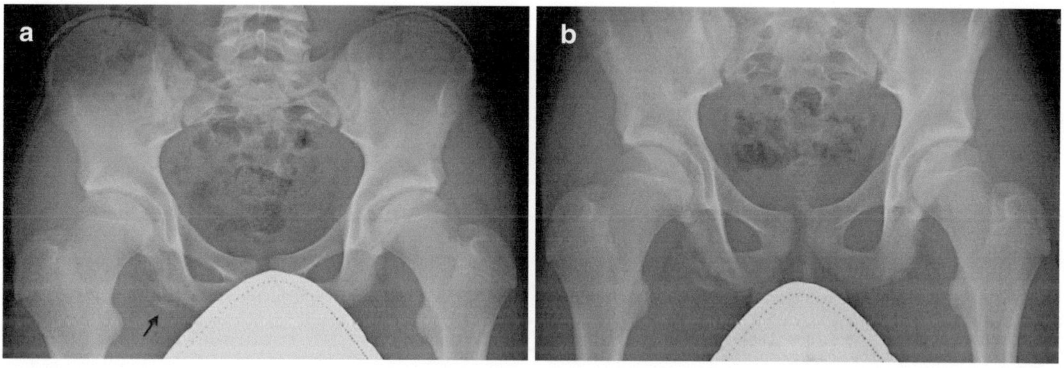

Fig. 17.42 Avulsion fracture of the ischial tuberosity in a 15-year-old male athlete. (**a**) Acute fracture of the right ischial tuberosity (*arrow*), attachment site of the hamstrings. (**b**) Four months later, abundant, irregular callus must not be mistaken for neoplasm

MRI is the best method for accurate diagnosis, with sensitivity and specificity close to 100 % [32]. Water-sensitive sequences typically show ill-defined, nonspecific hyperintense marrow and periosteal edema. Small T2-hyperintense foci or striations may be evident in the otherwise hypointense cortex due to osteopenia and bone resorption, suggesting stress injury (Fig. 17.52). A hypointense fracture line on T1-W, T2-W, or STIR sequences is diagnostic (Fig. 17.53). Fracture detection is improved with gradient echo (GRE) T1-W fat-suppressed (FS) images [32].

Repetitive injury from compressive forces may also lead to growth plate fractures. Typically

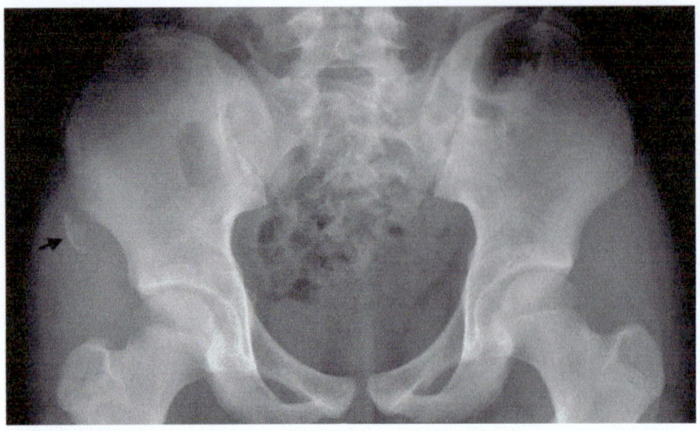

Fig. 17.43 Avulsion fracture of the right anterior-superior iliac spine (*arrow*), attachment site of the sartorius

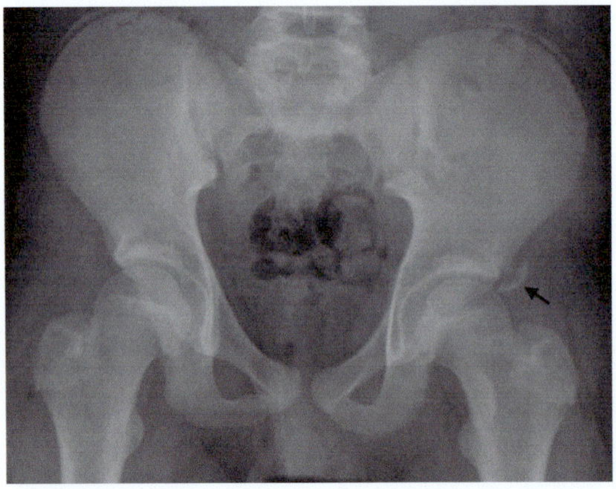

Fig. 17.44 Avulsion fracture of the left anterior-inferior iliac spine (*arrow*), attachment site of the rectus femoris

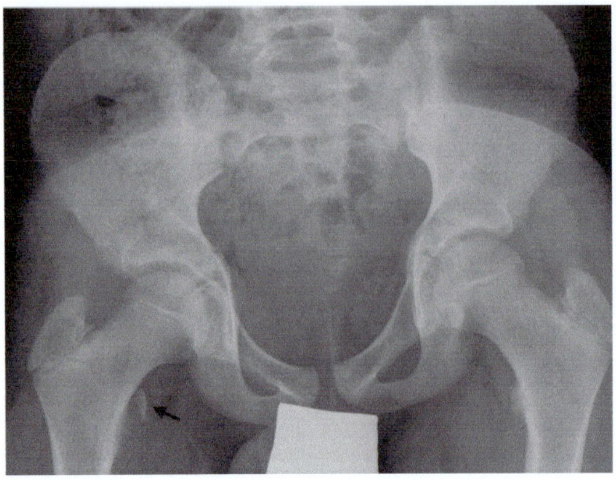

Fig. 17.45 Avulsion fracture of the lesser trochanter of the right femur (*arrow*), attachment site of the iliopsoas

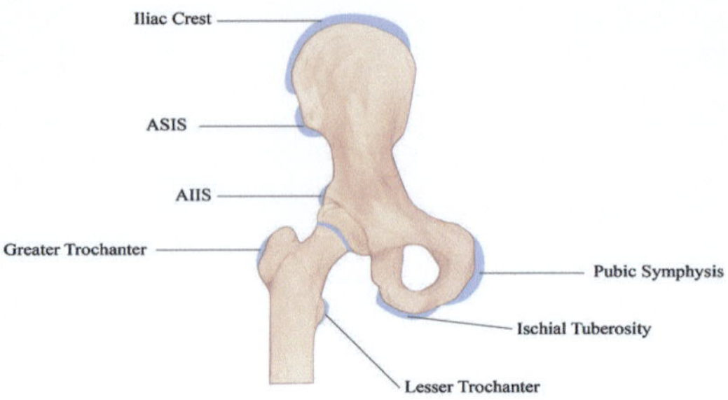

Fig. 17.46 Locations of pelvic avulsion fractures

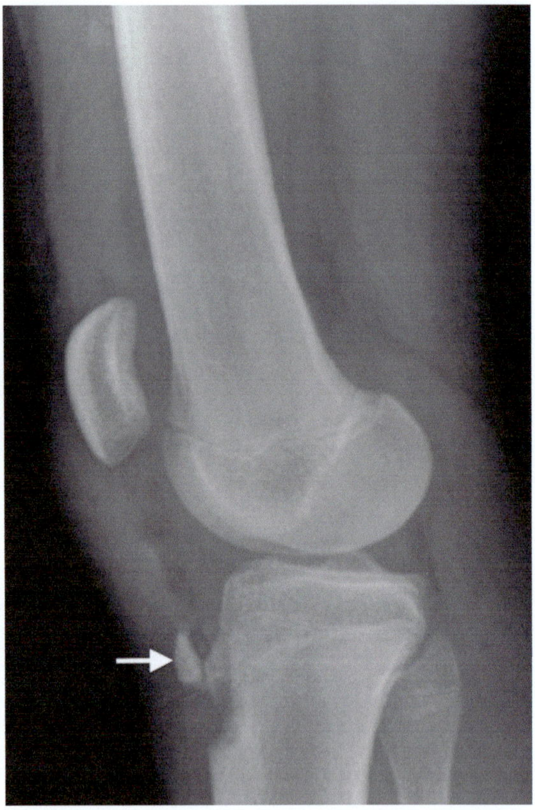

Fig. 17.47 Tibial tuberosity avulsion fracture. The fracture fragment is slightly displaced superiorly (*arrow*) and associated with patella alta and soft tissue swelling along the patellar tendon. Joint effusion

sports related, these are most common at the wrist, elbow, shoulder, and knee. The newly formed metaphyseal bone adjacent to the physis is less resistant to repetitive stress, which may alter microvascular perfusion in the metaphysis. This interferes with endochondral ossification, resulting in columns of physeal cartilage cells extending into the metaphysis [33]. The hypertrophic zone may also continue to increase in width

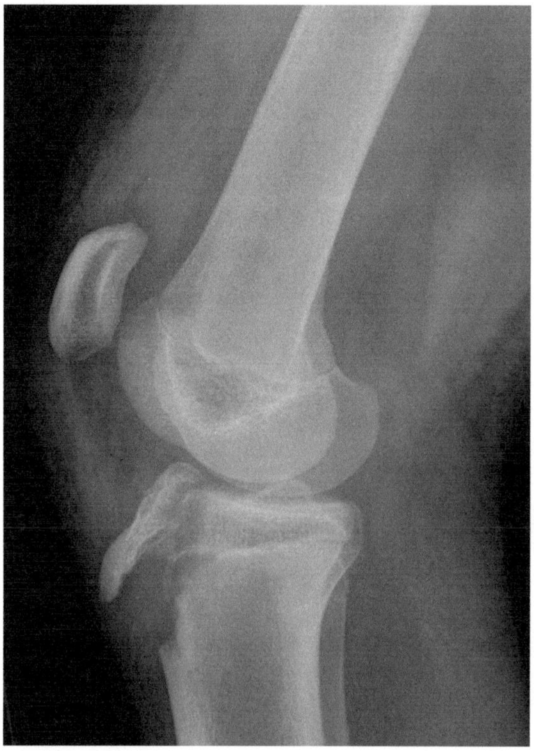

Fig. 17.48 Intra-articular fracture of tibial tuberosity. Displaced tibial tuberosity fracture, with superior extension to the articular surface. Joint effusion

due to continued growth in the germinal and proliferative zones, resulting in apparent growth plate widening. This process differs from Type I fractures, as there is no discrete fracture through the growth plate and no epiphyseal displacement. The physeal widening is usually temporary and typically heals with conservative treatment. However, there may be progressive growth plate changes, diminished growth, premature physeal closure, and resultant epiphyseal deformity [33].

These repetitive stress fractures are well documented in the distal radius in gymnasts, who often present with soft tissue swelling and wrist pain that are exacerbated by exertion. Radiographs may show bilateral distal radial growth plate widening with metaphyseal irregularity and sclerosis; similar changes may occur in the distal ulna in 20 % of cases [15]. MRI findings include diffuse growth plate thickening and irregularity, with focal areas of the physeal cartilage extending into the metaphysis (Fig. 17.54) [33]. Growth plate overuse injuries may also involve the proximal humerus of pitchers (Little Leaguer's shoulder) due to repetitive traction and rotational forces across the physis. Similar findings have been reported in other overhead sports, including cricket, gymnastics, badminton, swimming, and volleyball (adolescent athlete shoulder). Chronic physeal injuries may develop at the distal humerus and proximal radius of young baseball players and at the olecranon physis in gymnasts. Similar fractures in runners usually involve the physis of the distal femur and proximal tibia but may also occur in the distal tibia, distal fibula, and first metatarsal (Fig. 17.55). There are a few reported cases of subsequent premature closure of the proximal tibial growth plate resulting in genu varum deformity, but most of these injuries resolve with rest [33].

8 Fracture Healing and Remodeling (Box 17.4)

Box 17.4: Fracture Healing and Remodeling

Resorptive stage
- Peaks 2–3 weeks after injury
  - Widening of the fracture gap
  - Fracture becomes more ill defined

Reparative stage (temporary stabilization)
- First 2–3 months
  - Periosteal reaction
  - Early callus formation
  - Possible sclerosis along fracture margins (late)

Remodeling stage
- Begins at 8 weeks and lasts months to years
  - Increased density of callus compared to cortex
  - Incorporation of periosteal new bone
  - Bone bridging may begin

Pediatric fractures have remarkable potential to heal and remodel. Fracture healing is a continual process with overlapping histologic stages and corresponding radiographic findings, with slight

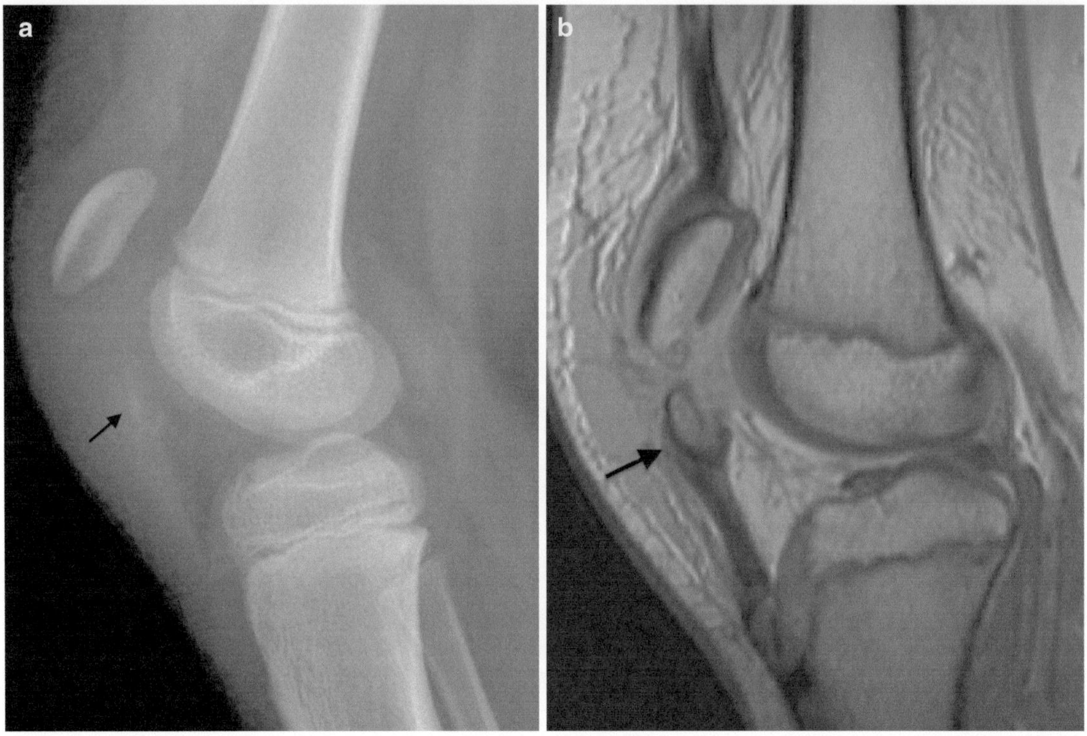

Fig. 17.49 Patellar sleeve injury. (**a**) Patella alta with marked soft tissue swelling. There is a tiny bone fragment (*arrow*). (**b**) Sagittal PD image shows a large osteochondral fragment avulsed from the inferior pole of the patella (*arrow*)

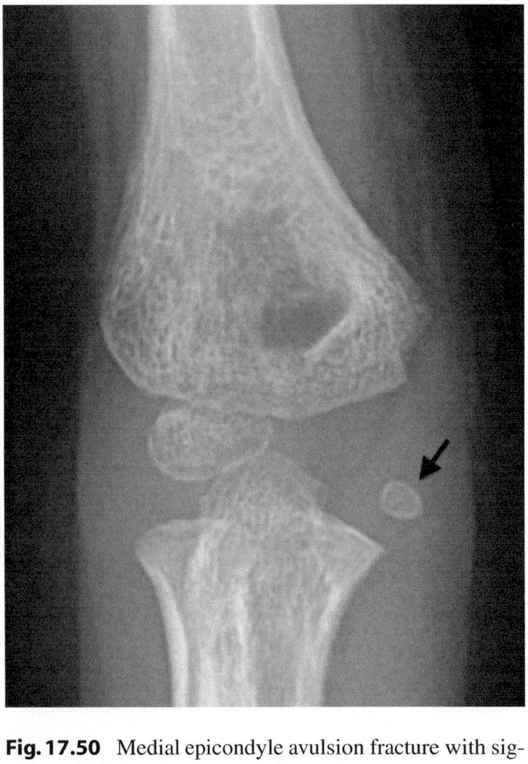

Fig. 17.50 Medial epicondyle avulsion fracture with significant inferior displacement (*arrow*)

differences in children compared to adults. During the initial resorptive phase (peaking 2–3 weeks post injury), bone disruption results in soft tissue swelling and hematoma. Fibrovascular tissue invades the hematoma, with subsequent mineralization to form primary woven bone. Since the pediatric bone is more vascular, the hyperemic response is greater in children than adults [4]. Radiographs during this stage may show widening of the fracture gap, and the fracture becomes more ill defined [34].

During the reparative phase (up to 2–3 months after injury), there is rapid bone formation, and the callus begins to develop, providing temporary stabilization [35]. Radiographic findings include periosteal reaction, early callus formation, and sclerosis along the fracture margins. The subsequent remodeling stage is the longest of the three phases, starting around 2 months and lasting months to years and sometimes until skeletal maturity. The provisional callus is gradually removed, and new compact bone is deposited along the lines of stress [4, 36]. The bone gradually remodels toward its original shape and strength [35, 36]. Radiographs show callus that may be denser than the cortex, incorporation of periosteal new bone, and osseous bridging.

Radiographic signs of bone healing have a wide variation in appearance and duration, with pediatric fractures generally healing twice as fast as adults [34]. The rate at which a fracture heals also depends on its location, with growth plate injuries healing faster than diaphyseal fractures. Growth plate fractures generally heal in 3 weeks, due to prominent vascularity and active osteogenesis in the adjacent metaphysis. In contrast, diaphyseal fractures heal more slowly, due to decreased vascularity and relatively dormant osteogenesis. Children with stable fractures are typically treated conservatively with a cast and short-term radiological follow-up to exclude displacement. Healing time and therefore immobilization time vary with age. Children younger than 10 years generally require a cast for 3–4 weeks for most fractures, whereas after age 10, 5–6 weeks of immobilization is generally necessary [7]. Indications for surgical treatment of pediatric fractures include displaced growth plate fractures or intra-articular fractures, unstable fractures, segmental fractures, open fractures, and failure to achieve adequate reduction in children older than age 10 [6].

Pediatric fractures can heal well despite striking malalignment, and fractures that initially unite with some deformity may completely remodeling phase (Fig. 17.56) [9]. The typical long bone fracture remodels primarily by reorientation of the physis (75 %) and also by appositional remodeling of the diaphysis (25 %) (Fig. 17.57) [1, 35]. Infants and young children, with more growth potential, can remodel significantly more than adolescents [7]. The potential for fracture remodeling also depends on the orientation to the joint axis, proximity to the growth plate, and specific bone involved. The so-called *bayonet displacement* (side to side displacement) corrects better than axial deviation (angulation deformity), and remodeling of rotation for practical purposes does not occur [7, 35]. The degree of angulation correction depends on fracture location: the closer the fracture is to the physis, the more angulation can be corrected. This is because the growth plate realigns to become perpendicular to the long axis of the diaphysis due to asymmetric growth of the physis [35]. The specific bone injured also determines the extent of fracture remodeling. The physes of the proximal humerus and distal radius are responsible for most growth in the upper extremity and have significant remodeling potential. In contrast, the distal humerus accounts for significantly less longitudinal growth, and its remodeling potential is limited. The lower extremities have less remodeling potential, especially at the distal femur or proximal tibia [35].

9 Complications of Pediatric Fractures (Box 17.5)

Box 17.5: Complications of Pediatric Fractures

Growth arrest	Most common sites: distal tibia, distal femur, proximal tibia
	Usually Type III to V
Malunion	Most common sites: distal humerus, diaphysis of radius and ulna
	More likely with displacement, rotation, and angulation
Nonunion	Most common site: lateral condyle
	More likely with missed fracture, inadequate reduction, late displacement
Synostosis	Most common sites: radius and ulna
	More common after high-energy trauma or surgical manipulation
	More common if joint line is offset
Osteoarthritis	Uncommon but can involve knee and ankle
	More likely with intra-articular Type III or IV fracture or OCD
Avascular necrosis	Most common site: proximal femur
	More likely with SCFE, acute femoral neck fracture, traumatic hip dislocation

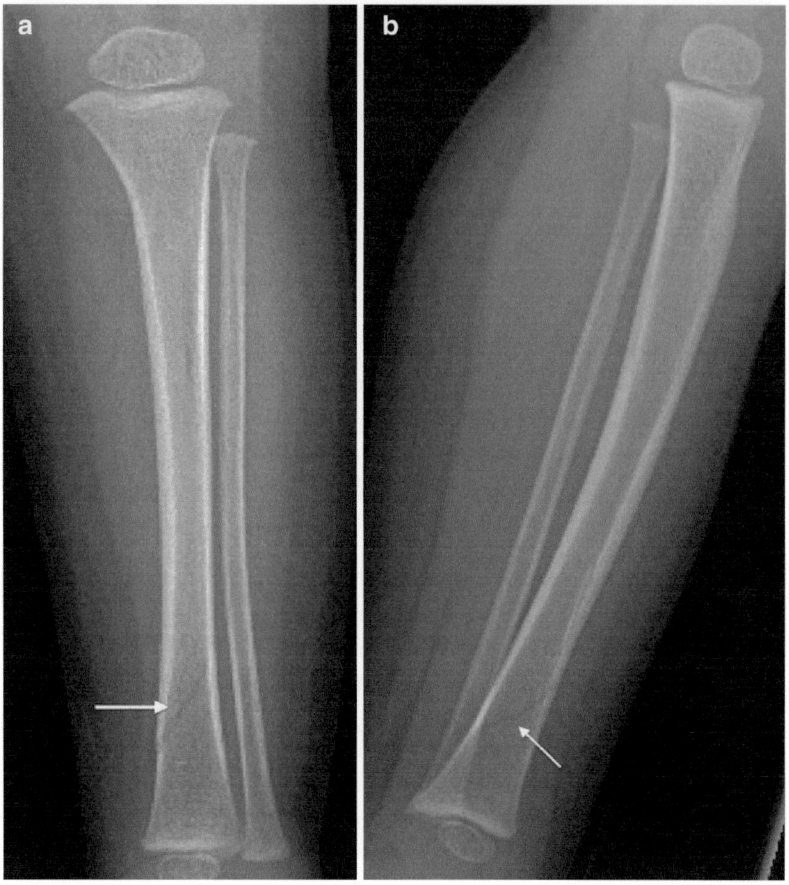

Fig. 17.51 Toddler's fracture. (**a**, **b**) Non-displaced fracture of the distal tibial diaphysis (*arrows*). Note pretibial soft tissue swelling

Malunion (Fig. 17.58) and growth arrest with resulting deformity or limb length discrepancy (Fig. 17.59) are the main complications of pediatric fractures. Nonunion and osteoarthritis are less common sequelae in children than adults [25, 35]. Of all pediatric fractures, those of the lateral condyle are most likely to result in nonunion (Fig. 17.60). Posttraumatic synostosis is rare in children but most common in the forearm, especially after high-energy trauma or surgical manipulation [3]. Other possible complications include avascular necrosis, compartment syndrome, infection, and neurovascular injury (Fig. 17.61).

Approximately 30 % of growth plate injuries will result in some form of growth arrest, but only 2 % interfere with function [15]. Premature physeal fusion usually begins 1–2 months after growth plate fracture [37]. Growth cartilage has a great capacity to recover from insults and can overcome small bony and fibrous bridges. Larger bone bridges, however, will tether the growth plate and terminate growth even in uninvolved areas. Central bridge formation generally prevents further longitudinal bone growth, whereas peripheral bridge formation may cause angular deformity.

In general, the incidence of growth arrest is highest in Type III to V fractures. Type I and II fractures tend to propagate horizontally through the hypertrophic zone, and growth usually continues without sequelae. Since in

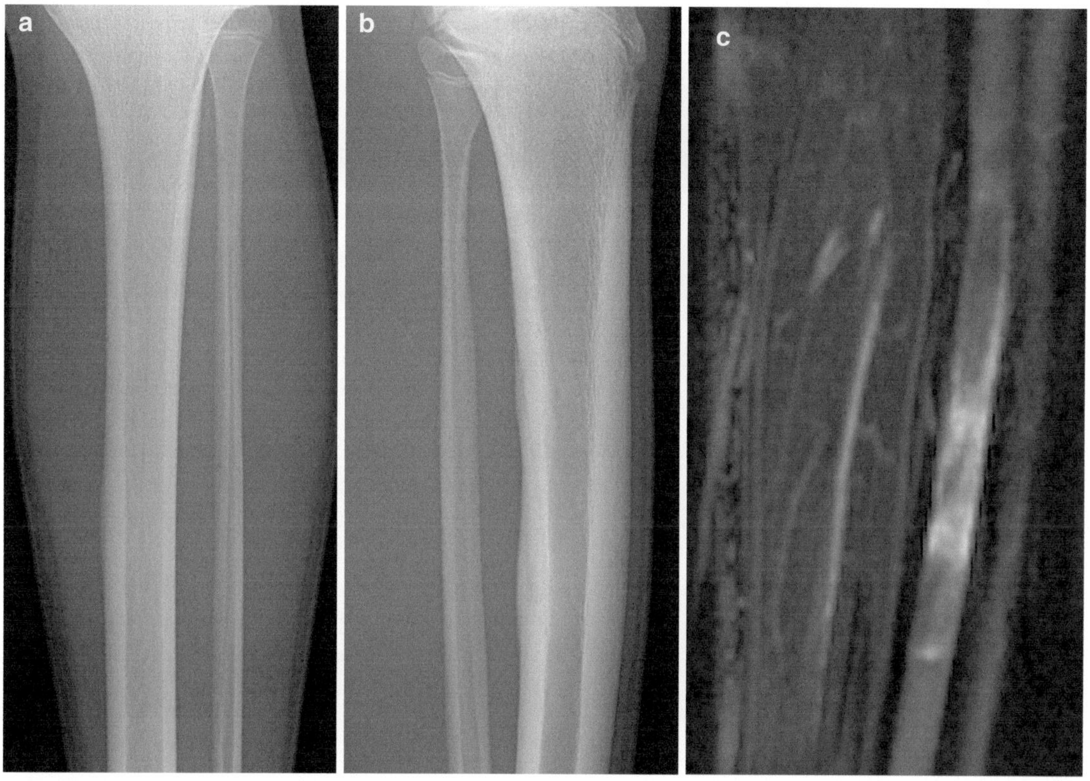

Fig. 17.52 Stress change at tibial diaphysis. (**a**, **b**) Radiographs show periosteal reaction at the medial and posterior tibial mid-diaphysis. (**c**) Sagittal T2-W FS image shows marrow edema but no discrete fracture line (Courtesy of Sandra L. Wootton-Gorges)

Type III and IV injuries the fracture extends vertically through the germinal layer of the physis to the articular surface, premature growth plate fusion and osteoarthritis may develop if anatomic reduction is not achieved. Vertical fractures extending perpendicularly through the growth plate result in bone bridge formation in 75 % of cases. This is related to development of transphyseal vessels that connect the normally separate epiphyseal and metaphyseal vessels. Osteoprogenitor cells associated with transphyseal vessels then form a bone bridge that acts as a tethering point and restricts growth [38]. In addition, unreduced step-offs in the growth plate permit direct bone-to-bone fusion between the epiphyseal ossification center and the metaphysis. In Type V fractures, severe compressive forces often cause significant increased pressure in the growth plate, leading to germinal cell death and subsequent growth arrest [2]. Type VI lesions, involving the perichondrium, may cause very peripheral bone bridging, resulting in early development of angular deformity. However, most peripheral bone bridges are due to Type I to IV injuries [39].

The prognostic implications of the Salter-Harris/Ogden classification have some limitations, as the risk of physeal arrest also depends on the child's age, fracture location, and severity of injury. Younger children have a worse prognosis because they have more growth

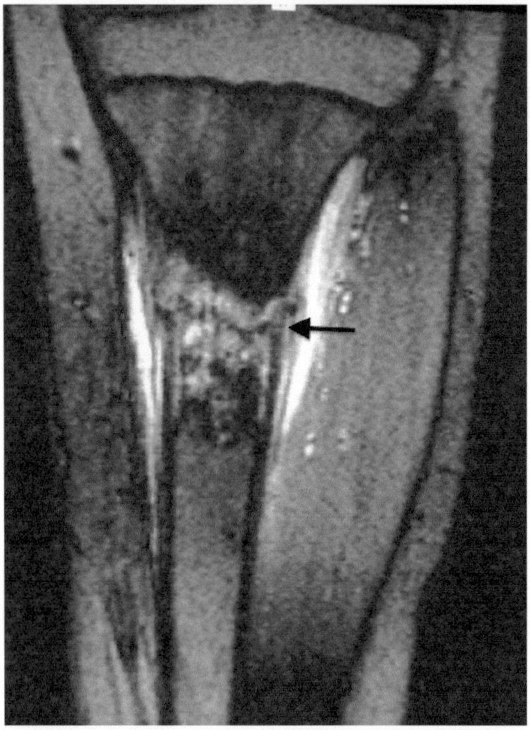

Fig. 17.53 Stress fracture of proximal tibial diaphysis. Coronal short tau inversion recovery (STIR) image shows transverse low signal line (*arrow*) with surrounding marrow edema and adjacent periosteal reaction

potential. Severe growth plate injuries, fragment displacement, and comminution are also associated with increased likelihood of growth disturbance. Physeal fractures of the distal long bones and those involving the lower extremities generally have a worse prognosis as well [6]. In the lower extremity, all physeal injuries affecting the tibia and femur have a guarded prognosis, especially fractures of the proximal femur which may develop avascular necrosis (AVN) [6].

The distal tibia is the most common site of bone bridge formation, usually at Kump's bump at the anterior-medial quadrant of the physis, where normal distal tibial physeal closure begins [13]. More than 10 % of physeal fractures involve the distal tibia, and about one third develop growth arrest. However, most of these injuries occur when the growth plate is partially closed, so they do not usually result in significant leg length discrepancy (see Chap. 16 for further discussion).

The proximal tibia and distal femur are also prone to significant complications of growth arrest. The distal femur in particular accounts

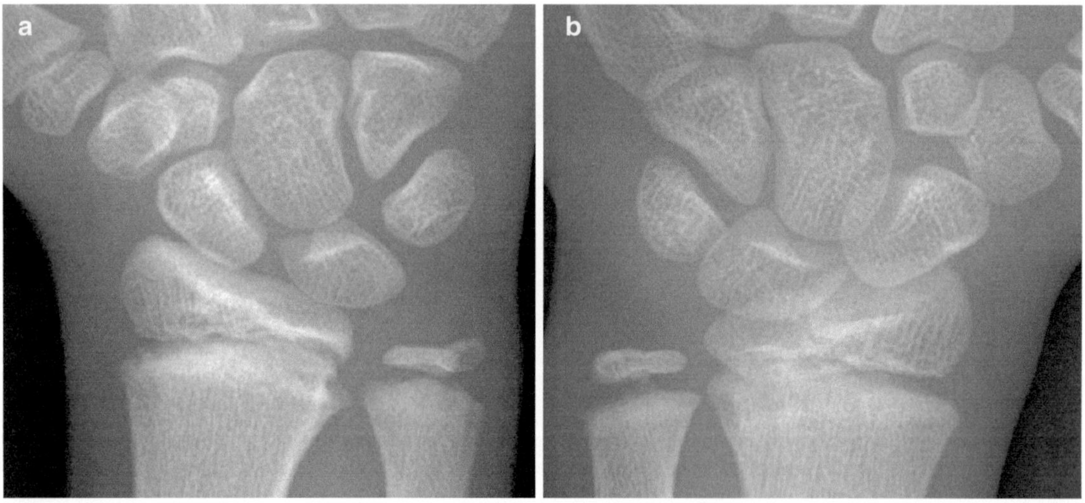

Fig. 17.54 Growth plate stress injury in gymnast. Radiographs of *right* (**a**) and *left* (**b**) wrists show bilateral irregularity, sclerosis, and growth plate widening of the distal radius and ulna. Corresponding coronal STIR images (**c**, **d**) show high signal along the growth plates and within the metaphyses

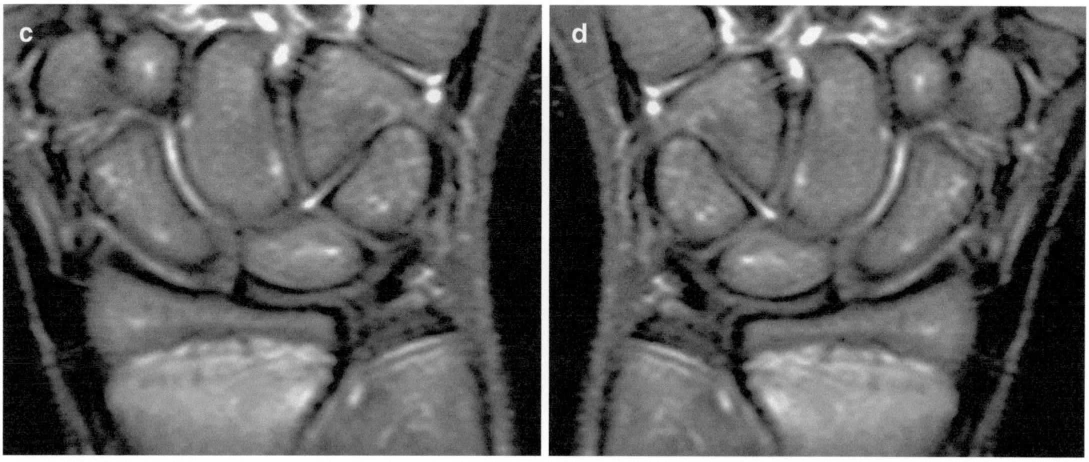

Fig. 17.54 (continued)

for only 1.4 % of growth plate fractures but has a 35 % incidence of posttraumatic bone bridge formation [27]. A central physeal undulation at the distal femoral physis is the most common site of posttraumatic closure. Even transverse distal femoral physeal fractures may affect the germinal and proliferative zones, usually at the central undulation, causing localized premature bone bridge formation. Since the distal femoral physis contributes to 70 % of longitudinal femoral growth, physeal fractures are often complicated by shortening or angular deformity (Fig. 17.62). These complications are more significant in the lower extremities. A maximum of 2 cm of limb length discrepancy is acceptable [27, 15]. Growth plate damage may become evident years after injury, and radiographic follow-up is therefore indicated until skeletal maturity [10]. Limb length discrepancy may also follow femoral diaphysis fractures, due to generalized increased blood flow to the affected limb. This stimulates the growth plates and may result in as much as 4 cm overgrowth. Long-term follow-up is usually necessary to monitor healing and growth, with radiographs of both limbs at 3–6 month intervals, for at least 2 years [4, 35].

10 Complications of Growth Plate Injury (Box 17.6)

Box 17.6: Imaging Findings of Growth Arrest

Radiographs	
Early	Physeal widening or narrowing
3 months post trauma	Bone bridge
	Loss of continuity of radiolucent growth plate
	Localized metaphyseal or epiphyseal sclerosis
	Tethered growth recovery lines
Long term	*Central bridge*
	Limb shortening
	Metaphyseal cupping
	Peripheral bridge
	Angulation deformity
MRI	Premature physeal bridges
	Appearance depends on size and composition
	Large bone bridge containing marrow fat: hyperintense on T1
	Small bone or fibrous bridges: usually hypointense on all sequences
	All bridges on GRE: hypointense segment interrupting hyperintense physis

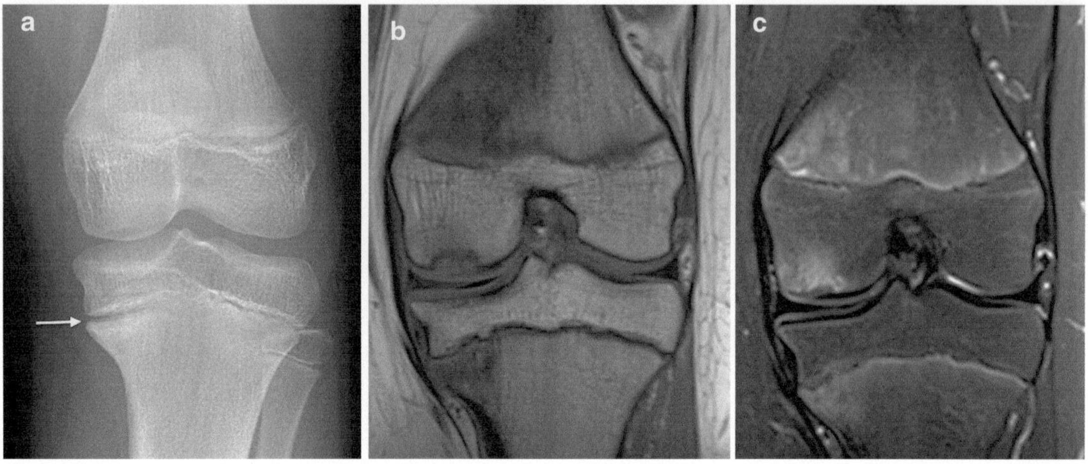

Fig. 17.55 Repetitive stress injury of the distal femur and proximal tibia in a runner. (**a**) Medial growth plate widening (*arrow*) and metaphyseal sclerosis of the proximal tibia. Coronal T1-W image (**b**) shows hypointensity at the medial physis and adjacent metaphysis of the distal femur and proximal tibia, with corresponding hyperintensity on STIR (**c**). Note OCD in the medial femoral condyle

Around 3 months after injury, radiographs often show initial findings suggesting growth arrest or bone bridging. These findings include growth plate narrowing and interruption of the radiolucent growth plate. Central bridge formation may progress to metaphyseal cupping and limb shortening (Fig. 17.63), and peripheral bridging may cause angulation of the growth plate and articular surface (Fig. 17.64) [7].

Bone bridges are also commonly associated with tethered growth recovery lines. Undistorted growth recovery lines appear as thin disks of transversely oriented bony trabeculae (unlike the usual longitudinally oriented trabeculae). These disks form at the physis during slowed growth because of fracture, immobilization, or illness and typically appear within 12 weeks of injury. If normal, symmetric growth resumes, growth recovery lines appear to move deeper into the metaphysis, away from—but staying parallel to—the physis. However, if a growth recovery line appears angled relative to the physis, its normal migration has been tethered by a bone bridge. This is an early radiographic indication of impending deformity. If growth recovery lines are tilted, curved, or absent, growth disturbance is likely (Fig. 17.65) [15].

Bone bridges may be missed on radiographs, and children at increased risk of growth arrest may benefit from cross-sectional imaging, preferably with MRI [11]. This technique is particularly helpful for precise determination of the location and extent of a bone bridge. The appearance depends on the composition of the bone bridge as well as its size. Larger bone bridges that contain marrow fat are hyperintense on T1-W and proton density (PD) images (Fig. 17.66). Smaller osseous or fibrous bridges have a variable appearance but are usually hypointense on all sequences. Bone bridges also demonstrate a hypointense segment that interrupts the hyperintense growth plate on T2-W and GRE images (Fig. 17.67). 3D volumetric images with axial maximum intensity projection (MIP) maps of the physis may be obtained using FS SPGR sequences with 1 mm or less slice thickness [39]. This helps demonstrate the exact location of the bridge as well as the percentage of the growth plate involved. Bridges involving less than 50 % of the physis have a good prognosis for growth resumption after surgical resection in children with 2 or more years of remaining growth [6, 29, 32]. A tethered growth recovery line is best seen on

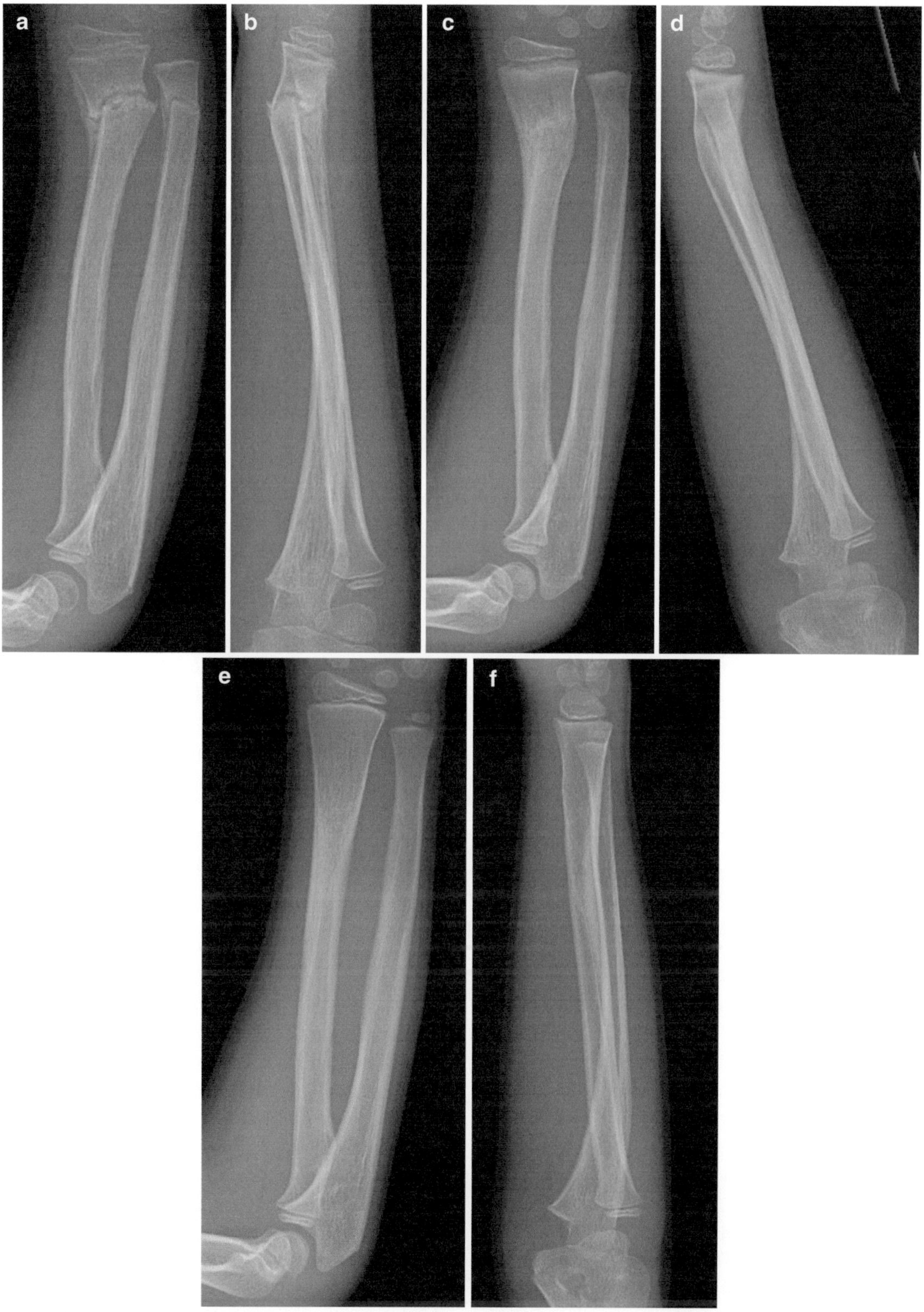

Fig. 17.56 Progressive healing and remodeling of displaced, angulated fracture. One month (**a**, **b**), 3 months (**c**, **d**), and 5 months (**e**, **f**) post injury

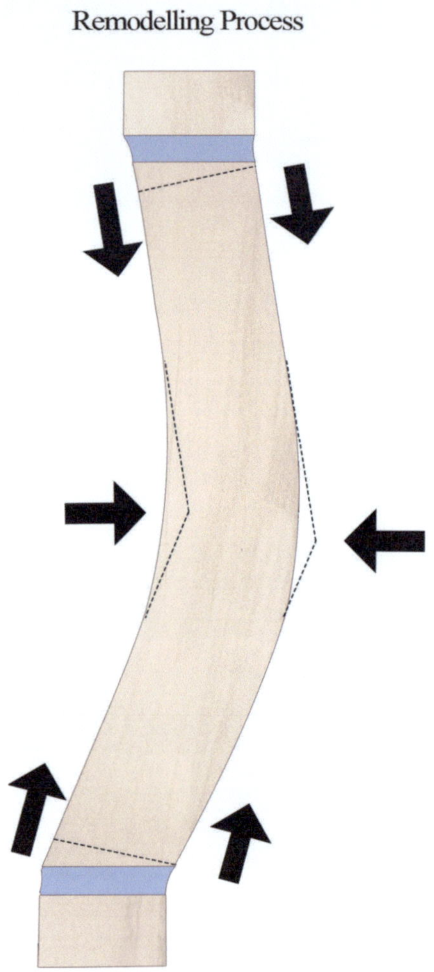

Fig. 17.57 Long bone fracture remodeling occurs by reorientation to the growth plate and appositional remodeling (Adapted from [1])

T1-W images as a thin, hypointense line contrasted with surrounding normal hyperintense fatty marrow (Fig. 17.68) [13].

Other abnormalities associated with posttraumatic growth arrest include cartilaginous rests and avascular necrosis. Cartilaginous rests represent persistent cartilage in abnormal locations, usually within the metaphysis. A consequence of vascular injury and secondary temporary disruption of endochondral ossification, they are most often associated with Type II and IV fractures. These cartilage rests appear as T2-hyperintense foci, with similar signal to the growth plate. Several different patterns are seen on MRI, including focal intrusions of the growth plate into the metaphysis, widening and irregularity of the growth plate, and small cartilage islands trapped within the epiphysis (Fig. 17.69) [37].

Devascularized bone fragments may be found in 15 % of patients with posttraumatic growth arrest, most often in the distal femur and proximal tibia. These areas of infarction typically appear as wedge-shaped regions of fatty marrow signal with hypointense peripheral sclerosis, positioned between the fracture line and the physis (Fig. 17.70) [27]. Avascular necrosis of metaphyseal bone fragments may cause persistent pain at the site of injury and also impair healing, resulting in growth disturbance [15]. Epiphyseal injury may lead to decreased epiphyseal size and avascular necrosis. If the vascular supply of the epiphysis is injured, the normally hyperintense fatty marrow of the epiphysis may become hypointense on T1-W imaging (Fig. 17.71).

Although delayed union or nonunion is often assessed only on radiographs, MRI may suggest abnormal fracture healing. Persistent hyperintensity along fracture margins suggests cartilage and granulation tissue within callus [10].

11 Patterns of Pediatric Articular Trauma

Lipohemarthrosis implies the presence of an intra-articular fracture that has allowed marrow fat to enter the joint, although this finding may alternatively be caused by capsular/ligamentous tears or extensive para-articular soft tissue trauma [40]. Lipohemarthrosis is most common in the knee, but can also be identified in the elbow and shoulder. A fat-blood level may be seen in about 35 % of intra-articular fractures at the knee, most often associated with tibial plateau fractures. A horizontal beam radiograph demonstrates a horizontal interface between lucent fat (above) and dense hemorrhagic fluid (below) (Fig. 17.72).

Ligament injury is relatively uncommon in children, as pediatric ligaments are elastic. Instead, avulsion fractures typically occur.

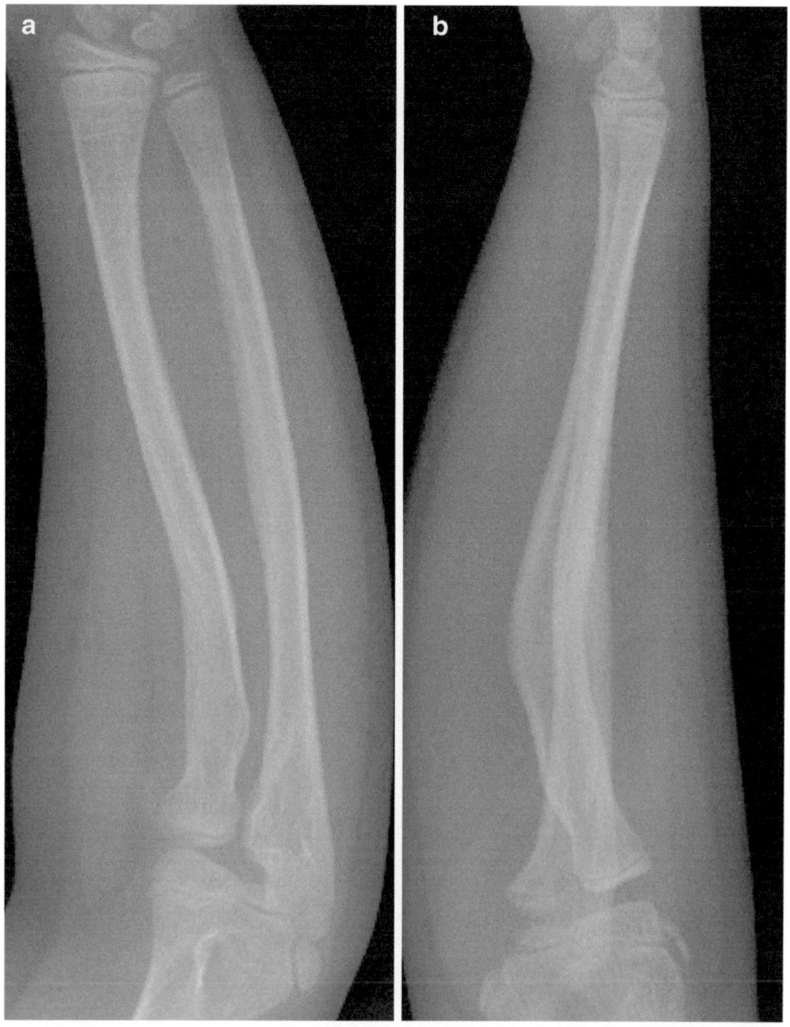

Fig. 17.58 Malunion. (**a**, **b**) A fracture of the radial diaphysis has healed with significant residual anterior-medial bowing. Mild medial bowing of the ulna

These are usually seen at the osseous insertion of ligaments, although if the fragment is unossified, it may be radiographically occult. This injury can occur in all joints but is most common in the knee, ankle, and elbow. The anterior cruciate ligament (ACL) is the most commonly injured ligament in the pediatric knee. In children less than 11 years old, ACL injury usually occurs at the ligament's insertion into the tibial spine, resulting from failure of the incompletely ossified tibial eminence. These subtle fractures may not be evident on standard radiographs, and a tunnel view may be helpful. MRI shows the fragment of the avulsed tibial spine (Fig. 17.73), attached to an abnormally T2-hyperintense ACL. True ACL tears occur later in adolescence and are much more common in girls (see Chap. 14). Posterior cruciate ligament (PCL) tears are uncommon in children and are usually associated with a tear of the ACL or collateral ligaments or with posterior-lateral injury (Fig. 17.74).

Dislocation of an otherwise normal joint is uncommon in children, as pediatric capsular and ligamentous structures are two to five times stronger than bones. The elbow is most often dislocated, with incidence peaking at 10–15 years of age. Elbow dislocations usually occur in a posterior or posterolateral direction and may be associated with medial epicondyle, coronoid, or radial neck fractures (Fig. 17.75). The Monteggia fracture-dislocation complex

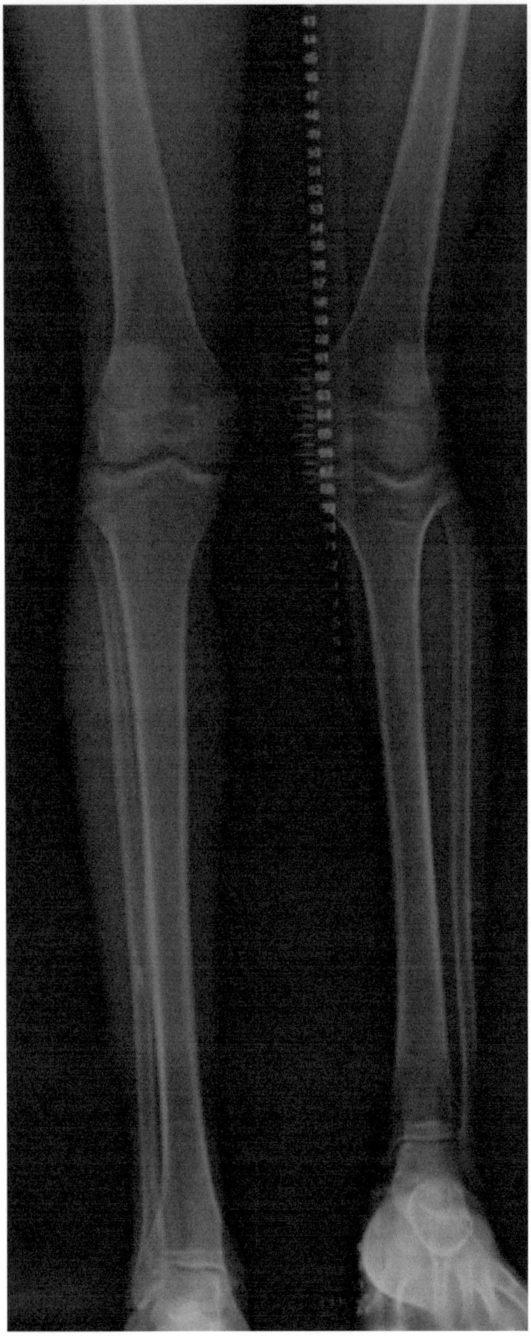

Fig. 17.59 Leg length discrepancy related to growth arrest from prior left proximal tibial growth plate fracture. Genu valgum deformity and shortening of the left leg

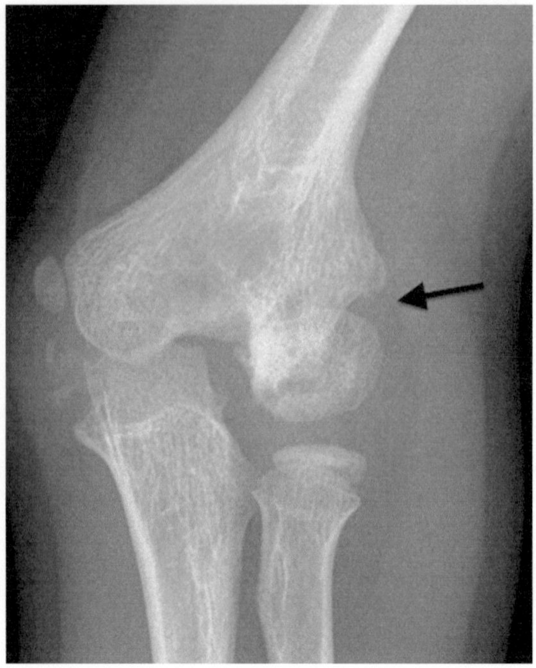

Fig. 17.60 Nonunion. There is a residual fracture cleft (*arrow*) through the lateral condyle and deformity of the distal humerus with cubitus valgus

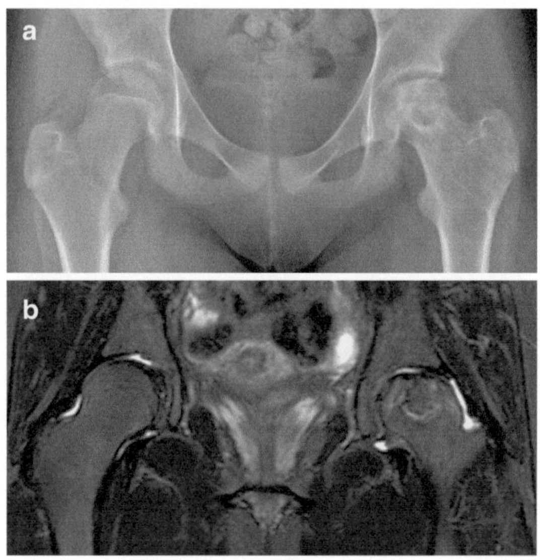

Fig. 17.61 Avascular necrosis (AVN) of the femoral head due to previous femoral neck fracture. (**a**) Lysis and sclerosis on the left, with subchondral collapse. Residual screw tracts from prior hardware. (**b**) Coronal STIR image shows hyperintense ringlike area, compatible with AVN

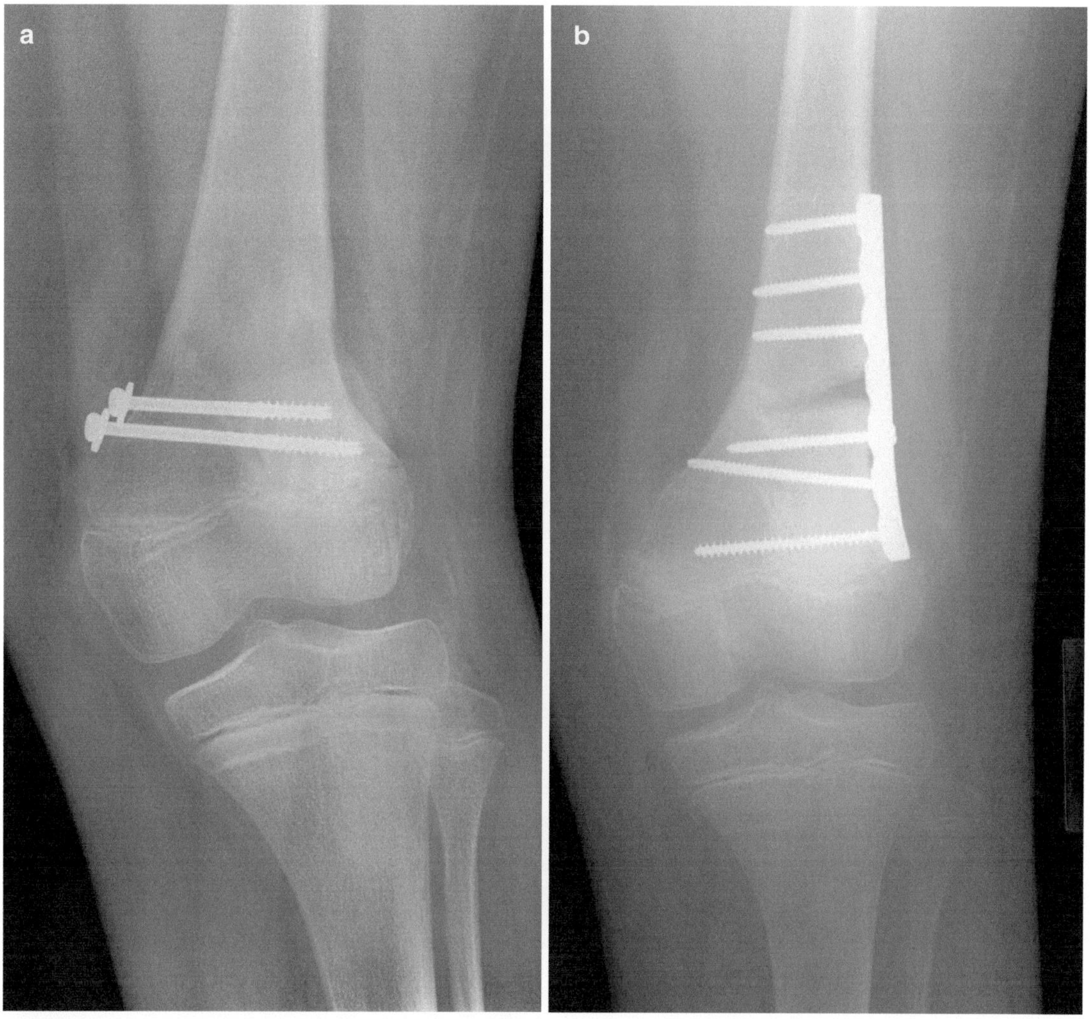

Fig. 17.62 Angular deformity after a 9-year-old girl suffered a Type II distal femoral fracture that was operatively reduced and fixated. (**a**) Growth arrest at the lateral femur causes valgus deformity at the physis. (**b**) Correcting wedge osteotomy (Courtesy of Sandra L. Wootton-Gorges)

(Fig. 17.76) is much more common in children than adults, with a peak incidence at 5–7 years of age [5]. This consists of radial head dislocation with a proximal ulnar fracture. Galeazzi fracture-dislocation is uncommon in children and usually occurs at a slightly older age, with a peak incidence at 9–12 years of age. It consists of dislocation of the distal radial-ulnar joint along with a radial fracture (see Chap. 8 for further discussion).

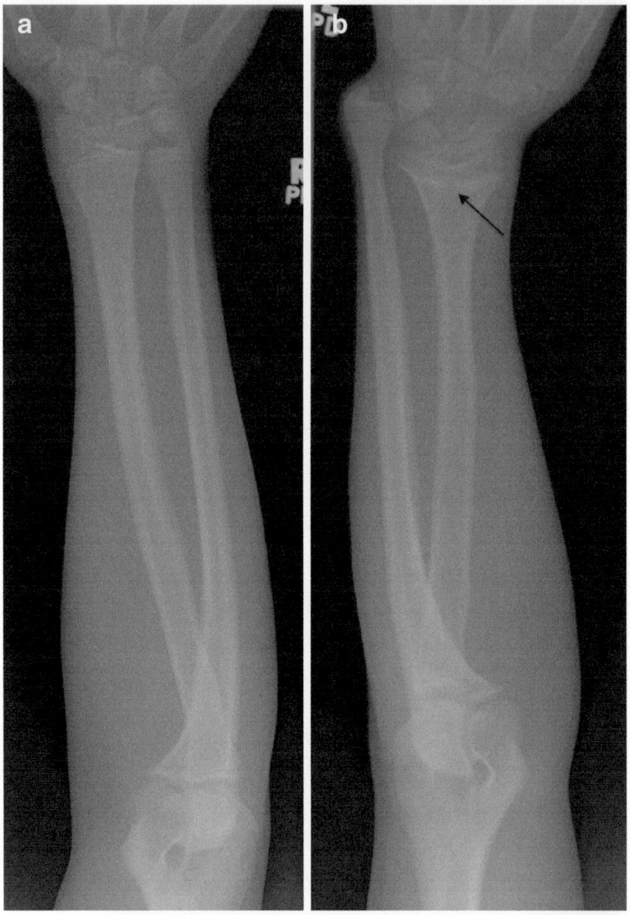

Fig. 17.63 Premature fusion of the central growth plate. (**a**) Normal left side (for comparison). (**b**) Metaphyseal cupping (*arrow*) with impaired growth of the right radius results in ulnar plus deformity

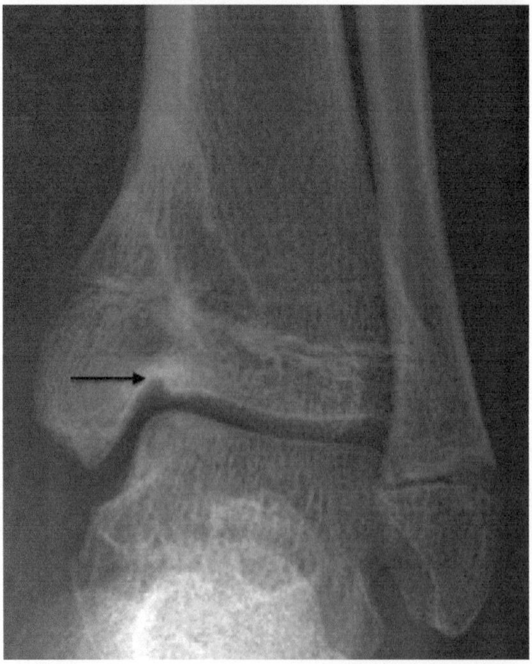

Fig. 17.64 Angular deformity at healed type IV fracture. Premature fusion of the medial physis causes varus deformity and irregularity (*arrow*) along the medial tibial plafond

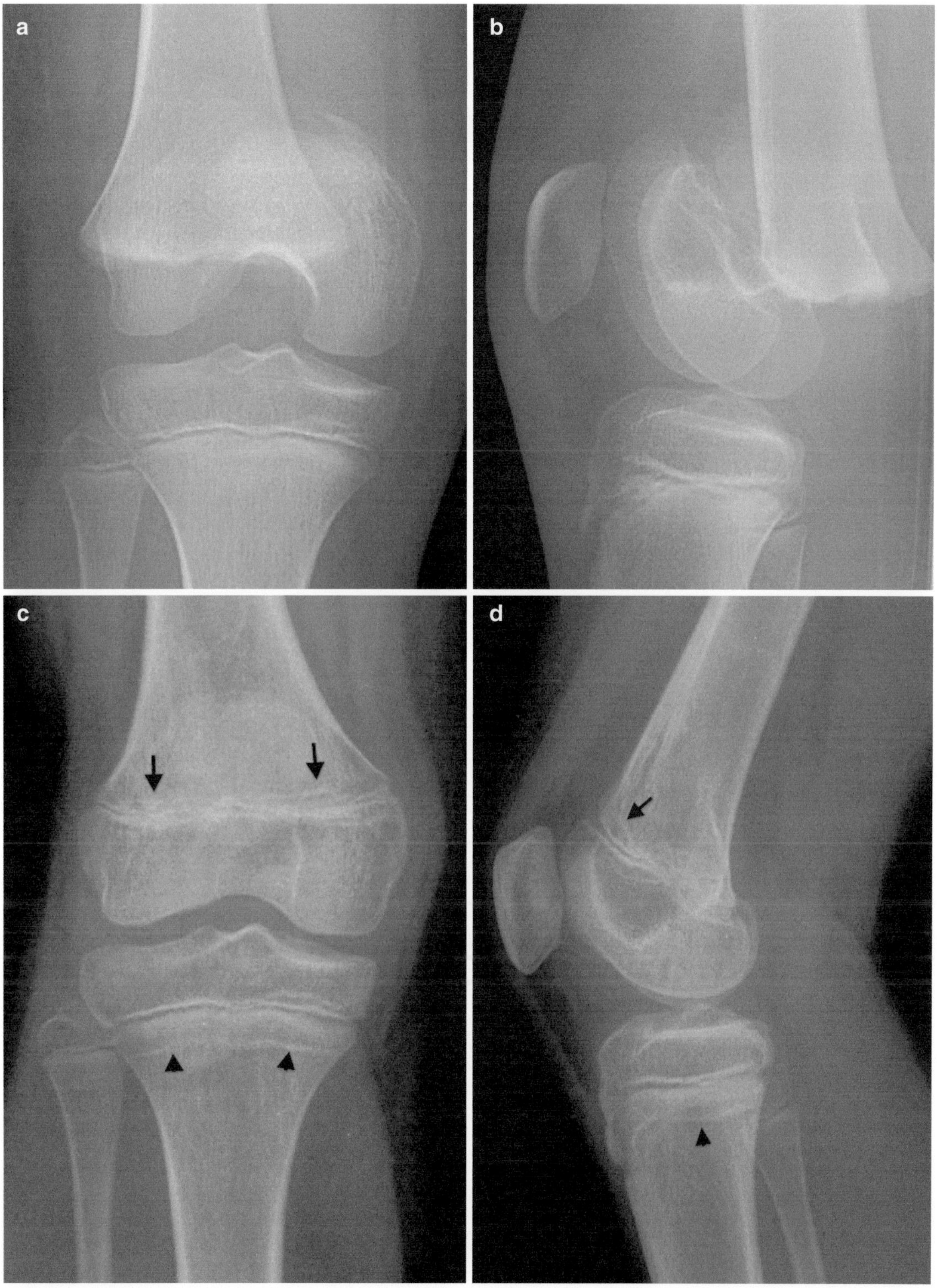

Fig. 17.65 Growth arrest after Type II fracture of the distal femur. (**a**, **b**) Immediately post trauma, there is significant angulation and displacement of the distal femoral epiphysis and metaphyseal fragment. (**c**, **d**) After reduction and healing, there is thinning and poor visualization of the central and posterior aspects of the distal femoral growth plate, suspicious for premature fusion. Compared to the growth recovery line at the proximal tibia (*arrowheads*), that at the distal femur is incomplete, slightly angulated, and closer to the physis (*arrows*)

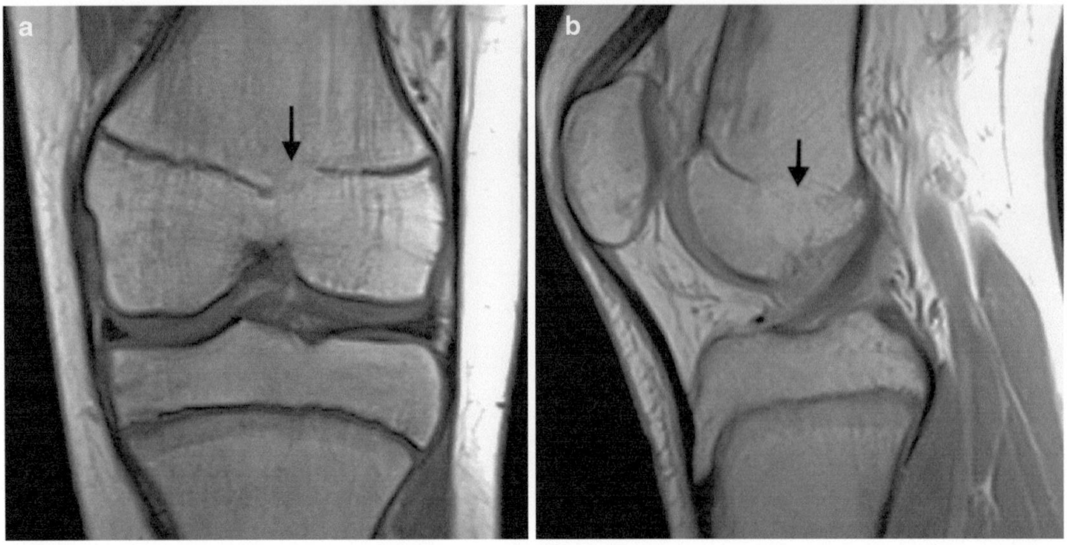

Fig. 17.66 Partial premature fusion of the distal femoral growth plate. Coronal T1-W (**a**) and sagittal PD (**b**) images show loss of the normal physis due to a bone bridge, hyperintense due to marrow fat (*arrows*)

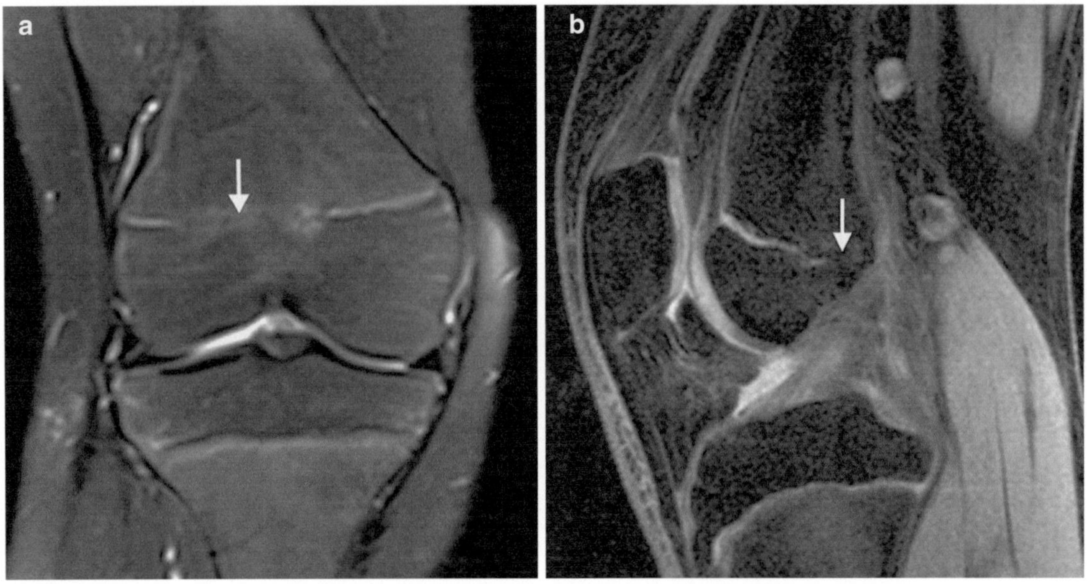

Fig. 17.67 Bone bridge formation at distal femur. Coronal FSE T2-W FS (**a**) and sagittal multi-echo data image combination (MEDIC) gradient echo (GRE) (**b**) images show interruption of the normal hyperintense growth plate, centrally and posteriorly (*arrows*)

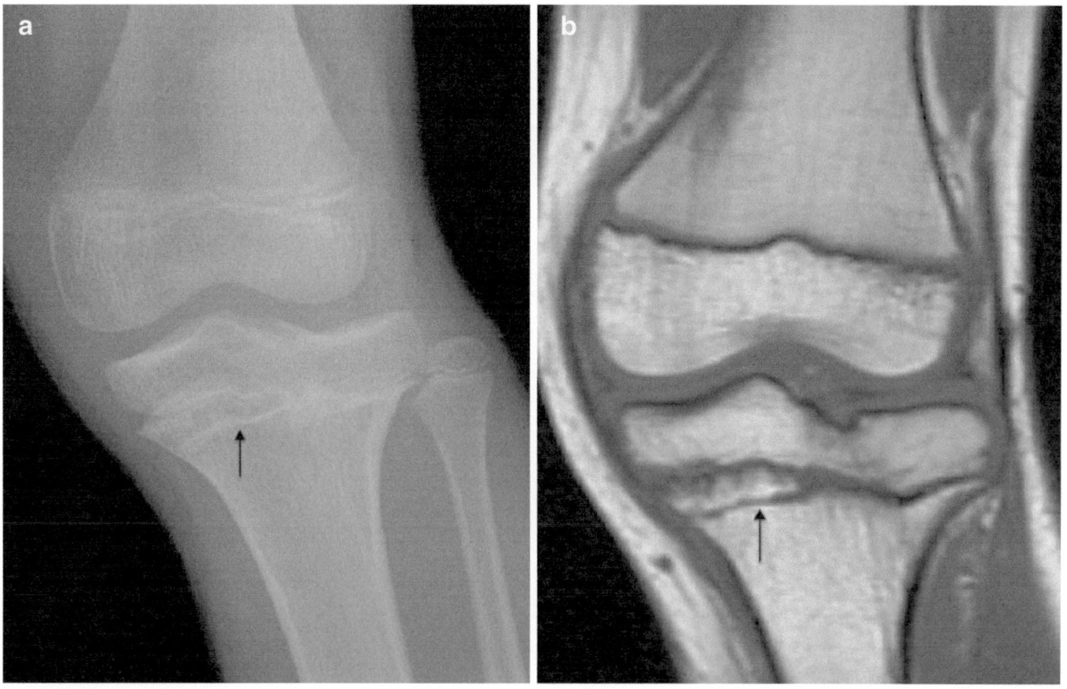

Fig. 17.68 Angular deformity of proximal tibia related to prior fracture. (**a**) Incomplete growth recovery line (*arrow*) with deformity of lateral tibial epiphysis. (**b**) Coronal T1-W MRI shows premature fusion of the lateral aspect of the proximal tibial growth plate and tethered growth arrest line (*arrow*)

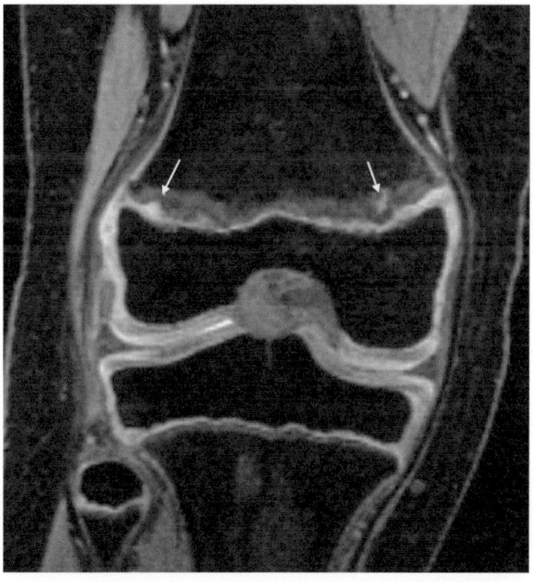

Fig. 17.69 Cartilage rests after Type I distal femoral fracture. Coronal dual echo steady state (DESS) MR image shows hyperintense cartilage intrusions into metaphysis (*arrows*)

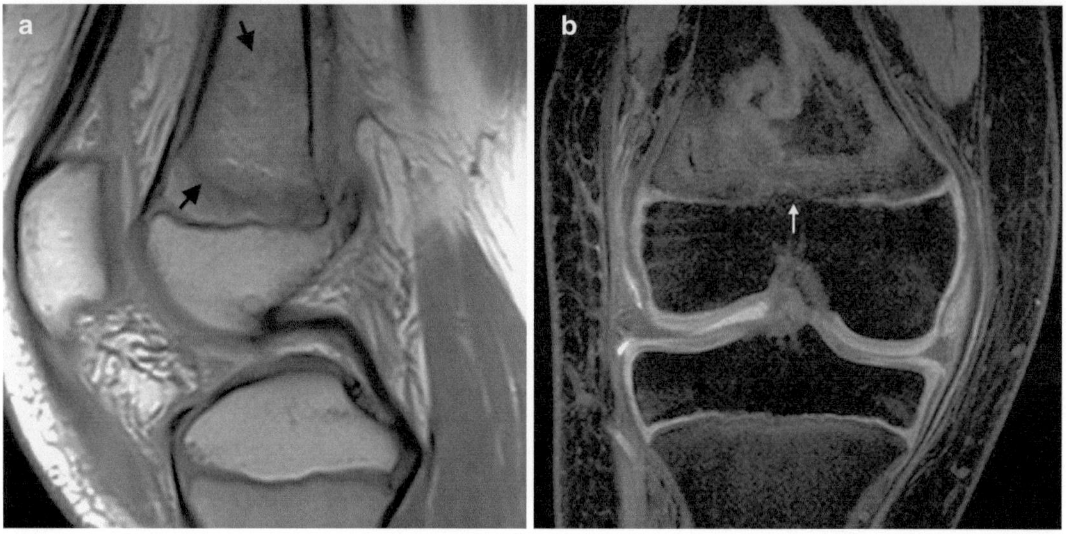

Fig. 17.70 Postfracture bone infarct. Sagittal PD (**a**) and coronal T2-W FS (**b**) images show an irregular, ringlike area in the distal femoral metaphysis with internal fatty signal, suggestive of infarction (*black arrows*). Note central bone bridge at distal femoral physis (*white arrow*)

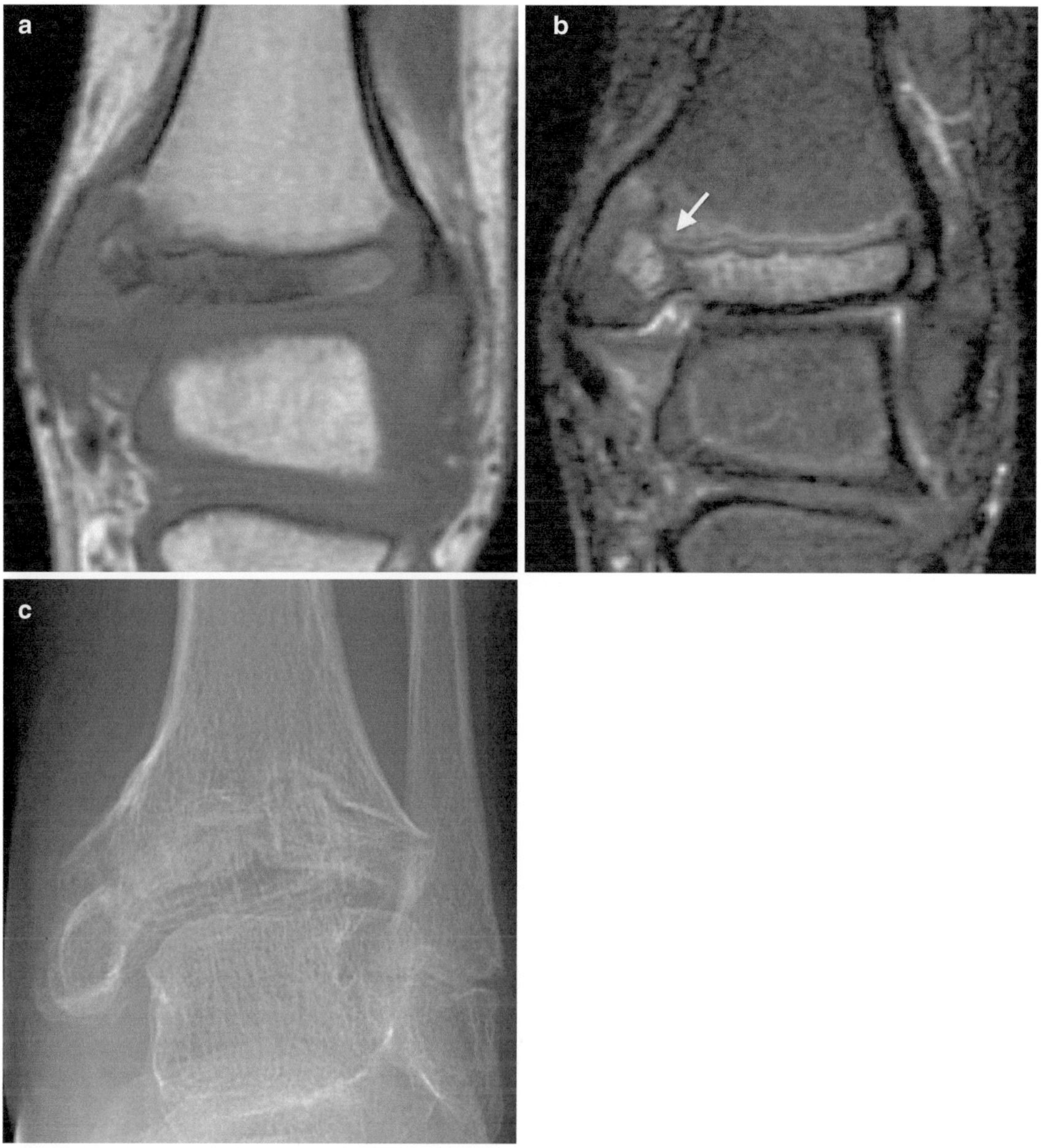

Fig. 17.71 Type IV fracture complicated by growth arrest and avascular necrosis. (**a**) Coronal T1-W MRI shows diffuse hypointensity at distal tibial epiphysis, with superior displacement of medial malleolus (reduction had been incomplete). (**b**) T2-W FS MRI shows corresponding hyperintensity, with a medial bone bridge (*arrow*) causing mild angular deformity. (**c**) Subsequent radiograph shows irregularity and collapse of the distal tibial epiphysis, compatible with AVN

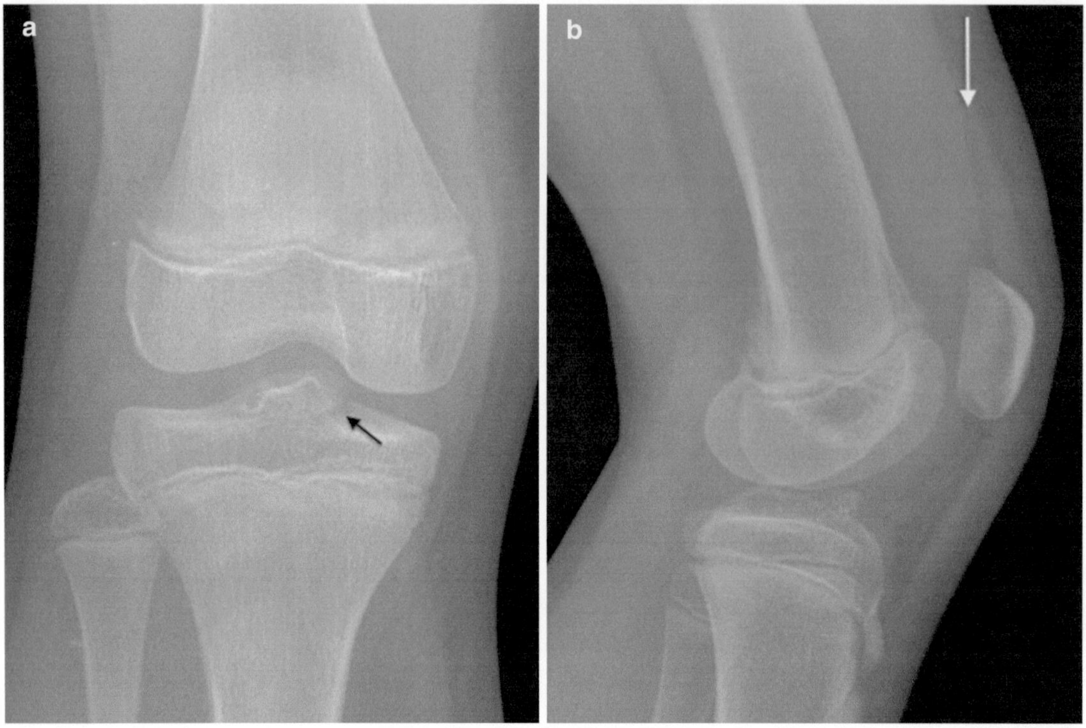

Fig. 17.72 Lipohemarthrosis. (**a**) Tibial spine avulsion fracture (*black arrow*). (**b**) Fat-fluid level (*white arrow*) on cross-table lateral, due to lipohemarthrosis (*white arrow*)

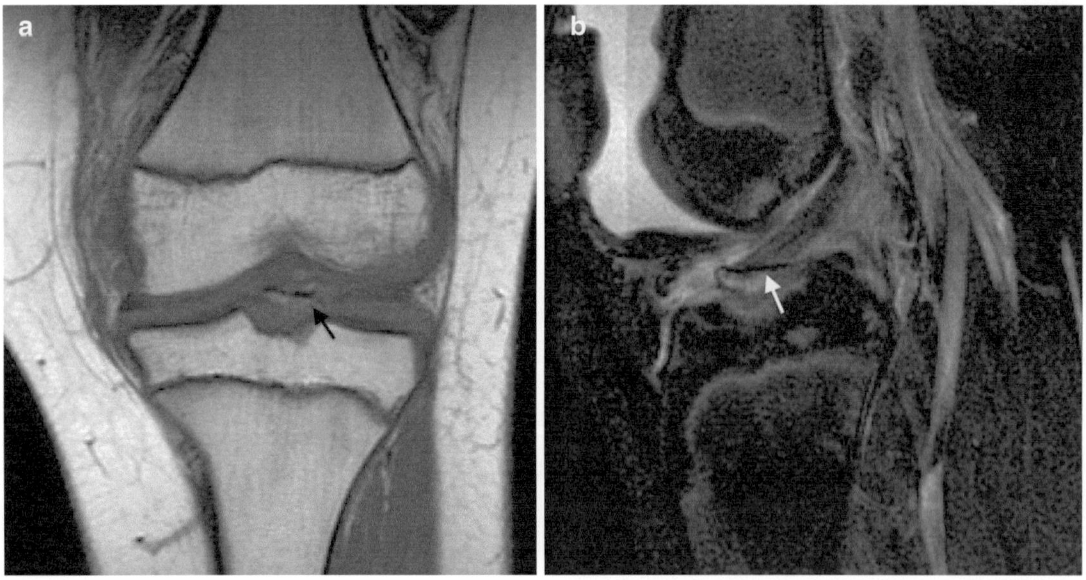

Fig. 17.73 Anterior cruciate ligament (ACL) injury at the tibial spine insertion. (**a**) Coronal T1-W image shows a small fracture fragment contiguous with the avulsed ACL (*arrow*). (**b**) Sagittal FSE T2-W FS MRI shows the fracture fragment (*arrow*), along with a fluid-fluid level due to hemarthrosis

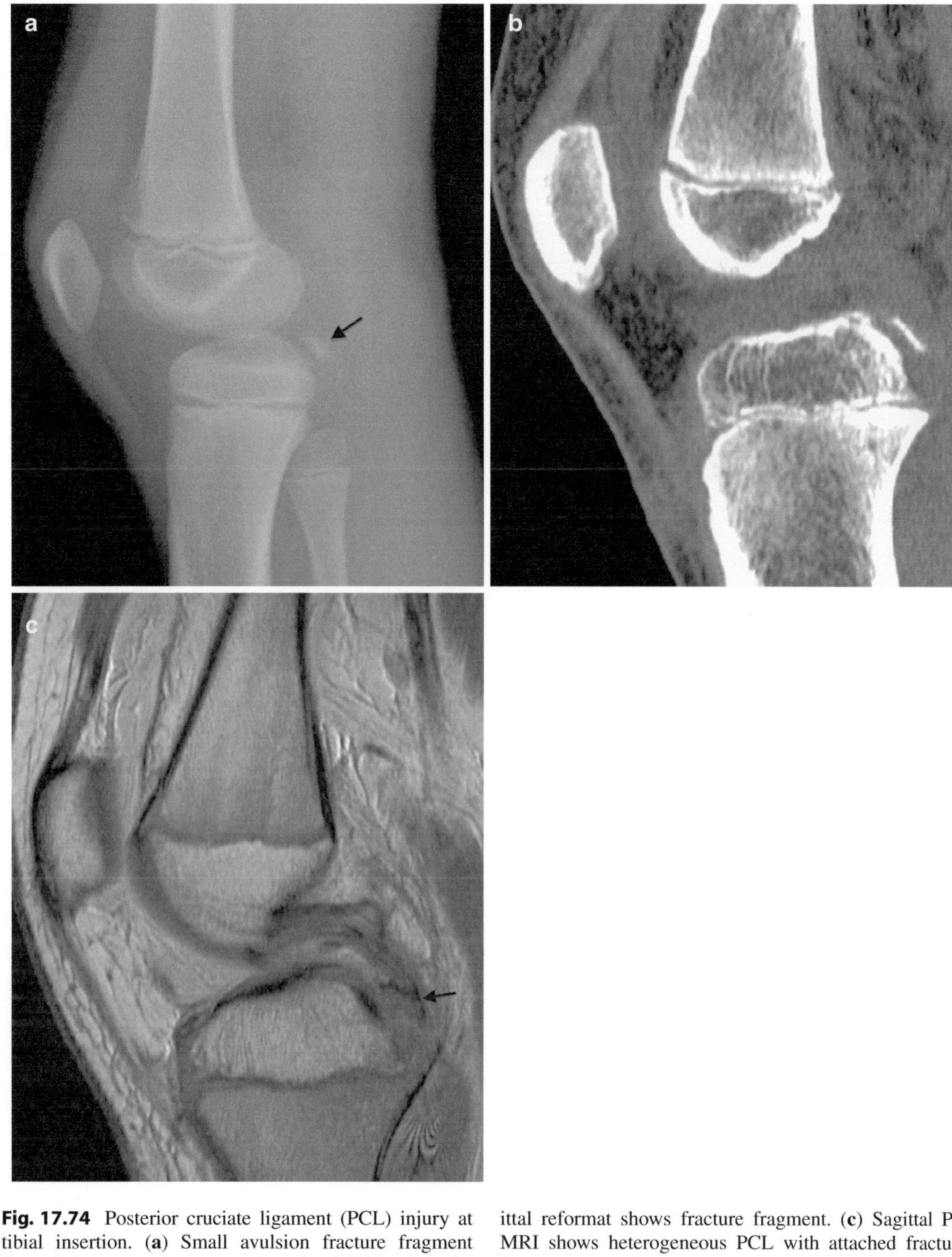

Fig. 17.74 Posterior cruciate ligament (PCL) injury at tibial insertion. (**a**) Small avulsion fracture fragment (*arrow*) from posterior aspect of proximal tibial epiphysis, with marked posterior soft tissue swelling. (**b**) 2D CT sagittal reformat shows fracture fragment. (**c**) Sagittal PD MRI shows heterogeneous PCL with attached fracture fragment (*arrow*)

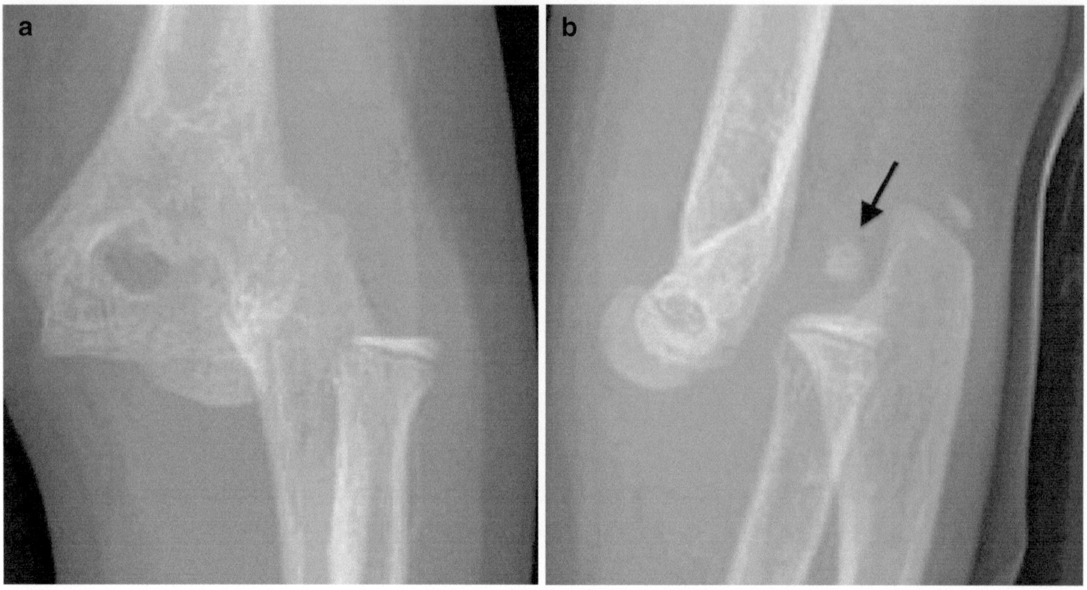

Fig. 17.75 Elbow dislocation with displaced avulsion fracture of the medial epicondyle (*arrow*) (**a**, **b**)

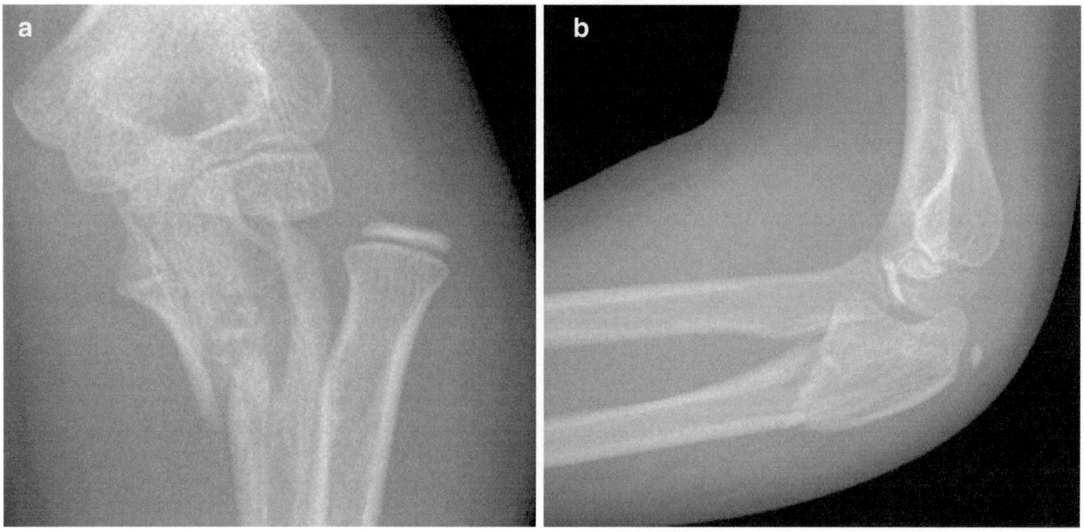

Fig. 17.76 Monteggia fracture-dislocation with radial head dislocation and proximal ulnar fracture (**a**, **b**)

References

1. Staheli JT. Fundamentals of pediatric orthopedics. 4th ed. Philadelphia: Lippincott Williams & Wilkins; 2008.
2. Brown JH, Deluca SA. Growth plate injuries: Salter Harris classification. Am Fam Physician. 1992;46: 1180–5.
3. Carson S, Woolridge DP, Colletti J, Kilgore K. Pediatric upper extremity injuries. Pediatr Clin North Am. 2006;53:41–67.
4. Lindaman LM. Bone healing in children. Clin Podiatr Med Surg. 2001;18:97–108.
5. Johnson KJ, Bache E. Imaging in pediatric skeletal trauma: techniques and applications. Berlin: Springer; 2007.
6. Rodriguez-Merchan EC. Pediatric skeletal trauma: a review and historical perspective. Clin Orthop Relat Res. 2005;432:8–13.
7. Slongo TF. The choice of treatment according to the type and location of the fracture and the age of the child. Injury. 2005;36(Suppl):A12–9.
8. Cho KH, Lee SM, Lee YH, Suh KJ. Ultrasound diagnosis of either an occult or missed fracture of an extremity in pediatric-aged children. Korean J Radiol. 2010;11:84–94.
9. Fayad LM, Corl F, Fishman EK. Pediatric skeletal trauma: use of multiplanar reformatted and three-dimensional 64-row multidetector CT in the emergency department. Radiographics. 2009;29:135–50.
10. Jaramillo D, Hoffer FA, Shapiro F, Rand F. MR imaging of fractures of the growth plate. AJR Am J Roentgenol. 1990;155:1261–5.
11. Jaramillo D, Kammen BF, Shapiro F. Cartilaginous path of physeal fracture-separations: evaluation with MR imaging—an experimental study with histologic correlation in rabbits. Radiology. 2000;215: 504–11.
12. Brighton CT. The growth plate. Orthop Clin North Am. 1984;15:571.
13. Ecklund K. Magnetic resonance imaging of pediatric musculoskeletal trauma. Top Magn Reson Imaging. 2002;13:203–17.
14. Jaramillo D, Villegas-Medina OL, Doty DK, Rivas R, Strife K, Dwek JR, et al. Age-related vascular changes in the epiphysis, physis, and metaphysic: normal findings on gadolinium-enhanced MRI of piglets. AJR Am J Roentgenol. 2004;182:353–60.
15. Rogers LF, Poznanski AK. Imaging of epiphyseal injuries. Radiology. 1994;191:297–308.
16. Laor T, Zbonjniewicz AM, Eismann EA, Wall EJ. Juvenile osteochondritis dissecans: is it a growth disturbance of the secondary physis of the epiphysis? AJR Am J Roentgenol. 2012;199:1121–8.
17. Salter RB, Harris WR. Injuries involving the epiphyseal plate. J Bone Joint Surg. 1963;45A:587.
18. Ogden JA. Current concepts review: the evaluation and treatment of partial physeal arrest. J Bone Joint Surg Am. 1987;69:1297–302.
19. Jacobsen S, Hansson G, Nathorst-Westfelt J. Traumatic separation of the distal epiphysis of the humerus sustained at birth. J Bone Joint Surg Br. 2009;91:797–802.
20. Schnetzler KA, Hoernschemeyer D. The pediatric triplane ankle fracture. J Am Acad Orthop Surg. 2008;15:738–47.
21. Badelon O, Bensahel H, Mazda K, Vie P. Lateral humeral condylar fractures in children: a report of 47 cases. J Pediatr Orthop. 1988;8:31–4.
22. Tejwani N, Phillips D, Goldstein RY. Management of lateral humeral condylar fracture in children. J Am Acad Orthop Surg. 2011;19:350–8.
23. Chapman VM, Grottkau BE, Albright M, Salamipour H, Jaramillo D. Multidetector computed tomography of pediatric lateral condylar fractures. J Comput Assist Tomogr. 2005;29:842–6.
24. John SD, Wherry K, Swischuk LE, Phillips WA. Improving detection of pediatric elbow fractures by understanding their mechanics. Radiographics. 1996;16:1443–60.
25. Schmittenbecher PP. What must we respect in articular fractures in childhood? Injury. 2005;36 Suppl 1: A35–43.
26. Brown SD, Kasser JR, Zurakowski D, Jaramillo D. Analysis of 51 tibial triplane fractures using CT with multiplanar reconstruction. AJR Am J Roentgenol. 2004;183:1489–95.
27. Ecklund K, Jaramillo D. Imaging of growth disturbance in children. Radiol Clin North Am. 2001; 39:823–41.
28. Dupuis CS, Westra SJ, Makris J, Wallace EC. Injuries and conditions of the extensor mechanism of the pediatric knee. Radiographics. 2009;29:877–86.
29. Zionts LE. Fractures around the knee in children. J Am Acad Orthop Surg. 2002;10:345–55.
30. Tepper KB, Ireland ML. Fracture patterns and treatment in the skeletally immature knee. Instr Course Lect. 2003;52:667–76.
31. Jaines C, Jimenez M, Shabshin N, Laor T, Jaramillo D. Taking the stress out of evaluating stress injuries in children. Radiographics. 2012;32:537–55.
32. Sanchez TR, Jadhav SP, Swischuk LE. MR imaging of pediatric trauma. Magn Reson Imaging Clin N Am. 2009;17:439–50.
33. Laor T, Wall EJ, Vu LP. Physeal widening in the knee due to stress injury in child athletes. AJR Am J Roentgenol. 2006;186:1260–4.
34. Islam O, Sobeleski D, Symons S, et al. Development and duration of radiographic signs of bone healing in children. AJR Am J Roentgenol. 2000;175:75–8.
35. Wilkins KE. Principles of fracture remodeling in children. Injury. 2005;36 Suppl 1:A3–11.
36. Prosser I, Lawson Z, Evans A, et al. A timetable for the radiologic features of fracture healing in young children. AJR Am J Roentgenol. 2012;198: 1014–20.
37. Craig JG, Cramer KE, Cody DD, Hearshen DO, Ceulemans RY, van Holsbeeck MT, et al. Premature

partial closure and other deformities of the growth plate: MR imaging and three-dimensional modeling. Radiology. 1999;210:835–43.
38. Shapiro F, Rand F. Traumatic fracture separations of the epiphysis: a pathophysiologic approach. Adv Orthop Surg. 1982;15:175–203.
39. Jaramillo D, Hoffer FA, Shapiro F. Growth cartilage: normal appearance, variant, and abnormalities. MRI Clin North Am. 1998;6:455–71.
40. Ahn JM, El-Khoury GY. Role of magnetic resonance imaging in musculoskeletal trauma. Top Magn Reson Imaging. 2007;18:155–68.

Non-accidental Trauma 18

Thomas Ray Sanchez, Angelo Don S. Grasparil II, and Kevin Coulter

Contents

Abstract

This chapter presents the different imaging modalities that may be used in the radiographic diagnosis of non-accidental trauma, with particular emphasis on the skeletal survey. The different fracture patterns related to non-accidental trauma are then reviewed, including high-, moderate-, and low-specificity lesions. Fracture aging is also presented. Finally, mimics of non-accidental trauma are discussed, with more detailed presentation of osteogenesis imperfecta and rickets.

Child abuse, as defined by the World Health Report 2002, "constitutes all forms of physical and/or emotional ill-treatment, sexual abuse, neglect or negligent treatment or commercial or other exploitation, resulting in actual or potential harm to the child's health, survival, development or dignity in the context of a relationship of responsibility, trust or power" [1]. In one study, child abuse has been classified into three different forms: battered child syndrome, sexual abuse, and neglect [2]. Imaging—and thus the radiologist—plays a vital role in cases of battered child syndrome and sometimes in cases of neglect. For

T.R. Sanchez, MD (✉)
Department of Pediatric Radiology,
University of California Davis Medical
Center and UC Davis Children's Hospital,
4860 Y Street, Suite 3100, Sacramento, CA 95817, USA

Department of Diagnostic Imaging,
Shriners Hospitals for Children Northern,
California, Sacramento, CA 95817, USA
e-mail: thomas.sanchez@ucdmc.ucdavis.edu

A.D.S. Grasparil II, MD
Department of Radiology,
Cardinal Santos Medical Center,
10 Wilson Street, Greenhills, San Juan,
NCR 1502, Philippines

Radiology Division,
Philippine Children's Medical Center,
Quezon Ave. cor. Agham Road, Quezon City,
NCR 1101, Philippines
e-mail: dgrasparil.pedrad@gmail.com

K. Coulter, MD
Department of Pediatrics,
University of California Davis Medical
Center and UC Davis Children's Hospital,
2516 Stockton Boulevard, Suite 336, Sacramento,
CA 95817, USA
e-mail: kevin.coulter@ucdmc.ucdavis.edu

R. Stein-Wexler et al. (eds.), *Pediatric Orthopedic Imaging*,
DOI 10.1007/978-3-642-45381-6_18, © Springer-Verlag Berlin Heidelberg 2015

the purpose of this discussion, the terms "battered child syndrome," "non-accidental trauma," and "child abuse" are used interchangeably.

Child abuse is probably underreported, and official reports probably also underestimate the extent of the problem [3]. There is an inverse relationship between non-accidental trauma and patient age [4]. Children aged 3 years and less are the most vulnerable, as they are least able to defend themselves or explain how they got their injuries; they are thus at greatest risk for fatal or near-fatal trauma. Infants less than 1 year old are at greatest danger [5].

Failure of physicians to properly diagnose child abuse has enormous consequences for the patient, the patient's family, and the physician. Children who have been intentionally injured must be identified, as they are likely to receive further injury if returned to the care of the perpetrator [6]. Misdiagnosis carries a high degree of morbidity and mortality, with a 50 % reinjury rate and 10 % mortality rate for unprotected children [7]. It is also extremely important to correctly diagnose fractures that arise from underlying bone abnormalities rather than from non-accidental trauma, as misdiagnosis of child abuse can also have devastating consequences. The radiologist must therefore be able to differentiate pathology from normal anatomic variants, differentiate traumatic from nontraumatic abnormalities, suggest a mechanism of injury, offer a reasonable estimate for time of injury, and identify or suggest an underlying abnormality that may predispose the child to fractures [6].

1 Imaging Techniques

The skeletal survey is the primary diagnostic imaging modality for the evaluation, documentation, and follow-up of suspected and confirmed cases of child abuse. High-quality skeletal survey protocol requires that the extremities be imaged in at least a frontal projection with coned views; images of the wrists, knees, and ankles may also be obtained, centered on each joint. The axial skeleton should be imaged in at least two projections. Additional right and left posterior oblique views of the ribs demonstrate additional fractures not routinely seen on standard frontal and lateral radiographs [8, 9] (Table 18.1). Additional views may be acquired, especially if equivocal abnormalities are identified. Coned views of the ankles are often helpful in addition to the routine skeletal survey.

Table 18.1 ACR-SPR imaging protocol for the skeletal survey of known or suspected child abuse

Axial skeleton	Appendicular skeleton
Chest (AP, lateral, and bilateral obliques to include the upper lumbar spine	Humeri (AP)
Pelvis (AP), to include the mid-lumbar spine	Forearms (AP)
Lumbosacral spine (lateral)	Femurs (AP)
Cervical spine (AP and lateral)	Lower legs (AP)
Skull (frontal and lateral)	Hands and feet (AP)

Reprinted from American College of Radiology (ACR), Society for Pediatric Radiology (SPR) [8]. Reprinted with permission of the American College of Radiology. No other representation of this material is authorized without expressed, written permission from the American College of Radiology

The *babygram*, which is a single image of the entire chest and abdomen as well as the extremities, is inadequate. Peripheral areas are incorrectly exposed, and subtle fractures can be missed. Proper radiographic technique, positioning, collimation, and shielding are vital to optimize visualization of osseous structures and allow diagnosis of pathology with high sensitivity while keeping radiation dose levels within acceptable limits. A follow-up skeletal survey, usually in 2 weeks, may increase the diagnostic yield, particularly if findings are equivocal on the initial study and there is strong clinical suspicion for abuse. The repeat study also helps with accurate dating of individual injuries.

Although the complete skeletal survey is almost always mandatory in suspected child abuse cases for patients under 2 years of age, its utility diminishes and provides little value after age 5. Between the ages of 2 and 5 years, imaging is guided by specific clinical indicators of abuse and should be individually prescribed [10].

Bone scintigraphy is generally limited in the evaluation of non-accidental injury. Its primary use is in the identification of subtle rib fractures, but it is not particularly good at demonstrating epiphyseal and metaphyseal fractures, as these areas are obscured by normal physiologic activity and high periphyseal uptake of radiopharmaceutical [11]. Skull fractures are notoriously difficult to visualize on routine bone scans [12]. Equally important, bone scans require sedation and expose the child to a relative high radiation dose [13]. They are mainly used if clinical suspicion is high and routine imaging fails to document acute or healing fractures.

There has been recent interest in computed tomography (CT) for initial imaging of rib fractures, especially if routine skeletal survey fails to document fractures in highly suspicious cases [14]. Magnetic resonance imaging is very sensitive for evaluating spine, pelvis, and long bone occult skeletal trauma in children [15] but is limited for evaluating rib and skull fractures. It may not show classic metaphyseal lesions [16]. Ultrasonography can be valuable for assessing epiphyseal separations that are suspected on routine radiographs. However, its operator dependence, lack of correlative data for dating fractures, and limited utility for follow-up imaging make it the least useful modality for evaluating non-accidental trauma.

2 Fracture Patterns

The classification of fractures into high, moderate, and low specificity for child abuse is well established (Box 18.1). High-specificity injuries include the classic metaphyseal lesion (CML) and rib, scapular, sternal, and spinous process fractures. Moderately specific fractures include multiple and/or bilateral fractures of varying ages and vertebral, digital, and complex skull fractures. Long bone diaphyseal fractures as well as clavicular and linear skull fractures are considered low-specificity injuries [17].

Box 18.1: Specificity of Skeletal Fractures

Specificity	Types of fractures
High	Classic metaphyseal lesions (CML)/corner fractures
	Rib fractures, especially posteromedial
	Scapular fractures
	Sternal fractures
	Multiple fractures of varying ages
	Vertebral body fractures
	Digital fractures
	Complex skull fractures
Low	Linear skull fractures
	Clavicular fractures
	Long bone shaft fractures especially in ambulatory children

Modified from Kleinman [17] and Dwek [11]

2.1 Classic Metaphyseal Lesions (CML)

The terms "corner fracture" and "bucket handle fracture" describe fractures at the metaphyses of the long bones that are highly specific for non-accidental trauma, since nonambulatory children cannot inflict this type of injury on themselves (Box 18.2). The fractures result from tractional and torsional force applied to an extremity and are virtually diagnostic of child abuse, particularly in children under 1 year of age. Violent shaking of an infant causes tearing and injury at the level of the zone of provisional calcification of the physis; the detached bone creates a curvilinear density that constitutes the bucket handle fracture [11] (Fig. 18.1). If this fragment is viewed in tangent, it appears as a detached corner, whereas if it is viewed partially en face it appears as a bucket handle. CMLs involve the metaphyses of long bones and are most common at the proximal or distal tibias, distal femurs, and proximal humeri; they are frequently bilateral [18]. They usually involve the posteromedial aspect of the distal femurs, proximal tibias, and distal tibias. At the proximal humeri, they are usually lateral and are best seen with external rotation.

Box 18.2: Corner Metaphyseal Lesions

Traction/torsion cause tearing at zone of provisional calcification

Bucket handle vs. corner fragment appearance results from difference in projection

Most common: proximal/distal tibias, distal femurs, proximal humeri

- Posteromedial: tibia, femur
- Lateral: humeri

Differential: birth trauma, orthopedic manipulation, normal metaphyseal spur

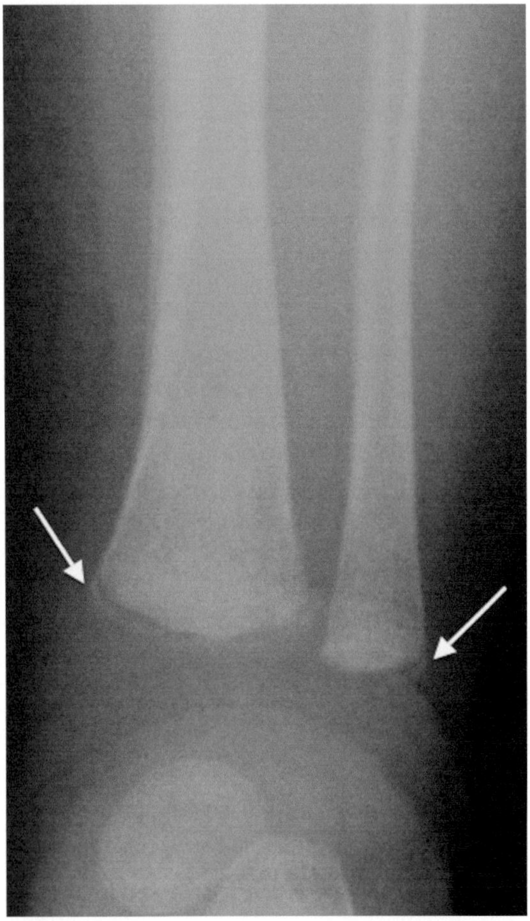

Fig. 18.1 Classic metaphyseal lesions (CML) showing bucket handle configuration at the distal tibia and fibula (*arrows*)

Rarely, a similar lesion may result from birth trauma [19] or from manipulation during orthopedic procedures. The timing of injury and the clinical history differentiate such fractures from abusive trauma. These fractures should also be differentiated from the normal subperiosteal bone collar and normal metaphyseal spur seen in rapidly growing long bones of young children, which are attached to the adjacent bone with no intervening lucency (Fig. 18.2) (see Chap. 2).

2.2 Rib Fractures

Rib fractures are the most common and highly specific injury found in abused children, with positive predictive values as high as 95 % in children less than 3 years of age [18]. Furthermore, in some patients, rib fractures are the only skeletal manifestation of child abuse. Although involvement can be anywhere along the rib, unilateral, bilateral, or multiple posteromedial rib fractures are most specific for child abuse (Fig. 18.3). This is in keeping with the mechanism of how these fractures are sustained when the chest is squeezed in the anteroposterior direction, levering the posteromedial ribs against the transverse processes. For similar fractures to occur in the setting of accidental trauma, massive forces must be generated, such as in deceleration dashboard injuries or high-velocity vehicular impact. Cardiopulmonary resuscitation does not cause posteromedial rib fractures [20].

Routine chest radiography may not clearly demonstrate rib fractures, particularly if they are acute, incomplete, and non-displaced or if they are posterior. For this reason, oblique views, follow-up imaging after 2 weeks, and bone scintigraphy have been suggested to improve detection of such fractures. CT of the chest has also been advocated in highly suspicious situations [14] (Fig. 18.4).

2.3 Skull Fractures

Skull fractures are common in both accidental and non-accidental injury and are therefore low-specificity lesions. Linear skull fractures occur most frequently, usually upon impact after low-velocity falls. However, complex fractures (such as concentric, star-shaped, or eggshell fractures)

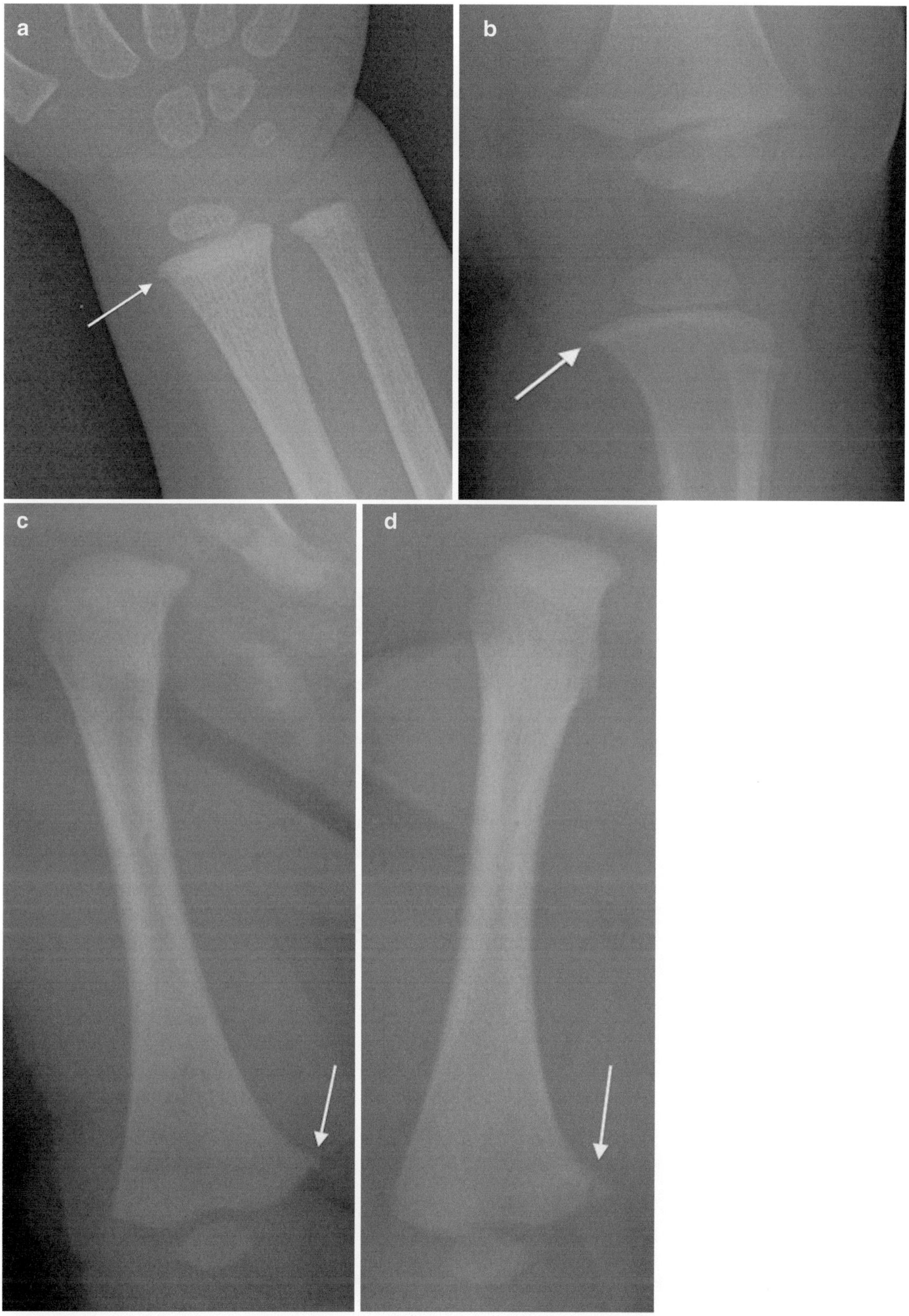

Fig. 18.2 Normal metaphyseal spurs and collars, contrasted with corner fracture. No lucency separates the metaphysis from the normal bone collar (*arrows*) at the distal radius (**a**) and proximal tibia (**b**), or the normal distal femoral spur (*arrow*, **c**). (**d**) Lucency separates the CML (with corner fracture configuration) (*arrow*) from the metaphysis

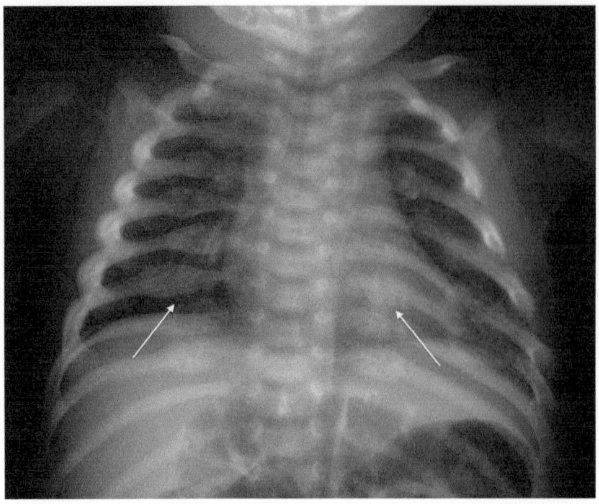

Fig. 18.3 Healing posteromedial rib fractures at almost every level are highly suggestive of child abuse (*arrows* indicate two of the many fractures). Multiple posterolateral rib fractures as well

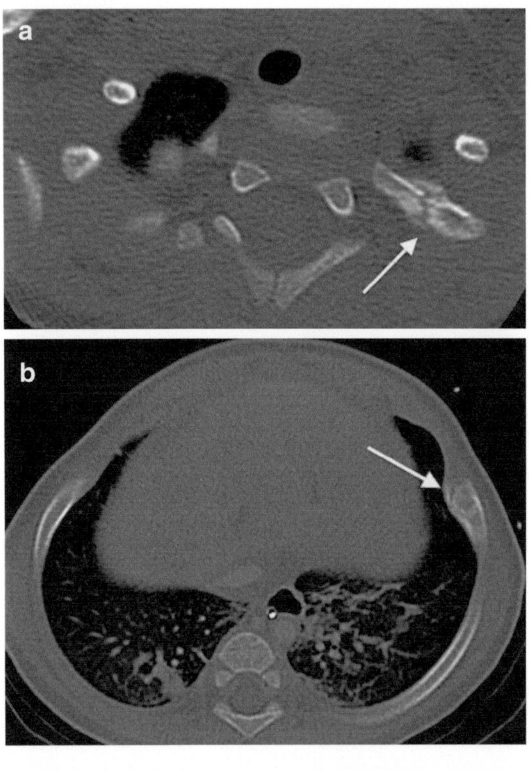

Fig. 18.4 Healing rib fractures on CT. (**a**) Axial CT shows healing second rib fracture that was not evident on contemporaneous radiograph. (**b**) Axial CT of a different patient with a healing left anterior rib fracture not evident even on oblique views (*arrow*)

imply high-velocity/high-energy trauma and carry a higher positive predictive value for abuse [21, 22] (Fig. 18.5).

A skull fracture is often the only evidence of abuse. It is therefore important that even these low-specificity lesions are accurately identified and correlated with the clinical history and reported mechanism of injury. This can sometimes present difficulties, especially in subtle cases, where the complex development of the infantile skull may make it difficult to differentiate between a linear fracture and an accessory suture. CT with three-dimensional (3D) reconstruction is very helpful in evaluating a suspicious fracture. Characteristics which favor fracture include a sharp lucency with nonsclerotic edges, fracture line widening as it approaches a suture, and associated soft tissue swelling [23] (Fig. 18.6).

2.4 Long Bone Diaphyseal Fractures

The presence of long bone diaphyseal fractures in a nonambulatory infant should raise concern for non-accidental injury. Such fractures usually result from application of a bending or rotational force, as the extremity is grabbed [22].

However, in older children, long bone fractures usually result from accidental trauma. These fractures are therefore generally of low specificity for abuse. Although spiral midshaft fractures have long been associated with abuse, more recent studies have concluded that the type (spiral, transverse, or oblique) as well as the location of the fracture (diaphyseal or metaphyseal) does not necessarily differentiate accidental from abusive injury. Given the appropriate mechanism of injury, these fracture types can occur in the setting of accidental trauma [24, 25].

2.5 Fractures in Unusual Sites

Fractures from child abuse have been described in virtually every bone [4]. However, spine fractures in the absence of documented high-energy trauma

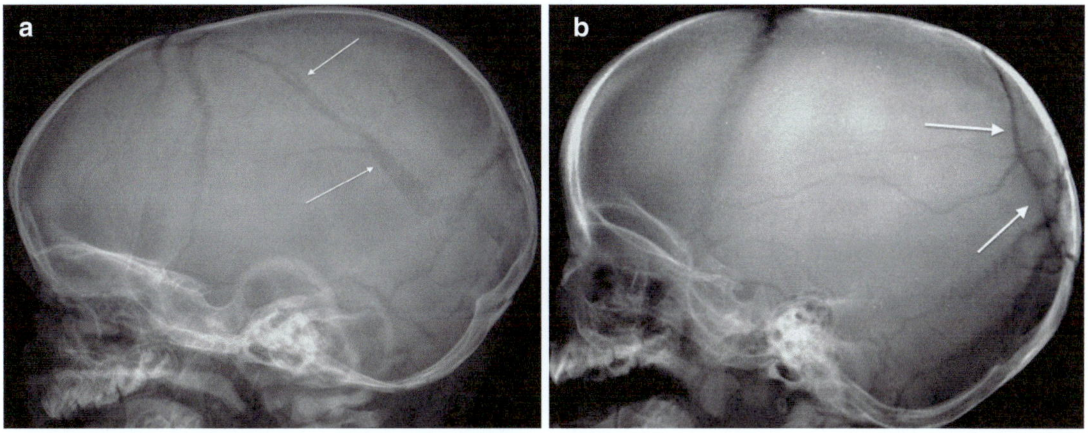

Fig. 18.5 Skull fractures. (**a**) Linear fracture of the parietal and occipital bones (*arrows*), a nonspecific fracture that can be accidental or result from abuse. However, diastasis, vague tangential fracture lines, and the fact that the fracture crosses a suture, all features that are less common in the typical fall from a low-height accidental injury, increase the suspicion for abuse. (**b**) Complex, star-shaped/eggshell fracture (*arrows*) of the parieto-occipital region indicates a high-impact injury, highly suggestive of abuse

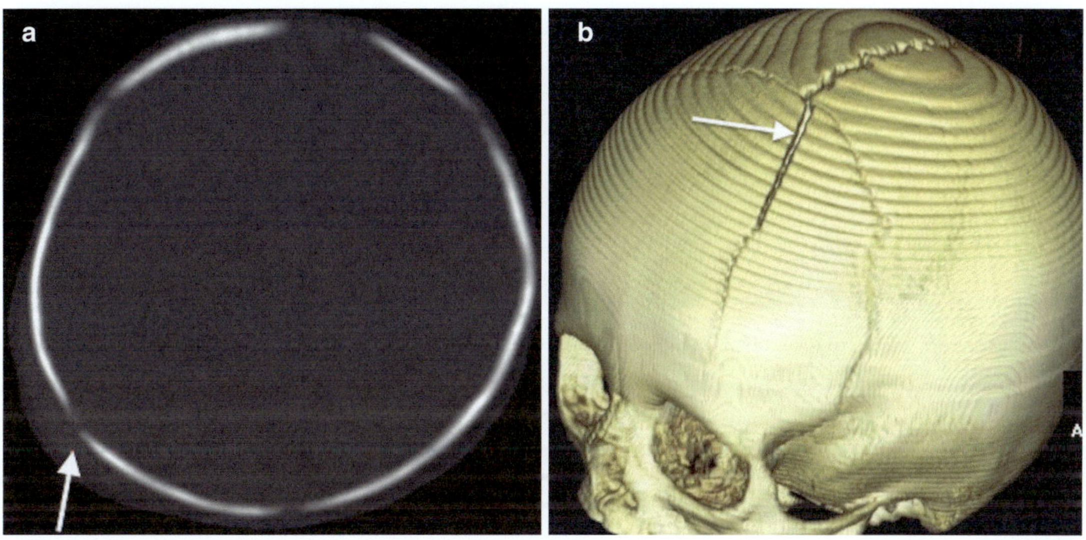

Fig. 18.6 Differentiating skull fractures from accessory cranial sutures. (**a**) Axial CT shows soft tissue swelling and step-off, which indicate that the lucency in the occipital bone represents fracture (*arrow*). (**b**) Three-dimensional CT reconstruction shows a linear lucency in the frontal bone which widens as it approaches the sagittal suture (*arrow*), also a feature of skull fracture

are rare in childhood and should suggest abuse. Mechanisms include hyperextension, hyperflexion, and/or axial loading from violent shaking, deliberate dropping, or throwing. Injury usually involves multiple vertebral levels, often near the thoracolumbar junction (see Chap. 4). Spinous process fractures, as well as vertebral body compression fractures with associated endplate defects, may be seen [26].

Other unusual fracture sites in infants and toddlers include the scapula (Fig. 18.7), sternum, phalanges, metacarpals, metatarsals, and pelvis. Fractures in these locations should also raise the possibility of non-accidental trauma, unless there

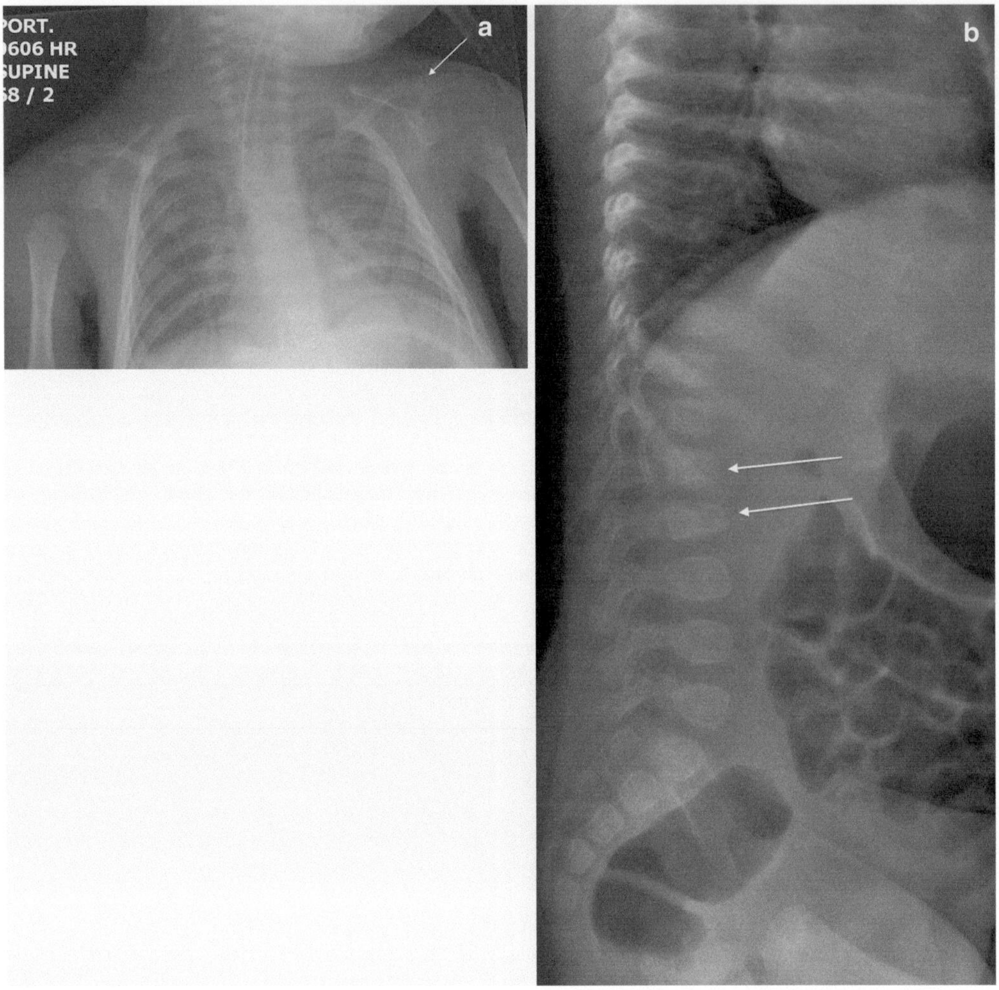

Fig. 18.7 Unusual fractures with high specificity for abuse. (**a**) Left acromion fracture (*arrow*), often a result of either non-accidental trauma or high-impact injury. (**b**) Lumbar vertebral body fractures (*arrows*) in a nonambulatory infant

is a legitimate history of an unusual mechanism of injury. Clavicular fractures—especially involving the middle third—are common and thus in general low-specificity lesions. They may also result from birth trauma but should be attributed to birth only if callus is apparent by age 11 days [11].

2.6 Multiple Fractures of Varying Ages

The presence of multiple fractures without a convincing history of accidental trauma should also raise suspicion for child abuse. There is a significant association between multiple unexplained fractures and child abuse: up to 74 % of abused children have two or more fractures [27]. Bilateral, symmetrical fractures involving the upper or lower extremities in non-ambulatory children are also associated with child abuse (Fig. 18.8).

The location and stage of healing of every fracture must be correlated with the clinical history, mechanism, and date of injury. Of course, the clinical history remains paramount in the final analysis, since children with metabolic abnormalities that predispose to bone fragility can present with multiple fractures of different ages.

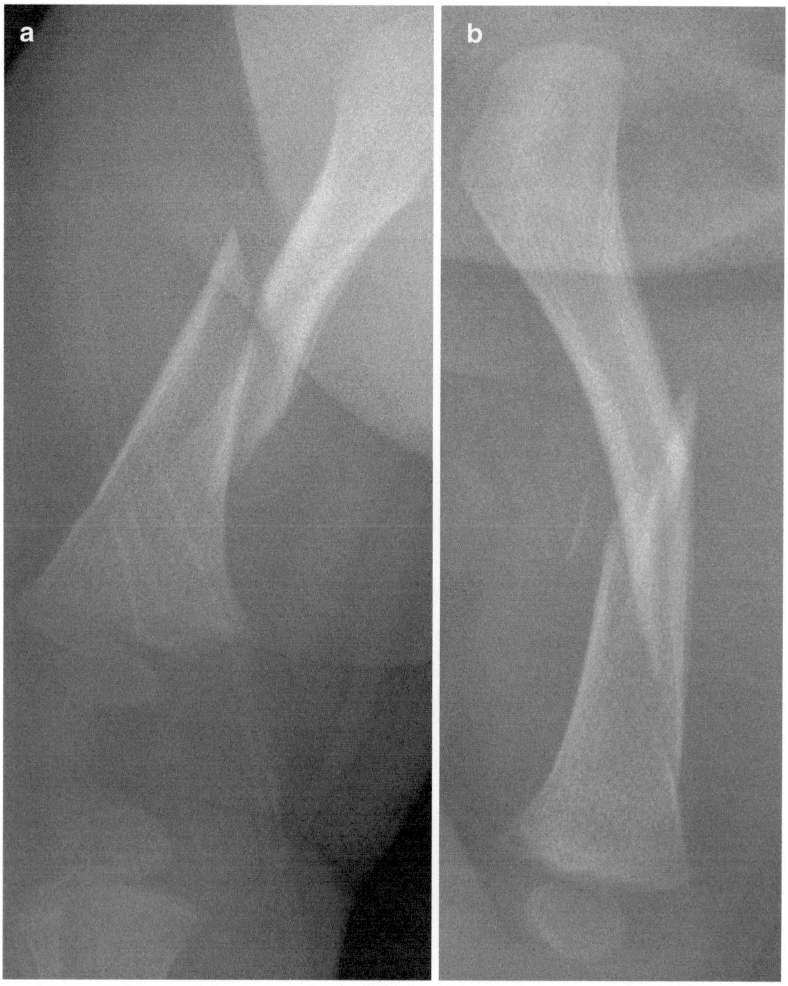

Fig. 18.8 Bilateral acute spiral fractures of the femurs in a 7-month-old victim of non-accidental trauma (**a**, **b**)

2.7 Subperiosteal New Bone Formation

Subperiosteal new bone forms when the periosteum separates from the underlying cortex. This may occur with trauma, as well as with infectious, metabolic, and neoplastic disease. Physiologic subperiosteal new bone formation is normal in long bones during the first 4 months of life, presumably due to rapid intramembranous ossification (see Chap. 2). It is usually bilateral but can be asymmetrical and should be no thicker than 2 mm [28]. Whereas posttraumatic subperiosteal new bone formation can extend to the metaphysis (Fig. 18.9), the physiologic process extends only as far as the metadiaphysis (see Chap. 2).

3 Fracture Dating

Fracture dating is important in the evaluation of child abuse injuries. Injury dating can unmask inconsistencies between the clinical history and radiographic findings and determine whether multiple fractures have been sustained over a period of time. Published material addresses the stages and timing of fracture healing [29–32], but the appearance at different time intervals overlaps considerably. Furthermore, the application of this data to non-accidental trauma may be inexact, since most studies deal with a wide age range of subjects and describe fractures that have been immobilized. Still, knowledge of the radiologic

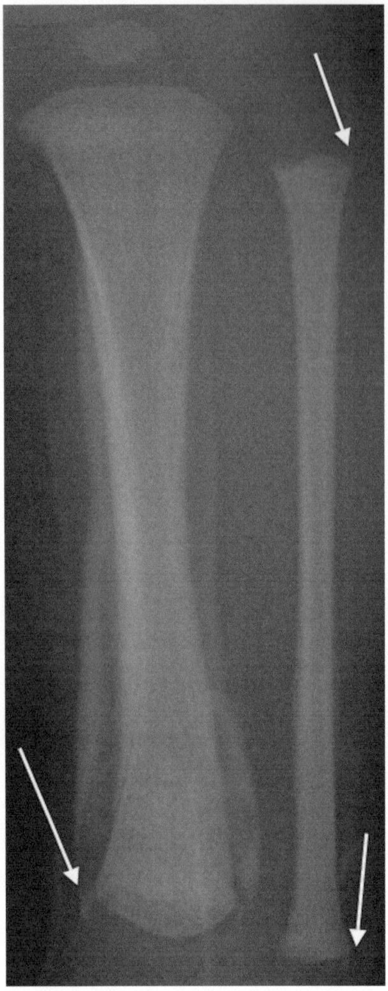

Fig. 18.9 Thick, wavy, posttraumatic subperiosteal new bone formation representing calcification of the periosteum, elevated likely due to subperiosteal hemorrhage. Corner fractures of the tibia and fibula (*arrows*)

features of fracture healing along with a general sense of timing can help the radiologist approximate fracture age.

Long bone fractures in children can be estimated as acute (less than 1 week old), recent (8–35 days), and old (more than 35 days), based on the appearance of periosteal reaction and callus [33] (Fig. 18.10). Rib fractures are more difficult to date, in part because they are never casted and can be subjected to repeated trauma. However, callus thickness can help guide assessment of rib fracture age [34] (Fig. 18.11).

4 Mimics of Child Abuse (Box 18.3)

Box 18.3: Mimics of Child Abuse

Osteogenesis imperfecta types I and IV
- Multiple accessory sutures (wormian bones)
- Osteoporosis
- Blue sclerae
- Associated long bone, lateral rib, diaphyseal fractures

Rickets
- Osteopenia
- Irregular/cupped metaphyses, wide physes
- Wrists and knees affected most severely

4.1 Osteogenesis Imperfecta

Osteogenesis imperfecta (OI) is a rare disorder of abnormal type 1 collagen quality and/or quantity, characterized by abnormal bone fragility and osteoporosis. Infants and children with OI manifest with multiple fractures and may resemble victims of non-accidental trauma. Other major characteristic features of OI that may suggest the diagnosis in infants include blue sclerae and multiple wormian bones; older children may demonstrate defective dentition, short stature, bowing deformities, and early onset hearing impairment [35]. Inheritance is autosomal dominant or autosomal recessive.

Types I and IV are most likely to be confused with non-accidental trauma (types II and III present with in utero or perinatal fractures). Type I is the most common and also the mildest form of OI; these patients usually have normal stature and few fractures or skeletal deformities. Their characteristically blue sclerae can facilitate diagnosis. Type IV is least common and has

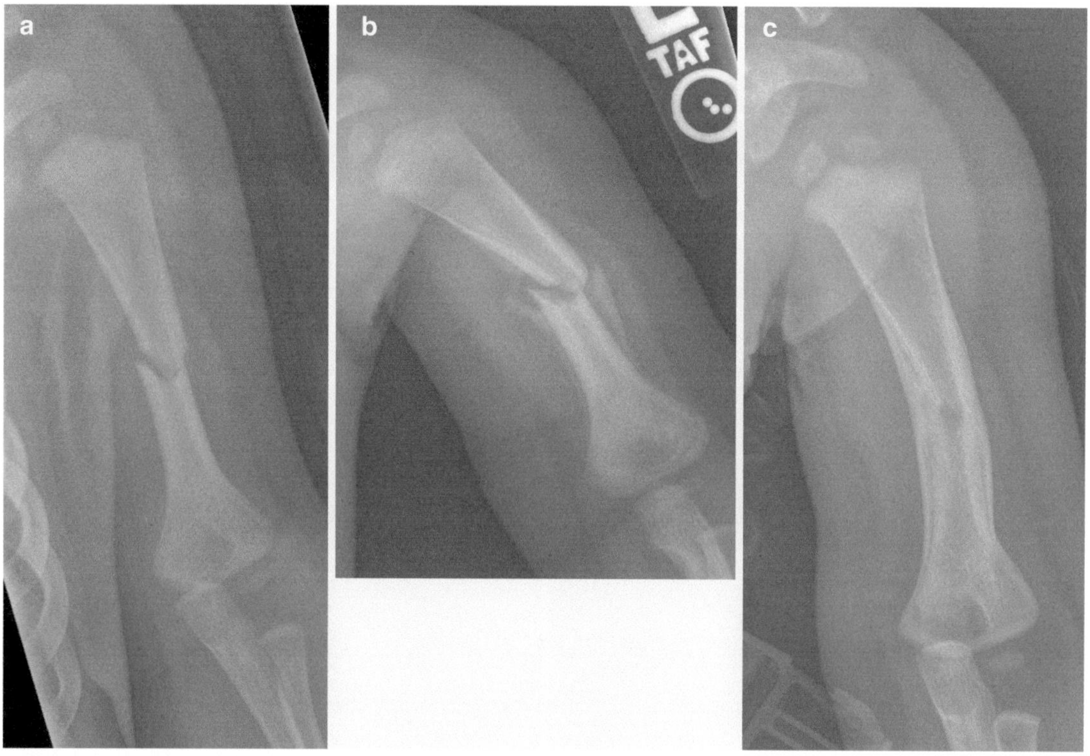

Fig. 18.10 Stages of long bone fracture healing. (**a**) Acute fracture without callus formation. (**b**) Two weeks later, there is early callus formation. (**c**) After 3 months, there are near total bridging of the fracture line and smooth cortical thickening

the mildest skeletal abnormalities. Biochemical analysis of collagen may help diagnose types I and IV but is not completely reliable. (See Chap. 23 for further discussion of the multiple subtypes of OI.)

It is important to recognize that the pattern of injury in OI differs from that encountered in non-accidental trauma. Patients with OI typically fracture the diaphyses of long bones and the lateral aspects of the ribs (Fig. 18.12). Therefore, if an infant with OI presents with fracture patterns that are typical of abuse (CMLs and posteromedial rib fractures), the possibility of abuse should still be entertained [11].

Temporary brittle bone disease has been proposed as a differential diagnosis for child abuse. As the name implies, affected infants are only transiently susceptible to fractures, and after spontaneous resolution of the condition, there is no further evidence of disease. The proponents of this entity suggest that it results from a transient defect in collagen synthesis or mineralization. However, extensive review of the scientific evidence has found no definitive proof that this condition exists, and it has largely been discredited as evidence against child abuse [36].

4.2 Rickets

Rickets is a common deficiency of bone mineralization that affects the zone of provisional calcification and is characterized radiographically

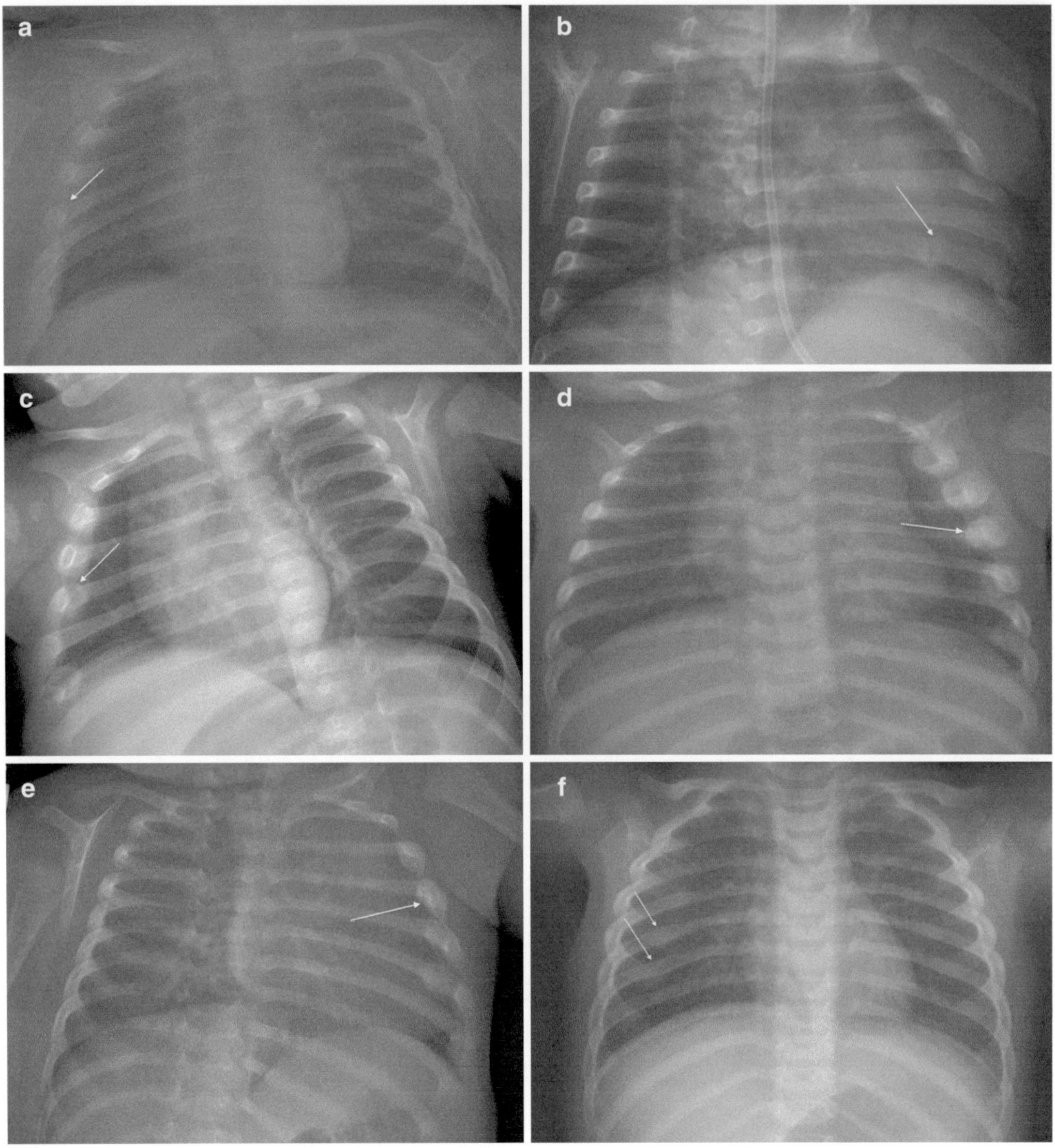

Fig. 18.11 Sequential healing of infantile rib fractures. (**a**) Acute injury with slight step-off (*arrow*) and absence of periosteal reaction (0–1 week). (**b**) Minimal periosteal reaction (*arrow*) and early resorption at the fracture site (1–3 weeks). (**c**) Progressive thickening of the callus (*arrow*) and widening of the fracture line (3–5 weeks). (**d**) Callus formation (*arrow*) is thickest at this stage (around 5–7 weeks). (**e**) Cortical thickening and remodeling of callus (*arrow*), with fracture line no longer visible (7–9 weeks). (**f**) After 9–11 weeks, the fracture is healed and the only indications of prior injury are cortical thickening and mild irregularity (*arrows*)

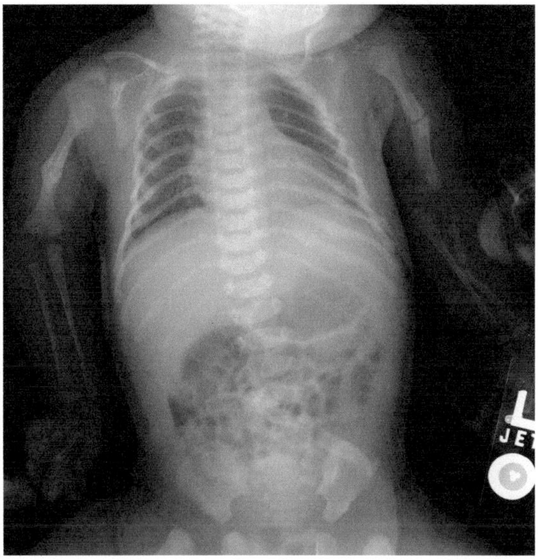

Fig. 18.12 Osteogenesis imperfecta in a newborn. The bones are diffusely osteopenic and thin, with fractures of both arms, the scapulae, and many ribs, at varying stages of healing. Multilevel platyspondyly

by osteopenia, metaphyseal irregularity and cupping, and physeal widening (Fig. 18.13). These changes are most evident in the faster growing areas of the appendicular skeleton, such as the wrists, ankles, and knees. Diffuse osteopenia precedes the classic metaphyseal findings, but radiographs are insensitive at evaluating bone mineralization since more than 30 % of bone must be lost before they demonstrate osteopenia [37]. The presence of osteopenia along with symmetrical involvement of the extremities makes differentiation from non-accidental trauma straightforward, even if corner fractures are present. However, it is important to recognize that in some patients nutritional deficiency results from neglect, which is also a form of child abuse, and that children with rickets can also suffer from physical abuse.

The existence of subclinical vitamin D deficiency is controversial. Some maintain that a

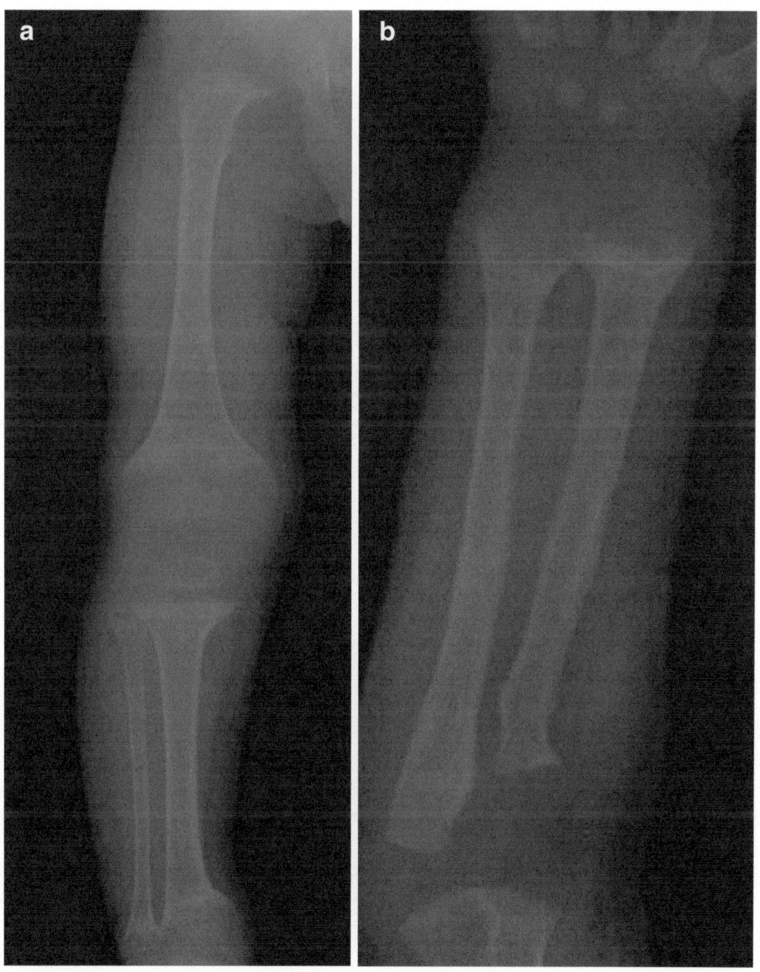

Fig. 18.13 Classic rickets showing metaphyseal flaring, fraying, and cupping (**a** lower extremity; **b** upper extremity). The hip and elbow contribute less to overall bone growth and are less severely affected

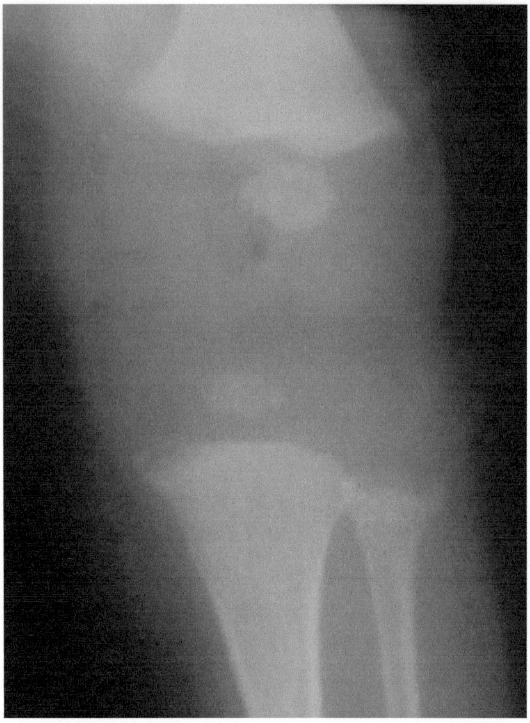

Fig. 18.14 Menkes kinky hair syndrome. Proximal tibial bony lesions mimic CMLs (Courtesy of Sandra L. Wootton-Gorges)

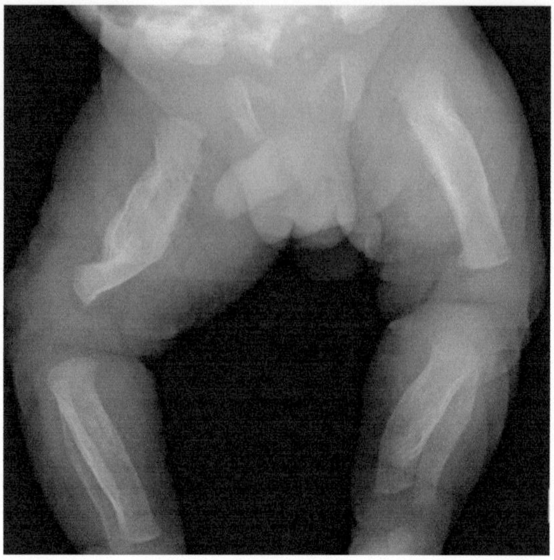

Fig. 18.15 Neonatal Caffey disease. Bowing deformity of the right femur and diffuse periosteal thickening of all long bones (Courtesy of Sandra L. Wootton-Gorges)

mild form of rickets typically seen in breast-fed infants results in multiple fractures, with some resembling CMLs [38]. However, there is no definite evidence at this time to support the existence of metaphyseal injuries characteristic of abuse in infants who have no clinical, laboratory, or radiographic evidence of rickets. Although CMLs can occur with rickets [39], these are usually seen only when there is already overt radiographic evidence of the disease. As with OI, the presence of posteromedial rib fractures in an infant with rickets strongly suggests abuse [38].

4.3 Other Less Common Mimics

Other conditions that may be considered in the differential diagnosis of child abuse include copper deficiency, fractures secondary to demineralization from paralysis, Menkes kinky hair syndrome (Fig. 18.14), scurvy, vitamin A intoxication, leukemia, congenital syphilis, Caffey disease (Fig. 18.15), metabolic storage diseases (Fig. 18.16), and prostaglandin administration (Fig. 18.17). Careful attention to history and physical examination, as well as correlation with distinctive laboratory parameters and radiographic findings, usually allows ready differentiation from non-accidental injury [40].

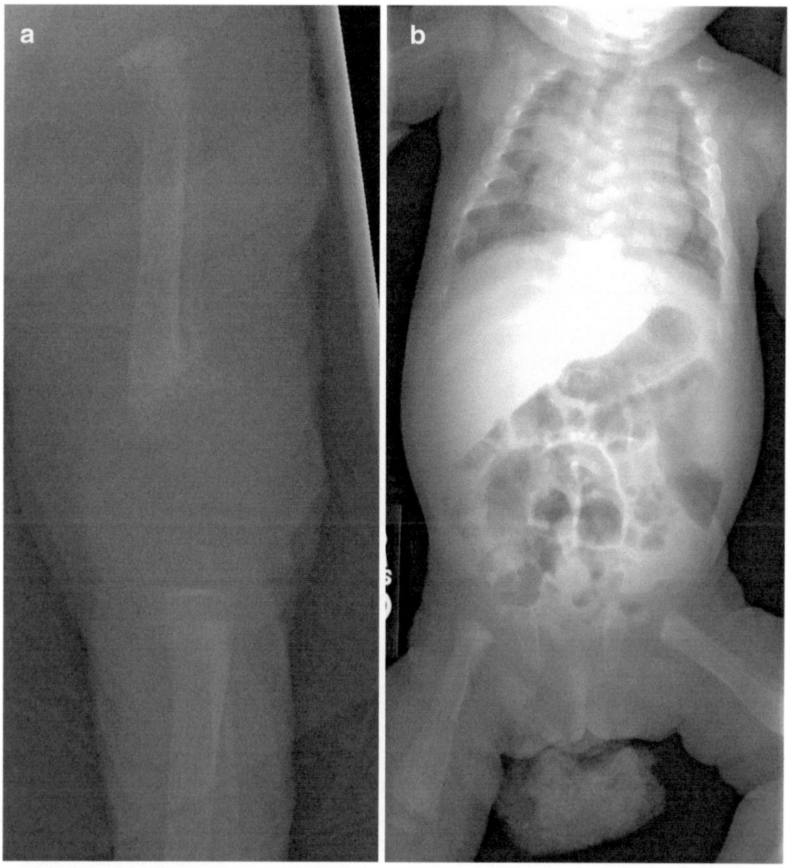

Fig. 18.16 Mucolipidosis in an infant. (**a**) Metaphyseal lytic lesions and diffuse periostitis in the lower extremity. These findings were also present at all long bones, suggesting either a metabolic abnormality (such as a storage disease) or infectious etiology (such as syphilis). (**b**) After several months of treatment, periosteal reaction is thicker and the metaphyses are reconstituted

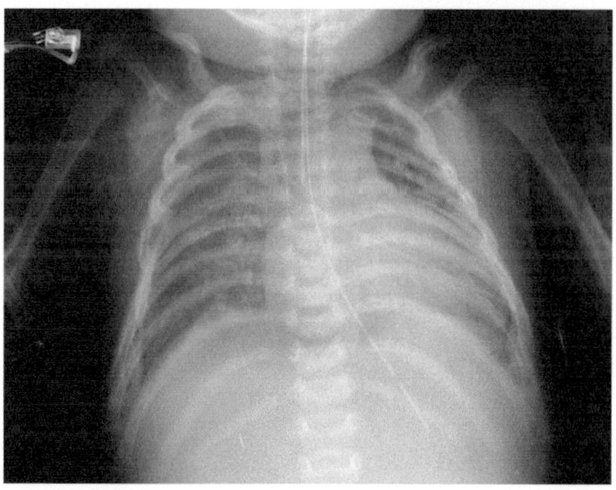

Fig. 18.17 Prostaglandin-induced periostitis in an infant with hypoplastic left heart syndrome. There is periosteal new bone formation along the humeri, clavicles, and ribs (Courtesy of Sandra L. Wootton-Gorges)

References

1. World Health Organization. World report on violence and health. Geneva: WHO; 2002.
2. Solarino M, De Filippi C, Solarino B. Radiological and forensic medicine aspects of traumatic injuries in child abuse. Radiol Med. 2009;114(8):1356–66. doi:10.1007/s11547-009-0501-8. Pubmed PMID: 19924509. Epub 2009. Nov 30. eng.
3. Hobbs C, Bilo R. Nonaccidental trauma: clinical aspects and epidemiology of child abuse. Pediatr Radiol. 2009;39(5):457–60. Pubmed PMID: 19198825. Epub 2009 Feb 7. Review. eng.
4. Kemp AM, Dunstan F, Harrison S, Morris S, Mann M, Rolfe K, Datta S, Thomas DP, Sibert JR, Maguire S. Patterns of skeletal fractures in child abuse: systematic review. BMJ. 2008;337:a1518. doi:10.1136/bmj.a1518. Pubmed PMID: 18832412. Review. eng.

5. Pierce MC, Bertocci GE, Vogeley E, Moreland MS. Evaluating long bone fractures in children: a biomechanical approach with illustrative cases. Child Abuse Negl. 2004;28(5):505–24. Pubmed PMID: 15206413. Review. eng.
6. Chapman S. Non-accidental injury. In: Johnson KI, Bache E, editors. Imaging in pediatric skeletal trauma. Berlin: Springer; 2008. eng.
7. Pandya NK, Baldwin K, Kamath AF, Wenger DR, Hosalkar HS. Unexplained fractures: child abuse or bone disease. A systematic review. Clin Orthop Relat Res. 2011;469(3):805–12. doi:10.1007/s11999-010-1578-z. eng. PubMed PMID: 20878560.
8. American College of Radiology (ACR), Society for Pediatric Radiology (SPR). ACR-SPR practice guideline for skeletal surveys in children [Online publication]. Reston: American College of Radiology (ACR); 2011. 6 p.
9. Hansen KK, Prince JS, Nixon GW. Oblique chest views as a routine part of skeletal surveys performed for possible physical abuse—is this practice worthwhile? Child Abuse Negl. 2008;32(1):155–9. Epub 2007 Dec 21. PubMed PMID: 18096227. eng.
10. Section on Radiology; American Academy of Pediatrics. Diagnostic imaging of child abuse. Pediatrics. 2009; 123(5):1430–5. doi:10.1542/peds.2009-0558. PubMed PMID: 19403511. eng.
11. Dwek J. The radiographic approach to child abuse. Clin Orthop Relat Res. 2011;469(3):776–89. doi:10.1007/s11999-010-1414-5. Review. PubMed PMID: 20544318; PubMed Central PMCID: PMC3032862. eng.
12. Kemp AM, Butler A, Morris S, Mann M, Kemp KW, Rolfe K, Sibert JR, Maguire S. Which radiological investigations should be performed to identify fractures in suspected child abuse? Clin Radiol. 2006;61(9):723–36. Review. PubMed PMID: 16905379. eng.
13. Erfurt C, Hahn G, Roesner D, Schmidt U. Pediatric radiological diagnostic procedures in cases of suspected child abuse. Forensic Sci Med Pathol. 2011;7(1):65–74. doi:10.1007/s12024-010-9148-y. Epub 2010 Feb 27. Review. PubMed PMID: 20195804. eng.
14. Wootton-Gorges SL, Stein-Wexler R, Walton JW, Rosas AJ, Coulter KP, Rogers KK. Comparison of computed tomography and chest radiography in the detection of rib fractures in abused infants. Child Abuse Negl. 2008;32(6):659–63. doi:10.1016/j.chiabu.2007.06.011. Epub 2008 Jun 17. PubMed PMID: 18562001. eng.
15. Sanchez TR, Jadhav SP, Swischuk LE. MR imaging of pediatric trauma. Magn Reson Imaging Clin N Am. 2009;17(3):439–50. doi:10.1016/j.mric.2009.03.007. Review. PubMed PMID: 19524195. eng.
16. Perez-Rossello JM, Connolly SA, Newton AW, Zou KH, Kleinman PK. Whole-body MRI in suspected infant abuse. AJR Am J Roentgenol. 2010;195(3):744–50. doi:10.2214/AJR.09.3364. PubMed PMID: 20729455. eng.
17. Kleinman P. Diagnostic imaging of child abuse. St. Louis: Mosby, Inc; 1998.
18. Barsness KA, Cha ES, Bensard DD, Calkins CM, Partrick DA, Karrer FM, Strain JD. The positive predictive value of rib fractures as an indicator of nonaccidental trauma in children. J Trauma. 2003;54(6):1107–10. PubMed PMID: 12813330. eng.
19. Snedecor ST, Wilson HB. Some obstetrical injuries to the long bones. J Bone Joint Surg Am. 1949;31A(2): 378–84. PubMed PMID: 18116571. eng.
20. Kleinman PK, Schlesinger AE. Mechanical factors associated with posterior rib fractures: laboratory and case studies. Pediatr Radiol. 1997;27(1):87–91. PubMed PMID: 8995179. eng.
21. Bilo R, Robben S, van Rijn R. Forensic aspects of pediatric fractures. Differentiating accidental trauma from child abuse. Berlin/Heidelberg: Springer; 2010.
22. Offiah A, van Rijn RR, Perez-Rossello JM, Kleinman PK. Skeletal imaging of child abuse (non-accidental injury). Pediatr Radiol. 2009;39(5):461–70. doi:10.1007/s00247-009-1157-1. Epub 2009 Feb 24. Review. PubMed PMID: 19238374. eng.
23. Sanchez T, Stewart D, Walvick M, Swischuk L. Skull fracture vs. accessory sutures: how can we tell the difference? Emerg Radiol. 2010;17(5):413–8. doi:10.1007/s10140-010-0877-8. Epub 2010 May 23. PubMed PMID: 20496093; PubMed Central PMCID: PMC2914264. eng.
24. Taitz J, Moran K, O'Meara M. Long bone fractures in children under 3 years of age: is abuse being missed in Emergency Department presentations? J Paediatr Child Health. 2004;40(4):170–4. PubMed PMID: 15009543. eng.
25. Bishop N, Sprigg A, Dalton A. Unexplained fractures in infancy: looking for fragile bones. Arch Dis Child. 2007;92(3):251–6. Review. PubMed PMID: 17337685; PubMed Central PMCID: PMC2083418. eng.
26. Boal D. Child abuse. In: Slovis EA, editor. Pediatric diagnostic imaging. Philadelphia: Mosby; 2008. p. 2816–30.
27. Worlock P, Stower M, Barbor P. Patterns of fractures in accidental and non-accidental injury in children: a comparative study. Br Med J (Clin Res Ed). 1986;293(6539):100–2. PubMed PMID: 3089406; PubMed Central PMCID: PMC1340839. eng.
28. Kwon DS, Spevak MR, Fletcher K, Kleinman PK. Physiologic subperiosteal new bone formation: prevalence, distribution, and thickness in neonates and infants. AJR Am J Roentgenol. 2002;179(4):985–8. PubMed PMID: 12239052.
29. Islam O, Soboleski D, Symons S, Davidson LK, Ashworth MA, Babyn P. Development and duration of radiographic signs of bone healing in children. AJR Am J Roentgenol. 2000;175(1):75–8. PubMed PMID: 10882250. eng.
30. Prosser I, Maguire S, Harrison SK, Mann M, Sibert JR, Kemp AM. How old is this fracture? Radiologic dating of fractures in children: a systematic review. AJR Am J Roentgenol. 2005;184(4):1282–6. Review. PubMed PMID: 15788611. eng.
31. Chapman S. The radiological dating of injuries. Arch Dis Child. 1992;67(9):1063–5. Review. PubMed PMID: 1417044; PubMed Central PMCID: PMC1793610. eng.
32. Yeo LI, Reed MH. Staging of healing of femoral fractures in children. Can Assoc Radiol J. 1994;45(1): 16–9. PubMed PMID: 8118709. eng.

33. Prosser I, Lawson Z, Evans A, Harrison S, Morris S, Maguire S, Kemp AM. A timetable for the radiologic features of fracture healing in young children. AJR Am J Roentgenol. 2012;198(5):1014–20. doi:10.2214/AJR.11.6734. PubMed PMID: 22528890. eng.
34. Sanchez TR, Nguyen H, Palacios W, Doherty M, Coulter K. Retrospective evaluation and dating of non-accidental rib fractures in infants. Clin Radiol. 2013;68(8):e467–71. doi:10.1016/j.crad.2013.03.017. Epub 2013 Apr 25. PubMed PMID: 23622800. eng.
35. Ablin DS, Greenspan A, Reinhart M, Grix A. Differentiation of child abuse from osteogenesis imperfecta. AJR Am J Roentgenol. 1990;154(5):1035–46. Review. PubMed PMID: 2108539. eng.
36. Mendelson KL. Critical review of 'temporary brittle bone disease'. Pediatr Radiol. 2005;35(10):1036–40. Epub 2005 Aug 24. Review. PubMed PMID: 16132899. eng.
37. Keller KA, Barnes PD. Rickets vs. abuse: a national and international epidemic. Pediatr Radiol. 2008;38(11):1210–6. doi:10.1007/s00247-008-1001-z. Epub 2008 Sep 23. PubMed PMID: 18810424. eng.
38. Chapman T, Sugar N, Done S, Marasigan J, Wambold N, Feldman K. Fractures in infants and toddlers with rickets. Pediatr Radiol. 2010;40(7):1184–9. doi:10.1007/s00247-009-1470-8. Epub 2009 Dec 9. Erratum in: Pediatr Radiol. 2010;40(7):1308. PubMed PMID: 20012034. eng.
39. Kleinman PK. Problems in the diagnosis of metaphyseal fractures. Pediatr Radiol. 2008;38 Suppl 3:S388–94. doi:10.1007/s00247-008-0845-6. Review. PubMed PMID: 18470447. eng.
40. Jenny C, Committee on Child Abuse and Neglect. Evaluating infants and young children with multiple fractures. Pediatrics. 2006;118(3):1299–303. Review. PubMed PMID: 16951031. eng.

Musculoskeletal Infection

19

Rebecca Stein-Wexler

Contents

R. Stein-Wexler, MD
Department of Radiology,
University of California Davis Medical
Center and UC Davis Children's Hospital,
4860 Y Street, Suite 3100, Sacramento, CA 95817, USA

Department of Diagnostic Imaging,
Shriners Hospitals for Children Northern California,
Sacramento, CA 95817, USA
e-mail: rebecca.steinwexler@ucdmc.ucdavis.edu

Abstract

Manifestation of musculoskeletal infection in children depends on the developmental anatomy of bones and in particular its changing vascular supply. Thus, it is essential to understand this process thoroughly. Osteomyelitis, septic arthritis, and cellulitis are relatively common. There are three accepted stages of osteomyelitis—acute, subacute, and chronic. Each has a unique presentation and imaging appearance, but they can be confused with other entities. Radiology, ultrasound, nuclear imaging, CT, and MRI each play a critical role depending on the clinical scenario and the suspected pathogen. Much of this discussion focuses on common bacterial infections (including methicillin-resistant *Staphylococcus aureus*), but meningococcemia, tuberculosis, fungal infections, and syphilis are also discussed. In addition, the chapter presents manifestations of osteomyelitis in unique locations, such as the epiphysis, the pelvis, and the spine, and in unique patient populations, such as those with sickle-cell disease. Although chronic recurrent multifocal osteomyelitis is auto-inflammatory rather than infectious, we include it here as well.

1 Osteomyelitis

Osteomyelitis and septic arthritis are relatively common, and their incidence is increasing. They occur in approximately 1 in 10,000 children per

R. Stein-Wexler et al. (eds.), *Pediatric Orthopedic Imaging*,
DOI 10.1007/978-3-642-45381-6_19,

year [1, 2]. However, diagnosis of musculoskeletal infection may be challenging. Although older children often present with fever, malaise, and localizing pain and tenderness, in infancy the only sign may be pseudoparalysis, or refusal to use a limb. Toddlers may present with a limp or with pseudoparalysis. Laboratory findings—such as elevated C-reactive protein (CRP) and erythrocyte sedimentation rate (ESR)—often suggest an inflammatory process but are otherwise nonspecific. Leukocytosis is not consistently encountered [3].

The peak age for septic arthritis is 2 years, and for osteomyelitis, the peak is 4 years [4, 5]. One third of osteomyelitis cases present before age 2 [6]. Osteomyelitis is twice as common in boys as in girls; there is no sex predilection for septic arthritis [6]. Both are more common in the immunocompromised. Multifocal disease is encountered in as many as 10 % of patients and is seen in up to 50 % of neonates [3].

Musculoskeletal infection in infancy and childhood usually results from hematogenous spread due to transient bacteremia [6, 7]; extension from adjacent cellulitis or direct inoculation is less common. In older children, however, direct implantation as a result of surgery or open fractures sometimes occurs. Preceding trauma may damage the periosteum, disrupting the natural barrier to infection. *Staphylococcus aureus* accounts for 70–90 % of cases in children [8]. Methicillin-resistant *Staphylococcus aureus* subtype (MRSA) is becoming increasingly common, in some studies accounting for 30 % of cases [1, 2]. Group A beta hemolytic *Streptococcus* is also a common pathogen. Group B *Streptococcus* and gram-negative *Enterococci* are important pathogens in newborns, and *Meningococcus* is encountered in infants as well as in sexually active teens. Patients with sickle-cell disease are prone to infection with *Salmonella species. Kingella kingae* is increasing in frequency and has a tendency to cause multifocal disease. Immunosuppressed patients—such as those with chronic granulomatous disease or human immunodeficiency virus (HIV)—are prone to fungal and mycobacterial infection. In countries with widespread immunization, *Hemophilus influenza* is no longer a common pathogen.

Osteomyelitis is most common at the more rapidly growing ends of long bones, and it also favors the lower extremities. The femur and tibia at the knee are the most common locations, followed by the wrist and shoulder. In infants, the femoral neck and capital femoral epiphysis are the most common sites of osteomyelitis and are often accompanied with septic arthritis of the hip. Metaphyseal equivalents such as synchondroses in the flat bones and apophyses of long bones are also prone to infection (especially the triradiate cartilage and ischiopubic synchondrosis in the pelvis) and—in 10 % of patients—the dorsal calcaneus [9]). Pelvic osteomyelitis is uncommon but important because it is often occult and therefore advanced when diagnosed; soft tissue abscesses are often present. Osteomyelitis of the spine must be recognized promptly to avoid cord compression due to epidural abscess.

A thorough understanding of bone development and resultant characteristics of musculoskeletal infection is essential to correct interpretation of imaging, discussed below:

1.1 Acute Osteomyelitis (Box 19.1)

Box 19.1 Acute Osteomyelitis

Radiography:
- Early: deep soft tissue swelling
- Mid: cortical fraying
- Late: moth eaten

MRI: positive 2 days after symptoms
- Overestimates extent
- T1 wide zone of transition
- Cortical destruction and periosteal elevation
- Intraosseous, subperiosteal, or soft tissue abscesses/edema

1. In most cases, organisms initially target the highly vascular metaphysis. Sluggish blood flow in the large, venous sinusoidal loops in this area allows bacteria to adhere to endothelium and penetrate capillaries to enter the extravascular space. Limited phagocytic activity in metaphyseal capillaries facilitates bacterial proliferation. Intraosseous pressure increases due to the inflammatory response

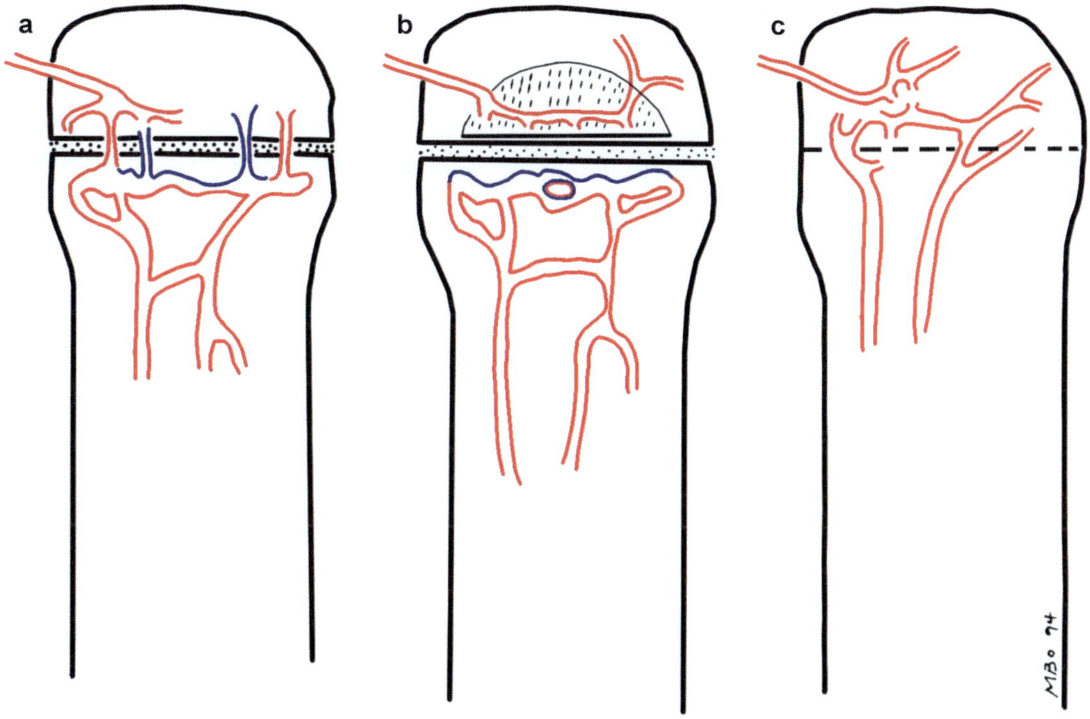

Fig. 19.1 The three stages of vascular development of the growth plate. (**a**) Until approximately 18 months, blood vessels from the epiphysis and the metaphysis cross the physis, allowing infection to easily spread. (**b**) From about 18 months until the physes close, the physis serves as a barrier to infection, since blood vessels do not traverse this area. Metaphyseal vessels terminate in sinusoids, where blood flow is sluggish. (**c**) After physeal closure, infection again spreads readily between the epiphysis and the metaphysis, via blood vessels that cross the physis as the bony scar is resorbed. (*Red* arterial supply, *Blue* venous drainage)

and exudate. Edema and vascular congestion progress to small vessel thrombosis, bone necrosis, and bone resorption. Subsequent spread of disease varies with patient age, as discussed below (Fig. 19.1).

2. In infancy (up to about 18 months), blood vessels penetrate the physis to extend from the metaphysis to the epiphysis. This allows infection to spread readily from the metaphysis to the epiphysis (Fig. 19.2). Septic arthritis is also very common, as infection can spread directly to the joint either by extension through the epiphysis or by perforating the metaphyseal cortex (which is intra-articular in the hip, shoulder, and elbow). Conversely, infection that begins within the joint may infrequently spread to the epiphysis and then the metaphysis. Avascular necrosis of the epiphysis is very common, as high pressure within the joint restricts blood flow. Septic arthritis of the hip frequently results in avascular necrosis of the femoral head, with eventual growth disturbance.
3. During childhood, contrasted with infancy, vessels do not penetrate across the physis, and thus the physis serves as a barrier to transphyseal spread to the epiphysis. Infection is initially confined to the metaphysis, but as intramedullary pressure increases, pus eventually penetrates the normal metaphyseal fenestrations to spread via Haversian and Volkmann canals. After reaching the subperiosteal space, it readily dissects along the diaphysis, as the periosteum is relatively loosely attached to bone in children. Subperiosteal abscesses may form. In addition, infection may penetrate the periosteum and spread into the soft tissues. Alternatively, septic arthritis may develop at joints with an intra-articular metaphysis.
4. After closure of the growth plate, osteomyelitis behaves as it does in adults. The metaphysis is still the most common location (due to

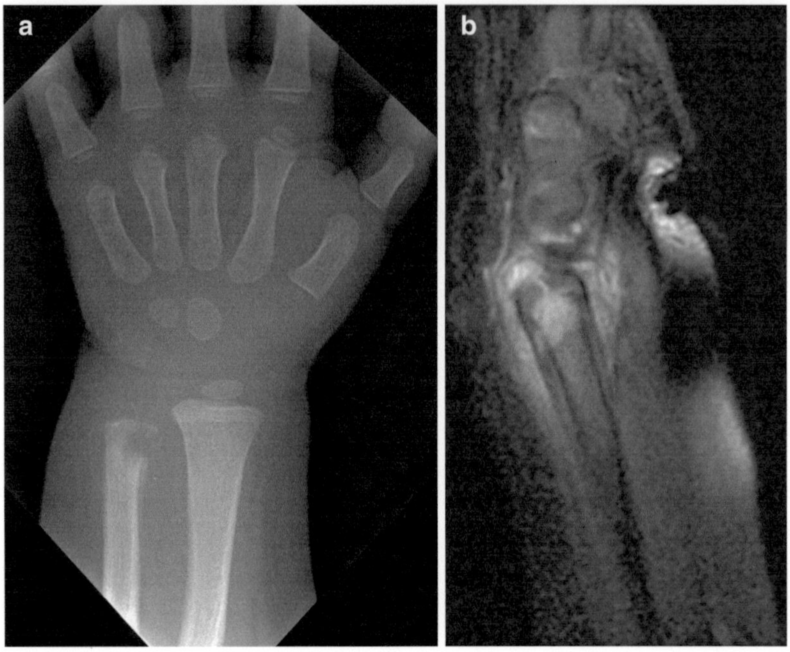

Fig. 19.2 Metaphyseal osteomyelitis in a 16-month-old. (**a**) Lytic defect in the distal ulna with very early periosteal reaction and extensive para-ulnar soft tissue swelling. (**b**) Sagittal T1-weighted (T1-W) gadolinium-enhanced fat-suppressed (FS) MRI shows a tract crossing the physis, with epiphyseal enhancement. Abnormal signal extends into the joint

its vascularity and the slow flow of blood in sinusoids), but epiphyseal spread is common, as vessels again cross the growth plate.

1.2 Subacute Osteomyelitis (Box 19.2)

> **Box 19.2 Brodie Abscess**
> Eccentric cortical or medullary abscess of subacute osteomyelitis
> Often drains to physis
> Radiography: central lucent focus, surrounding sclerosis, draining channel
> Mild periosteal reaction, localized
> MRI: penumbra

Subacute osteomyelitis develops if the host response or incomplete antibiotic therapy partially suppresses the infection or if the pathogen is indolent. Presentation is more insidious, with symptoms present for 2 weeks or longer [6]. Instead of the exuberant inflammatory process often encountered in acute osteomyelitis, the infection is more localized, usually confined to the metaphysis, and shows little periosteal thickening. The lower extremity is almost invariably involved, with over 90 % of lesions in the femur or tibia. Over 60 % are metaphyseal, and most occur at the distal tibia. Subacute osteomyelitis may occur in the epiphysis. Most common in adolescents and males, subacute osteomyelitis has not been described in patients younger than 6 years of age.

Subacute osteomyelitis may manifest as a Brodie abscess, which develops in the cortex or medulla and is usually eccentric. It usually drains to the physis and may extend to the epiphysis. Eburnated bone along with fibrous and granulation tissue encloses a central area of osseous necrosis. Staphylococcus is the usual pathogen [7].

1.3 Chronic Osteomyelitis (Box 19.3)

> **Box 19.3 Chronic Osteomyelitis**
> Involucrum: thick, ossified periosteal reaction
> Sequestrum: central sclerotic infarcted bone
> Cloaca: tract penetrating cortex, +/– to skin

Chronic osteomyelitis has been present for at least 6 weeks and is more common in developing nations. Periosteal thickening has typically progressed, thickened, and ossified, forming an involucrum (from the Latin, *involvere*, envelop) that isolates the more central infection. Meanwhile, increasing pressure causes cortical bone infarction and necrosis, forming a sequestrum, which may then serve as a nidus of infection. The central infection may break through the cortex or penetrate to the physis, forming a (from the Latin, *cloaca*, sewer), which then permits the inflammatory debris to drain to the skin via a sinus tract [7]. Formation of an involucrum and sequestrum is unusual if antibiotics are administered at an early stage.

Erythrocyte sedimentation rate and white blood cell count can be normal and also nonspecific. Blood cultures are positive in up to 60 % of cases, whereas cultures of aspirated material yield an organism in as many as 85 % [7].

1.4 Imaging

Radiographs

Radiographs are the initial imaging modality for acute osteomyelitis. While they help exclude such entities as tumors and fractures, they are often normal in cases of acute osteomyelitis. Deep soft tissue swelling may be apparent after 2 days of symptoms (Fig. 19.3), but bony findings are not evident for 1–2 weeks in the long bones and often much longer in the pelvis or spine. Demineralization of 30–50 % is necessary before bone lysis becomes apparent, but subtle cortical fraying due to subperiosteal resorption may be seen earlier (Fig. 19.4). Demineralization is usually due to disuse and confers a worse prognosis. In the appropriate clinical setting, osteolysis manifesting with a permeative or moth-eaten appearance, accompanied with periosteal reaction and surrounding subtle sclerosis, may allow diagnosis (Fig. 19.5). Physeal widening and epiphyseal destruction may occur in infants.

Brodie abscess, characteristic of subacute osteomyelitis, is composed of a central lucent focus in the metaphysis surrounded by sclerosis and accompanied by a tortuous channel that may drain to the physis (Figs. 19.6, 19.7, 19.8, and 19.9); identification of this channel confirms the diagnosis of subacute osteomyelitis [7]. Single or laminated periosteal new bone formation is typical, with little surrounding inflammation [6]. Epiphyseal subacute osteomyelitis usually appears as a lytic, cystic, intra-epiphyseal lesion.

Chronic osteomyelitis manifests with thick periosteum and cortex, forming the involucrum that encases the sclerotic sequestrum (Figs. 19.10 and 19.11). The prominent cortical thickening is termed "Garré sclerosing osteomyelitis."

Scintigraphy

Some centers advocate scintigraphy for diagnosis of osteomyelitis, performing magnetic resonance imaging (MRI) only in cases that involve the spine or pelvis or do not respond to treatment [10]. Three-phase bone scan may be easier to obtain and less expensive than other advanced imaging, and its sensitivity exceeds 80 %, but it is only 50 % specific [11]. Able to discern as little as 5 % change in bone turnover, a bone scan can be positive 24–48 h from onset of symptoms. The bone scan is especially useful in infants and other patients who cannot localize disease—such as neonates (Fig. 19.12) in whom 22 % of disease is multifocal [12]. Furthermore, in the 10 % of patients in whom the site of disease does not correspond to the painful locus, a whole-body bone scan should identify the disease (as will a whole-body MRI) [10].

A triple-phase bone scan should be performed. Osteomyelitis has increased uptake in all three phases (Fig. 19.13). However, the delayed images are most definitive, and excluding unusual locations such as the pelvis (see Fig. 19.18 below) normal delayed images usually exclude the diagnosis of osteomyelitis. Pinhole images are helpful. Single photo emission computed tomography (SPECT) improves spatial resolution but can be difficult to perform in children [13].

Bone scans may not show disease that abuts the physis, and ischemia or a weak inflammatory response can result in a false-negative examination. Increased pressure or marrow ischemia can lead to decreased blood flow resulting in

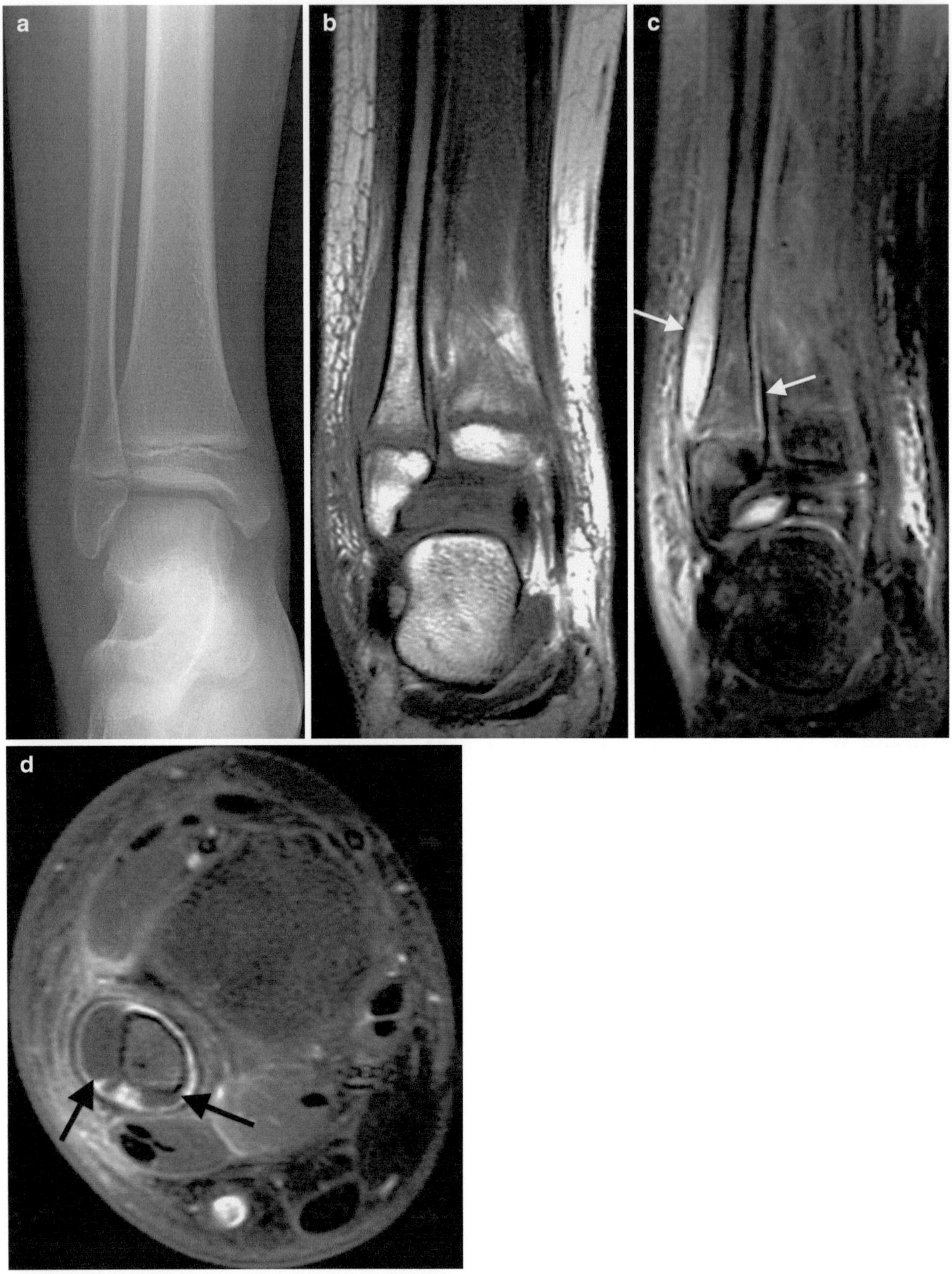

Fig. 19.3 Acute *Staphylococcus aureus* osteomyelitis with subperiosteal abscess. (**a**) Marked lateral soft tissue swelling and loss of subcutaneous fascial planes. (**b**) Contemporaneous T1-W coronal MRI shows periosteal thickening. (**c**) Coronal T2-weighted (T2-W) FS MRI shows subperiosteal fluid (*arrows*) with edema of the distal fibular metaphysis and epiphysis. (**d**) Gadolinium-enhanced FS T1-W axial image delineates subperiosteal abscesses (*arrows*) along the fibula

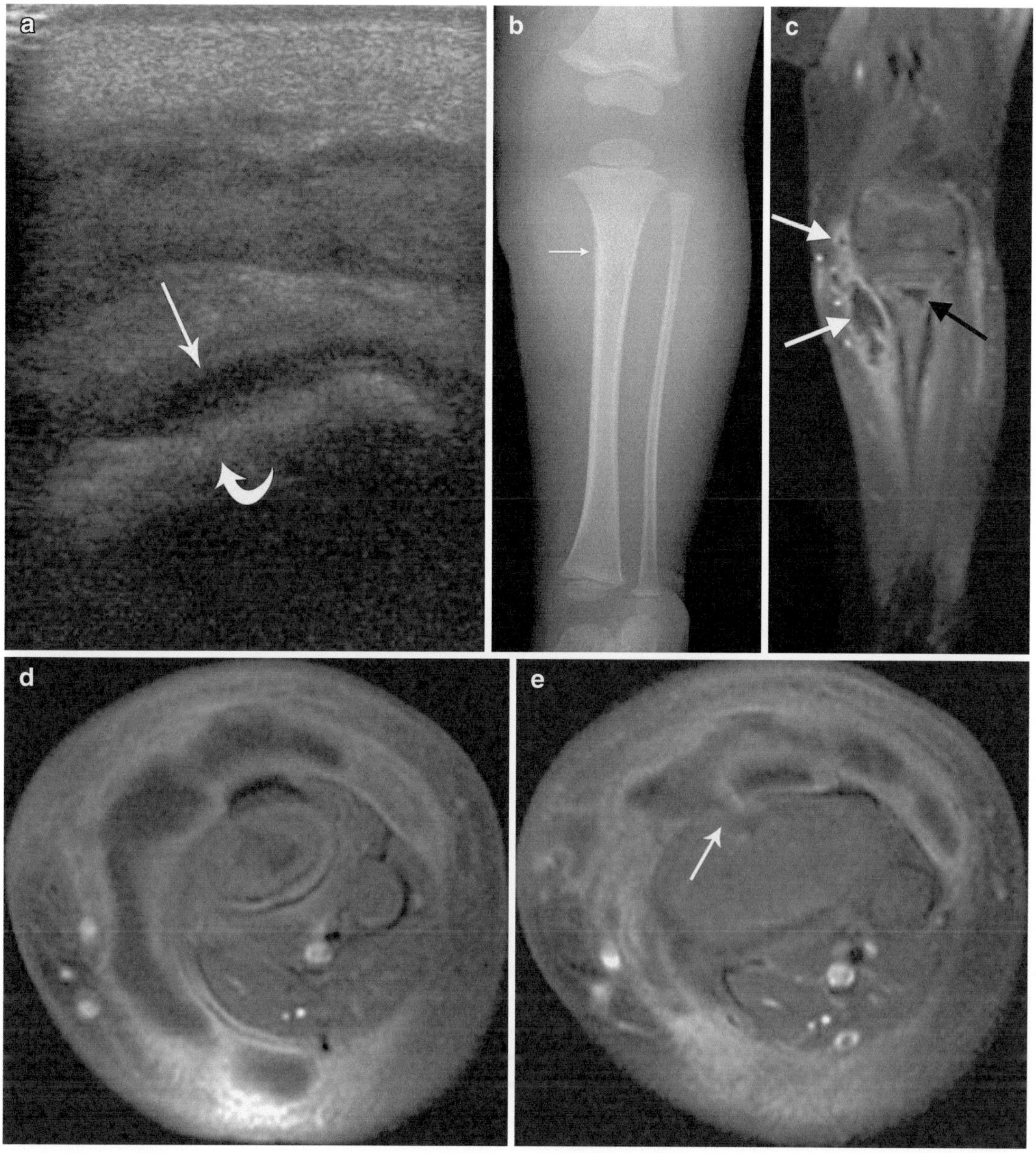

Fig. 19.4 *Staphylococcus aureus* osteomyelitis with subperiosteal, soft tissue, and intramedullary abscess formation. (**a**) Initial sagittal US shows cortical irregularity (*curved arrow*) along with subperiosteal fluid (*arrow*). (**b**) Four days later, proximal tibial bone density is slightly decreased, and there is a thin line of periosteal reaction (*arrow*). Soft tissues are edematous. (**c**) Coronal T1-W FS gadolinium-enhanced MRI shows marrow enhancement with intramedullary abscess (*black arrow*) and multiple soft tissue abscesses (*white arrows*). (**d**, **e**) Axial T1-W FS gadolinium-enhanced images better delineate multiple abscesses and periosteal fluid, along with the cloaca (*arrow*)

"cold" osteomyelitis and necrosis due to vascular thrombosis; both are more common with MRSA and might not be recognized at bone scan [14]. Findings of infection, tumor, and trauma can overlap. Gallium improves specificity to 80 % [6] and may delineate soft tissue abscesses, but it is less desirable than MRI, in part due to high radiation dose.

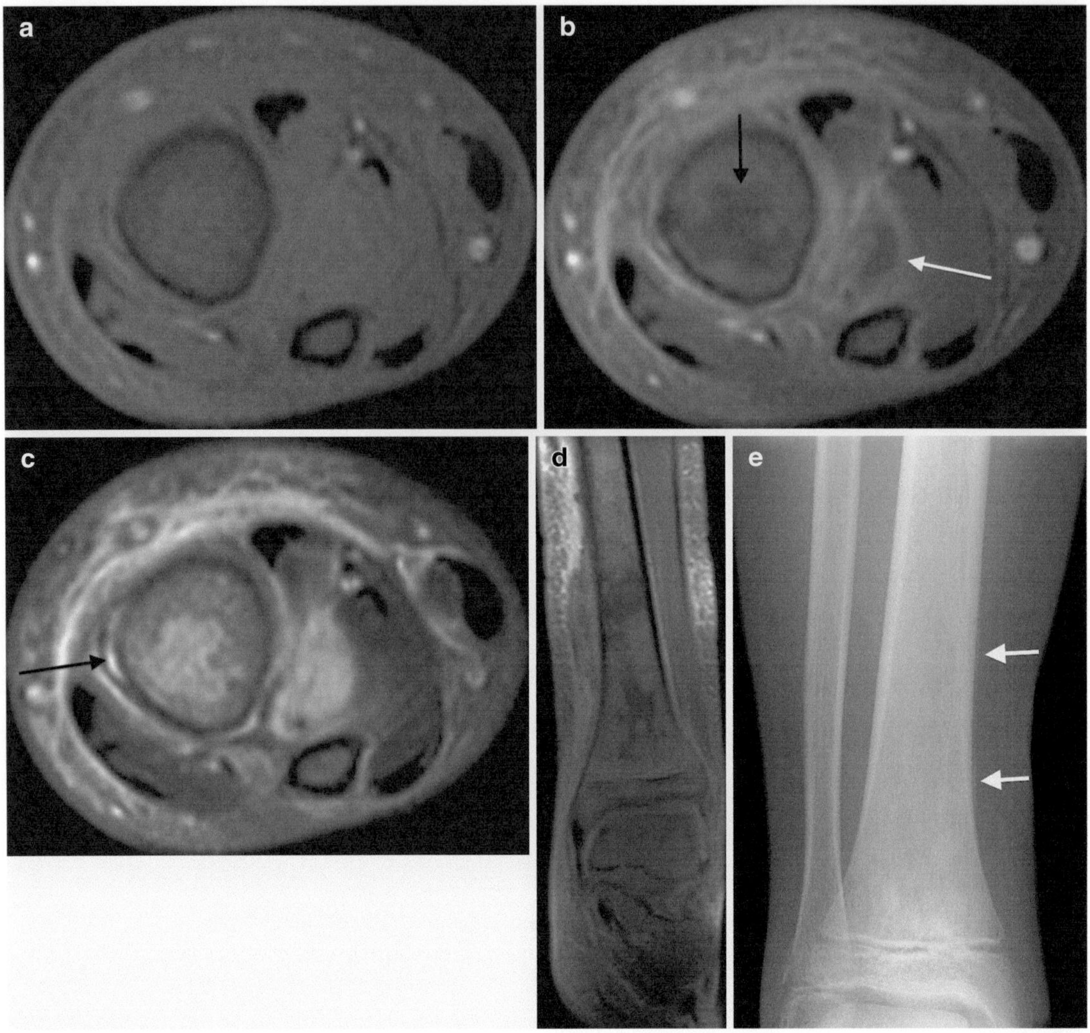

Fig. 19.5 Acute osteomyelitis with intraosseous, subperiosteal, and soft tissue abscesses in a 12-year-old. Axial T1-W FS (**a**) and gadolinium-enhanced T1-W FS (**b**) images show irregular tibial marrow enhancement and extensive soft tissue enhancement, with central nonenhancement both within the marrow (*black arrow*) and in the soft tissues lateral to the tibia (*white arrow*), indicating osseous and soft tissue abscesses. (**c**) The axial T2-W FS image shows increased signal in portion of marrow that does not enhance, with extensive soft tissue inflammation and a subperiosteal abscess (*arrow*). (**d**) Coronal gadolinium-enhanced FS T1-W image also shows intraosseous abscesses as well as the subperiosteal abscess. (**e**) Four weeks later, the distal tibia appears permeative, with a well-defined thin line of periosteal reaction (*arrows*)

Because scintigraphy cannot delineate abscesses, it is generally less useful in the spine and pelvis, where abscesses are especially common (again, gallium may be employed). In the spine, delineation of intraspinous abscesses and possible cord compression is essential. Abscesses are less often associated with osteomyelitis of the long bones. Scintigraphy may be sufficient in these cases, provided that if there is a poor response to antibiotic therapy, then MRI is performed [10].

Spatial resolution has improved with fludeoxyglucose photon emission tomography (FDG-PET) and SPECT, allowing better differentiation of osteomyelitis from septic arthritis and cellulitis; specificity of combined SPECT/CT exceeds 80 % [11, 15]. If complementary white blood cell scanning is performed, then

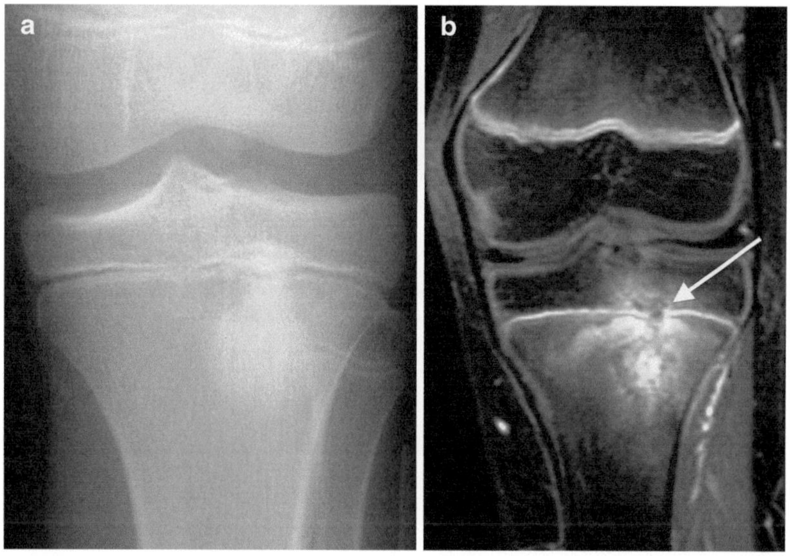

Fig. 19.6 Subacute osteomyelitis in a teenage boy. (**a**) Osteolysis surrounds sclerosis in this less classic case. (**b**) Coronal gadolinium-enhanced T1-W FS MRI shows layered enhancement, with a cloaca (*arrow*) breaking across the physis along with epiphyseal involvement. Note the relative lack of soft tissue enhancement

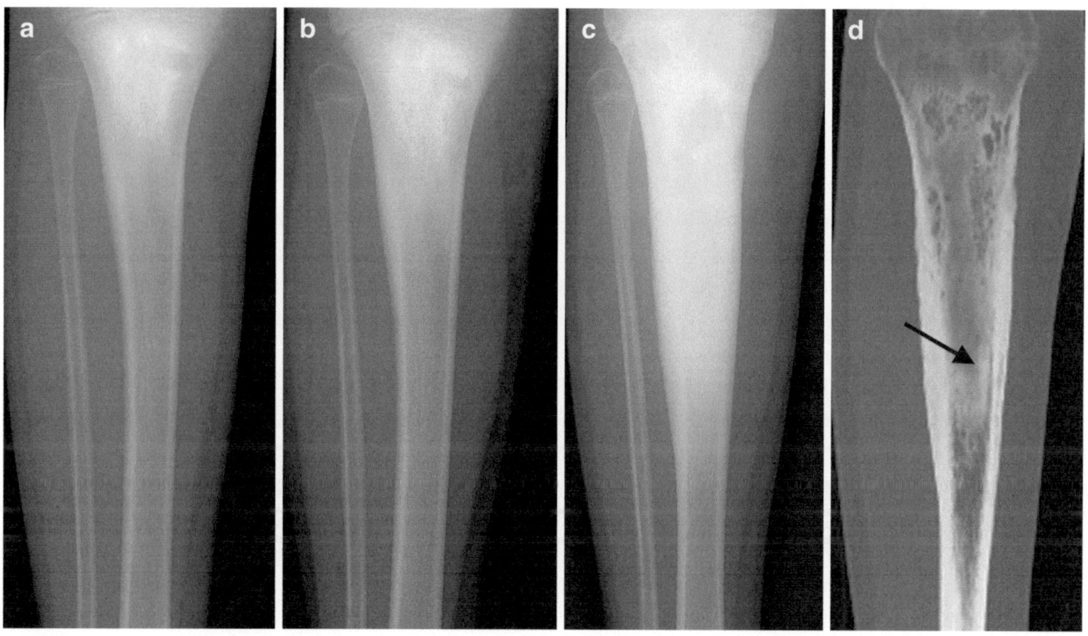

Fig. 19.7 Evolution of *Staphylococcus aureus* osteomyelitis. (**a**) Radiograph of subacute stage shows ill-defined decreased density with surrounding sclerosis in the proximal tibial metaphysis. (**b**) Several months later, there is diffuse sclerosis at the mid and proximal tibia with central lucency consistent with subacute to chronic osteomyelitis. (**c**) Three years later, sclerosis and thickening have progressed to chronic osteomyelitis. (**d**) Coronal reformatted CT shows a sequestrum (*arrow*)

sensitivity and specificity exceed 90 %, as the white blood cell (WBC) scan is positive in marrow that is cold on SPECT because the normal marrow has been replaced with an infectious process. However, the application of WBC scintigraphy to pediatric imaging is limited, as it usually requires at least 15 mL of blood [13]. PET/CT may be useful in follow-up of acute osteomyelitis, as it can differentiate between reparative activity and acute infection [16]. It may also allow identification of a focus of active infection within chronic osteomyelitis.

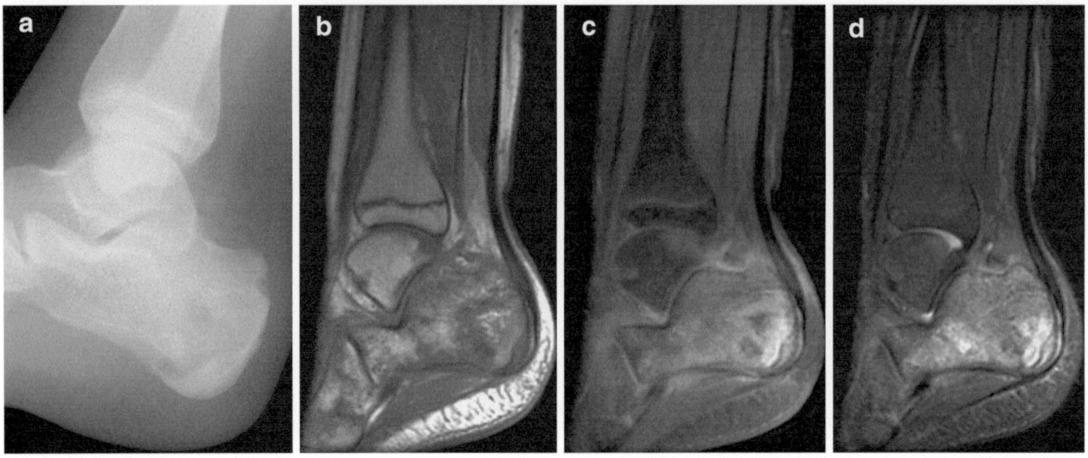

Fig. 19.8 Subacute osteomyelitis in a 12-year-old girl with 6 weeks' history of cellulitis and pain. (**a**) Lucent focus is seen posteriorly within the heterogeneous calcaneus. (**b**) Sagittal T1-W MRI shows a layered appearance to the calcaneus. (**c**) T1-W gadolinium-enhanced FS MRI shows osseous and limited soft tissue enhancement. (**d**) Short-tau inversion recovery sequence shows extensive calcaneal edema, which has a geographic appearance

Ultrasound

Ultrasound can depict juxtacortical soft tissue swelling as soon as 1 or 2 days after the onset of symptoms [17], well before radiographic changes are evident. In the early stages, soft tissue inflammation appears as loss of normal tissue planes along with interdigitating areas of decreased echogenicity. If subperiosteal fluid is present, bone is presumed to be involved [18]. Lentiform subperiosteal fluid collections measuring at least 2 mm in thickness, which may be of increased or decreased echogenicity, indicate disease progression and the development of subperiosteal abscesses [18] (Fig. 19.4). With further progression, superficial cortical bone defects, fistulas, and sequestra can become apparent [17, 18]. Color Doppler shows increased blood flow as soon as 4 days after the onset of symptoms [18] and may permit monitoring of disease progression by evaluating blood flow in soft tissues around infected periosteum [19]. It is important to recognize that a negative ultrasound does not exclude osteomyelitis.

CT

MRI has generally supplanted computed tomography (CT) for evaluation of acute osteomyelitis, but in cases of chronic osteomyelitis, CT is helpful, as it readily depicts foci of intraosseous gas, cortical thickening, sclerosis, encroachment on the medullary cavity, and draining sinus (Figs. 19.7 and 19.14). It also identifies not only large sequestra but also the smaller sequestra and foreign bodies that may not be appreciated at MRI but that must also be removed in order for antibiotic therapy to succeed [7].

MRI

MRI is widely used to assess musculoskeletal infection, as its inherent tissue contrast, multiplanar imaging, and ability to differentiate soft tissue from bone infection lead to high sensitivity and specificity. After screening radiographs, it is often the next diagnostic study. If symptoms of acute osteomyelitis persist for more than 48 h after initiation of antibiotic treatment, MRI is advisable to determine response to therapy, to evaluate for abscess formation, and to assist with surgical planning [20]. Locations with complex anatomy, such as the spine and pelvis, also benefit from early MRI.

The protocol includes T1, T2 with fat suppression, and short-tau inversion recovery (STIR) in orthogonal planes. Obtaining both pre- and postcontrast T1-weighted (T1-W) images facilitates correct interpretation of findings, but administration of gadolinium is somewhat

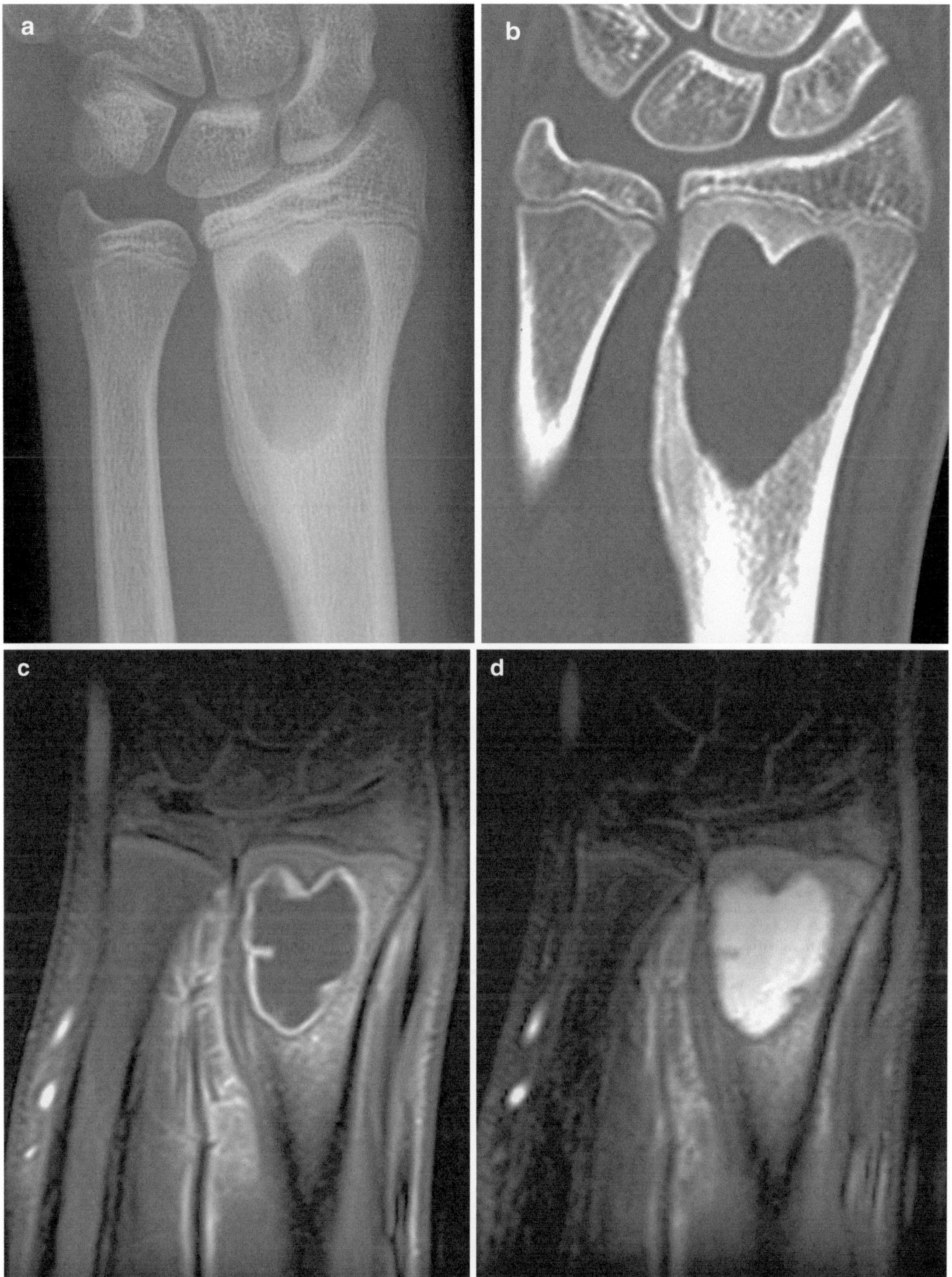

Fig. 19.9 Brodie abscess in a 14-year-old boy with wrist pain. (**a**) There is a well-circumscribed lucency in the distal radial metaphysis, with adjacent eburnated bone. (**b**) Coronally reformatted CT shows the abscess extending to the physis, with surrounding eburnation and maturing lamellar periosteal new bone. (**c**) T1-W gadolinium-enhanced FS image shows smooth marginal enhancement at the fluid collection and slight marrow and soft tissue enhancement. (**d**) Coronal T2-W FS MRI shows hyperintense fluid in the abscess but minimal marrow edema

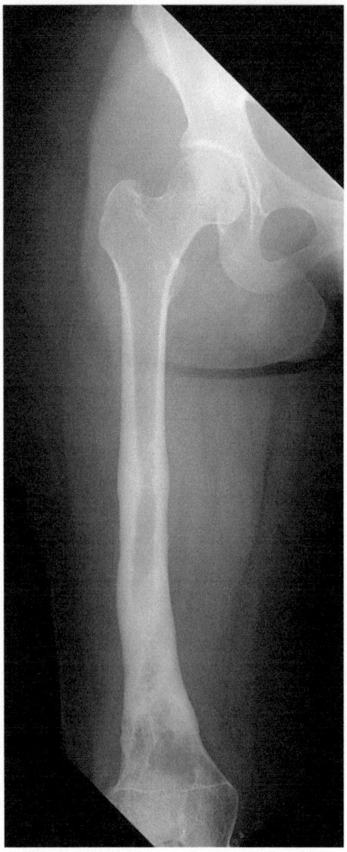

Fig. 19.10 Chronic osteomyelitis in a 15-year-old girl, refractory to treatment. There is marked endosteal sclerosis and a thick, undulating cortex

controversial. Diffusion-weighted imaging is useful, increasing conspicuity.

Marrow signal alters 1–2 days after onset of symptoms. However, signal changes are more subtle in children than in adults due to the higher water content in their bone marrow, and fluid-sensitive sequences can be misleading as both normal and abnormal marrow can be hyperintense. T1-W sequences better delineate marrow morphology [12], and a wide zone of transition is usually apparent. Edema, inflammatory cells, and exudate appear as ill-defined low T1 signal and as high-intensity signal on fluid-sensitive sequences (T2 and STIR) (Figs. 19.3, 19.4, 19.5, and 19.6). MRI may overestimate the extent of bony involvement, as reactive inflammation has a similar appearance [4]. Cortical bone may lose its normal low signal, and high T2 signal may be seen around the cortex, due to layering periosteal fluid. Epiphyseal and physeal involvement is readily seen on sagittal and coronal scans. If subperiosteal abscesses form, high T2/low T1 lentiform fluid collections are evident. Cortical thickening is not present in acute infection [7].

There has been considerable debate about whether gadolinium should be administered to assess osteomyelitis; many authors conclude that gadolinium is unnecessary if T1- and T2-weighted (T2-W) sequences are normal. However, if edema is present, the addition of contrast helps delineate epiphyseal involvement and also the presence of intraosseous, subperiosteal, and soft tissue abscesses. This both improves diagnostic confidence and affects management, as the presence of abscesses mandates surgical drainage [21, 22]. Devascularized bone due to septic thrombosis of nutrient channels also fails to enhance but does not demonstrate the typical rim enhancement of an abscess. Distribution of antibiotics mirrors that of gadolinium, with important implications for treatment [21]. MRI is especially useful in *Staphylococcus aureus* osteomyelitis, which tends to be more severe and is accompanied with a higher incidence of soft tissue complications [14].

Fat globules, larger than lipocytes, are seen in 70 % of cases of acute osteomyelitis, perhaps due to coalescence of lipid from lipocytes that have undergone necrosis. However, this is not pathognomonic for osteomyelitis, as fat globules can also be seen in sarcomas after treatment, in infarcts, and in Gaucher disease [23]. An extraosseous fat-fluid level may be pathognomonic for osteomyelitis [24]. Extraosseous fat is more common during and after puberty [25].

Although follow-up MRI is generally not necessary, it is useful in patients whose C-reactive protein does not fall within 14 days or in those with an otherwise worsening clinical course who may require repeat surgical drainage [26].

Differential Diagnosis

Aside from joint pathology such as soft tissue infection and arthritis, differential considerations for **acute osteomyelitis** include osteoid osteoma, osteosarcoma, Ewing sarcoma, leukemia/

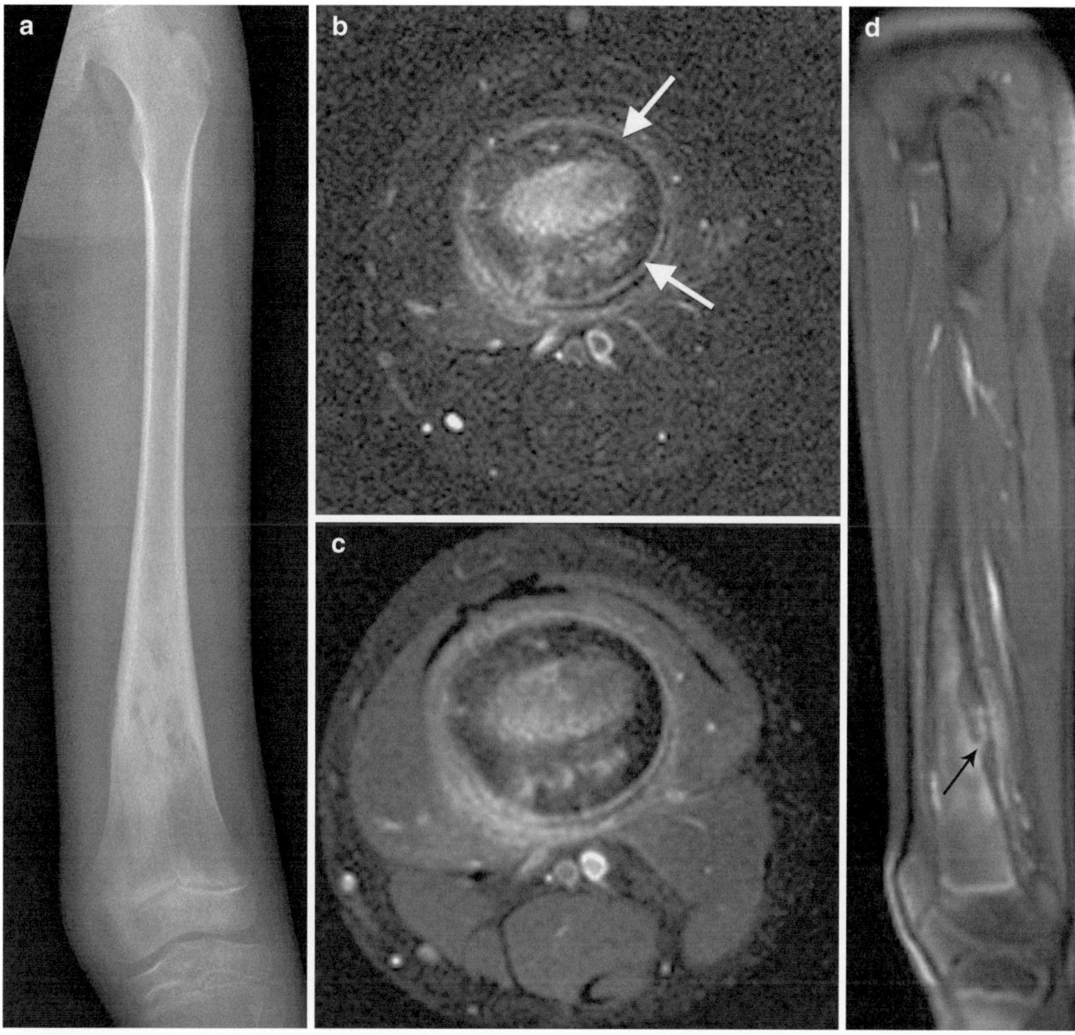

Fig. 19.11 Chronic osteomyelitis. (**a**) Diaphyseal and metaphyseal sclerosis in the distal femur. The thickened cortex is hypointense (*arrows*) on both axial T2-W fat-suppressed (**b**) and axial T1-W gadolinium-enhanced fat-saturated MRI (**c**), with relatively mild edema and enhancement in surrounding soft tissues. (**d**) Sagittal FS T1-W gadolinium-enhanced image shows a draining cloaca that enhances as it penetrates the posterior femoral cortex (*arrow*)

lymphoma, metastatic neuroblastoma, and Langerhans cell histiocytosis. The wide zone of transition on T1-W imaging helps differentiate osteomyelitis from these entities. It is also characterized by a more heterogeneous pattern of enhancement.

Subacute osteomyelitis bears some resemblance to tumor, having a more geographic appearance than does acute osteomyelitis at T1-W imaging. Several MRI characteristics help differentiate subacute osteomyelitis: the presence of multiple distinct layers and the so-called penumbra, where a central low T1/high T2 signal abscess cavity is surrounded by a two-layered rim (Figs. 19.6 and 19.8). The inner rim of granulation tissue is isointense to muscle on T1-W imaging and hyperintense on T2, whereas the outer fibrous rim is hypointense on all sequences. A halo of T1-hypointense edema surrounds the hypointense rim [27]. The penumbra consists of a thin layer of granulation tissue that surrounds the

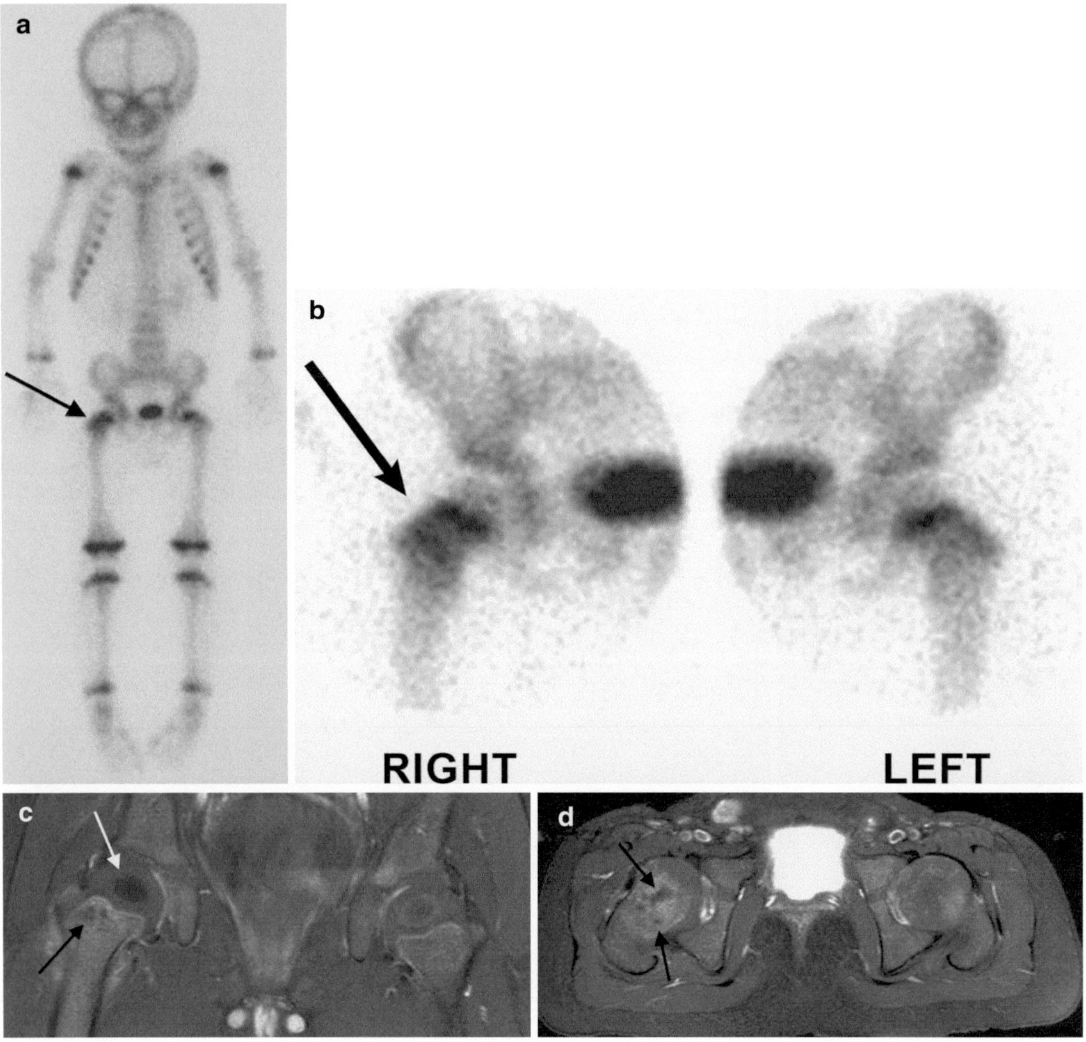

Fig. 19.12 Acute osteomyelitis in an infant. (**a**) Delayed whole-body Technetium-99m-labeled bone scan shows increased activity in the right hip (*arrow*). Pinhole views (**b**) localize the increased activity to the femoral neck and intertrochanteric region. Coronal (**c**) and axial (**d**) T1-W gadolinium-enhanced FS MRI show marrow and soft tissue enhancement. Non-enhancing foci in the femoral neck (*black arrows*) may represent abscesses, whereas the T1-hypointense right femoral head ossific nucleus (*white arrow*) is likely ischemic (Courtesy of Tal Laor, Cincinnati Children's Hospital)

abscess. On unenhanced T1-W sequences, it is slightly hyperintense, perhaps due to its relatively low water content compared to the more central abscess or the surrounding edema; it enhances intensely [28]. The penumbra is 75 % sensitive and specific for subacute osteomyelitis and can be useful for differentiation from tumor. Fat globules are not encountered in subacute osteomyelitis [23, 29].

Differential considerations include osteoid osteoma, stress fracture, and—less likely—Ewing sarcoma, lymphoma, or metastatic neuroblastoma. Epiphyseal subacute osteomyelitis may be mistaken for chondroblastoma.

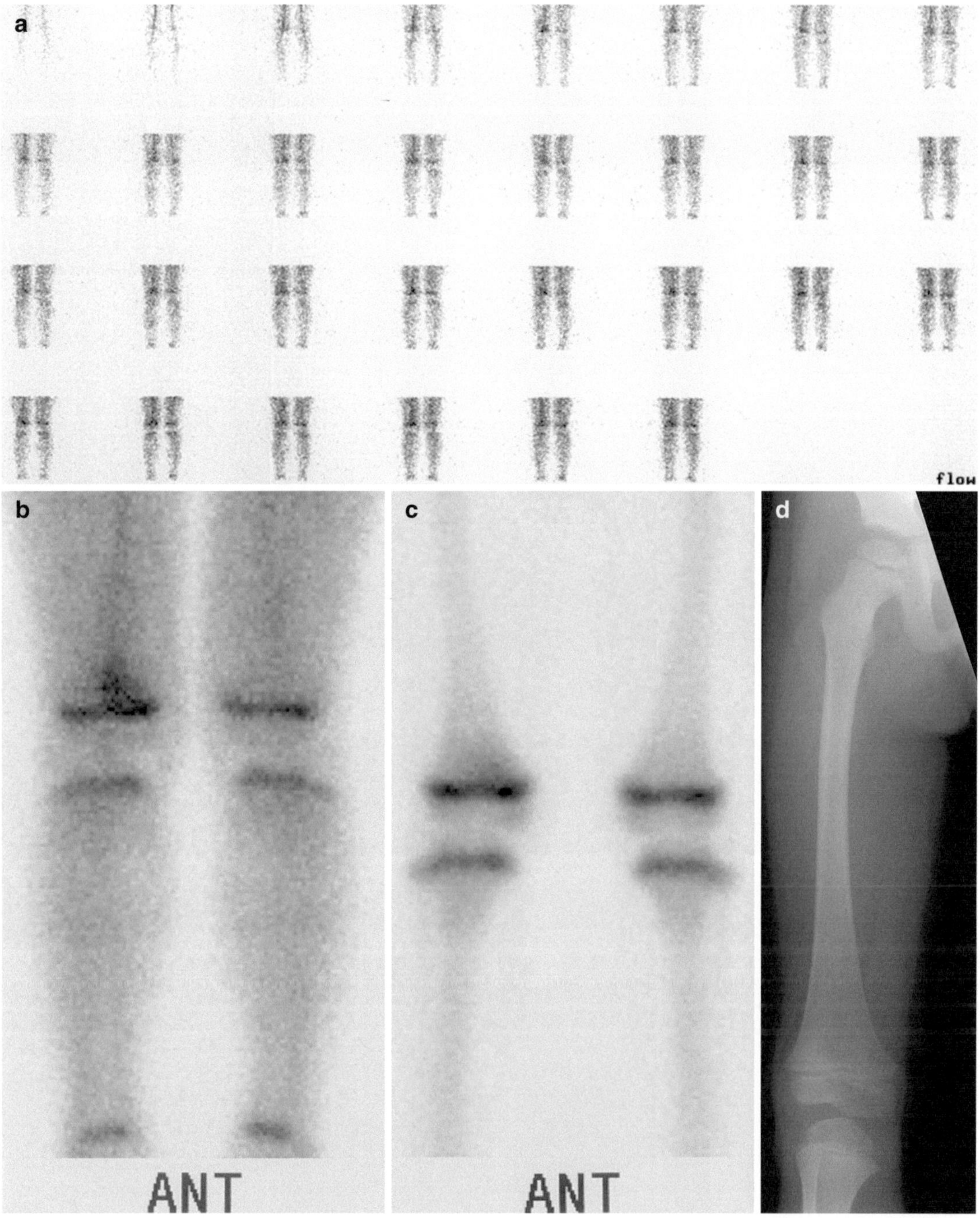

Fig. 19.13 Acute osteomyelitis in a 4-year-old boy with right knee pain after receiving a course of antibiotics for strep throat. (**a**) Blood flow image in a Technetium-99m-labeled three-phase bone scan shows increased flow to the right leg. (**b**) Blood pool shows focal increased activity at the distal right femur. (**c**) Delayed image shows persistent increased activity, localized to the distal femoral metaphysis. (**d**) The contemporaneous radiograph is normal (Courtesy of Alan H. Siegel, MD, Dartmouth Hitchcock Medical Center)

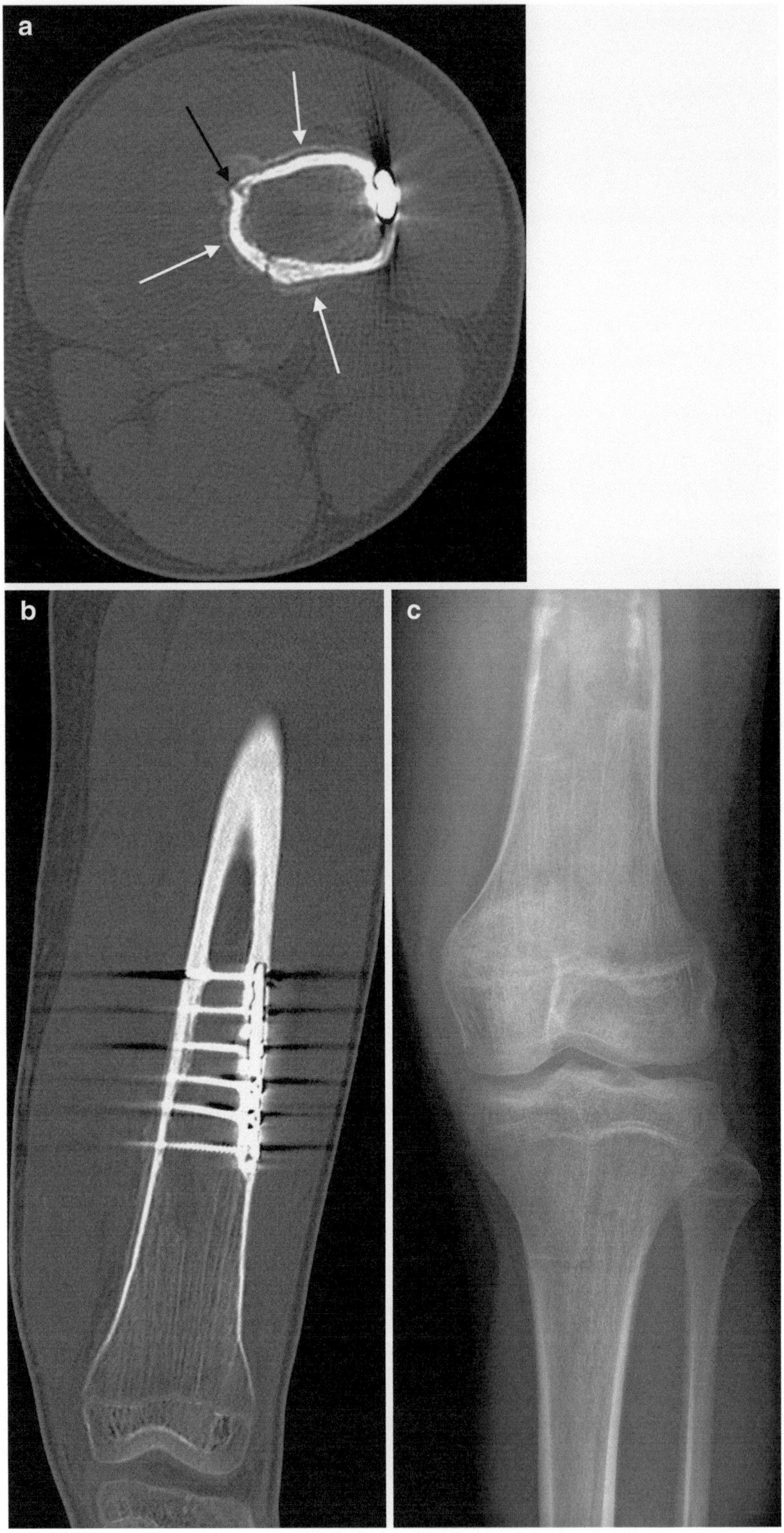

Fig. 19.14 Chronic osteomyelitis in a 15-year-old boy with knee pain 6 years after plate and screw fixation of a femoral fracture. (**a**) Axial CT shows periosteal new bone (*white arrows*) with a cloaca (*black arrow*). (**b**) Coronal reformatted CT reveals the extent of the abnormality. (**c**) One month later, hardware has been removed, and there is patchy lysis and sclerosis of the distal femoral diametaphysis

Bone sclerosis and cortical thickening in **chronic osteomyelitis** are hypointense on all sequences. The sequestrum and involucrum do not enhance but are surrounded by enhancing granulation tissue (Fig. 19.11). Sinus tracts are hypointense on T1 and hyperintense on T2, and their margins demonstrate enhancement. Marrow edema is present, with a sharp, well-defined margin between normal and abnormal marrow (in acute osteomyelitis, the zone of transition is ill-defined) [7]. Fat signal—if present—is due to the restoration of normal marrow [23]. Primary differential considerations are osteosarcoma and Ewing sarcoma.

Long-term sequelae include restricted or angular growth secondary to physeal damage and resultant early growth plate fusion. Alternatively, limb overgrowth can occur, as a result of hyperemia. Epiphyseal avascular necrosis or destruction decreases growth and produces severe deformity (Fig. 19.15). MRI or CT can be useful to analyze physeal damage as well as to assess the condition of the epiphysis. Long-term follow-up radiographs assess the impact on growth and angular deformity (Fig. 19.16).

2 Primary Epiphyseal Osteomyelitis

Involvement of the epiphyseal ossification center is common in infants, secondary to extension from the metaphysis. There is also an uncommon subacute primary form that occurs in early childhood; this follows direct hematogenous seeding of the epiphysis [30]. Pain and limp are often recurrent. The knee is affected almost exclusively, with distal femoral epiphyseal involvement more likely than proximal tibia. *Staphylococcus aureus* is the most common pathogen.

A well-circumscribed epiphyseal lucency is seen (Fig. 19.17), usually without any other bone involvement, and nuclear scintigraphy is positive. MRI demonstrates typical findings of osteomyelitis [30]. Differential diagnoses are limited and include chondroblastoma,

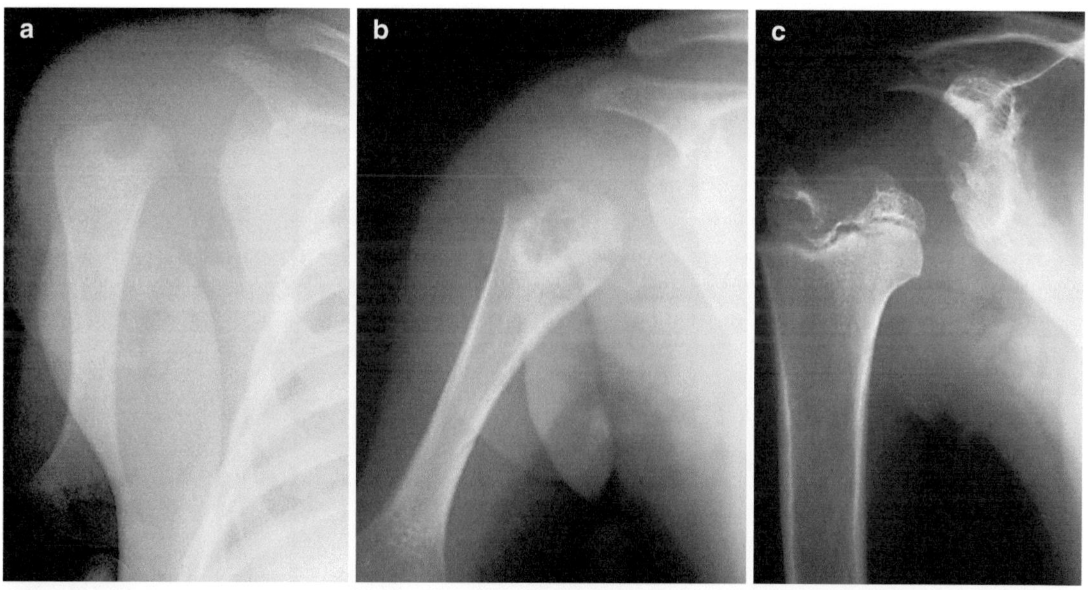

Fig. 19.15 Osteomyelitis in a premature infant. (**a**) There is lucency in the proximal humeral metaphysis. Although the epiphysis is not yet ossified, the humerus is displaced laterally by a joint effusion, suggesting epiphyseal involvement as well. (**b**) One month later, the lesion has enlarged, and surrounding sclerosis indicates reactive bone formation. Lateral displacement has resolved, and interval growth results in apparent distal migration of the lucent focus. (**c**) Several years later, the humeral head is small, deformed, and displaced laterally

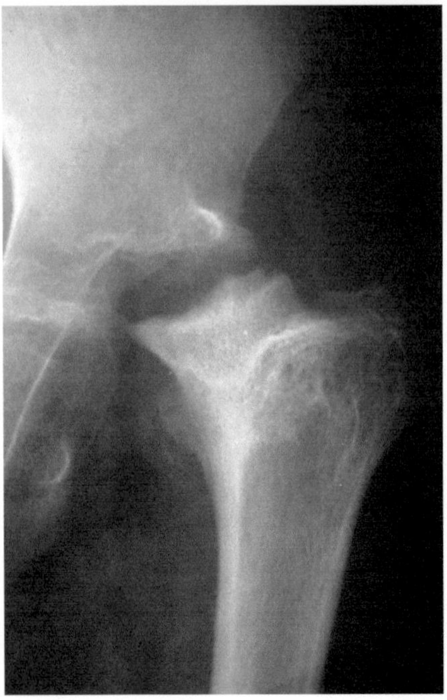

Fig. 19.16 Late sequelae of neonatal osteomyelitis of the hip. The femoral epiphysis has been destroyed, and there is very little space between the deformed acetabulum and the sclerotic, deformed metaphysis

epiphyseal osteoid osteoma, and normal developmental epiphyseal lucencies [31].

3 Pelvic Osteomyelitis

Pelvic osteomyelitis accounts for 10 % of cases of acute osteomyelitis and tends to occur in older males (average age 7–14 years) [32]. There is often a history of trauma [33]. Signs and symptoms vary, and as many as 50 % are afebrile; diagnosis is often delayed, with symptoms initially attributed to septic arthritis, slipped capital femoral epiphysis, Legg-Perthes disease, appendicitis, or tubo-ovarian abscess [32, 34]. Abscesses are especially common in pelvic osteomyelitis, perhaps because of the typical delay (average 12 days) in diagnosis [35]. An ESR of more than 55 may help predict the presence of an abscess [32].

Osteomyelitis in the pelvis occurs in metaphyseal equivalents that border cartilage, where—as in the metaphyses of long bones—sluggish blood flow in venous sinusoids favors bacterial deposi-

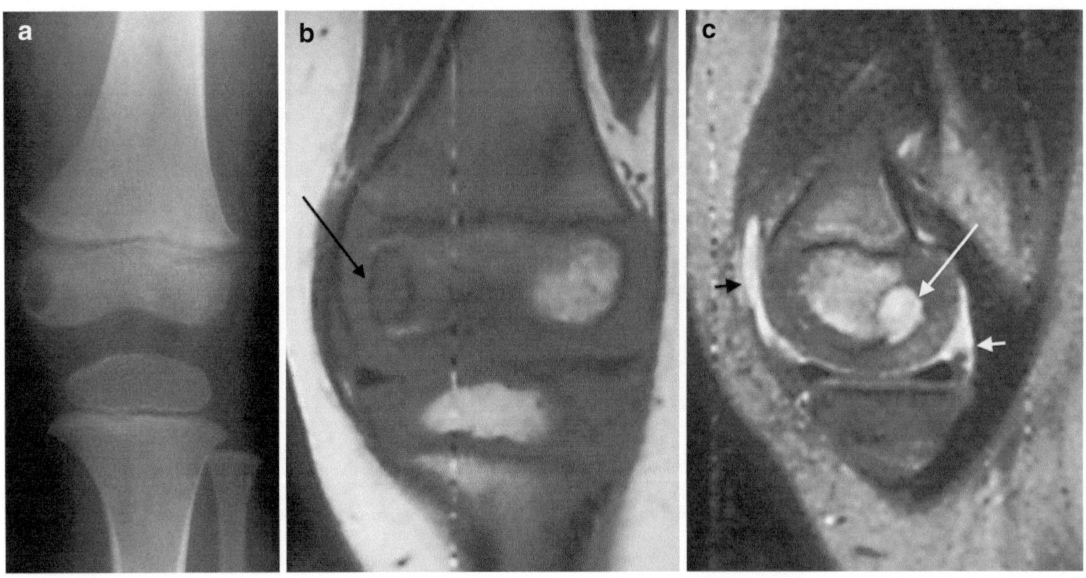

Fig. 19.17 Primary epiphyseal osteomyelitis. (**a**) Well-circumscribed lucency in the medial femoral condyle. (**b**) T1-W MRI shows hypointensity in the epiphysis, most pronounced in the medial condyle (*arrow*), sparing a portion of the lateral condyle. (**c**) Sagittal T2-W image shows fluid signal within the lesion (*long arrow*), which spans the ossified and cartilaginous portions of the epiphysis. Small joint effusion (*short arrows*)

tion and proliferation. Prior to skeletal maturation, the bony margins of the triradiate cartilage and ischiopubic synchondroses are common sites of pelvic osteomyelitis, followed by the sacroiliac joint, pubic symphysis, ischium, and iliac apophysis [32–34].

Imaging

Radiographs are usually negative, and ultrasound rarely succeeds in assessing deep osseous and soft tissue structures of the pelvis, although it may demonstrate a hip effusion in the setting of acetabular osteomyelitis. Scintigraphy is sensitive for osteomyelitis but fails to delineate abscesses and may underestimate disease (Fig. 19.18). It is therefore of especially limited utility in the pelvis, where abscesses are so common [10]. CT is more sensitive than radiography, but early findings are nonspecific. As infection progresses, intramedullary density increases due to reactive thickening of trabeculae [34].

MRI plays a critical role in diagnosing pelvic osteomyelitis and accompanying soft tissue infection (Figs. 19.18 and 19.19). Osseous increased signal intensity on T2-W and short-tau inversion recovery (STIR) sequences may be subtle, and gadolinium may be required to demonstrate bone enhancement and confirm osteomyelitis [33]. Gadolinium is also essential to delineate the abscesses that accompany pelvic osteomyelitis in up to half of patients

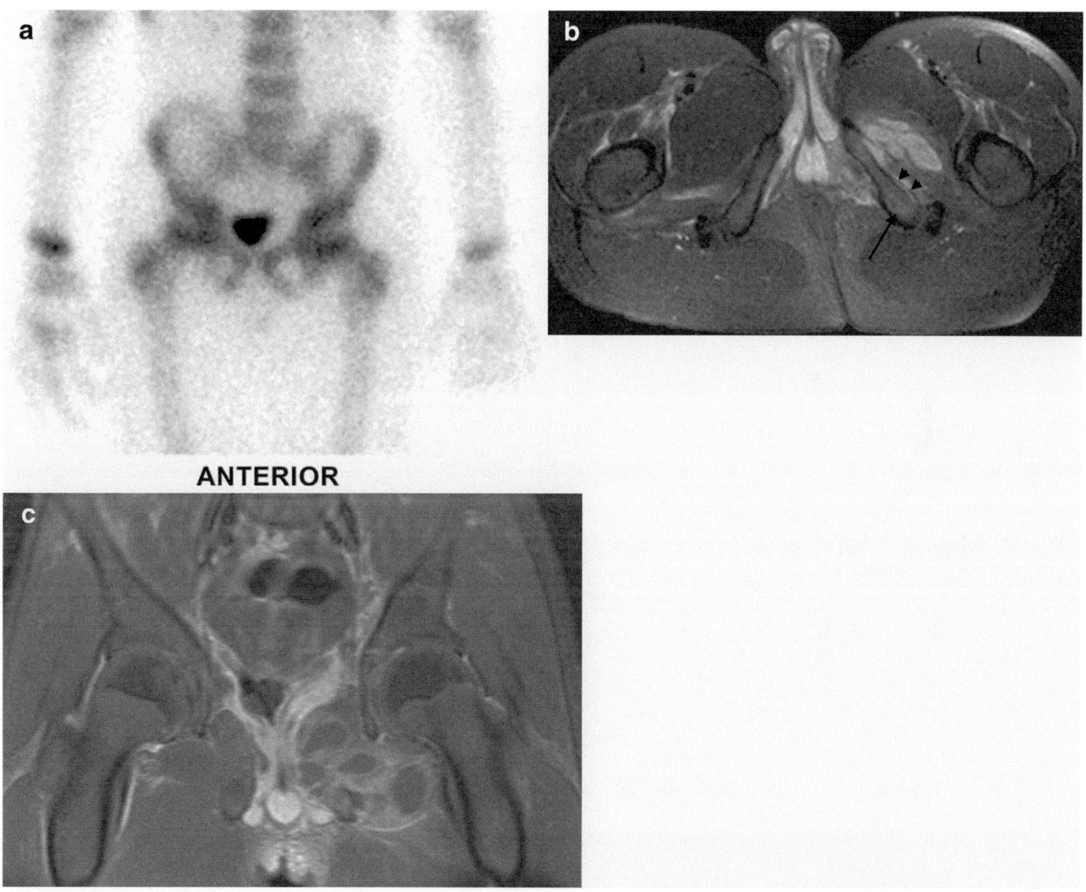

Fig. 19.18 Ischiopubic osteomyelitis with soft tissue abscesses, underestimated by bone scan. (**a**) Bone scan is normal. (**b**) Axial T2-W FS MRI shows slight edema of the left inferior ischiopubic ramus, (*arrow*) subperiosteal fluid (*short arrows*), and increased signal with fluid collections in the internal and external obturator muscles. (**c**) Coronal T1-W gadolinium-enhanced FS MRI shows multiple rim-enhancing intramuscular abscesses

[32–34]. Abscesses usually involve the soft tissues overlying bone, but intraosseous and subperiosteal abscesses are also encountered.

4 Discitis (Box 19.4)

Box 19.4 Discitis

Vessels in disc are terminal arterioles

Radiography: endplate irregularities after several weeks

MRI: early signal changes in disc

- Signal change in vertebral body usually reactive
- Destructive osteomyelitis unusual

Discitis in children is completely different from discitis in adults. In children, there is primary infection of the disc because—unlike adults—it is supplied with blood via terminal arterioles (whereas in adults, disease spreads from the adjacent vertebral body). Discitis is usually encountered between 6 and 48 months of age, although there is also a second peak in 10–14-year-olds [6, 36]. Children usually present with limp and local tenderness; systemic illness is unusual. The lumbar spine is most often involved.

Etiology is usually a low-grade bacterial infection acquired via hematogenous spread or—less often—via contiguous or direct implantation. Cultures are positive in only 50 %.

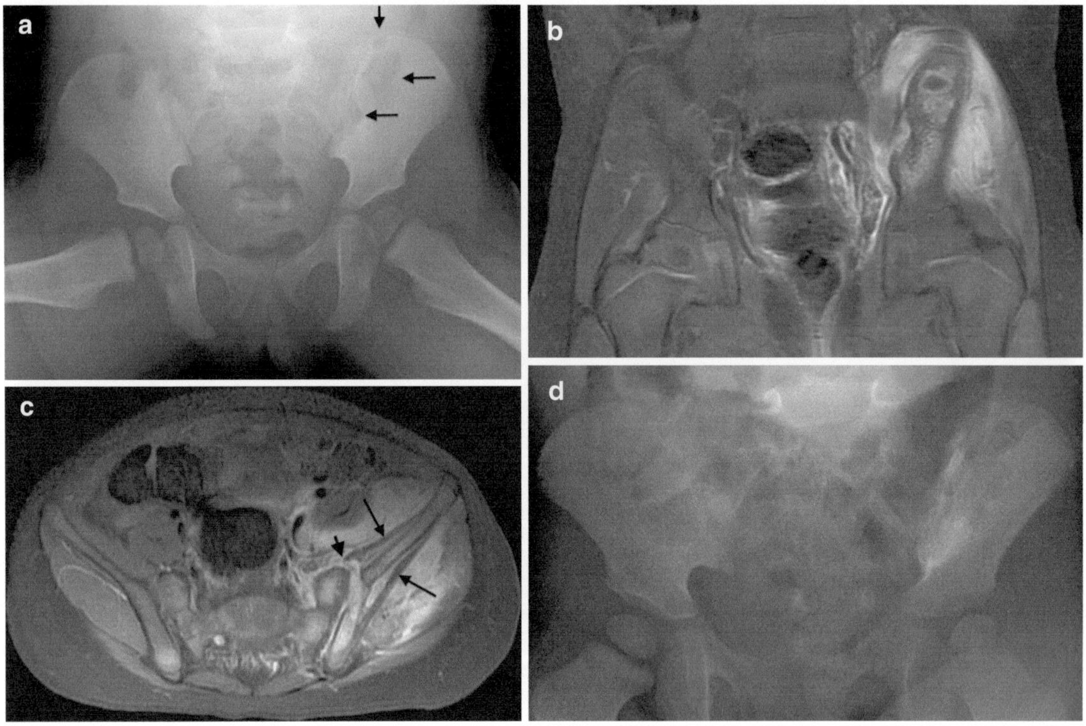

Fig. 19.19 Methicillin-resistant *Staphylococcus aureus* osteomyelitis in a 2-year-old, who refuses to walk. (**a**) Lucency over the left iliac wing could be attributed to bowel gas (*arrows*). (**b**) T1-W gadolinium-enhanced FS coronal MRI shows marrow enhancement, an intraosseous abscess, and intense muscle enhancement. (**c**) On T1-W FS gadolinium-enhanced MRI, enhancing inflammatory material drains anterior to the sacroiliac joint (*short arrow*), and the periosteum is markedly elevated (*long arrows*). (**d**) Six weeks later, symptoms have resolved, and there is sclerosis

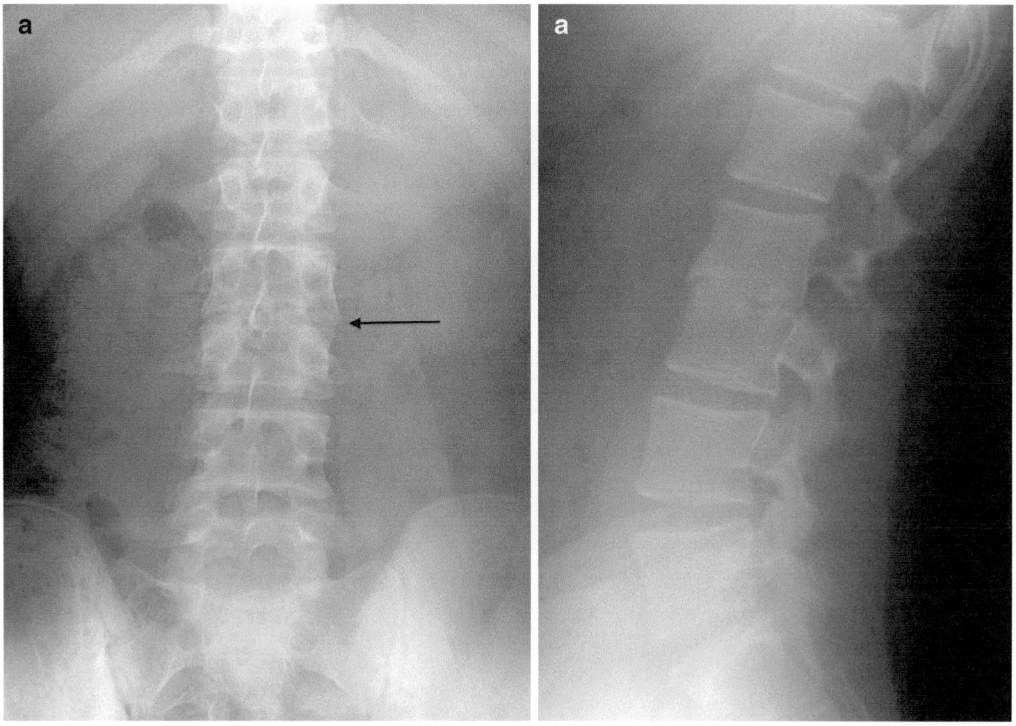

Fig. 19.20 Discitis in a 15-year-old. (**a**, **b**) There is marked narrowing of the intervertebral disc space at L2–3 (*arrow*), with severe endplate erosions and adjacent sclerosis

Imaging

Radiographs are normal for the first few weeks but eventually demonstrate vertebral endplate irregularities and narrowing of the intervertebral disc (Fig. 19.20). MRI is positive much earlier and—in addition to demonstrating signal change in the disc and adjacent vertebral body—delineates complications such as epidural abscess and cord compression. There may be mild reactive signal changes in the adjacent vertebral bodies; more intense signal alterations indicate accompanying osteomyelitis, but this is distinctly unusual (Fig. 19.21). White blood cell scanning is negative 50 % of the time, perhaps because leukocytes are unable to migrate into encapsulated infections [11].

5 Methicillin-Resistant *Staphylococcus aureus* (MRSA)

Community-acquired MRSA infections often carry the gene for Panton-Valentine leukocidin, a cytotoxin that destroys leukocytes by forming pores in their cell membranes. Panton-Valentine leukocidin (PVL)-positive MRSA osteomyelitis tends to be more severe and is often accompanied with bacteremia that can lead to systemic sepsis and multi-organ failure [37]. Other relatively common complications include deep venous thrombosis, septic thrombophlebitis, pulmonary embolism, septic emboli, necrotic pneumonia, empyema, and—locally—more intraosseous and subperiosteal abscesses, septic arthritis, and pyomyositis (Figs. 19.22 and 19.23) [14, 37]. MRSA often requires aggressive surgical debridement along with prolonged antibiotic therapy.

6 Meningococcemia

Encountered in infants and in sexually active teens, meningococcal osteomyelitis results from severe systemic infection complicated by septic microemboli to epiphyses and physes. Ischemia and infection result, progressing rapidly and, if

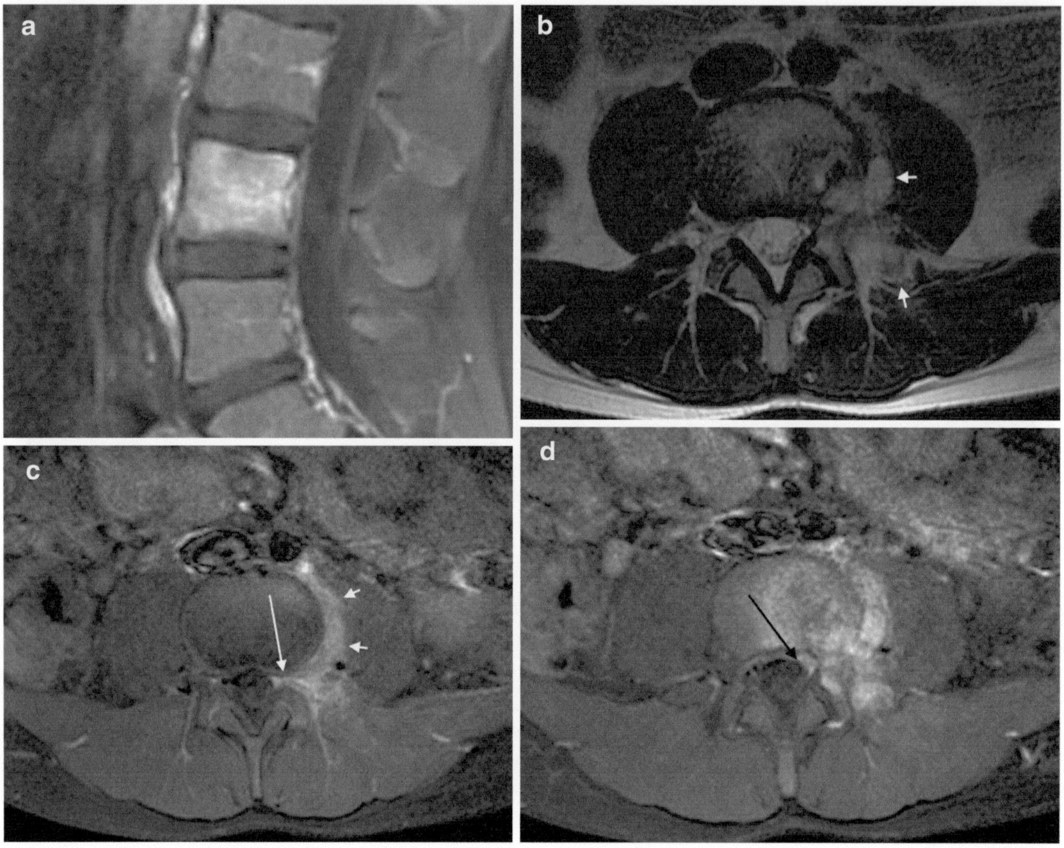

Fig. 19.21 Spinal osteomyelitis in a 14-year-old boy with back pain. (**a**) Sagittal T1-W FS gadolinium-enhanced image shows intense enhancement of L4 vertebral body, without significant involvement of the intervertebral disc. (**b**) Axial T2-W image shows soft tissue involvement (*short arrows*), with high signal between the vertebral body and the left psoas, extending into the left intervertebral foramen and to the paraspinous musculature. (**c, d**) Extension into the left intervertebral foramen (*long white arrow*) and slight encroachment on the thecal sac (*black arrow*) are confirmed by axial T1-W fat-suppressed gadolinium-enhanced images, also showing enhancement of paraspinous musculature (*short arrows*)

peripheral, sometimes leading to auto-amputation of digits (Fig. 19.24). Involvement of multiple sites is common, and physeal ischemia with subsequent fusion often results in long-term growth disturbance such as angular deformity and limb-length discrepancy (Fig. 19.25). Subluxation, pseudoarthrosis, and joint contractures also occur. Growth disturbance may be unapparent until many years after the septic insult, and therefore long-term follow-up is necessary.

7 Septic Arthritis (Box 19.5)

Box 19.5 Septic Arthritis

Cartilage destruction by 5 days

Imaging cannot differentiate septic from non-septic arthritis

- Soft tissue abscesses suggest septic arthritis

Ultrasound: effusion

MRI: thickly enhancing synovium

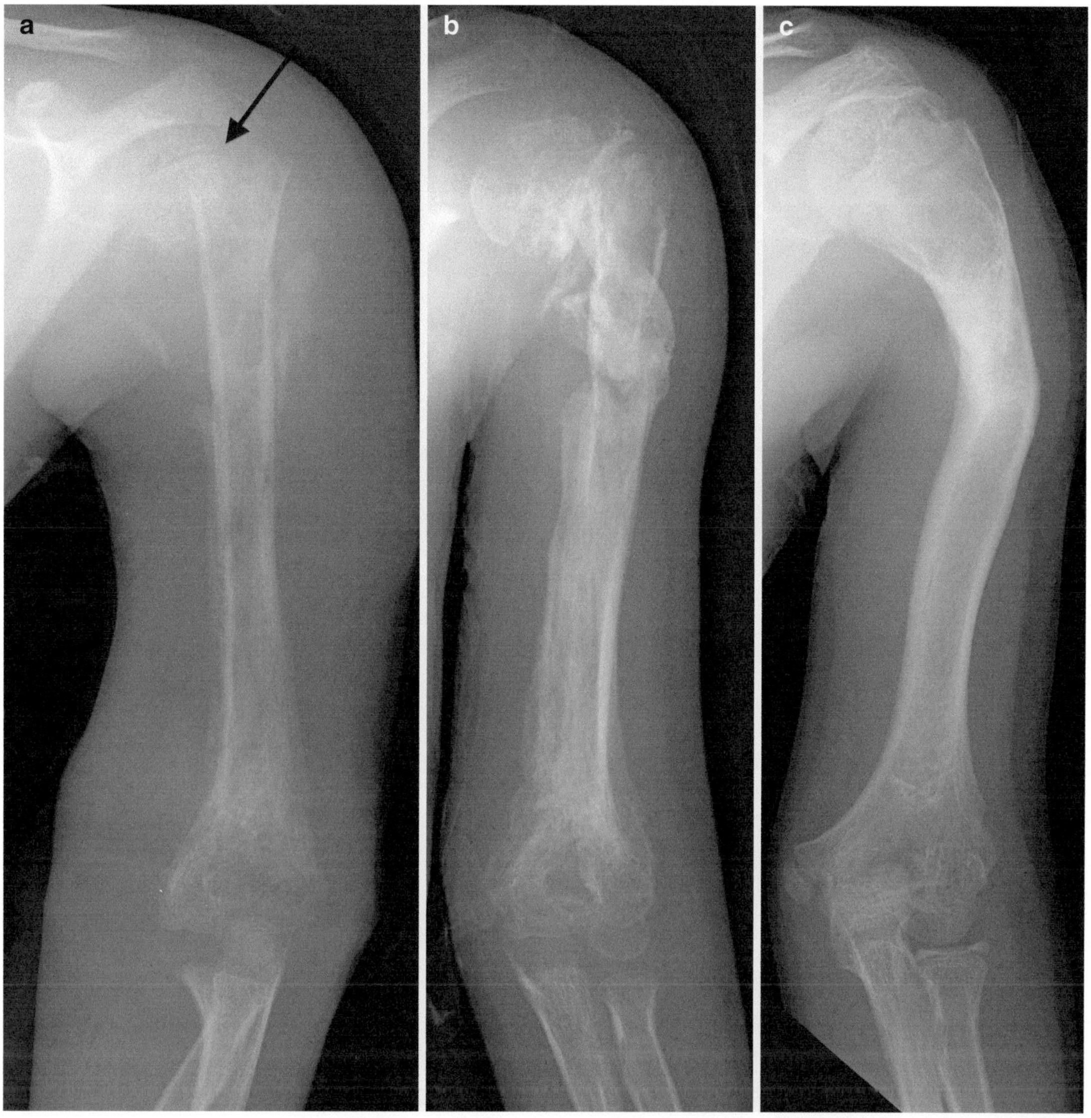

Fig. 19.22 Sequential radiographs of methicillin-resistant *Staphylococcus aureus* osteomyelitis show growth abnormalities resulting from extensive physeal, metaphyseal, and diaphyseal involvement. (**a**) At diagnosis, a permeative process extends the entire length of the humerus, with a proximal metaphyseal pathological fracture/dislocation. In addition to more mature periosteal reaction, cloudlike periosteal new bone is forming. (**b**) One month later, involucrum is well developed, and alignment essentially unchanged. (**c**) One year later, deformity persists despite extensive remodeling

The incidence of septic arthritis peaks around age 2, and this form of infection is especially common in neonates. During the neonatal period, septic arthritis usually accompanies osteomyelitis, although it can also develop due to spread of contiguous infection, a contaminated heel-stick, or seeding from implanted vascular catheters (Fig. 19.26). In older children, it often follows local soft tissue infection or trauma. It is more likely in children with hemophilia, immunodeficiency, or chronic arthritis. The joints of the lower extremity (especially hip and knee) are affected in more

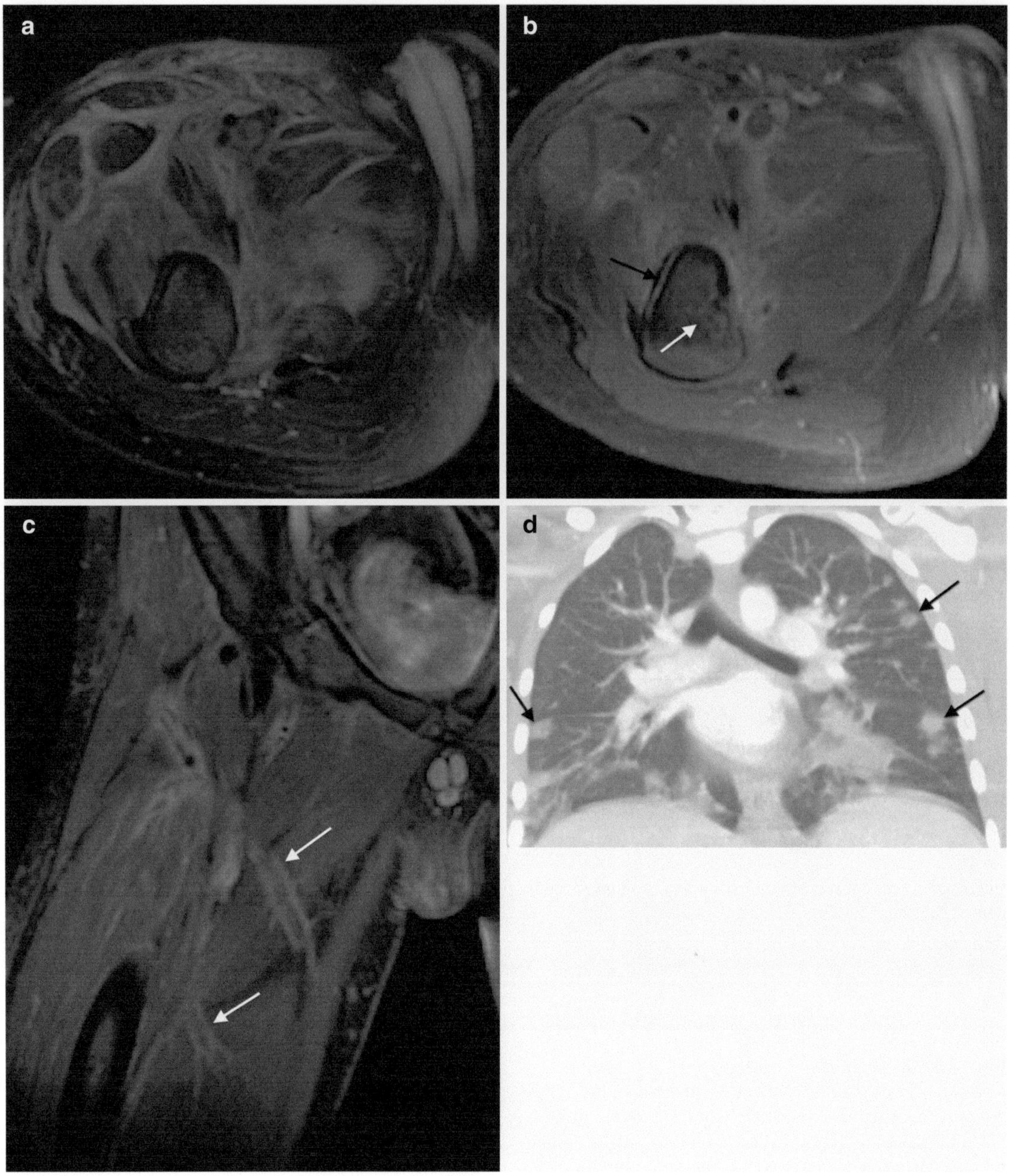

Fig. 19.23 Methicillin-resistant *Staphylococcus aureus* osteomyelitis in a 10 y/o boy. (**a**) Axial T2-W FS image shows mild marrow edema and extensive soft tissue edema. (**b**) Axial T1-W FS MRI shows multiple tiny intraosseous abscesses (*white arrow*) and a subperiosteal abscess (*black arrow*) as well as diffuse soft tissue edema. (**c**) Coronal T1-W gadolinium-enhanced FS image shows thrombophlebitis (*arrows*). (**d**) Contemporaneous CT (*coronal reformat*) shows bilateral septic emboli (*arrows*)

than 75 % of patients, and it is monoarticular in 90 %. In the hip, shoulder, ankle, and elbow, the joint capsule includes a portion of the metaphysis, so osteomyelitis can readily contaminate the joint if it breaks through the metaphyseal cortex.

Symptoms are more acute than with osteomyelitis, including fever, pain, edema, and erythema. There may be limp or refusal to bear weight. However, presentation in neonates is often nonspecific, including anorexia, irritability, and

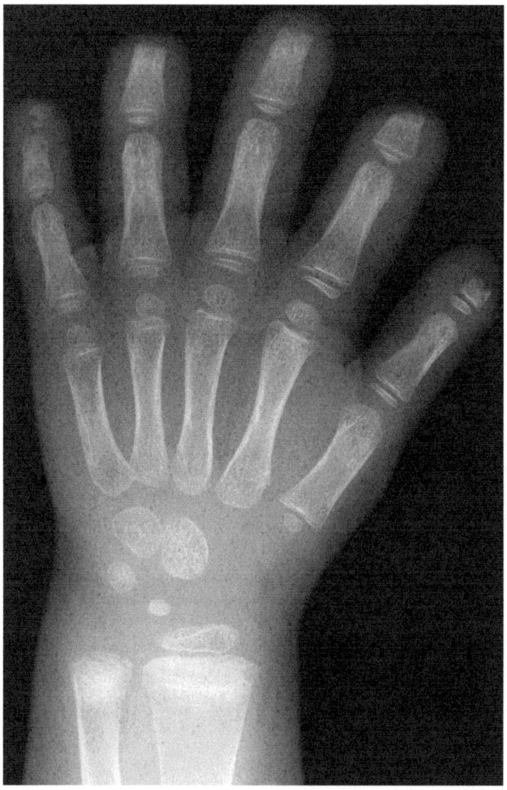

Fig. 19.24 Meningococcemia. Amputation of the tufts of the distal phalanges results from soft tissue necrosis

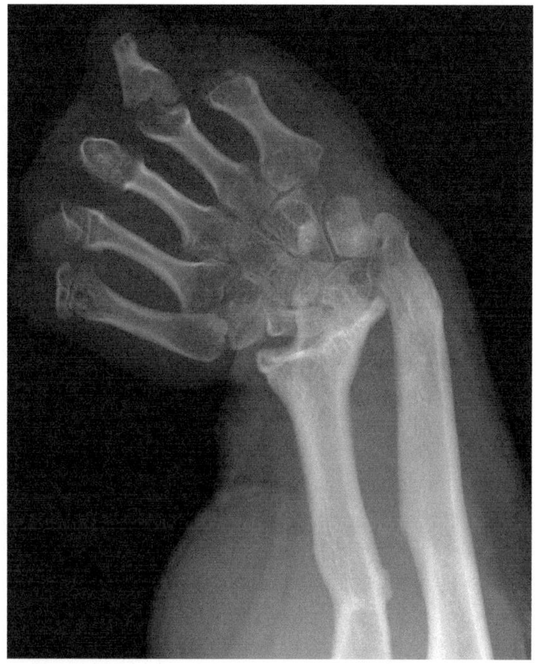

Fig. 19.25 Meningococcemia. Digit amputation as well as severe growth disturbance at the wrist results from prior damage to the physes and epiphyses

lethargy. As with osteomyelitis, young children may demonstrate pseudoparalysis. White blood cell count is usually elevated, and both erythrocyte sedimentation rate and C-reactive protein are elevated (the latter can be employed to track disease progression). Blood cultures are positive in only 30–50 % of patients. Joint aspiration and culture of synovial fluid are essential, yielding positive cultures in 50–80 % [38].

Septic arthritis usually results from *Staphylococcus aureus*, although, as in osteomyelitis, *Group A beta hemolytic streptococcus*, *Streptococcus pneumoniae*, and *Group B streptococcus* (in neonates) are also common. *Neisseria gonorrhoeae* in the mother can lead to infection in neonates, and adolescents may acquire the infection by sexual activity.

The synovium is very vascular, and lack of a basement membrane readily allows hematogenous seeding. Proteolytic enzymes rapidly destroy cartilage, with loss of proteoglycans by 5 days and collagen by 9 days [38]. Epiphyseal ischemia may result from pressure due to abundant purulent material, as well as thrombosis. Outcome is worse in premature infants, children younger than 6 months of age, if treatment is delayed by more than 4 days, or if there is concurrent osteomyelitis [39]. Resultant hip dislocation also confers a worse prognosis [38]. Prompt drainage is necessary to avoid sequelae of cartilage destruction or avascular necrosis. This may need to be repeated, especially for septic arthritis of the hip.

Imaging

As with osteomyelitis, radiographs must be performed initially, although they are usually normal except for possible deep soft tissue edema and joint fluid. In advanced disease, there are marginal erosions and joint space narrowing (Fig. 19.27). Epiphyseal ischemia may initially result in increased lucency of the epiphyseal center.

Technetium 99m methylene diphosphonate (MDP) bone scan demonstrates diffuse uptake in

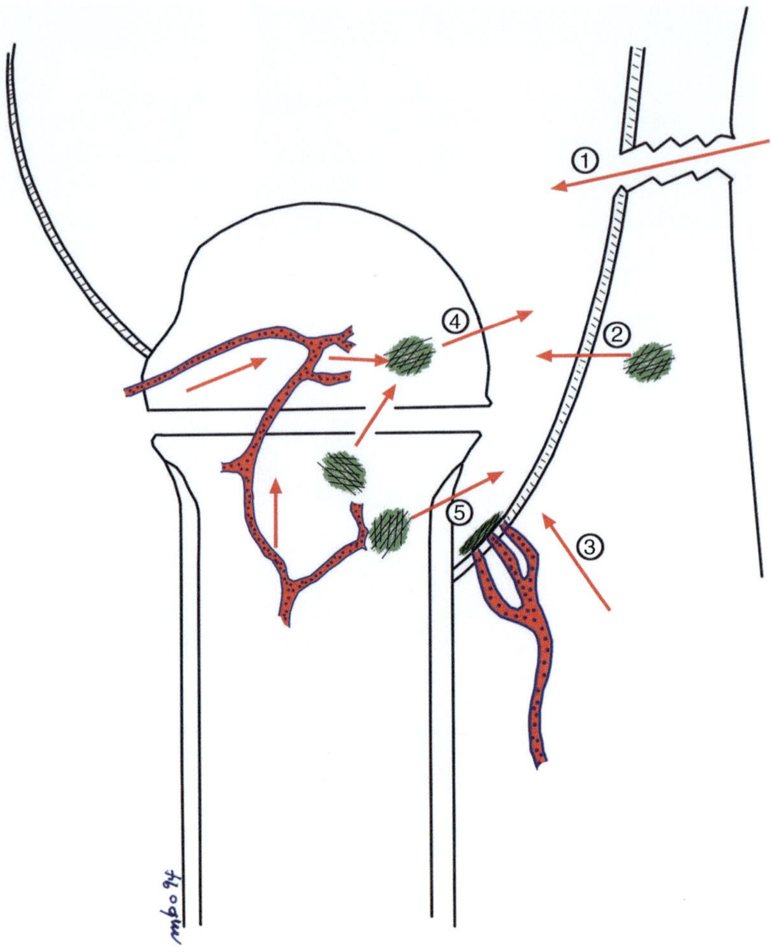

Fig. 19.26 Pathways for septic arthritis. The joint capsule may be breeched secondary to trauma (*1*), allowing direct inoculation of pathogens. A soft tissue infection may penetrate the joint capsule (*2*) or vascular seeding may occur (*3*). Alternatively, the infection may spread from bone directly to the joint. This can result from primary epiphyseal osteomyelitis (*4*), metaphyseal osteomyelitis that has crossed to the epiphysis in the infant or teen (*5*), or metaphyseal osteomyelitis that directly seeds the joint space (if the synovium includes a portion of the metaphysis)

the soft tissues and, to a lesser extent, in bone on either side of the joint. However, as with osteomyelitis, cross-sectional imaging provides important information.

Ultrasound offers excellent delineation of joint fluid, but it cannot characterize the fluid, as purulent fluid can appear anechoic, and non-infectious processes such as toxic synovitis may be associated with complex fluid [18, 40] (Figs. 19.27 and 19.28). The hip is interrogated from an anterior parasagittal approach, and when an effusion is present, the hip joint capsule bulges away from the cortex of the femoral neck [40]. The distance from the femoral neck cortex to the outer margin of the hip capsule should not exceed 5 mm, and it should be within 2 mm of the thickness of the contralateral hip [41]. Septic arthritis is rarely present in the absence of joint fluid [42].

Although MRI provides exquisite delineation of the extent of septic arthritis and associated soft tissue inflammation, it cannot differentiate septic from noninfectious arthritis and thus does not preclude aspiration. However, if abscesses have formed or if osteomyelitis is demonstrated, septic arthritis is likely.

At MRI, purulent joint fluid is, like simple fluid, typically dark on T1 and bright on fluid-sensitive sequences. There is thick synovial enhancement after administration of gadolinium. Reactive subchondral hyperemia and edema may result in mildly high T2 signal on both sides of the joint, but this is less intense than with osteomyelitis. Perisynovial edema and cartilage destruction are also seen (Fig. 19.27). If there is neither joint effusion nor synovial enhancement, septic arthritis can be excluded [43].

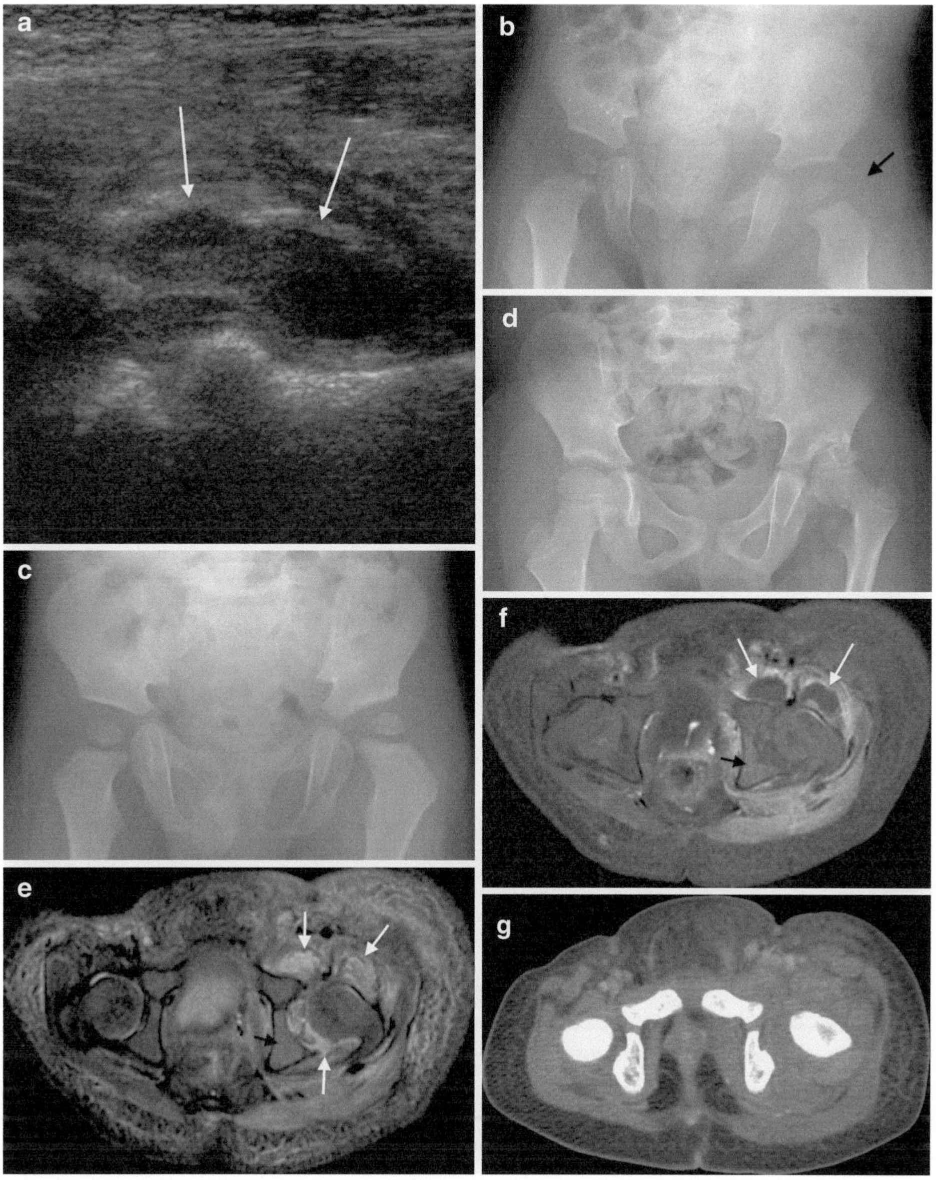

Fig. 19.27 *Staphylococcus aureus* septic arthritis and osteomyelitis in a 9-month-old boy, progressing to avascular necrosis and osteoarthritis. (**a**) At presentation, hip US shows a bulging joint capsule with synovial thickening (*arrows*). (**b**) The left femoral head is displaced laterally, with mild lateral convexity of the hip joint tissue plane (*arrow*), indicating a joint effusion. (**c**) Six months later, the femoral head is smaller and less dense, indicating avascular necrosis, with erosion of the acetabular roof. Note the growth arrest line on the right. (**d**) Six years later, there is remodeling of the femoral head, with marked joint space narrowing and developing osteoarthritis. (**e**) Axial short-tau inversion recovery (STIR) MRI (at presentation) shows a large joint effusion and synovial thickening (*white arrows*) as well as subtle increased fluid signal in the ischium (*black arrow*). (**f**) T1-W FS gadolinium-enhanced MRI delineates multiple soft tissue abscesses (*white arrows*) with faint enhancement of the ischium (*black arrow*). (**g**) CT with intravenous contrast shows extensive soft tissue thickening, subcutaneous edema, and joint fluid but fails to delineate either the multiple soft tissue abscesses or the osseous abnormalities

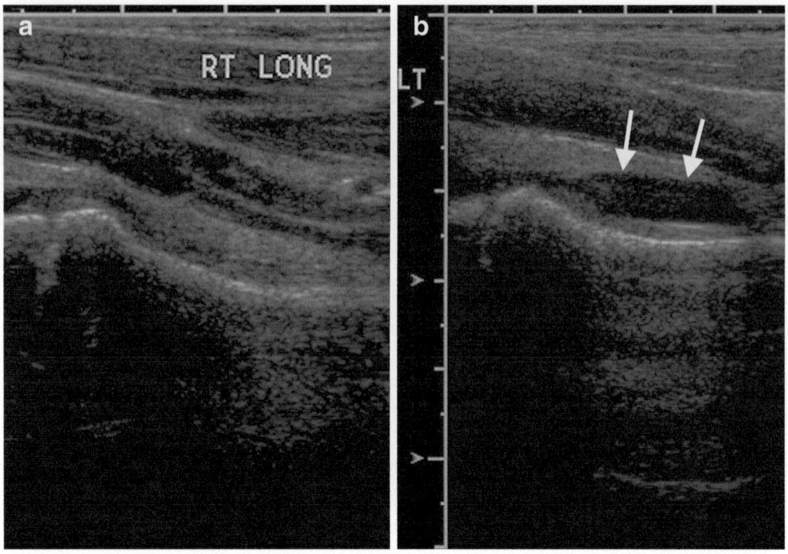

Fig. 19.28 Septic arthritis in an 8-year-old girl. Oblique sagittal US of the (**a**) left (normal for comparison) and (**b**) right hips show the capsule on the right is slightly convex (*arrows*) due to joint fluid

Limb-length discrepancy, avascular necrosis (especially of the femoral head), dislocation, arthritis, and ankylosis are some of the possible long-term sequelae (Fig. 19.27), and prompt open arthrotomy is essential to avoid these complications, which occur in as many as 40 % of patients. Growth disturbance is extremely common after neonatal septic arthritis, mandating long-term follow-up.

Differential Diagnosis

Differential considerations in septic arthritis in older children include tuberculous joint disease, juvenile idiopathic arthritis and other noninfectious arthritides, pigmented villonodular synovitis, hemophilia, synovial chondromatosis, and (in the hip) transient synovitis and Legg-Perthes disease.

An important differential consideration for hip pain is toxic synovitis, which is a self-limited inflammation of the hip common in children between 4 and 10 years of age. Clinical differentiation between septic arthritis and toxic synovitis is quite difficult; the latter is more likely if the patient is able to bear weight, is afebrile, has an erythrocyte sedimentation rate of less than 40 mm/h, and has fewer than 12,000 white blood cells per cubic millimeter [38]. Capsular distension and increased width of the hip joint may be apparent at radiography. Both septic arthritis and toxic synovitis demonstrate either complex or simple joint fluid at ultrasound, and diagnosis may rest on the results of aspirate. MRI may demonstrate synovial thickening and enhancement in both disorders. Signal changes in marrow and enhancement in surrounding soft tissues strongly favors septic arthritis [44] (see Chap. 12 for further discussion).

8 Soft Tissue Infection

The presenting signs for cellulitis, soft tissue abscess, and pyomyositis are similar to those for osteomyelitis and septic arthritis. Grouped together, soft tissue infections cause about 40 % of all musculoskeletal infections in children [39]. Superficial cellulitis may lead to deeper soft tissue infection or abscess formation. Abscesses are especially common in the buttock, groin, thigh, and foot. Cellulitis and soft tissue abscess are more common than pyomyositis, but the latter occurs with increasing frequency in regions with limited access to health care [45] and is common in the tropics and Africa. This suppurative infection of skeletal muscle usually involves the large muscle groups of the thigh and pelvis [18].

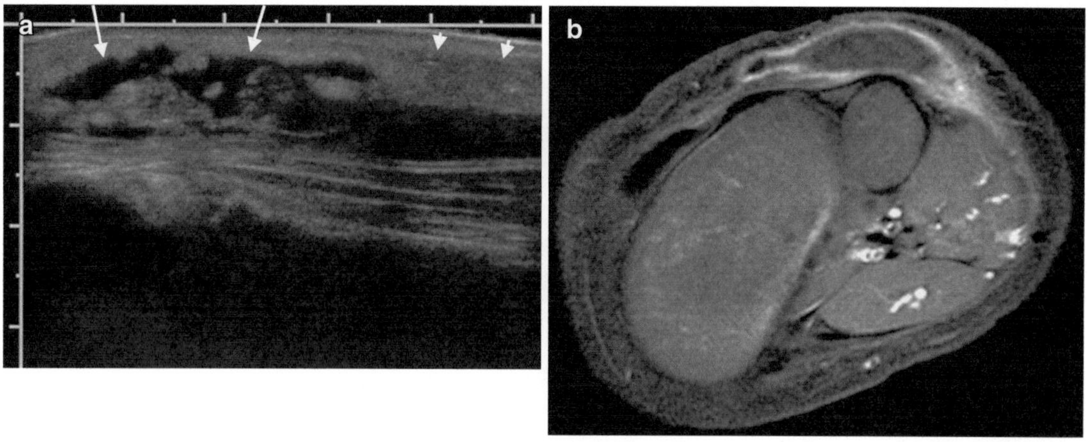

Fig. 19.29 Soft tissue abscess in a 3-year-old boy. (**a**) US over the fibula shows mildly heterogeneous thickened superficial soft tissues (*short arrows*). An adjacent abscess is more strikingly heterogeneous (*long arrows*). (**b**) Axial T1-W FS gadolinium-enhanced MRI shows an elliptical rim of enhancement in the subcutaneous adipose tissue, tracking along fascial planes but sparing musculature

Staphylococcus aureus and *Streptococcus pneumoniae* are also the most common pathogens for soft tissue infections in children, although mycobacterium, fungus, and *Bartonella henselae* (cat scratch fever) infections also occur. Skeletal muscle usually resists seeding by bacteria, and pyomyositis is often secondary to adjacent osteomyelitis or septic arthritis [45]; vigorous exercise or trauma can also predispose children to developing pyomyositis.

Imaging

Ultrasound (US) and MRI are the mainstays for diagnosis of soft tissue infection and play a major role in determining the optimal site for aspiration.

Grayscale ultrasound of cellulitis reveals thickening and increased echogenicity of subcutaneous fat along with blurring of tissue planes; a cobblestone appearance develops due to hypoechoic perifascial fluid (Fig. 19.29) [18, 19]. Hyperemia may be evident. If the process progresses, abscesses may appear as anechoic or hypoechoic fluid collections.

When there is question, pressure can be applied, causing particles in the fluid to move [18]. Color Doppler demonstrates peripheral hyperemia and no central flow. Pyomyositis appears as ill-defined intramuscular increased echogenicity, with or without focal areas of decreased echogenicity and increased blood flow. Focal fluid may become confluent and form well-defined intramuscular abscesses [19].

MRI initially demonstrates low T1/high T2 ill-defined feathery stranding in the superficial subcutaneous adipose tissue, thickening of the skin, and mild diffuse enhancement extending into muscle and fascial planes (Figs. 19.30 and 19.31). If soft tissue inflammation approaches bone, there may be marrow edema and enhancement, which can be reactive or due to osteomyelitis. More specific bone abnormalities such as periosteal reaction or focal destruction allow confident diagnosis of osteomyelitis. Abscesses appear as central fluid with peripheral enhancement (Figs. 19.29 and 19.31).

9 Sickle-Cell Disease

Osteomyelitis occurs in 18 % of patients with sickle-cell disease, but septic arthritis is much less common. Clinical differentiation of infarction from osteomyelitis can be difficult, as both present with pain, fever, swelling, and increased serum inflammatory markers. Blood cultures are positive in only 50 % of patients with osteomyelitis [46].

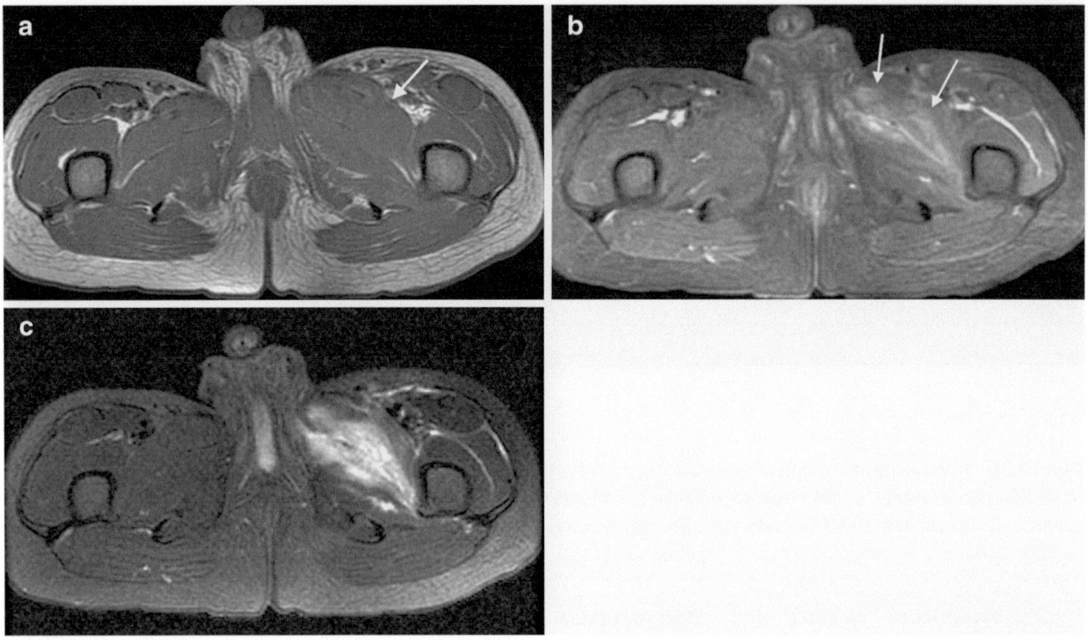

Fig. 19.30 Infectious myositis involving left adductor magnus in a 5-year-old boy. (**a**) T1-W image shows enlargement of the adductor magnus (*arrow*). (**b**) T1-W gadolinium-enhanced fat-suppressed image shows muscle enhancement (*arrows*). (**c**) T2-W MRI with fat saturation shows extensive muscular enhancement with mild accompanying soft edema. Fluid tracks between fascial planes

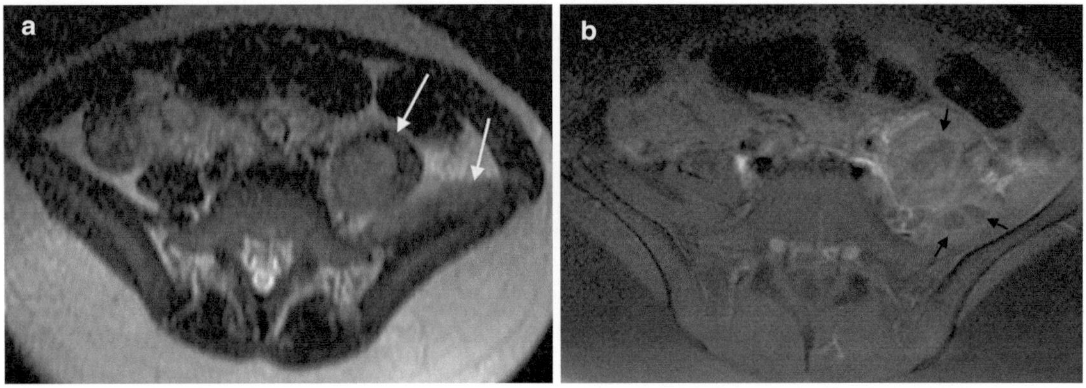

Fig. 19.31 Pyomyositis in a 16-year-old with recent trauma, presenting with hip pain. (**a**) Axial T2-W single-shot fast spin echo MRI shows mild increased signal in enlarged left iliacus and psoas muscles (*arrows*). Their margins are indistinct. Bone is normal. (**b**) T1-W gadolinium-enhanced FS image shows intense enhancement of musculature with several intramuscular abscesses (*arrows*)

Recurrent ischemia, functional hyposplenia, and impaired polymorphonuclearcyte function predispose patients with sickle-cell disease to osteomyelitis. Although these patients may become infected with common pathogens such as *Staphylococcus aureus*, *Salmonella* is encountered most often (as a result of impaired function of the reticuloendothelial system). Infection usually involves the diaphysis of long bones, and it is often more extensive than osteomyelitis in normal patients. Multifocal disease is more common.

Imaging

Scintigraphy employing a combination of Technetium 99m MDP 3-phase MDP bone scan and radiolabeled leukocytes or sulfur colloid may help differentiate osteomyelitis from infarction, as normal to increased uptake essentially rules out infarction [36]. MRI demonstrates typical findings of osteomyelitis, whereas in the setting of infarction marrow may appear hyperintense on non-enhanced T1-W fat-suppressed images.

10 Tuberculous Osteomyelitis (Box 19.6)

Box 19.6 Tuberculous Osteomyelitis

Spine: in 50 %, affects adjacent vertebrae, sparing disc

Spreads along anterior longitudinal ligament

Metaphyses: often spreads to epiphyses/apophyses

Caseating granulomas and debris in join appear dark on T2-W

Skeletal tuberculosis accounts for only 1–2 % of cases of tuberculosis but tends to occur in children, in whom tuberculosis is more common overall [47]. It typically results from hematogenous spread from a concomitant primary lung infection. Most children with osteoarticular disease are between 1 and 10 years of age [47]. Pain and fever are usually absent, and therefore disease is usually severe when finally diagnosed. Up to 10 % of cases are multifocal; about 50 % involve the spine [47]. Progression from osteomyelitis to septic arthritis is common, occurring in 50 % of long bone cases.

Tuberculous osteomyelitis is characterized by a more indolent course and relatively common extension across the physis and into the adjacent joint; osteoarticular involvement is five times more common than exclusively osseous disease [47]. Bone is eroded due to the direct action of bacilli as well as pressure necrosis from granulation tissue; cortical erosion may lead to soft tissue infection as well as joint involvement [47]. Compared with bacterial septic arthritis, tuberculous disease more frequently demonstrates erosions, but the joint space is preserved until late in the course of disease.

Although with bacterial osteomyelitis proteolytic enzymes rapidly destroy cartilage, with tuberculosis cartilage destruction occurs more slowly, usually due to erosion by granulomatous pannus. Both the erosions and the abscesses demonstrate marginal enhancement that is thinner and smoother than with bacterial infection. Marrow edema is also less pronounced [44]. Tuberculous lesions in children usually lack sclerosis or sequestra, although, in contrast to adult disease, layered periosteal reaction may occur [48].

Tuberculous involvement of the spine (or Pott disease) occurs in about 50 % of patients, most often involving the thoracic but sometimes the lumbar region; the cervical and sacral spine are usually spared. Hematogenous spread of bacilli occurs via the end arterioles that terminate adjacent to the anterior end plate [48, 49]. This initially causes destruction of anterior corners of vertebral bodies and progresses to frank fragmentation and collapse. Infection spreads deep to the anterior longitudinal ligament, typically involving several adjacent vertebrae, although skip lesions may occur. Because *Tuberculous bacillus*, unlike many bacteria, lacks the proteolytic enzymes that destroy cartilage, disc spaces are usually intact until the disease is extremely advanced [48]. Posterior elements are usually spared. As a result of intact posterior elements and infected vertebral bodies, anterior compressive forces lead to vertebral collapse and subsequent focal kyphosis with gibbus formation. Large paravertebral abscesses are characteristic. Intraspinal extension may result in cord compression due to formation of epidural abscesses, and paravertebral abscesses may spread to the psoas muscles. Discharging sinuses may drain to locations such as the buttocks, groin, and chest [49]. Calcifications develop in areas of chronic soft tissue infection.

When the long bones are involved, the metaphyses of the femur and tibia are the most common sites, whereas pelvic tuberculous osteomyelitis is centered at the sacroiliac joint or greater trochanter [47]. The flat bones such as the sternum, skull, and ribs may be affected.

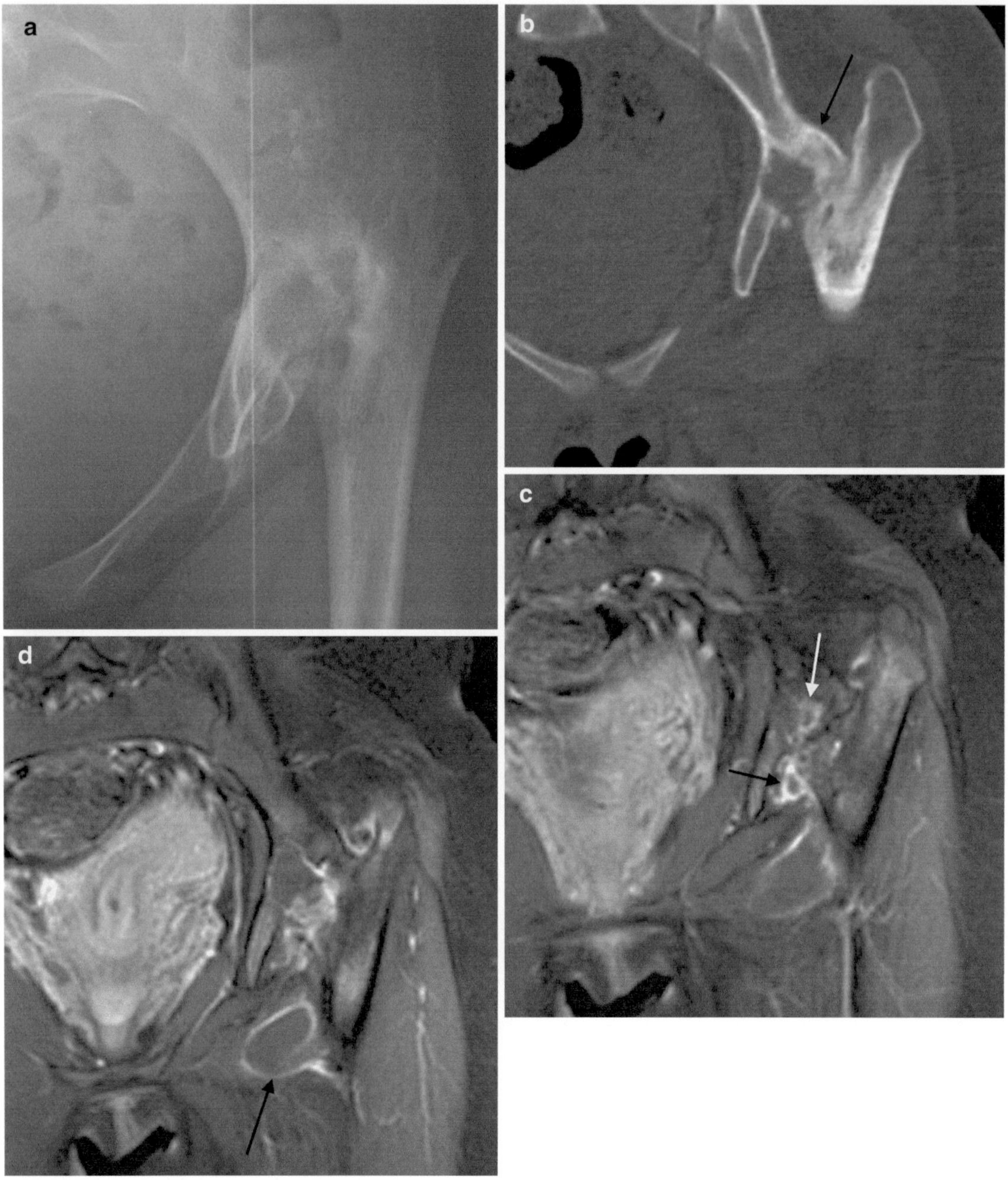

Fig. 19.32 Chronic tuberculous arthritis and osteomyelitis. (**a**) The left hip is eroded, subluxated, and possibly fused to the adjacent ileum. (**b**) Coronal-oblique reformatted CT confirms ankylosis (*arrow*) and shows a large erosion involving the ischium and femoral neck. (**c**, **d**) On coronal FS, gadolinium-enhanced T1-W images, thin, smooth focal areas of enhancement (*arrows*) indicate persistent active disease

Imaging

Initial radiographs are normal, but as disease progresses, lysis, metaphyseal expansion, and periosteal reaction occur. Lytic foci are usually sharply defined, and sclerosis is unusual (Fig. 19.32). Bone scans are not very helpful, as 35 % result in a false-negative examination [47]. CT is useful for showing soft tissue calcifications and to guide biopsy. However, as with bacterial osteomyelitis, MRI is generally more useful than CT.

MRI demonstrates marrow edema early in the course of disease. The caseous granulomas of tuberculous osteomyelitis demonstrate low to intermediate T2 signal, which can be helpful for diagnosis [50]. Abscesses may appear bright on unenhanced T1-W sequences, further differentiating tubercular from bacterial disease. Sinus tracts extending to the skin demonstrate linear T2 signal along with tram-track marginal gadolinium enhancement. Tubercular disease demonstrates a penumbra similar to bacterial osteomyelitis; this rim of slightly increased signal on T1-W imaging helps exclude neoplasm [50].

Tuberculous arthritis frequently accompanies bony involvement because lesions often extend from the metaphysis across the physis to the epiphysis or penetrate the cortex to directly involve the soft tissues. Direct hematogenous spread to synovium is less common [39, 48]. Transphyseal spread of infection through the intact growth plate is characteristic of tuberculous skeletal infection but is a feature of pyogenic infection only after growth plate closure [48].

Tuberculous osteoarticular disease usually affects only one joint, typically the hip or knee. Granulomatous involvement causes smooth synovial thickening and joint fluid; bony erosions result from pressure necrosis. Cortical and subcortical bone destruction occurs on both sides of the joint [48]. With progressive disease, cold abscesses and sinus tracts form in the periarticular soft tissues. However, the absence of destructive proteolytic enzymes results in preservation of articular cartilage and lack of joint space narrowing until disease is advanced. If caseous material calcifies, rice bodies may form.

MRI depicts high-T2 joint effusions along with low-T2 debris, hemosiderin, calcification, loose bodies, and septations [48]; synovial enhancement is relatively thin and smooth. Rice bodies appear as non-enhancing multiple tiny elliptical loose bodies that are dark on both T1- and T2-W MRI [39].

Late sequelae include epiphyseal overgrowth secondary to hyperemia, along with premature physeal fusion. End-stage tuberculous arthritis manifests with severe joint destruction, sclerosis, and—usually fibrous—ankylosis if articular cartilage was destroyed (bony ankylosis is more typical of pyogenic arthritis). These findings are best seen at CT.

Tuberculous dactylitis involves the small tubular bones of the hands and feet, usually in children younger than 5 years old. The metacarpal and proximal phalanges of multiple digits are usually affected. Periostitis and soft tissue swelling are common. Caseous granulation tissue may expand the bone, forming a cystlike cavity, known as "spina ventosa."

Differential considerations for multiple disseminated lytic lesions include other infections and such neoplastic processes as neuroblastoma and non-Hodgkin lymphoma.

11 Fungal Osteomyelitis

Incidence of fungal infections is increasing, especially in immunocompromised patients. However, infection is indolent and diagnosis often delayed. Candida infection is encountered in premature infants and in children being treated with antibiotics and/or chemotherapy. Aspergillus typically occurs in immunosuppressed patients as well, whereas Coccidioidomycosis, Histoplasmosis, and Blastomycosis (Fig. 19.33) are associated with typical geographic regions. Imaging characteristics are similar to bacterial disease, but the locations differ, with spine and flat bones involved more often than the long bones (Fig. 19.34).

12 Syphilis

Infants infected with *Treponema pallidum* present with rash, anemia, hepatosplenomegaly, ascites, and nephrotic syndrome. Skeletal findings become apparent during the first 2 months of life and are typically bilateral and symmetric. A dense band of sclerosis is seen between the growth plate and a metaphyseal lucent band (Fig. 19.35), and there may be foci of lytic destruction in the diaphyses. Wimberger sign, which is seen in 50 % of patients, consists of focal osteolysis at the upper medial tibial metaphysis. Pathologic fractures and periosteal new bone formation may be present.

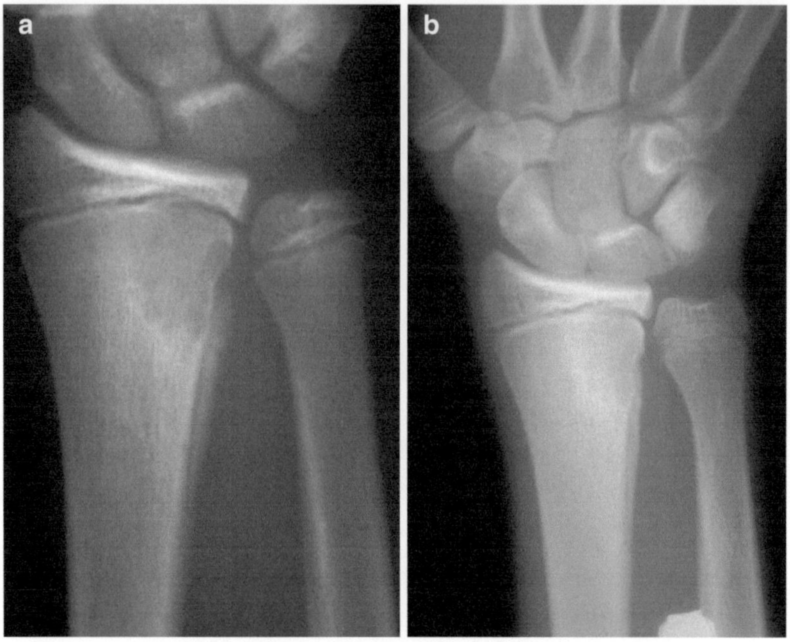

Fig. 19.33 Blastomycosis, resembling bacterial osteomyelitis. (**a**) A lucent focus in the distal metaphysis abuts the physis, with mild surrounding sclerosis and abundant periosteal reaction. (**b**) With healing, sclerosis has increased and periosteal reaction matured

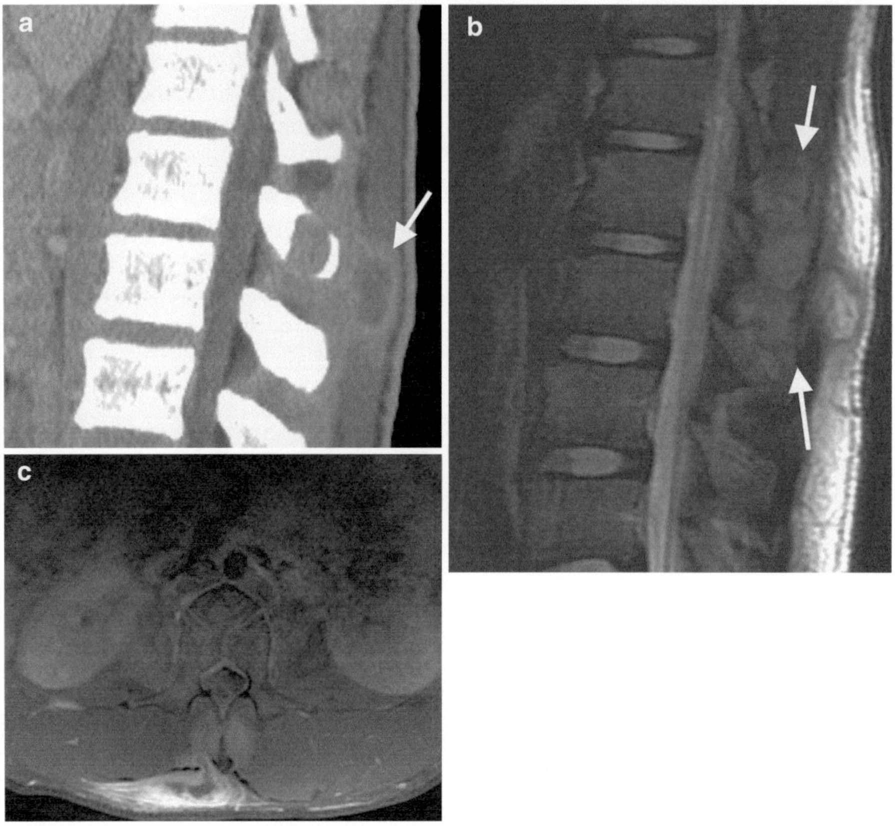

Fig. 19.34 Coccidioidomycosis. (**a**) Sagittal reformatted CT postcontrast shows a well-circumscribed lytic defect at the L1 spinous process, with a soft tissue rim-enhancing abscess (*arrow*). (**b**) Sagittal T2-W MRI shows inflammation as well (*arrows*). (**c**) Axial T1-W FS image shows intense enhancement (*arrows*) around both the abscess and the spinous process

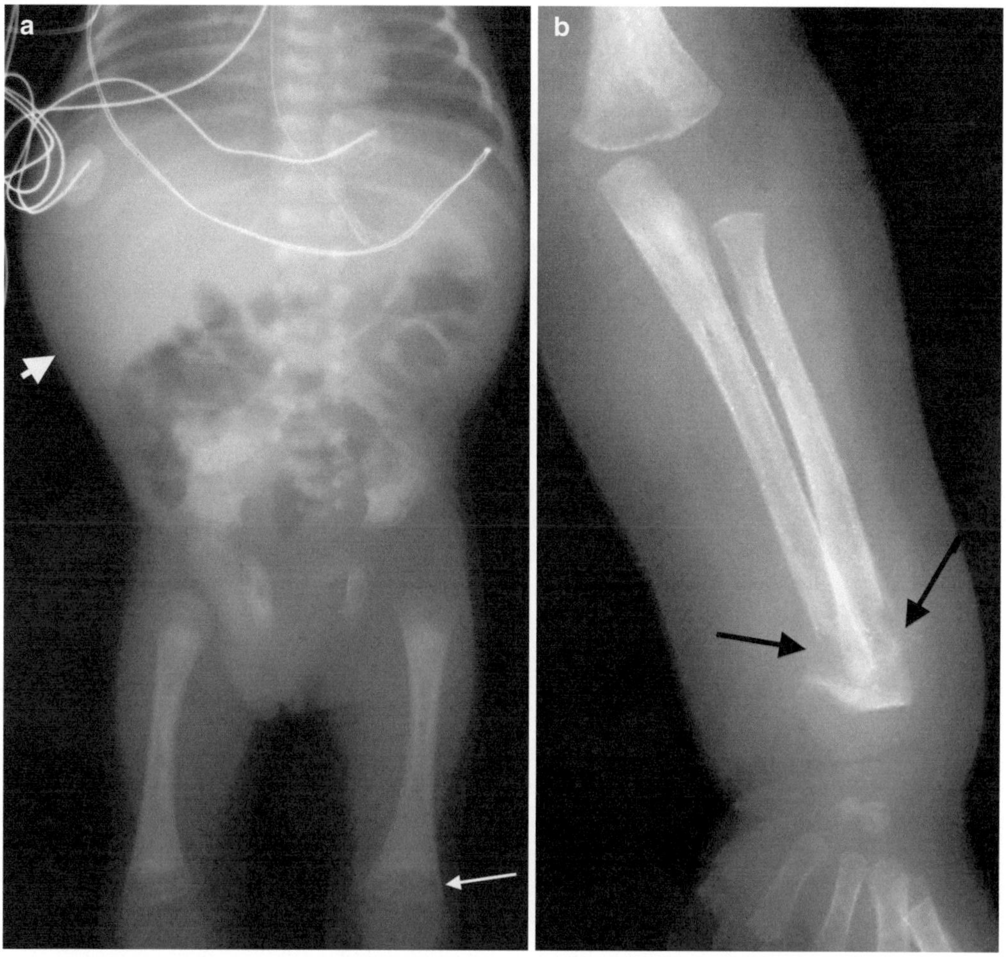

Fig. 19.35 Syphilis in an infant. (**a**) Metaphyses are lucent (*long arrow*), and there is hepatosplenomegaly (*short arrow*). The relatively dense bone is normal. (**b**) Focal osteolysis at the distal humerus, radius, and ulna, with pathological fractures (*arrows*) and periostitis

13 Chronic Recurrent Multifocal Osteomyelitis (Box 19.7)

Box 19.7 Chronic Recurrent Multifocal Osteomyelitis

Inflammatory, not infectious
Little soft tissue abnormality
Metaphysis, medial clavicle, spine
Whole-body MRI preferable to bone scan
MRI similar to osteomyelitis but no abscess, fistula, sequestrum

Chronic recurrent multifocal osteomyelitis (CRMO) is a poorly understood autoimmune/inflammatory disorder that is most common in females and occurs predominantly in older children and adolescents. Although this disease is not infectious, its appearance and evolution somewhat resembles osteomyelitis, and CRMO is therefore usually grouped with infectious musculoskeletal disease. It is predominantly a diagnosis of exclusion. The erythrocyte sedimentation rate and C-reactive protein are usually elevated, whereas the white blood cell count is normal. Histopathologically, the lesions are composed of fibrovascular material and inflammatory cells, predominantly lymphocytes.

After a lengthy waxing and waning clinical course, children present with insidious onset of local pain, swelling, and tenderness. There may be malaise and low-grade fever. It is sometimes accompanied with skin manifestations, most often pustulosis palmoplantaris; it is also associated with peripheral arthritis, inflammatory bowel disorders, psoriasis, and sacroiliitis [51]. In some patients, CRMO is part of the SAPHO syndrome (synovitis, acne, pustulosis, hyperostosis, osteitis). Human leukocyte antigen B27 (HLA B27) is usually negative [52].

Disease is almost always multifocal, but lesions may present at different phases of evolution [51]. Symmetry is common. The lower extremities (hip to ankle) are involved more often than the upper extremities; atypical locations include the clavicle, pelvis, mandible, sternum, ribs, and vertebrae. Metaphyses are usually affected [53]. Clinical course varies and is usually self-limited, but recurrence is (by definition) common.

Organisms have not been isolated. Thought to be an inflammatory process, CRMO responds to treatment with nonsteroidal anti-inflammatory drugs (NSAIDs) rather than antibiotics. NSAIDs more effectively reduce symptoms when fewer lesions are present [51].

Imaging

In the appropriate clinical setting, radiographs may be diagnostic in this often-indolent disease, but findings can be subtle and easily overlooked. There is typically very little soft tissue swelling or periosteal reaction, and the usual finding is an eccentrically located metaphyseal lytic lesion abutting the growth plate with a thin sclerotic rim. Lack of soft tissue changes can help steer the diagnosis away from bacterial or tuberculous osteomyelitis. Periosteal elevation and sequestra are absent. The bone eventually becomes thicker and more sclerotic, and the process often gradually spreads to involve the diaphysis.

MRI typically reveals more marrow involvement than is apparent on radiographs; increased signal at STIR sequences and with gadolinium administration is typical [51]. At MRI, the bony findings resemble osteomyelitis with edematous marrow and heterogeneous enhancement, but there is limited soft tissue involvement, and abscesses, fistulae, and sequestra do not form [51]. STIR/T2 high signal normalizes before T1 signal improves [51].

Whole-body MRI is preferable to bone scan in the pediatric population [53]. Short-tau inversion recovery sequences are useful to demonstrate multiple foci of disease; multifocal disease is essentially universal but often occult at radiography [53].

Although lesions usually resolve radiographically after 2 years [51], they may take years to heal and can recur locally; this disease can last as long as 25 years. During exacerbations, small cortical-based lytic lesions and periosteal new bone formation develop; these are more readily appreciated at MRI [52]. CRMO rarely results in premature physeal closure. Limb-length discrepancy, angular deformity, and kyphosis are less common than with bacterial or tuberculous osteomyelitis.

CRMO commonly affects the medial aspect of the clavicle (Fig. 19.36). Early findings of lytic medullary destruction and periosteal new bone formation are nonspecific at radiographs and MRI, but the location is suggestive. During remission, the lesion heals with sclerosis and organization of periosteal new bone [52]. Multiple episodes result in progressive sclerosis and hyperostosis of the clavicle. STIR or fat-suppressed T2 sequences are very useful to delineate active foci of high signal. Complete healing is rarc.

CRMO of the spine presents either as spondylodiscitis or as a predominantly lytic lesion; the former is more common [52] (Fig. 19.37). Erosive changes at the end plates may be accompanied with subchondral sclerosis and narrowed intervertebral disc spaces [51, 52]. MRI signal characteristics are similar to infectious spondylitis, but in CRMO, the process is usually limited to one end plate, rarely crosses the intervertebral disc, and is not accompanied with abscess formation [51]. These lesions usually heal with minimal sequelae.

Predominant lytic vertebral lesions probably represent progression of spondylodiscitis-like lesions with resultant severe bone destruction, collapse, and resultant vertebra plana. MRI assists in differentiation from eosinophilic granuloma and malignancies, as there is no accompanying mass. Kyphosis may develop if there is significant vertebral collapse [52].

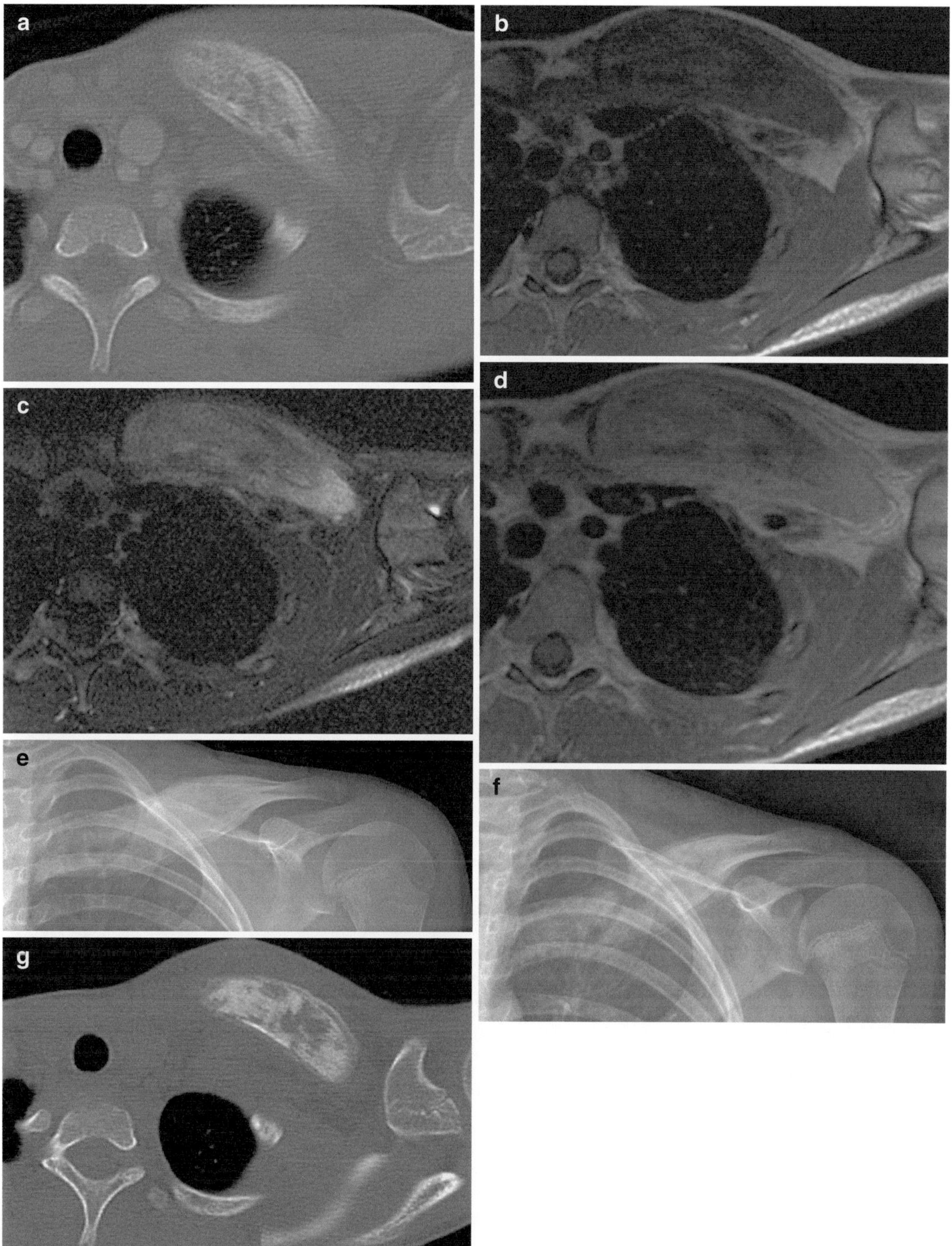

Fig. 19.36 Chronic recurrent multifocal osteomyelitis of the clavicle in a 13-year-old girl. (**a**) CT at diagnosis shows advanced disease, with sclerosis and thick periosteal reaction. (**b**) Near-simultaneous T1-W MRI shows heterogeneous well-circumscribed hypointensity that is hyperintense on (**c**) T2-W fat-saturated sequence. (**d**) With gadolinium, there is heterogeneous central enhancement, with more uniform periosteal enhancement. Note the absence of significant surrounding soft tissue enhancement. (**e**) Four months later, there is sclerosis and thickening. (**f**) One year later, new periosteal reaction and increased intralesional lysis denote recurrence, confirmed on CT (**g**)

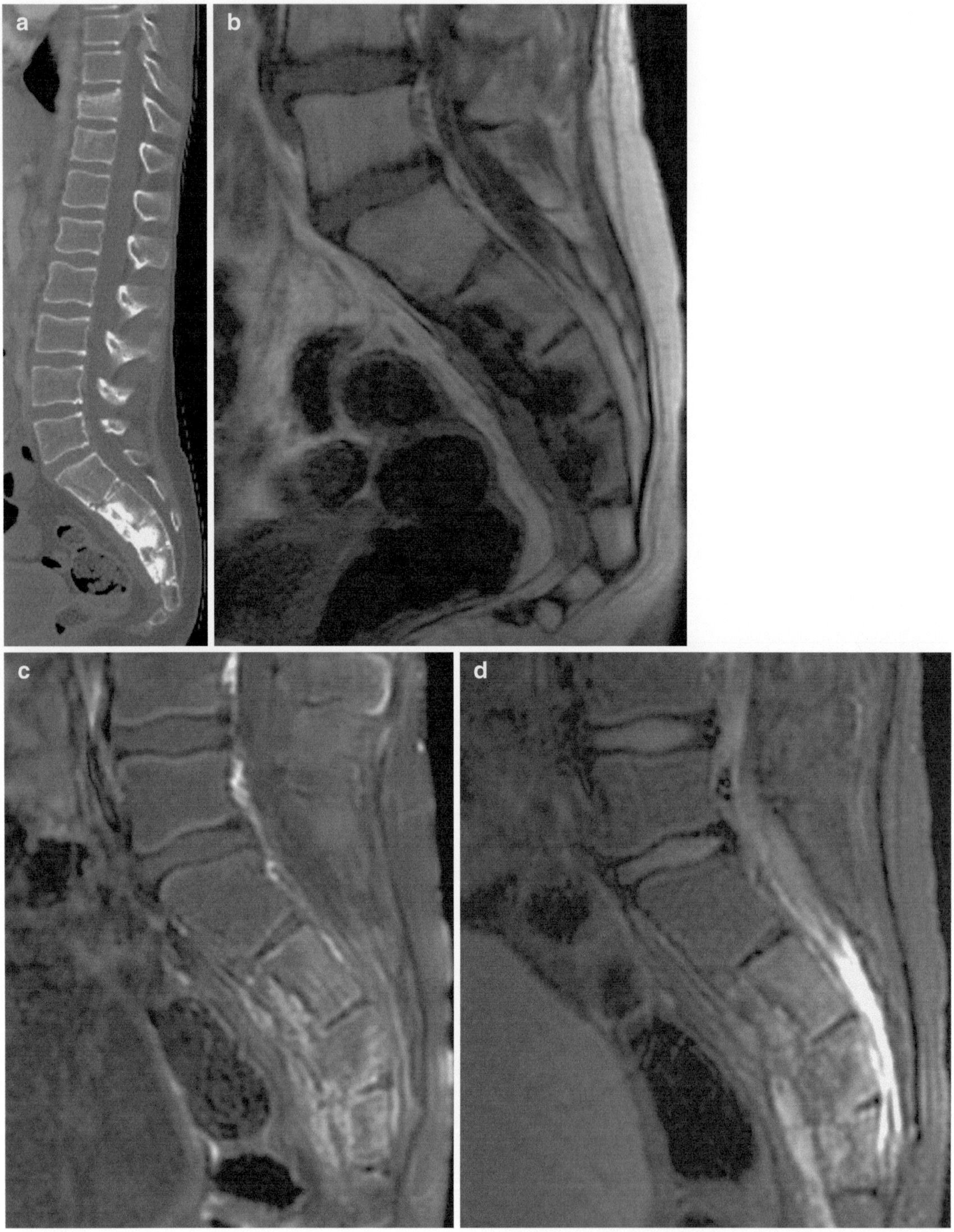

Fig. 19.37 Chronic recurrent multifocal osteomyelitis in a 12-year-old girl. (**a**) Sagittal reformatted CT shows sacral sclerosis and sclerosis and compression of T10. (**b**) On sagittal T1-W FS MRI, well-circumscribed ventral hypointense foci at S2–4, with diffuse enhancement on (**c**) T1-W gadolinium-enhanced sagittal image. (**d**) STIR sequence shows marrow edema and presacral soft tissue edema

Differential Diagnosis

This includes infectious osteomyelitis, juvenile idiopathic arthritis, and tumors as well as tumorlike lesions such as Ewing sarcoma, leukemia, and Langerhans cell histiocytosis. Clinical features assist with diagnosis: gradual onset of localized pain, multifocal lesions, skin disease, recurrent exacerbations, absence of an organism, and improvement with nonsteroidal anti-inflammatory treatment.

References

1. Arnold SR, Elias D, Buckingham SC, Thomas ED, Novais E, Arkader A, et al. Changing patterns of acute hematogenous osteomyelitis and septic arthritis: emergence of community-associated methicillin-resistant Staphylococcus aureus. J Pediatr Orthop. 2006;26(6):703–8. PMID: 17065930. Epub 2006/10/27. eng.
2. Gafur OA, Copley LA, Hollmig ST, Browne RH, Thornton LA, Crawford SE. The impact of the current epidemiology of pediatric musculoskeletal infection on evaluation and treatment guidelines. J Pediatr Orthop. 2008;28(7):777–85. PubMed PMID: 18812907. Epub 2008/09/25. eng.
3. Steer AC, Carapetis JR. Acute hematogenous osteomyelitis in children: recognition and management. Pediatr Drugs. 2004;6(6):333–46. PubMed PMID: 15612835, Epub 2004/12/23. eng.
4. Offiah AC. Acute osteomyelitis, septic arthritis and discitis: differences between neonates and older children. Eur J Radiol. 2006;60(2):221–32. PubMed PMID: 16971078Epub 2006/09/15. eng.
5. Riise OR, Kirkhus E, Handeland KS, Flato B, Reiseter T, Cvancarova M, et al. Childhood osteomyelitis-incidence and differentiation from other acute onset musculoskeletal features in a population-based study. BMC Pediatr. 2008;8:45. PubMed PMID: 18937840, Pubmed Central PMCID: 2588573, Epub 2008/10/22. eng.
6. Blickman JG, van Die CE, de Rooy JW. Current imaging concepts in pediatric osteomyelitis. Eur Radiol. 2004;14 Suppl 4:L55–64. PubMed PMID: 14752569, Epub 2004/01/31. eng.
7. Pineda C, Vargas A, Rodriguez AV. Imaging of osteomyelitis: current concepts. Infect Dis Clin North Am. 2006;20(4):789–825. PubMed PMID: 17118291, Epub 2006/11/23. eng.
8. Harik NS, Smeltzer MS. Management of acute hematogenous osteomyelitis in children. Expert Rev Anti Infect Ther. 2010;8(2):175–81. PubMed PMID: 20109047, Pubmed Central PMCID: 2836799, Epub 2010/01/30. eng.
9. Mellado Santos JM. Diagnostic imaging of pediatric hematogenous osteomyelitis: lessons learned from a multi-modality approach. Eur Radiol. 2006;16(9):2109–19. PubMed PMID: 16541223, Epub 2006/03/17. eng.
10. Connolly LP, Connolly SA, Drubach LA, Jaramillo D, Treves ST. Acute hematogenous osteomyelitis of children: assessment of skeletal scintigraphy-based diagnosis in the era of MRI. J Nucl Med. 2002;43(10):1310–6. PubMed PMID: 12368368, Epub 2002/10/09. eng.
11. Gotthardt M, Bleeker-Rovers CP, Boerman OC, Oyen WJ. Imaging of inflammation by PET, conventional scintigraphy, and other imaging techniques. J Nucl Med. 2010;51(12):1937–49. PubMed PMID: 21078798, Epub 2010/11/17. eng.
12. Pruthi S, Thapa MM. Infectious and inflammatory disorders. Magn Reson Imaging Clin N Am. 2009;17(3):423–38, v. PubMed PMID: 19524194. Epub 2009/06/16. eng.
13. DiPoce J, Jbara ME, Brenner AI. Pediatric osteomyelitis: a scintigraphic case-based review. Radiographics. 2012;32(3):865–78. PubMed PMID: 22582364. Epub 2012/05/15. eng.
14. Browne LP, Mason EO, Kaplan SL, Cassady CI, Krishnamurthy R, Guillerman RP. Optimal imaging strategy for community-acquired Staphylococcus aureus musculoskeletal infections in children. Pediatr Radiol. 2008;38(8):841–7. PubMed PMID: 18560822, Epub 2008/06/19. eng.
15. Parisi MT. Functional imaging of infection: conventional nuclear medicine agents and the expanding role of 18-F-FDG PET. Pediatr Radiol. 2011;41(7):803–10. PubMed PMID: 21607605, Epub 2011/05/25. eng.
16. Warmann SW, Dittmann H, Seitz G, Bares R, Fuchs J, Schafer JF. Follow-up of acute osteomyelitis in children: the possible role of PET/CT in selected cases. J Pediatr Surg. 2011;46(8):1550–6. PubMed PMID: 21843723, Epub 2011/08/17. eng.
17. Riebel TW, Nasir R, Nazarenko O. The value of sonography in the detection of osteomyelitis. Pediatr Radiol. 1996;26(4):291–7. PubMed PMID: 8677150, Epub 1996/01/01. eng.
18. Robben SG. Ultrasonography of musculoskeletal infections in children. Eur Radiol. 2004;14 Suppl 4:L65–77. PubMed PMID: 14752567, Epub 2004/01/31. eng.
19. Chao HC, Lin SJ, Huang YC, Lin TY. Color Doppler ultrasonographic evaluation of osteomyelitis in children. J Ultrasound Med. 1999;18(11):729–34. PubMed PMID: 10547104, quiz 35–6; Epub 1999/11/05. eng.
20. Kan JH, Hilmes MA, Martus JE, Yu C, Hernanz-Schulman M. Value of MRI after recent diagnostic or surgical intervention in children with suspected osteomyelitis. AJR Am J Roentgenol. 2008;191(5):1595–600. PubMed PMID: 18941107, Epub 2008/10/23. eng.

21. Averill LW, Hernandez A, Gonzalez L, Pena AH, Jaramillo D. Diagnosis of osteomyelitis in children: utility of fat-suppressed contrast-enhanced MRI. AJR Am J Roentgenol. 2009;192(5):1232–8. PubMed PMID: 19380545, Epub 2009/04/22. eng.
22. Kan JH, Young RS, Yu C, Hernanz-Schulman M. Clinical impact of gadolinium in the MRI diagnosis of musculoskeletal infection in children. Pediatr Radiol. 2010;40(7):1197–205. PubMed PMID: 20180105, Epub 2010/02/25. eng.
23. Davies AM, Hughes DE, Grimer RJ. Intramedullary and extramedullary fat globules on magnetic resonance imaging as a diagnostic sign for osteomyelitis. Eur Radiol. 2005;15(10):2194–9. PubMed PMID: 15864595, Epub 2005/05/03. eng.
24. Kumar J, Bandhu S, Kumar A, Alam S. Extra-osseous fat fluid level: a specific sign for osteomyelitis. Skelet Radiol. 2007;36 Suppl 1:S101–4. PubMed PMID: 16988800, Epub 2006/09/22. eng.
25. Mattis TA, Borders HL, Ellinger DM, Junewick JJ. Relationship between the clinical characteristics of osteomyelitis and the finding of extraosseous fat on MRI in pediatric patients. Pediatr Radiol. 2011;41(10):1293–7. PubMed PMID: 21553040, PubMed PMID: 21553040.
26. Courtney PM, Flynn JM, Jaramillo D, Horn BD, Calabro K, Spiegel DA. Clinical indications for repeat MRI in children with acute hematogenous osteomyelitis. J Pediatr Orthop. 2010;30(8):883–7. PubMed PMID: 21102217, Epub 2010/11/26. eng.
27. Marti-Bonmati L, Aparisi F, Poyatos C, Vilar J. Brodie abscess: MR imaging appearance in 10 patients. J Magn Reson Imaging. 1993;3(3):543–6. PubMed PMID: 8324315. Epub 1993/05/01. eng.
28. Davies AM, Grimer R. The penumbra sign in subacute osteomyelitis. Eur Radiol. 2005;15(6):1268–70. PubMed PMID: 15300398, Epub 2004/08/10. eng.
29. DA Grey AC, Mangham DC, Grimer RJ, Ritchie DA. The 'penumbra sign' on T1-weighted MR imaging in subacute osteomyelitis: frequency, cause and significance. Clin Radiol. 1998;53(8):587–92.
30. Hempfing A, Placzek R, Gottsche T, Meiss AL. Primary subacute epiphyseal and metaepiphyseal osteomyelitis in children. Diagnosis and treatment guided by MRI. J Bone Joint Surg Br. 2003;85(4):559–64. PubMed PMID: 12793564, Epub 2003/06/10. eng.
31. Johnson DP, Hernanz-Schulman M, Martus JE, Lovejoy SA, Yu C, Kan JH. Significance of epiphyseal cartilage enhancement defects in pediatric osteomyelitis identified by MRI with surgical correlation. Pediatr Radiol. 2011;41(3):355–61. PubMed PMID: 20936273, Epub 2010/10/12. eng.
32. Connolly SA, Connolly LP, Drubach LA, Zurakowski D, Jaramillo D. MRI for detection of abscess in acute osteomyelitis of the pelvis in children. AJR Am J Roentgenol. 2007;189(4):867–72. PubMed PMID: 17885058, Epub 2007/09/22. eng.
33. Kleinman PK. A regional approach to osteomyelitis of the lower extremities in children. Radiol Clin North Am. 2002;40(5):1033–59. PubMed PMID: 12462467, Epub 2002/12/05. eng.
34. McPhee E, Eskander JP, Eskander MS, Mahan ST, Mortimer E. Imaging in pelvic osteomyelitis: support for early magnetic resonance imaging. J Pediatr Orthop. 2007;27(8):903–9. PubMed PMID: 18209613, Epub 2008/01/23. eng.
35. Kumar J, Ramachandran M, Little D, Zenios M. Pelvic osteomyelitis in children. J Pediatr Orthop B. 2010;19(1):38–41. PubMed PMID: 19858750, Epub 2009/10/28. eng.
36. Schmit P, Glorion C. Osteomyelitis in infants and children. Eur Radiol. 2004;14 Suppl 4:L44–54. PubMed PMID: 14531001, Epub 2003/10/08. eng.
37. Vander Have KL, Karmazyn B, Verma M, Caird MS, Hensinger RN, Farley FA, et al. Community-associated methicillin-resistant Staphylococcus aureus in acute musculoskeletal infection in children: a game changer. J Pediatr Orthop. 2009;29(8):927–31. PubMed PMID: 19934711, Epub 2009/11/26. eng.
38. McCarthy JJ, Dormans JP, Kozin SH, Pizzutillo PD. Musculoskeletal infections in children: basic treatment principles and recent advancements. Instr Course Lect. 2005;54:515–28. PubMed PMID: 15948476, Epub 2005/06/14. eng.
39. Ranson M. Imaging of pediatric musculoskeletal infection. Semin Musculoskelet Radiol. 2009; 13(3):277–99. PubMed PMID: 19724994, Epub 2009/09/03. eng.
40. Zawin JK, Hoffer FA, Rand FF, Teele RL. Joint effusion in children with an irritable hip: US diagnosis and aspiration. Radiology. 1993;187(2):459–63. PubMed PMID: 8475290, Epub 1993/05/01. eng.
41. Chau CL, Griffith JF. Musculoskeletal infections: ultrasound appearances. Clin Radiol. 2005;60(2):149–59. PubMed PMID: 15664569, Epub 2005/01/25. eng.
42. Gordon JE, Huang M, Dobbs M, Luhmann SJ, Szymanski DA, Schoenecker PL. Causes of false-negative ultrasound scans in the diagnosis of septic arthritis of the hip in children. J Pediatr Orthop. 2002;22(3):312–6. PubMed PMID: 11961445. Epub 2002/04/19. eng.
43. Hopkins KL, Li KC, Bergman G. Gadolinium-DTPA-enhanced magnetic resonance imaging of musculoskeletal infectious processes. Skelet Radiol. 1995;24(5):325–30. PubMed PMID: 7570151, Epub 1995/07/01. eng.
44. Kim HK, Zbojniewicz AM, Merrow AC, Cheon JE, Kim IO, Emery KH. MR findings of synovial disease in children and young adults: part 2. Pediatr Radiol. 2011;41(4):512–24. PubMed PMID: 21336643, Epub 2011/02/22. eng.
45. Karmazyn B, Kleiman MB, Buckwalter K, Loder RT, Siddiqui A, Applegate KE. Acute pyomyositis of the pelvis: the spectrum of clinical presentations and MR findings. Pediatr Radiol. 2006;36(4):338–43. PubMed PMID: 16474970, Epub 2006/02/14. eng.
46. Ejindu VC, Hine AL, Mashayekhi M, Shorvon PJ, Misra RR. Musculoskeletal manifestations of sickle

cell disease. Radiographics. 2007;27(4):1005–21. PubMed PMID: 17620464. Epub 2007/07/11. eng.
47. Morris BS, Varma R, Garg A, Awasthi M, Maheshwari M. Multifocal musculoskeletal tuberculosis in children: appearances on computed tomography. Skelet Radiol. 2002;31(1):1–8. PubMed PMID: 11807585, Epub 2002/01/25. eng.
48. De Vuyst D, Vanhoenacker F, Gielen J, Bernaerts A, De Schepper AM. Imaging features of musculoskeletal tuberculosis. Eur Radiol. 2003;13(8):1809–19. PubMed PMID: 12942283, Epub 2003/08/28. eng.
49. Teo HE, Peh WC. Skeletal tuberculosis in children. Pediatr Radiol. 2004;34(11):853–60. PubMed PMID: 15278319, Epub 2004/07/28. eng.
50. Sharma P. MR features of tuberculous osteomyelitis. Skelet Radiol. 2003;32(5):279–85. PubMed PMID: 12679845, Epub 2003/04/08. eng.
51. Iyer RS, Thapa MM, Chew FS. Chronic recurrent multifocal osteomyelitis: review. AJR Am J Roentgenol. 2011;196(6 Suppl):S87–91. PubMed PMID: 21606238, Epub 2011/05/27. eng.
52. Jurik AG. Chronic recurrent multifocal osteomyelitis. Semin Musculoskelet Radiol. 2004;8(3): 243–53. PubMed PMID: 15478027, Epub 2004/10/13. en0067.
53. Fritz J, Tzaribatchev N, Claussen CD, Carrino JA, Horger MS. Chronic recurrent multifocal osteomyelitis: comparison of whole-body MR imaging with radiography and correlation with clinical and laboratory data. Radiology. 2009;252(3): 842–51. PubMed PMID: 19567645, Epub 2009/07/02. eng.

Arthritis

20

Rebecca Stein-Wexler and Mahesh M. Thapa

Contents

Abstract

Imaging plays a key role in the evaluation of patients with known or suspected arthritis. Following clinical and laboratory assessment, radiography is the traditional imaging starting point. Other potential modalities include ultrasound, computed tomography, nuclear medicine, and magnetic resonance imaging. This chapter will present the following conditions: juvenile idiopathic arthritis (JIA) along with the enthesitis-related arthritis (ERA) subtype, hemophilia, and pigmented villonodular synovitis (PVNS). Synovial chondromatosis and dermatomyositis are discussed in Chaps. 12 and 24, respectively.

The child with chronic joint pain often presents a diagnostic challenge. Radiographs constitute the initial imaging modality, but in children with arthritis, these studies are usually normal until relatively late in the disease—or they demonstrate only nonspecific soft tissue swelling and joint fluid. Only after chronic inflammation has destroyed the thick cartilage that covers the bone do findings such as joint space narrowing, osseous erosions, ankylosis, and growth disturbance become apparent. Diagnosis therefore often rests on clinical factors along with advanced imaging, typically gadolinium-enhanced magnetic resonance imaging (MRI) although Doppler ultrasound (US) may also contribute useful information.

R. Stein-Wexler, MD (✉)
Department of Radiology,
University of California Davis Medical
Center and UC Davis Children's Hospital,
4860 Y Street, Suite 3100, Sacramento, CA 95817, USA

Department of Diagnostic Imaging, Shriners Hospitals
for Children Northern California,
Sacramento, CA 95817, USA
e-mail: rebecca.steinwexler@ucdmc.ucdavis.edu

M.M. Thapa, MD
Department of Radiology, Seattle Children's Hospital,
4800 Sand Point Way NE, Seattle, WA 98105, USA
e-mail: thapamd@uw.edu

R. Stein-Wexler et al. (eds.), *Pediatric Orthopedic Imaging*,
DOI 10.1007/978-3-642-45381-6_20, © Springer-Verlag Berlin Heidelberg 2015

1 Juvenile Idiopathic Arthritis

Juvenile idiopathic arthritis (JIA) is the most common chronic rheumatic disease of childhood and encompasses all idiopathic arthritides that present before age 16 years and last at least 6 weeks. The disorder is further classified according to the number of joints involved (up to four being "oligoarticular"), the presence of systemic disease, and the results of serologic tests for rheumatic factor. Prevalence is 1 per 1,000 children [1], and the disease is most common in girls. Patients present with joint pain and swelling and sometimes with extraskeletal findings as well.

Etiology is multifactorial, with both environmental and genetic factors playing a role. The disease appears to develop when a genetically predisposed child mounts a particular immunological response to an infectious process. Pannus and inflammation develop within the synovium after an antigen-antibody cross-reaction [2]. Initial synovitis progresses to synovial hyperplasia and formation of highly cellular inflammatory pannus. This eventually erodes the overlying cartilage and bone and causes articular destruction, ankylosis, and growth disturbance.

The term JIA replaces older terminology, such as "juvenile chronic arthritis" and "juvenile rheumatoid arthritis." The newer term, with its subtypes, facilitates more accurate identification of homogeneous groups of children with distinct clinical features. The International League of Associations for Rheumatology (ILAR) identifies eight distinct subtypes of JIA [3], and this classification system will almost certainly undergo further refinement (Table 20.1).

The most common JIA subtype, "oligoarticular," affects no more than four joints during the first 6 months of presentation; it usually affects the knees and/or ankles, as well as the wrists and elbows, of girls less than 6 years old [1]. Up to

Table 20.1 ILAR classification of juvenile idiopathic arthritis

Arthritis	Inclusionary criteria
Systemic arthritis	Arthritis in at least one joint
	2 weeks' fever consecutive at least 3 days
	Rash, generalized lymphadenopathy, hepatomegaly/splenomegaly, or serositis
Oligoarthritis (persistent)	Arthritis of 1–4 joints during the first 6 months
	Never involves more than 4 joints
Oligoarthritis (extended)	Arthritis of 1–4 joints during the first 6 months
	Eventually affects at least 5 joints
Polyarthritis (RF negative)	Arthritis of more than 5 joints during the first 6 months
	RF test negative
Polyarthritis (RF positive)	Arthritis of more than 5 joints during the first 6 months
	RF test positive (at least twice, during the first 6 months)
Psoriatic arthritis	Arthritis and psoriasis
	Or arthritis and at least 2 in first-degree relative:
	Dactylitis, nail pitting, psoriasis
Enthesitis-related arthritis	Arthritis and enthesitis, with
	Sacroiliac joint tenderness and/or lumbosacral pain
	HLA-B27 antigen
	Male over 6-year-old
	Acute anterior uveitis
	First-degree relative with ankylosing spondylitis, enthesitis-related arthritis, sacroiliitis with inflammatory bowel disease, Reiter syndrome, or acute anterior uveitis
Undifferentiated arthritis	Arthritis that fulfills two or more of these categories or that fails to fall into one of these categories

Adapted from Wallace and Levinson [4]

30 % of these children also have iridocyclitis. "Polyarticular" arthritis presents with involvement of at least five joints within 6 months of presentation and is usually symmetric, involving the wrists, hands, and feet. Results of serologic testing allow further categorization: RF-positive cases typically occur in adolescent girls, and like rheumatoid arthritis in adults, the disease affects the small joints of the hands. RF-negative cases, which have a broad variety of manifestations, occur throughout childhood.

Arthritis is categorized as systemic if at least one joint is affected and if accompanied or recently preceded by at least 2 weeks of fever (consecutive for at least 3 days), a transitory rash, hepatomegaly, splenomegaly, lymphadenopathy, or serositis. Classic polyarticular and symmetric symptoms generally occur late in the course of disease. Systemic JIA may be life-threatening in a small subset of patients who develop pancytopenia, disseminated intravascular coagulation, and multiorgan failure ("macrophage activation syndrome").

Psoriatic arthritis and enthesitis-related arthritis (ERA) subtypes are based on the presence of dactylitis, psoriasis, symptoms related to the sacroiliac joints or lower back, presence of human leukocyte antigen (HLA)-B27, and additional findings. Juvenile psoriatic arthritis affects large or small joints, and joint findings may precede development of skin abnormalities. ERA (formerly termed juvenile spondyloarthritis) is unusual among the subtypes of JIA in that the hip is often affected. This disease tends to affect sites of tendinous and ligamentous insertion at the pelvis, knee, and calcaneus. Axial involvement is rare in children under 10 years of age, although the spine and sacroiliac joints may be affected in older children (see following section for further discussion of Sect. 1.1). Undifferentiated JIA encompasses cases with none of these features or with features that are present in at least two different subtypes.

Disease usually becomes inactive with anti-inflammatory medication. However, in many patients, disease progresses unabated, regardless of treatment. Between 28 and 55 % of patients develop cartilage or bone erosions, often leading to joint irregularity, within 7 years of initial diagnosis [4]. Ankylosis, most common in the carpal and tarsal bones as well as the cervical spine, may develop within 3–5 years of disease onset.

Imaging (Table 20.1)

General Considerations. Radiographs are often initially normal, but in the early phase there may be nonspecific consequences of hypervascularity and inflammation, including joint effusion, soft tissue swelling, epiphyseal widening, and periarticular osteopenia. This is partly because in the pediatric skeleton thick cartilage protects bone, so erosive change is encountered only with advanced disease. In addition, the synovial hypertrophy and cartilaginous changes typical of early JIA are radiographically occult. However, radiographs performed early in the course of disease do both allow exclusion of other causes of pain and establish a baseline. US and MRI are able to demonstrate early findings of synovial hypertrophy and hyperemia.

During the intermediate phase, cartilage destruction results in joint space narrowing, cortical erosions, and epiphyseal overgrowth; these findings are demonstrable on both radiographs and MRI and to a lesser extent US. Finally, ankylosis, muscle atrophy, growth disturbance, angular deformity at the joints, and contractures may be seen with late disease.

During active disease, clinical examination generally provides adequate assessment of articular synovitis. US and MRI are, however, useful for early staging and for monitoring response to therapy. Indeed, techniques such as T2 mapping may demonstrate progressive cartilage deterioration even when clinical findings are stable [5]. Numerous attempts have been made to develop radiographic scoring systems, none of which have been widely accepted [6, 7]. Radiographs therefore do not play an important role in monitoring progression, but they are important for evaluating deformities and growth abnormalities.

Radiographic Findings. Radiographs may demonstrate joint effusions early in JIA, especially at the knee (Fig. 20.1) The small joints of the hands and feet may show fusiform soft tis-

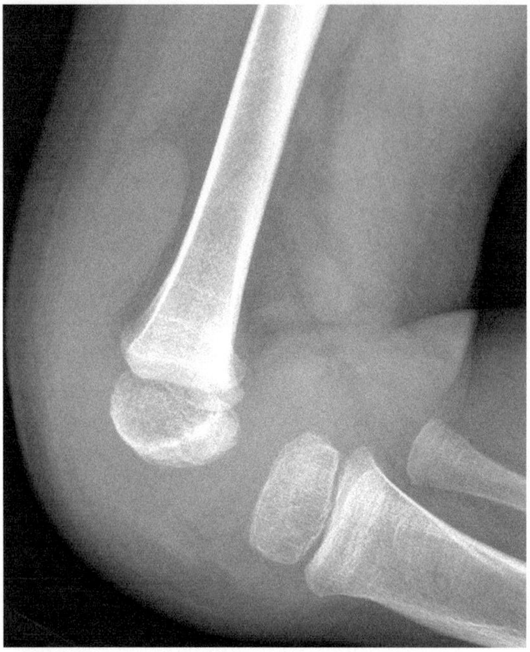

Fig. 20.1 Knee effusion in a 3-year-old boy with polyarticular juvenile idiopathic arthritis (JIA), symptomatic since age 1 year. There are also growth arrest lines and juxta-articular osteopenia. Findings were bilaterally symmetric (Same patient as Fig. 20.4) (Image copyright Shriners Hospital for Children Northern California)

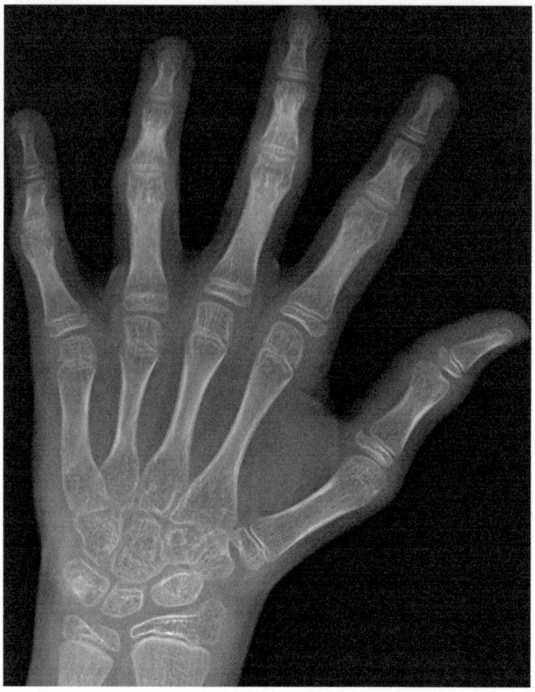

Fig. 20.2 Erosions and osteopenia in a 10-year-old girl with seronegative polyarticular JIA. In addition to the carpal erosions and juxta-articular demineralization/soft tissue swelling, there are flexion deformities at the third through fifth proximal interphalangeal (PIP) joints (Image copyright Shriners Hospital for Children Northern California)

sue swelling, especially common with psoriatic arthritis. US and MRI are more sensitive for evaluation of the small joints than are radiographs.

Osteopenia is another relatively early finding (Fig. 20.2). In the acute setting, this results from juxta-articular hyperemia and resultant trabecular resorption, whereas in chronic disease it is more generalized and results from steroid use and disuse atrophy.

Periostitis occurs at any stage of disease and in any long bone but is most common in the short tubular bones of the hands and feet (Fig. 20.3). This usually develops at para-articular locations, due to inflammation of the joint capsule and tendinous insertions. Bones may enlarge and become square as a result (especially common with psoriatic arthritis) (Fig. 20.4).

Erosions are evident relatively late, after thick protective cartilage has been destroyed by prolonged synovial proliferation (Fig. 20.5). Although erosions may occur anywhere along the articular surface, they are most common at locations where there is less cartilage—insertion sites of intraosseous ligaments and synovial reflections. Radiographs show decreased joint space due to cartilage loss before erosions become apparent, but they are relatively insensitive for showing trabecular bone loss [8]. In patients with systemic JIA, joint space narrowing and erosions may be found relatively early in the course of disease [9].

Growth disturbance, a relatively late finding, is both more common and more severe in children with early onset of disease. It may be generalized, resulting from chronic disease and long-term steroid use. Alternatively, localized growth disturbance may result from periarticular inflammation and localized hyperemia, which lead to early growth acceleration and subsequent epiphyseal enlargement as well as early physeal closure and accelerated maturation. This accounts

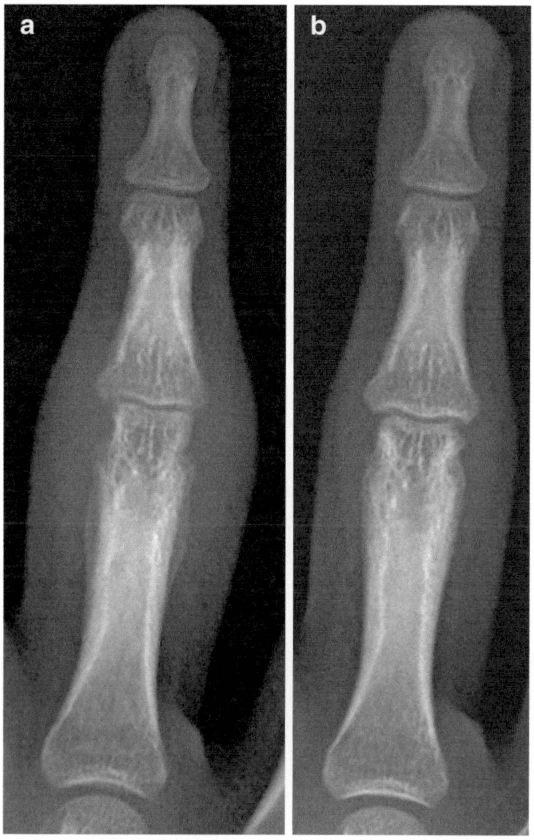

Fig. 20.3 Periostitis in a 15-year-old girl with psoriatic JIA. (a) Marked soft tissue swelling, moderate joint space narrowing, and erosions at the PIP joint of the right fourth digit. Periosteal reaction along the proximal phalanx. (b) Eight months later, after methotrexate therapy, findings have improved (Images copyright Shriners Hospital for Children Northern California)

for the typical appearance at the knee (Figs. 20.6 and 20.7): ballooned epiphyses, wide intercondylar notch, and squared inferior patella, which may in turn lead to subluxation. Although hyperemia leads to initial growth acceleration and longitudinal overgrowth, premature bone maturation and physeal fusion/epiphyseal destruction may eventually cause decreased limb length. A similar process takes place in the carpal and tarsal bones, which may demonstrate premature ossification and then osseous coalition (Fig. 20.8).

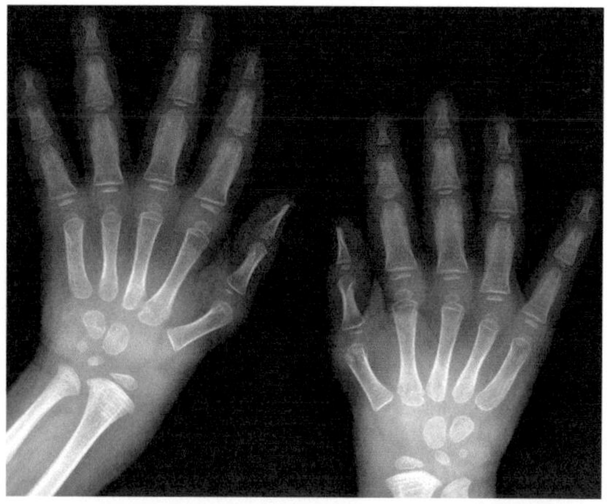

Fig. 20.4 Squaring of phalanges in a 3-year-old boy with polyarticular JIA. Findings are most striking in the proximal and middle phalanges, where periostitis causes thickening of phalanges. Diffuse soft tissue swelling (Same patient as Fig. 20.1) (Image copyright Shriners Hospital for Children Northern California)

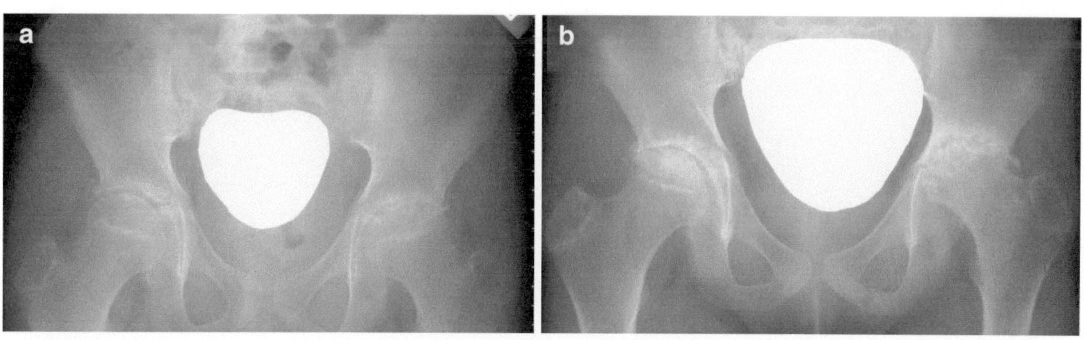

Fig. 20.5 Disease progression in a teenage girl with systemic JIA. (a) At age 15 years, there are small femoral head erosions and uniform joint space narrowing on the left, whereas the right is almost normal. (b) Two years later, the joint space on the left is barely evident, and there are more acetabular and femoral head erosions as well as sclerosis. The right femoral head is developing erosions (Images copyright Shriners Hospital for Children Northern California)

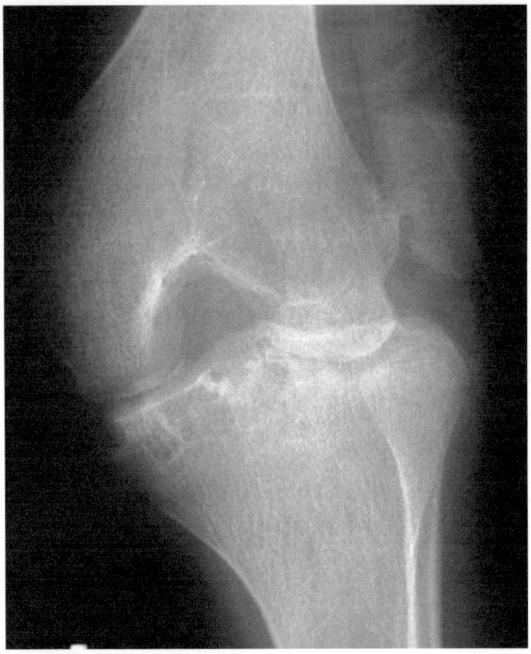

Fig. 20.6 Knee deformity in chronic JIA. Epiphyseal squaring, femoral notch enlargement, joint space narrowing, and subchondral cysts are typical of long-standing disease. Dislocated patella (Image copyright Shriners Hospital for Children Northern California)

Growth disturbance is also common in the mandible (see discussion below).

Ankylosis (Fig. 20.9), erosions, synovial hypertrophy, effusions, and muscle imbalance may cause abnormal stress at the joints and lead to flexion and extension deformities as well as joint subluxation and dislocation (see subsequent paragraph). The knee may develop varus or valgus deformity, in part due to asymmetric epiphyseal overgrowth (see Fig. 20.7). This may contribute to deformity at the hip, including enlargement of the femoral head, acetabular protrusion, coxa vara, and hip subluxation. A similar process may occur in the upper extremities, with asymmetric epiphyseal enlargement causing deformity at the elbow and shoulder (Figs. 20.10 and 20.11).

Deformities at the hand and wrist are most common with polyarticular JIA. These include such finger deformities as flexion at the proximal interphalangeal (PIP) and distal interphalangeal (DIP) joints, Boutonniere deformity (flexion at PIP with hyperextension at DIP) (Fig. 20.12), and swan neck deformity (extension at PIP and

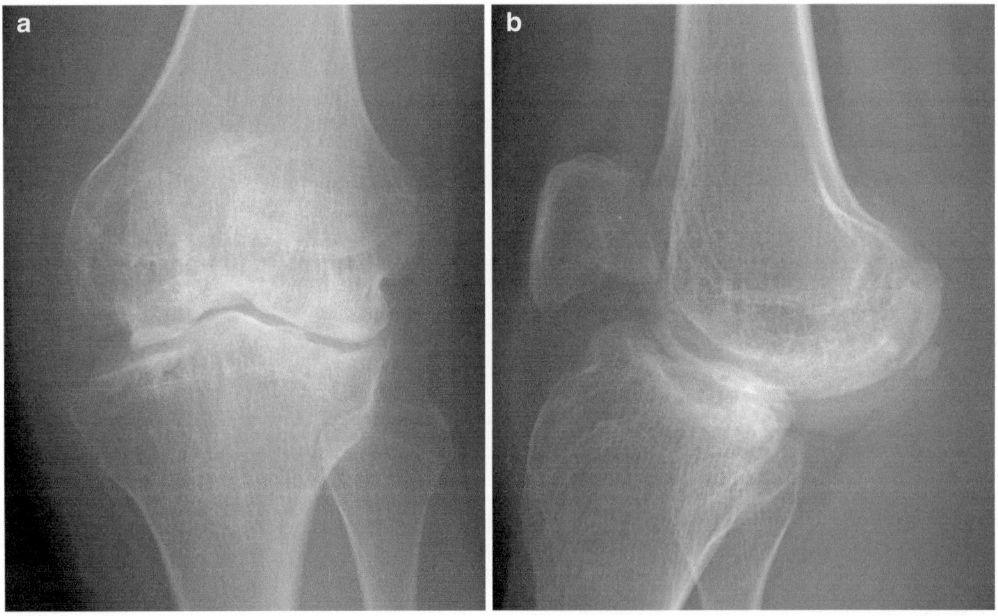

Fig. 20.7 Knee deformity and subluxation in an 18-year-old female with JIA. (**a**) Epiphyseal enlargement and asymmetric growth, joint space narrowing, subchondral cysts, and valgus deformity are characteristic of long-standing disease. (**b**) Squaring of the patella and subluxation at the tibiofemoral joint. Findings were bilaterally symmetric (Same patient as Fig. 20.17) (Images copyright Shriners Hospital for Children Northern California)

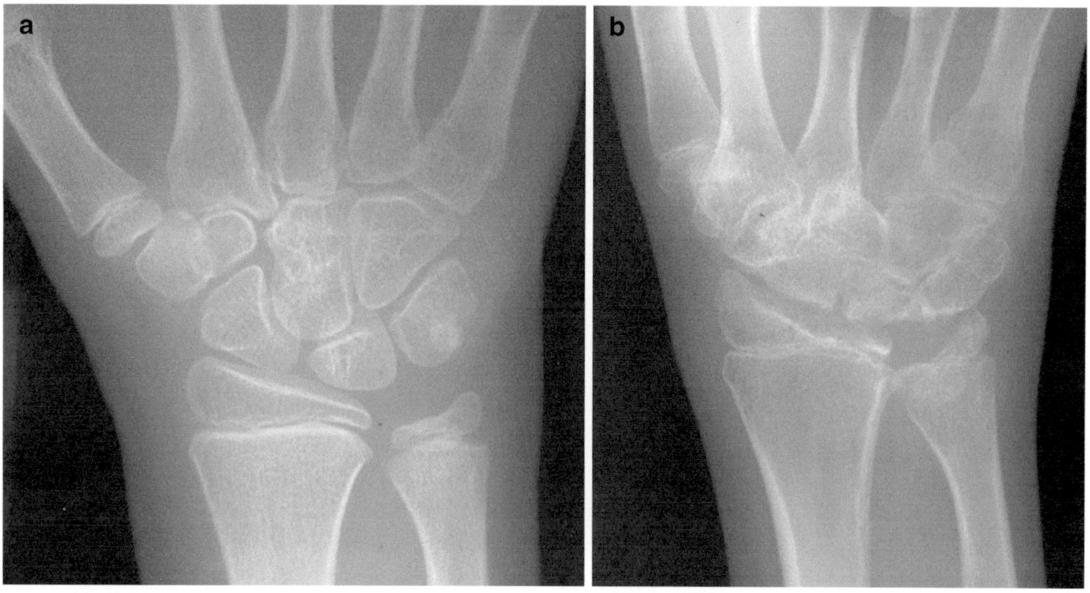

Fig. 20.8 Progression of carpal pathology in a girl with polyarticular JIA. (**a**) Slight intercarpal joint space narrowing at age 9 years. (**b**) At age 15 years, there is marked intercarpal narrowing, along with erosions and developing ankylosis. Note erosions and deformity of the distal radius and ulna. The gap at the radiocarpal articulation is likely due to hypertrophic pannus (Images copyright Shriners Hospital for Children Northern California)

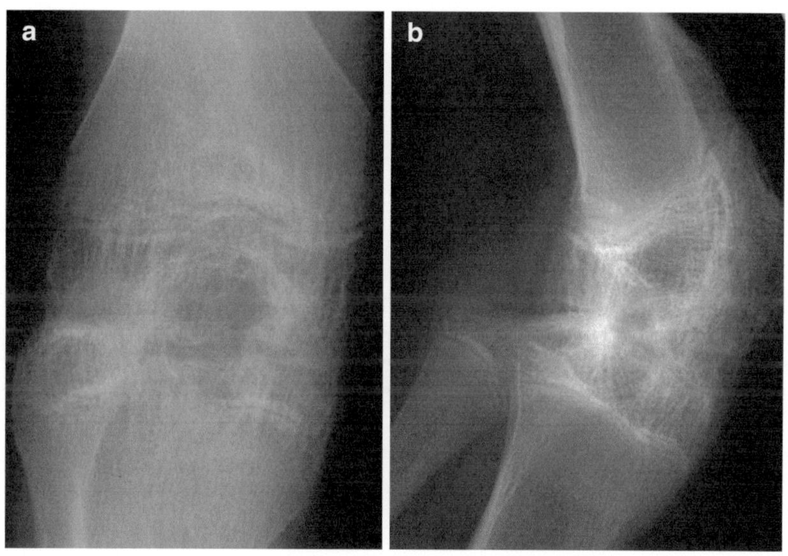

Fig. 20.9 Ankylosis at the knee in late-stage polyarticular JIA. (**a**, **b**) Growth plates are still open, and the femoral notch is enlarged (Images copyright Shriners Hospital for Children Northern California)

flexion at DIP). Ligamentous laxity and sometimes mass-like hypertrophied synovium may lead to carpal subluxation or dislocation, especially common at the hamate. The wrist may deviate in a radial direction [7].

Patients with the psoriatic or enthesitis-related subtypes may demonstrate overgrowth and inflammation of a digit (dactylitis) (Fig. 20.13). ERA may manifest with thickening of tendons and ligaments, showing wispy periostitis along their osseous attachments.

Ultrasound. Both US and MRI may be used for early assessment of the disease process (Fig. 20.14). US depicts the severity of disease

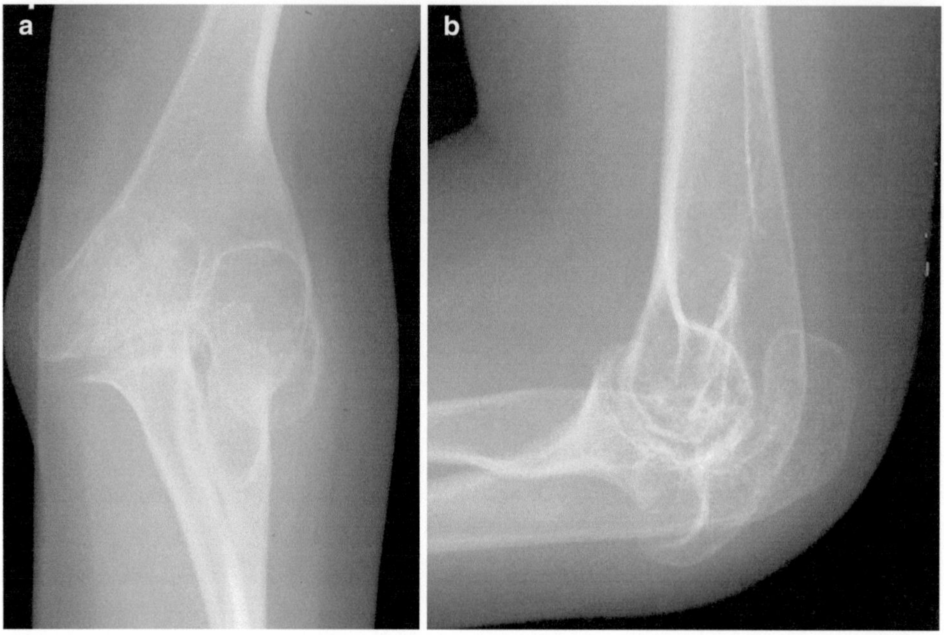

Fig. 20.10 Elbow deformity in a 13-year-old girl with polyarticular JIA. (**a, b**) Osteopenia, epiphyseal enlargement, and joint space narrowing (Images copyright Shriners Hospital for Children Northern California)

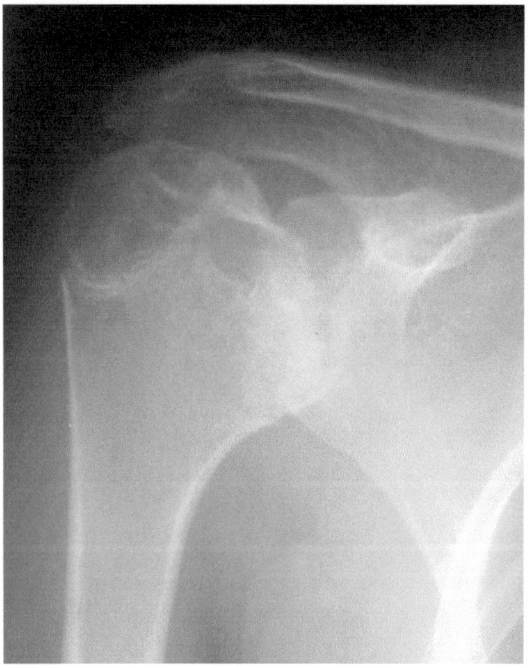

Fig. 20.11 Shoulder deformity in a 17-year-old girl with polyarticular JIA. There are erosions and deformity of the humeral head (Image copyright Shriners Hospital for Children Northern California)

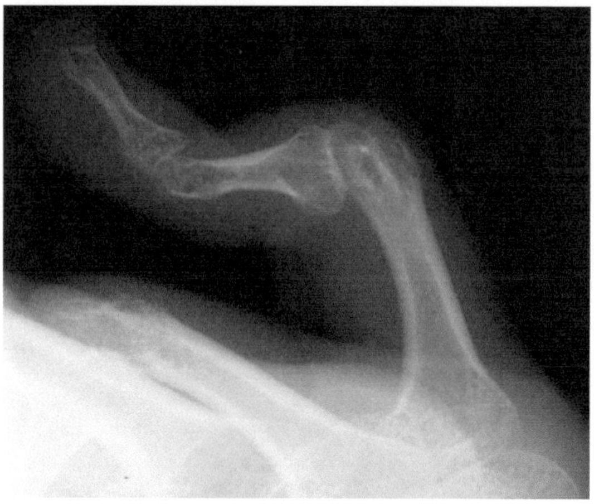

Fig. 20.12 Boutonniere deformity in a 19-year-old male with JIA (Image copyright Shriners Hospital for Children Northern California)

by allowing assessment of joint effusions, synovial thickening, cartilage destruction/thinning, associated synovial cysts, erosions, and tenosynovitis (Figs. 20.15 and 20.16). It may identify clinically occult knee effusions as well as subclinical synovitis in multiple joints [10, 11].

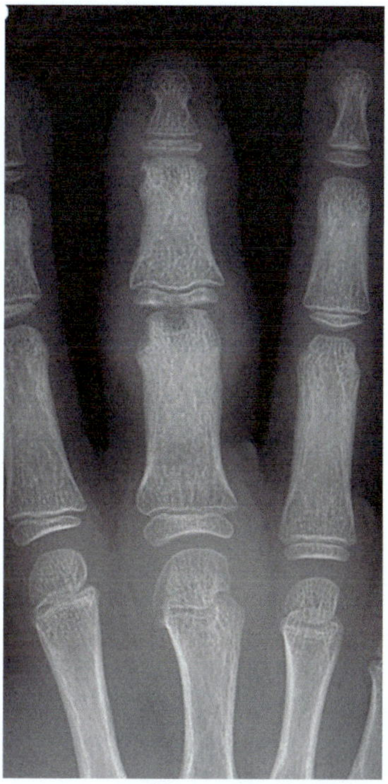

Fig. 20.13 Sausage digit in a child with psoriatic arthritis. There is soft tissue swelling at the PIP and DIP joints, along with central erosions. Increased width of the affected phalanges results in brachydactyly (Courtesy of J. Herman Kan)

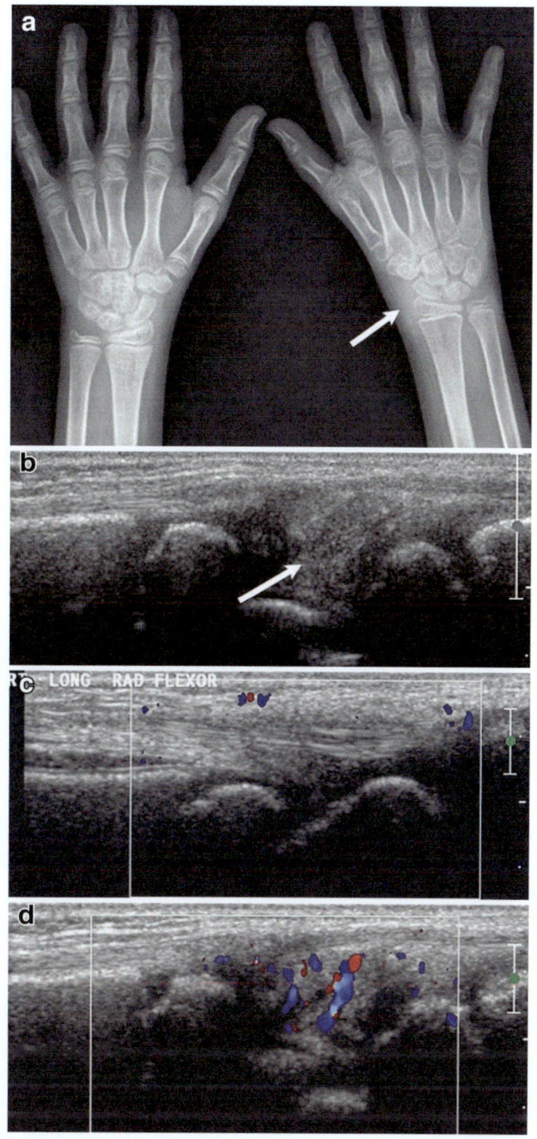

Fig. 20.14 New onset of significant left thenar atrophy, swelling around the wrist, and limited motion in a 7-year-old girl who subsequently received a diagnosis of antinuclear antibody (ANA)- and rheumatoid factor (RF)-negative JIA. (**a**) There is minimal lateral soft tissue swelling (*arrow*). (**b**) Longitudinal ultrasound (US) of the radial aspect of the wrist shows thickened, echogenic synovial tissue (*arrow*). (**c**) Color Doppler of the unaffected wrist shows normal flow (for comparison). (**d**) The affected side is hyperemic (Reprinted from Miller and Doria [37], with kind permission from Springer Science + Business Media) (Image courtesy of Andrea Doria)

Later on, it may identify enthesitis, inflammation of tendons or ligaments where they insert into the bone (most common at the calcaneal insertion of the Achilles tendon). US is especially useful for evaluating the joints of the hand and feet. It may be employed to guide joint aspiration or therapeutic injection, and it helps assess response to intra-articular treatment [7].

Synovial proliferation appears as hypoechoic, irregular synovial membrane thickening, easily distinguishable from joint fluid (see Chap. 22). With cartilage involvement, the normal smooth contour of hypoechoic cartilage is altered, and the typically sharp margins become blurred and obliterated [10]. Erosions appear as a break in the cortex that measures at least 2 mm; the floor is irregular, and adjacent marrow demonstrates acoustic enhancement [12].

If power Doppler demonstrates hypervascular pannus, disease is considered active (see Fig. 20.14). Serial US may then be used to monitor disease activity and demonstrate response to therapy, showing decreased thickness and vascularity of the synovium, as well as a decrease in joint fluid

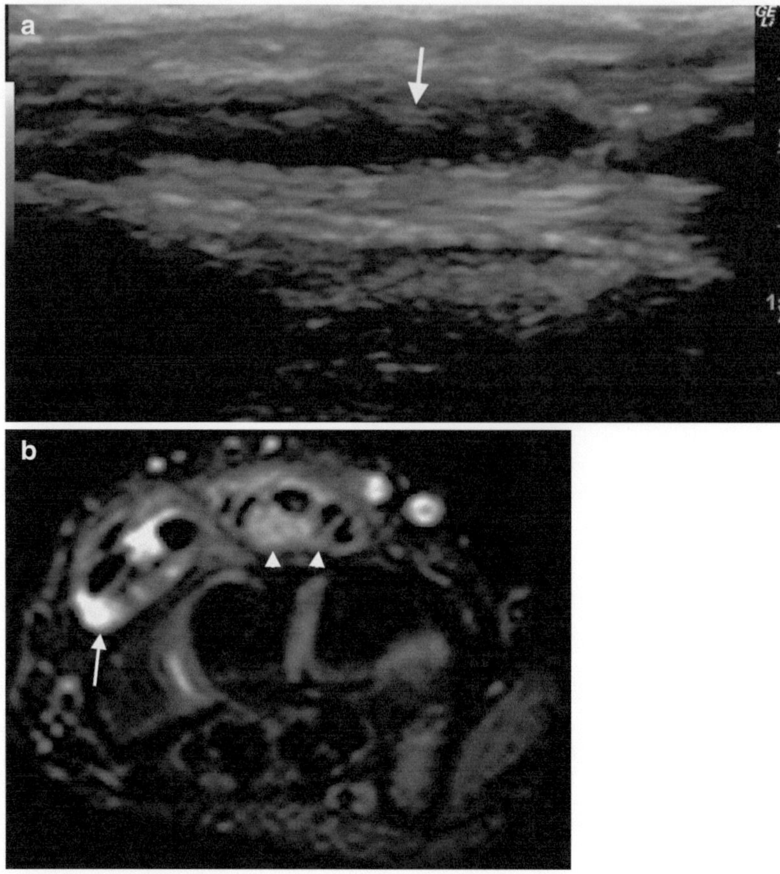

Fig. 20.15 Tenosynovitis in a 7-year-old girl with JIA. (**a**) Longitudinal US shows pannus along the tendon sheath (*arrow*). (**b**) Axial short tau inversion recovery (STIR) image of the wrist shows fluid (*arrow*) and pannus (*arrowheads*) surrounding thickened extensor digitorum tendons (Courtesy of J. Herman Kan)

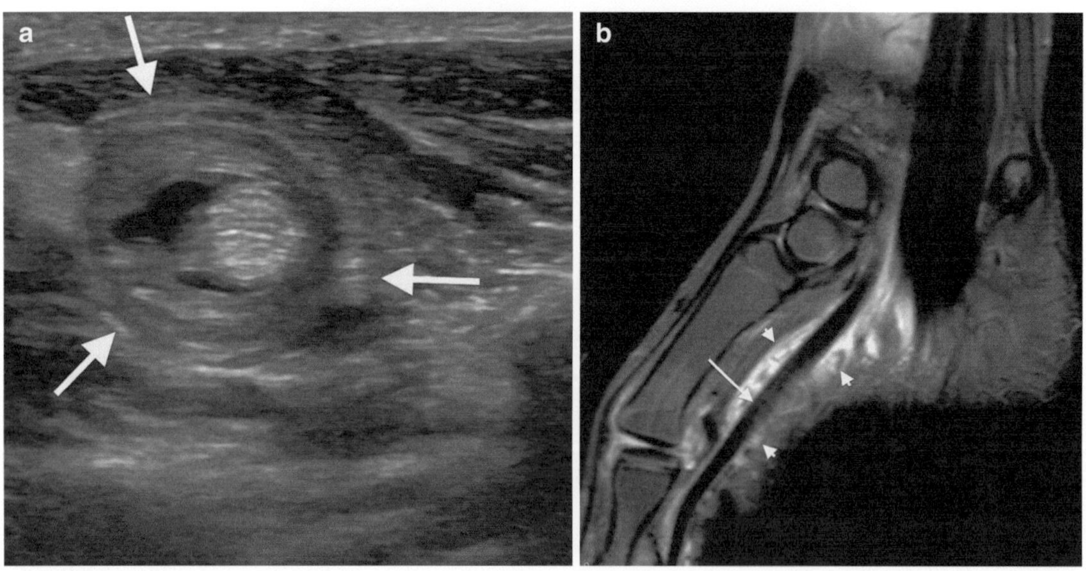

Fig. 20.16 Tenosynovitis in an 11-year-old boy. (**a**) Axial US of the flexor pollicis longus demonstrates circumferential thickening of the tendon sheath (*arrows*) and tenosynovial fluid. (**b**) Sagittal STIR image shows extensive tenosynovitis of the flexor pollicis longus. The tendon is thickened and mildly hyperintense (*arrow*), and there is surrounding fluid and soft tissue edema (*arrowheads*). Note fluid in the MTP joint (Courtesy of J. Herman Kan)

[13]. However, US provides only limited visualization of some joints (such as the sacroiliac and temporomandibular joints), and a narrow acoustic window may preclude complete assessment of large joints. The efficacy of US is also limited by difficulty in positioning and examining children whose joints are swollen and painful.

Magnetic Resonance Imaging. MRI offers optimal assessment of joint disease in JIA, and contrast-enhanced MRI is the most sensitive technique for detecting synovitis, demonstrating pathology even before the physical exam becomes abnormal. It is superior to US in depicting early inflammation and synovitis, as well as in evaluation of the cartilage. MRI readily shows marrow edema, which predicts future erosions [14]. It also accurately evaluates the late manifestations of the disease, including erosions, joint space loss, and ligamentous involvement (Figs. 20.17, 20.18, and 20.19) [7, 13, 15]. MRI thus plays an important role in determining prognosis.

Joint effusion and acute synovitis constitute the earliest MRI manifestations in JIA (Fig. 20.20) [16]. Joint fluid and thickened synovium appear similar on conventional spin echo images. However, heavily T2-weighted (T2-W) images and fast spin echo (FSE) techniques differentiate hyperintense joint fluid from relatively hypointense synovium [13]. Normal synovium (Fig. 20.21) is at most 2 mm thick and appears hypointense on T1-weighted (T1-W) and T2-W sequences. Abnormal synovium appears as a thick, irregular, wavy layer that is hypo- to isointense on T1-W and hyperintense on T2-W sequences (Fig. 20.22). T2-W sequences may delineate frond-like pannus, formed when progressive inflammation leads to synovial proliferation (Fig. 20.23). Hypertrophic synovium may slough and undergo fibrinoid necrosis, forming intra-articular loose bodies ("rice bodies"), readily apparent on heavily T2-W images (Fig. 20.24). These loose bodies preclude the use of intra-articular steroids.

The presence of enhancement also helps differentiate between normal and abnormal synovium. Normal synovium may show minimal enhancement on T1-W fat-suppressed (FS) imaging, but avid early enhancement indicates the presence of synovitis (see Fig. 20.24). Intense enhancement also helps differentiate thickened synovium from simple joint fluid (scanning should be performed within 5–10 min of administration of gadolinium, as contrast eventually diffuses into the joint). Administration of gadolinium is essential for distinguishing active, hypervascu-

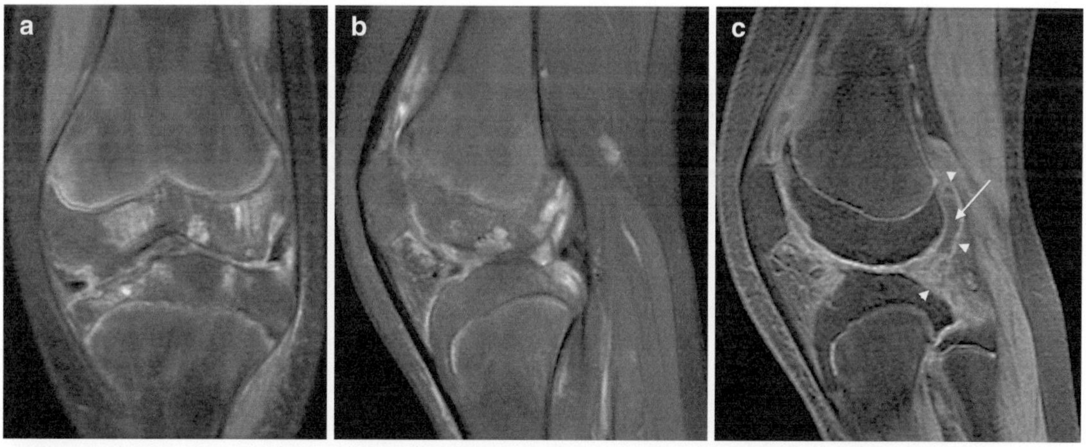

Fig. 20.17 JIA in a 14-year-old girl with polyarticular disease. (**a**) Coronal proton density (PD) FS image of the knee shows cartilage destruction with joint space narrowing, epiphyseal marrow edema, subcortical erosions and cysts, and deformity. Central menisci are compressed. (**b**) On sagittal T2-W image, synovial inflammation and joint fluid result in diffuse hyperintensity (*arrows*). (**c**) Enhancement on sagittal spoiled gradient (SPGR) gadolinium-enhanced image differentiates joint fluid (*arrow*) from the synovium (*arrowheads*) (same patient as Fig. 20.7)

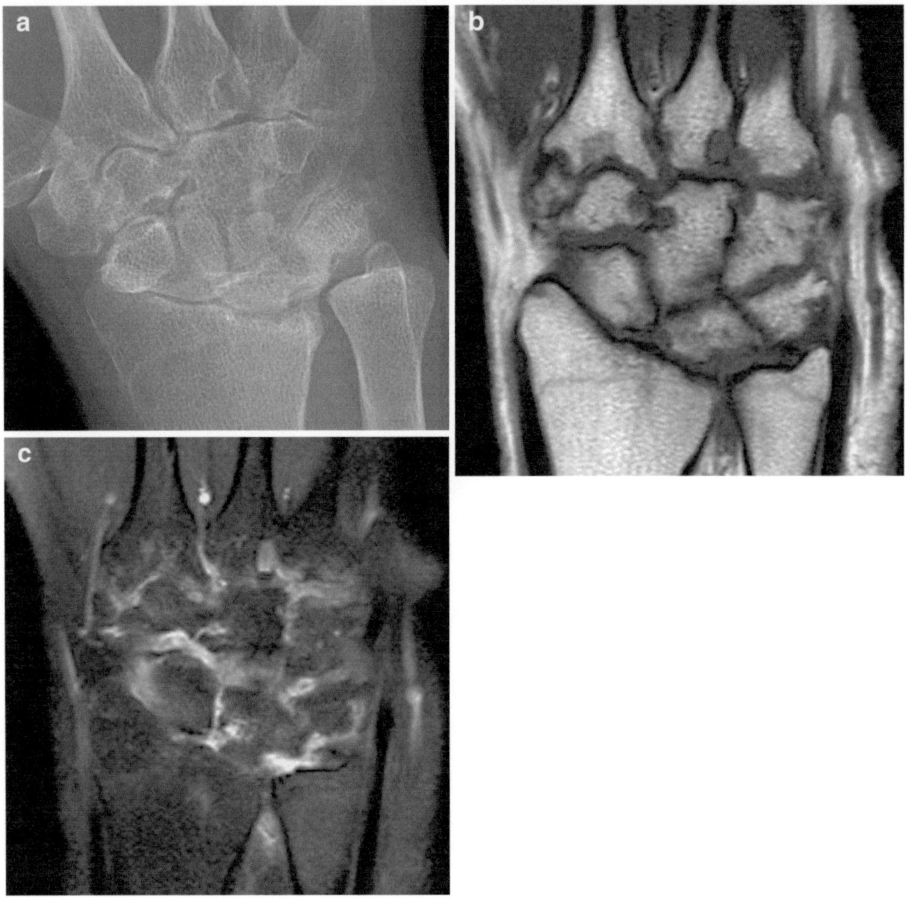

Fig. 20.18 Late manifestations of JIA in an 18-year-old female. (**a**) Radiograph shows extensive erosions, joint space narrowing, and ulnar overgrowth. (**b**) Coronal T1-W image better delineates multiple erosions. (**c**) Coronal T1-W FS gadolinium-enhanced image shows enhancing synovium throughout all carpal joint spaces and extending into the erosions (Courtesy of J. Herman Kan)

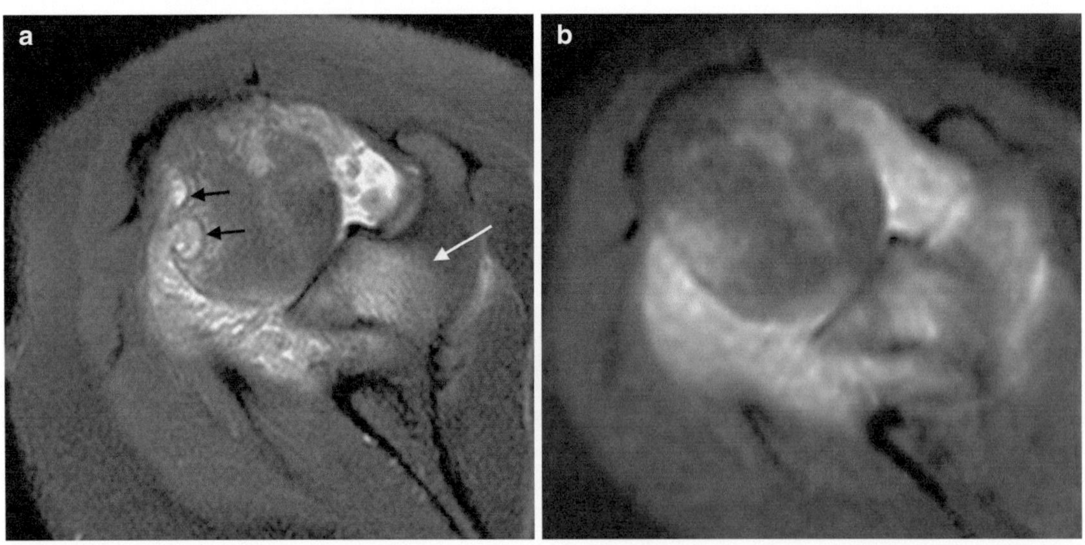

Fig. 20.19 Advanced JIA in a 16-year-old girl. (**a**) Axial T2-W image of the shoulder shows well-circumscribed hyperintense erosions (*black arrows*) in the humeral head, with osteitis (*white arrow*) in the adjacent scapula. (**b**) T1-W FS gadolinium-enhanced image shows pannus enhances diffusely (Courtesy of J. Herman Kan)

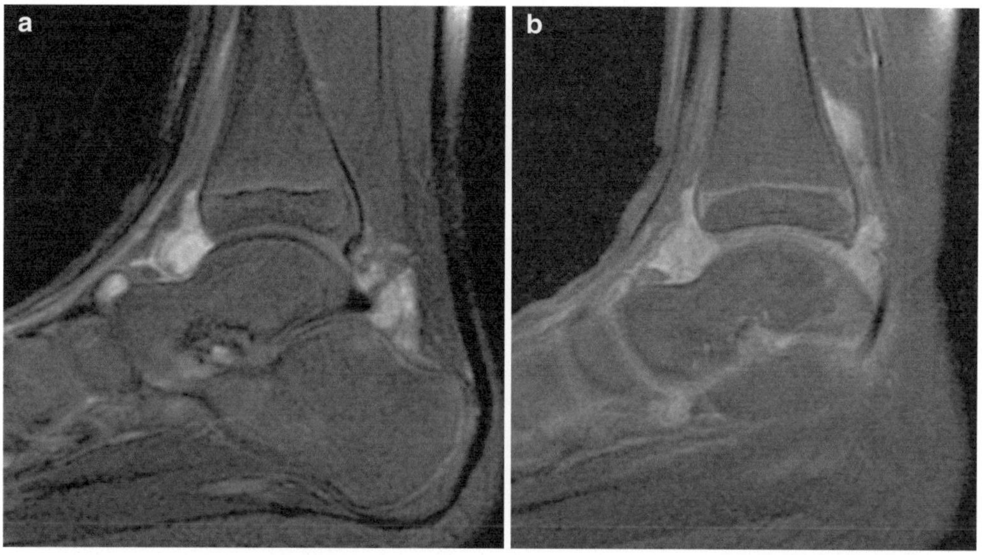

Fig. 20.20 Synovitis with enhancing pannus in a 6-year-old boy with JIA. (**a**) Sagittal T2-W image shows hyperintense thick material within the ankle joint. After administration of gadolinium (**b**, T1-W FS), all the hyperintense areas enhance, indicating they represent thickened synovium, not joint fluid. The cartilage appears intact (Courtesy of Tal Laor, Cincinnati Children's Hospital)

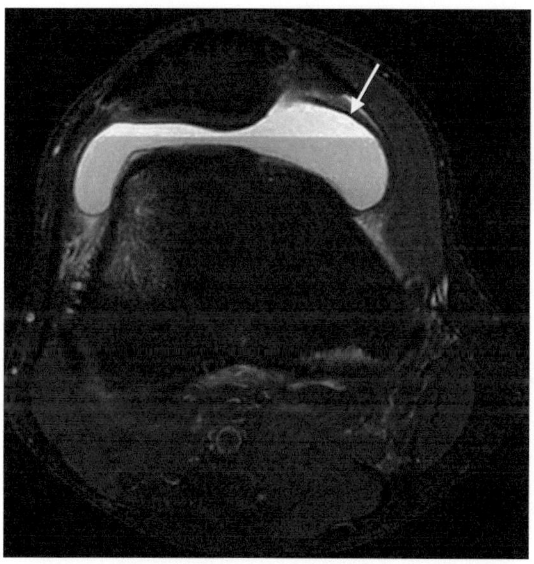

Fig. 20.21 Normal synovium. Axial PD FS image of a 17-year-old male after trauma shows normal hypointense non-thickened synovium (*arrow*). Note lipohemarthrosis and distal femoral marrow edema

lar synovium, which enhances, from inactive, fibrotic synovium, which does not [7, 13].

The rate of contrast enhancement and measurements of dynamic synovial enhancement may be used to assess the degree of inflammatory response, but this is not routinely performed in clinical practice. Quantitative MRI assessment of synovial volumes also assesses response to therapy [17].

MRI is the most sensitive modality for detecting morphologic alterations in articular cartilage. T1-W FS 3-dimensional (3D) gradient echo (GRE) techniques reliably assess cartilage loss with relatively high sensitivity and specificity. Normal cartilage is hyperintense, and defects appear as hypointense foci. Subtle irregularities, cystic changes, and underlying desiccation are readily recognized. 3D data can be further analyzed, allowing quantitative assessment of cartilage volume. Thickness and contour may be mapped, with important implications in assessing therapeutic response and determining long-term prognosis (Fig. 20.25) [18]. As articular cartilage degenerates, microstructural alterations cause T2 relaxation time to increase. Indeed, in patients with JIA, the cartilage may demonstrate degeneration on T2 mapping, even when disease is apparently clinically quiescent or improving [5].

Additional GRE techniques for imaging pediatric hyaline and in particular articular cartilage

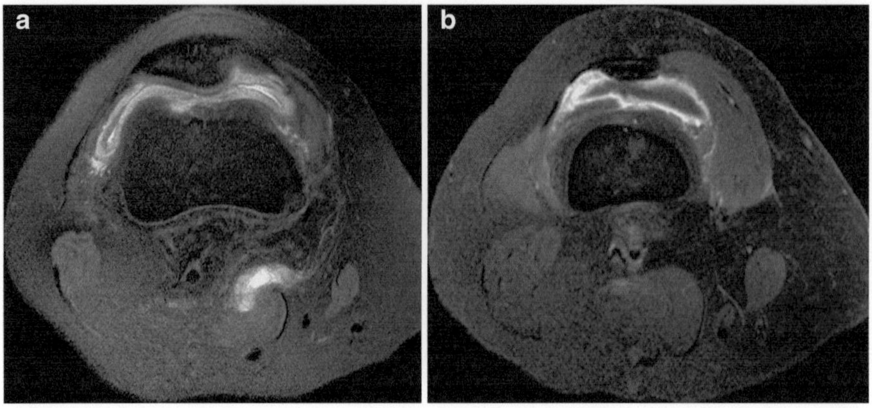

Fig. 20.22 Thickened synovium in a patient with JIA. (**a**) Axial PD FS image of the knee shows synovial thickening and hyperintensity along with a small amount of joint fluid. (**b**) T1-W FS gadolinium-enhanced image shows diffuse enhancement of the thickened synovium, along with hypointense joint fluid

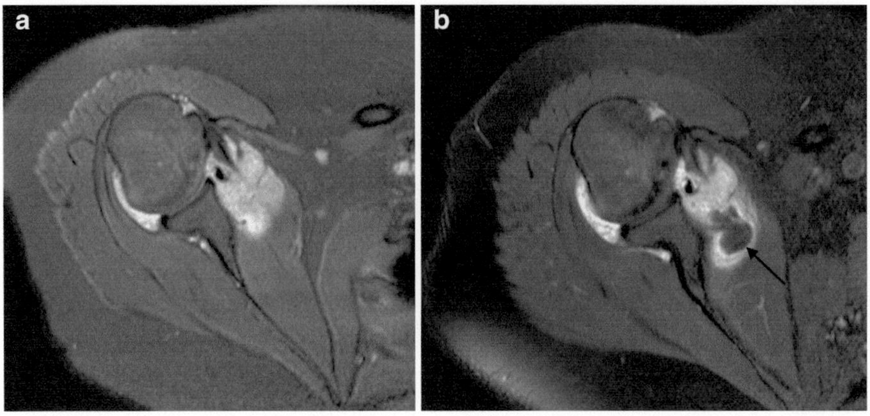

Fig. 20.23 Enhancing pannus in a 19-year-old girl with JIA. (**a**) T2-W FS axial image shows hyperintense fluid and pannus at the shoulder. (**b**) T1-W FS gadolinium-enhanced axial image contrasts non-enhancing joint fluid (*arrow*) and enhancing pannus (Courtesy of J. Herman Kan)

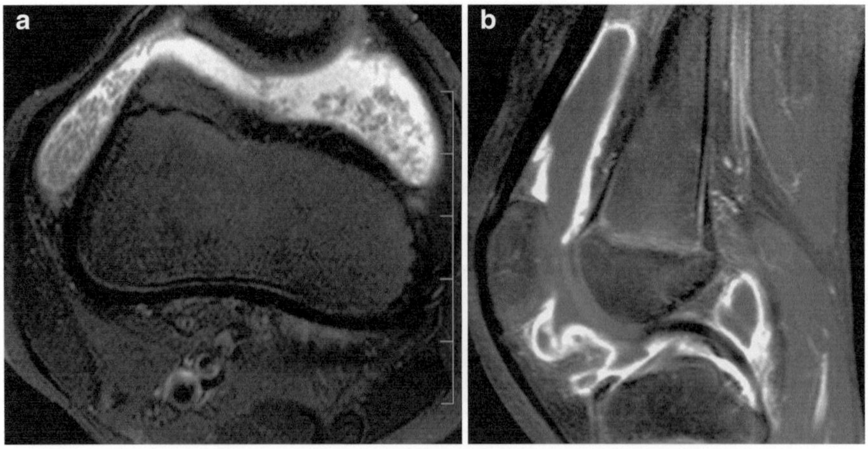

Fig. 20.24 Rice bodies in a 7-year-old girl. (**a**) Axial T2-W image demonstrates multiple intermediate-intensity rice bodies within hyperintense joint fluid. (**b**) Sagittal T1-W FS gadolinium-enhanced image shows thick, enhancing synovium, but the rice bodies are occult

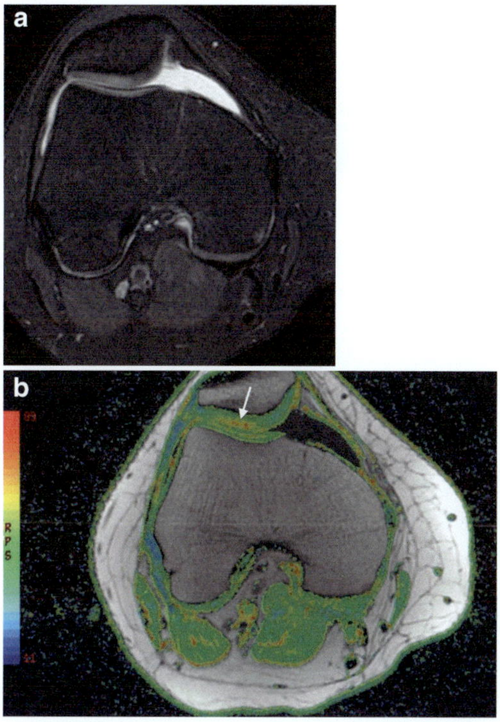

Fig. 20.25 T2 mapping of cartilage in a child with JIA. (**a**) Axial T2-W FS image shows that although the morphology is normal, there is relatively increased signal intensity in the articular cartilage of the lateral facet. (**b**) Corresponding T2 map at the same level. The hotter colors (*oranges* and *reds*) correspond to longer T2 relaxation times. There is replacement of the normal laminar configuration of the articular cartilage in the lateral facet by a focal area of abnormally increased T2 signal intensity (*arrow*). This likely reflects the effect of disease on cartilage microstructure, prior to morphologic change. The colors correspond to specific T2 relaxation times, which allows for quantitative, objective evaluation over time (Courtesy of Tal Laor, Cincinnati Children's Hospital)

include such steady-state sequences as dual echo steady state (DESS), refocused steady-state free precession (SSFP), and water selective balanced steady-state free precession (WS-bSSFP). The DESS sequence, which combines two gradient echoes, provides high T2 contrast and depicts joint morphology well [19].

Osteitis, which may precede the development of bone erosions, appears hypointense on T1-W imaging and hyperintense on short tau inversion recovery (STIR) and T2-W imaging (see Fig. 20.19). Although often mistakenly described as "edema," osteitis actually represents an inflammatory cellular infiltrate [20]. Erosions are also hypointense on T1-W and hyperintense on T2-W imaging, but their margins are well circumscribed, and there must be overlying cortical disruption. Enhancement within erosions indicates the presence of hypervascular pannus, implying active disease. Erosions and cartilage destruction are more common after skeletal maturity, when the cartilage has thinned [16].

Erosions are common at the wrist (see Fig. 20.18) and must be differentiated from normal carpal undulations. The latter, found in more than 50 % of children, are often seen in the capitate or hamate [21]. Erosion is more likely if there is edema, cartilage destruction, and synovial enhancement. In addition, erosions are more common at the bare areas of intra-articular bone (i.e., the nonarticular portions of metacarpal and metatarsal heads and bases), where there is no overlying cartilage) [21].

MRI also assesses joint deformities and growth disturbances, especially in locations where radiography and ultrasound provide limited information, such as the sacroiliac joints and temporomandibular joints.

Regional Findings (Box 20.1)

Mandible. The mandible is subject to erosions, joint space narrowing, and growth disturbance.

Box 20.1: Imaging Features of Juvenile Idiopathic Arthritis (JIA) by Anatomic Region

Mandible	Short body and ramus
	Flat condyle, wide intercondylar joint
	Concave undersurface of the mandibular body (antegonial notching)
Cervical spine	Ankylosis of the upper cervical spine
	Affected vertebrae hypoplastic
	Erosion of the odontoid process
Hands/feet	Premature ossification
	Ankylosis of the tarsals and carpals
	Subluxation
	Periostitis of the metatarsals and metacarpals
Knee	Epiphyseal enlargement
	Wide intercondylar notch
	Squared lower pole of the patella

The temporomandibular joint (TMJ) is affected in up to 87 % of patients with JIA, especially in patients whose initial presentation was before age 4 [14]. Common findings include shortening of the body and ramus, flattening of the condyle, widening of the intercondylar joint, narrowing of the joint space, and abnormal concavity of the undersurface of the mandibular body (*antegonial notching*, Fig. 20.26) [7]. If there is active inflammation, contrast-enhanced MRI demonstrates typical findings of effusion, synovial enhancement, and marrow edema. Open and closed mouth dynamic assessment may depict abnormal joint motion, disk abnormalities, and growth disturbances.

Cervical Spine. The cervical spine is affected in about 60 % of patients [14], and patients with polyarticular or systemic JIA are most likely to have cervical spine involvement. Ankylosis may occur within 3–5 years of disease onset and is most common at the apophyseal joints at C2–3, though multiple levels are often affected (see Fig. 20.26). The associated vertebral bodies are often hypoplastic in transverse and anteroposterior dimensions, and disk spaces are narrow. Synovial proliferation may cause erosions of the odontoid process, and ligamentous insufficiency may lead to atlantoaxial instability. Atlantoaxial impaction may occur in young adults with polyarticular JIA.

Hands and Feet. Ankylosis of the carpal and tarsal bones may develop within 3–5 years of onset of disease [14] (see Fig. 20.8). Carpal bones of the wrist may ossify prematurely (uni- or bilaterally). Subluxation, dislocation, and flexion/extension deformities are more common in the hands and feet than elsewhere (see Fig. 20.12); if the wrist is affected, it deviates in a radial direction. Periostitis may lead to a squared off appearance of the metacarpals and metatarsals (see Fig. 20.4).

Knee. Overall, the knee is the most commonly affected joint. Standing radiographs best assess for joint space narrowing and other complications. The knee may develop the classic appearance of epiphyseal enlargement, widened intercondylar notch, and squared lower pole of the patella (see Figs. 20.6 and 20.7). These findings are also sometimes seen with hemophilia.

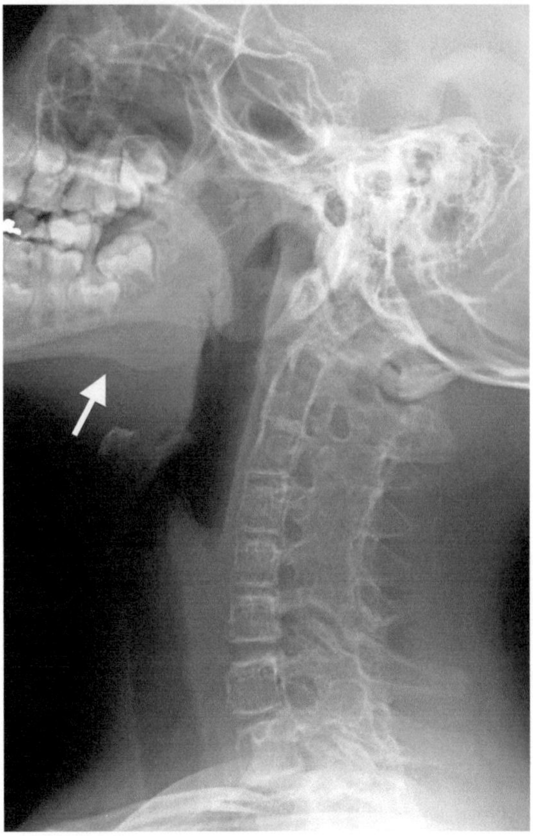

Fig. 20.26 Cervical spine deformity and fusion in a 10-year-old girl with systemic polyarticular JIA. The laminae are fused from C2 through C6, and the vertebral bodies are unusually tall and narrow. Intervertebral disks are narrowed, with fusion across C2–3. Antegonial notching (*arrow*) at the mandible

1.1 Enthesitis-Related Arthritis (ERA)

Several arthritides share the common feature of enthesopathy (inflammation of ligaments or tendons where they attach to bone). These include juvenile onset ankylosing spondylitis, reactive arthritis, and undifferentiated spondyloarthropathy. Diagnosis requires at least two of the following criteria: onset in a male age 8 or older, HLA-B27 positivity (or positive family history), spinal or sacroiliac pain, and anterior uveitis. The discussion below is predominantly limited to juvenile onset ankylosing spondylitis.

Ankylosing spondylitis usually manifests during adulthood. When encountered in children, it

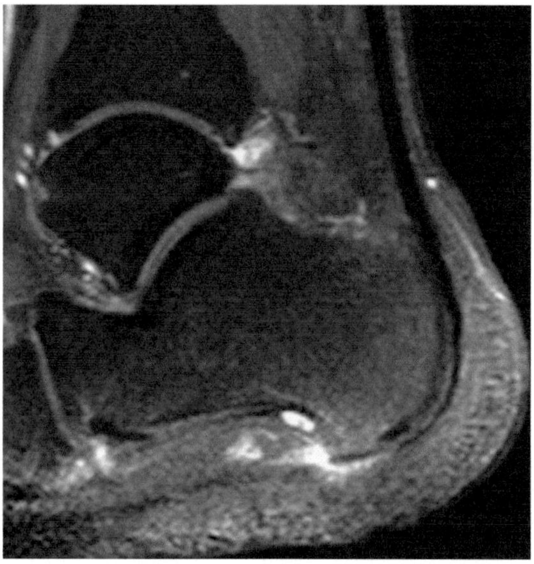

Fig. 20.27 Calcaneal spur in an 8-year-old boy with ERA. Sagittal T1-W FS gadolinium-enhanced image shows spur with enhancement at the insertion of the plantar aponeurosis (Courtesy of J. Herman Kan)

is commonly seen in male patients in late adolescence. Unlike in adults, it typically presents with early extra-axial involvement and a higher frequency of peripheral arthritis and enthesitis. The hips, knees, and shoulders are most frequently involved. Although a cause of long-term disability, sacroiliitis is often initially asymptomatic, and fewer than 25 % of children complain of spine or sacroiliac signs or symptoms [22].

Imaging (Box 20.2)

Radiographic findings include joint space narrowing and erosions, which, unlike in the adult population, do not typically evolve into severe joint destruction. Enthesitis, a common element, may present as a bony erosion, lucency, or spur. Spurs are especially common at the calcaneus, either at the insertion of the Achilles tendon or at the insertion of the plantar aponeurosis (Fig. 20.27). Not uncommonly, periostitis may be present along short tubular bones of the hand and, in some cases, along other bones.

However, radiographic abnormalities in the axial skeleton take much longer to appear than those in the peripheral skeleton. Radiographic evidence of sacroiliac arthritis is almost always seen well before any radiographic abnormality becomes apparent in the spine. Even this is seen only after clinical symptoms have progressed to an advanced stage, after disease has been present for 5–10 years. Bilateral asymmetrical involvement of the sacroiliac joints is the most common pattern (Fig. 20.28). Occasionally unilateral involvement mimics tuberculosis and subacute septic arthritis. Unlike in JIA, the cervical spine is usually normal. Syndesmophyte formation is rarely seen in children, and the "bamboo spine" typical of adults is generally not encountered in children. Sacroiliac arthritis is almost always seen well before any radiographic abnormality of the spine.

MRI evaluation of the sacroiliac joints allows earlier identification of sacroiliitis, making this a useful screening tool in patients with suspected ERA who have no spine or sacroiliac symptoms. Dynamic contrast-enhanced MRI is useful for

Box 20.2: Enthesitis-Related Arthritis (ERA)

Common	Enthesitis at calcaneus (at the Achilles tendon or plantar aponeurosis)
	Hips, knees, shoulders
	Joint space narrowing, erosions
<25 %	Spine or sacroiliac joints
	Radiographs positive after 5–10 years: bilateral, symmetric
	MRI positive sooner: T2 hyperintensity and enhancement

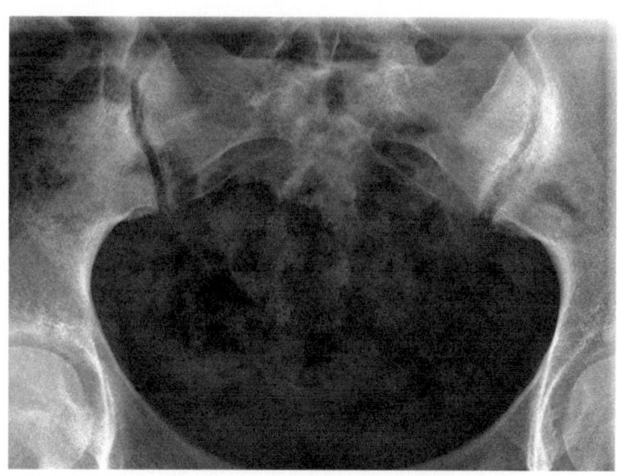

Fig. 20.28 Sacroiliitis in a 15-year-old girl with ERA. Asymmetrical (left worse than right) irregularity of the sacroiliac joints and iliac osteitis on the left

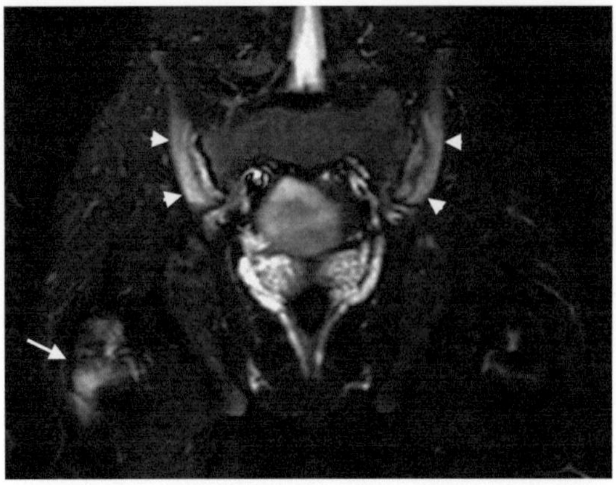

Fig. 20.29 Osteitis in a 16-year-old boy with ERA. Coronal T2-W image shows marrow hyperintensity consistent with enthesitis in the right greater trochanter (*arrow*). In addition, there is bilateral sacroiliitis, with hyperintense signal within the joints and juxtasynovial iliac bone osteitis (*arrowheads*) (Courtesy of J. Herman Kan)

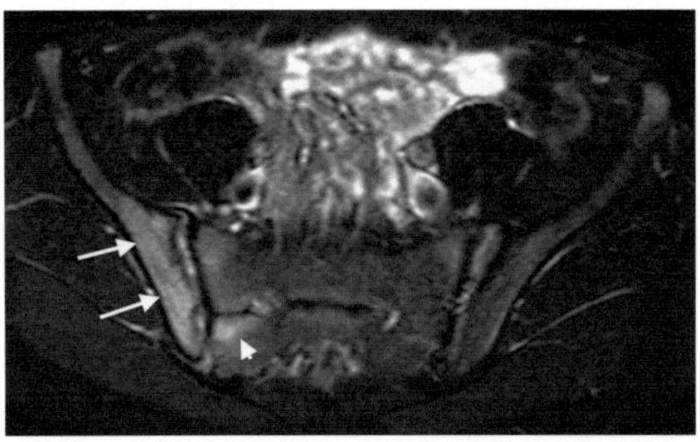

Fig. 20.30 Sacroiliitis in a 13-year-old boy with ERA. Axial T2-W image shows hyperintensity at the right and to a lesser extent left sacroiliac joints. In addition, there is right iliac osteitis present (*arrows*), as well as right greater than left sacral alar osteitis (*arrowhead*) (Courtesy of J. Herman Kan)

diagnosing both acute and chronic abnormalities in the sacroiliac joints [23, 24]. Typical findings include subarticular marrow edema or osteitis and T2 hyperintensity at the sacroiliac joints (Figs. 20.29 and 20.30). With more advanced disease, erosions on T1-W sequences and synovial enhancement may be evident.

US and MRI are both useful for assessing the small joints of the hands and feet. US demonstrates thickening of the tendons as well as peritendinous fluid. Typical MRI findings of enthesitis include swelling and T2 hyperintensity at the tendons and ligaments where they attach to bone. There may also be T2 hyperintensity within the adjacent bone, and bursae may be distended and soft tissues edematous [24]. MRI may delineate tenosynovitis and enthesitis (Fig. 20.31), along with subclinical ligament rupture.

2 Hemophilic Arthropathy

This X-linked autosomal recessive disorder affects 1 in 10,000 boys and typically presents before age 20. There are two subtypes, both due to an abnormal coagulation factor. Deficiency in clotting factor VIII leads to subtype A, and deficiency in plasma factor IV results in subtype B. Clinical presentation and imaging findings are similar for both forms of the disease. Patients have a propensity to bleed after minor trauma, especially into the joints. Indeed, 90 % of patients with severe hemophilia eventually develop joint disease [25]. The initial hemorrhagic episode often occurs before age 10.

The most commonly affected joints are the knee, ankle, and elbow. Bleeding usually begins in the synovium and extends to involve the joint space itself. Chondrocytes and macrophages absorb released iron, and hydrolytic enzymes then incite an inflammatory response. Inflamed synovium is prone to rebleed, and a vicious cycle of recurrent bleeding ensues. Epiphyseal overgrowth occurs as part of the inflammatory response.

Bleeding into the bone and soft tissues may lead to development of pseudotumors in up to 2 % of patients, generally in those with severe coagulopathy [26]. The resultant chronic, painless, encapsulated, slowly expanding mass may result from minor trauma and is usually an incidental finding. Bleeding into the subperiosteum occurs uncommonly.

Treatment of hemophilia generally involves replacing missing clotting factors, preferably prior to onset of joint damage. However, up to 30 % of patients produce antibodies to these clotting factors, leading to increased risk of uncontrolled bleeding [27]. Affected joints may be treated with radionuclide or open synovectomy [25].

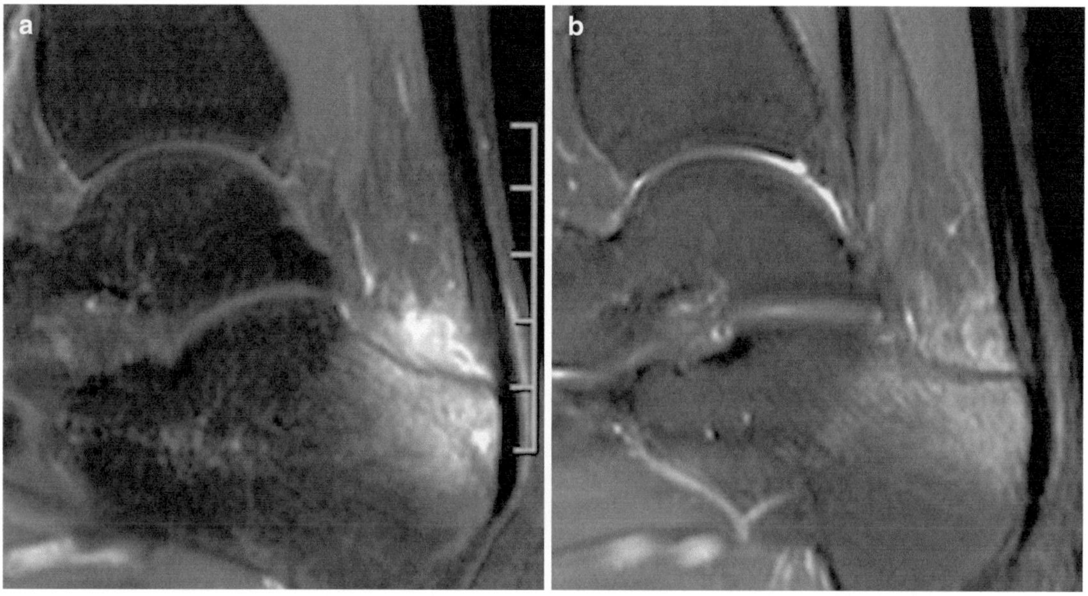

Fig. 20.31 Enthesitis in a 17-year-old girl with ERA. (**a**) Sagittal T1-W FS gadolinium-enhanced image shows enhancement in the calcaneal body and tuberosity at the Achilles insertion, as well as in Kager fat pad. (**b**) Sagittal PD FS image shows corresponding hyperintensity, as well as increased intrasubstance signal within the distal Achilles tendon (Courtesy of J. Herman Kan)

Imaging (Box 20.3)

Radiographs. Joint effusion and hemarthrosis are early findings (Fig. 20.32). Synovial hypertrophy and hemosiderin deposition appear as nonspecific soft tissue swelling. However, with progressive articular and periarticular pathology, osseous erosions and subchondral cysts become evident (Fig. 20.33). Joint space narrowing due to cartilage thinning may eventually become evident on radiographs. Inflammation and hyperemia may lead to epiphyseal overgrowth and osteopenia, with early growth plate closure. At the knee, epiphyseal overgrowth is common, with widening of the intercondylar notch, flattened contours of the condyles, squaring of the patella, and cartilage as well as subchondral bony destruction (Fig. 20.34).

The Arnold-Hilgartner system grades osteochondral and soft tissue radiographic findings on a scale of 0–5 and can predict the presence of synovial hypertrophy (Table 20.2). This system is commonly employed in the USA [28, 29]. The Pettersson scoring system provides a framework for analysis of radiographic findings, wherein a cumulative score is assigned based on the presence or absence of multiple findings. This scoring system has been adopted by the World Federation of Hemophilia [30].

Box 20.3: Imaging Features of Hemophilic Arthropathy

Hemarthrosis: knee, ankle, elbow

Radiographic stages described by Arnold-Hilgartner system (Table 20.2)

US	Evaluates synovial vascularity, hemarthrosis
MRI	
Early	Joint effusion with fluid-fluid level
	Synovial hypertrophy
	Focal cartilage erosion
	Synovial hemosiderin deposition
	Synovial T2 hyperintensity (inflammation)
Chronic	Hypointense fibrotic synovium
	Synovial hemosiderin deposition
	Cartilage thinning, bone erosion
	Subchondral cysts

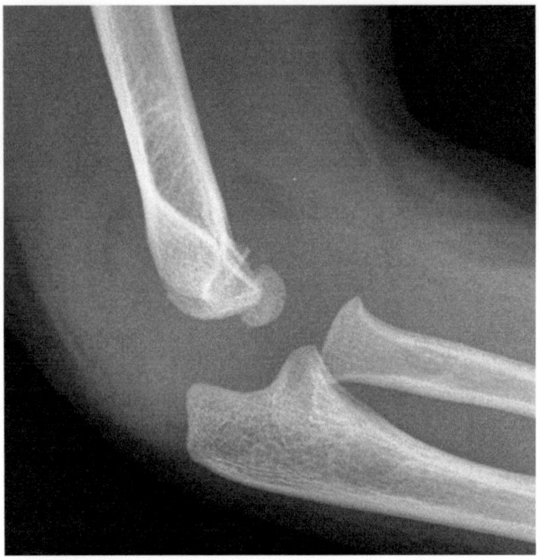

Fig. 20.32 Joint effusion in a young boy with hemophilia. Bones are normal (Courtesy of J. Herman Kan)

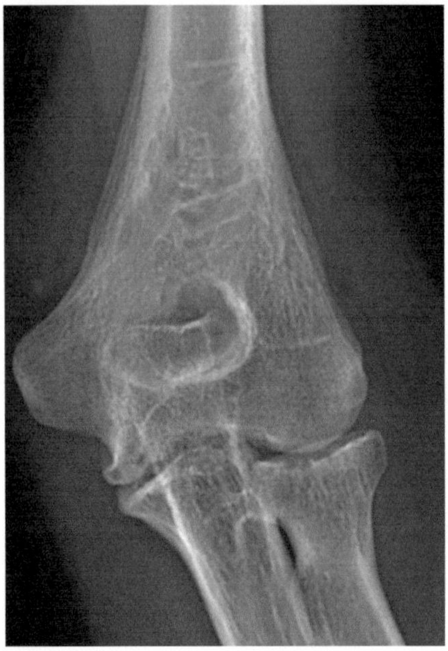

Fig. 20.33 Elbow joint space narrowing and osseous erosions at the trochlea, proximal ulna, and radial head in a 15-year-old boy with hemophilia

Pseudotumors are encountered most often in the soft tissues but also occur in the bone or subperiosteum. The femur, pelvis, tibia, and hand are the most common locations of osseous pseudotumors (in descending order of frequency) [26]. A soft tissue pseudotumor appears as a hemorrhagic soft tissue mass, sometimes eroding adjacent bone.

Bony pseudotumors appear as well-defined, expansile, lytic uni- or multilocular eccentric or intramedullary masses (Fig. 20.35). There may be cortical thinning and erosions, endosteal scalloping, peripheral sclerosis, and pathological fractures. Dystrophic calcification may be seen, along with subperiosteal new bone formation and aggressive periosteal reaction. Pseudotumors may completely replace affected bone. The differential is broad, including many lucent bone lesions. Peripheral curvilinear calcific struts extending into the soft tissues are characteristic.

US. Doppler US may be employed to evaluate synovial vascularity and to evaluate for hemarthroses (Fig. 20.36) [31]. US may also be used to follow soft tissue tumors.

CT. Computed tomography (CT) may demonstrate trabeculae crossing the radiolucent pseudotumor as well as characteristic calcific struts.

MRI. MRI allows more precise evaluation of joint involvement in early as well as advanced disease. Scoring systems (such as the semiquantitative Denver scale) facilitate assessment of treatment response [27]. Early MRI finding in joints affected by hemophilia include effusions with fluid-fluid levels, synovial hypertrophy, and focal areas of cartilage erosion. Synovial hemosiderin deposition is often apparent, with susceptibility artifact appearing dark on GRE sequences. Hemosiderin also appears markedly hypointense on T1- and T2-W sequences (Fig. 20.37). Cartilage destruction is best recognized on FS proton density (PD) or DESS sequences (Fig. 20.38) [31]. Synovial hypertrophy may be identified as hyperintense thickening on T2-W FS and on T1-W gadolinium-enhanced sequences (Fig. 20.39). In the chronic phase of disease, fibrotic synovium appears hypointense, and there may be cartilage thinning, bony erosions, and subchondral cysts (Fig. 20.40).

A pseudotumor appears as a hemorrhagic intraosseous and/or soft tissue mass with a rim that is hypointense on both T1- and T2-W imaging (Fig. 20.41). Enhancement is typically thin and nodular. Intralesional methemoglobin and

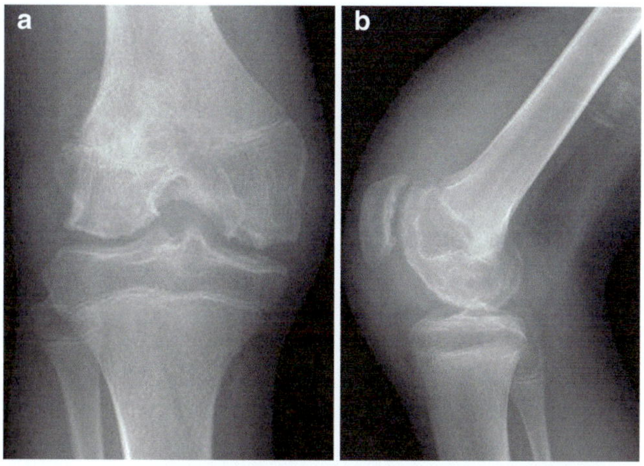

Fig. 20.34 Knee deformity in a boy with hemophilia. (**a**, **b**) The intercondylar notch is enlarged, the femoral condyles are overgrown, and there is joint space narrowing with bony erosions. Large, dense joint effusion (Courtesy of J. Herman Kan)

Table 20.2 Arnold-Hilgartner staging for hemophilia

Stage	Findings in joint
0	Normal
1	Soft tissue swelling; normal bones
2	Epiphyseal osteoporosis and overgrowth No erosions or joint space narrowing
3	Early subchondral bone cysts Knee and humerus: wide intercondylar notch Squared patella Joint space intact
4	Narrowed joint space Other findings of stage 3 more advanced
5	Narrowed joint space Fibrous joint contracture Marked epiphyseal enlargement Disorganization of joint

Adapted from Arnold and Hilgartner [28]

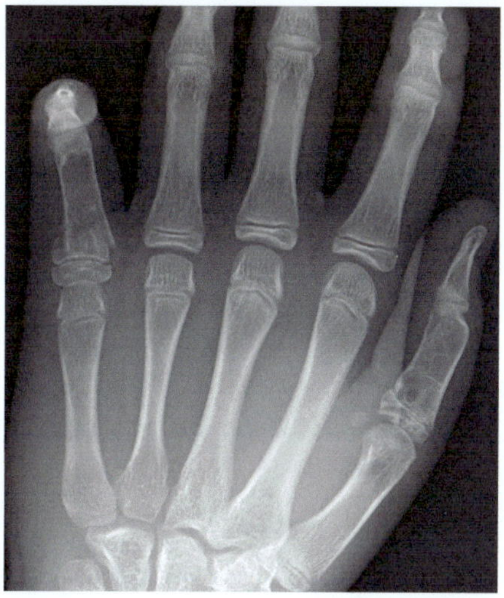

Fig. 20.35 Pathological fractures through pseudotumors in the first and fifth digits in a teen with hemophilia

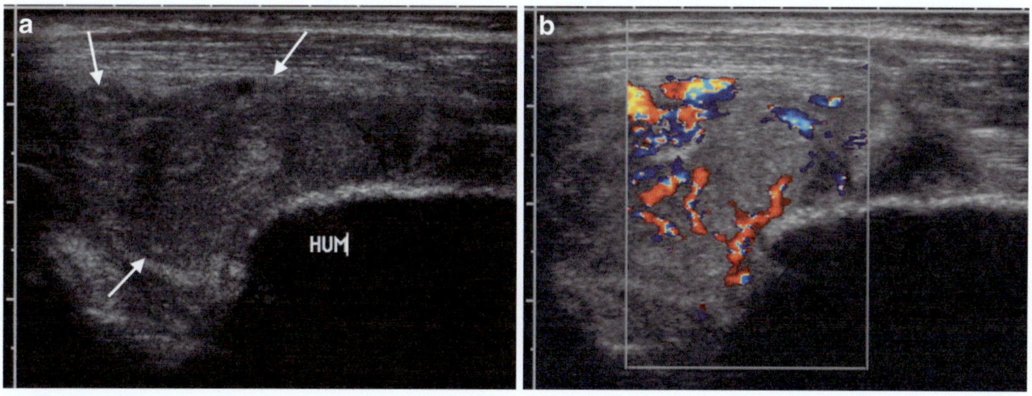

Fig. 20.36 Synovial proliferation in the elbow of a 14-year-old boy with factor VIII deficiency. (**a**) US demonstrates a heterogeneous mass (*arrows*) in the elbow joint with (**b**) increased vascularity. "Hum" denotes "humerus" (Same patient as Fig. 20.39)

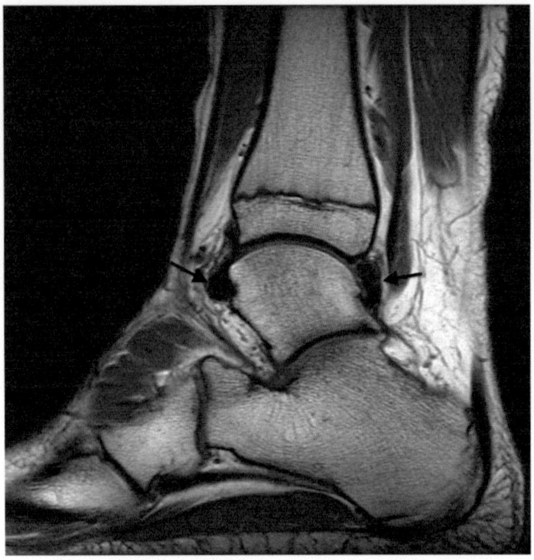

Fig. 20.37 Hemosiderin deposition in the ankle joint of a 16-year-old boy with hemophilia, without erosions. *Arrows* indicate hypointense hemosiderin

hemosiderin are evident, and there may be fluid-fluid levels.

3 Pigmented Villonodular Synovitis

Another relatively uncommon condition in children, pigmented villonodular synovitis (PVNS) is a benign, hypertrophic process that affects the synovium, bursas, and tendon sheaths. It usually presents in the third or fourth decade of life but has been reported in patients as young as 4 years of age [32]. Pediatric PVNS may be associated with vascular lesions, cherubism, lymphedema, Noonan and multiple lentigines syndrome, and jaw lesions [33]. In adults, lesions are usually solitary, but children are more likely to have polyarticular or multifocal involvement [33].

At any given location, either diffuse or localized disease may develop. The diffuse form typically affects the large joints, especially the knee (66–80 %) [33]. Other joints that may be affected include the hip, ankle, shoulder, and elbow, in decreasing order of frequency. The focal nodular form is more common in the distal extremities, typically the fingers. A similar process may also affect extra-articular spaces, such as tendon sheaths (PVNTS, or pigmented villonodular tenosynovitis) and bursas (PVNB, or pigmented villonodular bursitis). PVNTS, also termed giant cell tumor of the tendon sheath, is especially common in the hand and wrist. Patients with extra-articular PVNTS or PVNB present with a soft tissue mass and pain, whereas those with intra-articular PVNS usually complain of pain, joint swelling, and occasionally dysfunction.

Proliferation may be villous, nodular, or villonodular. The affected tissue in the diffuse intra-articular form of PVNS appears tan or yellow because of hemosiderin/fat deposition in the proliferative synovium. Epithelioid and giant cells are arrayed within a fibrous stroma that contains hemosiderin and lipid [34]. While the diffuse form is more infiltrative and demonstrates more prominent deposits of hemosiderin, the localized form tends to be well defined, with a collagenous pseudocapsule. Etiology is uncertain, but cytogenetic aberrations are evident in most cases of PVNS, suggesting a neoplastic origin [33].

Surgical resection is the mainstay of treatment for PVNS. If resection is incomplete, radiation or chemotherapy may be employed. However, incidence of local recurrence is as high as 50 % [2].

In the vast majority of cases, PVNS is limited to benign proliferation of the synovium (or bursas and tendon sheaths). However, a malignant form has been described in patients as young as 12 years old. Malignant PVNS is characterized by development of a sarcomatous tumor that histologically resembles PVNS within a joint that currently is or previously was affected by PVNS. The knee is most often involved [35].

Imaging (Box 20.4)

The classic early radiographic finding of PVNS is soft tissue swelling without calcification. Joint space is initially preserved. Extrinsic erosions with well-defined sclerotic borders develop on both sides of the joint, especially in joints where ligaments limit expansion or where joint capacity is small, such as the hip, shoulder, elbow, and ankle (Fig. 20.42). Erosive changes are less common at the more capacious knee (Fig. 20.43) [36]. As disease progresses and the cartilage

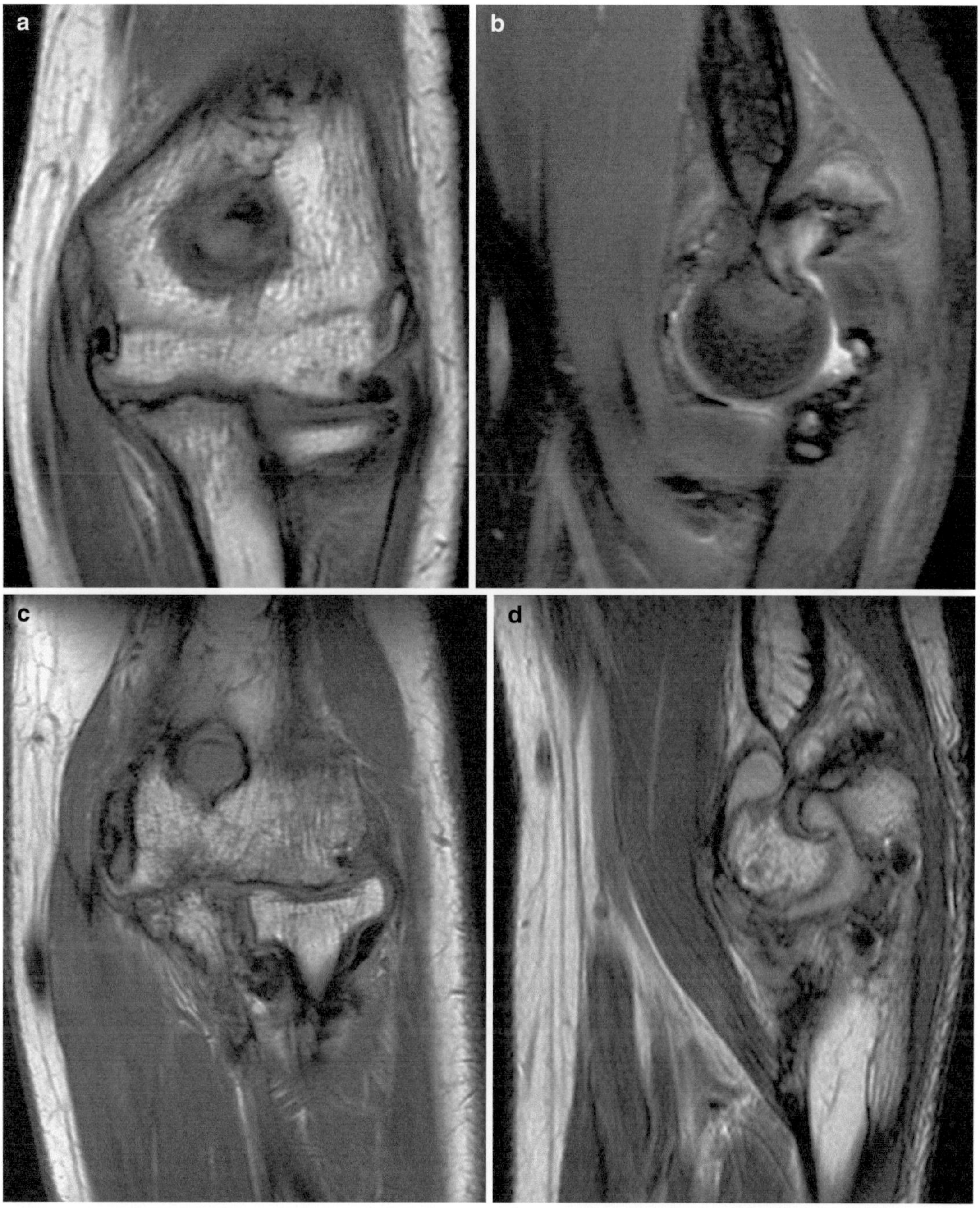

Fig. 20.38 Progressive arthropathy in a 12-year-old (**a**, **b**) and then 19-year-old (**c**, **d**) male with factor VIII deficiency. (**a**) Coronal T1-W image shows joint space narrowing and small subchondral cysts. (**b**) Sagittal PD FS image shows intra-articular joint fluid as well as fluid within the subchondral cysts and hemosiderin deposition along mildly thickened synovium. (**c**) Seven years later, coronal T1-W image shows high-grade chondral thinning with cortical irregularity, progressive joint space narrowing, periarticular marrow edema, and hemosiderin deposition. (**d**) Sagittal PD image shows susceptibility artifact from hemosiderin deposition within subchondral cysts

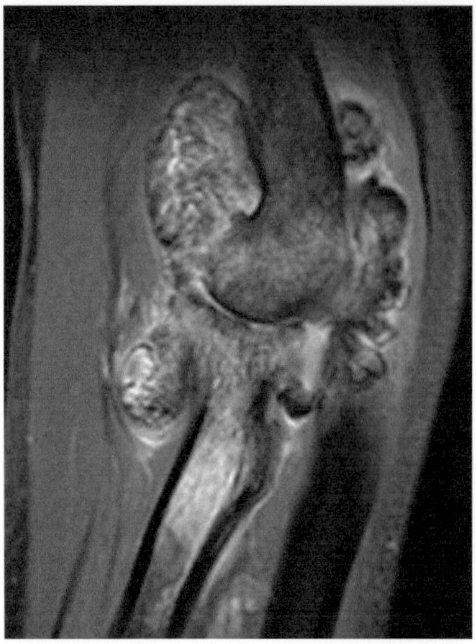

Fig. 20.39 Mass-like synovial proliferation in a 14-year-old boy with factor VIII deficiency. T1-W FS gadolinium-enhanced sagittal image demonstrates heaped up masses of synovium that demonstrate heterogeneous enhancement with peripheral hypointensity indicating hemosiderin deposition. There is joint space narrowing and marrow edema, as well as small cortical erosions (Same patient as Fig. 20.36)

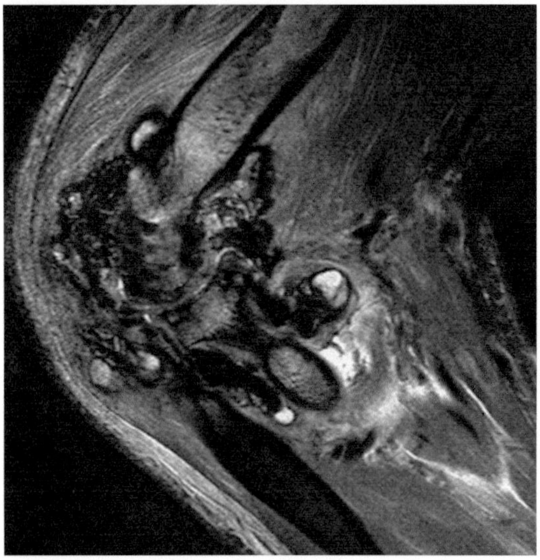

Fig. 20.40 Hemophilic arthritis in an 11-year-old boy. Sagittal T2-W FS image of the elbow demonstrates extensive susceptibility artifact related to hypertrophied and hemosiderin-laden synovium. There is subcutaneous and muscular edema, along with distal humeral and proximal radial marrow edema. (Courtesy of J. Herman Kan)

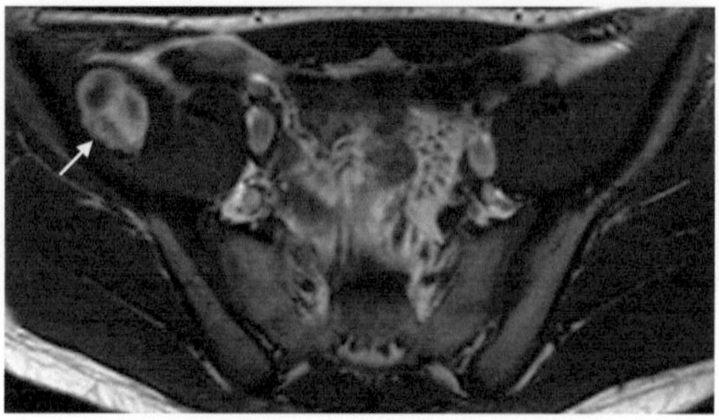

Fig. 20.41 Soft tissue pseudotumor in a patient with hemophilia. Axial T1-W image shows a large pseudotumor (*arrow*) within the right iliacus muscle. Note heterogeneous areas of T1 shortening within the pseudotumor, consistent with hemosiderin (Courtesy of J. Herman Kan)

Box 20.4: Imaging Features of Pigmented Villonodular Synovitis (PVNS)

Radiography

Early Soft tissue swelling
 Preservation of joint space
Mid Extrinsic erosions with sclerotic borders
 In tight joints (hip, shoulder, elbow, ankle)
 Less common in the knee
Late Cartilage erosion → joint space narrowing
 Loose bodies, geodes, osteophytes

Early findings on MRI

Focal or nodular synovial thickening
Hemosiderin deposition more with diffuse than localized form
Intermediate or low signal on all sequences
T2: linear hypointensity along periphery of the synovium

becomes eroded, joint space narrowing may develop, along with osteopenia, loose bodies, geodes, and osteophytes. These findings also are more common in relatively tight joints. US demonstrates vascular, hypoechoic, mass-like synovial proliferation (Fig. 20.44).

MRI demonstrates diffuse or focal nodular synovial thickening, depending on whether the patient has the diffuse or localized form of disease (Fig. 20.45). Synovium has low or intermediate signal on all pulse sequences; T2-W sequences reveal linear hypointense signal along

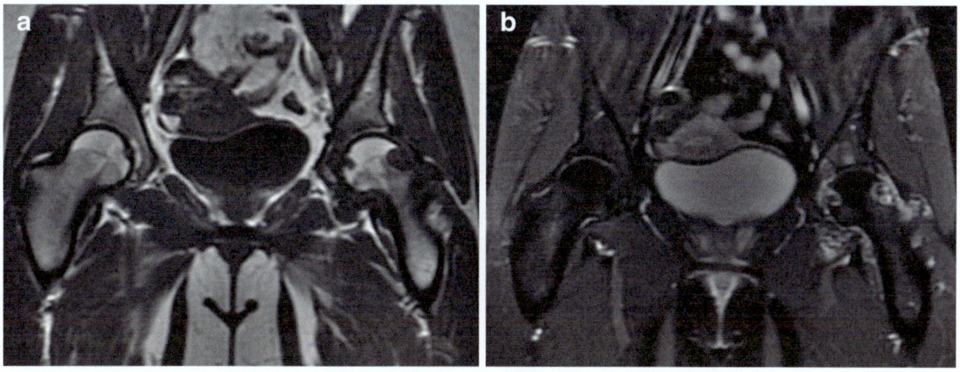

Fig. 20.42 Erosions in a 21-year-old female with PVNS. (**a**) Coronal T1-W image shows well-circumscribed erosions in the left femoral head. (**b**) Coronal T1-W FS gadolinium-enhanced image shows synovial enhancement extending into the erosions (Courtesy of J. Herman Kan)

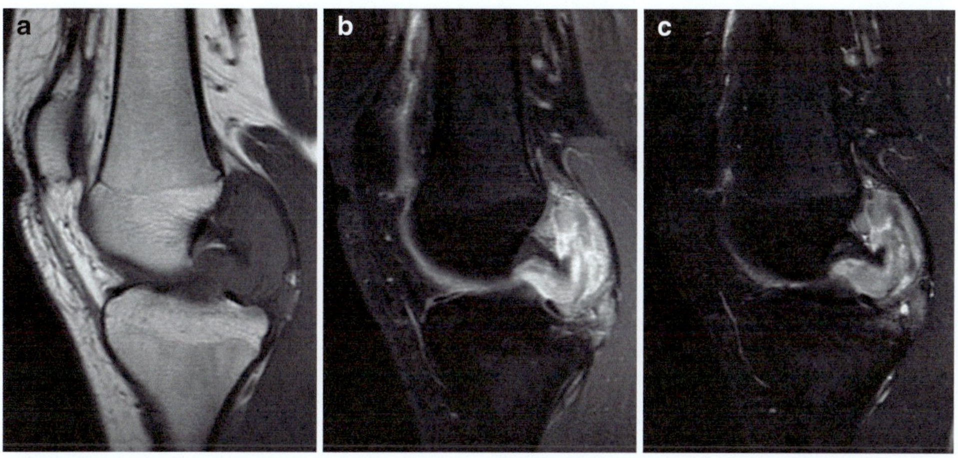

Fig. 20.43 Nodular PVNS in a 14-year-old girl. Sagittal T1-W (**a**), T1-W FS gadolinium-enhanced (**b**), and IR (**c**) images show that despite the presence of a large, heterogeneous mass encasing the posterior cruciate ligament, there are no significant osseous erosions. Peripheral hypointense hemosiderin deposition

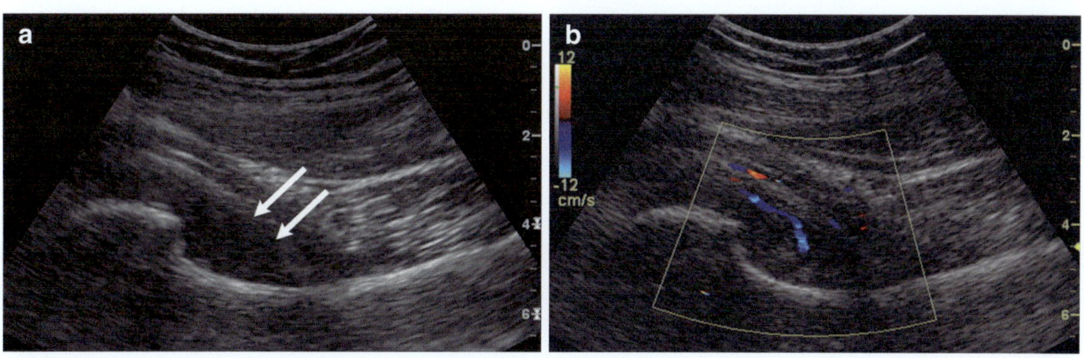

Fig. 20.44 PVNS in a 17-year-old girl. Longitudinal hip US (**a**) shows synovial thickening with fine internal solid echogenicity (*arrows*). There is internal vascularity on color Doppler (**b**) (Reprinted from Doria and Babyn [38], copyright Elsevier 2013) (Image courtesy of Andrea Doria)

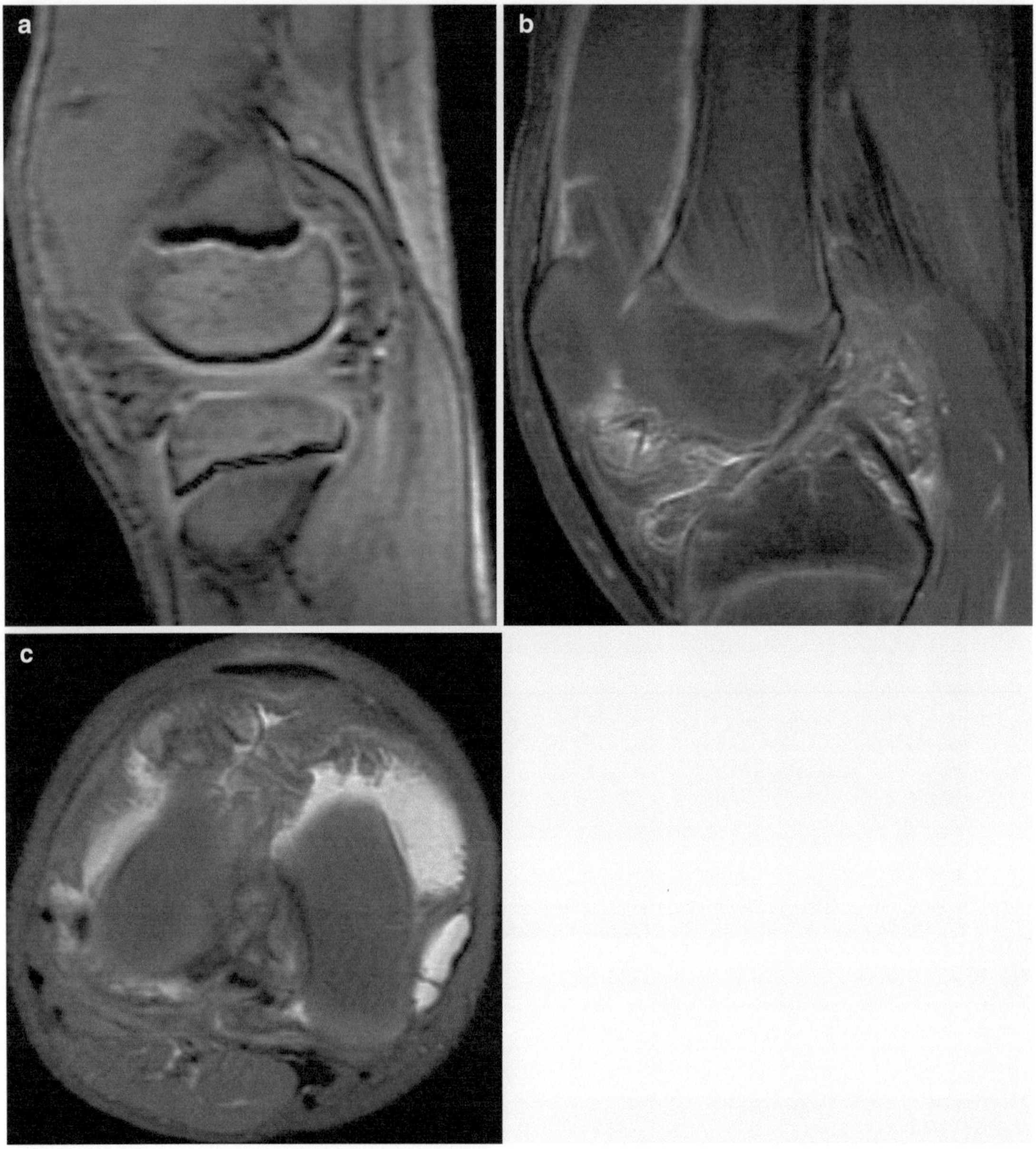

Fig. 20.45 Diffuse PVNS. (**a**) Sagittal GRE scout image demonstrates blooming artifact in the anterior and posterior knee joint. (**b**) Sagittal T1-W FS gadolinium-enhanced image shows corresponding diffuse serpiginous enhancement, with mild thickening of suprapatellar synovium. Large suprapatellar joint effusion. (**c**) Axial PD FS image shows diffuse nodularity with foci of hypointense hemosiderin (Courtesy of Tal Laor, Cincinnati Children's Hospital)

the periphery of thickened synovium, secondary to hemosiderin deposition. Hemosiderin deposition is more pronounced with the diffuse than with the localized form. "Blooming" of susceptibility artifact is apparent with GRE imaging. Enhancement is usually robust and homogeneous. A joint effusion is common in large joints.

Differential Diagnosis. Both hemophilia and hemangioma may also result in hemosiderin deposition within a joint as a result of repetitive intra-articular hemorrhage. However, the clinical history of hemophilia allows differentiation, as does the typical vascular appearance of hemangioma.

References

1. Jordan A, McDonagh JE. Juvenile idiopathic arthritis: the paediatric perspective. Pediatr Radiol. 2006; 36(8):734–42.
2. Kim HK, Zbojniewicz AM, Merrow AC, Cheon JE, Kim IO, Emery KH. MR findings of synovial disease in children and young adults: part 1. Pediatr Radiol. 2011;41(4):495–511; quiz 545–496.
3. Petty RE, Southwood TR, Manners P, Baum J, Glass DN, Goldenberg J, He X, Maldonado-Cocco J, Orozco-Alcala J, Prieur AM, Suarez-Almazor ME, Woo P, R. International League of Associations. International League of Associations for Rheumatology classification of juvenile idiopathic arthritis: second revision, Edmonton, 2001. J Rheumatol. 2004;31(2):390–2.
4. Wallace CA, Levinson JE. Juvenile rheumatoid arthritis: outcome and treatment for the 1990s. Rheum Dis Clin North Am. 1991;17(4):891–905.
5. Kim HK, Laor T, Graham TB, Anton CG, Salisbury SR, Racadio JM, Dardzinski BJ. T2 relaxation time changes in distal femoral articular cartilage in children with juvenile idiopathic arthritis: a 3-year longitudinal study. AJR Am J Roentgenol. 2010;195(4):1021–5.
6. Pettersson H, Rydholm U. Radiologic classification of knee joint destruction in juvenile chronic arthritis. Pediatr Radiol. 1984;14(6):419–21.
7. Johnson K. Imaging of juvenile idiopathic arthritis. Pediatr Radiol. 2006;36(8):743–58.
8. Reed MH, Wilmot DM. The radiology of juvenile rheumatoid arthritis. A review of the English language literature. J Rheumatol Suppl. 1991;31:2–22.
9. Lang BA, Schneider R, Reilly BJ, Silverman ED, Laxer RM. Radiologic features of systemic onset juvenile rheumatoid arthritis. J Rheumatol. 1995;22(1):168–73.
10. Sureda D, Quiroga S, Arnal C, Boronat M, Andreu J, Casas L. Juvenile rheumatoid arthritis of the knee: evaluation with US. Radiology. 1994;190(2):403–6.
11. Haslam KE, McCann LJ, Wyatt S, Wakefield RJ. The detection of subclinical synovitis by ultrasound in oligoarticular juvenile idiopathic arthritis: a pilot study. Rheumatology (Oxford). 2010;49(1):123–7.
12. Wakefield RJ, Gibbon WW, Conaghan PG, O'Connor P, McGonagle D, Pease C, Green MJ, Veale DJ, Isaacs JD, Emery P. The value of sonography in the detection of bone erosions in patients with rheumatoid arthritis: a comparison with conventional radiography. Arthritis Rheum. 2000;43(12):2762–70.
13. Lamer S, Sebag GH. MRI and ultrasound in children with juvenile chronic arthritis. Eur J Radiol. 2000;33(2):85–93.
14. Sheybani EF, Khanna G, White AJ, Demertzis JL. Imaging of juvenile idiopathic arthritis: a multimodality approach. Radiographics. 2013;33(5):1253–73.
15. Damasio MB, Malattia C, Martini A, Toma P. Synovial and inflammatory diseases in childhood: role of new imaging modalities in the assessment of patients with juvenile idiopathic arthritis. Pediatr Radiol. 2010;40(6):985–98.
16. Gylys-Morin VM, Graham TB, Blebea JS, Dardzinski BJ, Laor T, Johnson ND, Oestreich AE, Passo MH. Knee in early juvenile rheumatoid arthritis: MR imaging findings. Radiology. 2001;220(3):696–706.
17. Workie DW, Graham TB, Laor T, Rajagopal A, O'Brien KJ, Bommer WA, Racadio JM, Shire NJ, Dardzinski BJ. Quantitative MR characterization of disease activity in the knee in children with juvenile idiopathic arthritis: a longitudinal pilot study. Pediatr Radiol. 2007;37(6):535–43.
18. Kight AC, Dardzinski BJ, Laor T, Graham TB. Magnetic resonance imaging evaluation of the effects of juvenile rheumatoid arthritis on distal femoral weight-bearing cartilage. Arthritis Rheum. 2004;50(3):901–5.
19. Mosher TJ, Dardzinski BJ. Cartilage MRI T2 relaxation time mapping: overview and applications. Semin Musculoskelet Radiol. 2004;8(4):355–68.
20. Ostergaard M, Peterfy C, Conaghan P, McQueen F, Bird P, Ejbjerg B, Shnier R, O'Connor P, Klarlund M, Emery P, Genant H, Lassere M, Edmonds J. OMERACT Rheumatoid Arthritis Magnetic Resonance Imaging Studies. Core set of MRI acquisitions, joint pathology definitions, and the OMERACT RA-MRI scoring system. J Rheumatol. 2003;30(6):1385–6.
21. Kan JH. Juvenile idiopathic arthritis and enthesitis-related arthropathies. Pediatr Radiol. 2013;43 Suppl 1:S172–80.
22. Rosenberg AM. Juvenile onset spondyloarthropathies. Curr Opin Rheumatol. 2000;12(5):425–9.
23. Bollow M, Biedermann T, Kannenberg J, Paris S, Schauer-Petrowski C, Minden K, Schontube M, Hamm B, Sieper J, Braun J. Use of dynamic magnetic resonance imaging to detect sacroiliitis in HLA-B27 positive and negative children with juvenile arthritides. J Rheumatol. 1998;25(3):556–64.
24. Daldrup-Link HE, Steinbach L. MR imaging of pediatric arthritis. Magn Reson Imaging Clin N Am. 2009;17(3):451–67, vi.
25. Hilgartner MW. Current treatment of hemophilic arthropathy. Curr Opin Pediatr. 2002;14(1):46–9.
26. Park JS, Ryu KN. Hemophilic pseudotumor involving the musculoskeletal system: spectrum of radiologic findings. AJR Am J Roentgenol. 2004;183(1):55–61.
27. Maclachlan J, Gough-Palmer A, Hargunani R, Farrant J, Holloway B. Haemophilia imaging: a review. Skeletal Radiol. 2009;38(10):949–57.
28. Arnold WD, Hilgartner MW. Hemophilic arthropathy. Current concepts of pathogenesis and management. J Bone Joint Surg Am. 1977;59(3):287–305.
29. Ng WH, Chu WC, Shing MK, Lam WW, Chik KW, Li CK, Li CK, Ling SC. Role of imaging in management of hemophilic patients. AJR Am J Roentgenol. 2005;184(5):1619–23.
30. Kilcoyne RF, Nuss R. Radiological assessment of haemophilic arthropathy with emphasis on MRI findings. Haemophilia. 2003;9 Suppl 1:57–63; discussion 63–54.

31. Doria AS. State-of-the-art imaging techniques for the evaluation of haemophilic arthropathy: present and future. Haemophilia. 2010;16 Suppl 5:107–14.
32. Neubauer P, Weber AK, Miller NH, McCarthy EF. Pigmented villonodular synovitis in children: a report of six cases and review of the literature. Iowa Orthop J. 2007;27:90–4.
33. Murphey MD, Rhee JH, Lewis RB, Fanburg-Smith JC, Flemming DJ, Walker EA. Pigmented villonodular synovitis: radiologic-pathologic correlation. Radiographics. 2008;28(5):1493–518.
34. Goldman AB, DiCarlo EF. Pigmented villonodular synovitis. Diagnosis and differential diagnosis. Radiol Clin North Am. 1988;26(6):1327–47.
35. Bertoni F, Unni KK, Beabout JW, Sim FH. Malignant giant cell tumor of the tendon sheaths and joints (malignant pigmented villonodular synovitis). Am J Surg Pathol. 1997;21(2):153–63.
36. Dorwart RH, Genant HK, Johnston WH, Morris JM. Pigmented villonodular synovitis of synovial joints: clinical, pathologic, and radiologic features. AJR Am J Roentgenol. 1984;143(4):877–85.
37. Miller E, Doria A. Imaging for early assessment of peripheral joints in juvenile idiopathic arthritis. In: Medina LS, Applegate KE, Blackmore CC, editors. Evidence-based imaging in pediatrics: optimizing imaging in pediatric patient care. New York: Springer Science+Business Media; 2010.
38. Doria AS, Babyn P. Arthritides and other inflammatory disorders. In: Coley BD, editor. Caffey's Pediatric Diagnostic Imaging. Philadelphia: Elsevier; 2013.

Tumors and Tumor-Like Conditions of Bone

21

Sandra L. Wootton-Gorges

Contents

Abstract

This chapter first discusses general principles of tumor imaging, including both characteristics of benign and malignant tumors and utility of different imaging modalities. It then enters an in-depth discussion of benign tumors and tumor-like lesions, addressing cystic, cartilaginous, osseous, fibro-osseous, and vascular lesions, along with Langerhans cell histiocytosis. It concludes with a review of osteosarcoma and Ewing sarcoma, the more common malignant tumors, as well as chondrosarcoma, lymphoma, malignant fibrous histiocytoma, and metastatic disease.

1 General Principles of Imaging

Over 40 % of bone tumors arise during the first two decades of life [1, 2]. They can be categorized according to their pathological diagnosis (Table 21.1) [3]. Tumor location helps direct the differential diagnosis (Tables 21.2 and 21.3), and the appearance of the lesion and patient age provide important information [3].

For malignant tumors, imaging delineates the local extent of the tumor and the presence of distant metastases. It also helps determine the response to therapy and detect recurrent disease. The ALARA (as low as reasonably achievable) principle allows for optimal imaging while minimizing exposure to radiation [4].

S.L. Wootton-Gorges, MD
Department of Radiology,
University of California Davis Medical
Center and UC Davis Children's Hospital,
4860 Y Street, Suite 3100, Sacramento, CA 95817, USA

Department of Diagnostic Imaging, Shriners Hospitals
for Children Northern California, Sacramento, CA, USA
e-mail: sandra.gorges@ucdmc.ucdavis.edu

R. Stein-Wexler et al. (eds.), *Pediatric Orthopedic Imaging*,
DOI 10.1007/978-3-642-45381-6_21, © Springer-Verlag Berlin Heidelberg 2015

Table 21.1 Pediatric primary bone tumors and tumor-like lesions (organized according to histologic characteristics)

	Benign	Malignant
Bone-forming tumors	Osteoblastoma Osteoid osteoma	Osteosarcoma
Cartilage-forming tumors	Chondroblastoma Chondromyxoid fibroma Enchondroma Osteochondroma	Chondrosarcoma
Cystic lesions	Aneurysmal bone cyst Unicameral (simple) bone cyst	
Fibro-osseous lesions	Fibrous dysplasia Nonossifying fibroma	Fibrosarcoma Malignant fibrous histiocytoma
Giant cell tumors	Giant cell tumor	
Small round cell tumors	Lymphoma	Ewing sarcoma
Vascular tumors	Hemangioma Lymphangioma	Hemangiopericytoma
Other	Langerhans cell histiocytosis	

Reprinted with permission from Wootton-Gorges [3]

1.1 Radiography (Box 21.1)

Box 21.1: General Radiographic Characteristics of Bone Tumors

Benign
- Well-defined and often sclerotic borders
- Cortical expansion
- May produce solid periosteal reaction

Malignant
- Poor definition of margins
- Cortical destruction
- Spiculated, onion skin, or interrupted periosteal reaction
- Soft tissue mass

Radiography constitutes the initial imaging modality for characterizing primary bone tumors and tumor-like conditions. This modality determines the location of the lesion within the bone and assesses its interface with the adjacent normal bone, along with the presence and appearance of both mineralized matrix and periosteal reaction [5]. Benign neoplasms usually grow more slowly and have well-defined and often sclerotic borders. Slower-growing tumors result in cortical expansion and may produce solid periosteal reaction. Malignant lesions usually show poor marginal definition, along with cortical destruction, a soft tissue mass, and a spiculated or interrupted periosteal reaction. However, these general characteristics are not absolute.

Periosteal reaction may be classified as either linear (single or multiple), solid, or spiculated [6]. Single linear reaction, appearing as a thin layer of new bone adjacent to the cortex, may be seen with benign periosteal reaction of infancy, trauma, osteomyelitis, and benign or malignant tumors, including metastases (Fig. 21.1a). Multiple layers of linear or lamellated reaction, known as "onion skin," are frequently seen with aggressive tumors such as Ewing sarcoma or osteosarcoma but may also be seen with Langerhans cell histiocytosis and osteomyelitis (Fig. 21.1b). Spiculated periosteal reaction, oriented in the direction of rapid tumor growth, forms along vascular channels and Sharpey bands and appears in either a "hair on end" or "sunburst" form (Fig. 21.1b, c). Hair on end periosteal reaction is associated with Ewing sarcoma; a sunburst appearance is most often seen with osteosarcoma. The Codman triangle, or interrupted periosteal reaction, occurs when tumor, pus, or hemorrhage lifts or interrupts the periosteum. This may be seen with aggressive tumors (Fig. 21.1d), infection, or sometimes healing fractures. However, periosteal reaction has a broad range of appearances, and even with malignant tumors, it is not always visible.

Table 21.2 Typical skeletal locations of pediatric primary bone tumors

Small tubular bones	
	Enchondroma
	Osteoid osteoma
Long tubular bones	
	Metastases
	Most benign and malignant bone tumors and tumor-like lesions (see Table 21.3 for specific locations within tubular bones)
Ribs:	
	Cartilaginous tumors
	Ewing sarcoma
	Fibrous dysplasia
	Langerhans cell histiocytosis
	Metastases
Spine – vertebral body:	
	Chordoma
	Giant cell tumor
	Hemangioma
	Langerhans cell histiocytosis
	Lymphoma
	Metastases
Spine – posterior elements:	
	Aneurysmal bone cyst
	Osteoblastoma/osteoid osteoma
Skull and facial bones:	
	Fibrous dysplasia
	Langerhans cell histiocytosis
	Metastases
	Osteoma
Pelvis	
	Chondrosarcoma
	Ewing sarcoma
	Fibrous dysplasia
	Metastases
	Osteochondroma

Reprinted with permission from Wootton-Gorges [3]

Tumors may produce osseous, chondroid, or fibrous matrix (Fig. 21.2). Osseous matrix is usually cloud-like, while chondroid matrix is typically characterized by stippled rings and arcs [5]. Destruction, replacement, or resorption of bone by the tumor may produce a lytic appearance. This tends to be well marginated, or geographic, with benign tumors, and more aggressive (permeative or moth-eaten) with malignant tumors.

Ultrasound can assess associated soft tissue masses but has an otherwise limited role in imaging bone tumors.

Table 21.3 Tumor distribution within long bones

Epiphysis	Chondroblastoma
Metaphysis	Aneurysmal bone cyst
	Chondromyxoid fibroma
	Enchondroma
	Ewing sarcoma
	Fibrous dysplasia
	Giant cell tumor
	Lymphoma
	Malignant fibrous histiocytoma
	Metastases
	Nonossifying fibroma
	Osteochondroma
	Osteosarcoma
	Unicameral bone cyst
	Adamantinoma
Diaphysis	Ewing sarcoma
	Lymphoma
	Osteofibrous dysplasia
	Osteoid osteoma

Reprinted with permission from Wootton-Gorges [3]

1.2 Nuclear Medicine Imaging

Technetium-99m-methylene diphosphonate (^{99m}Tc-MDP) bone scintigraphy and positron emission tomography (PET) have a limited role in the evaluation of solitary benign-appearing bone lesions as the patterns of uptake are usually not specific. However, in the initial staging and treatment evaluation of osteosarcoma and Ewing sarcoma, scintigraphy can assess for bone metastases, synchronous tumor, and skip lesions [7, 8]. It is also useful for multifocal processes, such as fibrous dysplasia, Langerhans cell histiocytosis (LCH), and other metastatic diseases [5]. 18F-fluorodeoxyglucose positron emission tomography (FDG-PET) CT is a promising means to evaluate patients with bone sarcomas [9, 10]. This technique may help predict tumor grade and assess treatment response when coupled with histologic evaluation [9].

1.3 Computed Tomography

Computed tomography (CT) offers greater spatial and contrast resolution than radiography and thus provides more detailed information about the intra-

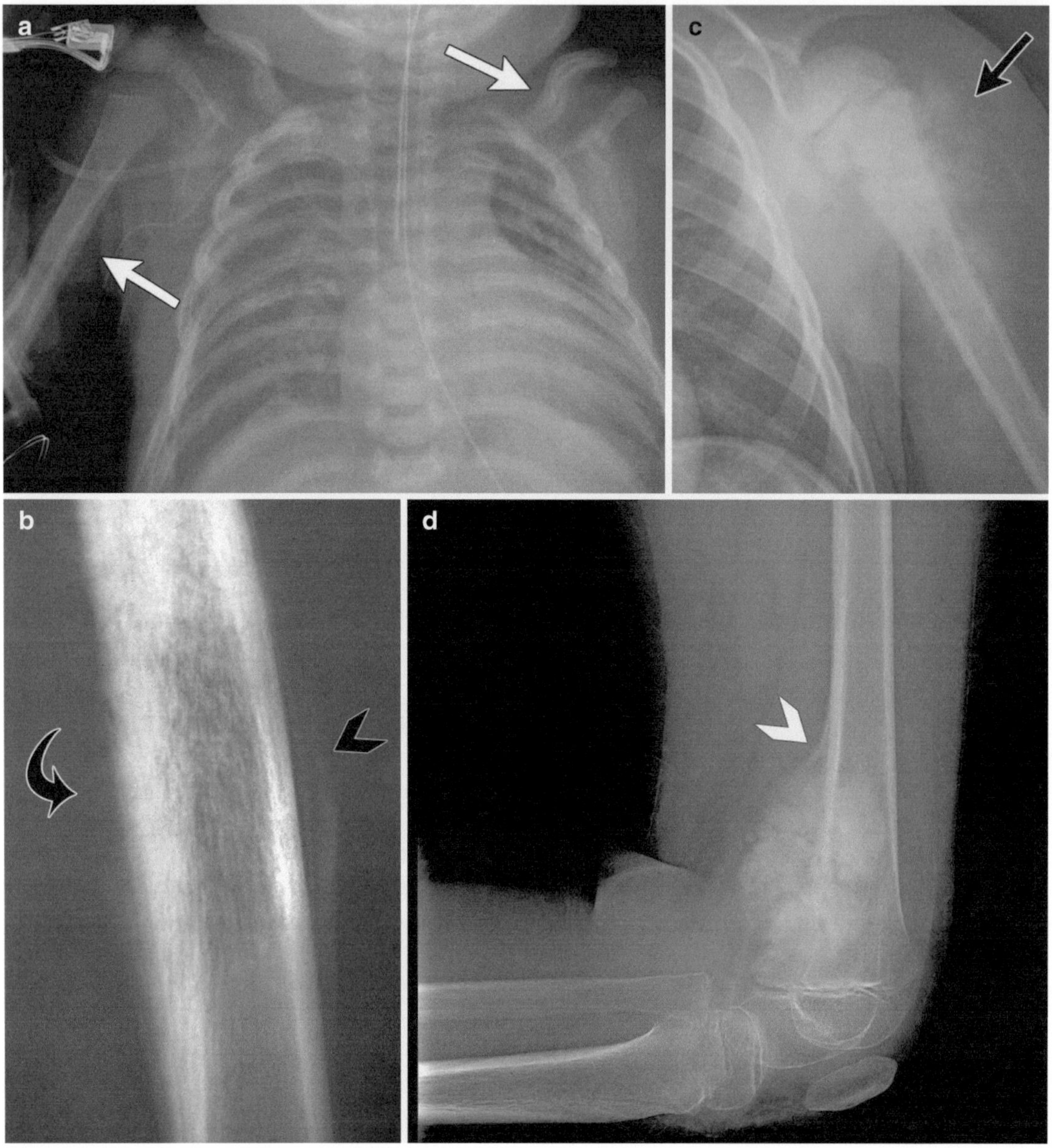

Fig. 21.1 Examples of different types of periosteal reaction. (**a**) Linear periosteal reaction (*white arrow*) in newborn with hypoplastic left heart syndrome and prostaglandin-induced periostitis. (**b**) Diaphyseal hair-on-end periosteal reaction (*curved black arrow*) and marginal onion skin periosteal reaction (*black arrowhead*) with Ewing sarcoma. (**c**) Sunburst periosteal reaction (*black arrow*) with osteosarcoma. (**d**) Codman *triangle* (*white arrowhead*) with distal femoral osteosarcoma

and extraosseous extent of tumor, the configuration of mineralization within the lesion, the type and location of tumor matrix, and the resultant cortical and periosteal changes [1, 5]. Furthermore, fat and fluid–fluid levels may sometimes be detected within the lesion, and the extent of contrast enhancement may be delineated [11]. CT may demonstrate periosteal reaction earlier than plain radiography [6].

1.4 Magnetic Resonance Imaging

Magnetic resonance imaging (MRI) exquisitely assesses the extent of cortical, intramedullary, joint, and soft tissue involvement by the neoplasm [8]. Important features such as fluid–fluid levels and tumor composition may lead to a more accurate diagnosis [11].

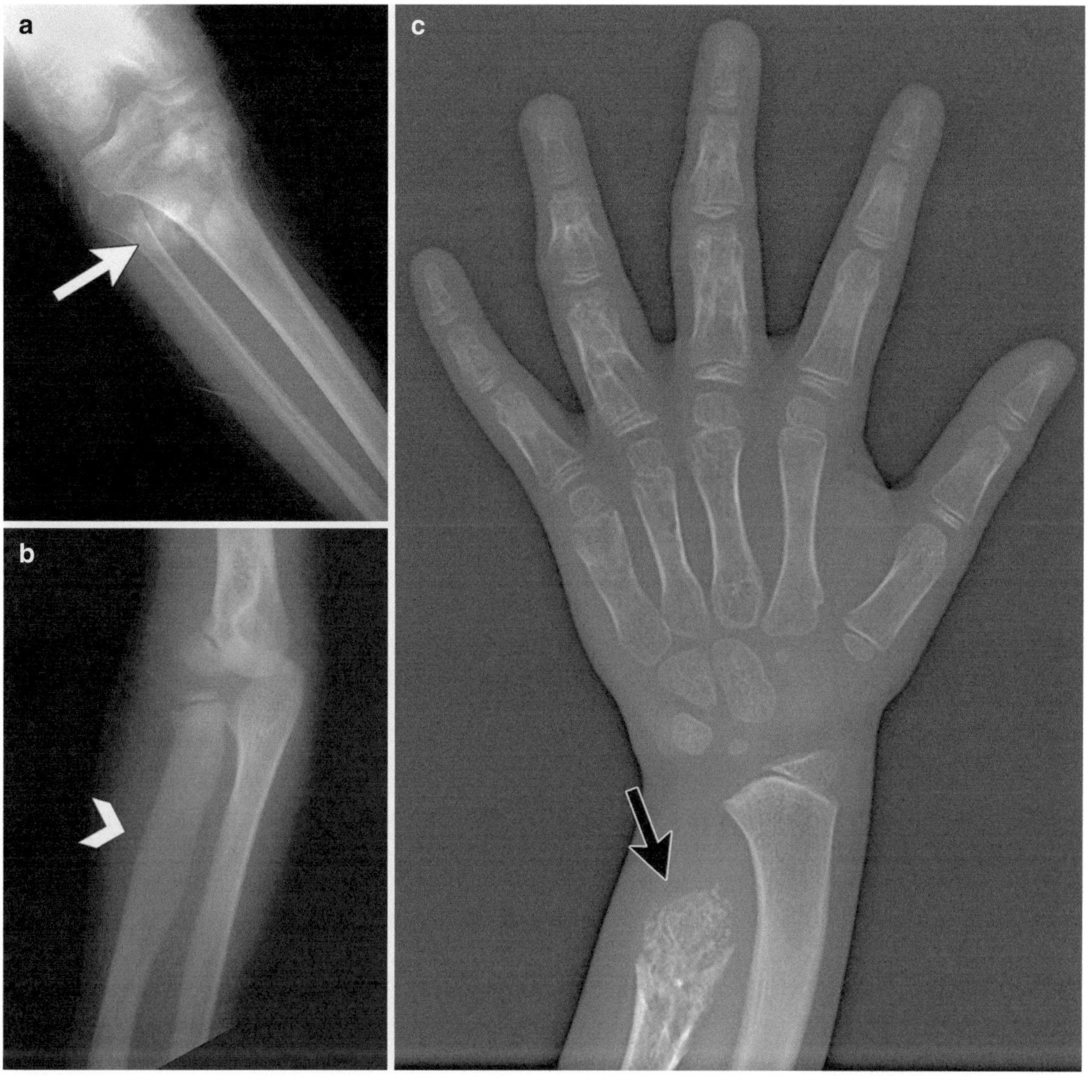

Fig. 21.2 Examples of different types of matrix. (**a**) Osseous matrix in osteosarcoma (*white arrow*). (**b**) Fibrous matrix in fibrous dysplasia (*white arrowhead*). (**c**) Chondroid matrix in enchondromatosis (*black arrow*) (**b**, **c** copyright Shriners Hospital for Children Northern California)

The primary tumor, adjacent soft tissues, and vascular, nerve, and joint involvement must be assessed. The MRI examination must include the entire bone to evaluate for skip lesions and assess the longitudinal extent of the tumor [8, 12]. T1-weighted (T1-W) images show the highest specificity for evaluating tumor extent: intraosseous tumor is typically hypointense and distorts the normal marrow architecture [12]. Short tau inversion recovery (STIR) images detect tumor with the highest sensitivity (the tumor is typically hyperintense). Small field-of-view phased-array coil axial fast spin echo (FSE) fluid-sensitive and fat-suppressed (FS) sequences help determine the relationship of tumor to adjacent muscle, nerve, and vascular structures. Gradient echo sequences can show flow within areas of neovascularity. Gadolinium-enhanced (GE) T1-W FS images define areas of viable tumor and areas of tumor necrosis [8]. Hypointensity on both T1-W and T2-weighted (T2-W) images may suggest either osteoblastic/fibrous matrix or chronic hemorrhage [13].

Peritumoral edema may be seen with either benign or malignant tumors and may be intraosseous or extraosseous [5, 13]. The signal

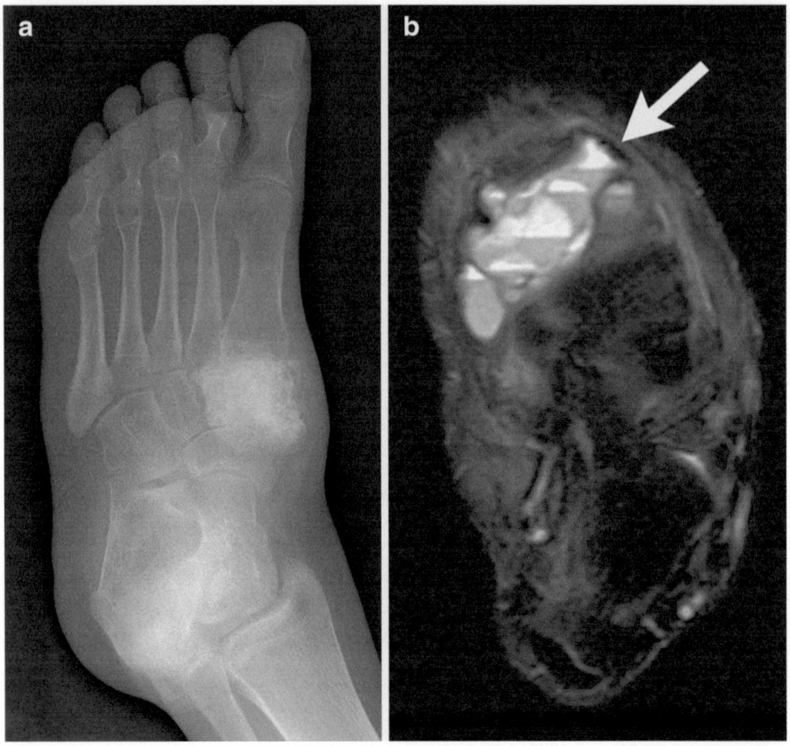

Fig. 21.3 Medial cuneiform aneurysmal bone cyst. (**a**) The bone is expanded and diffusely sclerotic, with scattered foci of dense sclerosis. (**b**) T2-weighted (T2-W) fat-suppressed (FS) axial MRI shows multiple fluid–fluid levels (*white arrow*)

characteristics of peritumoral edema resemble those of tumor, and care must be taken to distinguish between the two. Edema does not demonstrate mass effect or alter normal architecture [13]. Its margins within the bone are poorly defined, and it has a feathery appearance that follows muscle and fascial planes. Tumor margins are, in contrast, usually sharp. Like many tumors, signal intensity of marrow edema is intermediate between fat and muscle on T1-W sequences and high on T2 or STIR images. However, T2 hyperintensity due to marrow edema tends to be more heterogeneous than does that associated with tumor. The enhancement pattern also helps differentiate, as edema enhances less than tumor.

Fluid–fluid levels were first described in aneurysmal bone cysts (ABC) but occur in other benign and malignant tumors as well, including unicameral bone cyst, giant cell tumor, osteoblastoma, chondroblastoma, and telangiectatic osteosarcoma [5]. They are best evaluated with T2-W MRI (Fig. 21.3) [14]. Fluid–fluid levels in aneurysmal bone cysts result from separation of blood and serum in the cavernous spaces [13]. In other lesions, they may result from hemorrhage with breakdown of blood products or from tumor necrosis with sedimentation of cells and tissue fluid. The MRI appearance depends on the pulse sequences used as well as the composition of the fluid layers. On T1-W sequences, a high signal layer suggests methemoglobin. A layer that is isointense to slightly hyperintense to muscle on all sequences generally results from layering cellular debris or blood [13]. Although there are exceptions, as a general rule if more than two thirds of a lesion consists of fluid–fluid levels, it is benign, whereas if less than one third of it consists of fluid–fluid levels, it is malignant [15].

There are two major staging systems for malignant bone tumors, a surgical system developed by Enneking (Table 21.4) and a system

Table 21.4 Surgical staging of musculoskeletal tumors

Benign	
1	Latent
2	Active
3	Aggressive
Malignant	
IA	Low grade, intracompartmental
IB	Low grade, extracompartmental
IIA	High grade, intracompartmental
IIB	High grade, extracompartmental
III	Distant metastatic disease

Adapted from Jawad and Scully [17]

Table 21.5 American Joint Commission on Cancer (AJCC) bone tumor staging system

Stage IA	Primary tumor <8 cm in greatest dimension
	No regional nodes or metastases
	Low tumor histologic grade
Stage IB	Primary tumor >8 cm in greatest dimension (or discontinuous tumors at primary site)
	No regional nodes or metastases
	Low tumor histologic grade
Stage IIA	Primary tumor <8 cm in greatest dimension
	No regional nodes or metastases
	High tumor histologic grade
Stage IIB	Primary tumor >8 cm in greatest dimension
	No regional nodes or metastases
	High tumor histologic grade
Stage III	Discontinuous tumors at primary site
	No regional nodes or metastases
	High tumor histologic grade
Stage IVA	Primary tumor any size
	No regional nodes
	Lung metastases
	Any tumor histologic grade
Stage IVB	Primary tumor any size
	Regional lymph node spread
	Metastases
	Any tumor grade

Adapted from Edge et al. [79]

defined by the American Joint Commission on Cancer [16, 17] (Table 21.5) (AJCC). The former is useful for surgical planning, while the latter categorizes patient and monitor survival.

2 Benign Tumors and Tumor-Like Lesions

2.1 Cystic Lesions (Box 21.2)

Box 21.2: Cystic Lesions of Bone

Simple bone cyst: cyst with thin fibrous lining

Location	Metaphysis to diaphysis, central
	Proximal long bones (humerus, femur, tibia)
Appearance	Well-defined, ovoid, lytic, expansile
	± Multiloculated, especially after fracture (fallen fragment)
	No fluid–fluid levels

Aneurysmal bone cyst (ABC): large, giant cell-lined vascular spaces

Location	Pelvis, eccentric at metaphysis (femur, tibia, humerus)
	Posterior elements of the vertebrae
Appearance	Eccentric, radiolucent, bubbly, well-defined expansile mass
	Marked cortical thinning
	Fluid–fluid levels, septations, no osseous matrix
Caveat	If MRI shows soft tissue component, consider other diagnosis

Giant cell tumor: giant cells, usually after physes close

Location	Metaphysis, stops at physis (if open); eccentric
	Knee, the most common
	Also distal radius and tibia; proximal humerus and femur; pelvis
Appearance	Lucent, no matrix calcification
	Well-defined non-sclerotic wall
	Cortical thinning, no periosteal reaction
	Secondary aneurysmal bone cyst in about 14 %

Unicameral or Simple Bone Cyst

Most simple bone cysts occur in the long tubular bones, especially the proximal humerus, proximal femur, and proximal tibia. They are

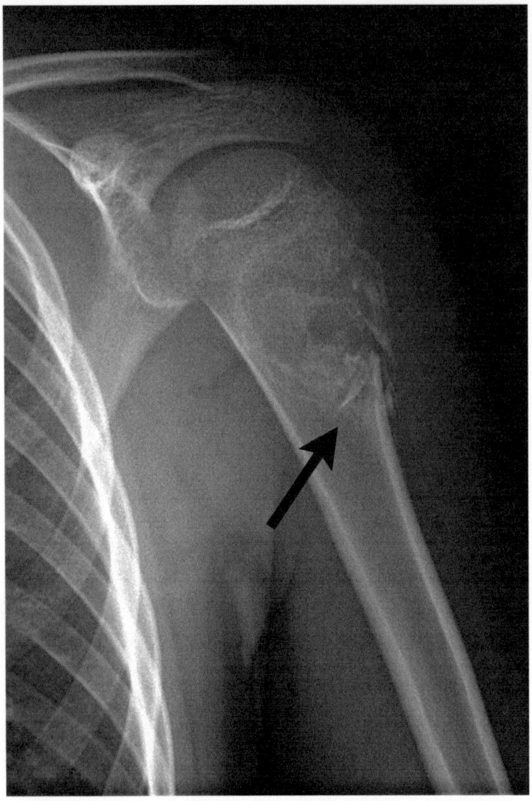

Fig. 21.4 Proximal humeral diametaphyseal simple bone cyst with pathological fracture and fallen fragment (*black arrow*)

usually encountered in children between nine and 15 years of age [18]. Discovery of the cyst may be incidental, or patients may present with pain after pathological fracture. Many simple bone cysts heal without treatment. Treatment may be indicated for cysts that do not heal on their own or that are at risk of fracture and includes disruption of the cyst wall, opening of the medullary canal, steroid injection, and/or filling the defect with a bone substitute [19]. Cysts of the lower extremity may also require structural support such as screw placement [20]. After treatment, cysts may recur (10–20 %), heal, and disappear completely or heal with residual deformity.

Imaging

This well-defined, elongated, lytic expansile lesion arises centrally in the metaphysis and may extend into the diaphysis. It may show internal trabeculation, especially after remote fracture. A fallen fragment, a pathognomonic sign of a unicameral bone cyst, may be seen in the dependent part of the cyst after fracture [1, 5] (Fig. 21.4). In the absence of fracture, there should be no periosteal reaction.

Nontraumatized simple bone cysts may be indiscernible at bone scan, or they may show a slight reactive margin surrounding a photopenic center [21].

CT or MRI may be useful to further define cysts that have an atypical appearance or location, such as multiloculated cysts or cysts in complex areas such as the pelvis. At MRI, the fluid-filled cyst is usually isointense on T1-W images and hyperintense on T2-W images. There may be a thin rim of enhancement. Simple bone cysts do not demonstrate fluid–fluid levels [18]. Hemosiderin deposition may be observed. Fatty change may be seen within the cyst and is most often encountered in the calcaneus [13]. Especially after prior fracture, unicameral bone cysts may be multiloculated and demonstrate heterogeneous signal, nodular enhancement, and fluid–fluid levels [22].

Aneurysmal Bone Cyst

Aneurysmal bone cysts (ABC's) are large, giant cell-lined vascular spaces filled with blood products. They are neither true cysts nor true aneurysms [18, 22]. ABCs may be primary or secondary, developing within a preexisting benign or malignant bone lesion such as giant cell tumor, osteoblastoma, chondroblastoma, fibrous dysplasia, hemangioma, or nonossifying fibroma (Fig. 21.3) [23]. Patients usually present during the second decade of life, with symptoms including escalating pain, bony mass, or pathological fracture. ABCs are most common in the pelvis; metaphyseal region of the femur, tibia, or humerus; or posterior elements of the vertebrae [18]. However, they may occur at any site in any bone. Treatment of ABC is typically surgical excision.

Imaging

Radiographs and CT demonstrate an eccentrically located, radiolucent, bubbly, well-defined expansile mass that causes marked cortical thinning. Septations are common, but there should be no osseous matrix. Rapidly expanding ABCs may have poorly defined margins and aggressive periosteal reaction [5].

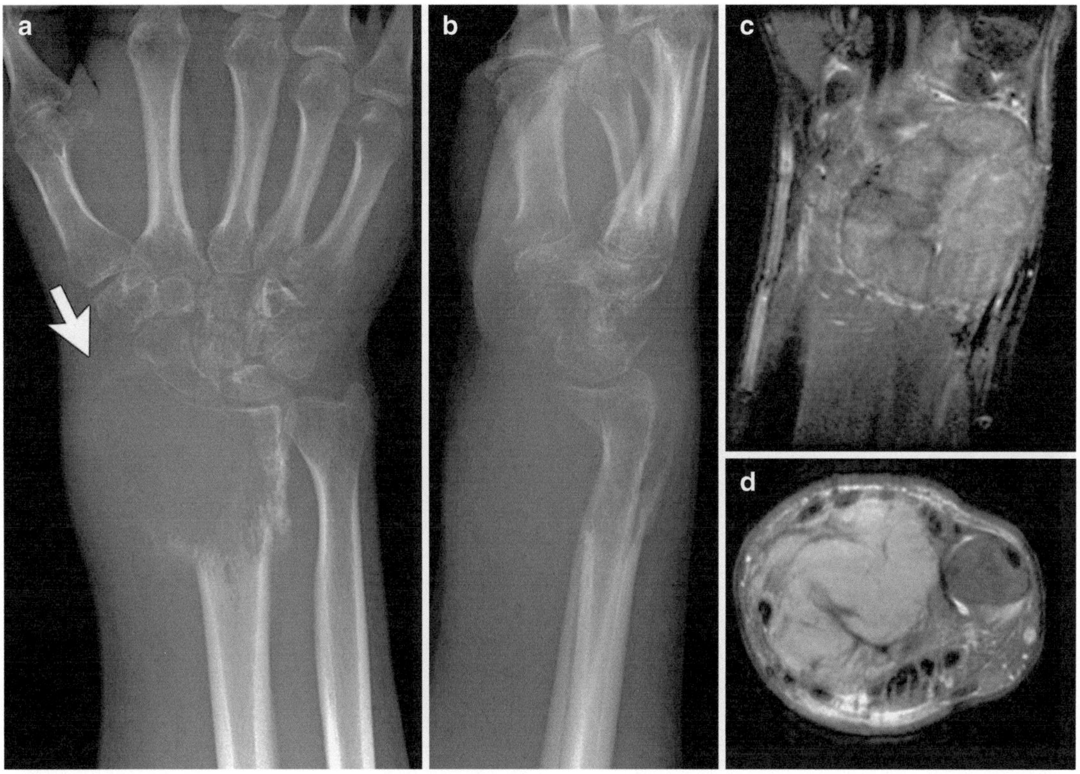

Fig. 21.5 Giant cell tumor in an 18-year-old male. (**a**, **b**) Expansile, ill-defined lytic bony mass extends to articular surface, and there is a large soft tissue mass (*white arrow*). Coronal T1-W FS (**c**) and axial proton density (PD) (**d**) images show a homogeneous lobulated mass that displaces adjacent structures. (Courtesy of John Hunter)

Bone scan typically shows a "donut sign," with moderate to intense uptake at the periphery and little activity in the center [21].

On MRI, ABCs are hypointense on T1-W images and hyperintense on T2-W images; septations are present, and low signal fibrous tissue lines the spaces [18, 24]. Fluid–fluid levels may be present, and there may be surrounding soft tissue edema. After gadolinium administration, the "cyst" walls and septations may enhance [25]. If solid tissue is present, the radiologist should consider a secondary ABC or an alternative diagnosis such as telangiectatic osteosarcoma [24].

Giant Cell Tumor

Giant cell tumors (GCTs) are very rare in children under 15 years of age and are more common in girls [1, 26]. They almost always develop after physeal closure. They are most often encountered at the knee but may also occur in the distal radius, distal tibia, proximal humerus, proximal femur, and pelvis [27]. GCTs are located in the metaphysis and do not cross the open physis [26] but may extend to the subchondral bone if the physis is closed. Patients may present with pain, swelling, limited range of motion, or pathological fracture. Treatment is usually surgical curettage/excision; occasionally, GCT may be treated with radiation therapy [28].

Imaging

On radiographs or CT, GCTs are solitary, well-defined, eccentric lytic lesions (Fig. 21.5). They lack matrix calcification and have well-defined but nonsclerotic margins. Cortical thinning is common, but periosteal reaction is unusual.

Scintigraphy shows increased radiotracer uptake on all three phases [21]. In nearly two-thirds of cases, delayed images show a nonspecific pattern of peripheral uptake with central decreased activity; diffuse increased uptake is sometimes evident [29]. Increased activity extends beyond the tumor margin.

At MRI, GCTs frequently demonstrate peripheral hypointensity on T1-W images and generalized hypointensity on T2-W images [26]. T2 hypointensity may result either from tumor cellularity or from recurrent intralesional hemorrhage. The solid portions of GCTs enhance diffusely after gadolinium administration, and cystic components demonstrate a delicate septal and peripheral enhancement pattern [26]. Reactive changes or edema at the outer cortical surface may mimic tumor extension [27]. Secondary ABC components are seen in about 14 % of GCTs.

2.2 Cartilaginous Lesions

Osteochondroma (Box 21.3)

Box 21.3: Osteochondroma

Most common pediatric benign tumor of the bone
Usually in long bones, especially about the knee
Metaphyseal, with growth away from epiphysis
Sessile or pedunculated
Continuity of periosteum, cortex, and medullary space from adjacent bone with osteochondroma
Growth during childhood, but should cease at skeletal maturity
Malignant transformation in about 1 % of solitary exostoses
Multiple hereditary exostoses (diaphyseal aclasis)
- Autosomal dominant
- Multiple osteochondromas
- Malignant transformation in 5–25 % of patients

Solitary osteochondroma is the most common benign bone tumor in children and is more common in males [30]. This tumor develops when a fragment of the epiphyseal growth plate cartilage separates and then herniates through the periosteum, or encoche of Ranvier, that normally surrounds the growth plate [31]. Osteochondromas develop only in the bone formed by enchondral ossification. They are an extension of normal bone and show continuity with the periosteum, cortex, and medullary space [5, 31].

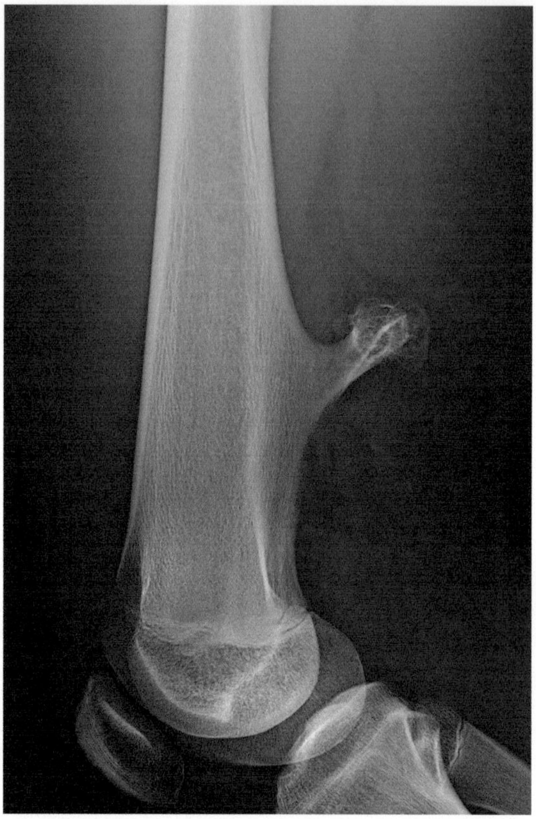

Fig. 21.6 Pedunculated osteochondroma in a teen. The cortex is intact, and the marrow trabeculae extend into the lesion

Osteochondromas are most common in the long bones, especially about the knee (Fig. 21.6). More unusual sites include the ribs, small bones of the hands and feet, scapula, pelvis, and spine [31]. Osteochondromas may develop in areas exposed to radiation therapy [1].

Osteochondromas may grow during childhood, but growth should cease at skeletal maturity. While lesions are usually asymptomatic, symptoms may result from osseous deformity, adjacent vascular injury, or neurologic compromise, fracture, or bursa formation. Osteochondromas may result in short stature. Malignant transformation, often to low-grade chondrosarcoma, occurs in about 1 % of patients with solitary osteochondroma and in 5–25 % of those with multiple hereditary extoses (MHE) [13, 24]. It is much more common in adults than in children.

Multiple hereditary exostoses (MHE, also known as diaphyseal aclasis) is an autosomal dominant disease characterized by multiple

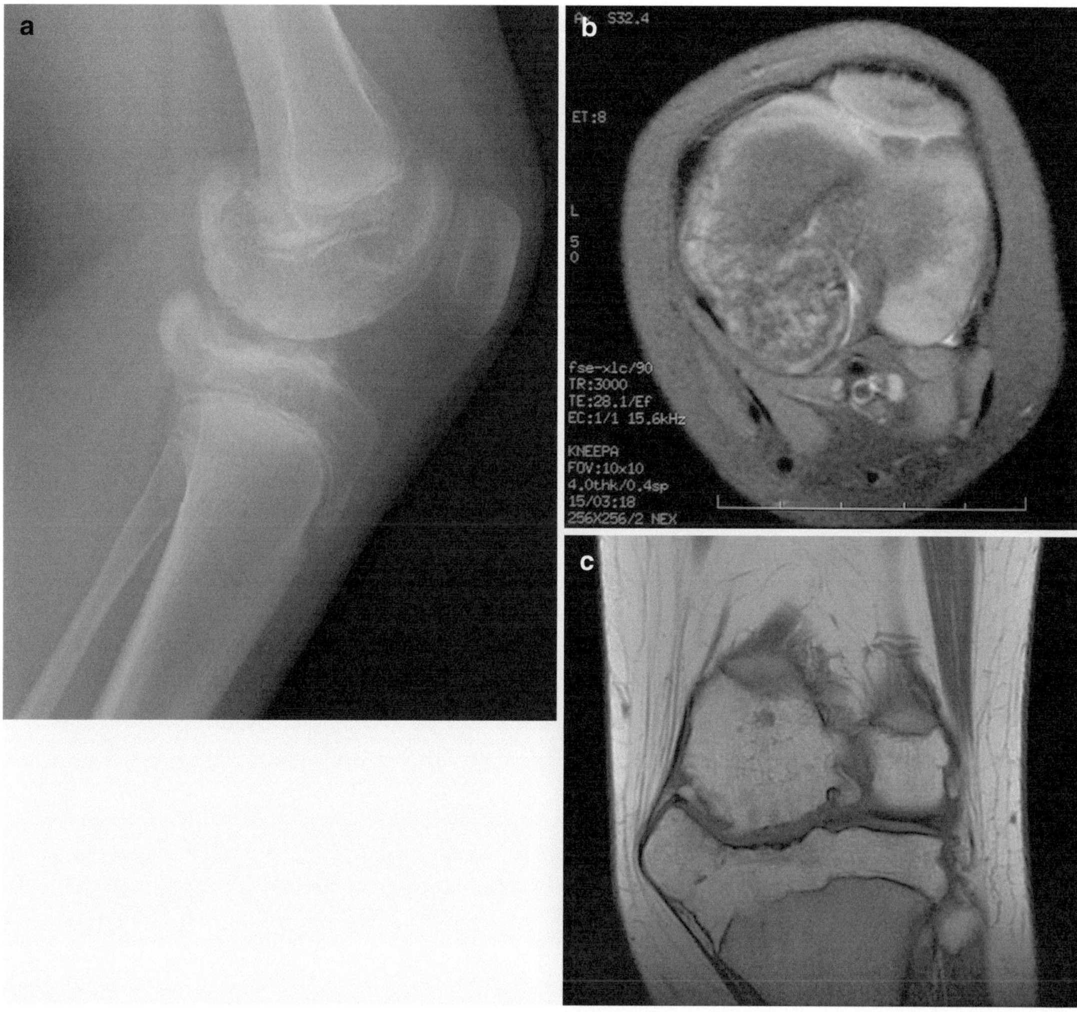

Fig. 21.7 Trevor disease. Radiograph (**a**), axial fast spin echo (*FSE*) MRI (**b**), and coronal T1-W image (**c**) show osteochondroma-like lesions at the epiphyses of the distal femur and proximal tibia (**a** copyright Shriners Hospital for Children Northern California)

osteochondromas, with genetic loci including exostosin EXT1 on chromosome 8, EXT2 on chromosome 11, and EXT3 on chromosome 19 [31]. MHE can be classified into three groups based on the extent of distal forearm involvement [32]. In Group I, the distal forearm is normal. Group II patients have exostoses at the distal forearm, but no deformity. Group III patients exhibit shortening of either the distal radius or ulna as a result of osteochondromas. Those in Group III present at an earlier age and are most likely to experience malignant transformation.

Trevor disease, also known as dysplasia epiphysealis hemimelica, is a rare, nonhereditary developmental disorder of the epiphysis of long bones, most commonly the distal femur, proximal tibia, and talus (Fig. 21.7) [33]. This most often initially manifests in boys under age 10. Cartilage growth is abnormal, and enchondral ossification results in osteochondroma-like epiphyseal lesions, usually on the medial side of the joint, limited to one side of the body [1]. The disorder may involve one or more bones of a single joint or it may be more generalized, affecting all the joints of an entire limb (e.g., hip, knee, and ankle) [34].

Treatment for symptomatic osteochondromas is surgical resection. The entire cartilage cap and perichondrium must be removed to prevent recurrence.

Imaging

In the long bones, osteochondromas initially arise on the surface of the metaphysis and grow away from the nearest epiphysis (with Trevor disease, these are epiphyseal). However, with somatic growth, the lesions appear to migrate away from the metaphysis. The lesions can be sessile or pedunculated; pedunculated lesions are more likely to deform adjacent bones. The cortex appears intact, and the trabecular pattern extends into the lesion. In the absence of fracture, there should be no periosteal reaction.

Bone scintigraphy shows increased activity in metabolically active osteochondromas. Once skeletal growth is complete, activity in the lesions should diminish to normal. Bone scan does not reliably determine malignant degeneration [31].

While most osteochondromas can be diagnosed by radiographs, CT and/or MRI may be useful for atypical cases or for preoperative planning when better anatomical definition is needed [5]. Three-dimensional (3D) CT images may be especially useful (Fig. 21.8). Thin section CT

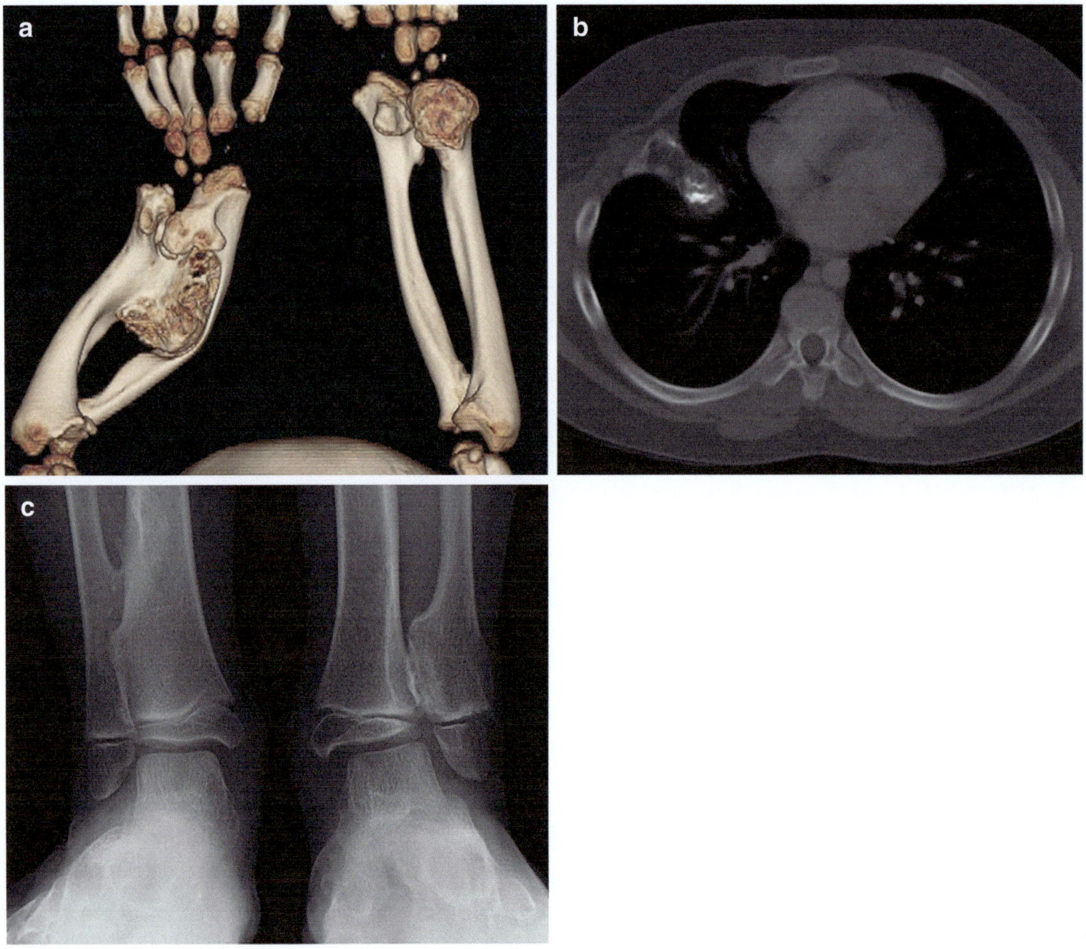

Fig. 21.8 Multiple osteochondromas in a 5-year-old boy. (**a**) 3-Dimensional (3D) CT reconstruction shows severe ulnar and radial deformity resulting from multiple osteochondromas. (**b**) Chest CT shows osteochondroma extending from the rib. (**c**) Multiple osteochondromas cause valgus angulation at the ankle

facilitates detection of intraspinal osteochondromas, which may cause spinal cord compression [31]. MRI also allows evaluation of the cartilage that covers the end of an osteochondroma (the "cartilage cap").

The cartilage cap should demonstrate intermediate signal intensity on T1-W images and hyperintensity on T2-W or STIR images. The perichondrium overlying the cartilage cap may appear as a thin, hypointense rim [13]. In children, the cap should be less than 3 cm thick.

The cartilage cap is the usual site of malignant transformation and is best assessed with fluid sensitive (T2-W or STIR) sequences. If the cartilage cap in a skeletally immature child exceeds 3 cm in thickness, the possibility of malignant degeneration should be considered (in adults, thickness greater than 2 cm should raise similar concern) [13, 23, 30]. Other features that suggest malignant change include growth of the cap after skeletal maturity, irregular cap contour, irregular lucencies or multiple foci of calcification within the lesion, soft tissue mass, irregular interface between cartilage and bone, and bony destruction [3].

Enchondroma (Box 21.4)

Box 21.4: Enchondroma

Second most common pediatric benign bone tumor

Abundant mature hyaline cartilage

Most often in small tubular bones of hands and feet

Can arise in any bone

Central, well-defined, lucent expansile mass with endosteal scalloping

Chondroid calcifications in about 50 %

Ollier disease (enchondromatosis): multiple enchondromas

Maffucci syndrome: multiple enchondromas and venous malformations

Enchondromas are the second most common benign pediatric bone tumor [1] and are characterized by the presence of abundant mature hyaline cartilage. They are most often encountered during the second decade and occur most frequently in the small tubular bones of the hands and feet (Fig. 21.9), although they can occur in

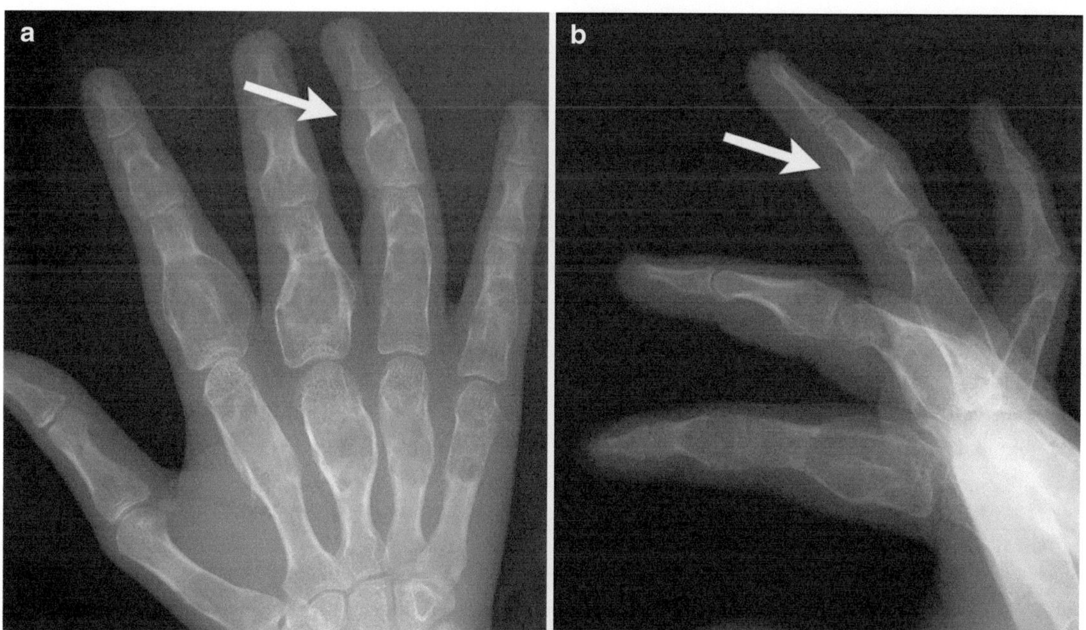

Fig. 21.9 Multiple enchondromas in the phalanges and metacarpals in a 13-year-old girl. There is a pathological fracture (*arrow*) through an enchondroma (Images courtesy of Shriners Hospital for Children Northern California)

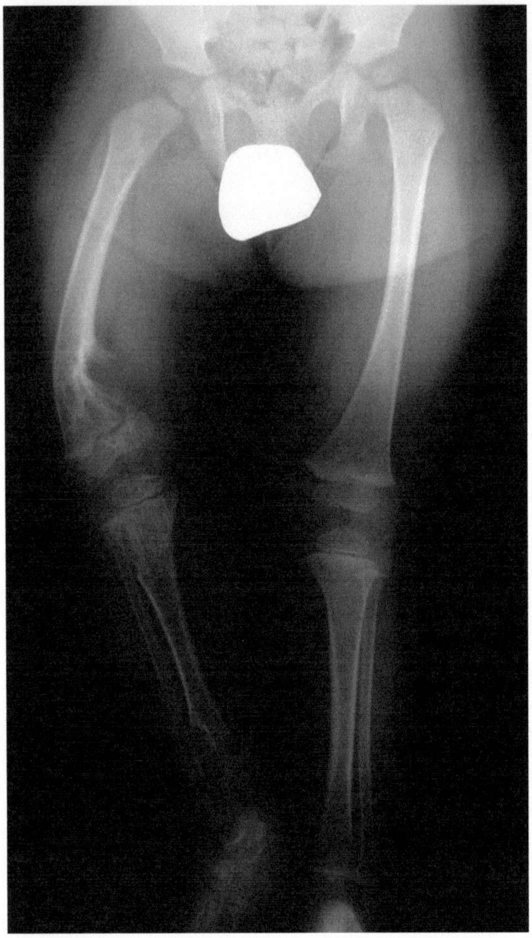

Fig. 21.10 Multiple enchondromas in a 1-year-old boy with Ollier disease. The right leg is shorter, and there is bowing of the distal right femur (Image courtesy of Shriners Hospital for Children Northern California)

any bone (Fig. 21.10). Patients may present with deformity or pain during times of rapid growth. Pain after skeletal maturity should raise the concern for malignant transformation or pathological fracture.

Ollier disease, or enchondromatosis, is a nonhereditary condition that occurs when abnormal growth plate cartilage leads to the development of multiple enchondromas. Patients may have leg length discrepancy due to asymmetrical involvement of the lower extremities. Maffucci syndrome consists of venous malformations in addition to multiple enchondromas. Malignant transformation of enchondroma to (usually) chondrosarcoma may occur in up to 30 % of patients with Ollier disease [1] and in up to half of those with Maffucci syndrome [35].

Imaging

Enchondromas are central, well-defined, expansile masses that cause endosteal scalloping. Chondroid calcifications are seen in about 50 % of cases [5]. At MRI, they appear as lobulated T1-hypointense and T2-hyperintense lesions that may contain hypointense foci of calcification [30]. Chemical shift artifact may be present, due to intralesional fat. Contrast-enhanced (CE) images may show a "ring and arc" pattern corresponding to fibrovascular tissue at the periphery of the avascular lobules of hyaline cartilage [24].

Chondroblastoma

Chondroblastoma is an uncommon and benign tumor of the primary cartilage that appears during the second and third decades of life [36]. Located eccentrically in the medullary space of the epiphysis or apophysis, this tumor usually occurs in the femur, humerus, or tibia (Fig. 21.11). It may extend into the adjacent joint, and in about half of cases, it extends into the metaphysis.

Imaging

On radiographs, chondroblastomas have a geographic-appearing contour, and there is marginal sclerosis. Stippled intralesional chondroid calcification may be present [5].

MRI shows a lobulated, heterogeneous lesion [37]. Matrix calcifications are very hypointense on both T1-W and T2-W sequences, while islands of cartilage are T1 hypointense and T2 hyperintense. A peripheral, thin (<1 mm), hypointense rim is characteristic but may be incomplete; this corresponds to marginal sclerosis that may be evident radiographically [37]. Associated marrow edema is common and may be extensive; soft tissue edema may be present as well. Associated synovitis may be seen [5]. After gadolinium administration, lobular enhancement is apparent in about 60 % of cases [36]. Septal enhancement suggests an associated ABC.

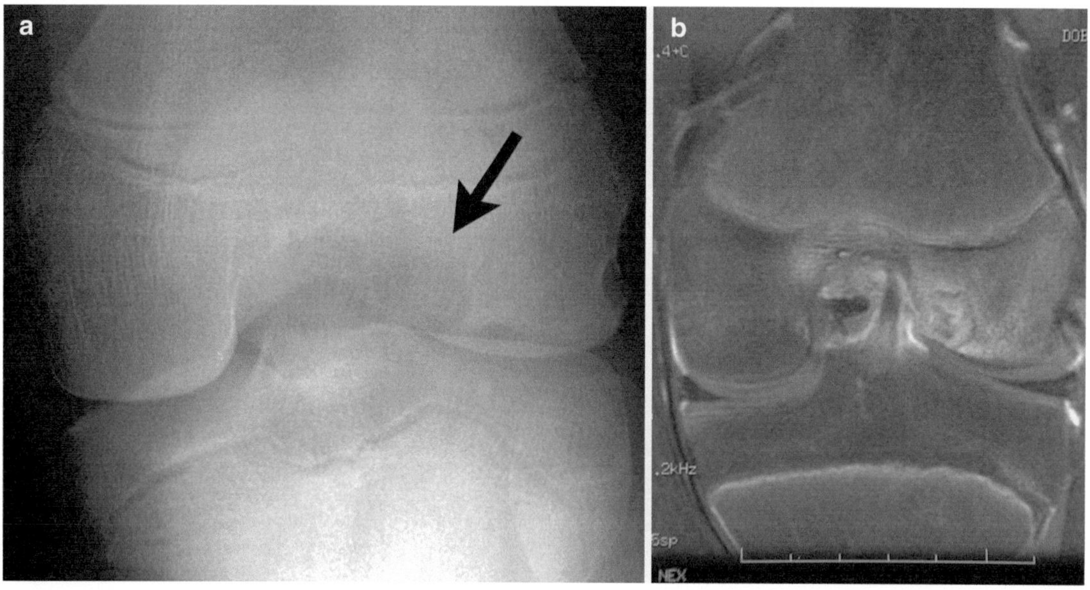

Fig. 21.11 Chondroblastoma. (**a**) Subtle rounded lytic lesion (*arrow*). (**b**). Coronal T1-W FS gadolinium-enhanced image shows inhomogeneous central enhancement, a surrounding hypointense rim, and adjacent epiphyseal hyperemia/enhancement

2.3 Osseous Lesions

Osteoid Osteoma

Osteoid osteoma is a benign tumor that is most common in boys in the second decade of life. Primitive woven bone and osteoid make up this hypervascular tumor. The tumor elicits a strong prostaglandin-mediated inflammatory response in the surrounding tissue [38], causing pain that is often more severe at night and relieved by aspirin [1, 39]. Osteoid osteoma occurs most often in the cortex of the shafts of tubular bones, especially the femur and tibia. It may also be seen in the posterior elements of the vertebrae (see Chap. 4) where it may cause painful scoliosis. Treatment of osteoid osteoma involves percutaneous ablation or surgical removal of the nidus.

Imaging

Radiographically, this tumor is characterized by intense, dense cortical thickening that contains a paracortical radiolucent nidus measuring less than 2 cm (Fig. 21.12).

CT best identifies the nidus and can differentiate the lesion from other intracortical processes, including stress fractures or intracortical abscesses [5]. It also helps plan image-guided intervention. At CT, the hypodense nidus contains a variable amount of mineralization and is surrounded by reactive sclerosis, periosteal reaction, and new bone formation [5].

Bone scintigraphy is very sensitive in detecting osteoid osteoma. The nidus demonstrates intense increased uptake, and there is moderately increased uptake in the surrounding reactive bone [40].

At MRI, cortical thickening appears hypointense on all pulse sequences [30]. The nidus varies in appearance, depending upon the amount of matrix and osteoid [23]. Its signal intensity ranges from T1 isointense and T2 hyperintense to hypointense on all pulse sequences. The nidus enhances with gadolinium. Edema may be quite prominent in the marrow or soft tissues, appearing hyperintense on STIR or T2-W sequences.

Less commonly, osteoid osteoma may be located in cancellous (medullary) bone and may be intra-articular (most often at the hip). Synovitis and joint effusion are often seen in such lesions, and reactive osteosclerosis is typically less intense and may not be centered about the

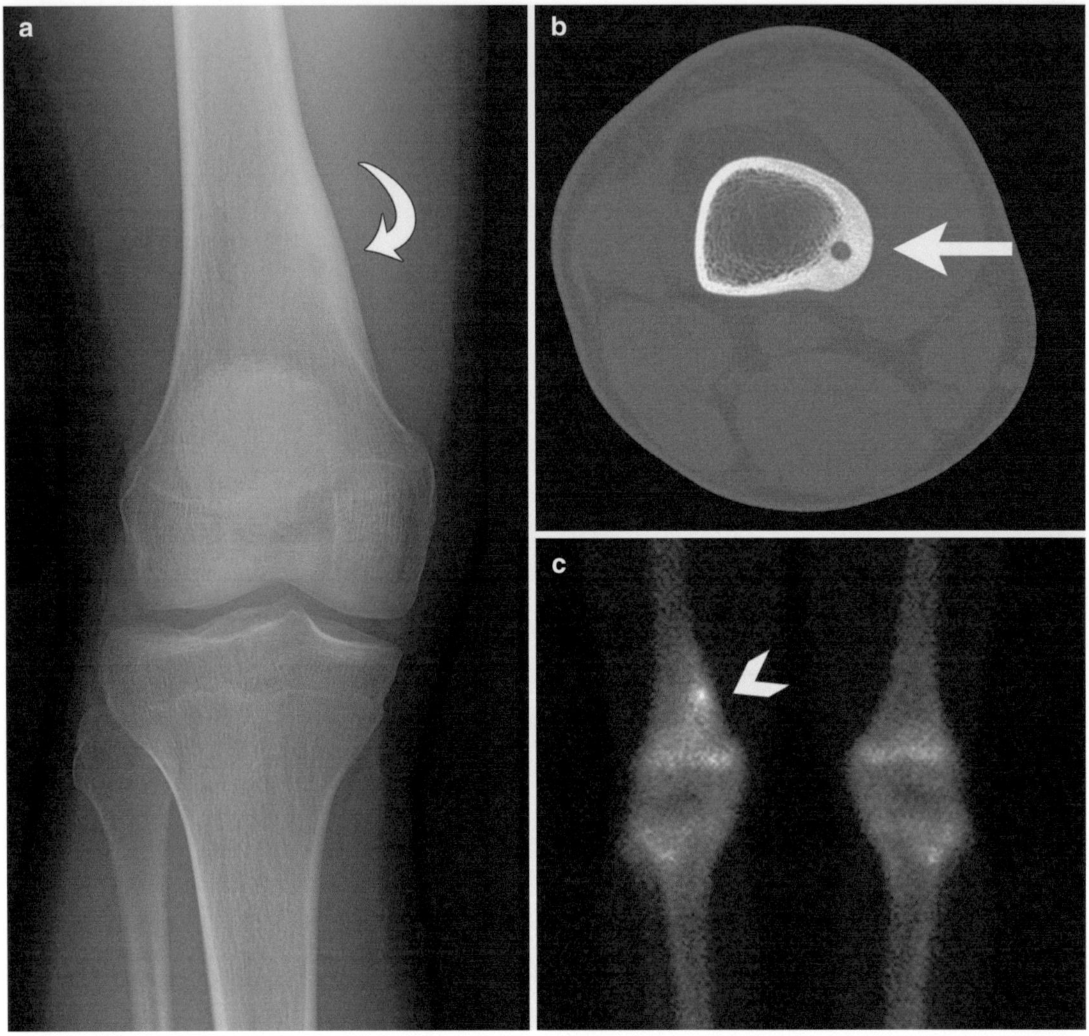

Fig. 21.12 Osteoid osteoma in a 16-year-old girl. (**a**) There is mature periosteal thickening (*curved arrow*), with the lucent nidus vaguely visible. (**b**) CT shows the hypodense nidus (*white arrow*). (**c**) Bone scintigraphy shows generalized increased uptake with more focal uptake at the nidus (*white arrowhead*)

nidus [41]. Occasionally, a cancellous osteoid osteoma may be located within the epiphysis, or within the small bones of the foot and hand. Subperiosteal osteoid osteoma is the rarest type and is usually found at the femoral neck or in the hands or feet (often talus). It is associated with an adjacent soft tissue mass; there may also be irregular bone resorption. Subperiosteal osteoid osteomas generally do not produce surrounding osteosclerosis. Scintigraphy, CT, and MRI are useful in identifying the tumor nidus in these unusual cases.

Osteoblastoma

Osteoblastomas are rare and differ from osteoid osteomas in that the nidus is larger than 2 cm in diameter (Fig. 21.13). This tumor also shows greater histologic variability [24]. It is most common in the posterior elements of the spine, where it may present as an osteolytic expansile tumor with shell-like periosteal reaction [5] (see Chap. 4). In the long bones, it is more commonly eccentrically positioned in the medullary bone of the diaphysis (followed by the metaphysis) [42]. Osteoblastoma may also be seen in the small bones of the hands

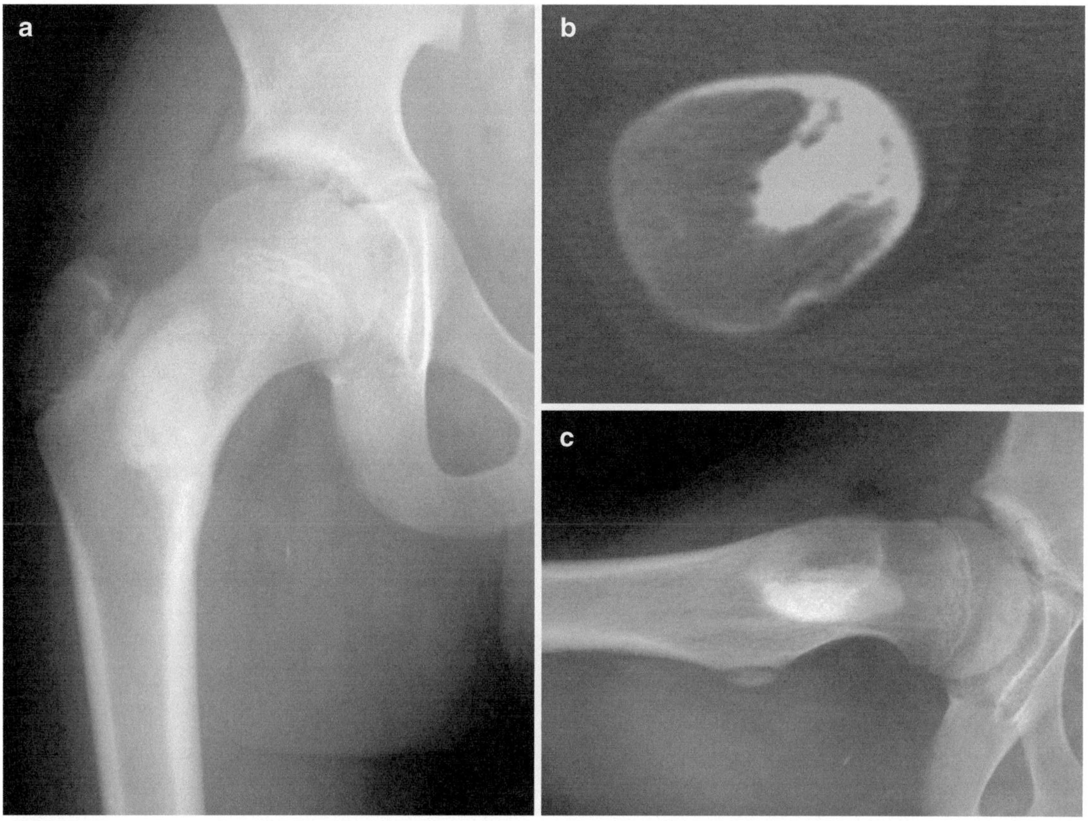

Fig. 21.13 Osteoblastoma. Radiographs (**a**, **c**) and CT (**b**) show a sclerotic intertrochanteric mass

and feet or in the pelvis, skull, or ribs. The pain with osteoblastoma is typically less intense than with osteoid osteoma and is not worse at night. Treatment involves removal of the tumor nidus.

The radiographic appearance of osteoblastoma varies. The tumor usually appears as a lucent, expansile mass with a rim of surrounding sclerosis, but it may be completely sclerotic. It is typically well defined and round or ovoid. Matrix calcification is common. Solid or lamellated periosteal reaction is usually present. Cortical thinning and bony expansion may be seen. There may be an associated soft tissue mass. Occasionally, this tumor has a more aggressive appearance, with moth-eaten borders and spiculated periosteal reaction [42].

As with osteoid osteoma, scintigraphy shows increased uptake within the nidus. CT typically demonstrates a lytic lesion with osteoid matrix and periosteal reaction, but again the appearance varies.

At MRI, the appearance depends upon the amount of matrix and osteoid. As with osteoid osteoma, there is often prominent surrounding edema [43]. MRI may overestimate the size and extent of the lesion since there may be extensive inflammatory response and enhancement [23, 44]. Secondary ABCs are associated with osteoblastomas and are suggested by the presence of fluid–fluid levels.

2.4 Fibro-osseous Lesions

Nonossifying Fibroma/Fibrous Cortical Defect

Nonossifying fibromas (NOFs) and fibrous cortical defects are common in children and adolescents and are usually painless, incidental findings. These lesions are differentiated by size: fibrous cortical defects measure less than 2 cm,

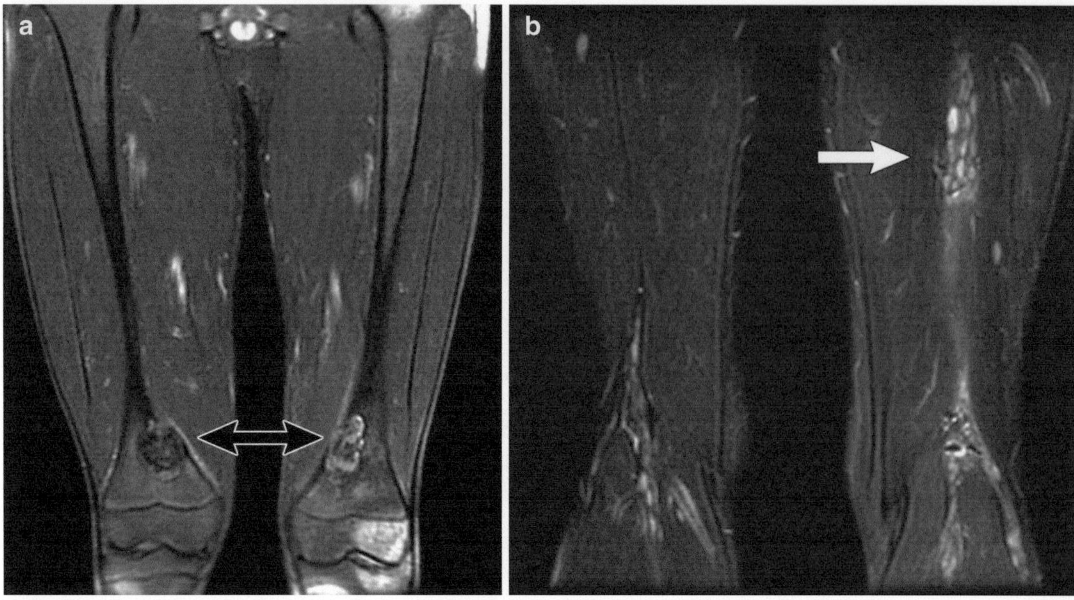

Fig. 21.14 Multiple nonossifying fibromas in a 15-year-old boy with Jaffe–Campanacci syndrome. (**a**, **b**) Coronal T2-W FS images show multiple nonossifying fibromas (*black arrows*) along with plexiform neurofibromas (*white arrow*) along the sciatic nerve

while NOFs are larger. They are eccentrically positioned in the metaphysis and metadiaphysis of long bones, usually in the lower extremities. Both regress over time and are not seen after 25 years of age [23]. Larger lesions may present with pain due to pathological fracture. Multiple nonossifying fibromas accompanied with café-au-lait spots characterize Jaffe–Campanacci syndrome; this may be a manifestation of neurofibromatosis type 1 (Fig. 21.14) [45, 46]. Most require no biopsy or treatment. If large, prophylactic curettage and bone grafting may be performed to avoid a pathological fracture.

Imaging

NOFs and fibrous cortical defects are eccentric, well-defined, cortically based lesions with marginal sclerosis [39] (Fig. 21.15). They are oriented longitudinally with respect to the axis of long bones, such that they are longer than they are wide. In narrow bones, such as the fibula, they may appear central rather than eccentric. No periosteal reaction is seen.

Fibrous cortical defects show mild peripheral uptake on bone scan, whereas NOFs show more diffuse increased uptake; the latter may mimic fibrous dysplasia. During healing, osteoblastic activity may lead to more intense increased uptake in NOFs [21].

At MRI imaging, both lesions are hypointense on T1-W images, whereas T2 signal varies depending on the extent of hypercellular fibrous tissue. Signal intensity is increased while the lesions are developing and decreases as they heal [5, 30]. A thin rim enhances after gadolinium administration [23]. (See Chap. 13 for additional discussion of NOFs and fibrous cortical defects.)

Fibrous Dysplasia

Fibrous dysplasia is a nonhereditary developmental abnormality characterized by fibrous cellular tissue and irregular bone trabeculae. Fibrous dysplasia can develop in any bone. Most cases are monostotic and asymptomatic, but about 20 % of cases are polyostotic. Symptoms may include bone pain, deformity, or pathological fracture. The combination of polyostotic fibrous dysplasia, café-au-lait skin lesions, precocious puberty, and endocrine dysfunction constitutes McCune–Albright syndrome. Fibrous dysplasia is usually a disease of young children, and lesions become quiescent with puberty [47]. The main complications of fibrous dysplasia are deformity and pathological fracture. Malignant sarcomatous

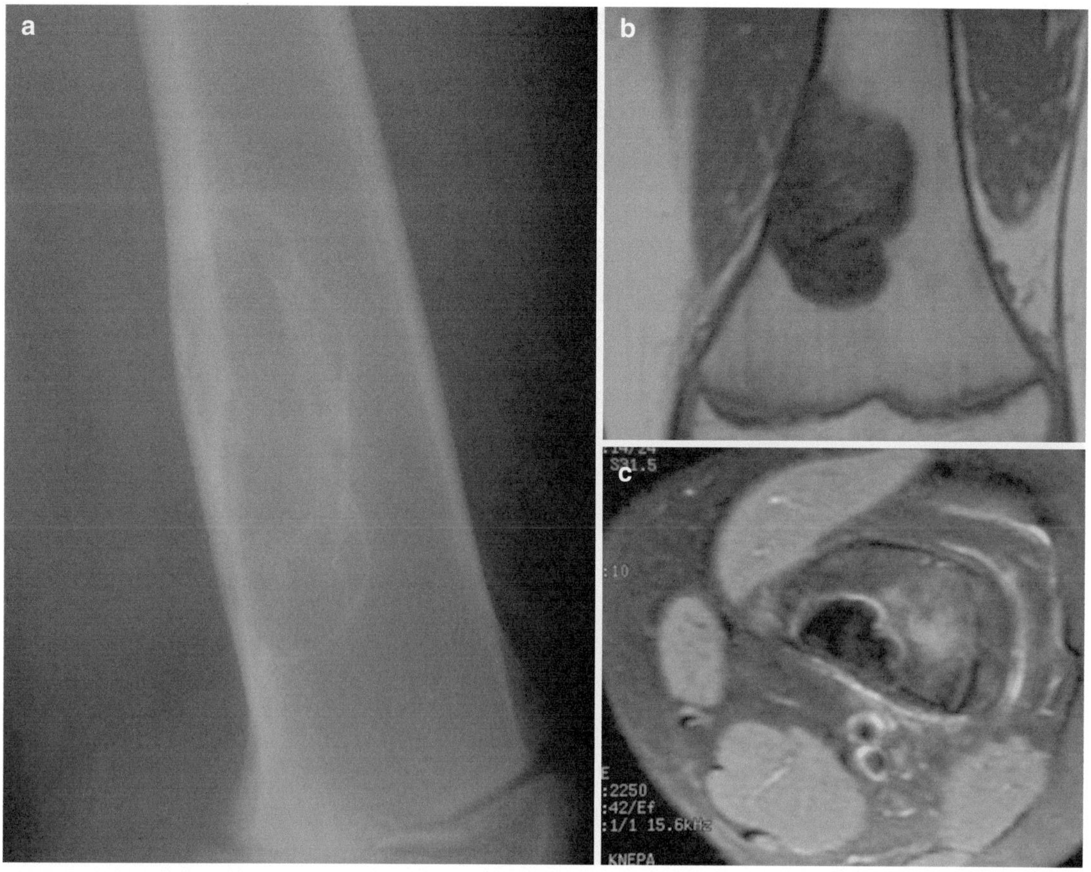

Fig. 21.15 Nonossifying fibroma. (**a**) Eccentric, scalloped, lytic lesion has a well-defined sclerotic margin, with the longest axis parallel to the diaphysis. It is hypointense on coronal T1-W (**b**) and axial fluid-sensitive (**c**) sequences

degeneration is rare. Treatment is symptomatic, such as fracture fixation or bisphosphonates for bone pain.

Imaging

Radiographically, fibrous dysplasia appears as a well-defined, expansile, ground-glass lesion with a sclerotic rim and sometimes endosteal scalloping [47] (Fig. 21.16). If the lesion contains a significant amount of cartilage, popcorn-like or more confluent calcification may be seen.

Fibrous dysplasia usually shows increased uptake on bone scintigraphy and is hypermetabolic at PET imaging [5, 7]. If the lesion is undergoing infarction, or becoming quiescent with maturation, it may appear normal on bone scan [21].

MRI readily demonstrates the extent of fibrous dysplasia. The lesion appears as a sharply defined intramedullary mass without cortical destruction. It is T1 hypo- to isointense and T2 hyperintense. Heterogeneity within fibrous dysplasia results from a combination of calcification, cysts, fatty areas, and/or septations. No matter the pulse sequence, a rim of hypointense signal typically surrounds the lesion, corresponding to the sclerotic rim evident on radiographs [47]. Enhancement may be patchy or homogeneous and may be limited to the rim.

Osteofibrous Dysplasia

Osteofibrous dysplasia presents with painless anterior bowing of the tibia (or rarely the fibula) and may be associated with a mass [23]. The lesion is usually limited to young children under age 10. Management varies from observation to surgical intervention, depending on the age of the patient and the extent of the lesion. The recurrence rate is relatively high if surgery is performed before skeletal maturity [48].

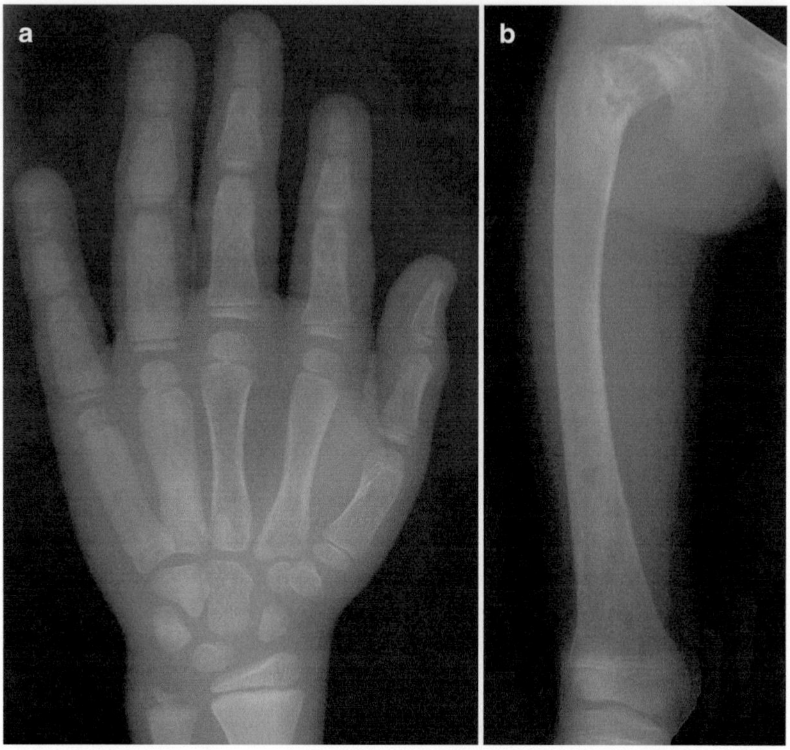

Fig. 21.16 Polyostotic fibrous dysplasia. (**a**) Ground-glass expansion of the fourth and fifth metacarpals and multiple phalanges. (**b**) Coxa vara deformity and lateral bowing with classic ground-glass opacity, focal lucencies, and mild metaphyseal and diaphyseal expansion (Images copyright Shriners Hospital for Children Northern California)

Imaging

The radiographic appearance of osteofibrous dysplasia is fairly pathognomonic. Arising on the anterior cortex of the diaphysis, the lesion slowly spreads longitudinally; there may be associated deformity (Fig. 21.17). It is cortically based, loculated, and expansile with sclerotic margins. Periosteal reaction only occurs in conjunction with pathological fracture. The lesion is hyperintense compared to muscle on T1-W imaging and hyperintense on T2-W imaging [49] (Fig. 21.18). Surrounding soft tissues appear normal.

2.5 Vascular Lesions

Vascular lesions are rarely confined to bone in children but instead present as soft tissue masses [1]. Intraosseous hemangiomas are the most common bony pediatric vascular lesion.

Hemangioma

Of all osseous hemangiomas, less than five percent are detected in children and adolescents [50]. Hemangiomas are often discovered incidentally and occur most frequently in the spine or skull [24]. In the spine, they are usually located within the vertebral body and infrequently in the posterior elements [51]. They are composed of capillaries and vascular spaces interposed between the bony trabeculae. Lipomatous tissue contributes to the expansile nature of this lesion. There is usually no evidence of prior hemorrhage within the lesion [51]. Hemangiomas of bone rarely require treatment.

Imaging

Radiographically, hemangiomas appear as a honeycomb pattern of thickened trabeculae and soft tissue stroma [51] (Fig. 21.19). On MRI, their appearance depends on the ratio of lipomatous tissue to vascular elements. Vascular elements are hypointense on T1-W sequences and hyperintense on fluid-sensitive sequences, while fatty elements are hyperintense on T1-W sequences and hypointense on STIR or fat-suppressed sequences [24, 50]. Hemangiomas enhance homogeneously after administration of contrast material.

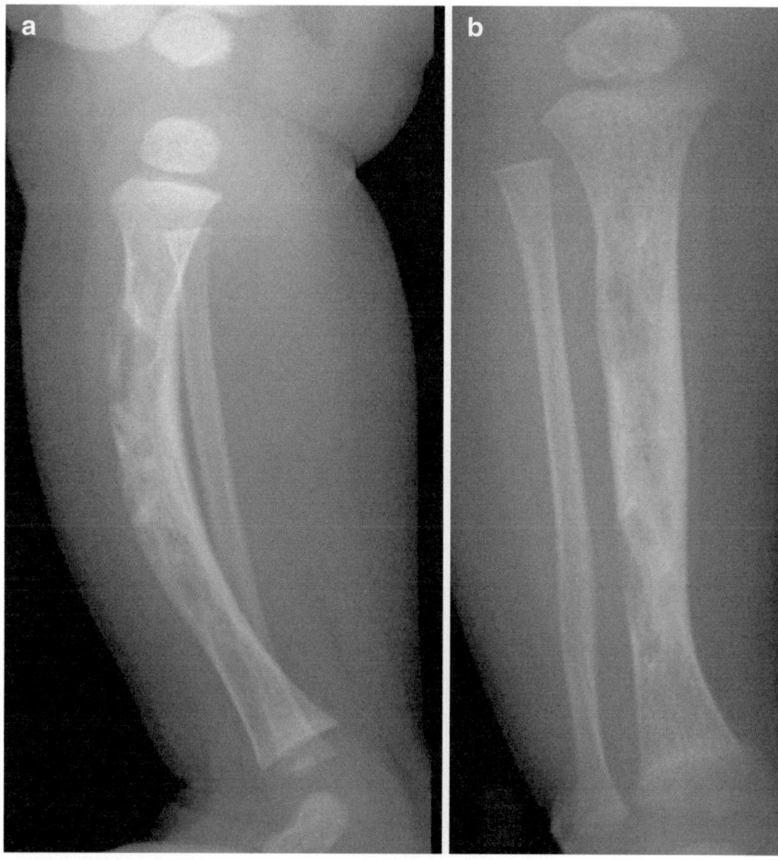

Fig. 21.17 Osteofibrous dysplasia in a 2-year-old. (**a**, **b**) There is anterior bowing of the tibia and a well-defined, septated, mildly expansile anterior lytic lesion

2.6 Langerhans Cell Histiocytosis (Box 21.5)

> **Box 21.5: Langerhans Cell Histiocytosis (LCH)**
>
> Prostaglandins produced by Langerhans cells cause medullary bone resorption
>
> Younger patients have more severe involvement
>
> Solitary bony lesions more common than multifocal disease
>
> Usually skull, jaw, ribs, vertebral bodies, and proximal long bones
>
> Extraskeletal involvement: liver, spleen, lymph nodes, lungs, and pituitary
>
> Early stage: poorly defined, permeative lesions ± lamellated periosteal reaction
>
> Late stage: well-defined, ovoid osteolytic lesions ± surrounding sclerosis
>
> Bony sequestration
>
> Skull lesions: beveled edge
>
> Spine: vertebra plana

Langerhans cell histiocytosis (LCH) results from an abnormal proliferation of antigen-presenting histiocytes, or Langerhans cells. These cells produce prostaglandins that cause resorption of medullary bone. It is unclear if the process is inflammatory or neoplastic. Early in the course of the disease, the lesion is characterized by inflammatory infiltration. This is followed by a granulomatous phase and finally a fibrous phase [52].

The lesions may arise in any hematopoietically active bone, but they are most common in the skull, jaw, ribs, vertebral bodies, and proximal long bones. Solitary bony lesions are more common than multifocal disease [1]. Extraskeletal involvement may include the liver, spleen, lymph nodes, and lungs [53]. Pituitary involvement may result in endocrine dysfunction (anterior pituitary) or diabetes insipidus (posterior pituitary) [54].

Patients usually present in the first decade and may be asymptomatic or have bone pain [1].

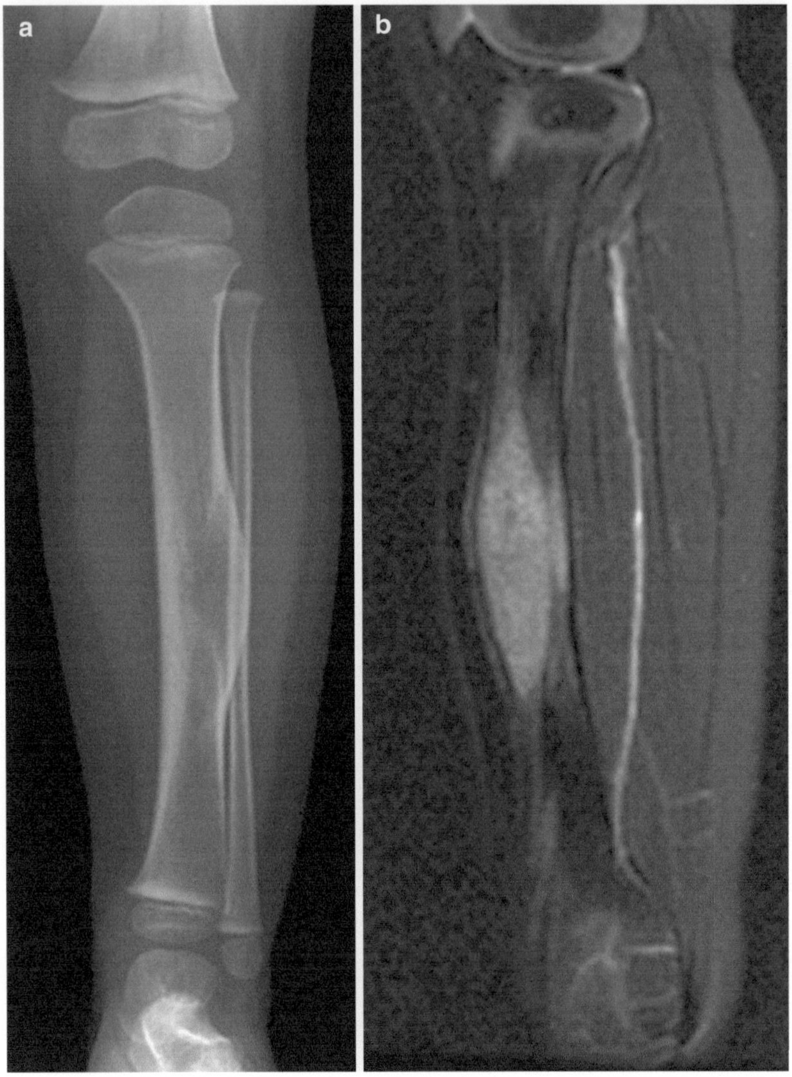

Fig. 21.18 Osteofibrous dysplasia in a 3-year-old. (**a**) Expansile lenticular lytic mass. (**b**) Mass is hyperintense on sagittal T2-W image

Girls are affected more commonly than boys, and younger patients tend to have more severe involvement than older children. Depending on the site and extent of disease, treatment of LCH may include chemotherapy, radiation therapy, and/or surgery.

Imaging

The appearance of LCH varies widely on radiographs and CT (Fig. 21.20). In the early stages, lesions may appear permeative and poorly defined, with lamellated periosteal reaction. In the later stage, they may appear ovoid, well-defined, and homogeneously lytic, with variable marginal sclerosis [1, 55]. Sometimes bone appears normal, although a lesion is known to be present. A bony sequestrum may be evident. Skull lesions often appear to have a beveled edge due to relatively more involvement of the inner table. Spinal lesions may present as vertebra plana. Absence of involvement of adjacent discs helps differentiate spinal LCH from osteomyelitis or discitis [52].

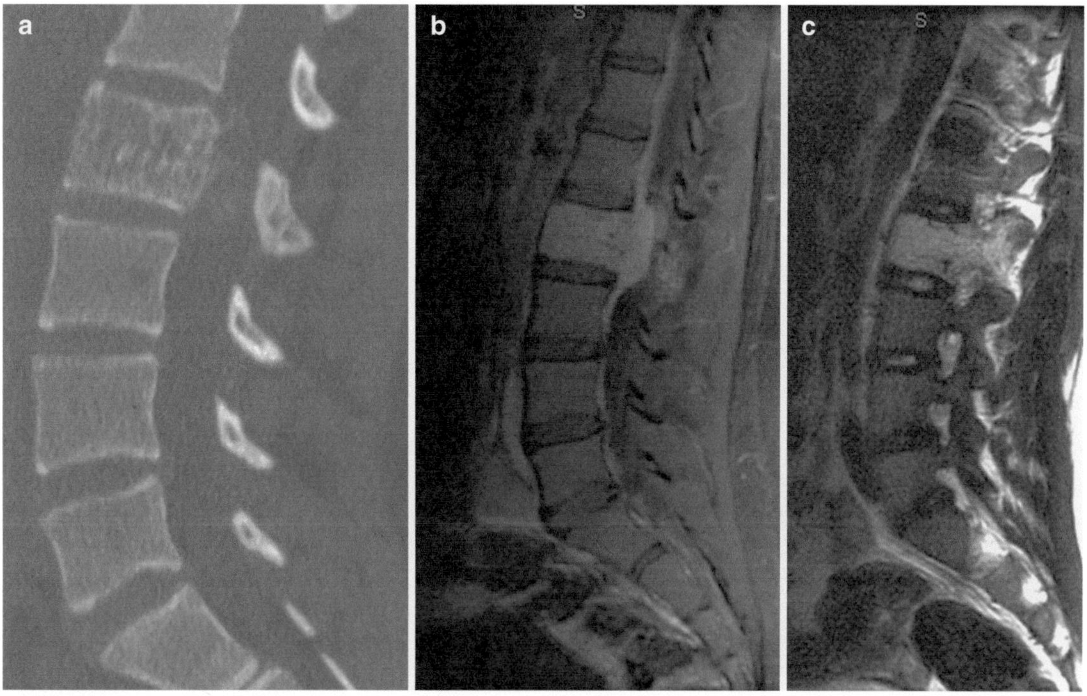

Fig. 21.19 Vertebral hemangioma in a 13-year-old girl. (**a**) Sagittal reformatted CT shows coarse trabeculae and mild expansion at L2 vertebral body. (**b**) Sagittal T1-W gadolinium-enhanced image shows the lesion enhances diffusely. (**c**) Sagittal T2-W image shows increased signal in the pedicle and vertebral body

On bone scan, lesions may show increased, decreased, or normal activity [7]. Bone scans and radiographic skeletal surveys are complementary, as some lesions are evident on only one of these imaging techniques [21]. Bone scan may be better than radiography for assessing response to treatment [21].

MRI best demonstrates bone marrow involvement, soft tissue mass, and surrounding inflammation [52, 56]. Lesions are focal, variable on T1-W images, and hyperintense on T2 and STIR images. Early in the course of the disease, the lesions markedly enhance after gadolinium administration. Lesions may show surrounding marrow and/or soft tissue edema, which are best seen on STIR images. Cortical breech and soft tissue masses may also be seen.

As lesions heal, MRI demonstrates decrease in lesion size, degree of T2 hyperintensity, and extent of contrast enhancement [53, 57]. On STIR imaging, an endosteal rim of decreased signal intensity denotes the marginal sclerosis that may develop with early healing [56]. Marrow and soft tissue edema also resolve.

Whole-body coronal MRI, including STIR and T1-W sequences, is better than skeletal survey or bone scintigraphy at showing the extent of disease [52, 53]. Post-gadolinium whole-body coronal imaging may also be useful.

3 Malignant Tumors

About 6 % of all childhood malignancies are malignant bone tumors, most commonly osteosarcoma and Ewing sarcoma (www.seer.cancer.gov/publications/childhood/bone.pdf). Imaging plays a major role in diagnosis. Radiographs provide essential information about the presence of bone forming elements, whereas MRI delineates tumor extent and its effect on adjacent structures.

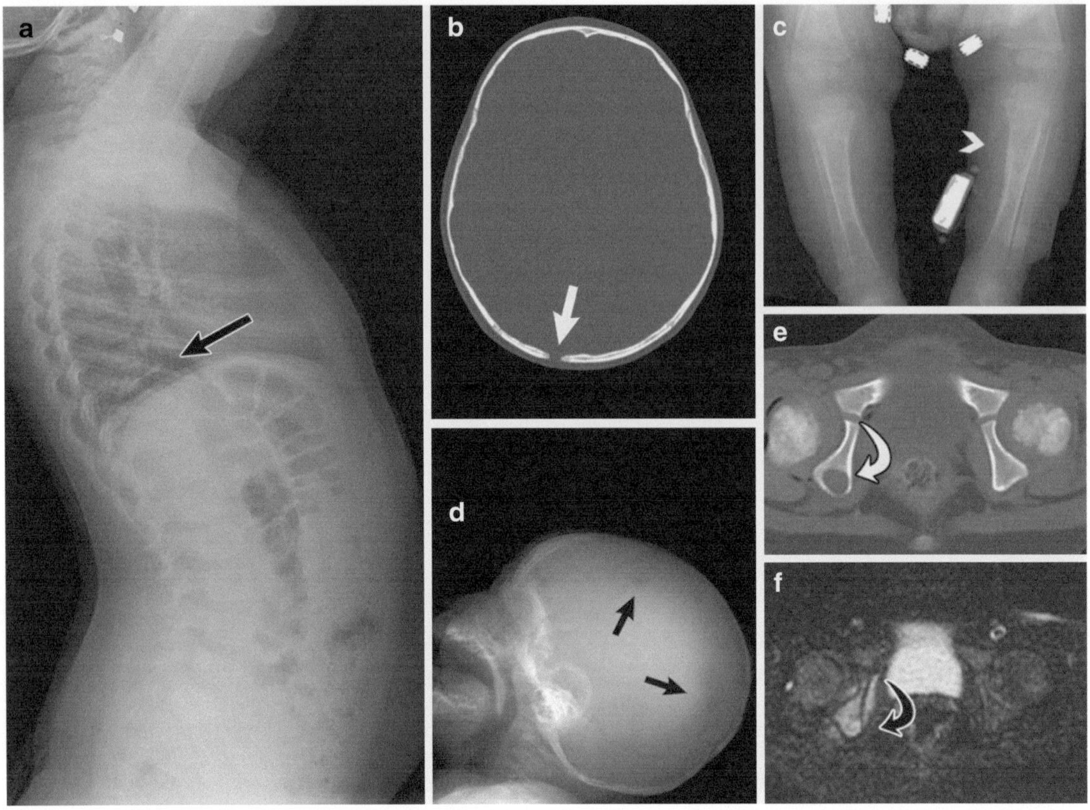

Fig. 21.20 Langerhans cell histiocytosis. (**a**) Vertebral plana (*black arrow*). (**b**) CT shows well-defined lytic lesion (*white arrow*) involving the inner and outer tables of the calvarium. (**c**) Geographic lytic lesion (*arrowhead*). (**d**) Multiple beveled skull lesions (*black arrows*). (**e**) CT shows a round, well-defined lytic lesion (*curved white arrow*), which is hyperintense on T2-W FS image (*curved black arrow*) (**f**)

3.1 Osteosarcoma (Box 21.6)

Box 21.6: Osteosarcoma

Most common primary malignant bone tumor in children

Origin usually metaphyseal, central medullary

Common sites: distal femur, proximal tibia, proximal humerus

Blastic, mixed, or lytic aggressive metaphyseal bony lesion

Indistinct margins, cortical destruction

Aggressive periosteal reaction, soft tissue mass

Metastases in about 20 % at presentation

Skip lesions in primary bone in 15 % (MRI)

Osteosarcoma is the most common primary malignant bone tumor in children, with an annual incidence of 4.4 per million children under age 20 [58]. About 400 children are diagnosed with osteosarcoma in the United States every year. Usually, the patient is in their second decade and presents with a painful mass. Due to its association with rapid longitudinal growth, on average girls present earlier than boys, at 12 years of age versus 16. However, the tumor is slightly more common in males and also slightly more common in black children than in white children [9]. Serum alkaline phosphatase levels are elevated in about half of cases [16]. While there is no generalized underlying etiology for the development of this tumor, there is

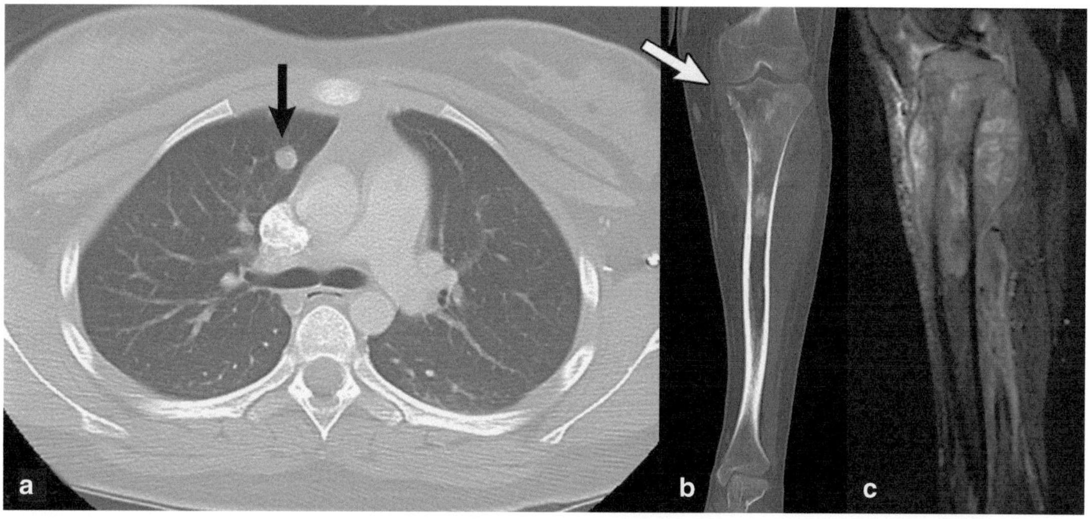

Fig. 21.21 Metastatic osteosarcoma in an 11-year-old. (**a**) CT shows a pulmonary mass (*black arrow*). (**b**) Coronally reformatted CT shows a destructive bone-forming tumor with epiphyseal involvement (*white arrow*) and a surrounding soft tissue mass. (**c**) Sagittal T2-W image further defines the inhomogeneous but predominantly hyperintense proximal tibial intramedullary and circumferential soft tissue mass. There is adjacent subcutaneous edema

an increased risk of osteosarcoma in patients with retinoblastoma and Li–Fraumeni syndrome and in those who have received radiation therapy.

Osteosarcomas derive from primitive bone-forming mesenchymal stem cells and may be pathologically described as osteoblastic, chondroblastic, or fibroblastic based on the tumor's predominant tissue type [1]. Children generally have conventional, high-grade osteosarcoma. Other subtypes include giant cell-rich, telangiectatic, and small cell [16]. Cytogenetic analysis of osteosarcomas frequently shows karyotypic abnormalities including gain in regions of chromosome 1 and loss in regions of chromosomes 6, 9, 10, 13, and 17 [59].

Osteosarcomas occur in both medullary and surface locations, and both locations are characterized by low-grade and high-grade subtypes. The "classic" central medullary osteosarcoma and the high-grade surface subtypes both have a worse prognosis than the parosteal and periosteal surface or the low-grade intraosseous subtypes [1, 9]. Pediatric osteosarcomas are usually metaphyseal and central medullary in origin. The most common sites in decreasing order of frequency are the distal femur (35 % of patients), proximal tibia (17 %), and proximal humerus (10 %), followed by the pelvis, jaw, fibula, and ribs [16]. Skip lesions are present in the primary bone in 15 % of patients.

Preoperative staging of osteosarcoma is important, as about 20 % of children with osteosarcoma have detectable metastases at presentation, usually within the lung (Fig. 21.21). Thus high-resolution chest CT is necessary for initial evaluation.

Following staging, treatment usually includes primary tumor wide resection, often with limb salvage surgery, and chemotherapy. Radiation therapy may be utilized in cases where the primary tumor cannot be completely resected.

Imaging

The tumor is characterized by production of bone and often appears blastic or mixed lytic/blastic, although it can appear purely lytic (Fig. 21.22). On radiographs and CT, it usually appears as a large, aggressive metaphyseal lesion with indistinct margins, cortical destruction, aggressive periosteal reaction, and a soft tissue mass. Pathological fracture is uncommon except with the rare telangiectatic osteosarcoma [16, 60].

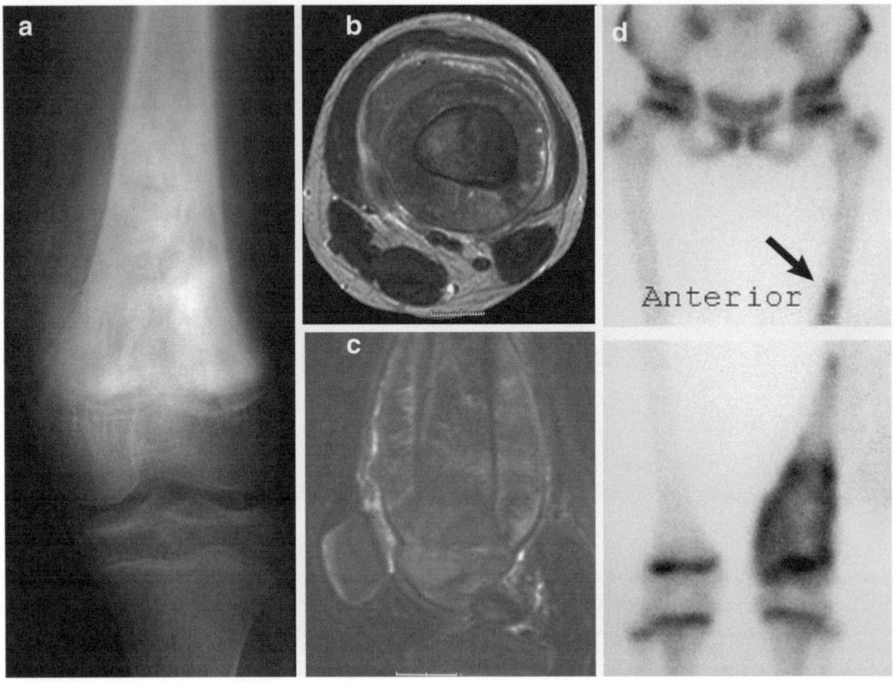

Fig. 21.22 Osteosarcoma in a 10-year-old girl. (**a**) Bone-producing mass with sunburst periosteal reaction. (**b**) Axial T1-W image shows the mass surrounds the distal femur. (**c**) Sagittal T1-W FS gadolinium-enhanced image shows the enhancing mass crosses the physis and extends into the epiphysis. (**d**) Bone scintigraphy shows increased uptake in the primary tumor, as well as a skip lesion in the proximal femur (*arrow*)

Bone does not have lymphatic drainage, and the rare presence of tumor in regional lymph nodes portends a worse prognosis [9].

FDG-PET has not been shown to be more sensitive than bone scan in the detection of bony metastases in osteosarcoma. Furthermore, it is less sensitive than dedicated chest CT in detecting pulmonary metastases [10, 61]. FDG-PET does help clarify cases in which MRI findings are equivocal, such as in detecting skip lesions in areas of red marrow, which is more cellular than fatty yellow marrow. It also helps determine response to therapy, as discussed below. FDG-PET/CT may be more useful than conventional imaging for detecting relapse [62].

MRI is crucial for staging and surgical planning. Images must encompass the primary tumor site as well as the entire affected bone [9]. Overall, osteosarcoma is usually hypointense on T1-W images and hyperintense on STIR and other fluid-sensitive sequences. However, the portions composed of neoplastic bone appear dark on all sequences [12]. Non-contrast longitudinal T1-W images best determine the extent of intramedullary tumor; the longitudinal extent of the soft tissue mass usually corresponds to that of the intramedullary tumor. Epiphyseal extension of tumor must be assessed to facilitate appropriate surgical planning [9] (Fig. 21.22). Skip lesions may be present in up to 15 % of patients and may occur proximal or distal to the primary lesion (Fig. 21.22). Marrow and soft tissue edema, sometimes massive, may be seen [63]. Fluid–fluid levels suggest intratumoral hemorrhage and are most often seen in telangiectatic osteosarcoma (Fig. 21.23).

The tumor burden, determined by size at diagnosis, correlates with the patient's response to chemotherapy and survival. High initial FDG-PET uptake values in the primary tumor, corresponding to glucose hypermetabolism, correlate with an overall worse prognosis. However, the histologic response to preoperative chemotherapy (indicated by percent

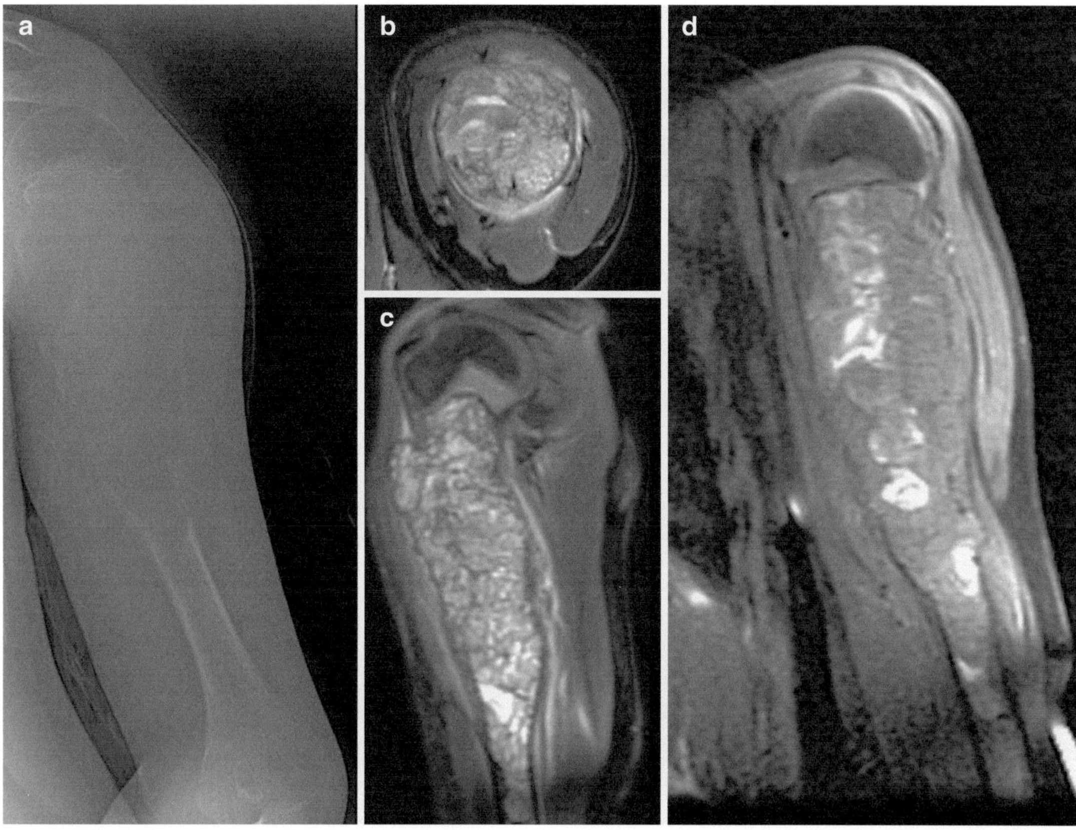

Fig. 21.23 Telangiectatic osteosarcoma in a 14-year-old boy. (**a**) Expansile, destructive, medullary-based mass with minimal periosteal reaction. Axial (**b**) and sagittal (**c**) PD along with coronal T1-W FS (**d**) images show the mass is multiloculated and contains multiple fluid–fluid levels

necrosis) is the strongest overall prognostic factor [64–66]. As the soft-tissue mass of an osteosarcoma tends to remain the same size but ossify with treatment, radiographs, CT, and conventional MRI do not assess the degree of tumor necrosis [67]. Thus, functional imaging studies (FDG-PET or advanced MRI) are necessary to quantify tumor response to neoadjuvant therapy. Decrease in uptake of FDG-PET correlates with tumor necrosis, and this helps determine response to therapy [10]. The apparent diffusion coefficient (ADC), determined with diffusion MRI, increases with tumor necrosis [68]. Dynamic contrast-enhanced MRI (DEMRI) uses the extent of gadolinium accumulation within a tumor to indicate tumor perfusion and microcirculation and thus viability [9].

3.2 **Ewing Sarcoma** (Box 21.7)

> **Box 21.7: Ewing Sarcoma**
>
> Second most common malignant primary bone tumor in children
>
> > 85 % of cases balanced t(11:22)(q24:12) translocation
>
> Most common in pelvis, followed by metadiaphysis of long bones
>
> Permeative, mixed sclerotic/lytic bony lesion
>
> Poorly marginated, cortical destruction
>
> Aggressive periosteal reaction
>
> Soft tissue mass larger than osteosarcoma
>
> Metastases: lungs, followed by bone and bone marrow

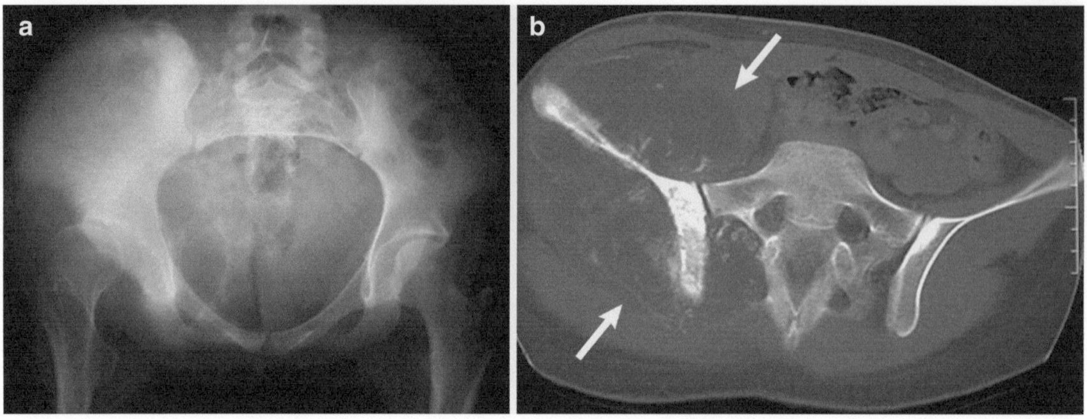

Fig. 21.24 Ewing sarcoma in a 15-year-old girl with Down syndrome and history of hip dysplasia. (**a**) Sclerotic right iliac wing and ischial bony mass with large adjacent soft tissue mass. (**b**) CT shows the sclerotic iliac mass with a large low-density partially calcified soft tissue mass displacing/invading adjacent musculature (*arrows*). The mass extends across the sacroiliac joint and erodes the sacrum

Ewing sarcoma is the second most common malignant bone tumor in children, with an annual incidence of 2.1 per million [9]. It usually appears during the second decade of life and is more common in Caucasian and Hispanic populations. Males and females are equally affected [69].

This highly malignant small blue round cell tumor probably develops from neural crest cells. A balanced t(11:22)(q24:12) translocation, which fuses the Ewing sarcoma (EWS) gene with the Friend leukemia virus integration 1 (FLI-1) gene, is found in over 85 % of cases, resulting in an abnormal transcription factor [70, 71].

Patients generally present with local pain and swelling and may have constitutional symptoms. A palpable mass is usually found, often with overlying erythema. An elevated white blood cell count and increased erythrocyte sedimentation rate may be present as well, sometimes leading to the clinical diagnosis of osteomyelitis. Ewing sarcoma is most commonly found in the pelvis, followed by the metadiaphysis of the long bones (of these, the femur is affected most often, followed by the tibia, humerus, and ribs) [69]. It rarely originates in the soft tissues (see Chap. 22).

Survival is less likely if the primary tumor is located in the axial skeleton or over 8 cm in diameter. In Caucasian patients, female sex predicts greater likelihood of survival [9]. Metastatic disease at diagnosis suggests a worse prognosis, and those with lung metastases alone do better than those with either bone or combined lung and bone metastases. If the tumor is centrally located or less than 90 % necrotic, there is a greater chance of local recurrence [9]. Children who are preteens at diagnosis do better overall than adolescents [9]. The type of dynamic enhancement at diagnosis does not correlate with the risk of metastatic disease [72].

Treatment of Ewing sarcoma includes systemic chemotherapy in conjunction with surgery and/or radiation therapy for local tumor control.

Imaging

Radiographs and CT show a permeative, poorly marginated, mixed sclerotic and lytic medullary mass with significant cortical destruction and a surrounding, often extensive, noncalcified soft tissue mass [69] (Figs. 21.24 and 21.25). Diaphyseal tumors are typically central, while those in the metaphysis are eccentrically located. Epiphyseal extension is rare. Aggressive periosteal reaction may have a spiculated or onionskin pattern.

Initial imaging is performed not only to assess the primary tumor site but also to evaluate for metastatic disease, which occurs most often in the lungs, followed by bone and bone marrow [8]. CT is the preferred modality to evaluate for lung metastases.

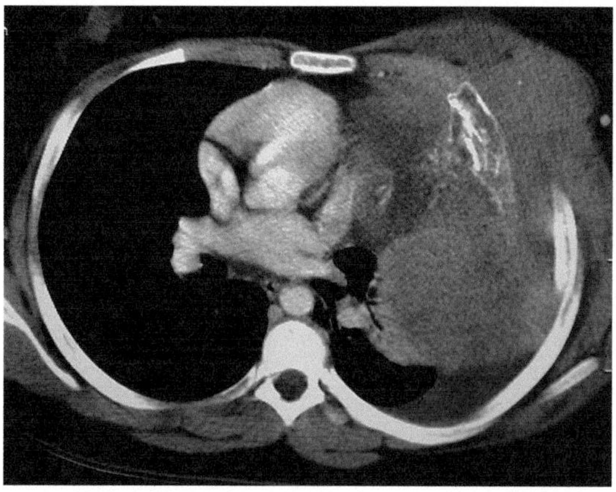

Fig. 21.25 Ewing sarcoma in a 12-year-old girl. contrast-enhanced CT shows a destructive rib mass with a large soft tissue component displacing the mediastinum and extending into and along the subcutaneous soft tissues. Malignant pleural effusion

Bone scan shows increased activity at the primary tumor site. Whole-body scanning may detect skip lesions or distant metastases. FDG-PET is more sensitive, specific, and accurate in detecting skeletal metastases in Ewing sarcoma than is bone scintigraphy [10]. FDG-PET is also useful in detecting local and distant tumor relapse.

MRI provides essential information about tumor configuration and extent. Longitudinal images that include the entire length of the affected bone as well as the adjacent joint are important, as skip lesions are present in about 14 % of patients at the time of diagnosis [69] and joint involvement is not uncommon. Transverse T2-W images best display the interface between tumor and adjacent soft tissues as well as its relationship with neurovascular structures.

The mass appears heterogeneous on MRI. It is usually iso- to mildly hypointense on T1-W imaging and hyperintense on T2-W sequences; the enhancement pattern varies [69, 73]. MRI may overestimate the extent of joint involvement, as minimal tumor involvement often incites an inflammatory response in the synovium.

Response of tumor to radiotherapy and/or chemotherapy can be assessed by conventional imaging, as the soft tissue mass should decrease in size while the intramedullary tumor undergoes myxoid degeneration. High FDG uptake following neoadjuvant chemotherapy portends a shorter period of disease-free survival [10]. In addition, DEMRI may be utilized to differentiate between tumor and necrosis [12]. Diffusion-weighted MRI shows that the ADC value increases where there is tumor necrosis [68].

3.3 Chondrosacroma

Chondrosarcoma is an uncommon tumor in the pediatric population, accounting for less than 5 % of primary bone tumors in young patients [1, 9]. Generally encountered in the pelvis or proximal femur, it may also be found in the shoulder girdle, ribs, spine, or metaphysis of long bones. Most chondrosarcomas are classified as "conventional" at pathology, but the clear cell variant may develop in the epiphyses of long bones [9]. Symptoms may include pain and/or mass.

Chondrosarcoma may be primary or secondary; secondary tumors generally arise in osteochondromas or enchondromas. Multiple lesions, an axial location, and a diameter over 5 cm are associated with a higher risk of osteochondroma or enchondroma degenerating into chondrosarcoma. Malignant degeneration should be suspected if either lesion develops a soft tissue mass, amorphous or chondroid heterogeneous mineralization, or ill-defined margins [9, 74]. (Additional characteristics of the cartilaginous cap that increase concern for malignant change are discussed earlier in this chapter, in the section on osteochondromas.)

Treatment includes wide surgical excision alone or in conjunction with chemotherapy and/or radiation therapy. Tumor grade and size, as well as successful wide surgical resection, are all of prognostic significance [9].

Imaging

On radiographs and CT, the tumor appears expansile, destructive, and osteolytic; it is often large at presentation (Fig. 21.26).

At bone scan, chondrosarcoma usually demonstrates intense, sometimes heterogeneous, uptake of radiotracer [21]. Bone scan may help evaluate for malignant degeneration of enchondromas,

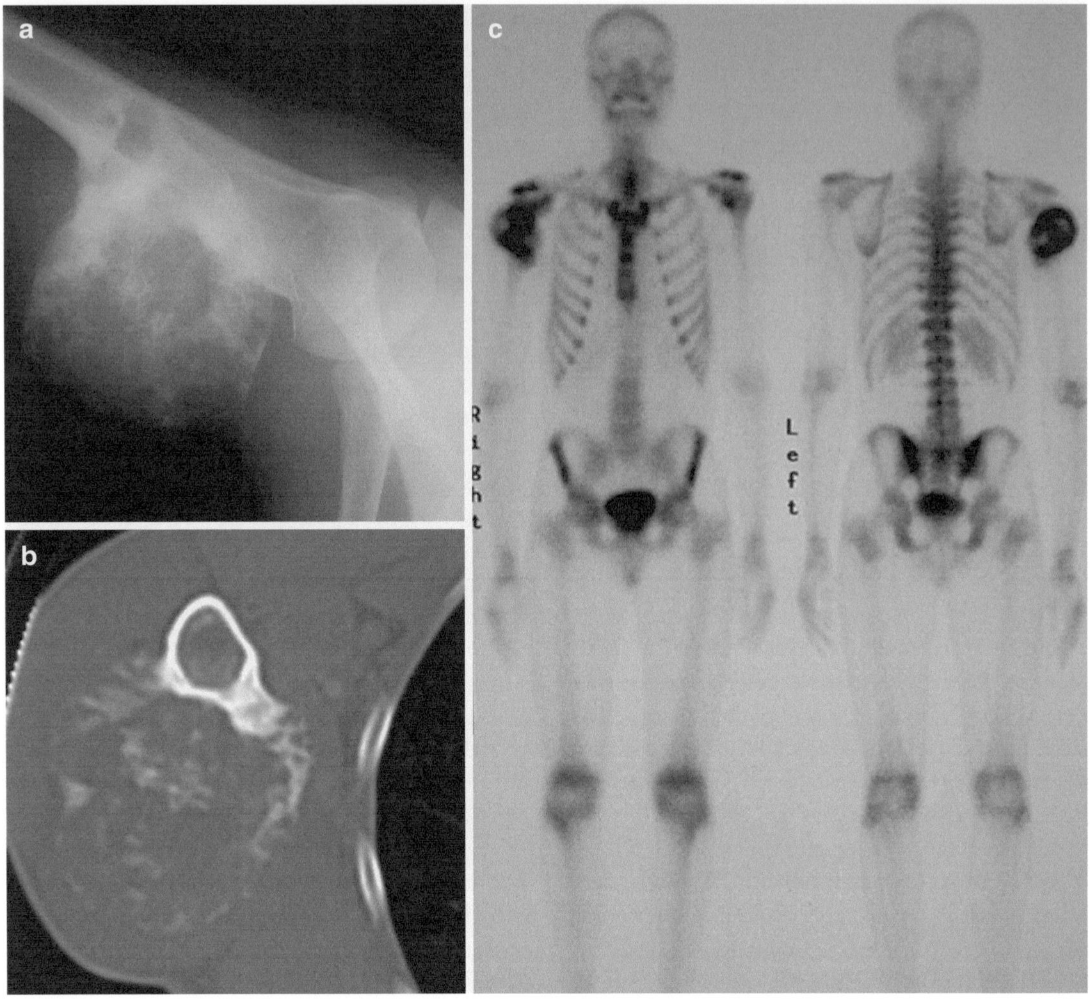

Fig. 21.26 Low-grade chondrosarcoma in a 19-year-old male. (**a**) Exophytic metaphyseal mass with chondroid matrix. (Image copyright Shriners Hospital for Children Northern California.) (**b**) CT demonstrates cortically based mass and intralesional patchy calcifications. (**c**) Increased activity on bone scintigraphy

as they normally show only mild to moderate uptake [21]. PET-CT may be useful in differentiating between benign lesions and malignant degeneration.

At MRI, it is heterogeneous due to intratumoral hemorrhage, foci of calcification, cystic change, and islands of cartilage [75, 76]. Soft tissue extension may occur, but marrow edema is often underwhelming [76]. The tumor enhances heterogeneously. DEMRI may prove useful in differentiating between benign lesions and malignant degeneration.

3.4 Lymphoma

About 5 % of children with lymphoma present with primary bone disease, generally high-grade and diffuse large B-cell lymphomas [1]. In children, the spine and long bone diaphyses are the most common locations for primary bone lymphoma. Symptoms may include pain, swelling, pathological fracture, and systemic symptoms such as fever, night sweats, and weight loss. Treatment includes chemotherapy and/or radiation therapy.

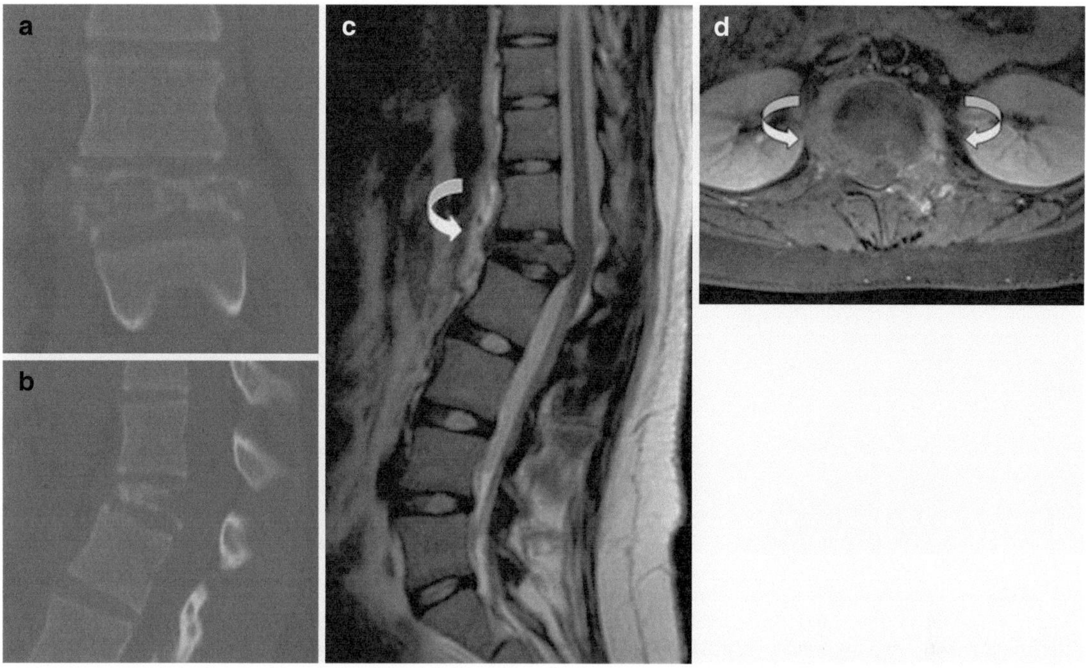

Fig. 21.27 Primary bony lymphoma in a 15-year-old girl. Coronal (**a**) and sagittal (**b**) reformatted CT images show vertebral collapse with an underlying permeative, lytic, destructive lesion and a small adjacent noncalcified soft tissue mass. (**c**) Sagittal T2-W image shows the collapsed vertebra is hypointense (*arrow*), and there is retropulsion of the vertebral body with mass effect on the spinal cord. (**d**) Axial T1-W FS gadolinium-enhanced image better defines the enhancing, circumferential soft tissue mass (*arrows*), which invades posterior soft tissues

Imaging

On radiographs and at CT, lymphomas commonly appear lytic and destructive, with an associated layered periosteal reaction (Fig. 21.27). However, osseous lymphoma, like other small round cell tumors such as Ewing sarcoma, may present with a soft tissue mass and no apparent cortical destruction (this occurs if the tumor cells grow along small cortical vascular channels to extend into the adjacent soft tissues). In this setting, bone lymphoma may be radiographically occult, but sequestra and cortical breakthrough are generally evident at CT.

Bony lymphoma typically shows increased uptake at bone scan and FDG-PET, and these modalities readily define multifocal disease. Both may be positive in cases of radiographically occult primary bone lymphoma. With treatment, FDG-PET activity decreases, but low-level activity may remain for a year post-therapy [77].

The affected marrow appears hypointense on T1-W imaging and hyperintense on T2-W imaging, and the tumor typically enhances after gadolinium administration. Peritumoral edema may also appear hyperintense on T2-W or STIR images. A soft tissue mass may be evident.

3.5 Malignant Fibrous Histiocytoma

Malignant fibrous histiocytoma (MFH) is rare in children, and most pediatric cases occur during adolescence. MFH usually occurs in the center of the metaphysis of a long bone. The tumor is lytic and ranges from geographic to permeative (Fig. 21.28). When geographic, MFH may mimic a nonaggressive tumor. When MFH occurs in the diaphysis, it tends to appear much more aggressive and permeative than its metaphyseal counterpart [78]. Unlike many other bone neoplasms,

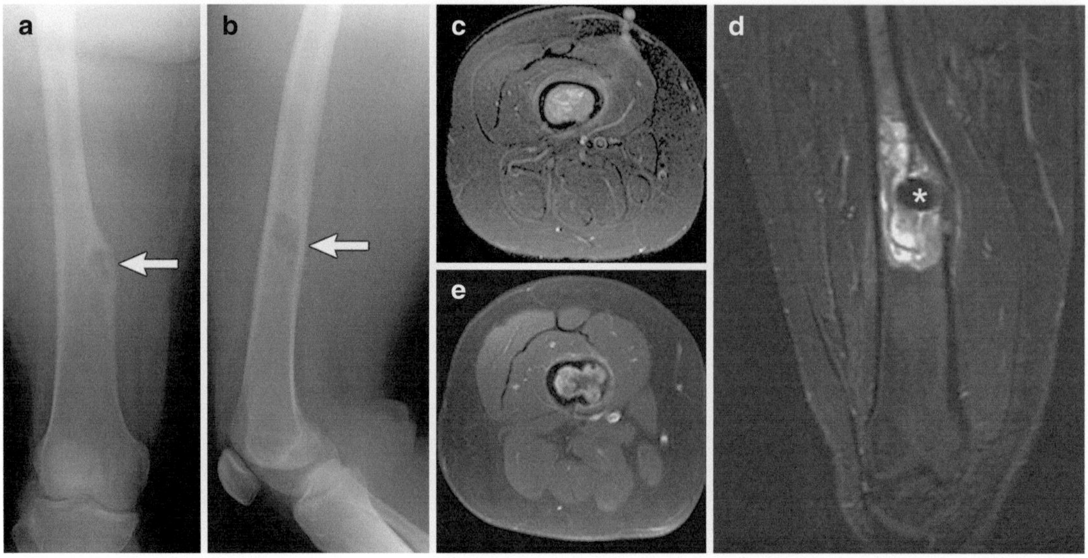

Fig. 21.28 Malignant fibrous histiocytoma in a 15-year-old girl. (**a**, **b**) Eccentric, lytic lesion (*arrows*) has a sclerotic margin with vague cortical destruction. (**c**) Axial short tau inversion recovery (*STIR*) image shows the mass fills the marrow cavity and breaks through the cortex. (**d**) Axial T1-W gadolinium-enhanced image better defines the intramedullary extent of the mass. (**e**) Coronal STIR image shows the extent of the lesion and demonstrates slight hyperintensity in the adjacent soft tissues. The hypointense focus (*) results from biopsy

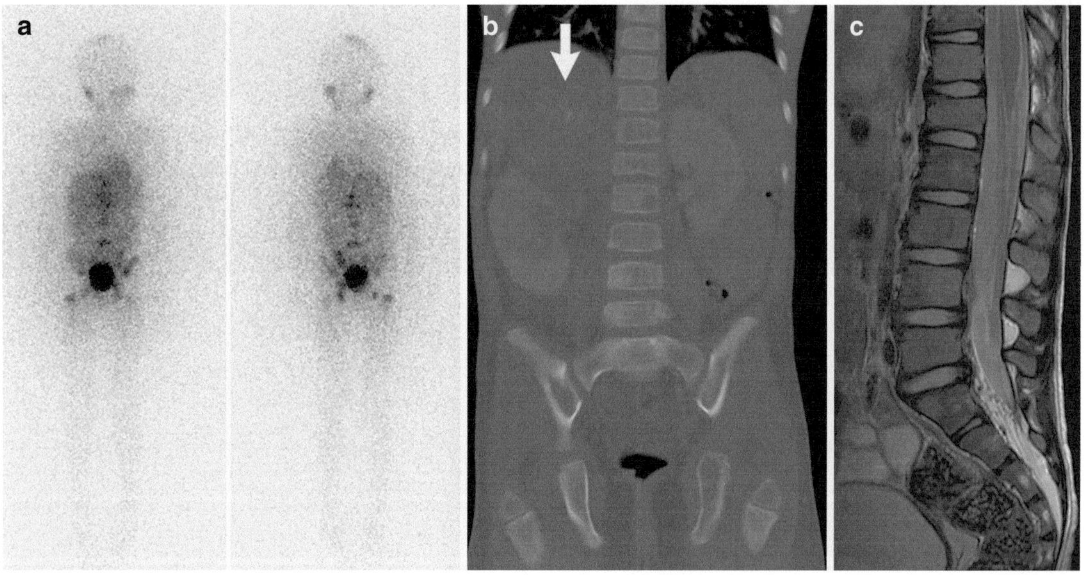

Fig. 21.29 Metastatic neuroblastoma in a 4-year-old. (**a**) Metaiodobenzylguanidine (MIBG) scan shows multiple areas of abnormal uptake in the skull, spine, pelvis, and proximal femurs. Increased uptake in the lower right chest results from subdiaphragmatic extension of the right suprarenal primary tumor. (**b**) Coronal CT shows multiple lytic bony lesions, as well as the primary calcified tumor (*arrow*). (**c**) Sagittal T2-W MRI shows inhomogeneous marrow signal in multiple vertebrae secondary to metastases

periosteal reaction is uncommon. MRI features of MFH are nonspecific: T1 signal is similar to muscle, and T2 signal is increased. However, MRI helps define tumor extent and involvement of adjacent structures.

3.6 Metastatic Disease

Neuroblastoma and leukemia are the most common primary pediatric malignancies that metastasize to the bone. Spread is hematogenous, as bone does not have lymphatics [1]. Bony metastases are poorly marginated and lytic; they may be associated with cortical destruction, periosteal reaction, and extraosseous extension [5]. Metastases in the long bones are most often metaphyseal; metastases are also encountered in the axial skeleton, including the skull (Fig. 21.29). Bone scan is extremely useful in detecting bony metastases, as it is highly sensitive and evaluates the entire skeleton [21]. Total body MRI also accurately assesses the extent of marrow involvement and bony metastases.

References

1. Vlychou M, Athanasou NA. Radiological and pathological diagnosis of paediatric bone tumours and tumour-like lesions. Pathology. 2008;40(2):196–216. PubMed PMID: 18203042. Epub 2008/01/19. eng.
2. Ademuyiwa FO, Edge SB, Erwin DO, Orom H, Ambrosone CB, Underwood 3rd W. Breast cancer racial disparities: unanswered questions. Cancer Res. 2011;71(3):640–4. PubMed PMID: 21135114. Epub 2010/12/08. eng.
3. Wootton-Gorges SL. MR imaging of primary bone tumors and tumor-like conditions in children. Magn Reson Imaging Clin N Am. 2009;17(3):469–87, vi. PubMed PMID: 19524197. Epub 2009/06/16. eng.
4. Voss SD, Reaman GH, Kaste SC, Slovis TL. The ALARA concept in pediatric oncology. Pediatr Radiol. 2009;39(11):1142–6. PubMed PMID: 19789861. Epub 2009/10/01. eng.
5. Khanna G, Bennett DL. Pediatric bone lesions: beyond the plain radiographic evaluation. Semin Roentgenol. 2012;47(1):90–9. PubMed PMID: 22166234. Epub 2011/12/15. eng.
6. Wenaden AE, Szyszko TA, Saifuddin A. Imaging of periosteal reactions associated with focal lesions of bone. Clin Radiol. 2005;60(4):439–56. PubMed PMID: 15767101. Epub 2005/03/16. eng.
7. Nadel HR. Pediatric bone scintigraphy update. Semin Nucl Med. 2010;40(1):31–40. PubMed PMID: 19958848. Epub 2009/12/05. eng.
8. Meyer JS, Nadel HR, Marina N, Womer RB, Brown KL, Eary JF, et al. Imaging guidelines for children with Ewing sarcoma and osteosarcoma: a report from the Children's Oncology Group Bone Tumor Committee. Pediatr Blood Cancer. 2008;51(2):163–70. PubMed PMID: 18454470. Epub 2008/05/06. eng.
9. Kaste SC. Imaging pediatric bone sarcomas. Radiol Clin North Am. 2011;49(4):749–65, vi-vii. PubMed PMID: 21807172. Epub 2011/08/03. eng.
10. Franzius C. FDG-PET/CT in pediatric solid tumors. Q J Nucl Med Mol Imaging. 2010;54(4):401–10. PubMed PMID: 20823808. Epub 2010/09/09. eng.
11. Fayad LM, Bluemke DA, Weber KL, Fishman EK. Characterization of pediatric skeletal tumors and tumor-like conditions: specific cross-sectional imaging signs. Skeletal Radiol. 2006;35(5):259–68. PubMed PMID: 16538462. Epub 2006/03/16. eng.
12. Hoffer FA. Primary skeletal neoplasms: osteosarcoma and Ewing sarcoma. Top Magn Reson ImagingTMRI. 2002;13(4):231–9. PubMed PMID: 12409691. Epub 2002/11/01. eng.
13. Alyas F, James SL, Davies AM, Saifuddin A. The role of MR imaging in the diagnostic characterisation of appendicular bone tumours and tumour-like conditions. Eur Radiol. 2007;17(10):2675–86. PubMed PMID: 17342487. Epub 2007/03/08. eng.
14. Van Dyck P, Vanhoenacker FM, Vogel J, Venstermans C, Kroon HM, Gielen J, et al. Prevalence, extension and characteristics of fluid-fluid levels in bone and soft tissue tumors. Eur Radiol. 2006;16(12):2644–51. PubMed PMID: 16612549. Epub 2006/04/14. eng.
15. O'Donnell P, Saifuddin A. The prevalence and diagnostic significance of fluid-fluid levels in focal lesions of bone. Skeletal Radiol. 2004;33(6):330–6. PubMed PMID: 15138727. Epub 2004/05/13. eng.
16. Yaw KM. Pediatric bone tumors. Semin Surg Oncol. 1999;16(2):173–83. PubMed PMID: 9988871. Epub 1999/02/16. eng.
17. Jawad MU, Scully SP. In brief: classifications in brief: enneking classification: benign and malignant tumors of the musculoskeletal system. Clin Orthop Relat Res. 2010;468(7):2000–2. PubMed PMID: 20333492. Pubmed Central PMCID: 2882012. Epub 2010/03/25. eng.
18. Sullivan RJ, Meyer JS, Dormans JP, Davidson RS. Diagnosing aneurysmal and unicameral bone cysts with magnetic resonance imaging. Clin Orthop Relat Res. 1999;366:186–90. PubMed PMID: 10627734. Epub 2000/01/11. eng.
19. Donaldson S, Wright JG. Recent developments in treatment for simple bone cysts. Curr Opin Pediatr. 2011;23(1):73–7. PubMed PMID: 21191299. Epub 2010/12/31. eng.
20. Hou HY, Wu K, Wang CT, Chang SM, Lin WH, Yang RS. Treatment of unicameral bone cyst: a comparative study of selected techniques. J Bone Joint Surg Am.

2010;92(4):855–62. PubMed PMID: 20360508. Epub 2010/04/03. eng.
21. Wang K, Allen L, Fung E, Chan CC, Chan JC, Griffith JF. Bone scintigraphy in common tumors with osteolytic components. Clin Nucl Med. 2005;30(10):655–71. PubMed PMID: 16166837. Epub 2005/09/17. eng.
22. Margau R, Babyn P, Cole W, Smith C, Lee F. MR imaging of simple bone cysts in children: not so simple. Pediatr Radiol. 2000;30(8):551–7. PubMed PMID: 10993540. Epub 2000/09/19. eng.
23. Azouz EM. Magnetic resonance imaging of benign bone lesions: cysts and tumors. Top Magn Reson ImagingTMRI. 2002;13(4):219–29. PubMed PMID: 12409690. Epub 2002/11/01. eng.
24. Woertler K. Benign bone tumors and tumor-like lesions: value of cross-sectional imaging. Eur Radiol. 2003;13(8):1820–35. PubMed PMID: 12700923. Epub 2003/04/18. eng.
25. Mahnken AH, Nolte-Ernsting CC, Wildberger JE, Heussen N, Adam G, Wirtz DC, et al. Aneurysmal bone cyst: value of MR imaging and conventional radiography. Eur Radiol. 2003;13(5):1118–24. PubMed PMID: 12695836. Epub 2003/04/16. eng.
26. Murphey MD, Nomikos GC, Flemming DJ, Gannon FH, Temple HT, Kransdorf MJ. From the archives of AFIP. Imaging of giant cell tumor and giant cell reparative granuloma of bone: radiologic-pathologic correlation. Radiogr Rev Publ Radiol Soc N Am Inc. 2001;21(5):1283–309. PubMed PMID: 11553835. Epub 2001/09/13. eng.
27. Purohit S, Pardiwala DN. Imaging of giant cell tumor of bone. Indian J Orthop. 2007;41(2):91–6. PubMed PMID: 21139758. Pubmed Central PMCID: 2989147. Epub 2007/04/01. eng.
28. Kriz J, Eich HT, Mucke R, Buntzel J, Muller RP, Bruns F, et al. Radiotherapy for giant cell tumors of the bone: a safe and effective treatment modality. Anticancer Res. 2012;32(5):2069–73. PubMed PMID: 22593490. Epub 2012/05/18. eng.
29. Van Nostrand D, Madewell JE, McNiesh LM, Kyle RW, Sweet D. Radionuclide bone scanning in giant cell tumor. J Nucl Med. 1986;27(3):329–38. PubMed PMID: 3712049. Epub 1986/03/01. eng.
30. Stacy GS, Heck RK, Peabody TD, Dixon LB. Neoplastic and tumorlike lesions detected on MR imaging of the knee in patients with suspected internal derangement: part I, intraosseous entities. AJR Am J Roentgenol. 2002;178(3):589–94. PubMed PMID: 11856679. Epub 2002/02/22. eng.
31. Murphey MD, Choi JJ, Kransdorf MJ, Flemming DJ, Gannon FH. Imaging of osteochondroma: variants and complications with radiologic-pathologic correlation. Radiographics Rev Publ Radiol Soc N Am Inc. 2000;20(5):1407–34. PubMed PMID: 10992031. Epub 2000/09/19. eng.
32. Taniguchi K. A practical classification system for multiple cartilaginous exostosis in children. J Pediatr Orthop. 1995;15(5):585–91. PubMed PMID: 7593567. Epub 1995/09/01. eng.
33. Wenger DR, Adamczyk MJ. Evaluation, imaging, histology and operative treatment for dysplasia epiphysealis hemimelica (Trevor disease) of the acetabulum: a case report and review. Iowa Orthop J. 2005;25:60–5. PubMed PMID: 16089075. Pubmed Central PMCID: 1888776. Epub 2005/08/11. eng.
34. Azouz EM, Slomic AM, Marton D, Rigault P, Finidori G. The variable manifestations of dysplasia epiphysealis hemimelica. Pediatr Radiol. 1985;15(1):44–9. PubMed PMID: 3969295. Epub 1985/01/01. eng.
35. Unger EC, Kessler HB, Kowalyshyn MJ, Lackman RD, Morea GT. MR imaging of Maffucci syndrome. AJR Am J Roentgenol. 1988;150(2):351–3. PubMed PMID: 3257324. Epub 1988/02/01. eng.
36. Jee WH, Park YK, McCauley TR, Choi KH, Ryu KN, Suh JS, et al. Chondroblastoma: MR characteristics with pathologic correlation. J Comput Assist Tomogr. 1999;23(5):721–6. PubMed PMID: 10524855. Epub 1999/10/19. eng.
37. Oxtoby JW, Davies AM. MRI characteristics of chondroblastoma. Clin Radiol. 1996;51(1):22–6. PubMed PMID: 8549042. Epub 1996/01/01. eng.
38. Ehara S, Rosenthal DI, Aoki J, Fukuda K, Sugimoto H, Mizutani H, et al. Peritumoral edema in osteoid osteoma on magnetic resonance imaging. Skeletal Radiol. 1999;28(5):265–70. PubMed PMID: 10424332. Epub 1999/07/29. eng.
39. Yildiz C, Erler K, Atesalp AS, Basbozkurt M. Benign bone tumors in children. Curr Opin Pediatr. 2003;15(1):58–67. PubMed PMID: 12544273. Epub 2003/01/25. eng.
40. Connolly LP, Treves ST. Assessing the limping child with skeletal scintigraphy. J Nucl Med. 1998;39(6):1056–61. PubMed PMID: 9627343. Epub 1998/06/17. eng.
41. Kransdorf MJ, Stull MA, Gilkey FW, Moser Jr RP. Osteoid osteoma. Radiographics Rev Publ Radiol Soc N Am Inc. 1991;11(4):671–96. PubMed PMID: 1887121. Epub 1991/07/11. eng.
42. Kroon HM, Schurmans J. Osteoblastoma: clinical and radiologic findings in 98 new cases. Radiology. 1990;175(3):783–90. PubMed PMID: 2343130. Epub 1990/06/01. eng.
43. Crim JR, Mirra JM, Eckardt JJ, Seeger LL. Widespread inflammatory response to osteoblastoma: the flare phenomenon. Radiology. 1990;177(3):835–6. PubMed PMID: 2243998. Epub 1990/12/01. eng.
44. Patel AJ, Fox BD, Fahim DK, Fulkerson DH, Whitehead WE, Curry DJ, et al. A clinicopathologic correlation in osteoblastoma of the spine in a child. J Clin Neurosci. 2011;18(12):1728–30. PubMed PMID: 21992740. Epub 2011/10/14. eng.
45. Hau MA, Fox EJ, Cates JM, Brigman BE, Mankin HJ. Jaffe-Campanacci syndrome. A case report and review of the literature. J Bone Joint Surg Am. 2002;84-A(4):634–8. PubMed PMID: 11940628. Epub 2002/04/10. eng.
46. Colby RS, Saul RA. Is Jaffe-Campanacci syndrome just a manifestation of neurofibromatosis type 1? Am J Med Genet A. 2003;123A(1):60–3. PubMed PMID: 14556247. Epub 2003/10/14. eng.

47. Shah ZK, Peh WC, Koh WL, Shek TW. Magnetic resonance imaging appearances of fibrous dysplasia. Br J Radiol. 2005;78(936):1104–15. PubMed PMID: 16352586. Epub 2005/12/15. eng.
48. Most MJ, Sim FH, Inwards CY. Osteofibrous dysplasia and adamantinoma. J Am Acad Orthop Surg. 2010;18(6):358–66. PubMed PMID: 20511441. Epub 2010/06/01. eng.
49. Dominguez R, Saucedo J, Fenstermacher M. MRI findings in osteofibrous dysplasia. Magn Reson Imaging. 1989;7(5):567–70. PubMed PMID: 2607907. Epub 1989/09/01. eng.
50. Ma LD. Magnetic resonance imaging of musculoskeletal tumors: skeletal and soft tissue masses. Curr Probl Diagn Radiol. 1999;28(2):29–62. PubMed PMID: 10088064. Epub 1999/03/24. eng.
51. Ropper AE, Cahill KS, Hanna JW, McCarthy EF, Gokaslan ZL, Chi JH. Primary vertebral tumors: a review of epidemiologic, histological, and imaging findings, part I: benign tumors. Neurosurgery. 2011;69(6):1171–80. PubMed PMID: 21725252. Epub 2011/07/05. eng.
52. De Schepper AM, Ramon F, Van Marck E. MR imaging of eosinophilic granuloma: report of 11 cases. Skeletal Radiol. 1993;22(3):163–6. PubMed PMID: 8480201. Epub 1993/01/01. eng.
53. Goo HW, Yang DH, Ra YS, Song JS, Im HJ, Seo JJ, et al. Whole-body MRI of Langerhans cell histiocytosis: comparison with radiography and bone scintigraphy. Pediatr Radiol. 2006;36(10):1019–31. PubMed PMID: 16896695. Epub 2006/08/10. eng.
54. Lanzkowsky P. Manual of pediatric hematology and oncology. 5th ed. London: Academic Press; 2010. 1058 p.
55. Stull MA, Kransdorf MJ, Devaney KO. Langerhans cell histiocytosis of bone. Radiogr Rev Publ Radiol Soc N Am Inc. 1992;12(4):801–23. PubMed PMID: 1636041. Epub 1992/07/01. eng.
56. Davies AM, Pikoulas C, Griffith J. MRI of eosinophilic granuloma. Eur J Radiol. 1994;18(3):205–9. PubMed PMID: 7957291. Epub 1994/08/01. eng.
57. Steinborn M, Wortler K, Nathrath M, Schoniger M, Hahn H, Rummeny EJ. Whole-body MRI in children with Langerhans cell histiocytosis for the evaluation of the skeletal system. RoFo Fortschritte auf dem Gebiete der Rontgenstrahlen und der Nuklearmedizin. 2008;180(7):646–53. PubMed PMID: 18561067. Epub 2008/06/19. Ganzkorper-MRT bei Langerhans-Zell-Histiozytose im Kindes- und Jugendalter zur Beurteilung des Skelettsystems. ger.
58. Longhi A, Errani C, De Paolis M, Mercuri M, Bacci G. Primary bone osteosarcoma in the pediatric age: state of the art. Cancer Treat Rev. 2006;32(6): 423–36. PubMed PMID: 16860938. Epub2006/07/25. eng.
59. Ragland BD, Bell WC, Lopez RR, Siegal GP. Cytogenetics and molecular biology of osteosarcoma. Lab Investig J Tech Methods Pathol. 2002;82(4):365–73. PubMed PMID: 11950895. Epub 2002/04/16. eng.
60. Weiss A, Khoury JD, Hoffer FA, Wu J, Billups CA, Heck RK, et al. Telangiectatic osteosarcoma: the St. Jude Children's Research Hospital's experience. Cancer. 2007;109(8):1627–37. PubMed PMID: 17351949. Epub 2007/03/14. eng.
61. Volker T, Denecke T, Steffen I, Misch D, Schonberger S, Plotkin M, et al. Positron emission tomography for staging of pediatric sarcoma patients: results of a prospective multicenter trial. J Clin Oncol. 2007;25(34):5435–41. PubMed PMID: 18048826. Epub 2007/12/01. eng.
62. Arush MW, Israel O, Postovsky S, Militianu D, Meller I, Zaidman I, et al. Positron emission tomography/computed tomography with 18fluoro-deoxyglucose in the detection of local recurrence and distant metastases of pediatric sarcoma. Pediatr Blood Cancer. 2007;49(7):901–5. PubMed PMID: 17252575. Epub 2007/01/26. eng.
63. Arndt CA, Crist WM. Common musculoskeletal tumors of childhood and adolescence. N Engl J Med. 1999;341(5):342–52. PubMed PMID: 10423470. Epub 1999/07/29. eng.
64. Reddick WE, Wang S, Xiong X, Glass JO, Wu S, Kaste SC, et al. Dynamic magnetic resonance imaging of regional contrast access as an additional prognostic factor in pediatric osteosarcoma. Cancer. 2001;91(12):2230–7. PubMed PMID: 11413510. Epub 2001/06/20. eng.
65. Bacci G, Ferrari S, Bertoni F, Picci P, Bacchini P, Longhi A, et al. Histologic response of high-grade nonmetastatic osteosarcoma of the extremity to chemotherapy. Clin Orthop Relat Res. 2001;386:186–96. PubMed PMID: 11347833. Epub 2001/05/12. eng.
66. Provisor AJ, Ettinger LJ, Nachman JB, Krailo MD, Makley JT, Yunis EJ, et al. Treatment of nonmetastatic osteosarcoma of the extremity with preoperative and postoperative chemotherapy: a report from the Children's Cancer Group. J Clin Oncol. 1997;15(1):76–84. PubMed PMID: 8996127. Epub 1997/01/01. eng.
67. McCarville MB. New frontiers in pediatric oncologic imaging. Cancer Imaging. 2008;8:87–92. PubMed PMID: 18390392. Pubmed Central PMCID: 2324372. Epub 2008/04/09. eng.
68. Hayashida Y, Yakushiji T, Awai K, Katahira K, Nakayama Y, Shimomura O, et al. Monitoring therapeutic responses of primary bone tumors by diffusion-weighted image: initial results. Eur Radiol. 2006;16(12):2637–43. PubMed PMID: 16909220. Epub 2006/08/16. eng.
69. Peersman B, Vanhoenacker FM, Heyman S, Van Herendael B, Stam M, Brys P, et al. Ewing's sarcoma: imaging features. JBR-BTR: organe de la Societe royale belge de radiologie. 2007;90(5):368–76. PubMed PMID: 18085191. Epub 2007/12/19. eng.
70. Szuhai K, Ijszenga M, Tanke HJ, Rosenberg C, Hogendoorn PC. Molecular cytogenetic characterization of four previously established and two newly established Ewing sarcoma cell lines. Cancer Genet Cytogenet. 2006;166(2):173–9. PubMed PMID: 16631476. Epub 2006/04/25. eng.

71. Caudill JS, Arndt CA. Diagnosis and management of bone malignancy in adolescence. Adolesc Med State Art Rev. 2007;18(1):62–78, ix. PubMed PMID: 18605391. Epub 2008/07/09. eng.
72. Miller SL, Hoffer FA, Reddick WE, Wu S, Glass JO, Gronemeyer SA, et al. Tumor volume or dynamic contrast-enhanced MRI for prediction of clinical outcome of Ewing sarcoma family of tumors. Pediatr Radiol. 2001;31(7):518–23. PubMed PMID: 11486808.
73. Mar WA, Taljanovic MS, Bagatell R, Graham AR, Speer DP, Hunter TB, et al. Update on imaging and treatment of Ewing sarcoma family tumors: what the radiologist needs to know. J Comput Assist Tomogr. 2008;32(1):108–18. PubMed PMID: 18303298. Epub 2008/02/28. eng.
74. Littrell LA, Wenger DE, Wold LE, Bertoni F, Unni KK, White LM, et al. Radiographic, CT, and MR imaging features of dedifferentiated chondrosarcomas: a retrospective review of 174 de novo cases. Radiographics Rev Publ Radiol Soc N Am Inc. 2004;24(5):1397–409. PubMed PMID: 15371616. Epub 2004/09/17. eng.
75. Kaim AH, Hugli R, Bonel HM, Jundt G. Chondroblastoma and clear cell chondrosarcoma: radiological and MRI characteristics with histopathological correlation. Skeletal Radiol. 2002;31(2): 88–95. PubMed PMID: 11828329. Epub 2002/02/06. eng.
76. Collins MS, Koyama T, Swee RG, Inwards CY. Clear cell chondrosarcoma: radiographic, computed tomographic, and magnetic resonance findings in 34 patients with pathologic correlation. Skeletal Radiol. 2003;32(12):687–94. PubMed PMID: 14530882. Epub 2003/10/08. eng.
77. Borst AJ, States LJ, Reilly AF, Rheingold SR. Determining response and recurrence in pediatric B-cell lymphomas of the bone. Pediatr Blood Cancer. 2013;60(8):1281–6. PubMed PMID: 23519982. Epub 2013/03/23. eng.
78. Murphey MD, Gross TM, Rosenthal HG. From the archives of the AFIP. Musculoskeletal malignant fibrous histiocytoma: radiologic-pathologic correlation. Radiographics Rev Publ Radiol Soc N Am Inc. 1994;14(4):807–26.
79. Edge SB, Byrd DR, Compton CC, Fritz AG, Green FL, Trotti A, editors. American Joint Commission on Cancer (AJCC) staging manual. 7th ed. New York: Springer; 2010.

Soft Tissue Masses

22

Glade E. Roper and Rebecca Stein-Wexler

Contents

Abstract

The chapter is divided in two parts: the first part discusses benign masses and the second addresses malignancies. Vascular lesions are discussed, differentiating between high-flow and low-flow lesions. Fatty lesions, neurofibromas, tumoral calcinosis, and myositis ossificans are described in detail, and hematomas, popliteal cysts, and other lesions are presented more briefly. The following section on malignant masses focuses on sarcomas and other fibrous tumors. The discussion of sarcomas includes infantile fibrosarcoma, synovial sarcoma, rhabdomyosarcoma, lymphoma/leukemia, as well as lesions such as epithelioid sarcoma, granulocytic sarcoma, liposarcoma, extraskeletal Ewing sarcoma/osteosarcoma, and hemangiopericytoma.

G.E. Roper, MD
Department of Musculoskeletal Imaging and Intervention, Kaweah Delta Medical Center, 400 W. Mineral King Avenue, Visalia, CA 93291, USA
e-mail: glade.roper@gmail.com

R. Stein-Wexler, MD (✉)
Department of Radiology, University of California Davis Medical Center and UC Davis Children's Hospital, 4860 Y Street, Suite 3100, Sacramento, CA 95817, USA

Department of Diagnostic Imaging, Shriners Hospitals for Children Northern California, Sacramento, CA 95817, USA
e-mail: rebecca.steinwexler@ucdmc.ucdavis.edu

Soft tissue tumors in infants and children are relatively rare and are usually benign. When a child presents with a palpable mass in an extremity, radiographs should be performed to determine whether the mass involves or arises from bone and whether there are associated calcifications [1]. The risk from the radiation dose of a single set of radiographs is minimal, and the presence of typical calcifications (e.g., phleboliths in a venous malformation) may lead to a specific diagnosis.

Ultrasound (US) is the most appropriate next study [2]. This valuable tool is nearly universally

R. Stein-Wexler et al. (eds.), *Pediatric Orthopedic Imaging*,
DOI 10.1007/978-3-642-45381-6_22, © Springer-Verlag Berlin Heidelberg 2015

available, requires no sedation, exposes the child to no radiation, and is relatively inexpensive to perform. It distinguishes between cystic and solid masses, usually provides good information about the extent of the mass, and can evaluate for invasion of surrounding structures. Doppler US can identify and characterize vascularity. US also provides real-time guidance during biopsy. Of note, biopsy should be undertaken only after a multidisciplinary discussion including the surgeon who will be managing the case, to ensure that the biopsy tract will be included in any potential resection [2].

The next imaging study of choice is magnetic resonance imaging (MRI), with its multiplanar capacity, lack of ionizing radiation, and excellent tissue contrast [1]. Images must include the entire mass, and it is helpful to include at least one T1-weighted (T1-W) and one fluid-sensitive sequence including the entire adjacent bone. Imaging with gadolinium contrast provides important information about tumor vascularity and viability [3].

Although MRI may suggest a diagnosis, it is less often definitive [1]. The lesions for which definitive diagnosis at MRI is possible include many benign lesions: hemangioma, lymphangioma, and other vascular tumors; lipoma, periarticular cysts, hematoma, giant cell tumor of the tendon sheath, benign neural tumors, and fat necrosis [4]. However, imaging characteristics of many benign and malignant lesions overlap considerably [1, 5, 6], as many appear iso- or hypointense to muscle on T1-W imaging and hyperintense on T2-weighted (T2-W) imaging.

Fortunately, only 1–6 % of soft tissue masses in children are malignant [4]. When the MRI appearance is nonspecific, the mass is more likely to be benign if the patient is less than 20 years old and the mass measures under 10 cm and is in a subcutaneous or fascial location. It is also more likely to be benign if it appears well circumscribed, homogeneous on T2-W imaging, and has no surrounding edema [7]. Malignant lesions tend to show less rapid enhancement and more rapid washout than benign lesions [3]. MRI can demonstrate that a lesion is a simple cyst, provided that T1 signal is homogeneous and lower than that of adjacent muscle, T2 signal is homogeneously bright and equal to fluid, and there is no peripheral nodularity [8]. Contrast should be administered in equivocal cases to ensure that there are no solid components [9]. However, although some have found MRI capable of determining the benignity of specific lesions based on the criteria discussed above, biopsy is often necessary.

1 Benign Masses

1.1 Vascular Lesions

The most common type of soft tissue tumor in childhood, vascular abnormalities encompass a wide spectrum of pathology, from the innocuous to the aggressive and disfiguring to the malignant. The fundamental defect is abnormal connections between or proliferation of various types of channels: artery, vein, capillary, and lymph [10]. Eighty-nine percent of vascular lesions in children are benign, 9 % have intermediate histology, and only 2 % are malignant [10]. Vascular lesions have a wide variety of imaging appearances, but a lesion that does not respect fascial planes and that extends into multiple different tissue types is likely to be vascular in origin [11].

Infantile Hemangioma (Box 22.1)

Box 22.1: Hemangioma

Usual course: 8–10 months of rapid growth shortly after birth followed by involution

US	High vascular density (5 vessels/cm^2)
	Many surrounding vessels have low-resistance waveforms
	Usually hypoechoic and well defined
MRI	Intense, diffuse enhancement until involution

No calcifications or phleboliths

Hemangiomas and vascular malformations were differentiated in 1982 [12]. Infantile hemangiomas are encountered in over 12 % of infants, most often in girls and more commonly in fair-haired children [10]. The infantile hemangioma is small or absent at birth and then enters a proliferative phase over the first 8–10 months, during which it grows rapidly (under the influence of vascular endothelial growth factor and fibroblast growth factor). It then enters a plateau phase that lasts for months to several years, followed by an involution phase, when it gradually shrinks. It usually involutes completely within 10–12 years, and 50 % are completely gone within the first 5 years of life [13]. Children with multiple cutaneous hemangiomas are more likely to have multiple visceral hemangiomas [13]. Lesions on the skin surface are usually clinically obvious due to their "strawberry" appearance, but deeper lesions may manifest only by bluish discoloration of the skin (due to overlying draining veins) or mass effect.

The most appropriate treatment for these lesions is usually watchful waiting and reassurance, unless the lesion interferes with the child's function, such as blocking the airway or eyes, and in cases of rapid growth, ulceration with hemorrhage, visceral involvement, or congestive heart failure. Up to 10 % of patients with infantile hemangiomas require treatment [14]. Initial treatment is usually with high-dose systemic corticosteroids; 30 % of hemangiomas respond dramatically, and 40 % have some response [15]. Some centers have begun using propranolol as a first-line agent to treat infantile hemangiomas, as it is safer and, in some studies, more effective [16]. Other treatment modalities include antiangiogenesis factors such as α-interferon and chemotherapeutic agents such as vincristine, though the side effects of these treatments are substantial. Embolization is used for life-threatening complications, such as bleeding, congestive heart failure, or airway compression [11].

Of note, Kasabach-Merritt syndrome does not occur in the typical infantile hemangioma. This syndrome, which consists of thrombocytopenia, anemia, and consumptive coagulopathy, is associated with the rare variant called tuft hemangioma (which resolves more slowly than the common infantile hemangioma) and with kaposiform hemangioendothelioma (see section below) [11].

Imaging

The initial imaging modality for a superficial infantile hemangioma is usually visual inspection, followed by expectant management. If the lesion is deep, or if the diagnosis is uncertain, US is the most appropriate first imaging study due to cost, speed, and availability. A hemangioma usually appears well defined, solid, and hypoechoic relative to subcutaneous fat [17] (Fig. 22.1). It occasionally appears hyperechoic or heterogeneous [18]. High vessel density, defined as more than five vessels per cm^2 in the part of the lesion with highest flow on Doppler imaging, is typical [17]. The lesions usually have multiple surrounding vessels demonstrating low-resistance Doppler flow [15]. A maximum Doppler shift of greater than 2 kHz has been proposed as a criterion for diagnosis of hemangioma, but the utility of this finding is unclear [17]. US can usually confirm the diagnosis of hemangioma, though it may not demonstrate the full extent of the lesion.

Extensive lesions or lesions that cannot be fully evaluated with US should be evaluated with MRI. The MRI appearance varies with the phase of the lesion. During proliferation and plateau phases, hemangiomas appear isointense to muscle on T1- and hyperintense on T2-W imaging. On T2-W imaging, the typical appearance is a focal, well-marginated, lobulated mass, but margins may be indistinct at T1-W imaging. Enhancement is homogeneous and diffuse. Large, high-flow vessels, representing both arteries and veins within and around the mass, demonstrate increased signal on gradient recall echo and signal voids on spin-echo sequences; these vessels are easily seen on MR angiography. Central low-signal-intensity dots are common, probably representing fibrofatty septa viewed in cross section or perhaps thrombosed vascular channels [19]. There should be no calcifications or phleboliths. The mass may cause smooth saucerization of adjacent bone. As the lesion involutes, the vascularity and enhancement decrease, and the lesion is replaced by fat until only a few scattered hyperintense vessels remain. It is important to evaluate neurovascular, visceral, muscular, and osseous involvement, especially if embolization is contemplated [11].

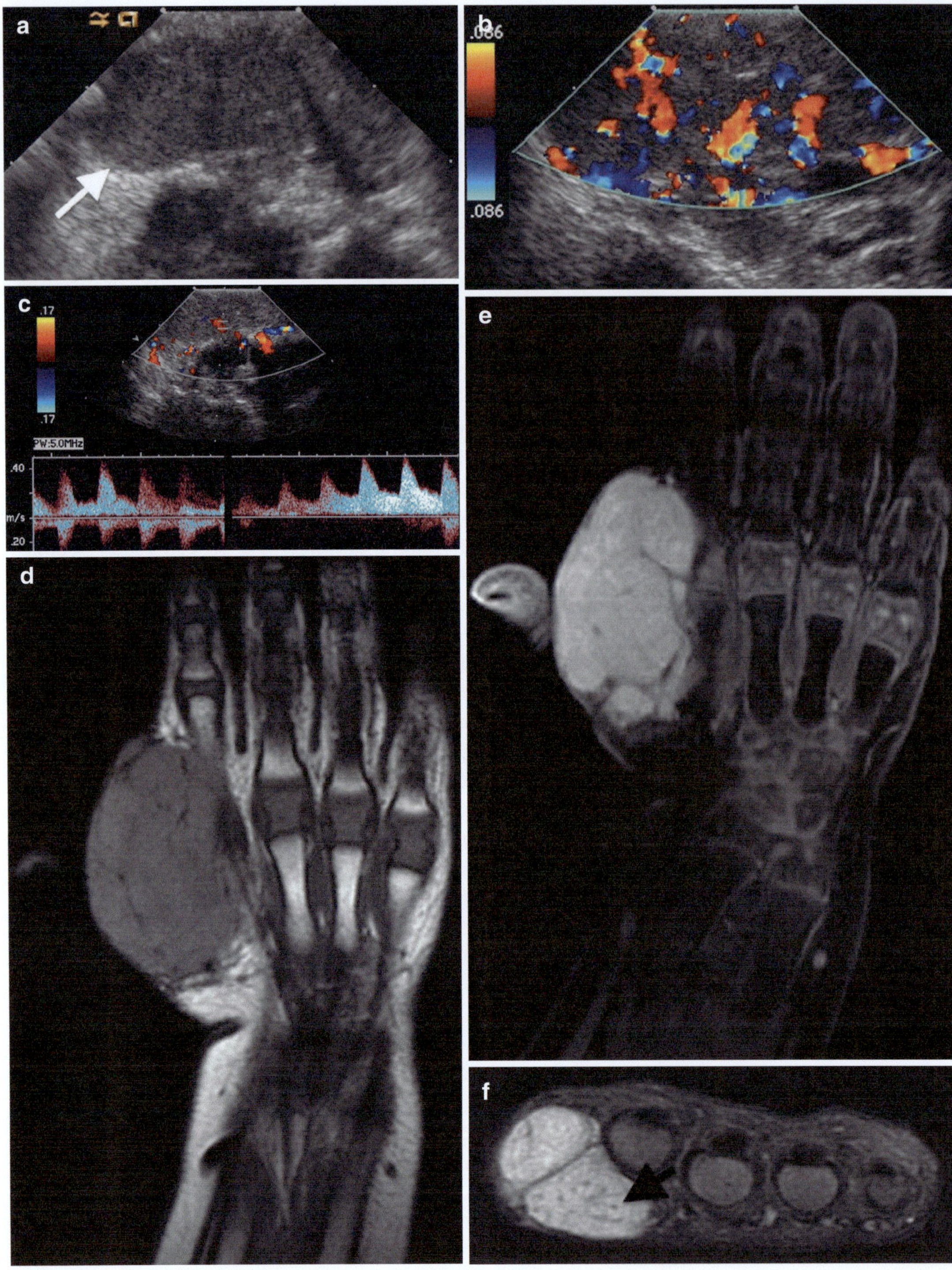

Fig. 22.1 Hemangioma of the hand in a 13-month-old boy. (**a**) Ultrasound (US) shows a hypoechoic, homogenous, and lobulated superficial soft tissue mass (*arrow*). (**b**) Doppler US shows high vessel density. (**c**) Spectral Doppler interrogation shows low-resistance arterial waveforms. The mass is intermediate signal on coronal T1-weighted (T1-W) magnetic resonance imaging (MRI) (**d**), and it enhances intensely (**e**, coronal T1-W FS gadolinium-enhanced image). (**f**) Proton density (PD) fat suppressed (FS) axial image shows central dots representing fibrofatty septa or thrombosed vessels (*arrow*). (**g**) Coronal magnetic resonance (MR) angiography shows adjacent large high-flow vessels

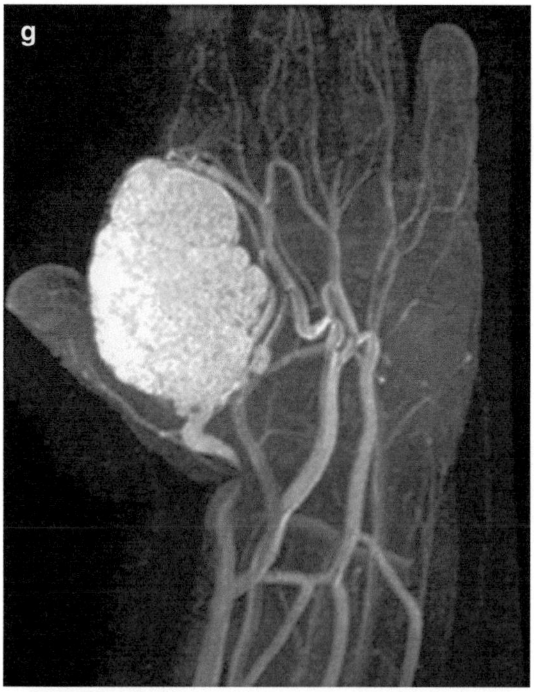

Fig. 22.1 (continued)

Differential Diagnosis

Differential considerations include neonatal soft tissue sarcomas, such as rhabdomyosarcoma and infantile fibrosarcoma. However, sarcomas tend to demonstrate more poorly defined margins and a more heterogeneous appearance both before and after contrast administration. The triad of lobulation, septation, and central low-signal-intensity dots is more common in hemangiomas [19]. Both T2 signal and enhancement are also generally more intense in hemangiomas than in soft tissue sarcomas [19]. Indeterminate masses require biopsy, but bleeding from a biopsied hemangioma can be profuse [20]. Unusual hemangiomas include rapidly involuting, non-involuting, and intramuscular subtypes.

Vascular Malformations

Vascular malformations, unlike classic infantile hemangiomas, are composed of dysplastic vessels, are present at birth, grow proportionally with the child, and do not spontaneously regress. The lesions are classified pathologically by what types of vessels are present, but a more practical differentiation is whether the lesion has high or low flow [11], as this determines treatment.

High-Flow Lesions

Arteriovenous Malformation

High-flow arteriovenous malformations (AVMs) occur when abnormal connections develop between arteries and veins, bypassing a capillary bed [21]. They are lined with nonproliferative endothelium [22]. The central feature of an AVM is the nidus (Latin for "knot") – a tangle of tortuous, dysplastic vessels, usually near the center of the AVM, where shunting of blood from the arterial to the venous system occurs [23].

The lesion presents as a soft, usually painless mass, often present at birth. Rarely, AVMs cause pain with exercise, warmth in the overlying skin, or distal ischemia due to steal phenomenon; compressive neuropathy, skin ulceration, high-output heart failure, or bleeding are even more unusual [22, 23]. Although most lesions grow proportionally with the child, some exhibit sudden, rapid growth in response to trauma, puberty, infection, or pregnancy [22].

The most effective treatment for an AVM is trans-arterial embolization, though surgery is occasionally necessary if embolization cannot be performed [22, 24]. An AVM may recur even after apparently successful embolization, ultimately requiring surgical resection or amputation [24].

Imaging

Radiographs may demonstrate overgrowth of adjacent bone and soft tissue due to increased blood flow (Fig. 22.2). US findings include multiple dilated vascular structures, some with high-velocity venous flow and others with low-resistance arterial flow. The nidus of the AVM may be difficult to identify [17]. The main differentiating factor between a hemangioma or venous malformation and an AVM on ultrasound is the lack of a discrete mass in an AVM.

MRI demonstrates multiple flow voids on spin-echo imaging and multiple surrounding venous structures, but there should be no discrete

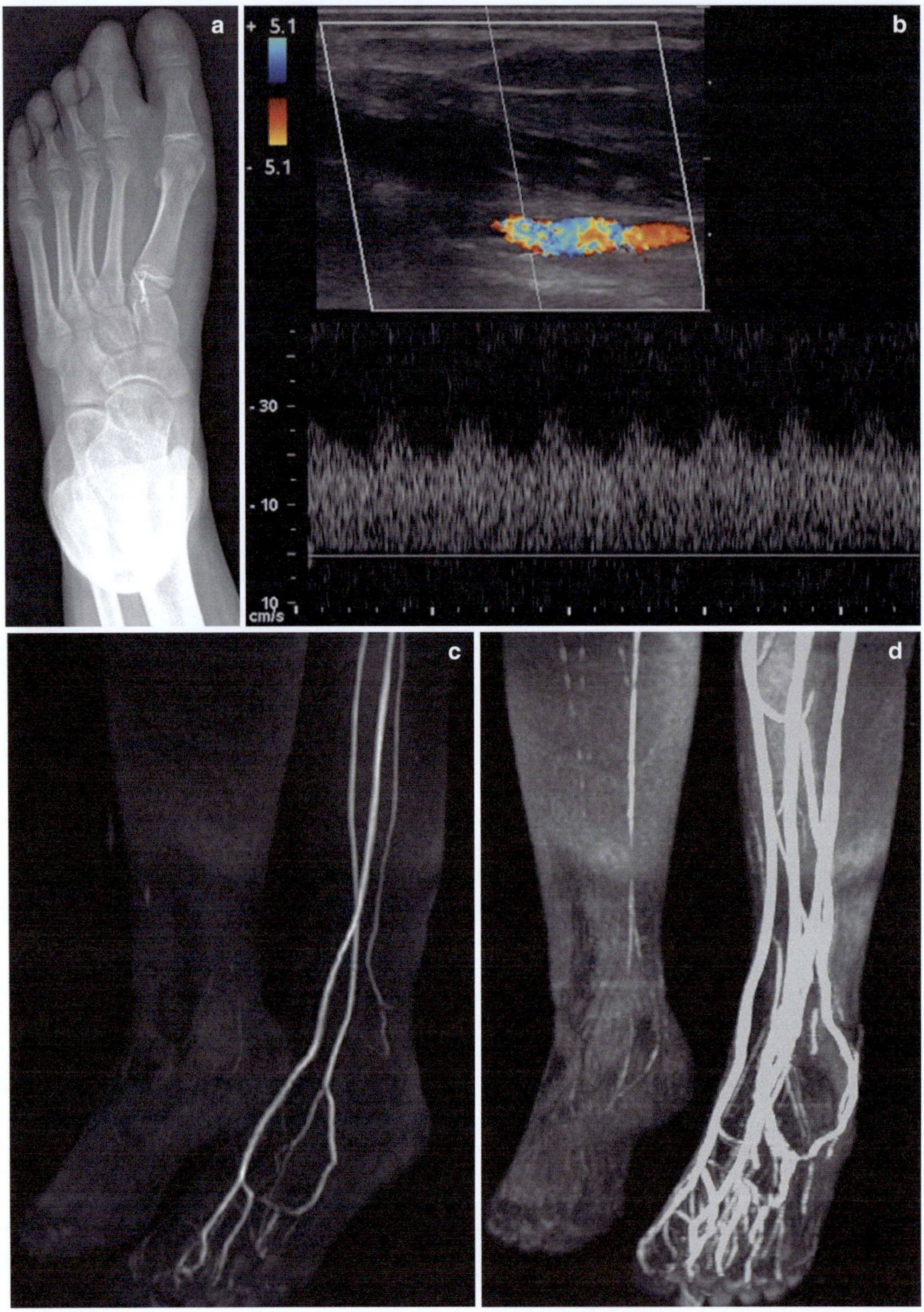

Fig. 22.2 Arteriovenous malformation (AVM) in a 10-year-old girl with a large second toe. (**a**) Soft tissue hypertrophy at medial foot (note hyperdense glue from attempted embolization). (**b**) Spectral Doppler US of the medial plantar artery shows low-resistance arterial waveform. (**c**) Maximum intensity projection (MIP) of gadolinium bolus MR angiography shows large feeding vessels, although the nidus is not identified. (**d**) Slightly delayed MIP image of gadolinium bolus MR angiography shows early draining veins. (**e**) Catheter digital subtraction angiography (DSA) shows complex, spiderweb-like nidus (*arrows*) with multiple early draining veins

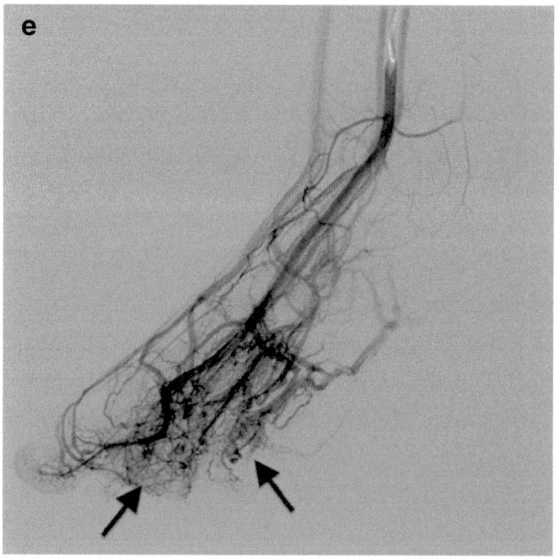

Fig. 22.2 (continued)

mass [22]. MR angiography can demonstrate high-flow feeding vessels. There may be overlying skin thickening or fatty overgrowth of the surrounding tissues, and there is occasionally surrounding soft tissue edema and enhancement that may simulate a mass [23]. When the lesion is confined to a muscle sheath, it closely mimics the appearance of a vascular tumor [23]. Angiography demonstrates arteriovenous shunting and demonstrates the nidus of the lesion to best effect. However, this modality is usually reserved for intervention and pre-intervention planning.

Arteriovenous Fistula

An arteriovenous fistula (AVF) consists of a direct connection between an artery and a vein. In the child it is usually iatrogenic or caused by fracture or blunt trauma [25, 26]. Clinical exam reveals a mass with a palpable thrill. US interrogation shows dilated venous structures with high-velocity flow and low-resistance arterial waveform on Doppler imaging [26]. Angiography with arterial injection reveals sudden filling of dilated veins at the level of the fistula without an intervening capillary phase. There may be associated pseudoaneurysms or other evidence of vascular trauma [26].

Low-Flow Lesions

Venous Malformation (Box 22.2)

Box 22.2: Venous Malformation

Most common soft tissue tumor in infants and children

Phleboliths pathognomonic

Most lesions contain both venous and lymphatic tissue

Speed of flow is more important than histology

Doppler US	Low-resistance arterial and venous flow
MRI	Dilated tubular structures may enhance
	Phleboliths hypointense on all sequences

Venous malformations (synonymous with cavernous hemangioma and phlebangioma) are the most common soft tissue tumor in infants and children [27]. These collections of dilated venous structures that lack mural smooth muscle cells [23] are also the most common type of vascular tumor overall.

This lesion may present as a soft, easily compressible bluish mass that enlarges with the Valsalva maneuver or if positioned dependently. It may involve only the skin or may extend into underlying fat, muscle, and bone [23]. The venous malformation often causes pain that increases from infancy into adulthood [11], along with deformity and decreased range of motion. A limb with a venous malformation is more likely to demonstrate undergrowth than overgrowth [23], but there may be associated fatty overgrowth. When the mass extends into a joint, recurrent hemorrhage may result in hemosiderin arthropathy, similar to that associated with hemophilia. The mass consists of multiple thin-walled venous channels without smooth muscle cells in the walls and possibly areas of organizing thrombus [10].

Treatment may include elastic compression garments, percutaneous injection with sclerosing agents, or surgical resection [11]. Percutaneous sclerosis often requires a staged procedure with

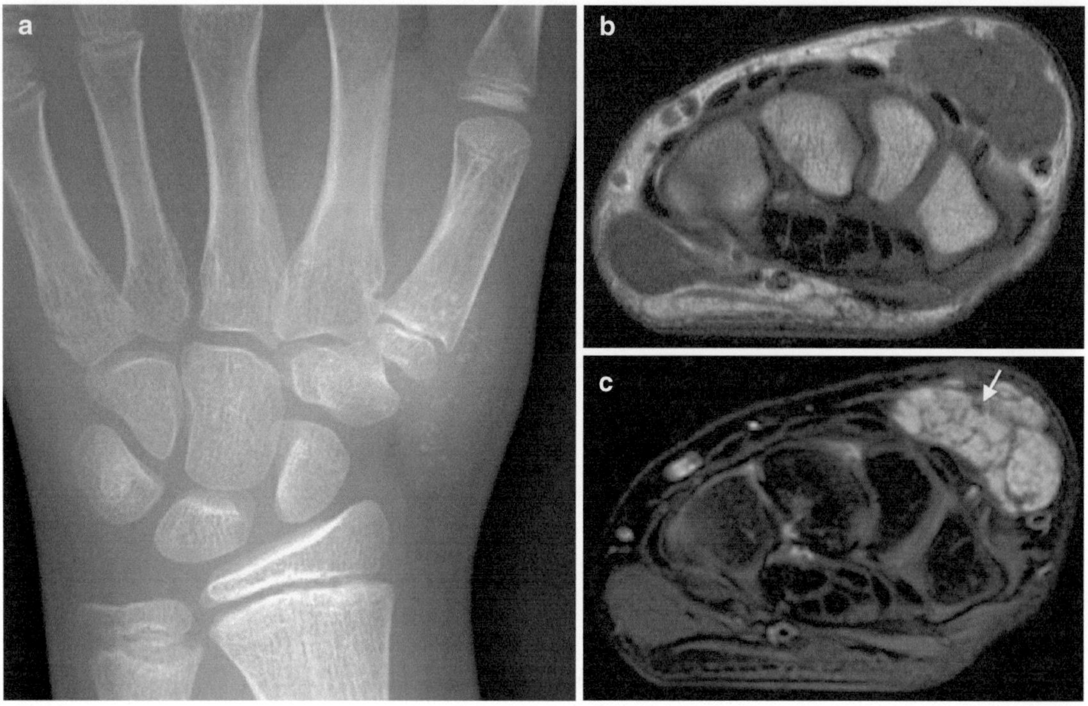

Fig. 22.3 Venous malformation in a 12-year-old boy with a wrist mass. (**a**) There are multiple round calcifications and ill-defined increased soft tissue density at the radial aspect of the wrist. (**b**) Axial T1-W image shows a lobulated, homogeneous mass of intermediate signal intensity. (**c**) Axial T2-weighted (T2-W) FS image shows homogeneous high signal intensity with septations and a few focal, round hypointensities (*arrow*) that correspond to calcifications

multiple sequential treatments. Only 20 % of patients will have complete relief from a single treatment, though in an additional 60 % symptoms and quality of life do improve [11].

Imaging

Phleboliths are the most specific radiographic finding of a venous malformation and allow definite differentiation from the classic infantile hemangioma [23] (Fig. 22.3). However, they occur in only 9–16 % of venous malformations [17]. If the lesions involve adjacent bone, the bone demonstrates lacy lytic changes that weaken trabeculae, predisposing to pathologic fractures [23].

US demonstrates a complex mass, often with multiple slow-flowing channels with intervening septations. There may be areas of low-resistance arterial flow, with antegrade flow both at systole and diastole (Figs. 22.4 and 22.5). Large phleboliths demonstrate acoustic shadowing [27]. Computed tomography (CT) reveals a soft tissue mass with multiple enhancing serpentine vascular structures [27]. There may be associated fatty overgrowth.

Small lesions appear homogeneous at MRI, with intermediate- to high-signal intensity on T1-W imaging and high signal on T2-W imaging (Fig. 22.5). Especially if the lesion is large, there is often overgrowth of surrounding fat. Fluid-fluid levels are rare and may correspond to areas of hemorrhage [23] (Fig. 22.6). Surrounding enlarged low-flow vessels may appear as dilated, fluid-filled (high T2, intermediate to low T1), tubular structures. After gadolinium administration, these vessels may enhance due to their low-velocity flow, unlike the high-flow vessels in AVMs and AVFs, which appear as flow voids [23]. Phleboliths appear as rounded areas of low signal on all sequences [21]. However, it should be noted that both venous and lymphatic components can coexist within a single malformation – in fact, more lesions demonstrate mixed histology than exist as pure venous or lymphatic malformations [11]. The lymphatic components do not enhance after contrast administration. Fortunately, the exact histology is less important than the speed of flow.

It is important to evaluate the extent to which the mass involves adjacent neurovascular bundles when planning for surgery, and if the lesion involves a joint, it is important to carefully assess the articular cartilage for evidence of arthropathy [23].

Lymphatic Malformation (Box 22.3)

Box 22.3: Lymphatic Malformation

Invasive	
Microcystic	Nonspecific solid mass
Macrocystic	Multiloculated cystic structure
MRI	Complex signal denotes prior hemorrhage or infection
	Fluid-fluid levels
	Enhancement of septations but not of cysts

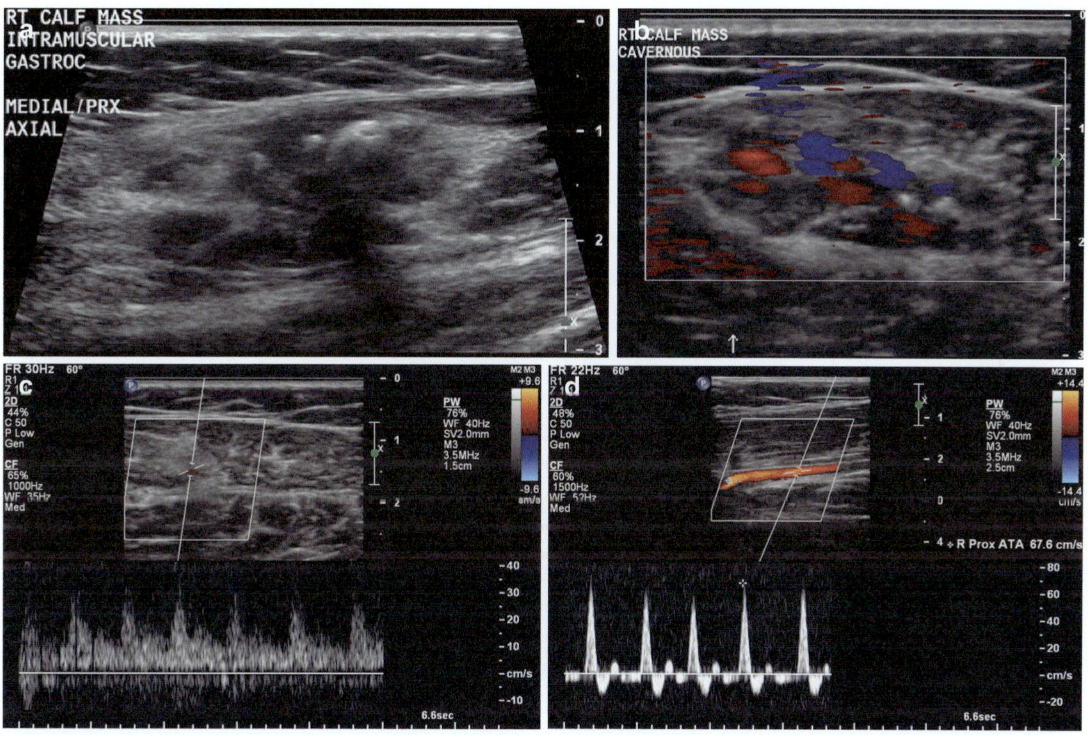

Fig. 22.4 Venous malformation in a 12-year-old girl complaining of calf pain. (**a**) US shows a heterogenous mass with shadowing, echogenic phleboliths. (**b**) Color Doppler US shows high vessel density. (**c**) Spectral Doppler waveform shows low-resistance arterial flow, compared with (**d**) normal triphasic arterial waveform of the anterior tibial artery. (**e**) Axial T1-W image shows a mass of intermediate signal intensity in the medial head of the gastrocnemius. Note phlebolith (*arrow*). (**f**) T2-W FS image shows heterogeneous hyperintensity. (**g**) Axial T1-W FS image shows homogeneous enhancement (except at the phlebolith)

Fig. 22.4 (continued)

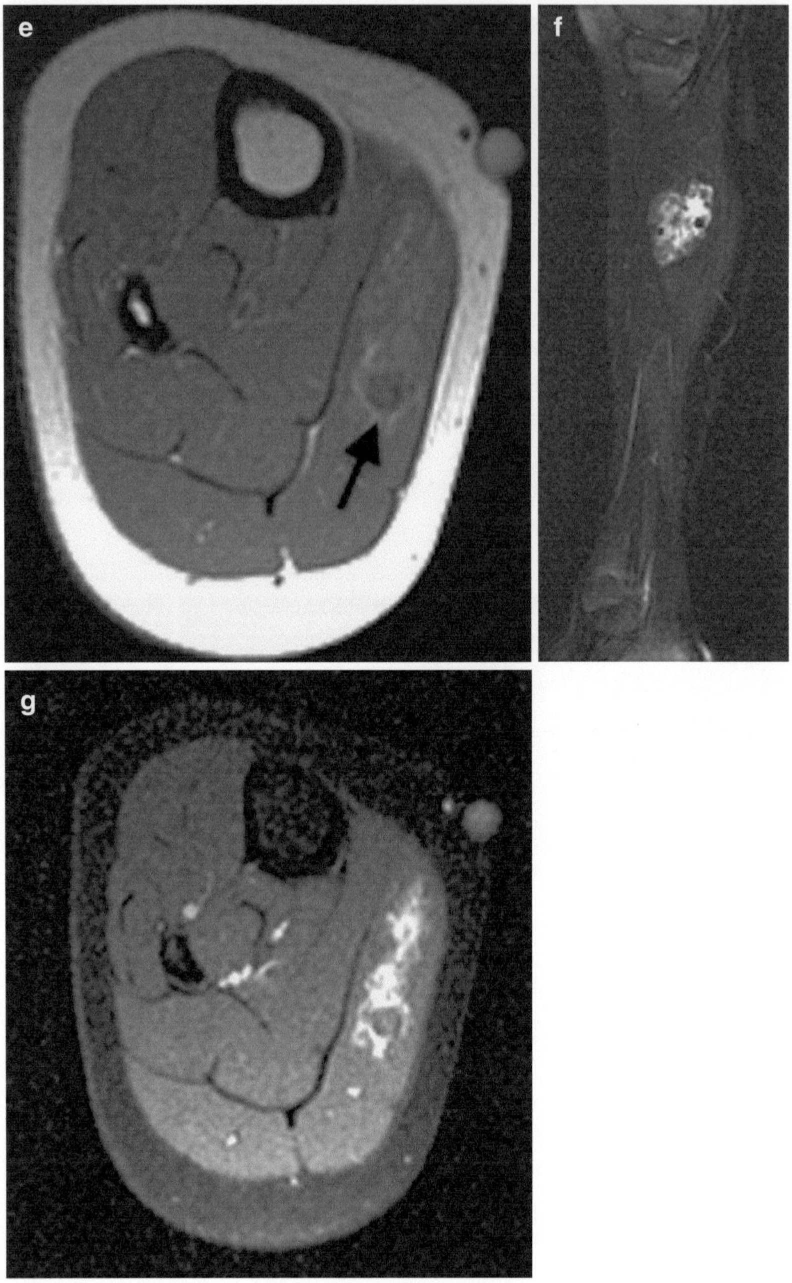

Lymphatic malformations are composed of dilated endothelium-lined channels containing lymphatic fluid [11]. Older terms for lymphatic malformations include lymphangioma and cystic hygroma. Seventy-five percent of lymphatic malformations involve the head and neck [23]. The lesions present as a soft mass with either diffuse or localized swelling and

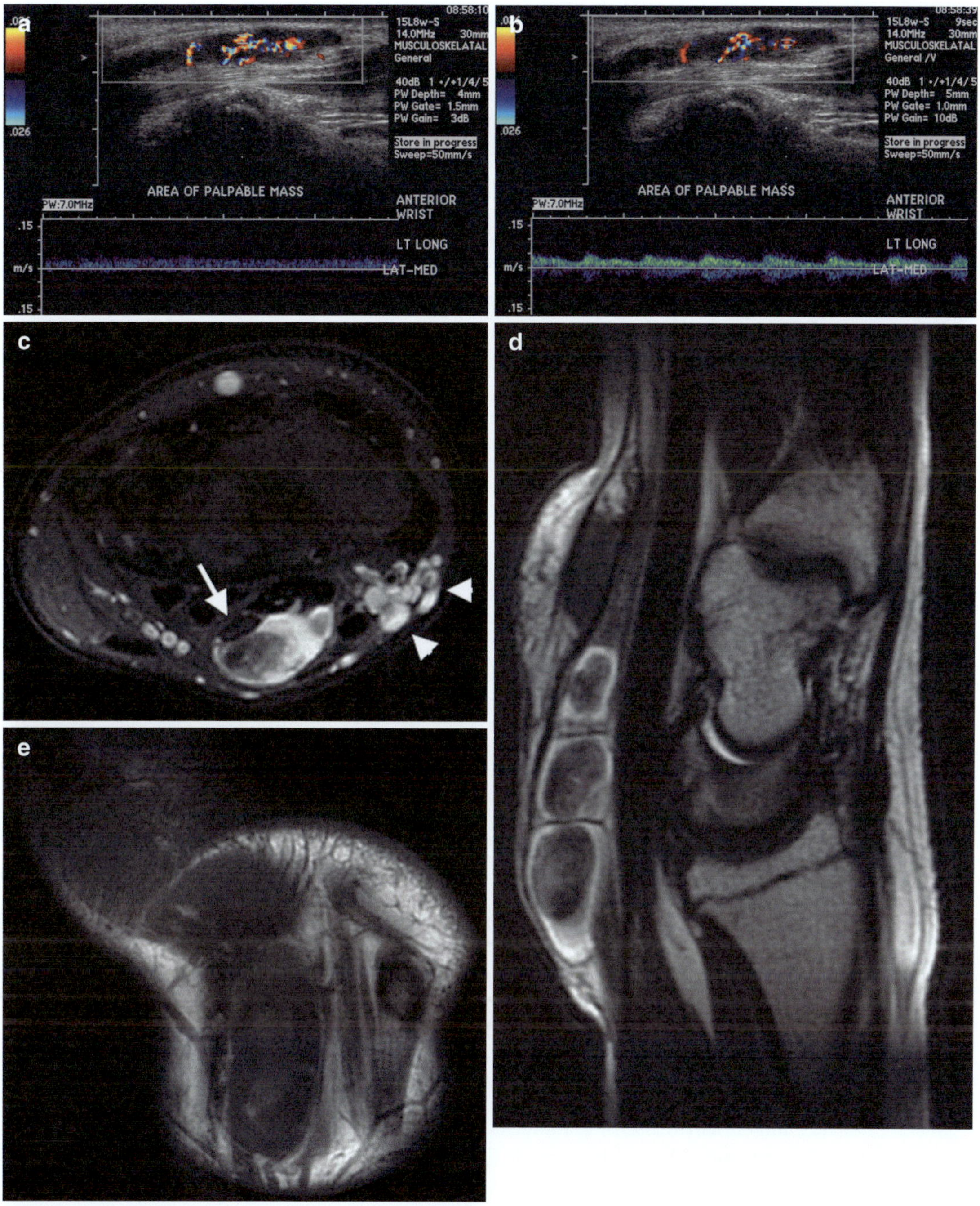

Fig. 22.5 Venous malformation of the wrist in a 15-year-old boy. The mass had multiple dilated vessels and foci of organizing thrombus and was intimately related with the median nerve. Spectral Doppler images demonstrate low-resistance venous (**a**) and arterial (**b**) flow within the mass. (**c**) Axial T2-W FS image shows central low signal, which corresponded to organizing thrombus. Note proximity to median nerve (*arrow*), which might suggest the diagnosis of nerve sheath tumor. There are enlarged vessels at the radial aspect of the wrist (*arrowheads*). (**d**) Sagittal T2-W FS image shows striking central hypointensity. (**e**) Coronal T1-W image shows multiloculated hypointense mass

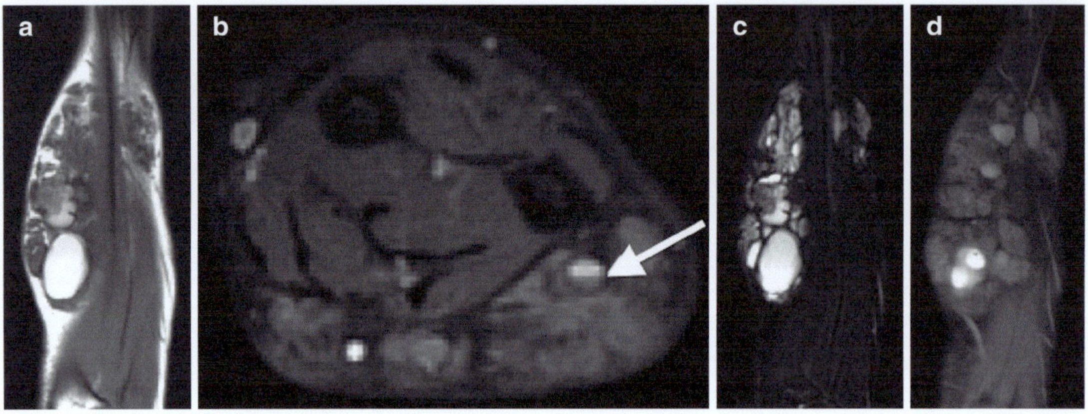

Fig. 22.6 Venous malformation involving the forearm in an 11-year-old boy. (**a**) Coronal T1-W image of the forearm shows a complex mass, predominantly isointense to muscle, with rounded areas of high signal and a hypointense rim corresponding to hemorrhage. Subcutaneous fat is overgrown. (**b**) Axial T2-W FS image shows high signal and septations with a fluid-fluid level (*arrow*). (**c**) Coronal T2-W FS image shows hyperintensity with multiple septations. (**d**) Coronal T1-W FS gadolinium-enhanced image shows diffuse low-level enhancement with areas of hyperintense hemorrhage and intervening lobules of overgrown subcutaneous fat

adjacent soft tissue and skeletal overgrowth [23]. Most present in infancy or childhood, 90 % before age 2 [11]. Although usually treated with surgical excision, percutaneous sclerotherapy is occasionally employed.

Imaging

Radiographs may demonstrate lacy infiltration of adjacent bones, along with soft tissue edema and hypertrophy. At US, macrocystic lesions appear multiloculated and cystic, with thin septations (Fig. 22.7); microcystic lesions appear solid and hyperechoic. CT demonstrates a nonspecific soft tissue mass.

The size of the cysts determines the appearance of the lesion at MRI. Lesions with microscopic cysts appear solid, with low signal on T1, high signal on T2, and either diffuse or complete absence of enhancement [21]. Macrocystic lesions have a more typical appearance, with multiple well-defined cysts that have low signal on T1 (unless there has been previous hemorrhage or infection) and high signal on T2 (Fig. 22.8). There may be fluid-fluid levels (Fig. 22.9). Although the septa may enhance, the cystic components do not enhance unless there has been prior treatment [21]. Like most vascular

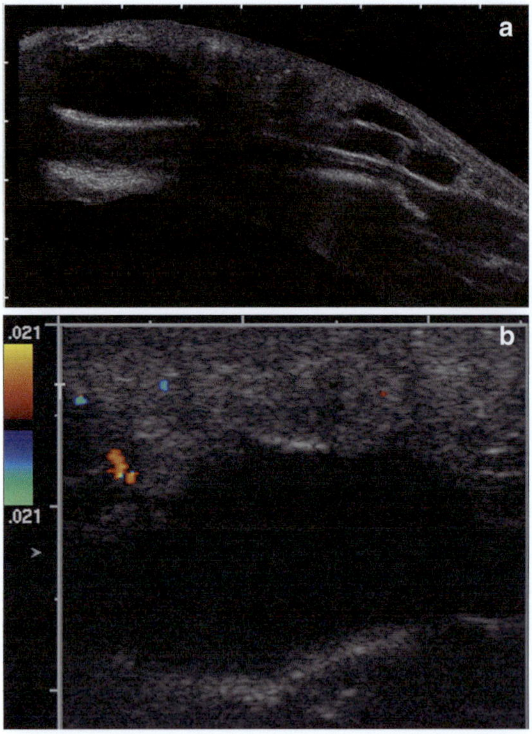

Fig. 22.7 Lymphatic malformation of the thigh in a 2-year-old girl. (**a**) Composite longitudinal US shows an elongated subcutaneous cystic mass with a few thick septations. (**b**) Color Doppler interrogation shows it is essentially avascular

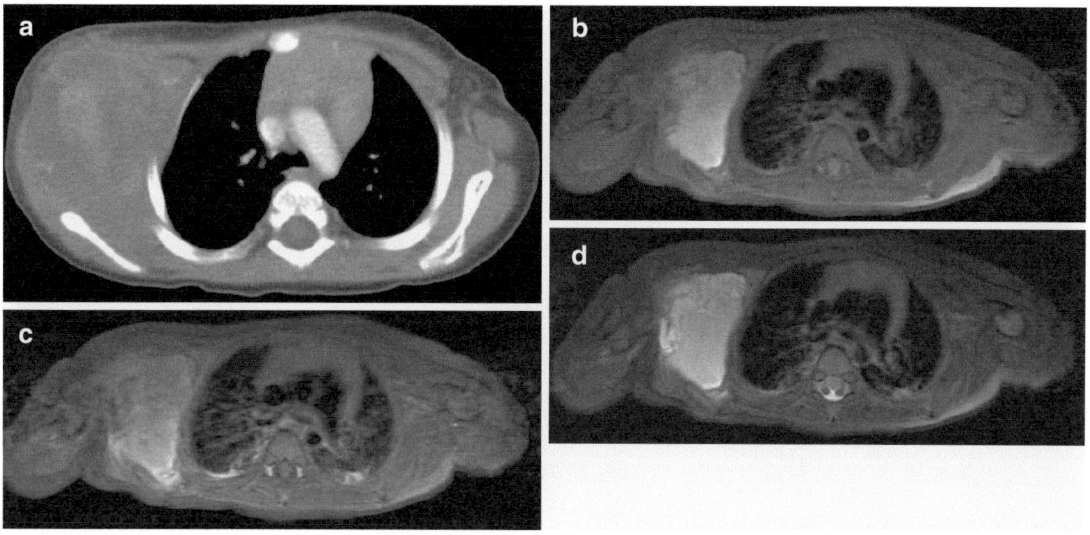

Fig. 22.8 Lymphatic malformation in the axilla of a 13-month-old boy. (**a**) Axial CT shows a nonspecific lobulated soft tissue mass. Axial T1-W FS (**b**) images demonstrate homogenous hyperintensity, indicating protein or hemorrhage. (**c**) Axial T1-W FS gadolinium-enhanced image shows no intralesional enhancement. (**d**) T2-W FS image shows moderately increased signal, consistent with complex fluid. Focal hypointensity likely represents hemosiderin

lesions, lymphatic malformations do not respect fascial planes and extend into multiple different tissue types (Fig. 22.10).

Syndromes Associated with Vascular Malformations

Klippel-Trenaunay-Weber syndrome (Fig. 22.11) consists of the triad of cutaneous hemangioma (manifesting as a port-wine stain), overgrowth of a limb or part of a limb, and varicose veins [27]. When the lesion is associated with an AVF, it is known as Parkes Weber syndrome. Both lesions usually demonstrate bony overgrowth, with increased fat and atrophy of the musculature. There is often associated fibromuscular dysplasia.

Maffucci syndrome consists of multiple enchondromas and multiple soft tissue venous malformations – the characteristic phleboliths and enchondromas clinch the diagnosis on radiographs [27]. The enchondromas eventually transform into chondrosarcomas in 15–20% of cases, and the venous malformations transform into vascular sarcoma in 3–5 % of cases [27].

Blue rubber bleb nevus syndrome causes multiple cutaneous vascular lesions and venous malformations of the gastrointestinal tract.

Osler-Weber-Rendu syndrome is a systemic fibrovascular dysplasia that causes AVMs in multiple organs as well as in the extremities, along with aneurysms and telangectasia [27].

Kaposiform Hemangioendothelioma

This rare tumor is intermediate in the continuum between infantile hemangioma and angiosarcoma – more aggressive than a hemangioma, but not malignant [10]. Its clinical features resemble those of a proliferative infantile hemangioma, but it does not regress and responds poorly to standard treatments for infantile hemangiomas [11, 28]. It usually requires surgical excision with or without preoperative embolization [10]. The histologic appearance of this densely cellular tumor resembles Kaposi sarcoma, but kaposiform hemangioendothelioma is not associated with human herpes virus-8 infection [15]. Immunohistochemical stains can confirm the diagnosis [10].

Imaging

On US, kaposiform hemangioendothelioma appears as an infiltrative mass with variable echogenicity and both high- and low-resistance waveforms on color Doppler imaging [15]. Although quite

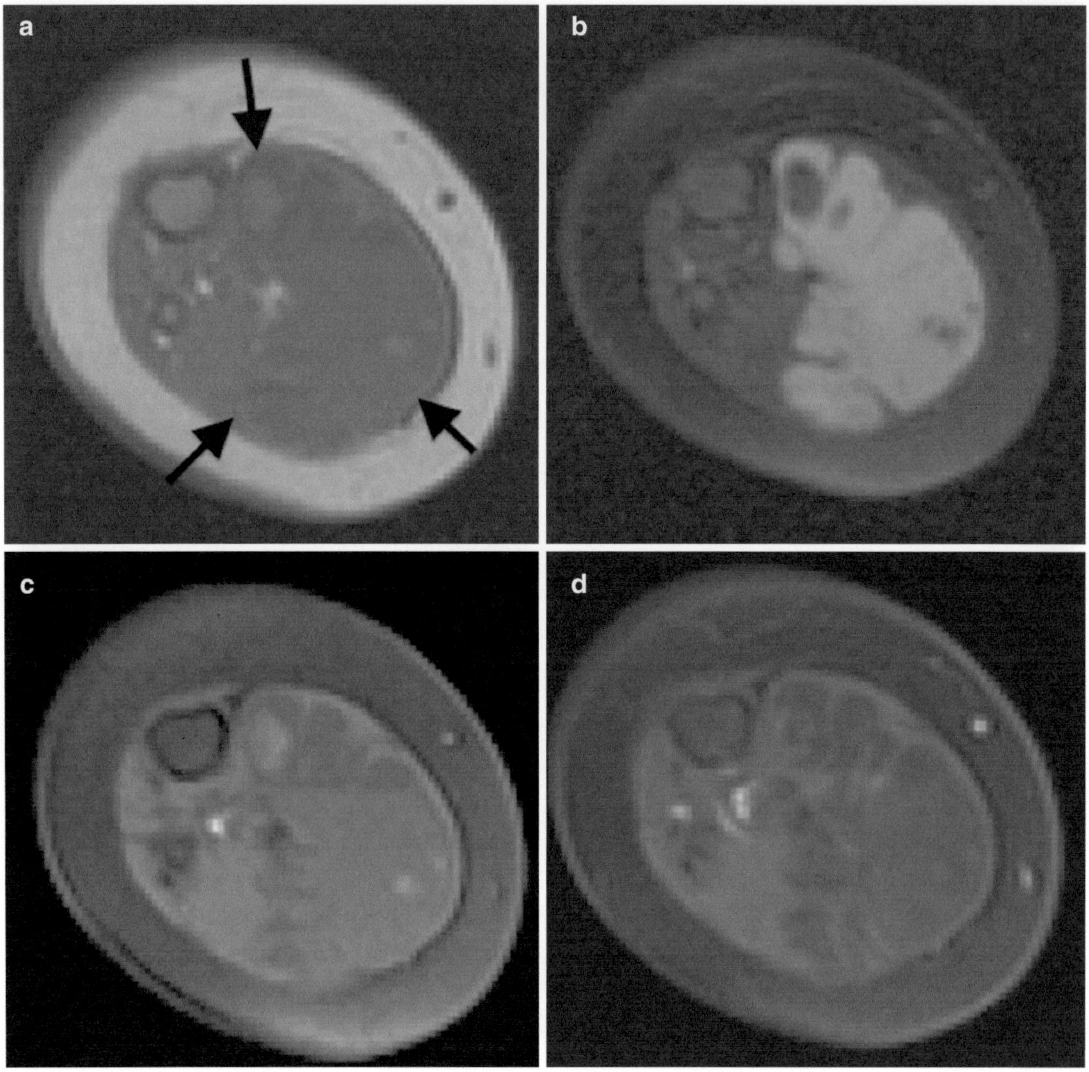

Fig. 22.9 Lymphatic malformation of the calf in a 5-month-old girl. (**a**) Axial T1-W image shows a fairly homogeneous mass in the medial head of the right gastrocnemius muscle (*arrows*), predominantly isointense to muscle, with several fluid-fluid levels and a few septations. Scattered areas of hyperintensity are probably fat. (**b**) Axial T2-W FS image shows a diffusely hyperintense mass with a few thin septations and a rounded area of decreased signal (likely hemorrhage). Axial T1-W FS (**c**) and T1-W FS gadolinium-enhanced (**d**) images show fluid-fluid levels and septal enhancement

vascular, it is typically less vascular than hemangioma [17]. The MRI appearance is nonspecific, with heterogeneous signal on T1, generally high signal on T2, and multiple surrounding vessels. There is usually subcutaneous stranding on T2-W sequences. The tumor enhances intensely. Unlike the infantile hemangioma, kaposiform hemangioendothelioma usually involves multiple tissue planes, causes skin thickening, and has abundant surrounding edema. There are fewer superficial feeding and draining vessels than with an infantile hemangioma, and adjacent bone destruction is more common [23].

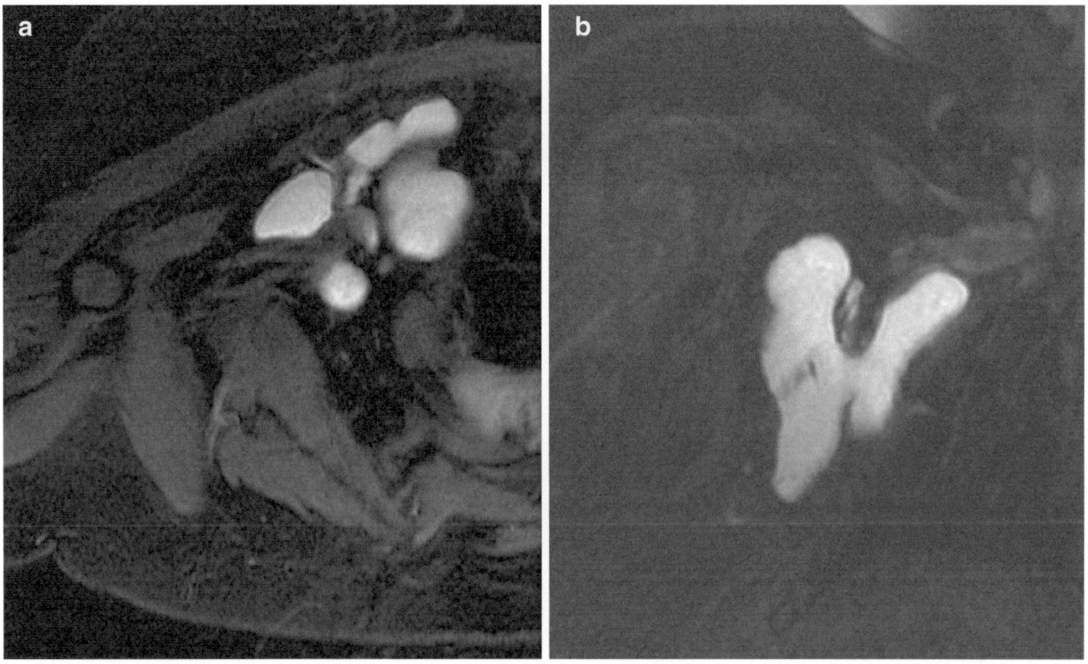

Fig. 22.10 Infiltrative lymphatic malformation in the axilla of a 4-year-old girl. Axial (**a**) and coronal (**b**) T2-W FS images show a multiloculated bilobed mass that wraps around soft tissue structures

Hematoma (Box 22.4)

> **Box 22.4: Hematoma**
>
> May present as palpable mass with no recollection of antecedent trauma.
>
> Even with history of trauma, evaluate an intramuscular hematoma with contrast-enhanced MRI to exclude underlying hemorrhagic tumor.
>
> Signal progression in soft tissue hematomas differs from CNS.

Children are very active but relatively uncoordinated and therefore suffer a lot of bumps, bruises, and falls. Although most of these insults cause no appreciable damage, some result in soft tissue hematomas. The acute but transient discolored, palpable mass with overlying bruising is usually managed without imaging, but occasionally a child presents with questionable history or indeed years after the initial trauma with no recollection of a specific injury. Histology reveals a mass composed of blood clot, fibrin, and amorphous debris in a central cavity. There is a fibrous pseudocapsule that may contain foreign body giant cells, cellular scarring, xanthogranulomatous inflammation, cholesterol clefts, and possibly dystrophic calcifications.

Treatment usually consists of watchful waiting, though resection is sometimes performed when imaging findings are nonspecific or if the mass fails to resolve.

Imaging

Radiographs demonstrate nonspecific swelling (Fig. 22.12). If the hematoma has liquefied, a fluid-fluid level may be evident.

US shows a heterogeneous mass with either well-defined or irregular margins. Acute hematomas appear hyperechoic, whereas in later stages

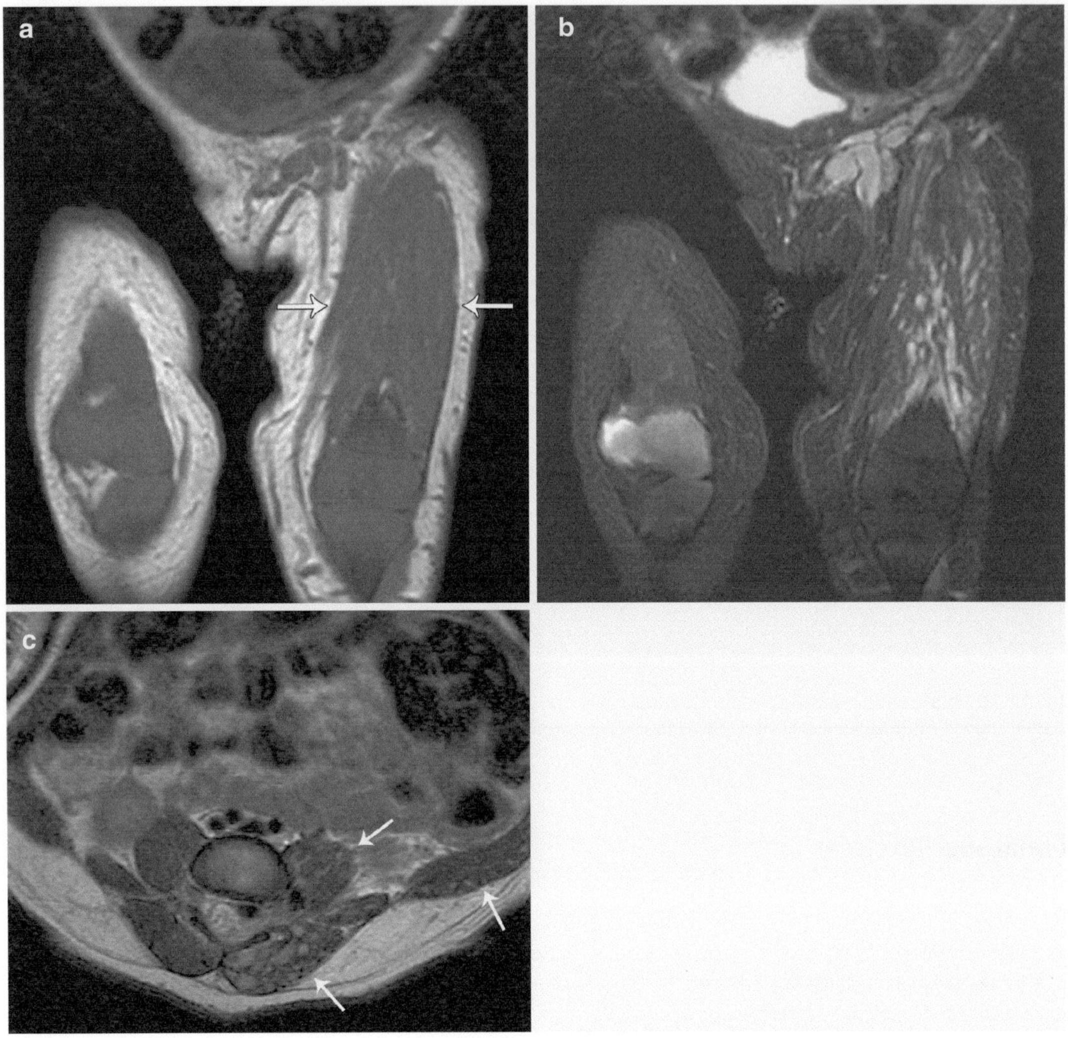

Fig. 22.11 Klippel-Trenaunay-Weber syndrome in a newborn. (**a**) Coronal T1-W image shows an isointense lymphaticovenous malformation insinuated within atrophic musculature (*arrows*). (**b**) Coronal T2-W FS image shows the mass extends to the inguinal area. (**c**) Axial T2-W image shows hyperintense cystic infiltration of the left erector spinae and other musculature (*arrows*), with enlargement of spinal veins (Reprinted from Stein-Wexler [98], copyright 2009, with permission from Elsevier)

they appear hypoechoic [29]. Furthermore, clotted blood appears more echogenic when evaluated with a higher frequency transducer. There may be internal septations. If the hematoma is associated with a muscle tear, dynamic imaging with passive flexion and extension may show retraction of muscle with increased size of the lesion [29]. There should be no internal Doppler signal in a benign hematoma, although there may be increased flow around it; vascular flow within a hematoma suggests there is an underlying lesion.

The CT appearance depends on the lesion's age. Acute blood is hyperdense, but subacute hematomas demonstrate mixed density, reflecting clot lysis. The rim may enhance after contrast

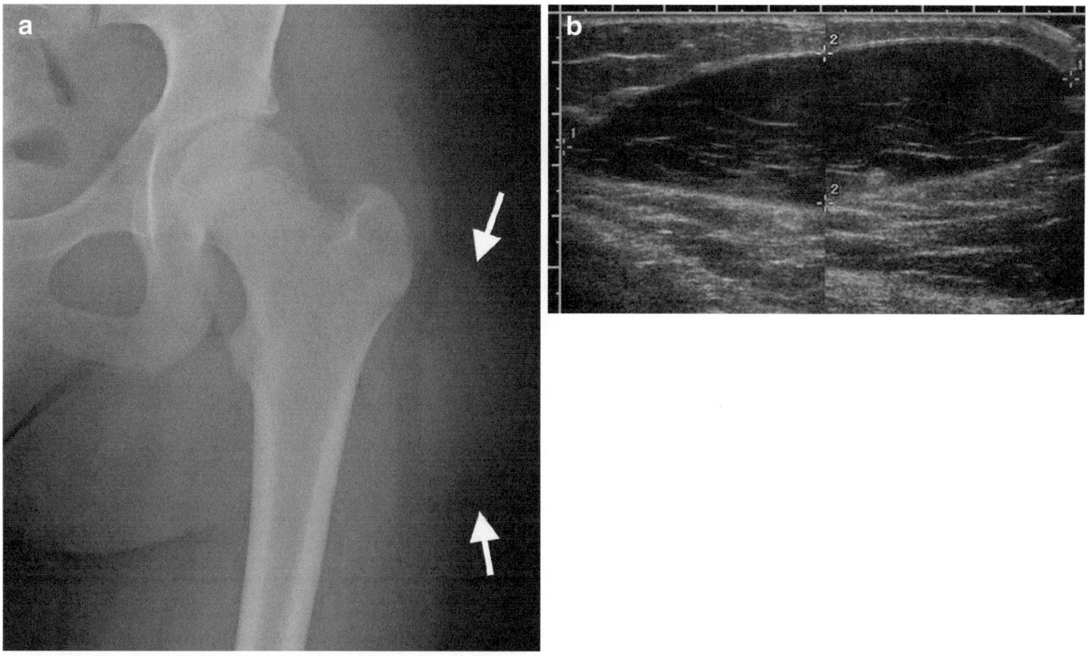

Fig. 22.12 Hematoma in a 13-year-old girl with a painful hip mass after trauma. (**a**) There is a lentiform soft tissue mass (*arrows*). (**b**) Composite US image shows a well-circumscribed, hypoechoic, subcutaneous lentiform mass, with internal septations. Color Doppler interrogation demonstrated no blood flow (not shown)

administration [30]. Chronic hematomas are well-defined, homogeneous, and of water density. The fibrous pseudocapsule of a chronic hematoma may calcify.

The MRI appearance is variable and changes as lesions evolve. It is important to recognize that the absence of a blood-brain barrier in the soft tissues causes hemorrhage to behave differently there than in the brain. Blood products degrade more rapidly, and signal intensity progresses differently [31]. When intramuscular hematomas were experimentally induced in rats, the low T2 signal ascribed to intracellular deoxyhemoglobin in the acute and subacute phases of brain hemorrhage never materialized, perhaps because blood flow in skeletal muscle allowed red blood cells to break down more rapidly than within the brain. However, at late stages hypointense hemosiderin did develop [31].

The internal signal of a hematoma may be heterogeneous, reflecting blood in various stages of evolution. Acute blood products tend to be bright on T1-W images (Fig. 22.13). In the acute and subacute stages, edema may surround the hematoma, but this resolves as the hematoma matures (Fig. 22.14). As early as 4 days after injury, a hypointense rim may be present at T2-W images, although no hemosiderin is present at histology; this may result from a boundary effect between two areas with different magnetic susceptibility [31]. The chronic hematoma often has a hypointense hemosiderin rim that may enhance. A mass with signal characteristics consistent with blood products most likely represents a benign hematoma, but short-term follow-up with contrast-enhanced MRI may be warranted to exclude an underlying neoplasm.

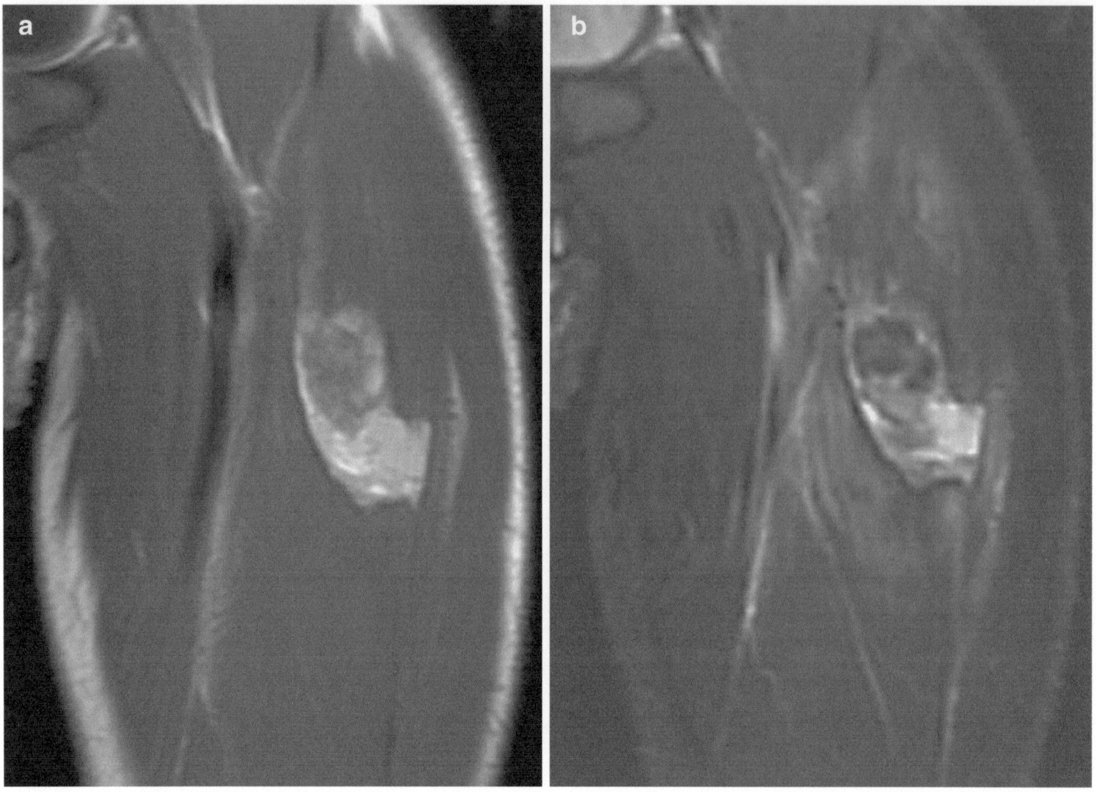

Fig. 22.13 Hematoma in a 14-year-old boy with sudden thigh pain while running. (**a**) Coronal T1-W image shows a moderately heterogenous. Mostly hyperintense mass within the rectus femoris muscle, with a thin hypointense rim. (**b**) Coronal T2-W FS image shows heterogenous, predominantly hyperintense mass with surrounding intramuscular edema

Differential diagnosis is broad and includes abscess and a wide variety of sarcomas.

1.2 Fibrous Lesions

Desmoid Tumor

Also known as aggressive fibromatosis and as desmoplastic fibroma when it arises in or extends into bones, this non-metastasizing and histologically benign but locally aggressive tumor consists of intertwining fibroblasts and myofibroblasts [32, 33]. It arises most often in muscles in the extremities. Although cases are most common in the third decade, up to 30 % occur before age 20 (mean age 13 years) [32]. Predisposing conditions include antecedent trauma to the area, radiation, and, in between 1 and 2 % of cases, Gardner syndrome [32].

Clinical presentation includes pain, mass, and (if the tumor crosses a joint) limited mobility. Interlacing bundles of spindle cells with entrapped skeletal muscle and surrounding soft tissue on a background of abundant collagen are apparent at histology [32]. If there are nuclear atypia and multiple mitotic figures, the pathologist is more likely to render a diagnosis of sarcoma. The tumor has infiltrative borders and is usually tan white, with a whorled appearance and firm texture.

Treatment is difficult, as the tumor invariably extends beyond the margins evident at imaging and palpable at surgery, so despite aggressive, wide resection about 60 % of tumors recur [34]. Tumors that involve the neurovascular bundle and/or bone are more difficult to resect completely and consequently have a higher risk of recurrence [33]. Treatment often includes radiation and chemotherapy, though radiation occasionally induces

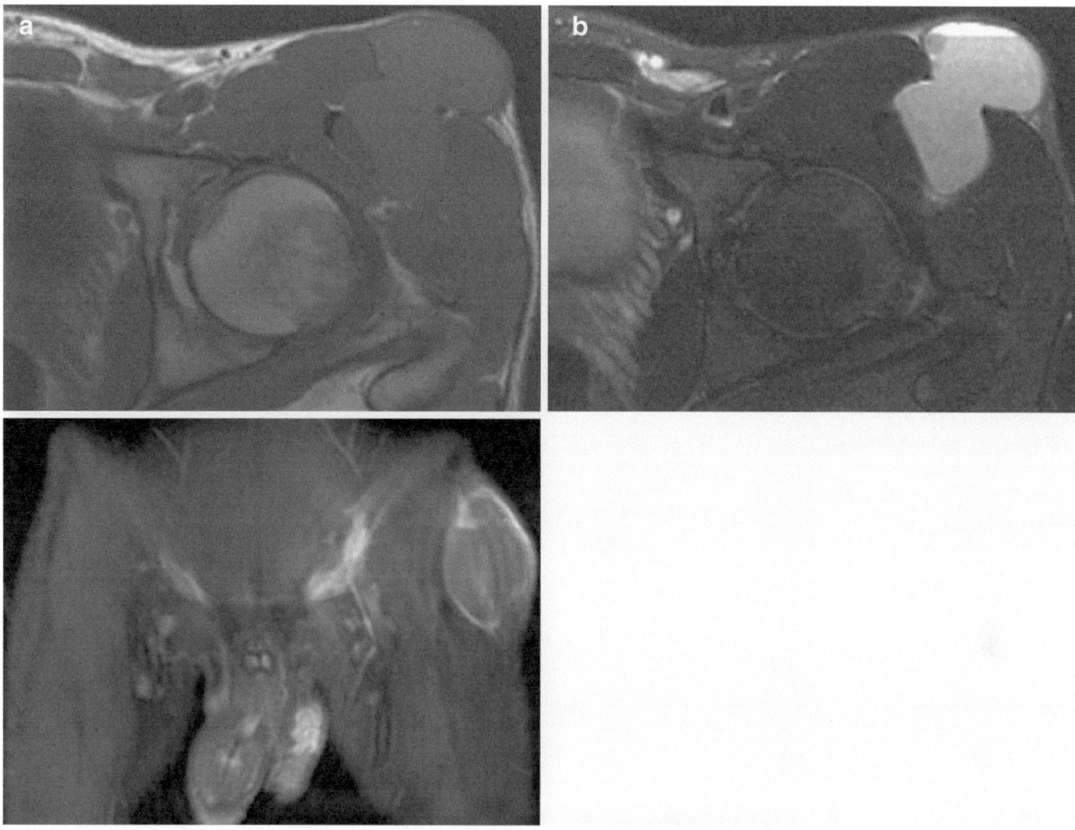

Fig. 22.14 Hematoma in a 15-year-old boy with chronic hip pain. (**a**) Axial T1-W image shows a bilobed, homogeneous, slightly hyperintense mass extending from intramuscular fascia to subcutaneous adipose tissue. (**b**) Axial T2-W FS image shows a fluid-fluid level and no surrounding edema. (**c**) Coronal T1-W FS gadolinium-enhanced image shows only a thin enhancing rim

additional desmoid tumors in the adjacent tissue [33]. Early experience suggests that cryoablation of desmoid tumors that do not involve vital structures provides long-term disease-free response in adults [35]; this may warrant further investigation in children.

Imaging

US appearance is variable and nonspecific [34]. At CT this tumor is similarly variable, but tends to be isodense to skeletal muscle [34]. There is no consistent relationship between CT appearance of the tumor and its histology. Intravenous contrast helps evaluate the relationship between the tumor and vessels.

MRI appearance (Fig. 22.15) varies with the extent of cellular, collagen, and myxoid material, though the tumor tends to be iso- to hyperintense to muscle on T1 and heterogeneously hyperintense to muscle on T2 [33]. It usually demonstrates avid enhancement. Linear and curvilinear strands of non-enhancing low-signal-intensity tissue that cross the tumor correspond to strands of collagen and may suggest the diagnosis [4]. Even if the margins of the tumor appear well circumscribed, there is usually microinvasion beyond the pseudocapsule at surgery. It is therefore essential to comment on adjacent important structures, such as the neurovascular bundle and joints. Features that have been reported to differentiate desmoid tumors from sarcomas include an infiltrative growth pattern, crossing of fascial planes, and lack of central necrosis even in very large lesions [36].

Infantile Myofibromatosis

The nodules of infantile myofibromatosis usually present in the neonatal period and are rare after age 2 years. They are composed of spindle cells,

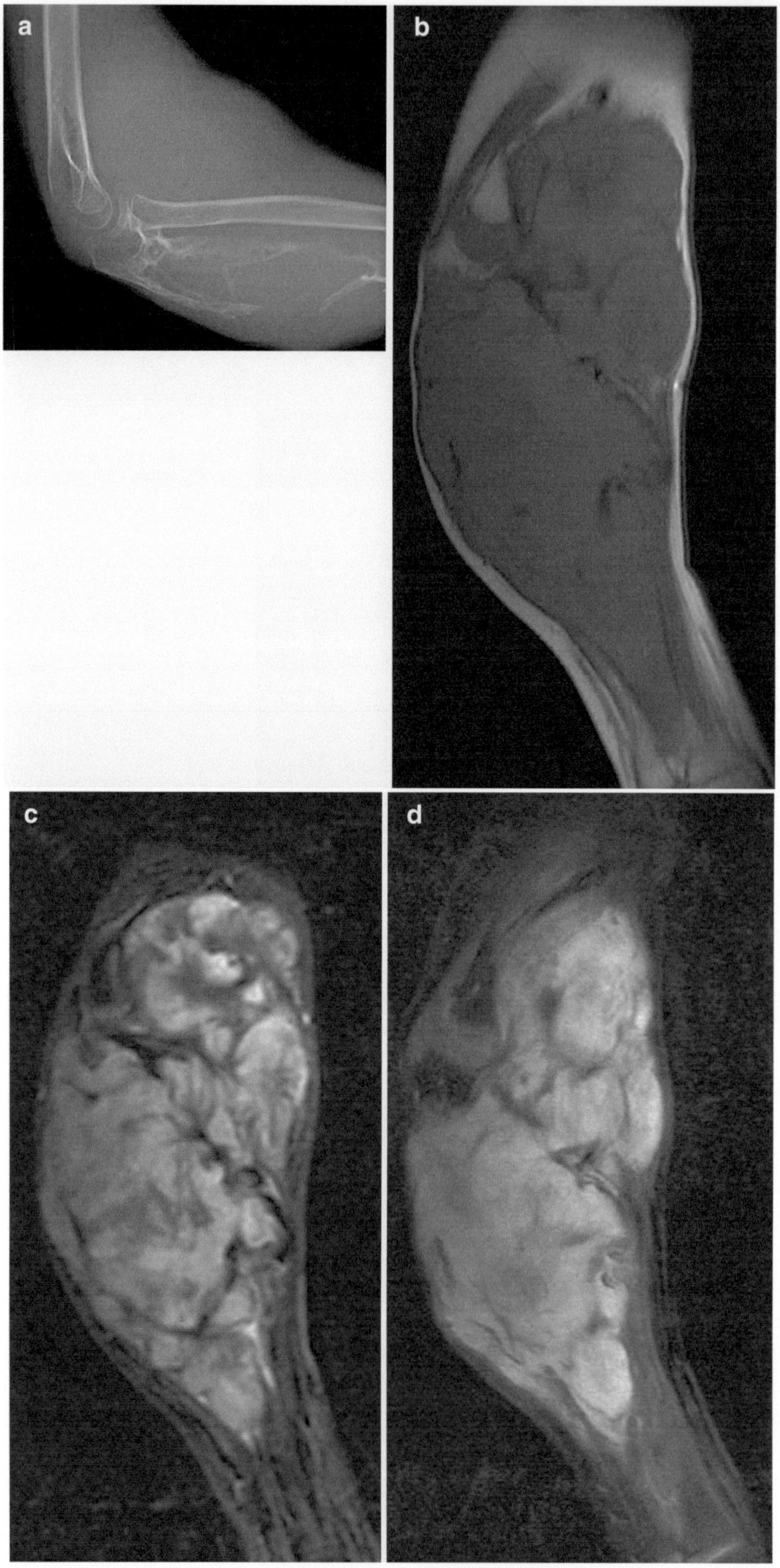

Fig. 22.15 Desmoid in a 9-year-old boy with an enlarging forearm mass. (**a**) A large mass expands and destroys the ulna. (**b**) Coronal T1-W image shows hypointense fibrous strands traversing a lobulated mass that is slightly hyperintense to skeletal muscle. (**c**) Coronal short tau inversion recovery (STIR) image shows it is heterogeneous, with hypointense strands. (**d**) Coronal T1-W FS gadolinium-enhanced image shows homogeneous enhancement (except for the fibrous strands)

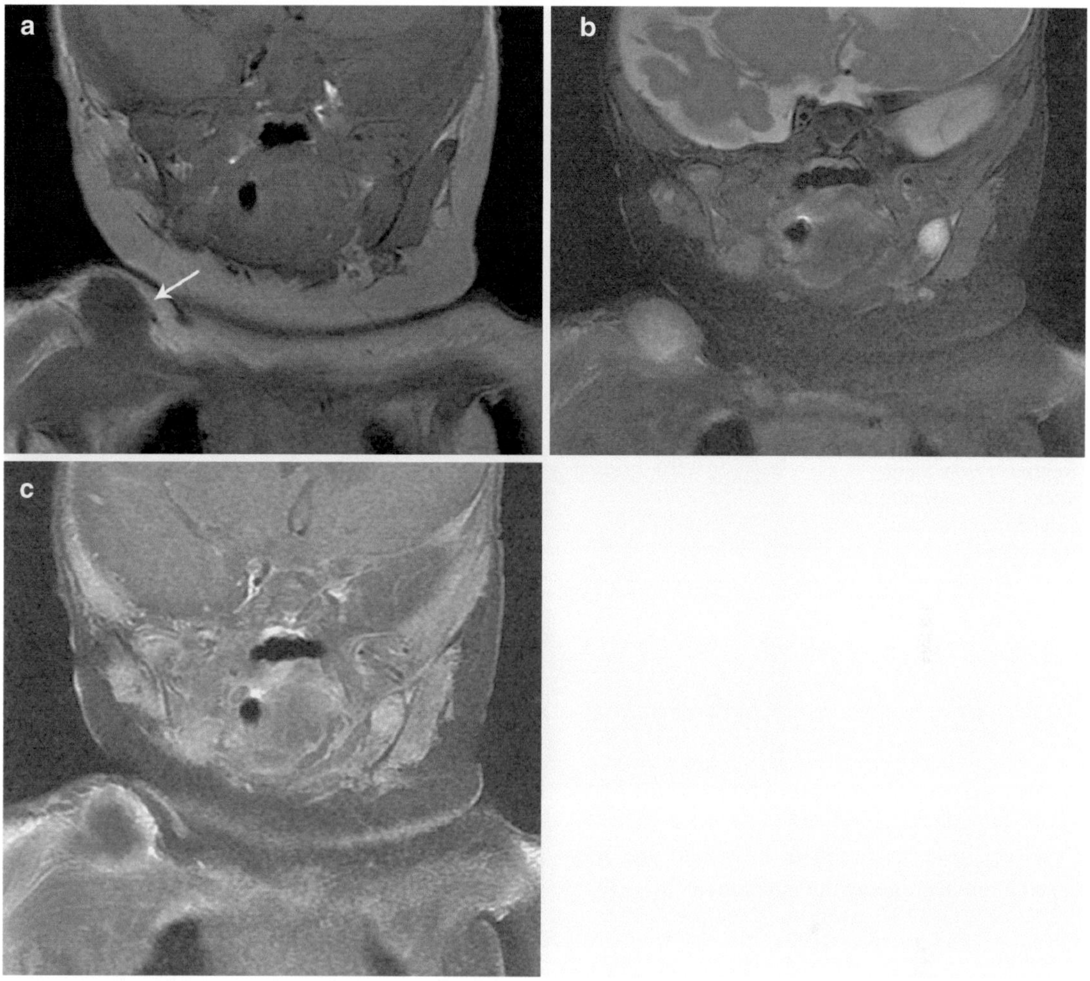

Fig. 22.16 Infantile myofibromatosis of the shoulder. (**a**) T1-W coronal image shows a rounded, well-defined, slightly hypointense right shoulder mass (*arrow*). The center is hyperintense on T2-W MRI (**b**), and there is marginal enhancement, resulting in a target appearance (**c**, T1-W FS gadolinium-enhanced) (Reprinted from Stein-Wexler [98], copyright 2009, with permission from Elsevier)

with features of fibroblasts and smooth muscle. Rarely unifocal, multiple soft tissue nodules in the subcutaneous soft tissues of the head, neck, or trunk are typical. Occasionally the skeleton, gastrointestinal tract, heart, or lungs are involved. Spontaneous regression occurs in 30 %, although if there is visceral involvement this disease is lethal in 70 % [37]. Multifocality is more likely in girls.

Imaging

These lesions are round and can be well circumscribed or ill defined. Signal intensity varies, but they are typically isointense to muscle on T1-W imaging, although the center can be mildly hyperintense (Fig. 22.16). They are usually uniformly hyperintense on T2-W sequences. After administration of gadolinium, a target appearance is common, with lack of central enhancement but with intense enhancement in the periphery [21].

Popliteal Cyst

Two percent of asymptomatic children and 6 % of children referred for MRI due to knee pain demonstrate a popliteal cyst at imaging [38].

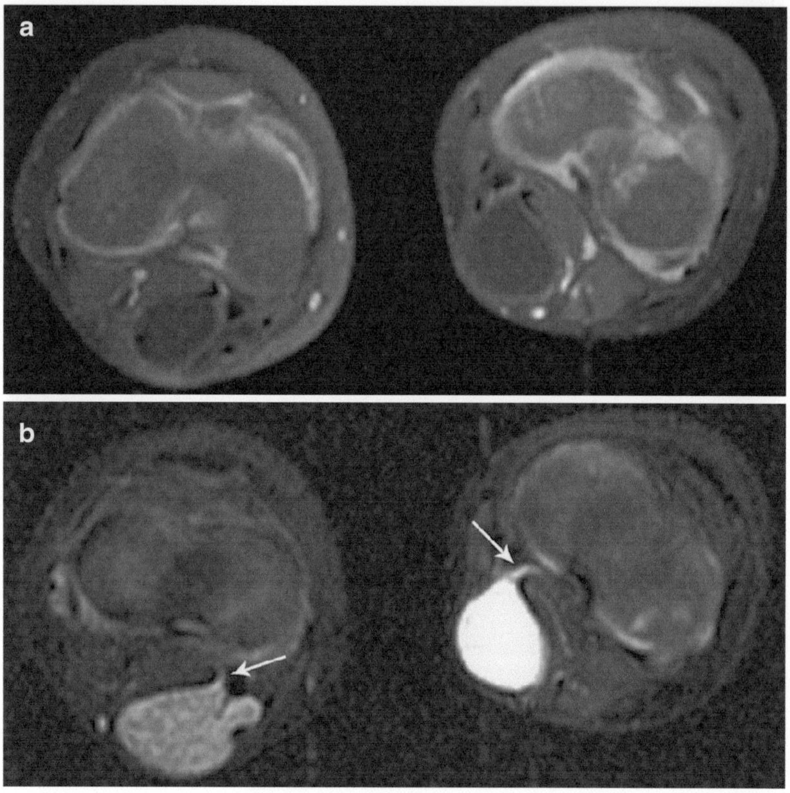

Fig. 22.17 Bilateral popliteal cysts in a 3-year-old girl. (**a**) Axial T1-W FS gadolinium-enhanced image shows bilateral cystic structures in the popliteal fossae. (**b**) Axial STIR image shows hemorrhage in the lesion on the *right* and simple fluid in that on the *left*. Both have tails (*arrows*) between the medial head of the gastrocnemius tendon and that of the semitendinosus, directed to the joint capsule. Both resolved spontaneously (Reprinted from Stein-Wexler [98], copyright 2009, with permission from Elsevier)

Cysts are more common in boys and are diagnosed at an average age of 8 years [39].

Imaging

On US, CT, and MRI, popliteal cysts present as well-delineated lesions extending through the space between the tendons of the medial head of the gastrocnemius muscle and the semimembranosus tendon (Fig. 22.17). Popliteal cysts in adults are almost always accompanied with joint pathology, but only 33 % of a series of patients referred from a pediatric rheumatologist had a knee-related risk factor for developing popliteal cysts (risk factors included juvenile idiopathic arthritis and Lyme arthritis) [40]. Other causes include unclassified oligoarthritis, gonoarthritis, trauma, benign joint hypermobility syndrome, hypophosphatasia, and a remote history of trauma [39]. However, any process within the joint that leads to an effusion can result in a popliteal cyst, including osseous lesions (Fig. 22.18). Some pediatric popliteal cysts may develop when seated children dangle their legs over the edge of a chair, irritating a weak portion of the posterior joint capsule; the presence of bursal thickening, as well as acute and chronic inflammation, supports this theory [41].

Popliteal cysts are an important entity to keep in mind solely to keep from confusing them with significant pathology. Usually asymptomatic, they require no specific treatment other than treating the underlying predisposing condition, if any.

1.3 Fatty Lesions

Lipoblastoma/Lipoblastomatosis

Lipoblastoma and its infiltrative form, lipoblastomatosis, are rare, benign tumors of embryonal white fat that usually occur before the age of 4 years. They are approximately three times more

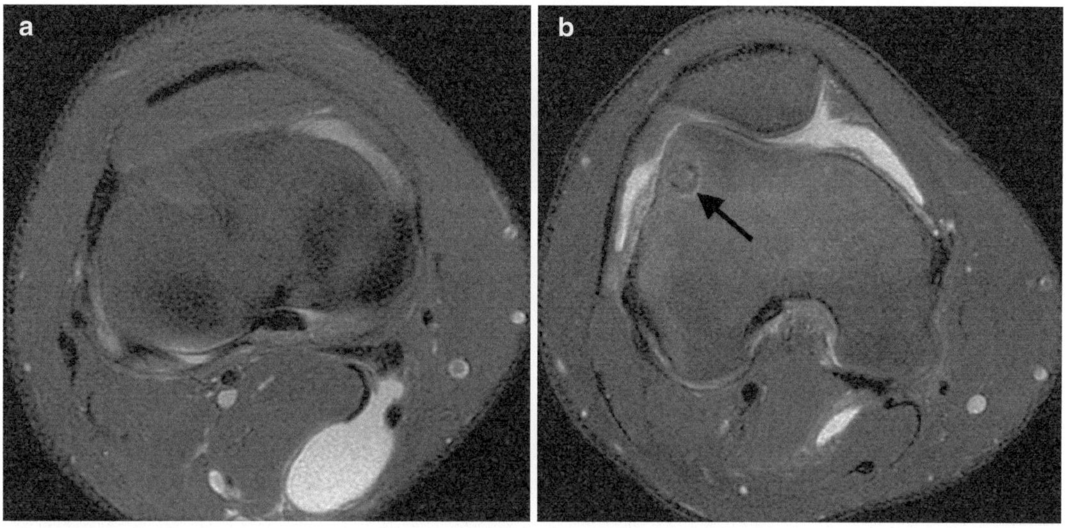

Fig. 22.18 Popliteal cyst in a 15-year-old boy with knee pain. (**a**) Axial PD FS images demonstrate (**a**) a cyst extending between the tendons of the medial head of the gastrocnemius and the semimembranosus tendon and (**b**) a joint effusion due to an osteoid osteoma (*arrow*)

common in boys [42]. The presenting symptoms relate to the size and location of the mass, but the mass itself is not painful [42]. Left alone, they mature into a benign lipoma [43].

Histologic evaluation reveals a spectrum of fat cells in various stages of maturation, ranging from lipoblasts to mature adipocytes, embedded in a variable amount of myxoid stroma; the myxoid component is anecdotally more prominent in very young patients [42]. There is a rich capillary network. Grossly, lipoblastoma ranges from red to pink to bright yellow and is composed of lobulated masses of fat with fibrous septations. Lipoblastomatosis has a similar appearance, but infiltrates the muscle and surrounding tissues.

The treatment for both lipoblastoma and lipoblastomatosis is gross total surgical resection. Lipoblastomatosis, an infiltrative lesion more difficult to completely resect, is more likely to recur.

Imaging

Imaging reflects the proportion of fat to myxoid material. Radiographs can demonstrate a lesion more lucent than muscle. US, CT, and MRI demonstrate a mass with echogenicity, density, and signal intensity identical to that of the adjacent subcutaneous fat (Fig. 22.19). The rich capillary network in some tumors can result in intense enhancement [44].

Differential Diagnosis

A predominantly fatty lesion in a child below age 10 is almost always lipoblastoma [42] and much less likely a hibernoma or fibrous hamartoma of infancy, which can occasionally contain fat. In patients over age 10, angiolipoma and lipoma are additional considerations [44]. An intensely enhancing lipoblastoma resembles a myxoid liposarcoma, but this lesion is rare in children [42].

Other Fatty Tumors: Lipoma and Hibernoma

Lipomas in older children and teens resemble those in adults, consisting of a well-circumscribed, homogeneous mass with signal, density, and echogenicity identical to subcutaneous fat [17, 42].

Hibernomas are composed of brown fat, which has an unusually rich blood supply and many mitochondria. They are relatively rare, and only 5 % occur in children [45]. They present as a soft, mobile mass, most common in the thigh. The hibernoma may feel warm relative to sur-

Fig. 22.19 Lipoblastomatosis of the leg in a 7-month-old boy. (**a**) Axial T1-W image shows a large, infiltrative mass with signal intensity identical to that of fat. (**b**) Signal intensity is completely suppressed on axial T1-W FS image. (**c**) Coronal T1-W and corresponding (**d**) T1-W FS gadolinium-enhanced images show the mass does not enhance

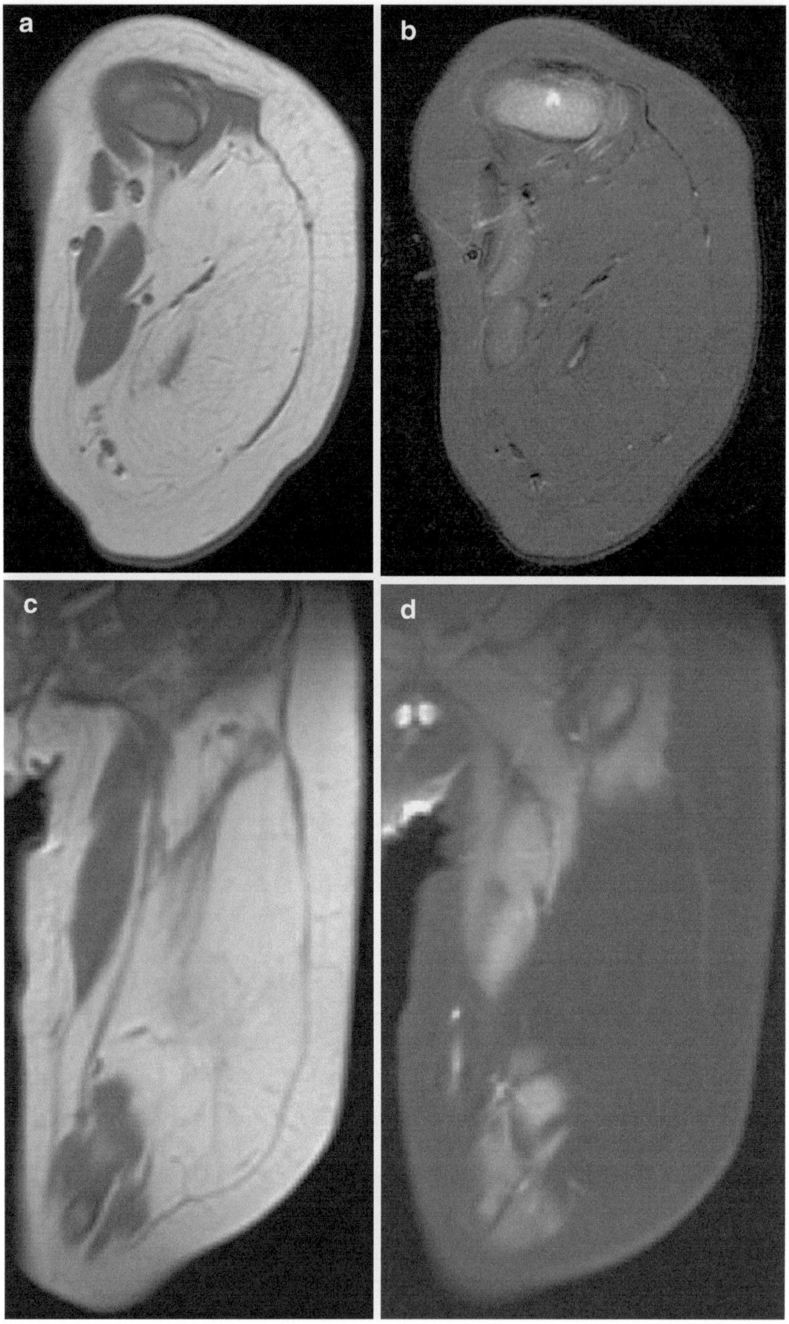

rounding tissues [42]. Surgical excision is definitive, with no reports of metastases or recurrence.

Imaging

The hibernoma appears lucent on radiographs. US demonstrates an echogenic, well-circumscribed mass that may have increased flow on Doppler imaging [42]. CT and MR appearance varies with the myxoid content of the tumor but is usually similar although not identical to fat. Enhancement is intense, which might raise concern for liposarcoma, but characteristic branching and serpentine high-flow vessels in and around the mass with additional low-flow vessels (never seen in liposarcoma) should suggest the diagnosis [42].

Bone scan with Tc-99m MDP demonstrates radiotracer uptake on flow and blood pool images. Positron emission tomography (PET) scan demonstrates intense fluorodeoxyglucose (FDG) uptake due to the lesion's high glucose metabolism [42].

Fat Necrosis

Trauma, injections, cold exposure, sickle cell disease, and vasculitis can injure the subcutaneous fat, usually in the hips, thighs, back, shoulders, and cheeks – areas with protuberant bones [17]. Neonates are particularly prone to fat necrosis, due to obstetrical injury, hypoxia, and hypothermia [46]. On histology, the lesion consists of necrotic adipose tissue with either admixed granulation tissue and lymphocytes or intense vasculitis [46, 47].

Fat necrosis presents as a firm mass in the subcutaneous tissues with possible overlying erythema; it may be mildly tender or asymptomatic [48]. The patient often does not recall antecedent trauma. A focus of fat necrosis usually enlarges slowly over weeks to months and then resolves over additional weeks to months, possibly leaving a subtle depression in the overlying skin. An important side effect of fat necrosis is hypercalcemia, which may develop up to 6 months after the insult. The current theory is that excess production of vitamin D by histiocytes infiltrating the necrotic fat causes increased uptake of dietary calcium; the serum calcium levels in neonates with fat necrosis should therefore be monitored for 6 months [46]. Treatment is either watchful waiting or, in equivocal cases, surgical resection.

Imaging (Fig. 22.20)

Radiographs demonstrate subtle stranding of the subcutaneous fat. The appearance varies at US, but all lesions are located in the subcutaneous fat. Fat necrosis can appear as a hyperechoic nodule in the subcutaneous fat, with poorly defined margins and very little vascularity on Doppler imaging [17]. Other appearances include well-defined nodules that are isoechoic to surrounding fat, with a hypoechoic rim, and heterogeneously hyperechoic and ill-defined lesions with increased flow on Doppler imaging [47].

CT may demonstrate a discrete soft tissue density nodule in the subcutaneous fat or diffuse stranding of the subcutaneous fat without extension beyond the superficial fascia [46]. On PET scans [49], these nodules may be FDG avid [47].

MRI appearance varies as well. There may be intermediate signal on T1-W and T2-W sequences, with diffuse contrast enhancement, or there may be heterogeneous signal on both sequences, with intense ring enhancement [47]. Linear signal intensity in the subcutaneous fat with heterogeneous T2 signal and no focal mass has also been reported [17]. The lack of a focal mass is reported to be the most distinguishing imaging feature [50].

Differential Diagnosis

This includes cellulitis and, for heterogeneous, ill-defined lesions, soft tissue sarcomas and aggressive fibromatosis.

1.4 Neurofibroma (Box 22.5)

Box 22.5: Neurofibroma

90 % are NOT associated with neurofibromatosis I

Localized: fusiform mass with true capsule, around nerve

- Split fat sign on MRI/CT: rim of fat around small neurofibroma

Target sign: hypointense center, T2 hyperintense surrounding myxomatous tissue

Diffuse: infiltrate subcutaneous fat and perineural soft tissue, plaque like

Plexiform: infiltrative, nodular ropelike mass along nerves

Malignant degeneration (5–10 % of plexiform neurofibromas):

- More likely if growth, pain, neurological symptoms

A neurofibroma is a benign proliferation of the connective tissue of the nerve sheath [51]. Neurofibromas may grow in three different patterns – localized, diffuse, and plexiform.

Localized neurofibromas are most common, representing 90 all percent of neurofibromas. These tumors involve superficial cutaneous nerves. *Diffuse neurofibromas* primarily occur in children and young adults, most often in the head and neck [52]. Even though neurofibromas are classically associated with neurofibromatosis type 1 (NF1), 90 % of all neurofibromas are solitary lesions not associated with the syndrome [52, 53].

Localized neurofibromas present as fusiform soft tissue masses. When they involve a large peripheral nerve, they may be deep seated. On imaging and at surgery they are well circumscribed and have a true capsule. When they involve a small peripheral nerve, they maintain a true capsule even if they extend beyond the borders of the nerve [52]. Diffuse neurofibromas, in contrast, infiltrate into the subcutaneous fat and other soft tissues around the nerve, resulting in a poorly defined lesion that presents as a plaque-like elevation of the overlying skin and subcutaneous soft tissues.

Histologic evaluation of both localized and diffuse neurofibromas reveals interlacing fascicles of elongated cells with abundant internal collagen, although diffuse neurofibromas contain a larger amount of uniform, fibrillary collagen. Immunohistochemical staining for S-100 protein is positive for both types [51].

Treatment of localized and diffuse neurofibromas is surgical resection, although at surgery the

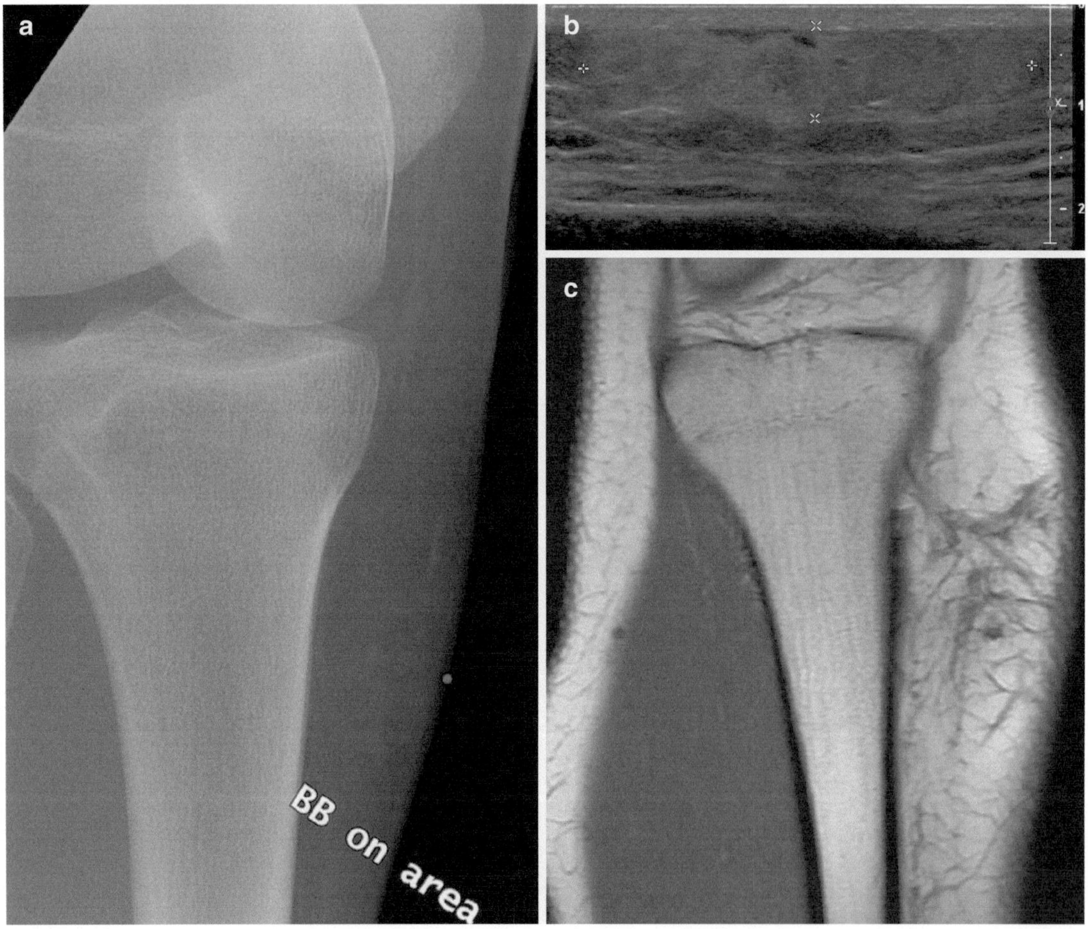

Fig. 22.20 Fat necrosis in a 16-year-old girl with a palpable, tender mass 2 weeks after being kicked in the shin. (**a**) There is hazy stranding in the subcutaneous fat. (**b**) Longitudinal US shows a hyperechoic, ill-defined subcutaneous mass (almost avascular at color Doppler (not shown)). (**c**) Coronal T1-W MRI shows linear hypointense stranding, hyperintense at (**d**) T2-W FS image. (**e**) Coronal T1-W FS gadolinium-enhanced image shows the strands enhance slightly, and there is no mass

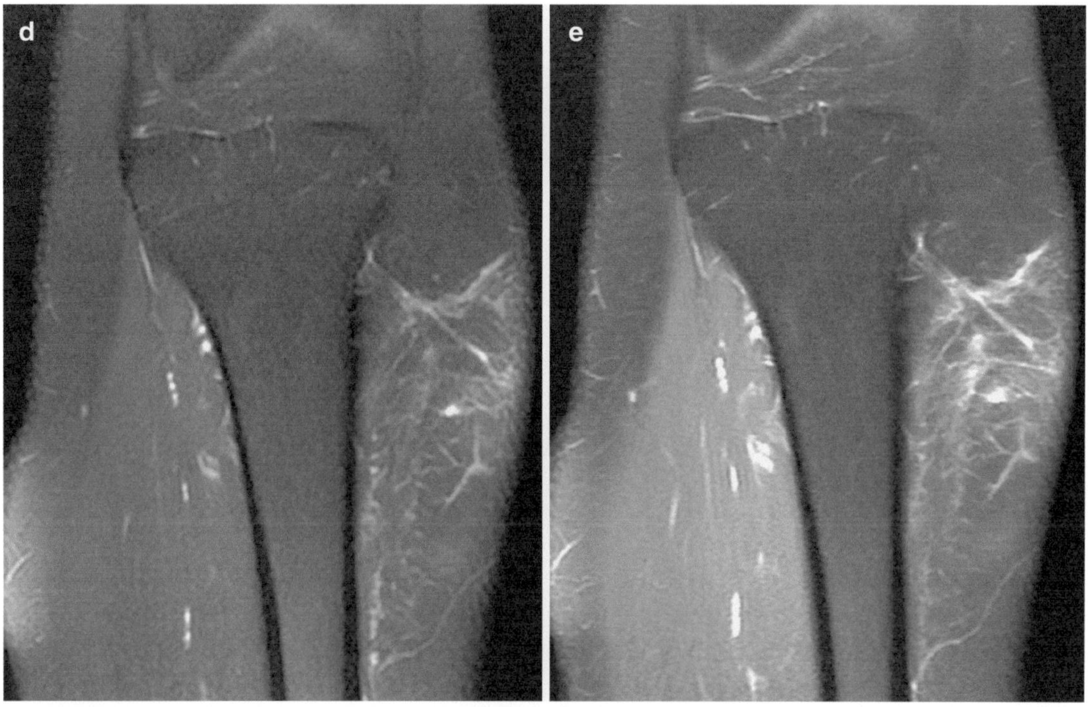

Fig. 22.20 (continued)

lesions cannot be separated from normal neural tissue, meaning that normal nerves must be sacrificed to achieve a complete resection. Often, patients and surgeons will opt for debulking of the tumor or conservative management with observation to avoid disabling symptoms from nerve damage. Malignant transformation of either diffuse or localized neurofibromas is extraordinarily rare.

Plexiform neurofibromas are essentially pathognomonic for NF1. However, the most common type of neurofibroma in a patient with NF1 is still the localized neurofibroma, which is more likely to be large, deep, or multiple in patients with NF1 [52]. Plexiform neurofibromas begin growing in early childhood, before the classic cutaneous neurofibroma develops. The plexiform neurofibroma consists of diffuse involvement of a peripheral nerve and its branches, with extension into the surrounding tissues beyond the perineurium. It may be associated with massive, disfiguring enlargement of the soft tissues surrounding the neurofibroma, termed *elephantiasis neuromatosa*.

Treatment is problematic; the sheer number of infiltrative lesions means that surgery is reserved for lesions that are severely disabling or disfiguring. Furthermore, the infiltrative nature of these lesions means that, even after resection, recurrence is common [52]. In patients with NF1, 5–10 % of plexiform neurofibromas will degenerate into malignant peripheral nerve sheath tumors (discussed later in this chapter).

Imaging

Radiographs may demonstrate bony and soft tissue overgrowth associated with elephantiasis neuromatosa but will only rarely demonstrate a fusiform mass with surrounding fat density [52].

US, CT, and MRI demonstrate findings consistent with the gross appearance – a mass composed of fusiform bundles of homogeneous neural tissue. *Localized neurofibromas* that arise within a neurovascular bundle may be associated with the "split fat" sign (Fig. 22.21): the neurovascular bundle is surrounded by fat, and a tumor growing within the bundle – usually a neurogenic tumor – has a small surrounding rim of fat unless it becomes large and infiltrative [52]. The split fat sign is more easily seen on CT and MRI.

MRI best demonstrates the tumors. These nerve sheath tumors have signal isointense to muscle on T1 and hyperintense on T2; they

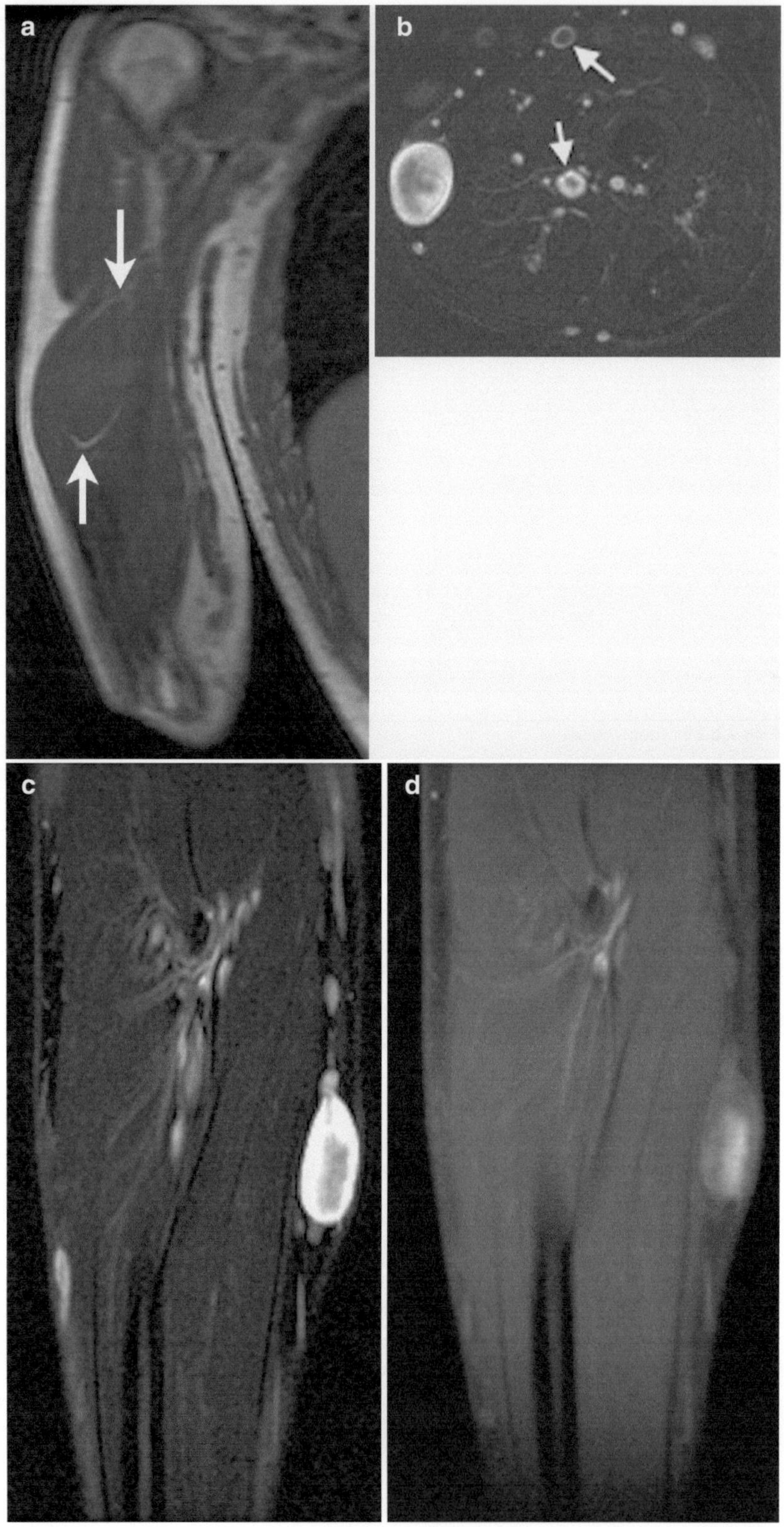

Fig. 22.21 Multiple neurofibromas in a sixteen-year-old boy with neurofibromatosis type I. (**a**) Coronal T1-W image of the arm shows a thin rim of fat around the fusiform mass, the split fat sign. (**b**) Axial T2-W FS image shows the typical target sign – central low signal and a hyperintense rim. Note multiple small neurofibromas (*arrows*). (**c**) Sagittal T2-W FS image shows a fusiform hyperintense mass with the target sign. (**d**) Sagittal T1-W FS gadolinium-enhanced image shows ill-defined enhancement

demonstrate avid, diffuse enhancement, which may be limited to the central portion of the tumor. The "target sign" of nerve sheath tumors, seen on cross section on T2-W imaging (Fig. 22.21), is caused by tightly packed central tissue surrounded by hyperintense myxomatous tissue [54].

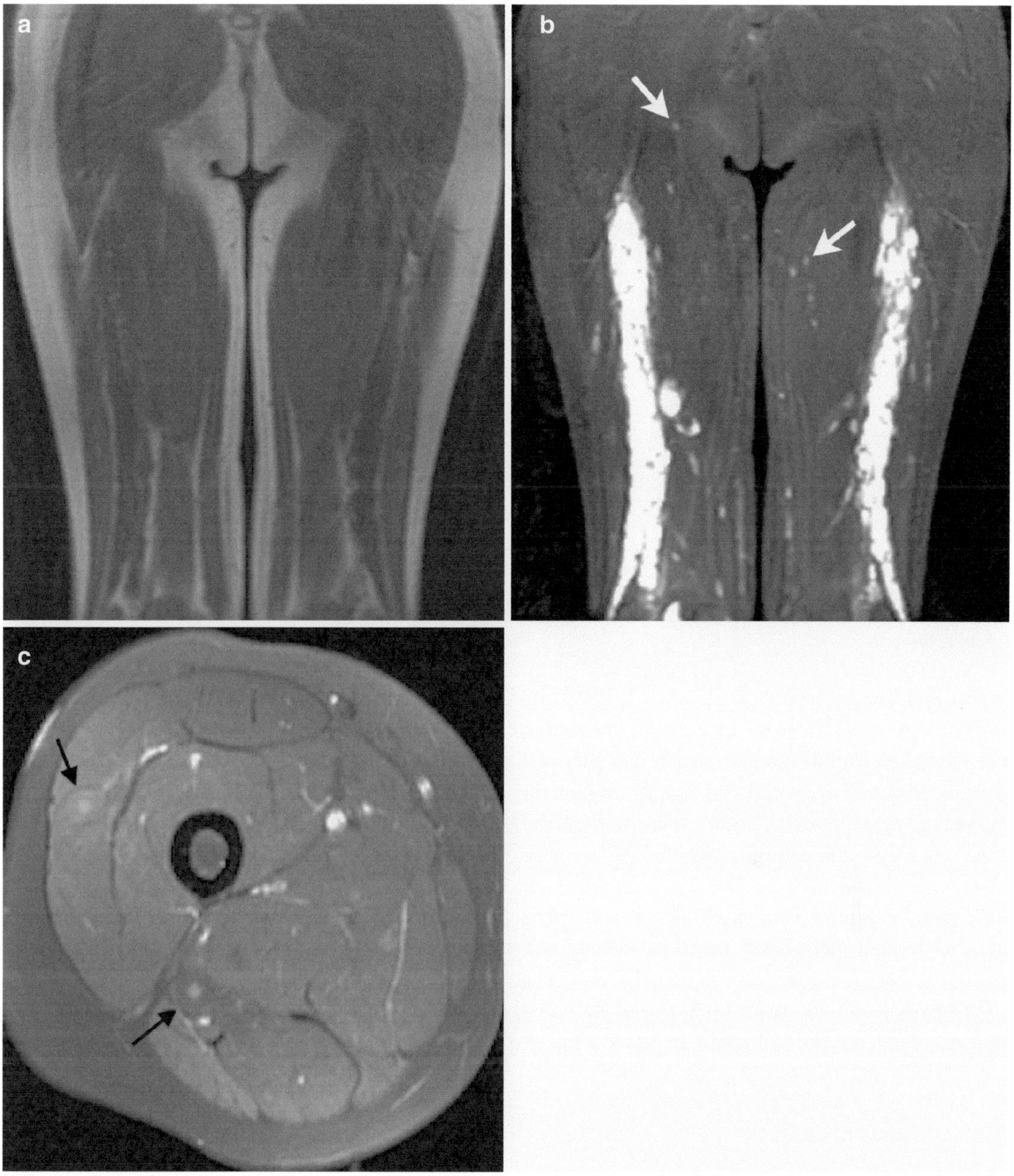

Fig. 22.22 Multiple plexiform neurofibromas in a twelve-year-old boy with neurofibromatosis type 1. (**a**) Coronal T1-W image shows bilateral enlargement of the sciatic nerves, isointense to muscle. (**b**) Coronal STIR images shows they are thick, ropy, nodular, and hyperintense. Note multiple smaller neurofibromas (*arrows*). (**c**) Axial T1-W FS gadolinium-enhanced image shows central enhancement

Diffuse neurofibromas present as reticulated material isointense to muscle on T1, replacing the subcutaneous fat, with a honeycomb appearance [52].

Plexiform neurofibromas appear as thick, ropy masses with low signal on T1 and high signal on T2 along the course of a nerve, often a major peripheral nerve (Fig. 22.22). They are slightly hypodense to muscle on CT and often extend into and widen the neuroforamina. The "target sign" is still present in each individual fascicle of the plexiform neurofibroma (Fig. 22.23).

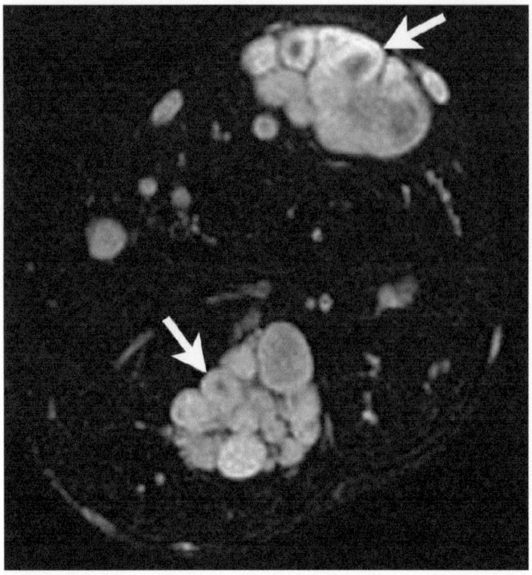

Fig. 22.23 Plexiform neurofibromas of the thigh in a 13-year-old boy with neurofibromatosis type 1. Axial T2-W FS image shows a target appearance (*arrow*) within multiple fascicles

Differential Diagnosis

Differential considerations include schwannoma, Charcot-Marie-Tooth disease (which has enlarged peripheral nerves with high T2 signal), malignant peripheral nerve sheath tumors, sarcomas (in the case of localized neurofibromas), and – very rarely – metastasis to the nerve. The only practical differential diagnosis of a plexiform neurofibroma is a malignant peripheral nerve sheath tumor, though a plexiform neurofibroma adjacent to a joint may superficially resemble synovial chondromatosis or a venous or lymphatic malformation.

1.5 Calcific Lesions

Tumoral Calcinosis

This condition is familial and most common in those of African descent. Patients with normal serum calcium levels, normal renal function, and elevated serum phosphate levels present with painless, calcified masses adjacent to the joints. Patients present in the first two decades of life with masses usually near the hip, elbow, shoulder, foot, and wrist, in descending order of frequency [55]. The masses tend to enlarge over time and may recur after excision [56]. They are more common on the extensor surfaces of the joints and may eventually ulcerate through the skin and exude chalky white material. They may envelop adjacent normal structures, such as nerves and vessels, but are not painful unless they directly impinge on a nerve. Mass effect may restrict joint mobility. Tumoral calcinosis is associated with dental abnormalities and intracranial and peripheral aneurysms [55].

The term "tumoral calcinosis" has been used imprecisely to describe any soft tissue deposition of calcium but is most appropriately reserved for this familial condition. It is distinct from the dystrophic calcifications associated with renal failure, connective tissue diseases, and other abnormalities of serum calcium homeostasis.

Tumoral calcinosis can be treated with phosphate depletion by giving the patient oral phosphate binders (such as aluminum hydroxide) in conjunction with acetazolamide. Densely encapsulated lesions may be resistant to this treatment, in which case surgical excision combined with phosphate depletion is generally effective [55]. At surgery, the masses are composed of chalky white or yellow material within cystic structures. Histologic evaluation reveals foreign body inflammatory cells, giant cells, and fibrosis surrounding calcifications [55].

Imaging

On radiographs, tumoral calcinosis presents as amorphous, cystic, multilobulated calcifications adjacent to a joint, without erosion of adjacent bony structures (Fig. 22.24). CT better demonstrates cystic structures and may demonstrate fluid-fluid levels. If there is no fluid-fluid level, the lesion is probably less metabolically active and thus less likely to grow [55]. At MRI, the lesion falls into one of two patterns – homogeneously intermediate signal intensity or alternating bright signal interposed with areas of signal void. It is brighter on T2 than would be expected based on the amount of calcium present [55].

Differential Diagnosis

The calcifications associated with chronic renal failure are identical to those of tumoral calcinosis, but can be distinguished because they occur in patients on hemodialysis. Calcinosis universalis occurs in autoimmune disease such as polymyositis and dermatomyositis and is associated with sheet-like deposits of calcium at the level of the superficial fascia, as opposed to the mass-like calcifications of tumoral calcinosis. Calcinosis circumscripta is, like calcinosis universalis, associated with autoimmune disease and can be distinguished by erosion of the underlying bone and by the location of the calcifications in the subcutaneous tissue rather than a bursal distribution. Myositis ossificans has mature bone rather than amorphous calcification. Calcific tendonitis is rare in children and is located in tendons. Synovial sarcoma and osteosarcoma can be distinguished by the presence of an associated soft tissue mass on MRI.

Myositis Ossificans (Box 22.6)

Box 22.6: Myositis Ossificans

Ossification of soft tissues 6–8 weeks after injury

Avoid biopsy–may mimic malignancy on histology

US: earliest specific finding, thin hyperechoic rim with surrounding hyperemia

Radiographs: thin peripheral calcification at 6–8 weeks (centripetal)

CT: thin calcific rim around hypodense mass

MRI: nonspecific and aggressive appearing with extensive edema early

Myositis ossificans (also known as heterotopic ossification and, if post-traumatic, myositis ossificans traumatica) is a benign, self-limited, non-neoplastic, proliferative mesenchymal response to soft tissue injury, in which the injured tissue gradually ossifies over the course of 6–8 weeks. The initial trauma is well documented in 60–75 %

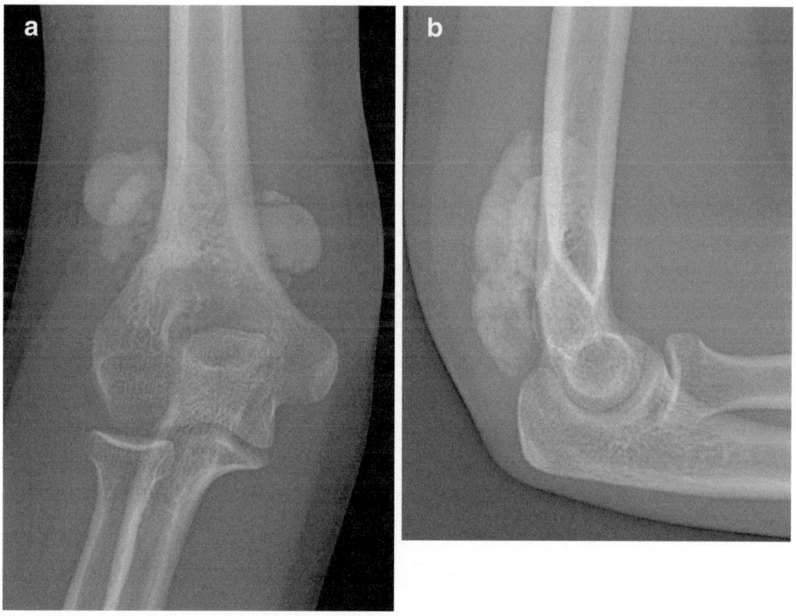

Fig. 22.24 Tumoral calcinosis in a 15-year-old girl with an elbow mass and a positive family history. (**a**, **b**) Multilobulated calcified masses, without joint erosion. T1-W axial (**c**) and sagittal (**d**) images show multiple hypointense lobulated masses. (**e**) Coronal T2-W FS image shows moderate adjacent edema

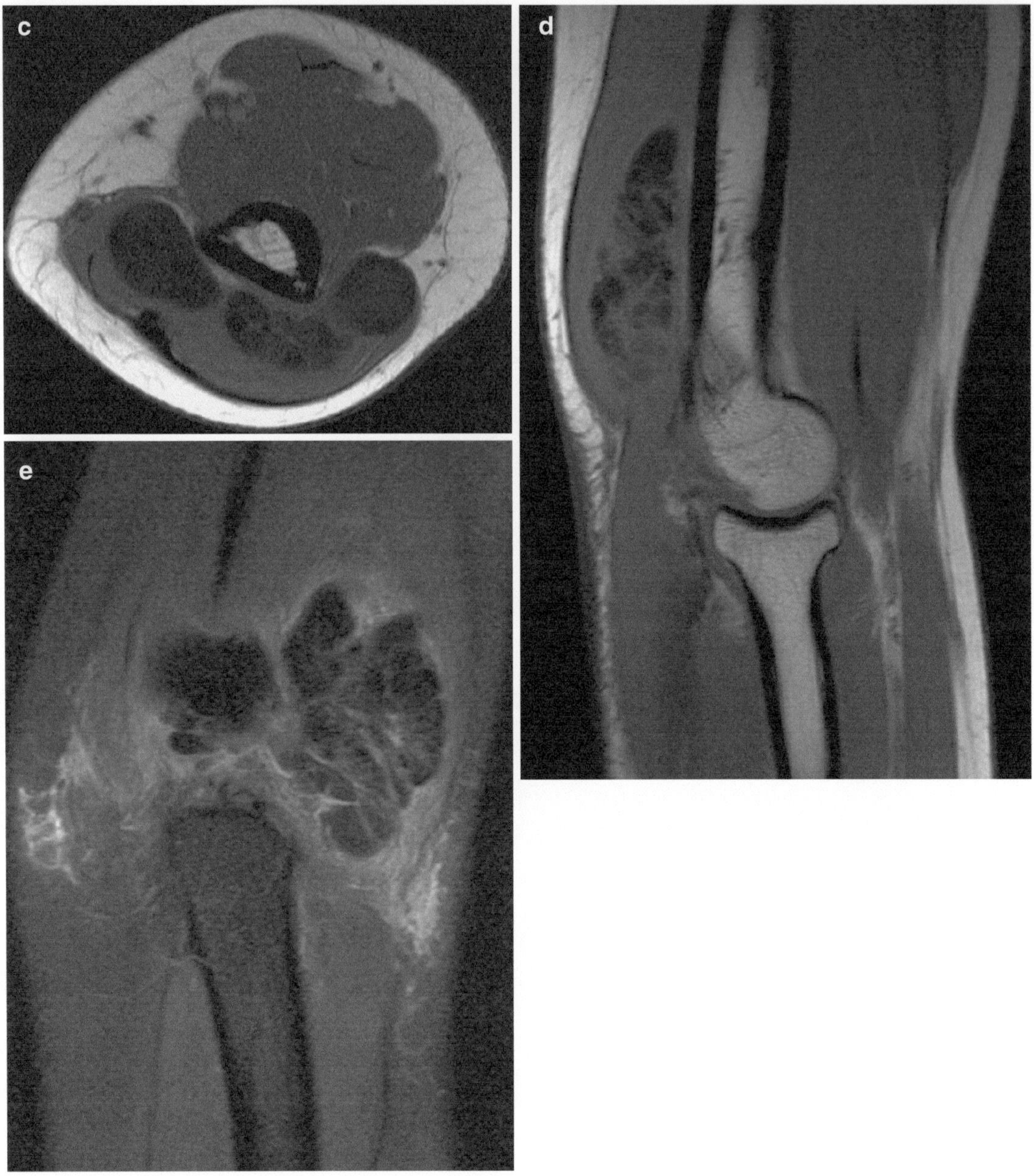

Fig. 22.24 (continued)

of cases [36]. However, children often do not remember any specific injury; pain and swelling may raise concern for infection or soft tissue neoplasm. Myositis ossificans is most common during the second and third decades and is extremely rare before age 10 [57]. It usually occurs in the large muscles of the anterior thigh or, less often, the upper arm. As the lesion matures, it shrinks, and 30 % of cases resolve entirely [57].

Myositis ossificans demonstrates increased cellularity at histologic evaluation. The cells have atypical features such as hyperchromasia and distinct nucleoli, though they lack atypical mitotic figures and have surrounding osseous or cartilaginous matrix. These features can easily lead to a diagnosis of osteosarcoma or chondrosarcoma. Correct imaging diagnosis of myositis ossificans avoids biopsy.

Imaging

US demonstrates the earliest findings specific to myositis ossificans: a thin, hyperechoic rim around a mass (representing the peripheral calcification), with surrounding hyperemia on Doppler imaging [58]. US findings appear when symptoms are maximal and prior to the characteristic radiographic findings.

By 6–8 weeks, radiographs demonstrate a thin peripheral rim of calcification around the mass, which is often close to an adjacent bone [59]. The calcification then proceeds in a centripetal fashion – the edges calcify prior to and more densely than the middle (Fig. 22.25).

CT demonstrates a well-defined, geometric, hypodense mass, with a thin rim of peripheral calcification in the earlier phases [57]; when mature, the calcification can be very dense.

MRI does not evaluate myositis ossificans well. Early myositis ossificans often appears nonspecific and aggressive until the chronic phase, with high T2 signal and intermediate T1 signal. Surrounding edema is extensive and more pronounced than would be expected for a primary malignancy [6]. There may be fluid-fluid levels and avid enhancement. During this time, a radiograph or US may show characteristic features and obviate the need for biopsy. After 6–8 weeks, myositis ossificans is completely mature. The mass then resembles a bone, with a hypointense cortical rim, trabeculae, and a fatty center.

Differential Diagnosis

The main differential diagnosis for a mass adjacent to a bone with early osseous matrix is a surface osteosarcoma, making the diagnosis of myositis ossificans somewhat nerve wracking. However, time, statistics, and biology are on the side of the radiologist, as parosteal and periosteal osteosarcomas are low- to intermediate-grade lesions with little propensity to metastasize, and high-grade surface osteosarcomas are very rare [60]. Profuse edema around myositis ossificans distinguishes it from low-grade surface osteosarcomas [6] and should prompt a short course of observation. Observing the lesion for 2 months to confirm that the ossification is maturing and that the lesion is shrinking will not appreciably delay the diagnosis of osteosarcoma and will, more often than not, confirm the benign diagnosis.

2 Malignant Masses (Box 22.7)

Box 22.7: Malignant Soft Tissue Tumors

0–5-year-old	Infantile fibrosarcoma
	Rhabdomyosarcoma
6–15-year-old	Rhabdomyosarcoma
	Synovial sarcoma
Imaging features	Deep location
	Larger than 5 cm
	Heterogeneous with necrosis
	Pseudocapsule common

The vast majority of malignant soft tissue masses are sarcomas, and these account for 4–8 % of childhood cancers. Of malignant tumors in the extremities, in those up to 5 years old, fibrosarcoma is most common, followed by rhabdomyosarcoma. From 6 to 15 years of age, malignant fibrous histiocytoma (MFH) has been reported to be the most common, followed by synovial sarcoma and rhabdomyosarcoma [61]. However, the term MFH has fallen out of favor as the use of immunohistochemistry has enabled pathologists to identify a cell of origin in most sarcomas [62]. In 2002 the World Health Organization revised the classification system for soft tissue tumors and reclassified MFH as "undifferentiated pleomorphic sarcoma," effectively making MFH a diagnosis of exclusion. Fortunately, only 1–6 % of soft tissue masses in children are malignant [4].

The treatment for most sarcomas is wide resection with or without neoadjuvant chemotherapy and/or radiation, followed by postsurgical radiation and chemotherapy. The first surgery is the best chance at cure; subsequent attempts at resection are less likely to succeed. It is therefore

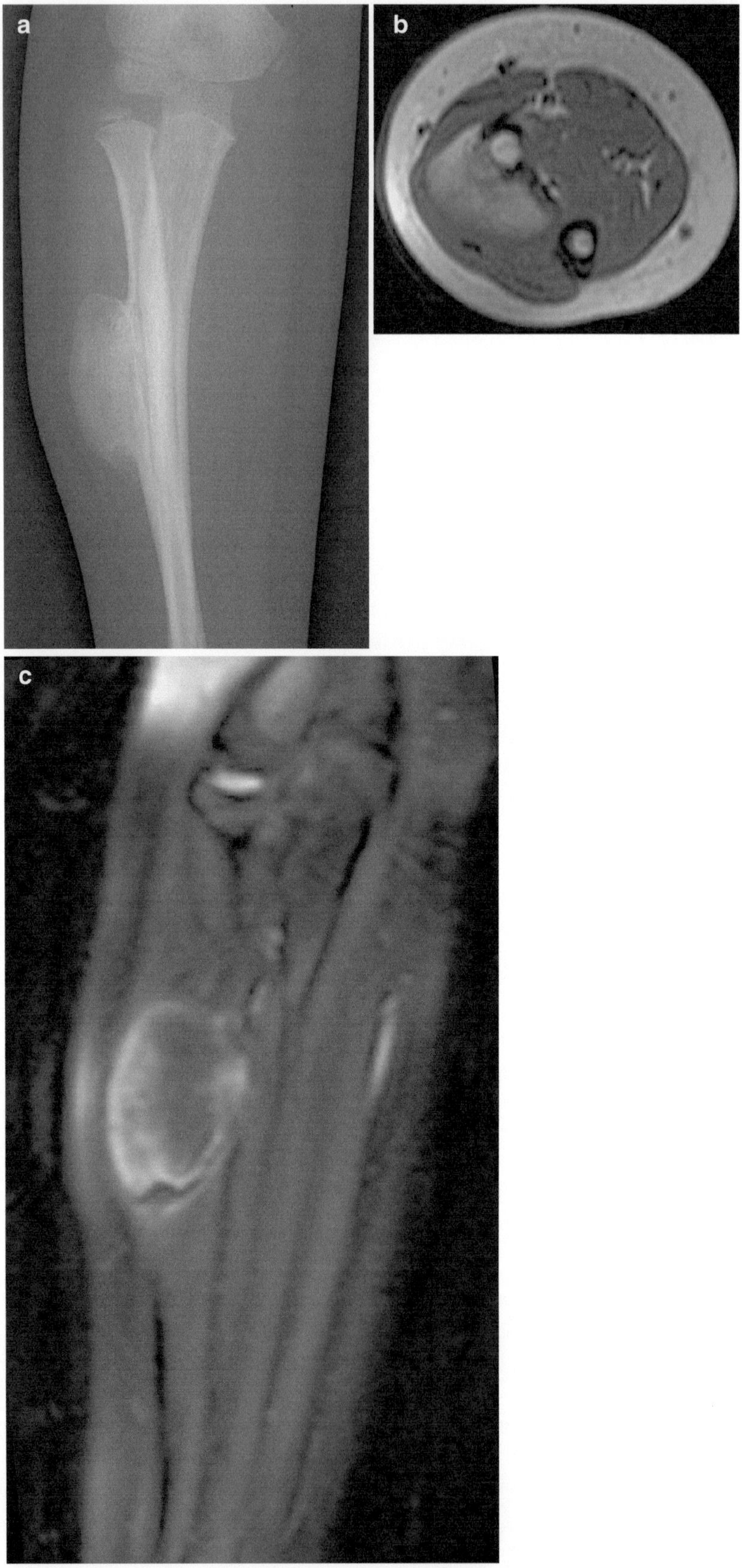

Fig. 22.25 Mature myositis ossificans at the forearm. (**a**) A well-circumscribed, smoothly corticated osseous density overlying the ulna has a well-defined trabecular pattern. (**b**) Axial T1-W image shows central hyperintense matrix similar to adjacent marrow, with a thin, hypointense rim of cortical bone. (**c**) T2-W FS fast spin-echo (FSE) sagittal image shows a hyperintense rim, with central hypointensity similar to marrow (Images courtesy of Leslie E. Grissom) (Reprinted from Stein-Wexler [98], copyright 2009, with permission from Elsevier)

imperative that the initial workup and treatment, including biopsy, are performed at a center with experienced orthopedic oncologists.

Deep location, size greater than 5 cm, and heterogeneous signal with areas of necrosis suggest malignancy. Most soft tissue sarcomas have a nonspecific appearance hyperintense on T2 and isointense to muscle on T1, with a pseudocapsule.

Even when MRI does not provide a definitive diagnosis, it offers valuable staging and presurgical planning information, including the most likely location within the tumor from which to obtain a diagnostic biopsy and involvement of neurovascular structures, adjacent lymph nodes, limb compartments, bone, skin, and joints. It is also useful in assessing response to therapy, although differentiation of residual or recurrent tumor from postoperative edema, hemorrhage, or inflammation is often difficult [63]. Sensitivity and specificity of MRI for residual tumor after incomplete resection have been shown to be 78 and 86 %, respectively [64]. If high T2 signal is present in the operative bed, but there is no mass effect, differential considerations include seroma, hematoma, postradiation change, packing material, fat necrosis, or hygroma [4]. If there is mass effect or gadolinium enhancement, recurrent or residual tumor becomes more probable. Correlation with pretreatment imaging is helpful, as signal characteristics of residual or recurrent tumor are likely to resemble those of the primary tumor [49].

Computed tomography (CT) exposes the child to ionizing radiation and is therefore less desirable than MRI or US. It is also generally considered less helpful for characterizing soft tissue masses, though at least one study found no significant difference between CT and MRI at staging the extent of musculoskeletal tumors [65], indicating that for patients who are unable to tolerate MRI, CT is a reasonable alternative. CT can also complement MRI by allowing identification of subtle calcifications in the mass, foci of fat, or other clues about the density of the tumor, subtle scalloping of adjacent bone, and the relationship of a mass to adjacent structures [66]. It can also be used to guide biopsy when the tumor is deep or obscured by overlying tissues.

2.1 Fibrous Tumors

Infantile Fibrosarcoma

Infantile fibrosarcoma is histologically similar to adult-type fibrosarcoma, but clinical features differ widely. It arises in infants and children under age 5, with about 30 % of cases present at birth and 74 % arising in the extremities [36]. Twelve percent of soft tissue tumors in infants are infantile fibrosarcoma [17]. The lesions grow rapidly, often becoming disproportionately large.

The mass initially resembles infantile hemangioma and kaposiform hemangioendothelioma, with purplish overlying skin and dilated superficial veins [36]. However, it grows rapidly and may soon assume a dome shape [17]. The lesion may be associated with disseminated intravascular coagulation, creating confusion with Kasabach-Merritt syndrome seen in kaposiform hemangioendothelioma. It may ulcerate, especially during its rapid proliferation phase and if exposed to friction. Metastases to the lung occur in 5–10% of cases, but the overall 5-year survival rate is greater than 80 % [36]. The tumor has multiple small ovoid tumor cells arranged in sheets and sharp intersecting bands, with frequent mitotic figures [36].

Imaging

On radiographs, a huge soft tissue mass is usually apparent, with deformity and reactive change in adjacent bones (Fig. 22.26). The appearance at US, CT, and MR is nonspecific, but flow voids and surrounding vessels are less prominent than in kaposiform hemangioendothelioma or infantile hemangioma [36]. US may demonstrate increased flow on color Doppler imaging [17]. MR demonstrates heterogeneous hyperintense T2 signal and T1 signal that is isointense to skeletal muscle (Fig. 22.27). Enhancement is heterogeneous. The patient's age should suggest the diagnosis.

Malignant Fibrous Histiocytoma

After the World Health Organization revised the diagnostic classification of soft tissue sarcomas in 2002, malignant fibrous histiocytoma became

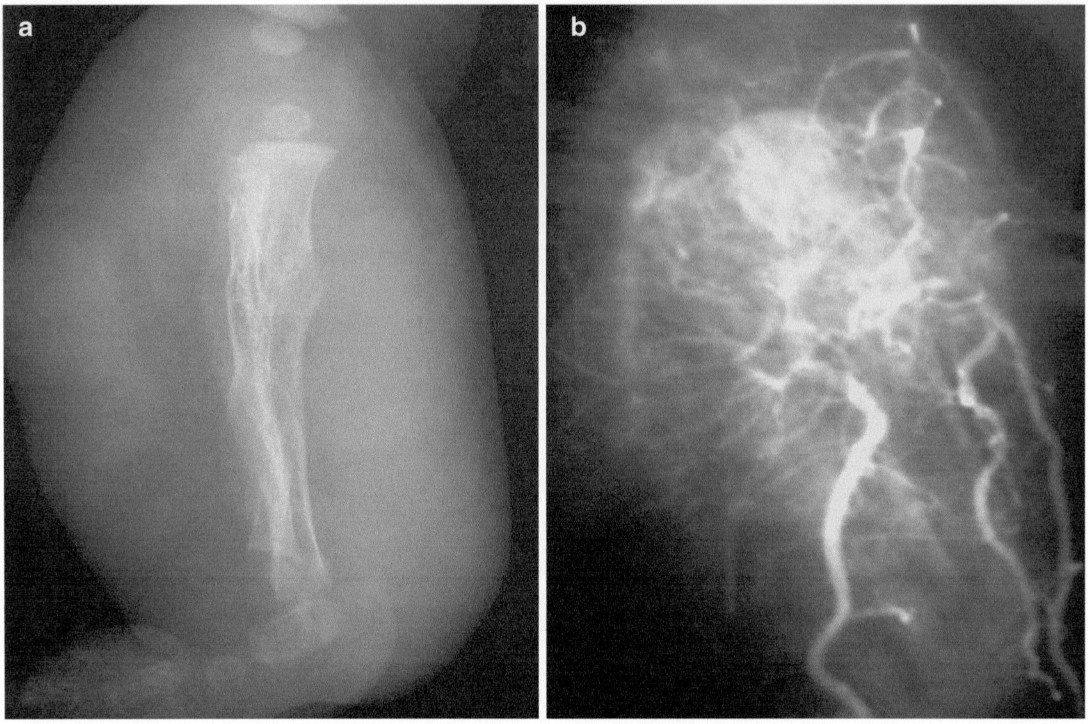

Fig. 22.26 Congenital/infantile fibrosarcoma of the calf in a 2-month-old. (**a**) There is an enormous soft tissue mass with bowing deformity and cortical thickening of the tibia and fibula. (**b**) Angiogram shows the mass is very vascular (Reprinted from Stein-Wexler [99], copyright 2011, with permission from Elsevier)

a diagnosis of exclusion, used to describe a noncohesive, heterogeneous group of poorly differentiated neoplasms. It now accounts for less than 7 % of non-rhabdomyosarcomatous pediatric tumors [36]. The tumor usually presents as a painless lump on the extremities, often larger than 5 cm at the time of presentation [36]. Imaging appearance is nonspecific.

Synovial Sarcoma (Box 22.8)

> **Box 22.8: Synovial Sarcoma**
>
> Often appears benign
>
> Painless mass present for weeks to years, chronic contracture
>
> Within 7 cm of joint; hands and feet, knee
>
> Calcifications in one third
>
> Small well-defined mass that appears encapsulated
>
> Triple signal sign in one third on T2:
>
> - Hyperintense hemorrhage, isointense necrosis, and hypointense fibrosis

Synovial sarcoma is a highly malignant, high-grade tumor that arises from primitive mesenchymal tissue; contrary to its name, it does not arise from synovial tissue. It is the second most common sarcoma in children after rhabdomyosarcoma, and half of all cases of synovial sarcoma arise in children or teenagers [67]. The tumor is slightly more common in boys. Eighty-six percent of synovial sarcomas arise within 7 cm of a joint [68, 69], with 71 % being intimately related with bone. Fifty percent abut the bone, and an additional 21 % either scallop the cortex or invade the medullary cavity [68]. The most classic clinical history is a painless mass that has been present for weeks to years, but the mass may also present as a chronic contracture. It may alternatively present in the pre-tumor phase with pain and swelling, but no focal mass, as acute arthritis or occasionally as a mass coming to attention because of minor trauma. Synovial sarcoma is most common in the hands and feet and about the knee.

The prognosis depends on whether the tumor is metastatic at the time of presentation.

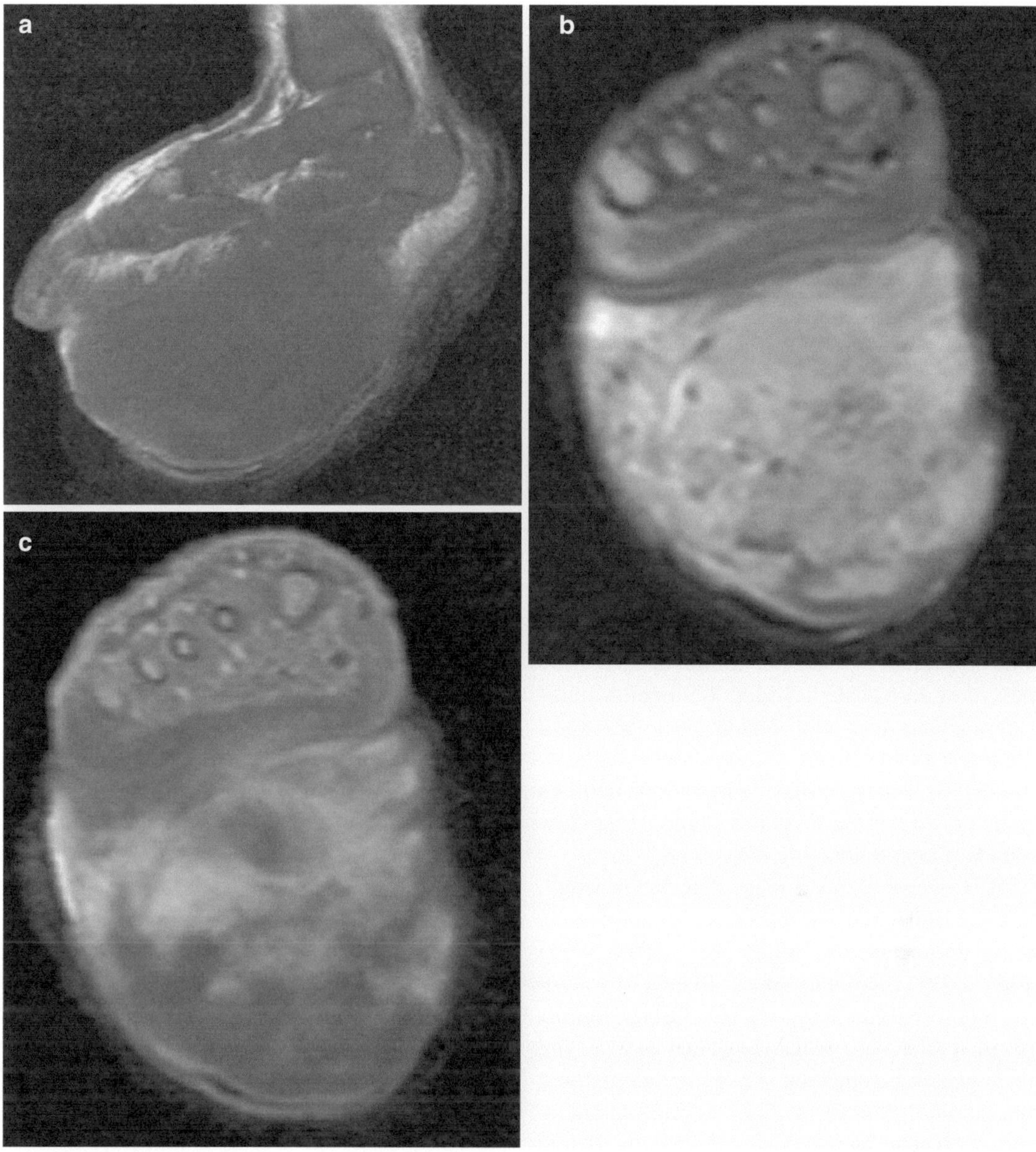

Fig. 22.27 Congenital/infantile fibrosarcoma in a 2-week-old boy with a large mass on the bottom of his foot, present since birth. (**a**) Sagittal T1-W image shows exophytic mass, isointense to muscle. (**b**) Coronal T2-W FS image shows the mass is heterogeneously hyperintense. (**c**) Coronal T1-W FS gadolinium-enhanced image shows heterogeneous enhancement (Courtesy of Mark Halverson)

Resectable disease has an excellent outcome, with 89 % 5-year survival [69]. Overall 5-year survival rate is 83 % in children [70]. Patients with metastases will usually die of their disease. The tumor metastasizes to the lung, bone, and lymph nodes.

There are two distinct histologic subtypes – monophasic, composed only of spindle cells, and biphasic, with spindle cells and epithelial cells. Almost all synovial sarcomas demonstrate a characteristic t(X; 18) (p11; q11) reciprocal transformation that results in two different fusion genes: SYT-SSX1 and SYT-SSX2 [70]. The SYT-SSX1 gene product correlates to biphasic histology and more malignant behavior, including shortened metastasis-free survival [67].

Treatment includes surgical resection, postsurgical radiation, and often chemotherapy. Patients who undergo postsurgical radiation have a better prognosis. Young patients whose tumors are small, in the hand, knee or foot, and without metastases have a better prognosis [69]. The prognosis is worse for boys [70].

Imaging

Radiographs demonstrate a soft tissue mass. About one third of the time, the mass has calcifications (Fig. 22.28), which are rare in other sarcomas and should suggest the diagnosis [71]. The adjacent bone may demonstrate periosteal reaction [71]. The mass is usually well defined and distinct from the surrounding tissue, giving it – particularly when small – a deceptively nonaggressive appearance [68]. Even though the mass appears encapsulated and appears to displace surrounding structures, histology usually demonstrates microinvasion.

CT and US demonstrate a mixed cystic and solid appearance when the tumor is large. CT may show microcalcifications. US demonstrates a nonspecific mass with mixed cystic and solid characteristics [72]. There is intense vascularity on US [73], and there may be septations within a cystic portion of the mass that demonstrate flow on color Doppler imaging [71].

MRI demonstrates a mass that, when small, appears well circumscribed and nonaggressive, with homogeneous high T2 signal [71] (Fig. 22.29). There may appear to be a surrounding low-signal-intensity capsule. Larger tumors are often lobulated, with areas of hemorrhage and heterogeneous signal on T2-W imaging; there may be fluid-fluid levels [71]. Foci of calcification, if present, have low signal on both T1 and T2. The "triple signal" sign (signal that is hyperintense, isointense, and hypointense to fat due to areas of hemorrhage, necrosis, and fibrosis) on T2-W sequences occurs in about one third of patients [72]. Enhancement is inhomogeneous.

Synovial sarcoma, when small, is often mistaken for a ganglion cyst or bursitis due to its homogeneous high signal on T2-W imaging, smooth, rounded appearance, and position near the joint [74]. It is the malignant lesion most likely to be misdiagnosed as benign [5]. It is therefore imperative to examine any suspected ganglion cyst very carefully to identify its connection to the joint and to have a low threshold for contrast-enhanced MR to confirm that the lesion does not enhance.

The differential diagnosis includes hematoma, abscess, vascular malformation, desmoid tumor, and other sarcomas. When adjacent to a joint, the mass mimics nodular synovitis, popliteal cyst, and ganglion cyst. Differentiating features include calcifications, inhomogeneous enhancement within the mass (differentiating from ganglion cyst, popliteal cyst, hematoma, and abscess), and the "triple signal" sign. Ultimately, the diagnosis requires biopsy.

2.2 Rhabdomyosarcoma (Box 22.9)

> **Box 22.9: Rhabdomyosarcoma**
> Most common pediatric soft tissue sarcoma.
> Twenty percent occur in extremities, not restricted to skeletal muscle.
> Usually alveolar subtype
> Imaging: nonspecific soft tissue mass with intense enhancement.

Fifty percent of childhood soft tissue sarcomas are classified as rhabdosarcoma, although, as discussed above, other types of sarcoma are more common in the extremities [61, 70]. Even though rhabdomyosarcoma represents the most common variety of pediatric soft tissue sarcoma, it is worthwhile to maintain perspective – only 350 cases of rhabdomyosarcoma are diagnosed each year in the United States [70], and only about 20 % of these occur in the extremities [75].

Rhabdomyosarcoma of the extremity is more likely to occur in older children and is usually the more aggressive alveolar subtype, as opposed to head and neck or genitourinary tumors, which are often the more favorable embryonal histology [76]. The tumor is not restricted to skeletal muscle but may arise essentially anywhere except within bone [77].

Rhabdomyosarcoma patients fare best if surgical resection is complete [76], as a patient with a nonresectable rhabdomyosarcoma has only a 50 % chance of survival. If the tumor is metastatic to lung, bone marrow, or bone, the survival rate drops

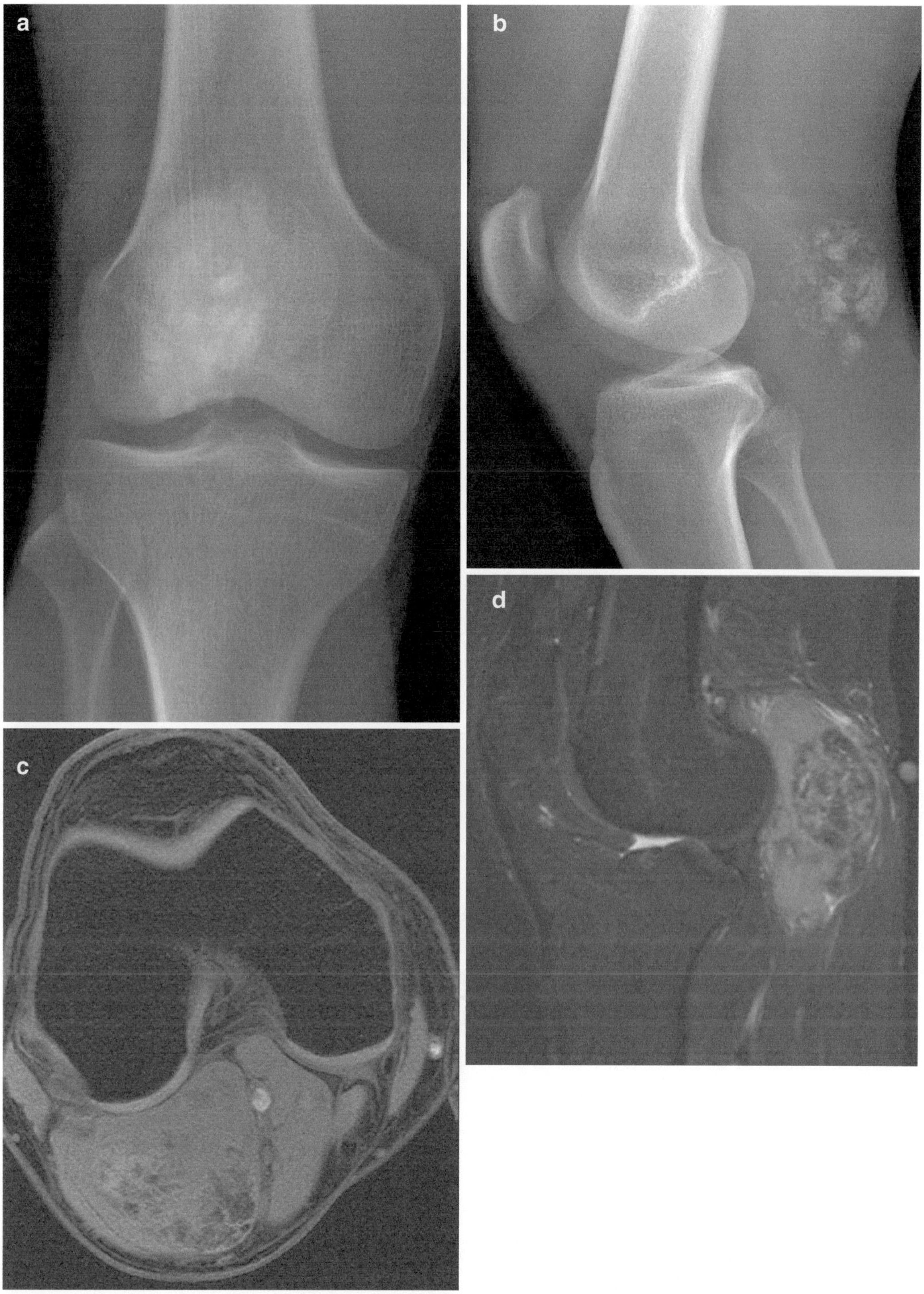

Fig. 22.28 Synovial sarcoma in a 17-year-old boy with a mass behind his right knee. (**a**, **b**) Flocculent calcifications cluster in the soft tissues (**a**, reprinted from Stein-Wexler [99], copyright 2011, with permission from Elsevier). (**c**) T1-W FS image localizes the mass to the lateral head of the gastrocnemius. Focal decreased signal corresponds to calcifications. (**d**) Sagittal STIR image shows heterogeneous hyperintense signal with scattered hypointensity. (**e**) Axial T1-W FS gadolinium-enhanced image shows heterogeneous, predominantly peripheral enhancement. (**f**) Axial T1-W FS gadolinium-enhanced image at a slightly higher level shows two enhancing lymph nodes. (**g**) Contemporaneous chest CT shows lung metastases, which progressed despite treatment (**h** chest radiograph) (Courtesy of John Hunter)

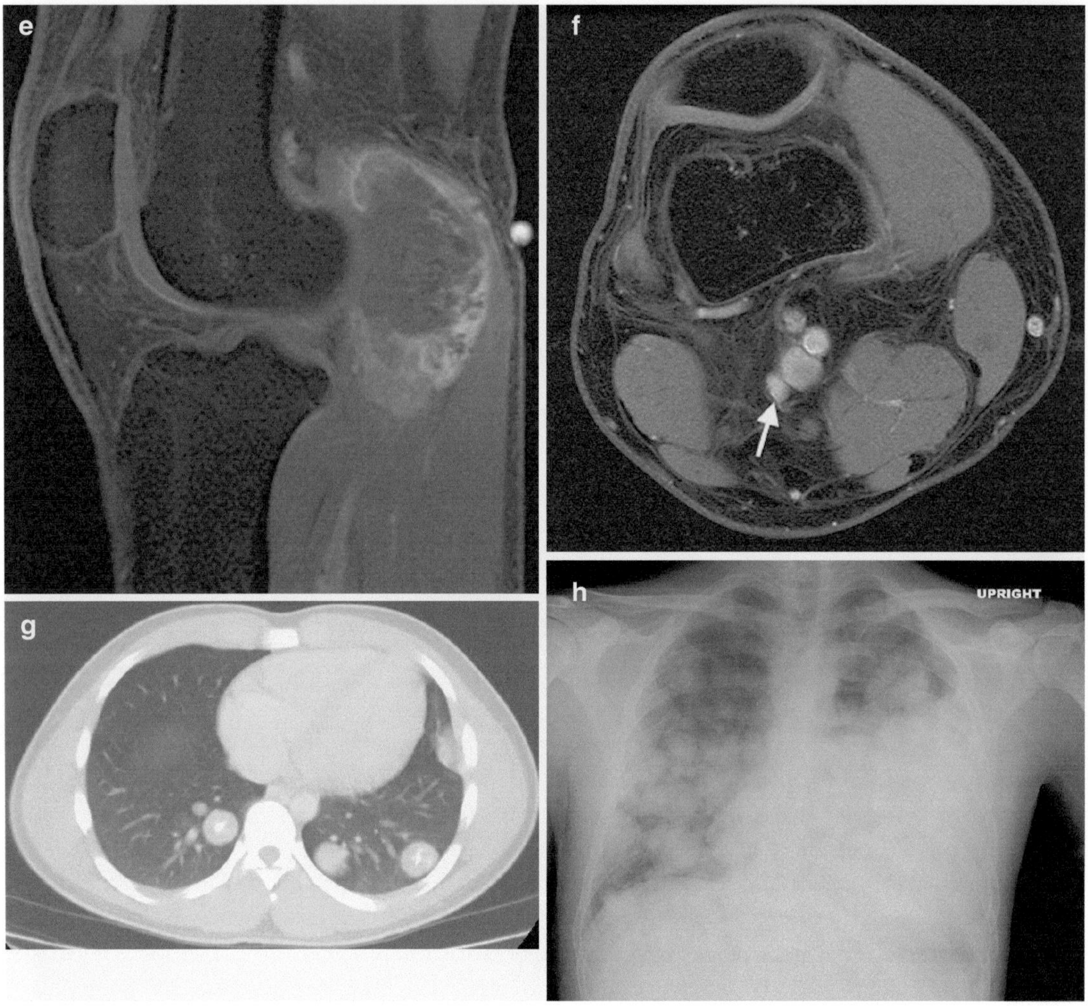

Fig. 22.28 (continued)

to 20 %, even with aggressive therapy. Fortunately, with modern surgical techniques, combined with chemotherapy and radiation, 70–80% of patients achieve local control [76, 77]. There is some evidence that primary radiotherapy to treat tumors in the hands and feet, where surgery would be severely disfiguring, is as efficacious as surgery [78]. All patients are offered chemotherapy, as the tumor is assumed to be metastatic at presentation.

Prognosis is based on tumor size (less than 5 cm diameter fares better), local invasiveness (worse), nodal metastasis (worse), and distant metastases (much worse). The imaging report should therefore comment on these factors. Newly diagnosed patients should also be staged with chest CT scan, nuclear medicine bone scan, and bilateral bone marrow aspiration and biopsy [77].

Imaging

Radiographs demonstrate a nonspecific soft tissue mass. The appearance on US, CT, and MRI is nonspecific. US may demonstrate a well-defined, slightly hypoechoic, heterogeneous mass with adjacent high-flow vessels, though cases with low vascular density have also been reported [17]. The mass is moderately dense on CT and enhances

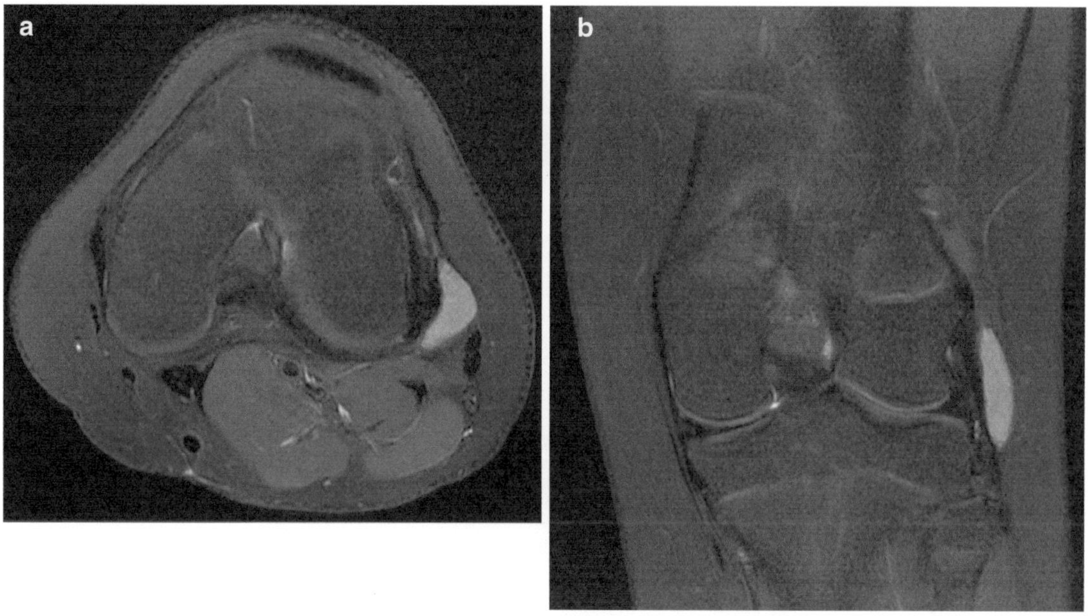

Fig. 22.29 Synovial sarcoma in a 15-year-old girl with knee pain. Axial (**a**) and coronal (**b**) PD FS images show a deceptively benign-appearing, homogenous, well-circumscribed mass adjacent to the fibular collateral ligament (Courtesy of John Hunter)

avidly (Fig. 22.30). MRI demonstrates intermediate to high signal on T2-W sequences and signal isointense to muscle on T1 (Fig. 22.31). The mass enhances intensely, and there are often signal voids due to high-velocity flow in surrounding vessels. MRI is useful to evaluate the site of origin, local extent including adjacent neurovascular structures or bone, and nodal spread.

2.3 Lymphoma/Leukemia

Lymphoma

Lymphoma is a heterogeneous disease that can affect essentially any part of the body at any age. When it arises in the soft tissues, it may mimic sarcoma or other small round blue cell tumors, requiring analysis of cell surface markers for diagnosis [79]. The distinction between lymphoma and other entities is critical, as lymphoma, unlike sarcomas, is curable with chemotherapy and radiotherapy alone; correct diagnosis obviates unnecessary surgery [80, 81].

Lymphomatous infiltration of the soft tissues can occur as primary disease or may represent either contiguous or distant spread. B-cell, T-cell, natural killer cell, and other types of non-Hodgkin lymphoma are most likely to present as a soft tissue mass; Hodgkin lymphoma is unlikely to do so [80]. The soft tissue mass often crosses fascial planes and surrounds, rather than displaces, adjacent vessels [81]. Distal limb swelling and subcutaneous edema may result [80].

Imaging

US demonstrates a homogeneously hypoechoic mass crossing fascial planes that often demonstrates increased flow on Doppler imaging; the different subtypes of lymphoma are not distinguishable on imaging. CT demonstrates a homogeneous mass that often has abundant adjacent subcutaneous stranding, reflecting the infiltrative nature of the tumor [82]. PET scan demonstrates avid radiotracer uptake [79].

On MRI, lymphoma of the soft tissues appears as an infiltrative mass, crossing fascial planes and

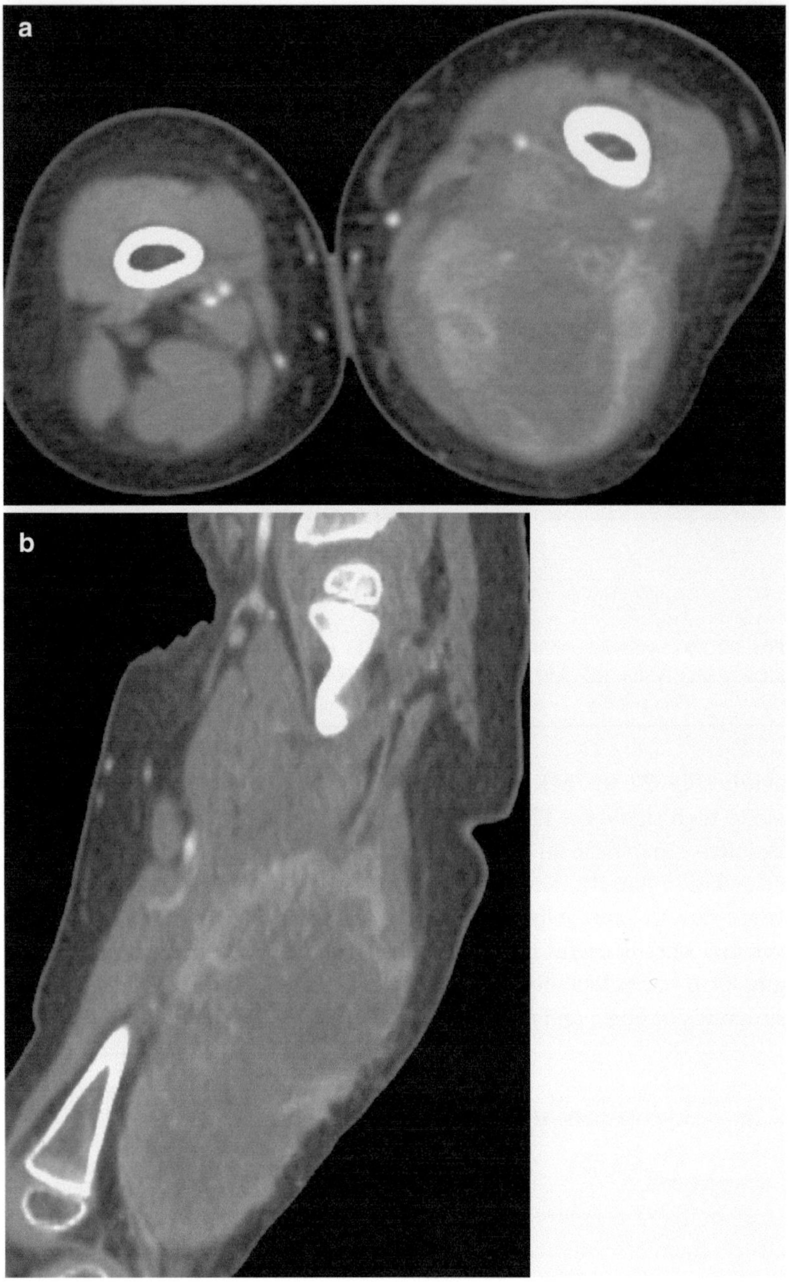

Fig. 22.30 Rhabdomyosarcoma in a 20-month-old girl with a thigh mass. Axial (**a**) and sagittal (**b**) contrast-enhanced CT images show a large, irregular mass with peripheral, heterogenous enhancement

surrounding, rather than displacing, neurovascular structures [81]. The mass has intermediate to high signal on T2-W imaging and intermediate signal on T1 [79, 81]. When lymphoma involves the muscle, it often involves more than one compartment and extends along the entire muscle length [79, 81]. The most important distinguishing features of lymphoma include surrounding fascial, subcutaneous, and cutaneous edema-like high signal on T2. Confluent lymphadenopathy in adjacent nodal regions is also reported to be a distinguishing feature of lymphoma that is rare in sarcoma [80].

Granulocytic Sarcoma

Granulocytic sarcoma (also known as chloroma or myeloid sarcoma) is a solid collection of

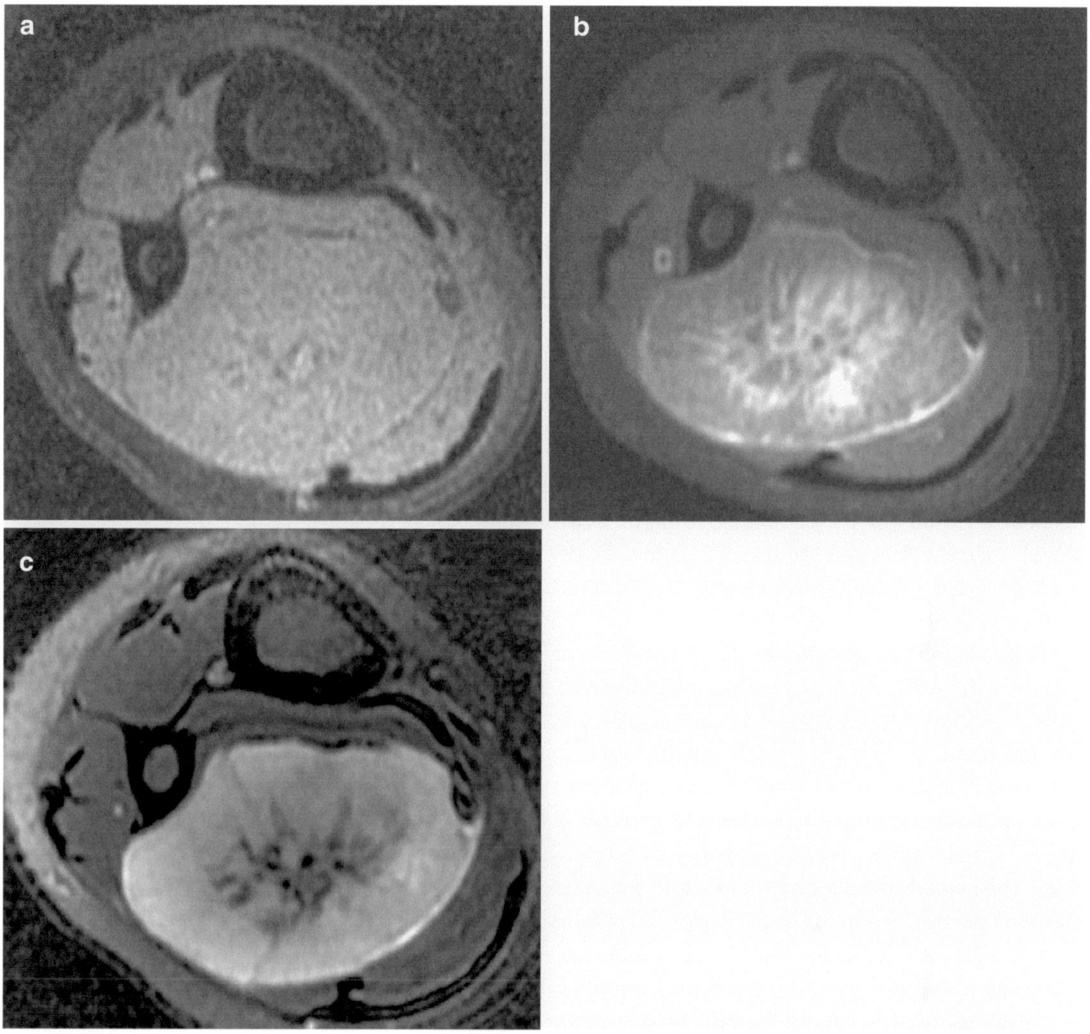

Fig. 22.31 Alveolar rhabdomyosarcoma of the calf in a 7-year-old boy. (**a**) Axial T1-W image shows a solid mass, isointense to muscle. (**b**) T1-W FS gadolinium-enhanced image shows central and peripheral enhancement. (**c**) T2-W FS image shows central serpiginous hypointensity, possibly due to large vascular channels (Courtesy of Leslie E. Grissom) Reprinted from Stein-Wexler [99], copyright 2011, with permission from Elsevier

leukemic cells outside the bone marrow. It develops in about 5 % of cases of acute myelogenous leukemia (AML). The tumors may arise concurrently with the diagnosis of leukemia, precede the diagnosis by up to 8 years, or arise during periods of remission as a manifestation of relapse [83]. They may arise in any organ of the body and in multiple locations, either concurrently or sequentially. The tumor is often found near a bone, as the myeloid precursor cells initially develop in the marrow and then extend into the surrounding soft tissues through Haversian canals [84].

At surgery or biopsy, granulocytic sarcoma tends to be green in color, owing to high levels of myeloperoxidase within the immature myeloid cells – though 30 % of tumors may be white, gray, or brown, depending on the amount and oxidation state of the myeloperoxidase in the various cell types [83].

Treatment is concurrent with the treatment of the leukemia with chemotherapy, and most lesions resolve completely within 3 months of initiating treatment [83]. Granulocytic sarcoma is radiosensitive, and radiation therapy can treat local symptoms.

Imaging

Radiographs reveal a nonspecific soft tissue mass, though there may be adjacent bone destruction or periosteal reaction. The US appearance varies. Solid hyperechoic masses have been reported in four cases [83]. In adult testes, the tumor has been reported to be homogeneously hypoechoic, with intense vascular flow [85], but the appearance in the adult breast varies from hyperechoic to hypoechoic relative to subcutaneous fat and from homogeneous to heterogeneous [86]. On CT, the mass is isodense or slightly hyperdense compared to skeletal muscle and demonstrates more avid enhancement [83]. MR shows a mass that is isointense to skeletal muscle on both T1- and T2-W sequences, though occasional cases with hyperintense T2 signal have been reported. The mass enhances avidly and uniformly [83].

The differential diagnosis of a mass in a patient with AML includes hematoma, abscess, and secondary neoplasm. The homogeneous enhancement of granulocytic sarcoma should help distinguish it from hematoma and abscess, since neither demonstrates central enhancement. Furthermore, the homogeneous signal equal to skeletal muscle on both T1 and T2 may suggest the diagnosis. In those cases in which the mass arises prior to the diagnosis of AML or when the mass fails to resolve within 3 months of initiating therapy for AML, biopsy is necessary. The pathologic differential diagnosis includes lymphoma; special stains are usually necessary.

2.4 Hemangiopericytoma

Hemangiopericytoma is a rare tumor, similar to kaposiform hemangioendothelioma, along the spectrum toward malignant angiosarcoma; it is intermediately aggressive, with both benign and malignant varieties [27]. Thirty to fifty percent develop in the extremities, and about 10 % are congenital [87]. The tumor arises from the vascular pericytes of Zimmermann. Unlike adults, children with this disease do well, with rare reports of recurrence and with distant metastases reported in only three cases of congenital hemangiopericytoma [27, 87].

Patients present with a palpable mass that may be tender and cause discoloration of the overlying skin. There should be no palpable thrill or bruit [87]. The mass is treated with surgical resection with or without radiation and chemotherapy.

Imaging

Radiographs demonstrate a homogeneous soft tissue mass. When a bone is (rarely) involved, the appearance resembles hemangioma, with a "hole within a hole" appearance. US may demonstrate a complex soft tissue mass with areas of cystic degeneration resulting from hemorrhage, though homogeneous soft tissue masses have been reported in infants [27, 87]. Doppler US reveals arteriovenous shunting. CT demonstrates a homogeneously enhancing, nonspecific soft tissue mass.

MR usually demonstrates prominent serpentine vessels in the periphery of the mass. These aggressive vascular masses have intermediate signal on T1-W imaging and high signal on T2 (Fig. 22.32). Unlike benign hemangiomas, they demonstrate invasion of surrounding tissues. There should be no surrounding fatty overgrowth, although there may be fluid-fluid levels and areas of T1 hyperintense hemorrhage or hemosiderin [27].

The differential diagnosis includes rhabdomyosarcoma, extraosseous Ewing sarcoma, alveolar soft part sarcoma, and kaposiform hemangioendothelioma.

2.5 Epithelioid Sarcoma

Epithelioid sarcoma is a curious lesion that tends to form within fascial planes, aponeuroses, and tendon sheaths of the distal extremities in teens and young adults – the fingers are a favorite location. The tumor may present as a nodule in the subcutaneous tissue or as a skin ulcer without an associated palpable mass. It has another, more aggressive manifestation as a more proximal, deep-seated lesion in the inguinal, genital, or perineal region [88, 89].

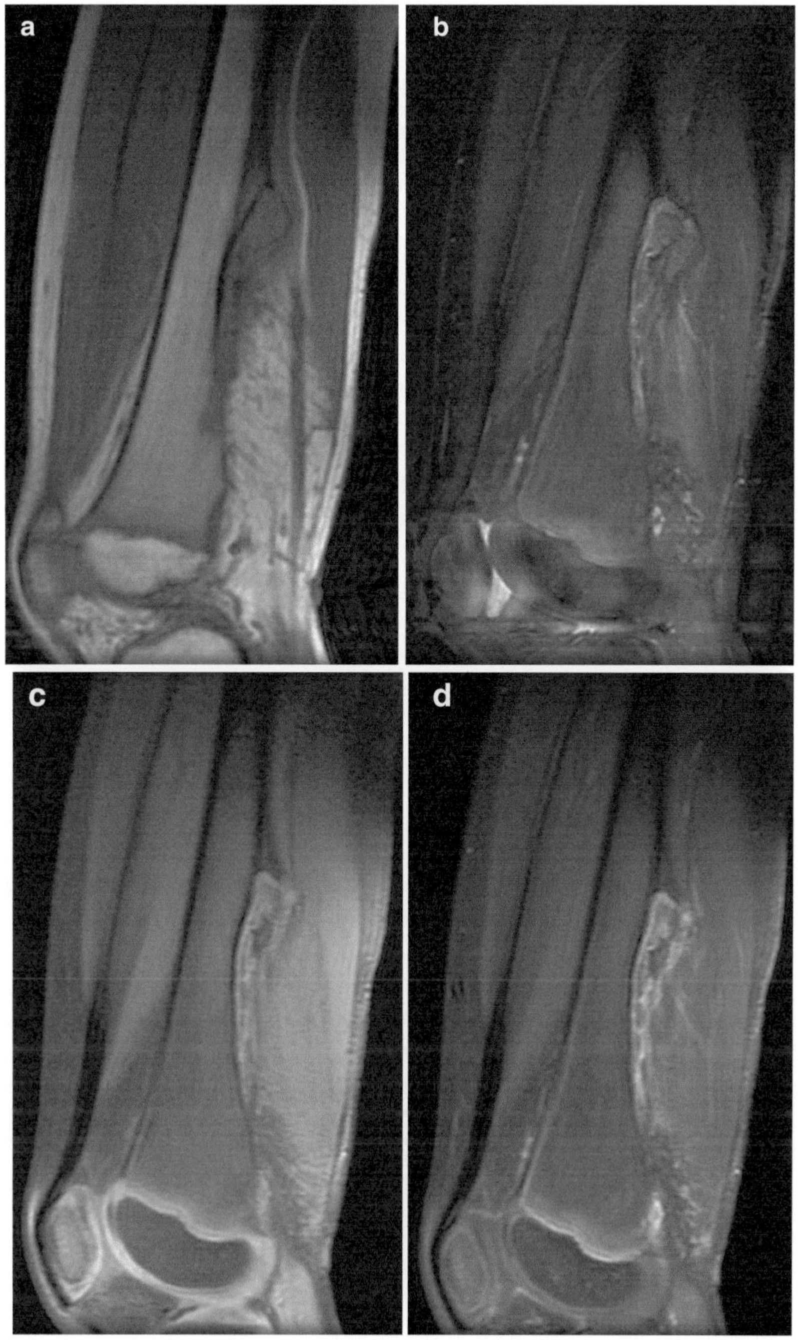

Fig. 22.32 Recurrent hemangiopericytoma adjacent to the femur in a 7-year-old boy. (**a**) Sagittal T1-W image shows postoperative changes at the distal femur and adjacent soft tissues, with an ill-defined recurrent soft tissue mass posterior to the femur that is isointense to muscle. (**b**) Sagittal STIR image shows heterogeneous mildly increased signal within the mass. T1-W FS (**c**) and T1-W FS gadolinium-enhanced (**d**) images show avid enhancement and confirm extensive residual mass

The distal variant can be completely cured with radical resection if caught early. In general, it has an indolent course, but incomplete resection results in inexorable progression of the tumor despite chemotherapy. Five-year survival is good, over 90 % in one study, but 10- and 15-year survival decreases to about 85 and 70 %, respectively [88]. Spread to local and regional lymph nodes is unfortunately common and confers a poor prognosis. Proximal lesions are more aggressive and have a worse prognosis, with about 60 % disease-specific mortality [89].

Evaluation of gross pathology reveals a lobulated mass with necrosis, hemorrhage, and hyalinized portions [69]. It is composed of sheets of large atypical epitheliod cells with vesicular nuclei, large nucleoli, and a rhabdoid phenotype. Immunohistochemical stains can confirm the diagnosis [88].

Imaging (Fig. 22.33)

MRI of both proximal and distal subtypes of epithelioid sarcoma demonstrates heterogeneous T1 and T2 signal due to a mixture of hemorrhage, necrosis, inflammation, hyalinization, and fibrosis [90]. The lesions may be multilobulated and either well or poorly circumscribed, with inhomogeneous enhancement after contrast administration. Regional lymph nodes are often involved in the proximal-type lesions [89]. The proximal-type lesion is inhomogeneous on CT and can demonstrate foci of calcification.

Differential diagnosis is broad, including most other types of sarcoma.

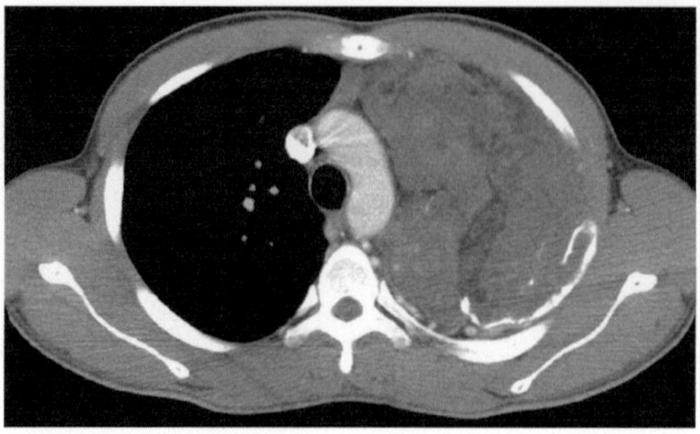

Fig. 22.33 Epithelioid sarcoma of the chest in a 24-year-old man. Axial CT contrast-enhanced image shows a lobulated, heterogeneously enhancing mass filling the left chest and destroying a rib (Reprinted from Stein-Wexler [99], copyright 2011, with permission from Elsevier)

2.6 Liposarcoma

Liposarcoma is an extraordinarily rare lesion in children, occurring mostly in teenagers. It cannot be differentiated from lipoblastomatosis by imaging or histology [17]. The most common liposarcoma in children is the myxoid subtype [91]. Liposarcomas are more heterogeneous than lipomas, with admixed myxoid components that may appear cystic; some liposarcomas have no recognizable fat at all. Molecular imaging techniques, including karyotype, are necessary to find the characteristic t(12;16) translocation specific for myxoid liposarcoma [91].

2.7 Alveolar Soft Part Sarcoma

Alveolar soft part sarcoma is a rare tumor, accounting for 5 % of non-rhabdomyosarcoma sarcomas in children [92]. Though it may arise from striated muscle cells, the cell of origin is unclear [69]. Alveolar soft part sarcoma is somewhat atypical among sarcomas in that it is more common in girls than boys, particularly during childhood. It usually arises in the striated muscles of the extremities and rarely in the head and neck [92]. The tumor may have an indolent course, and there are reports of metastases appearing after decades of complete remission [69]. Metastases to bone are common, often near the tumor. The tumor is treated with radical resection, as chemotherapy and radiation are ineffective [69].

The tumors consist of nests ("alveoli") of large cells with abundant granular cytoplasm separated by a rich capillary network. The histologic appearance could easily be mistaken for metastatic hepatocellular carcinoma, adrenal carcinoma, or renal cell carcinoma, requiring special stains to differentiate the tumor from these mimics [93].

Imaging

US demonstrates a well-circumscribed hypoechoic mass [93] (Fig. 22.34). Surrounding vascular structures may demonstrate brisk flow on color Doppler imaging, with low resistive index [94]. On CT, the tumor is hypoattenuating relative to adjacent skeletal muscle and demonstrates intense contrast enhancement. MR typically demonstrates flow voids around a tumor that is hyperintense on both T1- and T2-W imaging, with avid contrast enhancement. The T1 hyperintensity is a distinguishing feature.

Differential diagnosis is broad, including most other types of sarcoma, though the high signal on T1 should suggest the diagnosis.

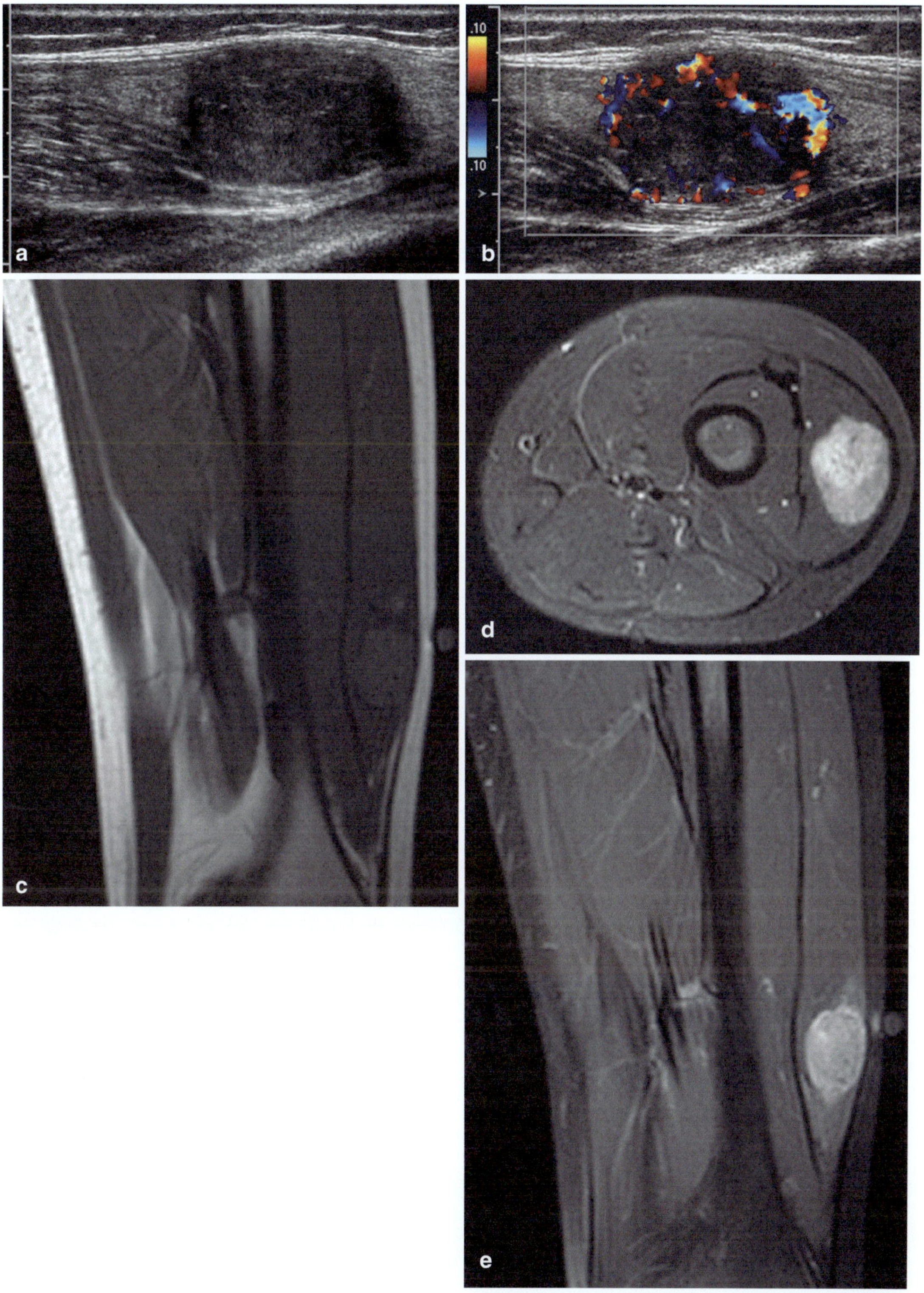

Fig. 22.34 Alveolar soft part sarcoma in an 8-year-old girl with a painful mass at the lateral thigh. (**a**). Sagittal US shows the mass is well circumscribed and heterogeneously hypoechoic. (**b**) There is exuberant Doppler flow. (**c**) Coronal T1-W image shows it is slightly hyperintense. (**d**) Axial STIR image shows the mass is heterogeneous and hyperintense. (**e**) Coronal T1-W FS gadolinium-enhanced image demonstrates exuberant, homogeneous enhancement (Courtesy of Leslie E. Grissom)

2.8 Malignant Peripheral Nerve Sheath Tumor (Box 22.10)

Box 22.10: Malignant Peripheral Nerve Sheath Tumor

Arises in plexiform neurofibroma or in irradiated tissues

Common in patients with NF1

Clues
- Symptoms more severe than with benign neurofibroma
- New-onset pain, neurologic symptoms
- Enlargement of quiescent neurofibroma
- More heterogeneous/ill defined than plexiform neurofibroma
- Disappearance of "central dot"

Patients with NF1 suffer from plexiform neurofibromas, as described above. In an unfortunate 5–10 % of these patients, a plexiform neurofibroma degenerates into a malignant peripheral nerve sheath tumor (MPNST). However, MPNST is not limited to those with NF1; 30–75 % of MPNST occur in patients who do not have NF1. MPSNT can arise as a secondary tumor in tissues that have been irradiated. The tumor has a male predilection, with 80 % of patients with MPNST and NF1 being male [52]. MPNST usually does not occur before age 10.

Patients present with pain and weakness in the distribution of the affected nerve, and the symptoms are much more severe than with benign nerve sheath tumors [52]. Sudden growth in a plexiform neurofibroma or sudden development of neurologic symptoms in a limb distal to a plexiform neurofibroma in a patient with NF1 should arouse suspicion of malignant degeneration and lead to prompt biopsy.

Treatment is wide surgical resection with or without adjuvant chemotherapy and radiation. Unfortunately, since the entire involved peripheral nerve must be sacrificed in the resection, the morbidity of surgery from nerve damage is considerable.

Imaging

On US, CT, and MRI, MPNST appear more heterogeneous and less well defined than plexiform neurofibromas, though heterogeneity is not necessarily sensitive or specific for malignant degeneration [21] (Fig. 22.35). The disappearance of the "central dot" on MR is not specific, but the presence of a "central dot" in the largest portion of a plexiform neurofibroma is a reassuring sign of the absence of malignant degeneration [52]. However, clinical symptoms are paramount – enlargement of a previously quiescent plexiform neurofibroma, localized pain, or any other neurologic symptoms should be viewed with suspicion.

The differential diagnosis includes benign plexiform neurofibroma and metastases to the nerve.

2.9 Soft Tissue Tumors That Usually Arise in the Bone

Extraskeletal Ewing Sarcoma

Extraskeletal Ewing sarcoma (EES)/peripheral primitive neuroectodermal tumor (pPNET) is an intermediate-grade malignant tumor that can arise anywhere. It has a predilection for the skeleton, but 20–40 % arise in the soft tissues [95] (most often in the chest wall, lower extremities, and paraspinal region). When skeletal and extraskeletal tumors are considered together, Ewing sarcoma is the third most common tumor in children and teens, with most cases diagnosed in the second decade. It is rare in children of Asian and African descent [70]. To keep the tumor in perspective, only about 300 cases (skeletal plus extraskeletal) occur per year in the United States [70].

Children with EES present with a mass that is often painful. They may also have systemic symptoms – fever, chills, and leukocytosis – that respond to antibiotic therapy, making EES a particularly good mimic of infection.

The tumor consists of homogeneous small round blue cells. Immunohistochemical features may overlap with those of other small round blue cell tumors, but genetic analysis detects the characteristic chromosomal abnormality (most cases demonstrate an EWS/FLI1 t(11;22) translocation) [70].

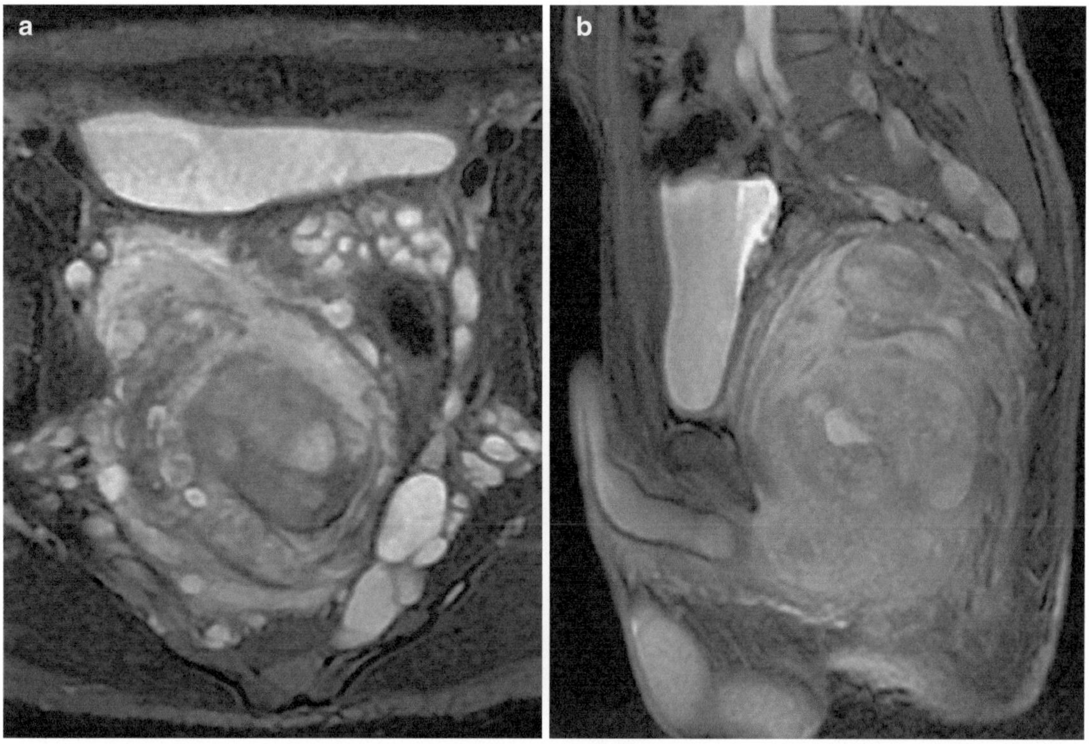

Fig. 22.35 Malignant peripheral nerve sheath tumor arising from a plexiform neurofibroma in a 19-year-old male with NF1. Axial T1-W FS gadolinium-enhanced (**a**) and sagittal T2-W FS (**b**) images show a huge, inhomogeneous, partially enhancing mass that infiltrates the posterior bladder wall

Treatment is initially with systemic multi-agent chemotherapy, as the disease is assumed to be metastatic at presentation. Local control of the tumor is imperative, with surgery being the most commonly recommended treatment. However, some series have demonstrated equivalent outcomes between radiation and surgery [70]. The most reasonable approach seems to be to perform surgery if the site is easily accessible and will cause minimal residual deformity or disability and to opt for radiation if surgery will be overly morbid, taking into consideration the 2–5 % risk of postradiation secondary malignancy [70].

Imaging

Radiographs of EES are nonspecific, demonstrating a soft tissue mass that does not calcify. US shows a well-circumscribed, hypovascular mass with mixed hypoechoic and anechoic areas [17]. Central necrosis may be evident at CT, and the mass appears heterogeneous, with possible rim enhancement. Adjacent marrow appears normal, although there may be bony erosion or periosteal new bone. MRI demonstrates a nonspecific, well-defined mass with heterogeneously hyperintense T2 signal and intermediate to decreased T1 signal (Fig. 22.36). Enhancement is variable but usually heterogeneous [17]. There may be cortical erosion and both cortical and periosteal thickening, but there should be no subperiosteal mass.

The differential diagnosis of this mass includes most other types of soft tissue sarcoma; diagnosis may only be made at histology.

Extraskeletal Osteosarcoma

Less than 4 % of osteosarcomas arise outside the skeletal system, most commonly as a mass in the soft tissues of the thigh or buttock [51]. Only a few cases have been reported in children [96]. The tumor can arise essentially anywhere, but 5–10 % of cases occur in a site that has received radiation therapy [51]. However, the latency

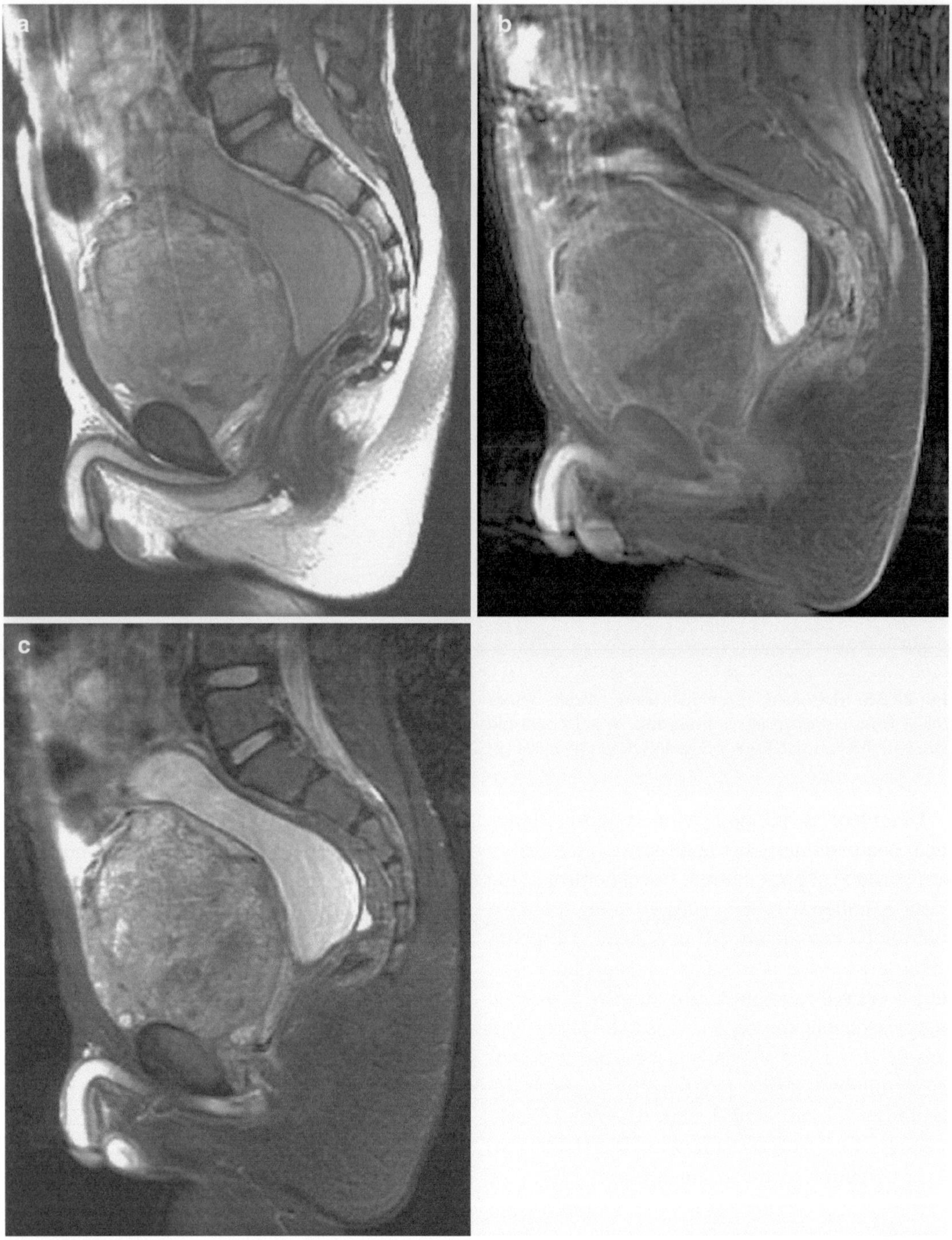

Fig. 22.36 (**a**) Sagittal T1-W image shows a fairly well-circumscribed moderately heterogeneous mass. (**b**) Fast spoiled gradient gadolinium-enhanced MRI shows moderate heterogeneous enhancement. (**c**) STIR image shows more marked heterogeneity. The urinary bladder is displaced posteriorly (Reprinted from Stein-Wexler [99], copyright 2011, with permission from Elsevier)

period for radiation-induced extraskeletal osteosarcoma (between 4 and 22 years) is long enough that patients are often adults when the tumor develops.

The mass typically grows slowly and is large at presentation. Metastases are common, usually to the lung [51]. Tumors may be predominantly of the fibroblastic subtype or may produce osteoid; fibroblastic tumors are less likely to have visible calcifications. They can be distinguished from other sarcomas with immunohistochemical stains [97]. Adults with extraskeletal osteosarcoma fare poorly, but, as with most tumors, children have a better prognosis [96].

Imaging

Half of these tumors have radiographically visible calcifications. The calcifications have the typical fluffy pattern of osteoid rather than the rings and arcs characteristic of chondroid matrix. They are positioned in the center of the tumor, unlike the peripheral calcifications of heterotopic ossification, for which it could possibly be mistaken [96]. US may demonstrate shadowing due to calcifications but cannot further characterize them. CT delineates central fluffy calcifications, but if the tumor is not calcified, it appears nonspecific.

MRI demonstrates a soft tissue mass, usually deep to the fascia, with heterogeneous T1 signal that is mostly isointense to muscle and heterogeneously hyperintense on T2. There is diffuse and avid enhancement throughout the lesion, unlike in heterotopic ossification, which enhances only peripherally. Central calcification may cause susceptibility artifact.

References

1. Kransdorf MJ, Murphey MD. Radiologic evaluation of soft-tissue masses: a current perspective. AJR Am J Roentgenol. 2000;175(3):575–87. PubMed PMID: 10954433. Epub 2000/08/23. eng.
2. Brisse HJ, Orbach D, Klijanienko J. Soft tissue tumours: imaging strategy. Pediatr Radiol. 2010;40(6):1019–28. PubMed PMID: 20432021.
3. Mutlu H, Silit E, Pekkafali Z, Basekim CC, Ozturk E, Sildiroglu O, et al. Soft-tissue masses: use of a scoring system in differentiation of benign and malignant lesions. Clin Imaging. 2006;30(1):37–42. PubMed PMID: 16377483. Epub 2005/12/27. eng.
4. Bissett 3rd GS. MR imaging of soft-tissue masses in children. Magn Reson Imaging Clin N Am. 1996;4(4):697–719. PubMed PMID: 8832851. Epub 1996/11/01. eng.
5. Berquist TH, Ehman RL, King BF, Hodgman CG, Ilstrup DM. Value of MR imaging in differentiating benign from malignant soft-tissue masses: study of 95 lesions. AJR Am J Roentgenol. 1990;155(6):1251–5. PubMed PMID: 2122675.
6. Jelinek J, Kransdorf MJ. MR imaging of soft-tissue masses mass-like lesions that simulate neoplasms. Magn Reson Imaging Clin N Am. 1995;3(4):727–41. PubMed PMID: 8564692.
7. Moulton JS, Blebea JS, Dunco DM, Braley SE, Bisset 3rd GS, Emery KH. MR imaging of soft-tissue masses: diagnostic efficacy and value of distinguishing between benign and malignant lesions. AJR Am J Roentgenol. 1995;164(5):1191–9. PubMed PMID: 7717231. Epub 1995/05/01. eng.
8. Ma LD, McCarthy EF, Bluemke DA, Frassica FJ. Differentiation of benign from malignant musculoskeletal lesions using MR imaging: pitfalls in MR evaluation of lesions with a cystic appearance. AJR Am J Roentgenol. 1998;170(5):1251–8. PubMed PMID: 9574596. Epub 1998/05/09. eng.
9. van Rijswijk CS, Geirnaerdt MJ, Hogendoorn PC, Taminiau AH, van Coevorden F, Zwinderman AH, et al. Soft-tissue tumors: value of static and dynamic gadopentetate dimeglumine-enhanced MR imaging in prediction of malignancy. Radiology. 2004;233(2):493–502. PubMed PMID: 15459325.
10. Bruder E, Alaggio R, Kozakewich HP, Jundt G, Dehner LP, Coffin CM. Vascular and perivascular lesions of skin and soft tissues in children and adolescents. Pediatr Dev Pathol. 2012;15(1 Suppl):26–61. PubMed PMID: 22420724.
11. Donnelly LF, Adams DM, Bisset 3rd GS. Vascular malformations and hemangiomas: a practical approach in a multidisciplinary clinic. AJR Am J Roentgenol. 2000;174(3):597–608. PubMed PMID: 10701595.
12. Mulliken JB, Glowacki J. Hemangiomas and vascular malformations in infants and children: a classification based on endothelial characteristics. Plast Reconstr Surg. 1982;69(3):412–22. PubMed PMID: 7063565.
13. Fishman SJ, Mulliken JB. Hemangiomas and vascular malformations of infancy and childhood. Pediatr Clin North Am. 1993;40(6):1177–200. PubMed PMID: 8255621.
14. Enjolras O, Gelbert F. Superficial hemangiomas: associations and management. Pediatr Dermatol. 1997;14(3):173–9. PubMed PMID: 9192407.

15. Ballah D, Cahill AM, Fontalvo L, Yan A, Treat J, Low D, et al. Vascular anomalies: what they are, how to diagnose them, and how to treat them. Curr Probl Diagn Radiol. 2011;40(6):233–47. PubMed PMID: 21939817.
16. Sans V, de la Roque ED, Berge J, Grenier N, Boralevi F, Mazereeuw-Hautier J, et al. Propranolol for severe infantile hemangiomas: follow-up report. Pediatrics. 2009;124(3):e423–31. PubMed PMID: 19706583.
17. Navarro OM. Soft tissue masses in children. Radiol Clin North Am. 2011;49(6):1235–59, vi-vii. PubMed PMID: 22024297.
18. Derchi LE, Balconi G, De Flaviis L, Oliva A, Rosso F. Sonographic appearances of hemangiomas of skeletal muscle. J Ultrasound Med. 1989;8(5):263–7. PubMed PMID: 2654417.
19. Teo EL, Strouse PJ, Hernandez RJ. MR imaging differentiation of soft-tissue hemangiomas from malignant soft-tissue masses. AJR Am J Roentgenol. 2000;174(6):1623–8. PubMed PMID: 10845496.
20. Robinson JL, Learch TJ. Vascular lesions presenting as musculoskeletal neoplasms. AJR Am J Roentgenol. 2011;197(1):W141–8. PubMed PMID: 21700975.
21. Stein-Wexler R. MR imaging of soft tissue masses in children. Magn Reson Imaging Clin N Am. 2009; 17(3):489–507, vi. PubMed PMID: 19524198.
22. Madhusudhan KS, Sharma R, Kandpal H, Kumar A, Gamanagatti S, Jain V, et al. A rare case of combined soft-tissue and intraosseous arteriovenous malformation of the hand with diffuse periosteal elevation: imaging appearances. Br J Radiol. 2009;82(983):e219–24. PubMed PMID: 19890114.
23. Konez O, Burrows PE. Magnetic resonance of vascular anomalies. Magn Reson Imaging Clin N Am. 2002;10(2):363–88, vii. PubMed PMID: 12424951.
24. White Jr RI, Pollak J, Persing J, Henderson KJ, Thomson JG, Burdge CM. Long-term outcome of embolotherapy and surgery for high-flow extremity arteriovenous malformations. J Vasc Interv Radiol JVIR. 2000;11(10):1285–95. PubMed PMID: 11099238.
25. Delaney RA, Burns A, Emans JB. Arteriovenous fistula formation after a closed proximal tibial fracture in a child. J Bone Joint Surg. 2011;93(10):1424–6. PubMed PMID: 21969446.
26. Yu PT, Rice-Townsend S, Naheedy J, Almodavar H, Mooney DP. Delayed presentation of traumatic infrapopliteal arteriovenous fistula and pseudoaneurysm in a 10-year-old boy managed by coil embolization. J Pediatr Surg. 2012;47(2):e7–10. PubMed PMID: 22325419.
27. Murphey MD, Fairbairn KJ, Parman LM, Baxter KG, Parsa MB, Smith WS. From the archives of the AFIP. Musculoskeletal angiomatous lesions: radiologic-pathologic correlation. Radiographics. 1995;15(4): 893–917. PubMed PMID: 7569134.
28. Lisle JW, Bradeen HA, Kalof AN. Kaposiform hemangioendothelioma in multiple spinal levels without skin changes. Clin Orthop Relat Res. 2009;467(9):2464–71. PubMed PMID: 19381744. Pubmed Central PMCID: 2866913.
29. Kaplan PA, Matamoros Jr A, Anderson JC. Sonography of the musculoskeletal system. AJR Am J Roentgenol. 1990;155(2):237–45. PubMed PMID: 2115246.
30. Heiken JP, Lee JK, Smathers RL, Totty WG, Murphy WA. CT of benign soft-tissue masses of the extremities. AJR Am J Roentgenol. 1984;142(3):575–80. PubMed PMID: 6607649.
31. Lee YS, Kwon ST, Kim JO, Choi ES. Serial MR imaging of intramuscular hematoma: experimental study in a rat model with the pathologic correlation. Kor J Radiol. 2011;12(1):66–77. PubMed PMID: 21228942. Pubmed Central PMCID: 3017886.
32. Coffin CM, Dehner LP. Fibroblastic-myofibroblastic tumors in children and adolescents: a clinicopathologic study of 108 examples in 103 patients. Pediatr Pathol Int Paediatr Pathol Assoc. 1991;11(4):569–88. PubMed PMID: 1946077.
33. McCarville MB, Hoffer FA, Adelman CS, Khoury JD, Li C, Skapek SX. MRI and biologic behavior of desmoid tumors in children. AJR Am J Roentgenol. 2007;189(3):633–40. PubMed PMID: 17715111.
34. Kingston CA, Owens CM, Jeanes A, Malone M. Imaging of desmoid fibromatosis in pediatric patients. AJR Am J Roentgenol. 2002;178(1):191–9. PubMed PMID: 11756119.
35. Kujak JL, Liu PT, Johnson GB, Callstrom MR. Early experience with percutaneous cryoablation of extra-abdominal desmoid tumors. Skeletal Radiol. 2010;39(2): 175–82. PubMed PMID: 19768644.
36. Laffan EE, Ngan BY, Navarro OM. Pediatric soft-tissue tumors and pseudotumors: MR imaging features with pathologic correlation: part 2. Tumors of fibroblastic/myofibroblastic, so-called fibrohistiocytic, muscular, lymphomatous, neurogenic, hair matrix, and uncertain origin. Radiographics. 2009;29(4):e36. PubMed PMID: 19448107.
37. Robbin MR, Murphey MD, Temple HT, Kransdorf MJ, Choi JJ. Imaging of musculoskeletal fibromatosis. Radiographics. 2001;21(3):585–600. PubMed PMID: 11353108. Epub 2001/05/16. eng.
38. De Maeseneer M, Debaere C, Desprechins B, Osteaux M. Popliteal cysts in children: prevalence, appearance and associated findings at MR imaging. Pediatr Radiol. 1999;29(8):605–9. PubMed PMID: 10415188.
39. Neubauer H, Morbach H, Schwarz T, Wirth C, Girschick H, Beer M. Popliteal cysts in paediatric patients: clinical characteristics and imaging features on ultrasound and MRI. Arthritis. 2011;2011:751593. PubMed PMID: 22046524. Pubmed Central PMCID: 3199937.
40. Magee TH, Segal LS, Ostrov B, Groh B, Vanderhave KL. Lyme disease presenting as popliteal cyst in children. J Pediatr Orthop. 2006;26(6):725–7. PubMed PMID: 17065933.
41. Lang IM, Hughes DG, Williamson JB, Gough SG. MRI appearance of popliteal cysts in childhood. Pediatr Radiol. 1997;27(2):130–2. PubMed PMID: 9028844.
42. Murphey MD, Carroll JF, Flemming DJ, Pope TL, Gannon FH, Kransdorf MJ. From the archives of the AFIP: benign musculoskeletal lipomatous lesions.

Radiographics. 2004;24(5):1433–66. PubMed PMID: 15371618.
43. Ha TV, Kleinman PK, Fraire A, Spevak MR, Nimkin K, Cohen IT, et al. MR imaging of benign fatty tumors in children: report of four cases and review of the literature. Skeletal Radiol. 1994;23(5):361–7. PubMed PMID: 7939836.
44. Chen CW, Chang WC, Lee HS, Ko KH, Chang CC, Huang GS. MRI features of lipoblastoma: differentiating from other palpable lipomatous tumor in pediatric patients. Clin Imaging. 2010;34(6):453–7. PubMed PMID: 21092875.
45. Furlong MA, Fanburg-Smith JC, Miettinen M. The morphologic spectrum of hibernoma: a clinicopathologic study of 170 cases. Am J Surg Pathol. 2001;25(6):809–14. PubMed PMID: 11395560.
46. Norton KI, Som PM, Shugar JM, Rothchild MA, Popper L. Subcutaneous fat necrosis of the newborn: CT findings of head and neck involvement. AJNR Am J Neuroradiol. 1997;18(3):547–50. PubMed PMID: 9090421.
47. Walsh M, Jacobson JA, Kim SM, Lucas DR, Morag Y, Fessell DP. Sonography of fat necrosis involving the extremity and torso with magnetic resonance imaging and histologic correlation. J Ultrasound Med. 2008;27(12):1751–7. PubMed PMID: 19023001.
48. Aljaser F, Weinstein M. A 1-week-old newborn with hypercalcemia and palpable nodules: subcutaneous fat necrosis. CMAJ Can Med Assoc J. 2008;178(13): 1653–4. PubMed PMID: 18559800. Pubmed Central PMCID: 2413302.
49. Garner HW, Kransdorf MJ, Bancroft LW, Peterson JJ, Berquist TH, Murphey MD. Benign and malignant soft-tissue tumors: posttreatment MR imaging. Radiographics. 2009;29(1):119–34. PubMed PMID: 19168840.
50. Tsai TS, Evans HA, Donnelly LF, Bisset 3rd GS, Emery KH. Fat necrosis after trauma: a benign cause of palpable lumps in children. AJR Am J Roentgenol. 1997;169(6):1623–6. PubMed PMID: 9393177.
51. Cates JM, Coffin CM. Neurogenic tumors of soft tissue. Pediatr Dev Pathol. 2012;15(1 Suppl):62–107. PubMed PMID: 22420725.
52. Murphey MD, Smith WS, Smith SE, Kransdorf MJ, Temple HT. From the archives of the AFIP. Imaging of musculoskeletal neurogenic tumors: radiologic-pathologic correlation. Radiographics. 1999;19(5): 1253–80. PubMed PMID: 10489179.
53. Abreu E, Aubert S, Wavreille G, Gheno R, Canella C, Cotten A. Peripheral tumor and tumor-like neurogenic lesions. Eur J Radiol. 2013;82(1):38–50. PubMed PMID: 21561733.
54. Bhargava R, Parham DM, Lasater OE, Chari RS, Chen G, Fletcher BD. MR imaging differentiation of benign and malignant peripheral nerve sheath tumors: use of the target sign. Pediatr Radiol. 1997;27(2):124–9. PubMed PMID: 9028843. Epub 1997/02/01. eng.
55. Olsen KM, Chew FS. Tumoral calcinosis: pearls, polemics, and alternative possibilities. Radiographics. 2006;26(3):871–85. PubMed PMID: 16702460.
56. Smack D, Norton SA, Fitzpatrick JE. Proposal for a pathogenesis-based classification of tumoral calcinosis. Int J Dermatol. 1996;35(4):265–71. PubMed PMID: 8786184.
57. Gindele A, Schwamborn D, Tsironis K, Benz-Bohm G. Myositis ossificans traumatica in young children: report of three cases and review of the literature. Pediatr Radiol. 2000;30(7):451–9. PubMed PMID: 10929363.
58. Thomas EA, Cassar-Pullicino VN, McCall IW. The role of ultrasound in the early diagnosis and management of heterotopic bone formation. Clin Radiol. 1991;43(3):190–6. PubMed PMID: 1901533.
59. McCarthy EF, Sundaram M. Heterotopic ossification: a review. Skeletal Radiol. 2005;34(10):609–19. PubMed PMID: 16132978.
60. Cesari M, Alberghini M, Vanel D, Palmerini E, Staals EL, Longhi A, et al. Periosteal osteosarcoma: a single-institution experience. Cancer. 2011;117(8):1731–5. PubMed PMID: 21472720.
61. Kransdorf MJ. Malignant soft-tissue tumors in a large referral population: distribution of diagnoses by age, sex, and location. AJR Am J Roentgenol. 1995;164(1): 129–34. PubMed PMID: 7998525. Epub 1995/01/01. eng.
62. Fletcher CD. Pleomorphic malignant fibrous histiocytoma: fact or fiction? A critical reappraisal based on 159 tumors diagnosed as pleomorphic sarcoma. Am J Surg Pathol. 1992;16(3):213–28. PubMed PMID: 1317996.
63. Siegel MJ. Magnetic resonance imaging of musculoskeletal soft tissue masses. Radiol Clin North Am. 2001;39(4):701–20. PubMed PMID: 11549166.
64. Kaste SC, Hill A, Conley L, Shidler TJ, Rao BN, Neel MM. Magnetic resonance imaging after incomplete resection of soft tissue sarcoma. Clin Orthop Relat Res. 2002;397:204–11. PubMed PMID: 11953612.
65. Panicek DM, Gatsonis C, Rosenthal DI, Seeger LL, Huvos AG, Moore SG, et al. CT and MR imaging in the local staging of primary malignant musculoskeletal neoplasms: report of the Radiology Diagnostic Oncology Group. Radiology. 1997;202(1):237–46. PubMed PMID: 8988217.
66. Subhawong TK, Fishman EK, Swart JE, Carrino JA, Attar S, Fayad LM. Soft-tissue masses and mass-like conditions: what does CT add to diagnosis and management? AJR Am J Roentgenol. 2010;194(6):1559–67. PubMed PMID: 20489097. Pubmed Central PMCID: 2884142. Epub 2010/05/22. eng.
67. McCarville MB, Spunt SL, Skapek SX, Pappo AS. Synovial sarcoma in pediatric patients. AJR Am J Roentgenol. 2002;179(3):797–801. PubMed PMID: 12185067. Epub 2002/08/20. eng.
68. Jones BC, Sundaram M, Kransdorf MJ. Synovial sarcoma: MR imaging findings in 34 patients. AJR Am J Roentgenol. 1993;161(4):827–30. PubMed PMID: 8396848. Epub 1993/10/01. eng.
69. Alaggio R, Coffin CM, Vargas SO. Soft tissue tumors of uncertain origin. Pediatr Dev Pathol. 2012;15(1 Suppl): 267–305. PubMed PMID: 22420732.

70. Wolden SL, Alektiar KM. Sarcomas across the age spectrum. Semin Radiat Oncol. 2010;20(1):45–51. PubMed PMID: 19959030.
71. Bixby SD, Hettmer S, Taylor GA, Voss SD. Synovial sarcoma in children: imaging features and common benign mimics. AJR Am J Roentgenol. 2010;195(4):1026–32. PubMed PMID: 20858835. Epub 2010/09/23. eng.
72. O'Sullivan PJ, Harris AC, Munk PL. Radiological features of synovial cell sarcoma. Br J Radiol. 2008;81(964):346–56. PubMed PMID: 18250123.
73. Jin W, Kim GY, Park SY, Chun YS, Rhyu KH, Park JS, et al. The spectrum of vascularized superficial soft-tissue tumors on sonography with a histopathologic correlation: part 2, malignant tumors and their look-alikes. AJR Am J Roentgenol. 2010;195(2):446–53. PubMed PMID: 20651203.
74. Blacksin MF, Siegel JR, Benevenia J, Aisner SC. Synovial sarcoma: frequency of nonaggressive MR characteristics. J Comput Assist Tomogr. 1997;21(5):785–9. PubMed PMID: 9294576. Epub 1997/09/19. eng.
75. Miser JS, Pizzo PA. Soft tissue sarcomas in childhood. Pediatr Clin North Am. 1985;32(3):779–800. PubMed PMID: 3889805.
76. Rao BN, Rodriguez-Galindo C. Local control in childhood extremity sarcomas: salvaging limbs and sparing function. Med Pediatr Oncol. 2003;41(6):584–7. PubMed PMID: 14595726.
77. McCarville MB, Spunt SL, Pappo AS. Rhabdomyosarcoma in pediatric patients: the good, the bad, and the unusual. AJR Am J Roentgenol. 2001;176(6):1563–9. PubMed PMID: 11373233. Epub 2001/05/25. eng.
78. La TH, Wolden SL, Su Z, Linardic C, Randall RL, Hawkins DS, et al. Local therapy for rhabdomyosarcoma of the hands and feet: is amputation necessary? A report from the Children's Oncology Group. Int J Radiat Oncol Biol Phys. 2011;80(1):206–12. PubMed PMID: 20646853. Pubmed Central PMCID: 3075377.
79. Lee VS, Martinez S, Coleman RE. Primary muscle lymphoma: clinical and imaging findings. Radiology. 1997;203(1):237–44. PubMed PMID: 9122401.
80. O'Neill JK, Devaraj V, Silver DA, Sarsfield P, Stone CA. Extranodal lymphomas presenting as soft tissue sarcomas to a sarcoma service over a two-year period. J Plast Reconstr Aesth Surg JPRAS. 2007;60(6):646–54. PubMed PMID: 17485053.
81. Chun CW, Jee WH, Park HJ, Kim YJ, Park JM, Lee SH, et al. MRI features of skeletal muscle lymphoma. AJR Am J Roentgenol. 2010;195(6):1355–60. PubMed PMID: 21098195.
82. Hermann G, Yeh HC, Schwartz I. Computed tomography of soft-tissue lesions of the extremities, pelvic and shoulder girdles: sonographic and pathological correlations. Clin Radiol. 1984;35(3):193–202. PubMed PMID: 6713795.
83. Pui MH, Fletcher BD, Langston JW. Granulocytic sarcoma in childhood leukemia: imaging features. Radiology. 1994;190(3):698–702. PubMed PMID: 8115614. Epub 1994/03/01. eng.
84. Stein-Wexler R, Wootton-Gorges SL, West DC. Orbital granulocytic sarcoma: an unusual presentation of acute myelocytic leukemia. Pediatr Radiol. 2003;33(2):136–9. PubMed PMID: 12557072. Epub 2003/01/31. eng.
85. Chiou SY, Chiou HJ, Chou YH, Tiu CM, Pan CC, Chang CY. Sonographic features of primary testicular granulocytic sarcoma. J Ultrasound Med. 2003;22(12): 1413–6. PubMed PMID: 14682435.
86. Lim HS, Park MH, Heo SH, Kim JW, Chang NK, Song SG, et al. Myeloid sarcoma of the breast mimicking hamartoma on sonography. J Ultrasound Med. 2008;27(12):1777–80. PubMed PMID: 19023005.
87. O'Donnell TM, Devitt AT, Kutty S, Fogarty EE. Recurrent congenital haemangiopericytoma in a child. J Bone Joint Surg. 2001;83(2):269–72. PubMed PMID: 11284579.
88. Casanova M, Ferrari A, Collini P, Bisogno G, Alaggio R, Cecchetto G, et al. Epithelioid sarcoma in children and adolescents: a report from the Italian Soft Tissue Sarcoma Committee. Cancer. 2006;106(3):708–17. PubMed PMID: 16353216. Epub 2005/12/15. eng.
89. Tateishi U, Hasegawa T, Kusumoto M, Yokoyama R, Moriyama N. Radiologic manifestations of proximal-type epithelioid sarcoma of the soft tissues. AJR Am J Roentgenol. 2002;179(4):973–7. PubMed PMID: 12239049. Epub 2002/09/20. eng.
90. Hanna SL, Kaste S, Jenkins JJ, Hewan-Lowe K, Spence JV, Gupta M, et al. Epithelioid sarcoma: clinical, MR imaging and pathologic findings. Skeletal Radiol. 2002;31(7):400–12. PubMed PMID: 12107573.
91. Navarro OM, Laffan EE, Ngan BY. Pediatric soft-tissue tumors and pseudo-tumors: MR imaging features with pathologic correlation: part 1. Imaging approach, pseudotumors, vascular lesions, and adipocytic tumors. Radiographics. 2009;29(3):887–906. PubMed PMID: 19448123.
92. Casanova M, Ferrari A, Bisogno G, Cecchetto G, Basso E, De Bernardi B, et al. Alveolar soft part sarcoma in children and adolescents: a report from the Soft-Tissue Sarcoma Italian Cooperative Group. Ann Oncol. 2000;11(11):1445–9. PubMed PMID: 11142485.
93. Lorigan JG, O'Keeffe FN, Evans HL, Wallace S. The radiologic manifestations of alveolar soft-part sarcoma. AJR Am J Roentgenol. 1989;153(2):335–9. PubMed PMID: 2750619. Epub 1989/08/01. eng.
94. Lai YC, Chiou HJ, Wu HT, Chou YH, Wang HK, Chen PC. Ultrasonographic and MR findings of alveolar soft part sarcoma. J Chin Med Assoc JCMA. 2009;72(6):336–9. PubMed PMID: 19541571.
95. Tsokos M, Alaggio RD, Dehner LP, Dickman PS. Ewing sarcoma/peripheral primitive neuroectodermal tumor and related tumors. Pediatr Dev Pathol. 2012;15(1 Suppl):108–26. PubMed PMID: 22420726.
96. Beall DP, Ly J, Bell JP, Parker EE, John CM, Babb JC, et al. Pediatric extraskeletal osteosarcoma. Pediatr Radiol. 2008;38(5):579–82. PubMed PMID: 18214458.

97. Lidang Jensen M, Schumacher B, Myhre Jensen O, Steen Nielsen O, Keller J. Extraskeletal osteosarcomas: a clinicopathologic study of 25 cases. Am J Surg Pathol. 1998;22(5):588–94. PubMed PMID: 9591729.
98. Stein-Wexler R. MR imaging of soft tissue masses in children. Radiol Clin North Am. 2009;47:977–95.
99. Stein-Wexler R. Pediatric soft tissue sarcomas. Semin Ultrasound CT MRI. 2011;32(5):470–88.

Generalized Disorders and Syndromes of Orthopedic Importance

23

Karen Rosendahl

Contents

Abstract

This chapter discusses selected generalized orthopedic disorders, focusing on those that are relatively common and that are often targets of surgical intervention. The four most common subtypes of osteogenesis imperfecta are presented first, followed by discussion of neurofibromatosis. The chapter then addresses typical problems encountered in arthrogryposis, as well as Down syndrome, sickle cell disease, and the many forms of mucopolysaccharidosis. Gaucher disease is reviewed, and then several brief sections address VACTRL/VATER association, limb-body wall defects, achondroplasia, multiple epiphyseal dysplasia, pseudoachondroplasia, and brachyolmia.

Skeletal dysplasias, metabolic disorders, and syndromes can have significant orthopedic implications. Although patients with skeletal dysplasias often present with disproportional short stature, some may present with a focal joint problem (stiffness, pain, deformity, contractures, dislocations, swelling, laxity) alone or in combination with spine problems (pain, stiffness, deformity) in childhood or adolescence. For example, patients with mild forms of multiple epiphyseal dysplasia (without significant limb shortening) may present only with hip problems, leading to misdiagnoses of Meyer dysplasia or bilateral Legg-Perthe disease [1]. Similarly,

K. Rosendahl, MD, PhD
Section of Paediatric Radiology,
Department of Clinical Medicine,
Faculty of Medicine and Dentistry,
University of Bergen, Haukeland University Hospital,
Jonas Liesvei 65, Bergen 5021, Norway
e-mail: karen.rosendahl@helse-bergen.no

R. Stein-Wexler et al. (eds.), *Pediatric Orthopedic Imaging*,
DOI 10.1007/978-3-642-45381-6_23, © Springer-Verlag Berlin Heidelberg 2015

patients with diastrophic dysplasia may initially present with clubfoot deformity, and those with brachyolmia may present simply with spine deformity. Thus, an understanding of the variety of manifestations of common syndromes and other generalized disorders is important.

To assist in diagnosing the broad spectrum of genetic skeletal disorders, a list has been developed, grouping these conditions by their cardinal features (Nosology and Classification of Genetic Skeletal Disorders) [2]. In the 2010 revision, 456 conditions were included and placed in 40 groups, of which 316 are associated with mutations in one or more of 226 genes. Groups 1–8 are based on a common underlying gene or pathway and include achondroplasia. Groups 9–17 are based on the location of radiographic abnormalities within specific bones (such as the epi-, meta-, and/or diaphysis of the long bones, or within the vertebrae) or how the changes are distributed within an extremity (rhizo, meso, or acro); multiple epiphyseal dysplasia (MED), pseudoachondroplasia, and brachyolmia are included within this cluster. Groups 18–20 are defined by macroscopic criteria combined with clinical features (bent or slender bones, multiple dislocations). Groups 21–25 and 28 take into account features of mineralization and include osteogenesis imperfecta. Group 27, the dysostosis multiplex group, includes the mucopolysaccharidoses. Group 29 (disorganized development of skeletal components) includes neurofibromatosis type 1, and groups 32–40 encompass the dysostoses [2]. In contrast to the dysplasias, the dysostoses often arise from embryonic morphogenic defects and are thus more closely related to multiple malformation syndromes [2].

In addition to the disorders highlighted above, this chapter will also discuss some metabolic/systemic disorders with significant skeletal manifestations (Gaucher disease, sickle cell disease), as well as arthrogryposis, VACTERL/VATER (vertebral-anorectal-cardiac-tracheoesophageal fistula-renal-limb/vertebral-anorectal-tracheoesophageal fistula-radial) association, and limb-body wall defects. Excellent texts can be reviewed for additional information [1, 3–5].

1 Osteogenesis Imperfecta

Osteogenesis imperfecta (OI) is a genetic disorder characterized by increased bone fragility, decreased bone mass, and abnormal connective tissues. Typical extraskeletal manifestations include blue sclera, dentinogenesis imperfecta, hyperlaxity of skin and ligaments, and hearing impairment. The prevalence is reported at 6 or 7 per 100,000 births. Severity varies from in utero presentation with multiple fractures and perinatal lethality to very mild forms manifesting in adulthood with few if any fractures [6, 7]. In around 90 % of patients, the disorder is caused by a mutation in one of the two genes that encode the α-chains of collagen type 1 (COL1A1 (chromosome 17) and COL1A2 (chromosome 7) genes); over 800 specific mutations have been identified to date. The remaining 10 % of cases are due to recessive variants in eight other genes or in others that are not yet recognized [8]. Diagnosis is based on family history and clinical findings but can be difficult if fractures are not associated with extraskeletal manifestations. When non-accidental injury is a consideration, analysis of the procollagen in fibroblasts (skin biopsy) or analysis of collagen type 1 genes can provide helpful information. The mainstay for medical management includes physiotherapy, rehabilitation, orthopedic surgery, and bisphosphonate treatment for moderate and severe forms of OI.

OI is characterized by an insufficient quantity and quality of bone, as type 1 collagen forms the latticework for mineralization of enchondral bone. Trabeculae are abnormally thin and relatively few in number, resulting in thin, osteoporotic bones (Fig. 23.1). Although individual osteoblasts produce less bone than normal, the overall rate of bone formation in the trabecular compartment is amplified, due to an increased number of osteoblasts. However, this increase does not lead to a net gain in trabecular bone mass, because the rate of bone resorption is also enhanced [7]. Moreover, although mineralized OI bone may be harder than normal bone at the material level, it breaks more easily when deformed and fatigues much faster on repetitive loading [7, 9, 10].

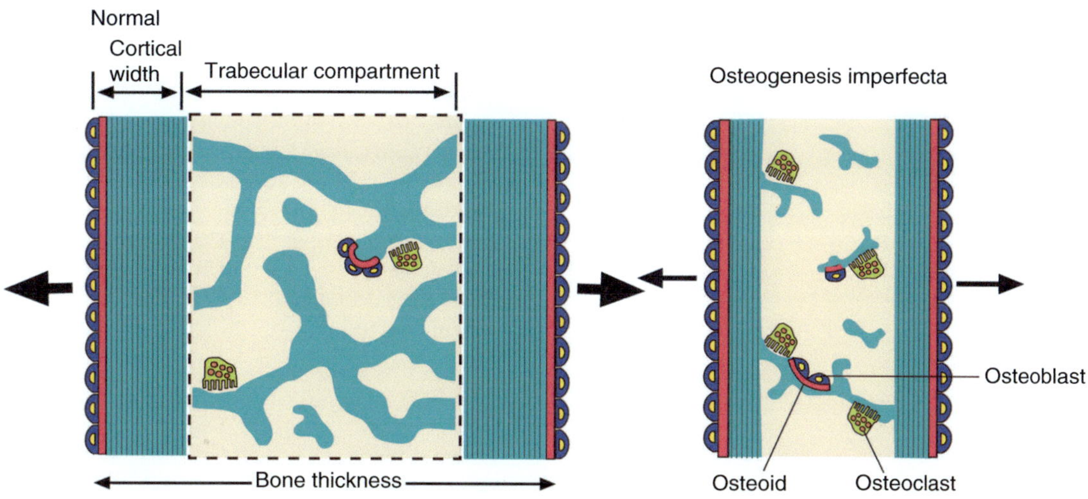

Fig. 23.1 Diagram demonstrating histological abnormalities in bone with osteogenesis imperfecta (OI). (**a**) Normal bone for comparison. (**b**) Diminished thickness due to impaired periosteal bone formation in OI. Trabeculae are reduced in number and are abnormally thin

Clinical diagnosis is based on increased bone fragility combined with the appropriate signs and symptoms (Table 23.1). A positive family history or the presence of several typical features simplifies diagnosis. However, diagnosis can be challenging in those with only a moderate increase in number of childhood fractures or in those who have gracile bones with thin cortices but no extraskeletal manifestations. Many of these patients have a family history of similar borderline skeletal abnormalities. Analysis of the collagen type 1 genes, either by screening for coding mutations in DNA extracted from the patient's white blood cells or by analyzing the amount and structure of type 1 procollagen molecules derived from the patient's cultured fibroblasts, can confirm the diagnosis in around 90 % of cases [7]. However, not all OI genes have been sequenced, and therefore negative chromosomal analysis cannot rule out OI. This has significant social and legal implications in the setting of suspected non-accidental trauma [11, 12] (see Chap. 18).

Many but not all patients with OI have abnormal sclera, ranging in color from faint gray-blue to deep blue. However, healthy infants can also have dark or bluish sclera, so this finding is not helpful in this age group [7]. Coloration is attributed to scleral thinning or other abnormalities that render visible the vascular layer of the choroid. The cornea may be abnormal as well.

Teeth are abnormal in over one third of patients. They range in color from amber brown to bluish-gray and have an opalescent character. The basic problem lies in the dentin, which is abnormally friable and induces cracking of normal enamel. Permanent teeth are usually less affected than primary teeth. Radiological or histological examination frequently shows abnormalities, even in individuals with apparently normal teeth [13]. Occasionally the disease is completely restricted to the teeth; this condition is termed dentinogenesis imperfecta.

Skin may be thin and translucent; it may bruise easily. The head may be large, with a prominent occipital overhang and eventually a characteristic triangular face. Peripheral joints are hypermobile and lax. Congenital hernias are described in some patients. A defect in homeostasis may precipitate hyperthermia during anesthesia and also cause these children to sweat easily and rarely feel chilled. Conductive or sensorineural deafness occurs occasionally. Arthrogryposis and osteopoikilosis infrequently accompany osteogenesis imperfecta, and several cases of osteogenic sarcoma have been described.

Table 23.1 Modified Sillence classification of osteogenesis imperfecta

Type	Inheritance	Clinical severity	Typical features	Affected gene(s)
I	AD	Mild nondeforming	Normal height/mild short stature Normal teeth (except type I) Hearing loss	COL1A1, COL1A2
II	AD, AR	Perinatal lethal	Multiple rib/long bone fractures at birth Pronounced deformities Lucent skull bones Dark sclera Very short	COL1A1, COL1A2, CRTAP, LEPRE1, PPIB
III	AD, AR	Severely and progressively deforming	Triangular face Severe scoliosis Grayish sclera, may normalize Dentinogenesis imperfecta Moderately short Fractures usually by age 2	COL1A1, COL1A2, CRTAP, LEPRE1, PPIB, FKBP10, SERPINH1
IV	AD, AR	Moderately deforming	Mild to moderate scoliosis Grayish or white sclera Dentinogenesis imperfecta	COL1A1, COL1A2, CRTAP, FKBP10, SP7
V	AD	Moderate to severe bone fragility	Mild to moderate short stature Mineralized interosseous membrane White sclera Normal teeth	Unknown

Adapted from [2, 7]
AD autosomal dominant, *AR* autosomal recessive

Fractures can occur with the least provocation in some patients and only rarely in others. However, fracture frequency decreases before puberty in severe cases and during and after puberty in all patients. The average number of fractures per individual ranges from less than 1 to 20–30 per year.

Short stature results from several factors. Multiple fractures with resultant bowing may shorten the legs, and repetitive trauma to the growth plate may induce growth plate dysfunction. Most patients also have an intrinsic growth defect.

Classification System

OI was first described in 1788 by a Swedish army surgeon [14]. In 1906, OI was classified into the now obsolete congenita and tarda forms [1, 8]. In 1978, Sillence and coworkers provided the first systematic classification into four clinical types, which were correlated with inheritance patterns: type I (mild OI, blue sclerae, autosomal dominant inheritance), type II (lethal perinatal OI, autosomal recessive inheritance, later subdivided in II-A, -B, and -C based on radiographic features), type III (progressively deforming, sclerae initially blue, autosomal recessive inheritance), and type IV (mild to moderate OI, normal sclerae, autosomal dominant inheritance) [15, 16].

New research unraveling the genetic and clinical complexity of OI has made additional classification possible, but the Sillence scheme is still clinically useful [17]. After the discovery of heterozygous collagen type I gene mutations in all types of OI [18, 19], the Sillence criteria were used mainly to describe the severity of disease and differences in clinical expression, rather than the inheritance pattern. With the subsequent discovery that some patients with lethal or severe

OI have normal type I collagen [20], the Sillence classification was expanded, first to include seven genetic types [7] and then to include eight [21]. Type V was added because of its characteristic clinical and radiological features, whereas the histology of type VI is unique. Types VII and VIII are genetically distinct, both with autosomal recessive inheritance and mutations in, respectively, the CRTAP and LEPRE1 genes [17]. The Nosology Group of the International Skeletal Dysplasia Society has retained the Sillence classification as the prototypic and universally accepted way to classify OI and avoids direct molecular reference (see Table 23.1).

The relatively mild types I and IV comprise considerably more than half of patients with OI. It is difficult to predict exactly what form this disease will take. About 20 % of patients with mild OI (especially those with type IV) have fractures at birth. Type III accounts for around 15 % of patients with OI, while type V accounts for between 4 and 5 % of all cases. The incidence of type II is reported at 1–2 per 100,000 [7, 8].

Management of OI is multidisciplinary. Subspecialty management of hearing, dental, and pulmonary abnormalities may be necessary. Skeletal abnormalities are addressed with medications such as bisphosphonates and recombinant human growth hormone, as well as surgical procedures and physical rehabilitation. Although some form of bisphosphonate therapy constitutes standard treatment, the specific drug and duration of treatment are subject to debate. Furthermore, it is difficult to predict which patients will respond with increased bone density and decreased incidence of fracture. Promising cellular therapies and new drug regimens are being developed.

Orthopedic treatment includes casting, rod placement, and osteotomies (cutting and realigning the bone); choice of procedure depends on the fracture type, disease severity, and patient's functional status. If routine casting is unsuccessful, intramedullary rods may be placed. Fragmentation may be required for difficult cases and is usually successful. This involves cutting a bowed and deformed bone into segments and then realigning them on a rigid or expandable rod. Complications following this and other procedures include rod breakage, uncoupling, extrusion, interference with growth plate function, and fracture at the end of a metallic device. Nonunion occasionally occurs, but in general fractures and osteotomies heal well. Management of scoliosis is complicated by extreme bone fragility.

Imaging

An excessive number of Wormian, or intrasutural, bones (exceeding the upper normal of eight to ten) are a typical feature in the skull [7, 22] (Fig. 23.2). Bones may be diffusely osteoporotic,

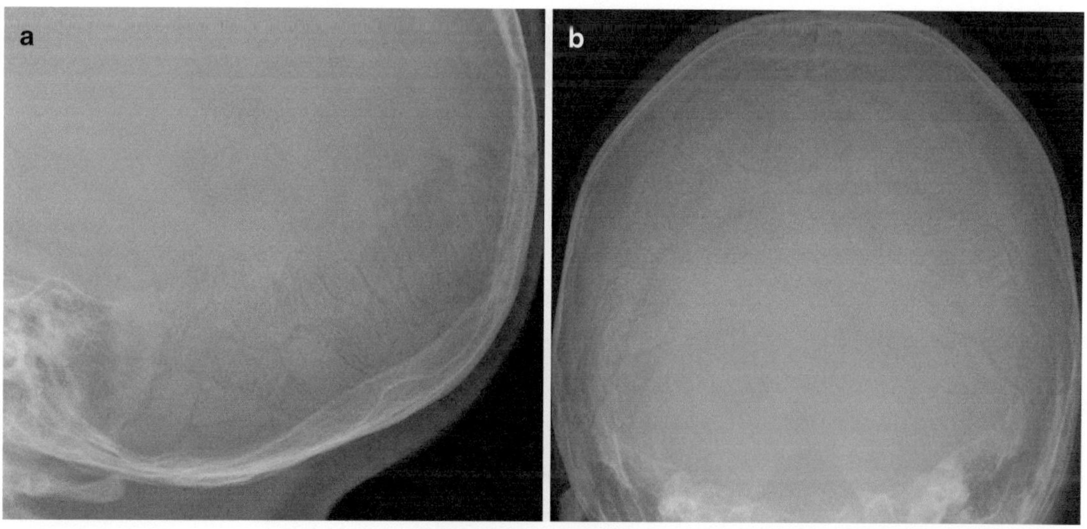

Fig. 23.2 (**a**, **b**) Multiple Wormian bones in the lambdoid suture in a 17-month-old boy with OI type I

with healing or healed fractures. Joint abnormalities such as genu valgum and coxa vara can result from both laxity and fracture deformity, while loss of structural strength can lead to acetabular protrusion (see Chap. 3).

Although there is considerable overlap, some imaging manifestations are more specific to the type of OI and are discussed below (Box 23.1).

Box 23.1: Osteogenesis Imperfecta: Radiographic Features

All	Excessive number of Wormian bones (>8–10)
	Diffuse osteoporosis
I	*Mild nondeforming*
	Slender ribs/long bones, no major bone deformity, normal or mild short stature
	Fractures after 2–3 years old (may be preceded by bowing)
	Diaphyseal, transverse, nondisplaced; often lower extremity
	Decreased frequency after puberty
	Vertebral fractures common
II	*Perinatal lethal*
	Beaded ribs, crumpled femurs, severely short stature
	Short, broad long bones
	Severe biconcave vertebrae
III	*Severely and progressively deforming*
	Gracile, mildly short long bones, very short stature
	Angulation at metadiaphysis
	Codfish vertebrae, progressive severe kyphoscoliosis
	Popcorn metaphyseal calcifications in up to 50 %
	Usually fractures at birth
IV	*Moderately deforming*
	Mild to moderate bone fragility, variable short stature
	Up to ¼ have fractures at birth
	Radiographs resemble type I but may have popcorn calcifications in metaphyses
V	*Moderate to severe bone fragility*
	Hyperplastic callus resembles osteosarcoma
	Variable short stature
	Calcification of interosseous membrane at the forearm, causing dislocation of the radial head

OI Type I (Mild Nondeforming)

This is the mildest and most common form of OI (see Table 23.1). It is associated with blue sclerae that persist throughout life, hearing loss in half of patients by 40 years of age, joint hypermobility, postfracture deformity, and easy bruising. Fracture incidence and severity vary. They often occur only after initiation of weight bearing, around 2 or 3 years of age. Children with OI who are younger than 5 years of age usually have diaphyseal, transverse, nondisplaced, and often lower extremity fractures, whereas normal children of the same age tend to fracture in the dia/metaphyses of the upper extremities [23]. Fractures continue throughout childhood but decrease in frequency after puberty. The “A” subtype is associated with dentin abnormality.

Radiographs usually demonstrate osteoporosis and slender ribs and long bones (Fig. 23.3).

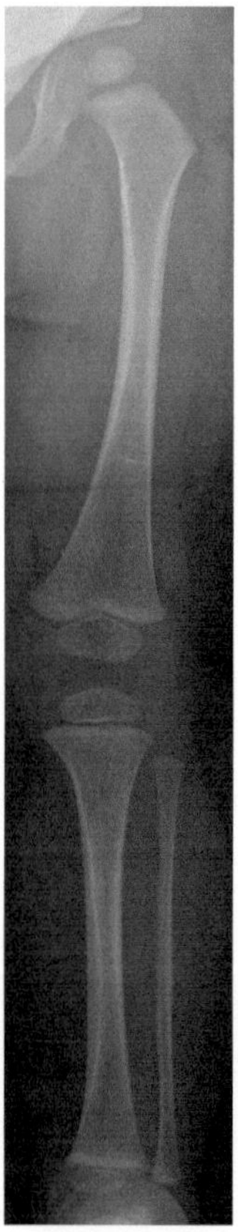

Fig. 23.3 Osteoporosis and slender long bones in a 2-year-old girl with OI type I

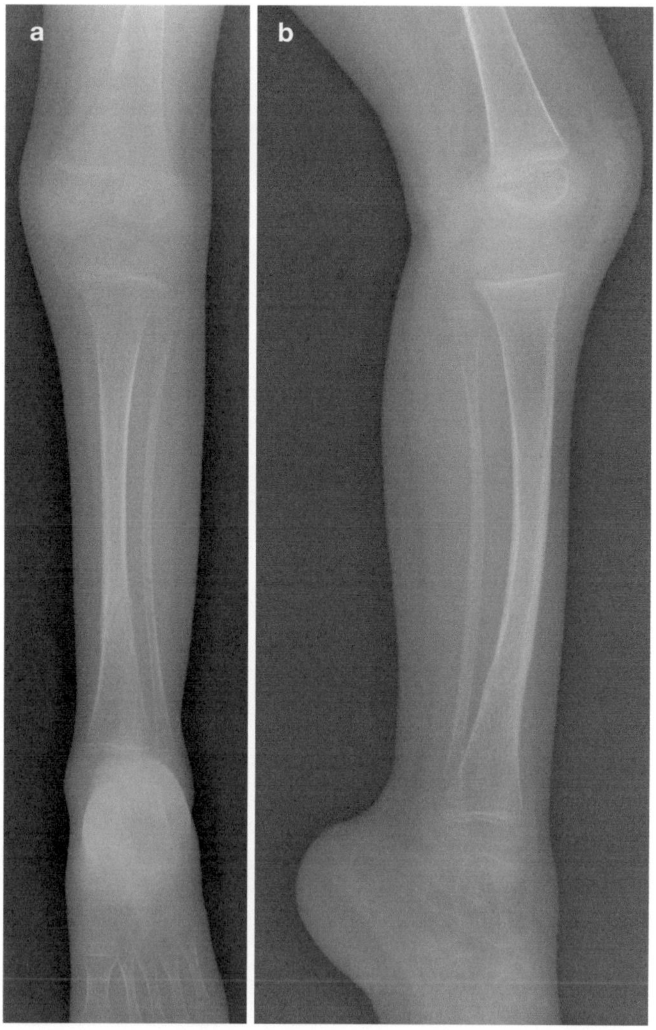

Fig. 23.4 OI type I in a 3-year-old. (**a**, **b**) The bones are gracile and show mild tibial bowing. Healing distal tibial fracture

Mild anterolateral bowing can precede fractures (Fig. 23.4). Vertebral fractures are common and can lead to mild scoliosis (see Chap. 3) (Fig. 23.5). As with other forms of OI, Wormian (or intrasutural) bones are common (see Fig. 23.2).

OI Type II (Perinatal Lethal)

This is characterized by blue sclerae and represents the most common second trimester ultrasound diagnosis of short, bent limbs [1]. Healing intrauterine fractures result in a beaded appearance of the ribs and crumpled femurs; deformity is obvious at birth (Fig. 23.6). Ribs are small and dysplastic due to multiple fractures, and this may result in a hypoplastic thorax with reduced lung volume and eventual respiratory failure and death. The bones of the extremities are short and wide, with evidence of periosteal new bone formation, callus, and healing and unhealed fractures. The increased bone width is largely due to remodeling after fracture healing, resulting in a blocklike, rectangular shaft. Impacted and torus fractures lead to wrinkled, crumpled, and thick cortices. Femoral and tibial bowing is typical. Severe biconcave compression deformity of the vertebral bodies may become so severe that the flattened, diminutive, osteoporotic vertebrae can barely be recognized between the intervertebral discs.

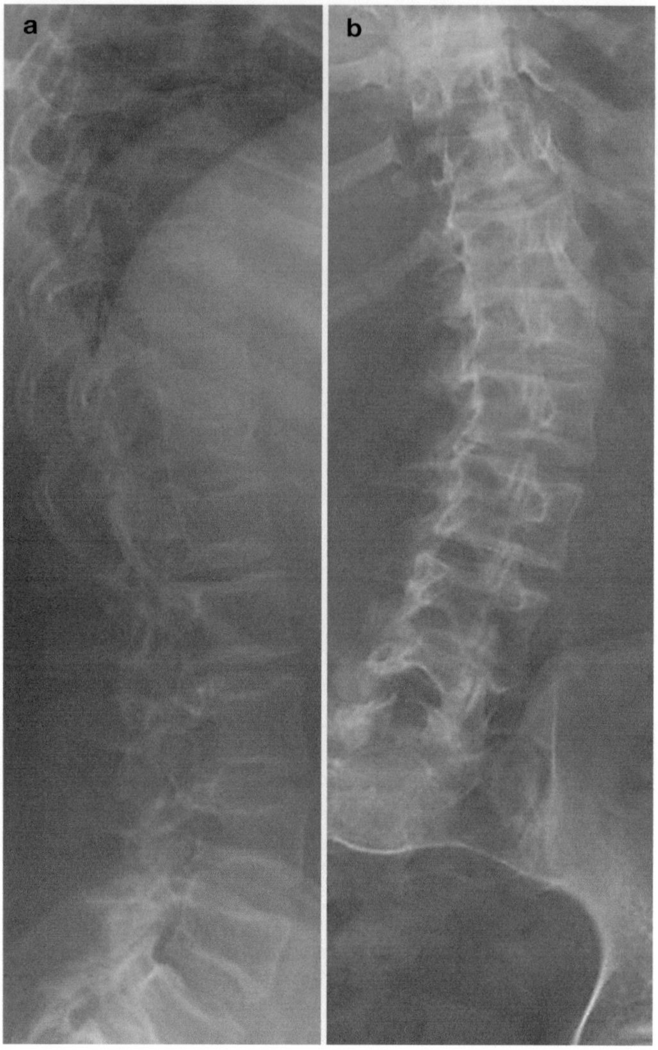

Fig. 23.5 OI type I in a 12-year-old girl. (**a**) Osteoporosis and multiple vertebral fractures. (**b**) Mild scoliosis

Radiographs of the most severe type A subgroup demonstrate absent ossification of the skull vault (Fig. 23.7), marked osteoporosis, broad ribs from multiple fractures, short and crumpled femurs with no metadiaphyseal differentiation, vertebral collapse, and angulated tibias [24]. The type B subgroup, which must be differentiated from type III in the perinatal period, has beaded ribs from discrete healing fractures, along with angulated tibias, but there is recognizable distinction between the metadiaphysis and the diaphysis. The type C subgroup is rare. It too lacks skull vault ossification but has unusually dense stippling throughout the skeleton, possibly secondary to healing fractures.

OI Type III (Severely and Progressively Deforming)

This is the most severe form in children that survive the neonatal period. The bones are extremely slender at birth, often with fractures and poor growth. By 2 years of age, numerous fractures are evident. Blue sclerae at birth and infancy later normalize. Hearing loss occurs early, teeth are abnormal, and the face is triangular with frontal bossing.

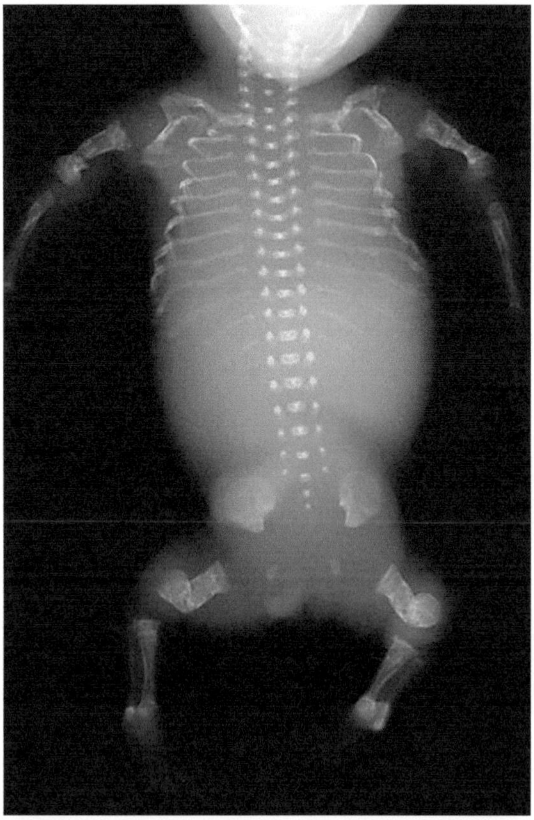

Fig. 23.6 OI type II in a fetus, whose gestation was terminated at 24 weeks. Multiple old and recent fractures of the extremities and ribs. Squaring of long bones due to periosteal callus in response to intrauterine fractures

Radiographs demonstrate severe osteoporosis, poor ossification of the skull with wide sutures, multiple Wormian bones, and large fontanelles (Fig. 23.8). The long bones are gracile and mildly shortened, with marked angulation and subsequent widening of the meta- and diaphyses (Figs. 23.9 and 23.10). The vertebral bodies develop a characteristic codfish shape, and there is progressive kyphoscoliosis.

"Popcorn" metaphyseal calcifications are encountered in up to one half of older children with type III OI and are occasionally seen in type IV. Resembling accumulations of popcorn, these lesions consist of multiple discrete conglomerations of small cystic lucencies, demarcated by sclerotic borders and sometimes containing central calcifications (Fig. 23.11) [25]. They are characteristically located in the lower extremities, especially at the knees, and can cause severe growth dysfunction. The metaphysis is typically expanded, and the growth plates partially or completely disrupted, with popcorn nodules extending into the epiphysis. Popcorn calcifications are not present at birth but develop as the patient grows, remodeling and disappearing with maturity. Their location and evolution suggest they may result from trauma to abnormal bone.

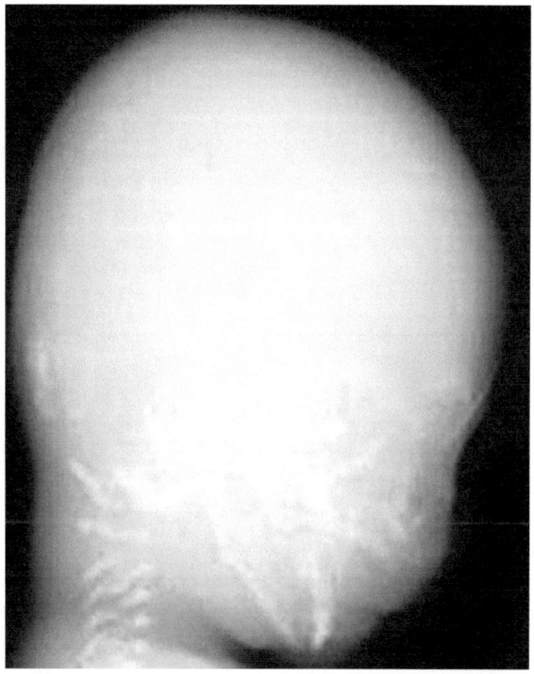

Fig. 23.7 Defective calvarial ossification in OI type IIA

OI Type IV (Moderately Deforming)

This represents a heterogeneous group characterized by mild to moderate osseous fragility and mild to moderate bone deformities. Sclerae are usually grayish or white (although they can be blue in infancy and childhood), and hearing is normal. Dental problems, osteoporosis, and fracture incidence vary, and the initial fractures occur at birth in up to one fourth of patients. Radiographs of these patients resemble those with type I OI

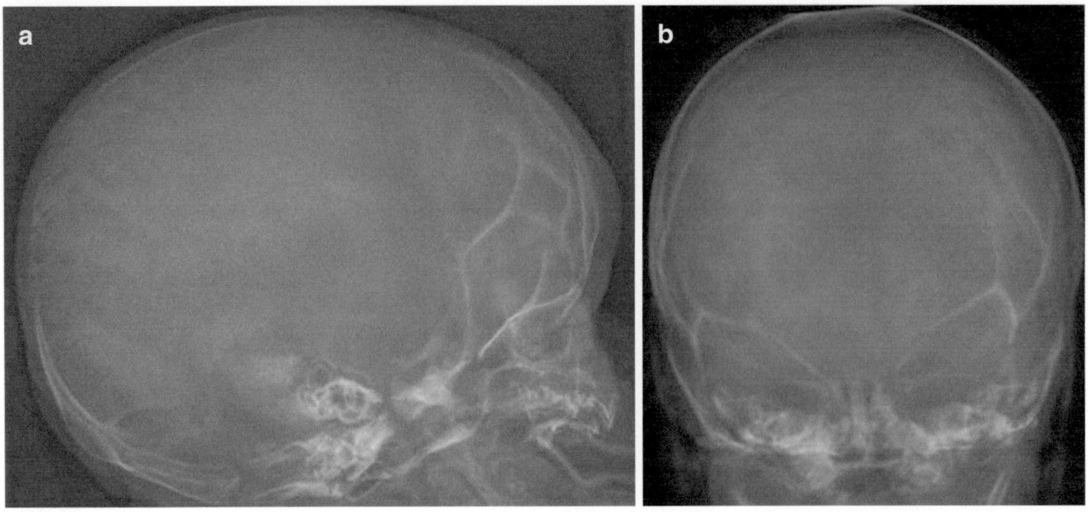

Fig. 23.8 OI type III in a 3-week-old boy. (**a**, **b**) Under-mineralized skull with wide sutures and multiple Wormian bones

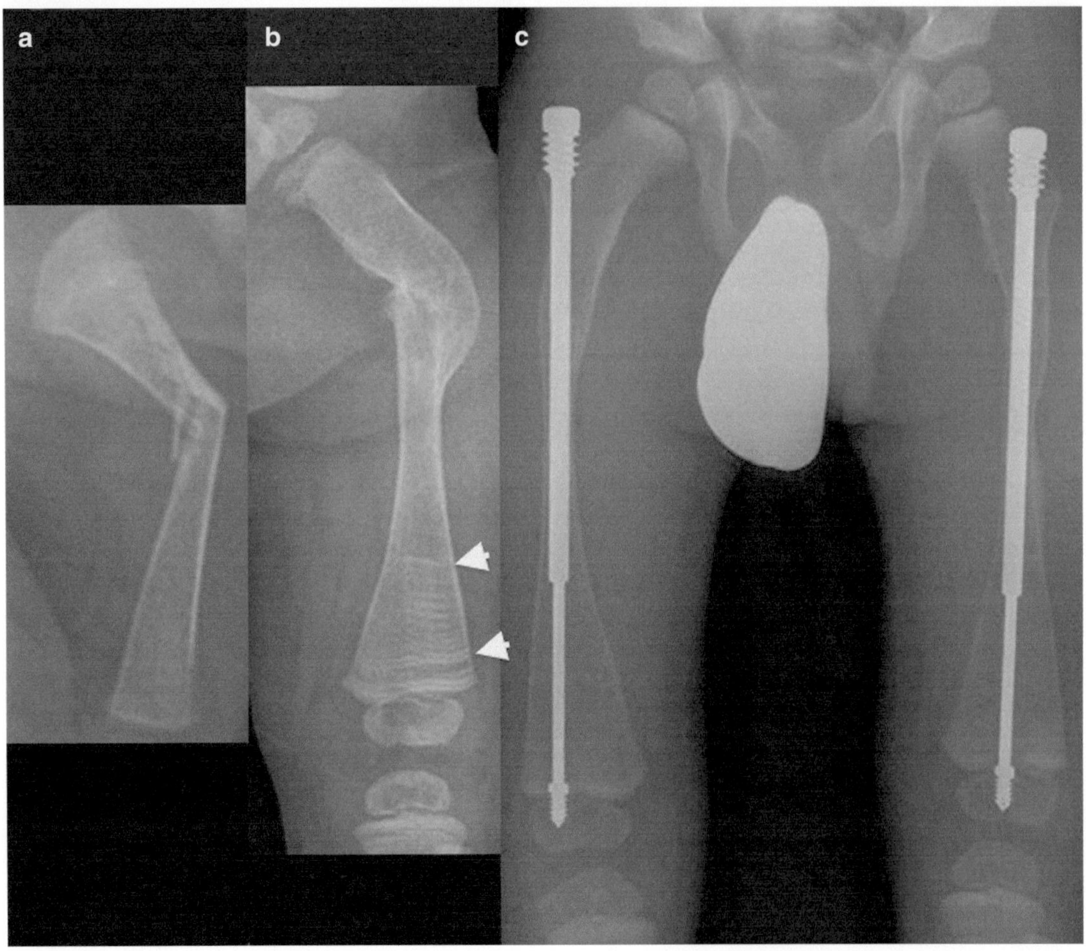

Fig. 23.9 Progressive changes in the femur of a boy with OI type III. (**a**) Recent femoral fracture when 3 weeks old. (**b**) At age 1.5 years, the fracture has healed with deformity. (**c**) At age 4 years, both femurs have been pinned, and bones are osteoporotic. Horizontal metaphyseal lines (*arrowheads*) due to bisphosphonate treatment

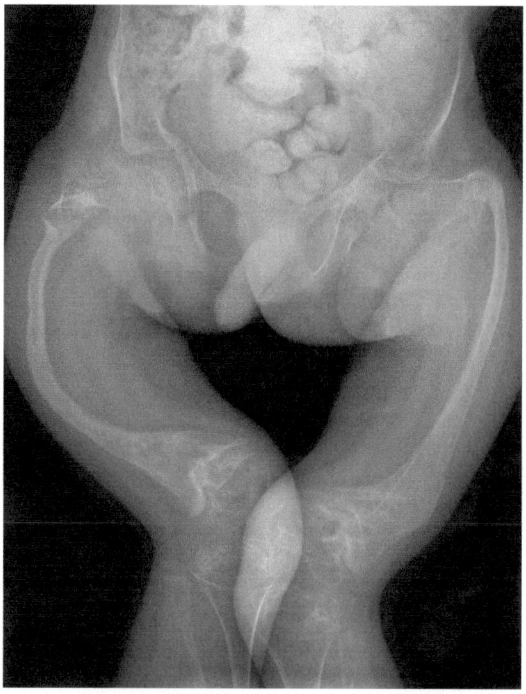

Fig. 23.10 Marked osteoporosis and deformity in a 9-year-old boy with OI type III, who was born with multiple fractures. The femurs are gracile, curved, and irregular due to numerous incomplete fractures

(Fig. 23.12). However, popcorn calcifications are encountered in about 10 % of patients with type IV OI.

OI Type V (Moderate to Severe Bone Fragility)

This form is characterized by calcification of interosseous membranes and/or hypertrophic callus [26]. Patients may be somewhat short but have normal teeth and sclerae. There is no evidence of a collagen type 1 abnormality [17]. The interosseous membrane at the forearm calcifies early in life, limiting hand movements and eventually causing the radial head to dislocate. After fractures or surgical procedures, hyperplastic callus can mimic osteosarcoma [27] (Fig. 23.13).

Differential Diagnosis

Several primary skeletal disorders can be confused with OI (Table 23.2), although chromosomal analysis will often differentiate between them. Radiographs of patients with Bruck syndrome resemble OI, but elbow contractures are present at birth and cubital webs develop [24]. Osteoporosis-pseudoglioma syndrome is similar to OI and was previously called ocular OI. Panostotic fibrous dysplasia involves all bones and is the extreme form of polyostotic fibrous dysplasia. Idiopathic hyperphosphatasia (juvenile Paget disease) is characterized by severe bone fragility and strikingly increased bone turnover [7], along with very high alkaline phosphatase activity. The presentation of

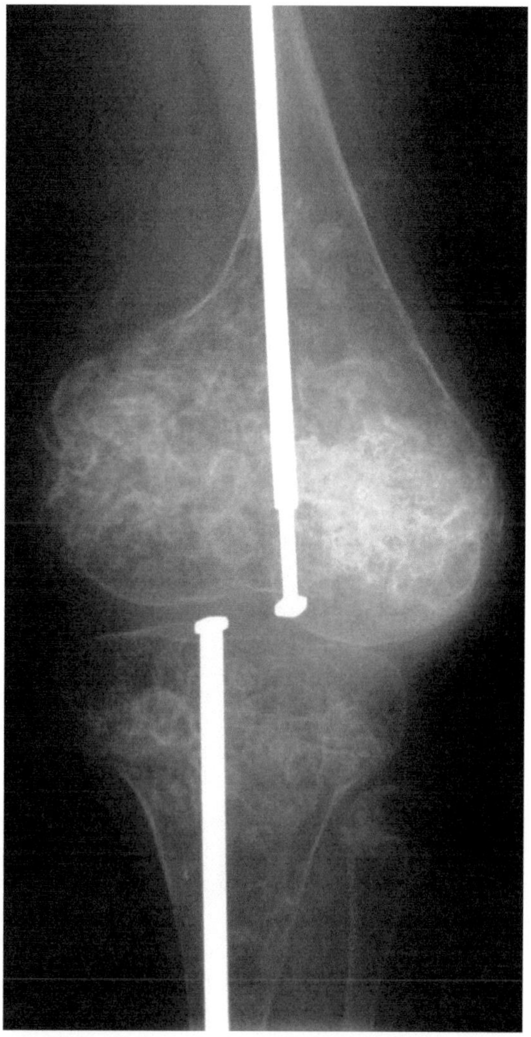

Fig. 23.11 Metaphyseal "popcorn" calcifications in a 12-year-old boy with OI (Courtesy of Sandra L. Wootton-Gorges)

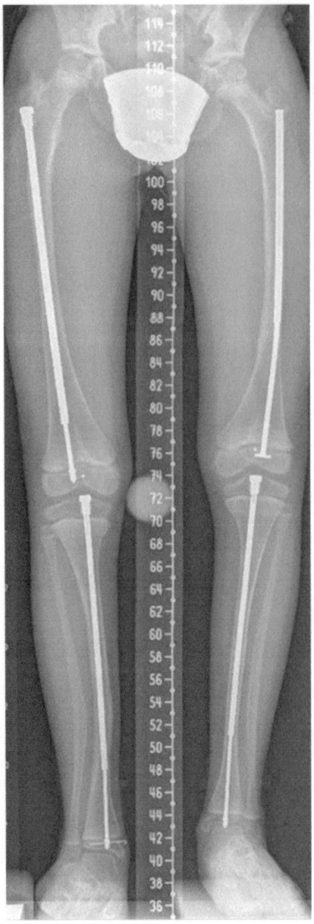

Fig. 23.12 Multiple healed fractures in an 11-year-old boy with OI type IV and resultant mild leg length discrepancy. Bones are severely osteopenic, with thin cortices and trabeculae. Impaired periosteal growth has led to thin diaphyses with relatively normal metaphyses

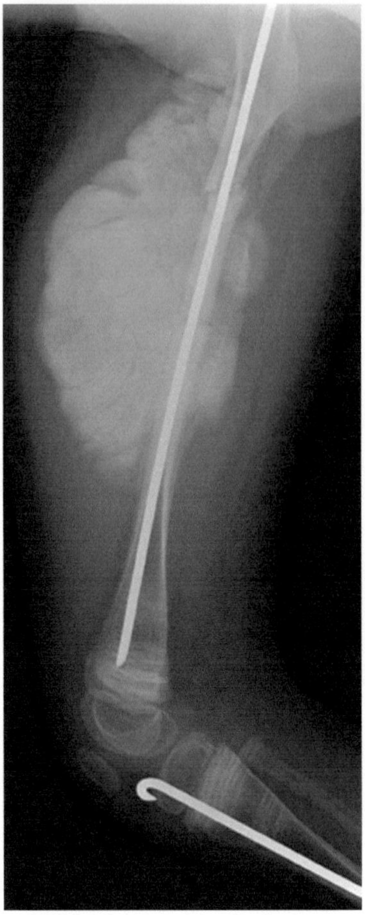

Fig. 23.13 Hyperplastic callus formation in a 13-year-old boy with OI type V and an upper femoral fracture

hypophosphatasia varies widely, from a severe perinatally lethal form with absent mineralization to pathological fractures that develop only in late childhood [28]. Cole-Carpenter syndrome is characterized by severe bone fragility and is distinguished from OI by the presence of craniosynostosis. In idiopathic juvenile osteoporosis, osteoporosis leads to fractures and collapse of vertebral bodies around age 5, with spontaneous improvement around puberty.

Non-accidental trauma can produce a variety of injuries and injury patterns in children, but none are completely pathognomonic [29]. Fractures are observed in approximately 30 % of abused children and are even more common in infants [29] (see Chap. 18). Collagen type 1 analysis can be useful if positive, but a negative test is by no means evidence for child abuse. Differentiating mild OI from non-accidental trauma is challenging if genetic analysis is normal, there is no family history, and teeth and sclerae are normal. Measurement of bone-mineral density with dual-energy X-ray absorptiometry (DXA) has been proposed to help in the differential diagnosis, but technical issues, difficulties with interpretation, and lack of normative data limit its use in children (see Chap. 26) [30].

Table 23.2 Skeletal disorders that resemble osteogenesis imperfecta

Disorder	Inheritance	Severity of bone fragility/deformity	Characteristics	Genetic defect
Bruck syndrome	AR	Moderate to severe	Congenital joint contractures	Telopeptide lysyl hydroxylase deficiency
Osteoporosis-pseudoglioma syndrome	AR	Moderate	Congenital blindness	*LRP5*
Panostotic fibrous dysplasia	None (somatic mutation)	Severe	Cystic or ground-glass lesions in all bones	*GNAS*
Idiopathic hyperphosphatasia	AR	Severe	Raised alkaline phosphatase activity Wide diaphyses Thick calvarium	*TNFRSF11B*
Hypophosphatasia	AR, AD	Mild to severe	Low alkaline phosphatase activity	*ALPL*
Cole-Carpenter syndrome	Unknown	Severe	Craniosynostosis Ocular proptosis	Unknown
Idiopathic juvenile osteoporosis	None	Mild to moderate	No extraskeletal abnormalities	Unknown

Adapted from [7]

2 Neurofibromatosis

Neurofibromatosis is a multisystem disorder with both tumor and non-tumor manifestations. Although anecdotal descriptions of neurofibromatosis date back centuries, von Recklinghausen and Wishart were the first to categorize neurofibromatosis type 1 (NF1) and neurofibromatosis type 2 (NF2) [31]. Based on genetic and molecular studies, three distinct forms have been recognized: NF1, NF2, and schwannomatosis.

NF1, previously known as von Recklinghausen or peripheral neurofibromatosis, is most common, with an estimated worldwide prevalence of 1 in 3,500 [32, 33]. An autosomal dominant disorder, it is caused by mutations in the NF1 gene that encodes the tumor suppressor protein neurofibromin [34–36]. This gene is located on chromosome 17 and has 100 % penetrance [36]. Around 50 % of patients with NF1 have inherited the mutation, while the rest have a de novo NF1 mutation. The disorder affects neuroectoderm, mesoderm, and possibly also endocrine organ systems, resulting in abnormalities of skin, nervous system, bones/cartilage, and select solid organs. Musculoskeletal abnormalities are found in about 50 % of patients and principally result from mesodermal dysplasia. Neurofibromas are also very common.

Neurofibromatosis type 2 (bilateral acoustic neurofibromatosis, central neurofibromatosis) is an autosomal dominant inherited tumor predisposition syndrome that occurs in around 1 in 40–60,000. It is caused by mutations in the NF2 gene on chromosome 22. Bilateral vestibular schwannomas are the hallmark NF2 lesions and are seen in nearly all affected individuals by age 30.

Schwannomatosis is a rare disorder that may be associated with the SMARCB1 gene on chromosome 22 (different from the NF2 gene), with an estimated prevalence of about 1 in 40,000 [37]. Most cases are thought to represent new mutations, and only 15 % are familial. In contrast to NF1 and NF2, penetrance is incomplete [31]. With schwannomatosis, patients develop multiple schwannomas everywhere except the vestibular nerve. Neurofibromas are absent.

Hallmarks of *neurofibromatosis type 1* are café-au-lait macules and multiple benign cutaneous neurofibromas, but the disorder can affect nearly every organ system. Clinical manifestations are highly variable between unrelated individuals and within the same family and are classified as tumor or non-tumor [31].

Non-tumor manifestations of NF1 commonly affect the skin, central nervous system, vessels, and bones. Café-au-lait macules are hyperpigmented, well-circumscribed lesions that can be present at birth but usually increase in number during the first 2 years of life and then increase in size as the child grows. Although 15 % of the general population has one or two café-au-lait pigmentations, very few people have more than two. Skinfold freckling, which is seen in most patients by age 10, occurs at sites of skin friction, such as the axilla, groin, and neck. High-signal-intensity lesions on T2-weighted (T2-W) images, referred to as (unidentified) bright objects, are frequently observed, typically in the basal ganglia and cerebellar white matter. Most are well demarcated and non-enhancing and diminish with age. They may show mass effect. Learning disabilities are fairly common, and seizures occur in around 5 % of patients. Additional central nervous system findings include aqueductal stenosis, Chiari type 1 malformation, and macrocephaly. Glaucoma, congenital heart disease, hypertension secondary to renal arterial dysplasia, and cerebrovascular disease (stenosis or aneurysms) are also encountered.

Neurofibromas can infiltrate the bladder, gastrointestinal tract, or retroperitoneum. The incidence of pheochromocytoma is increased, and pulmonary fibrosis as well as pulmonic stenosis and other congenital heart lesions have been reported. Skeletal findings include scoliosis, short stature, pseudarthrosis of long bones, sphenoid wing dysplasia, focal osseous lesions, pseudarthrosis, and osteopenia.

The most common tumor in NF1 is the neurofibroma (Box 23.2). This benign hamartomatous tumor is composed of Schwann cells, perineural cells, mast cells, and fibroblasts. The lesions are classified as cutaneous or plexiform, with marked differences in growth patterns and size. Cutaneous neurofibromas are small masses often associated with a single nerve ending. The localized neurofibroma is the most common form of neurofibroma encountered in patients with NF1, but most localized neurofibromas occur in patients who do not have NF1. When associated with a larger nerve, a neurofibroma may infiltrate the dermis and appear as a diffuse mass. Plexiform neurofibromas (Fig. 23.14) are much larger tumors and are usually associated with major nerve trunks and plexi. About one third of patients with NF1 develop clinically detectable plexiform neurofibromas [36]. These bulky masses may cause disfigurement, erode adjacent bones, or cause respiratory or gastrointestinal obstruction. Locally invasive, they are composed of an acid mucopolysaccharide myxomatous matrix that infiltrates normal axonal structures. They can become very large and have a marked potential for malignant transformation. The lifetime risk of malignant degeneration of a peripheral plexiform neurofibroma is estimated at 10–13 % [38] (see Chap. 22).

Box 23.2: Imaging Features of Neurofibromas

Localized	Well-circumscribed, fusiform mass continuous with nerve
Diffuse	Infiltrative or plaquelike, elevating skin/thickening dermis
Plexiform	Ropelike mass along major nerve trunks
Likely to be benign if	
Target sign on T2	Hypointense center, hyperintense periphery
Reverse target sign on enhanced T1	Enhancing center, hypointense periphery

Other tumors encountered in NF1 include Lisch nodules, optic gliomas, and various other malignancies. Lisch nodules (hamartomas that affect the iris) are specific to NF1. Fifteen percent of patients with NF1 develop optic pathway gliomas, but only around 5 % are symptomatic, usually during childhood. Additionally, patients with NF1 have an increased incidence of malignancies such as Wilms tumor, liposarcoma, medullary carcinoma of the thyroid, and hepatocellular carcinoma.

The National Institutes of Health (NIH) has established diagnostic criteria for NF1. These require at least two of the following for diagnosis:

1. Six or more café-au-lait macules (>5 mm in children and >15 mm in adults)

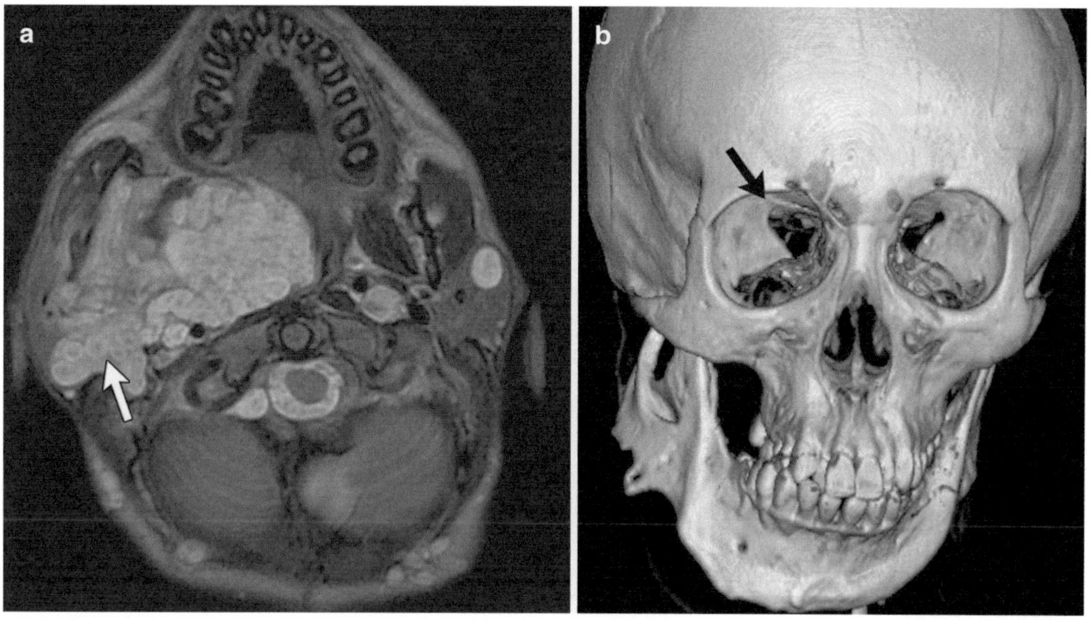

Fig. 23.14 Plexiform neurofibroma and sphenoid wing dysplasia in a 16-year-old male with neurofibromatosis type 1 (NF1). (**a**) Axial T2-W image shows plexiform neurofibroma involving infratemporal, pterygopalatine, and masticator spaces. Note multiple target signs (*white arrow*). There are multiple additional smaller neurofibromas in the subcutaneous tissues and left parotid gland. (**b**) 3D-CT shows mandibular remodeling from the plexiform neurofibroma, and also sphenoid wing dysplasia (*black arrow*)

2. Two or more neurofibromas of any type or one plexiform neurofibroma
3. Axillary or groin freckling
4. Optic pathway glioma
5. Two or more Lisch nodules
6. Bony dysplasia
7. First-degree relative diagnosed with NF1 according to the preceding criteria [31]

Comprehensive NF1 mutation screening detects mutation in more than 92 % of patients fulfilling the criteria outlined above. Molecular testing for NF1 can be helpful in equivocal cases, particularly in very young children with a negative family history and in whom the clinical criteria are incomplete. Molecular testing is also useful for adults with a mild phenotype, such as café-au-lait macules and axillary freckles but no neurofibromas.

Management of patients with NF1 includes active surveillance for non-tumor and tumor manifestations of the disease. Surgery is reserved for tumors that cause severe symptoms and for those that become malignant. Complete resection of plexiform neurofibromas is usually not possible, and recurrence is common.

Neurofibromatosis type 2 is characterized by schwannomas, which typically affect both vestibular nerves and are associated with symptoms of hearing loss, tinnitus, and impaired balance [39]. The average age of onset is 18–24 years, but about 15 % of patients present earlier with a wide variety of complications. These include orbital meningiomas, retinal hamartomas, and visual loss due to cataracts; seizures due to intracranial meningiomas; and myelopathy due to spinal tumors or cutaneous schwannomas. Childhood mononeuropathy frequently presents as a persistent facial palsy, a squint (third nerve palsy) or hand/foot drop [31].

Manchester diagnostic criteria for NF2 [40] include:

1. Bilateral vestibular schwannoma
   (a) First-degree relative with NF2 and unilateral vestibular schwannoma or any two of the following: meningioma, glioma,

neurofibroma, schwannoma, posterior subcapsular lenticular opacities

Or

(b) Unilateral vestibular schwannoma and any two of the following: meningioma, glioma, neurofibroma, schwannoma, posterior subcapsular lenticular opacities

Or

(c) Multiple meningiomas (at least two) and unilateral vestibular schwannoma or any two of the following: glioma, neurofibroma, schwannoma, cataract

Imaging (Box 23.3)

Box 23.3: Radiographic Features of NF1

Dystrophic scoliosis	4–6 vertebral levels
	Kyphosis
	Neural foraminal widening, scalloped vertebrae
	Spindled transverse processes, penciled ribs
Concave vertebral scalloping	
Paravertebral mass: neurofibroma, meningeal ectasia, lateral meningocele	
Ribs	Penciled or ribbonlike
Fractures	Narrowed or cystic/hourglass expansion of medullary canal
	Sclerotic, tapered ends of bone
	Segmental sclerosis at fracture site
Anterolateral bowing, pseudarthrosis of tibia	
Numerous nonossifying fibromas/fibrous cortical defects	

Neurofibromas

These are best imaged with magnetic resonance imaging (MRI). Cutaneous neurofibromas may be localized or diffuse. Localized neurofibromas are well-circumscribed, elongated, or fusiform masses that are continuous with the affected nerve. They usually demonstrate nonspecific signal intensity and variable enhancement. The classic target sign (see Fig. 23.14), which is almost pathognomonic, is evident on T2-W images: hyperintense myxoid peripheral material surrounds a relatively hypointense fibrous center. The "reverse target" sign may be seen on T1-W gadolinium-enhanced images and demonstrates an enhancing center and relatively little peripheral enhancement [41]. Diffuse neurofibromas (Fig. 23.15) grow in either an infiltrative/reticulated branching pattern or as a plaque-like area that elevates the skin and thickens the underlying dermis. These lesions enhance.

Plexiform neurofibromas are bulky, ropelike masses that extend along the sympathetic chain, vagus and phrenic nerves, and major nerve trunks of the extremities. Radiographs play little role in imaging, except in the chest, where they appear as mediastinal or paravertebral soft tissue masses. On MRI, they are best appreciated on fat-suppressed (FS) T2-W sequences, where they appear as multinodular, confluent masses, often with multiple target signs (see Chap. 22 for additional discussion of these tumors). Plexiform neurofibromas are almost pathognomonic for NF1.

Spine

The spine is abnormal in up to 50 % of patients with NF1, and of those with spinal involvement, the thoracic segment is affected in 40 % and the cervical in 30 % [42, 43]. Scoliosis is common, occurring in about 10–69 % of patients. Cervical or upper thoracic kyphosis is another feature of NF1. Vertebral bodies may demonstrate scalloping, and individual vertebrae may demonstrate abnormal pedicles and transverse processes.

Two forms of scoliosis are found in NF1: nondystrophic and dystrophic. Nondystrophic scoliosis is usually radiographically indistinguishable from the idiopathic condition [44], except that the curve typically affects younger patients and may progress to the dystrophic form. Dystrophic scoliosis is often accompanied with neuroforaminal widening, scalloped vertebrae, spindled transverse processes, and penciled ribs; it typically affects only four to six vertebrae and is often associated with kyphosis (which may be more pronounced than the scoliosis) (Figs. 23.16 and 23.17). Dystrophic scoliosis is a hallmark of NF1 and has a poor prognosis. Over 40 % of those with scoliosis also have cervical spine abnormalities. The severity of the curve is

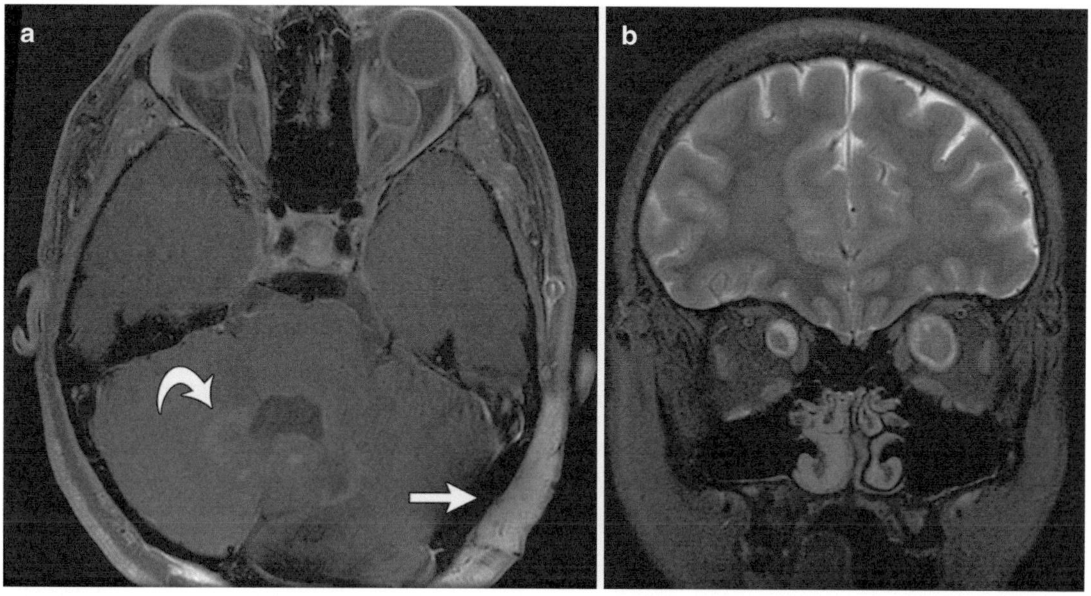

Fig. 23.15 Diffuse neurofibroma and bilateral optic gliomas in a 16-year-old with NF1. (**a**) Axial T1-W FS GE image shows optic glioma on the left and a diffuse, enhancing, neurofibroma (*straight arrow*). There are also NF spots (*curved arrow*) in the cerebellar white matter. (**b**) Coronal T2-W FS image shows optic nerve gliomas are bilateral, left larger than right (Courtesy of Sandra L. Wootton-Gorges)

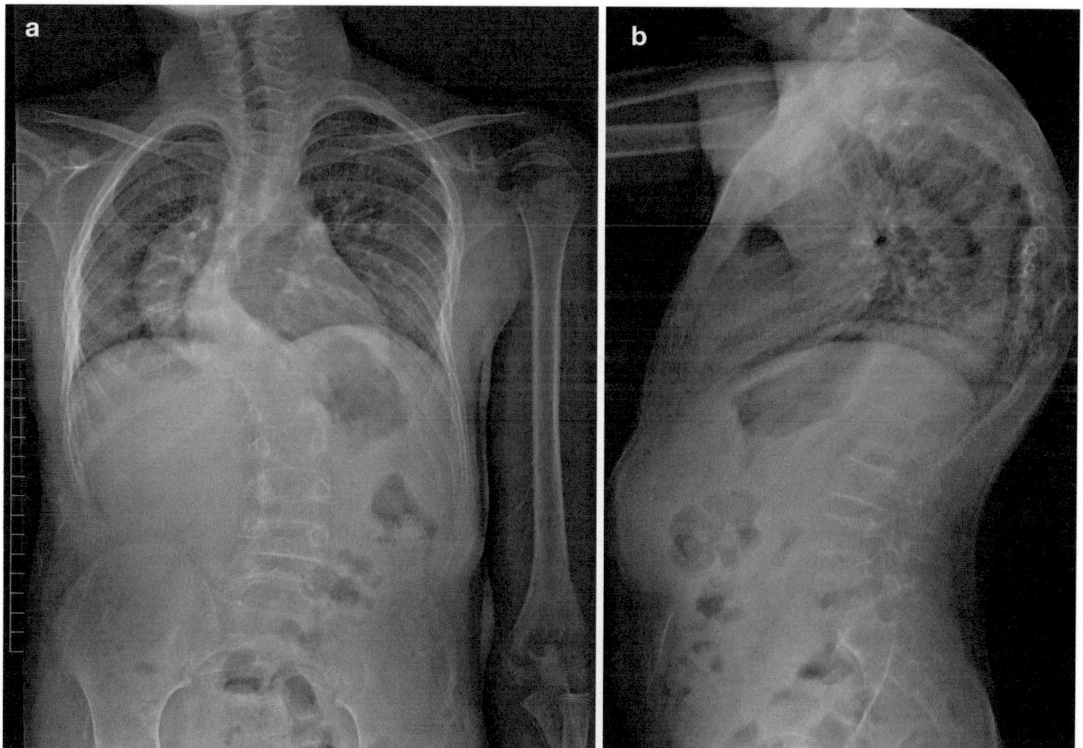

Fig. 23.16 Dystrophic kyphoscoliosis in a teenager with NF1. Short-segment thoracic curvature is associated with narrow posterior ribs (Courtesy of Rebecca Stein-Wexler)

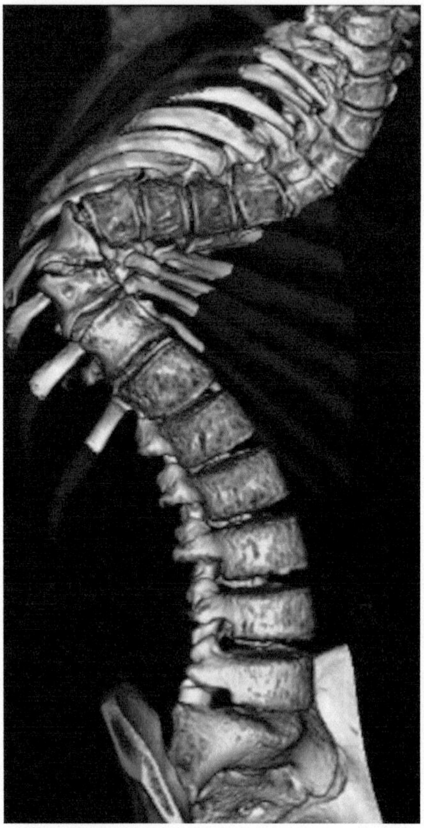

Fig. 23.17 Dystrophic kyphoscoliosis in a patient with NF1. 3D-reformatted CT shows short-segment kyphoscoliosis with dysmorphic vertebrae at the apex of the curve (Courtesy of Sandra L Wootton-Gorges)

unrelated to the degree of skin pigmentation or the presence of subcutaneous tumors.

The kyphosis associated with neurofibromatosis is often severe but is unusually flexible when traction is applied. In the cervical spine, the anterior aspects of the vertebrae at the apex of the kyphosis are often sharp and pointed, surrounded by hamartomatous tissue.

Concave scalloping of the vertebral body may occur on the anterior, posterior, or lateral surfaces. Dural ectasia and transmitted pulsations are thought to cause most posterior vertebral body scalloping (Fig. 23.18), although if only one or two levels are involved, an intradural mass may be responsible. The scalloped, dysplastic vertebral body of NF1 must be differentiated from that caused by intraspinal cysts or neoplasms, hydrosyringomyelia, hydrocephalus, achondroplasia, Melnick-Needles syndrome, and the dural ectasia of the Marfan and Ehlers-Danlos syndromes.

Agenesis or hypoplasia of the vertebral pedicles has been described in NF1 but also occurs in otherwise normal spines. The anomaly may be unilateral or bilateral and may involve multiple levels. Pedicle thinning, elongation, sclerosis, and hypoplasia result from mesodermal dysplasia, and the transverse processes are often abnormal. Generalized trabecular coarsening is common, but spondylolisthesis is rare.

Paravertebral masses generally represent either neurofibromas or lateral meningeal ectasia. If the latter enlarge, they may become lateral meningoceles. Foraminal widening or pediculate erosion is seen in 13 % of patients with NF1, usually secondary to primary dysplastic underdevelopment of the pedicles, dumbbell neurofibromas (Fig. 23.19), or lateral meningeal ectasia/meningoceles (see Fig. 23.18). Increased intraspinal volume, hydrosyringomyelia, dural ectasia, and intraspinal neoplasm may alternatively be present. Paraplegia in children usually results from spinal deformity, whereas in adults it tends to result from a tumor.

Computed tomography (CT), especially with its potential for three-dimensional (3D) reconstructions, allows exquisite delineation of dystrophic kyphoscoliosis (see Fig. 23.17). Spine MRI plays an important role in patients with NF1, as it can delineate dystrophic elements and may also disclose the presence of unrecognized neurofibromas, lateral thoracic meningoceles (see Fig. 23.18), and protrusion of ribs into the thecal sac in patients with dystrophic curves. Curves that appear non-dystrophic on radiographs may be shown to have dystrophic features on MRI. It is important to recognize this, as rapid curve progression is then more likely [45].

Ribs

Rib dysplasia occurs in about 60 % of patients with scoliosis and is most marked at the apex of

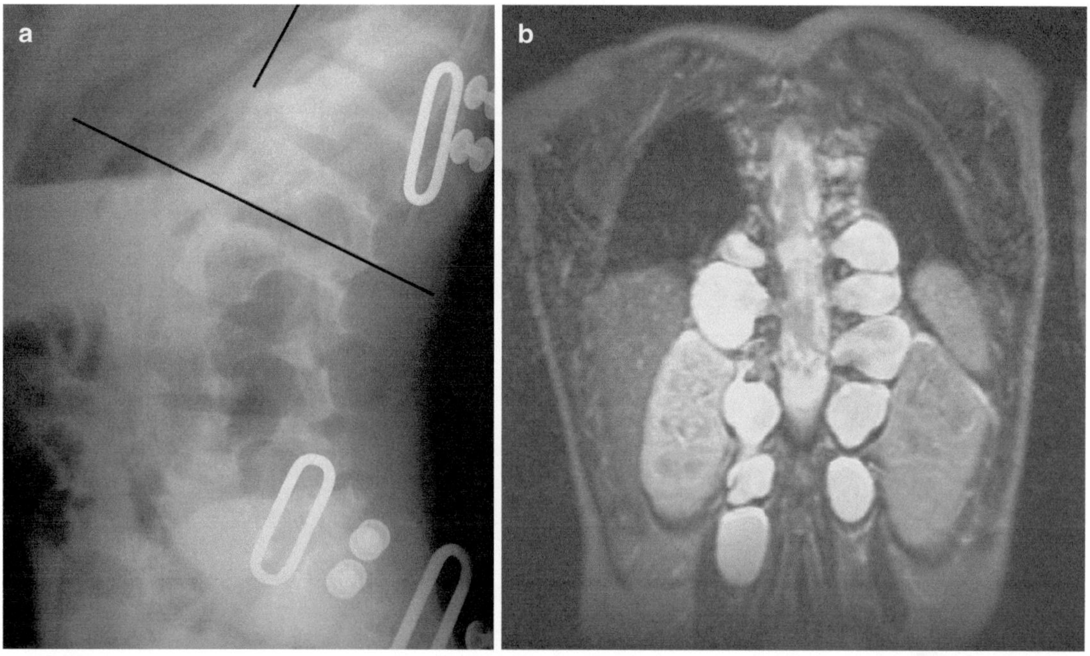

Fig. 23.18 Lateral meningoceles in a patient with NF1. (**a**) Lateral radiograph demonstrates enlargement of multiple neural foramina along with posterior scalloping of multiple vertebral bodies. (**b**) Coronal T2-W MRI shows fluid-filled sacs protruding laterally from every neural foramen (Courtesy of Rebecca Stein-Wexler)

the scoliosis on the convex side. Rib penciling is defined as the rib width being narrower than the narrowest part of the second rib [41]. Ribs may initially appear normal but develop undulations and become irregularly sclerotic and twisted as patients mature. The medial rib ends may appear pointed and if associated with pediculate thinning can protrude into the spinal canal [46]. Dysplasia must be differentiated from notching due to inter costal neurofibromas (Fig. 23.20), which resembles the small, discrete impressions produced by collateral vessels in aortic coarctation.

Skull and Facial Bones

Macrocephaly is common, with almost half of patients having a skull volume over the 95th percentile. Partial (see Fig. 23.14) or complete absence of the greater or lesser sphenoid wings may lead to pulsating exophthalmos. There may be round or ovoid osseous defects in the lambdoid suture near its bifurcation at the mastoid. Eighty percent of these defects occur on the left; this may be associated with poor aeration of the ipsilateral mastoid air cells. Facial bone dysplasia takes the form of osseous deformity and sclerosis, often with grotesque results. Plexiform neurofibromas may distort facial bones and contribute to development of sphenoid dysplasia (see Fig. 23.14).

Acoustic neuromas, optic gliomas, astrocytomas, ependymomas, meningiomas, and trigeminal nerve tumors are of course assessed by MRI, but mass effect or secondary foraminal enlargement may be evident on radiographs. MRI may also show clinically silent focal areas of increased T2 signal (Fig. 23.15), considered to be areas of heterotopia or hamartoma in the cerebellum, basal ganglia, and other cerebral structures.

Extremities

Fractures are more common in patients with NF1, occurring in bone that appears normal or only slightly osteoporotic, or through an underlying fibrous lesion. Features that suggest neurofibromatosis include segmental osseous

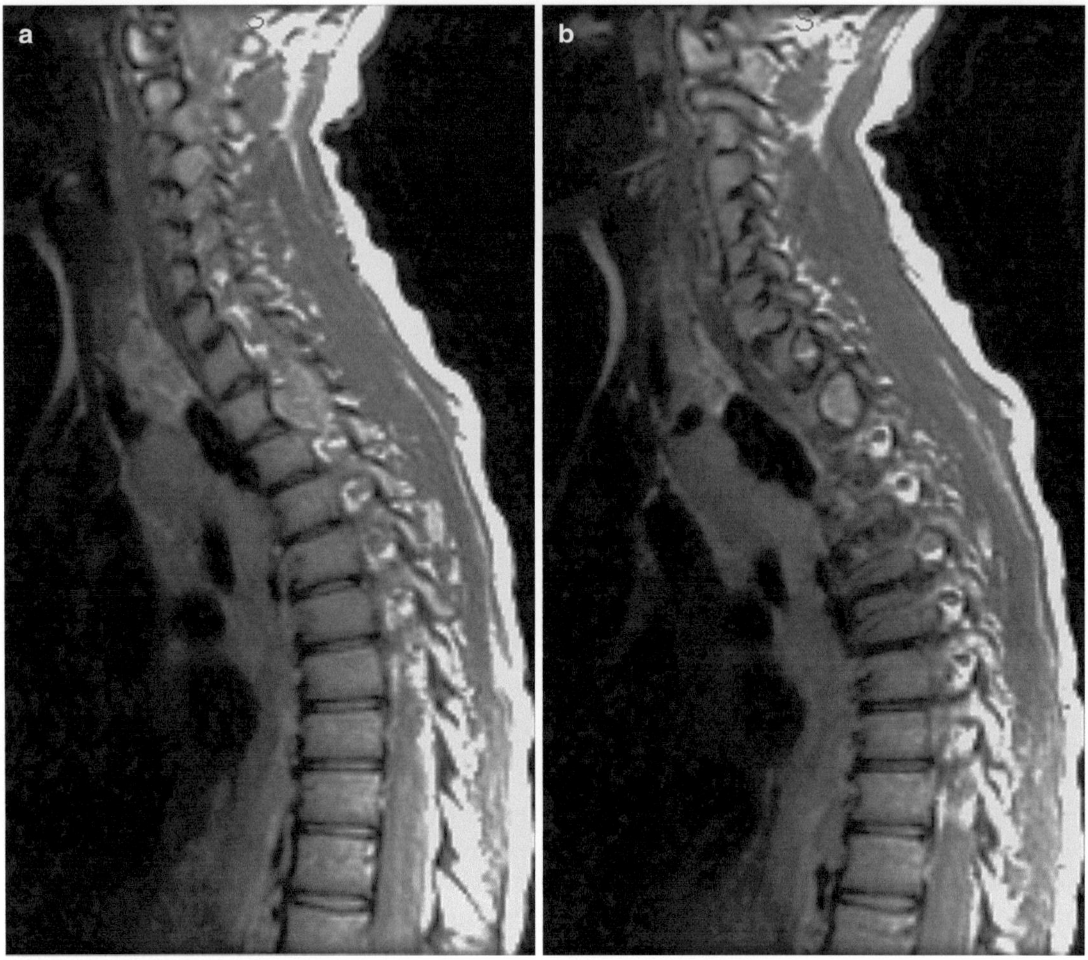

Fig. 23.19 Dumbbell neurofibroma in a patient with NF1. (**a**, **b**) Sagittal T2-W images show focal posterior scalloping secondary to a neurofibroma with both intraspinal and neural foraminal components (Courtesy of Rebecca Stein-Wexler)

sclerosis adjacent to the fracture site, narrowed medullary canal, cystic or hourglass expansion of the medullary canal, and sclerosis and tapering of the ends of the bones at the fracture site. However, fractures with subsequent nonunion can occur in radiographically normal bone.

Nonunion and pseudarthrosis complicate fracture healing in as many as 13 % of patients. Pseudarthrosis may result from dystrophic healing of fractured previously normal bone or follow a pathologic fracture. Histological evaluation of nonunion reveals a hamartomatous mass of connective tissue (not a neurofibroma), and the histology resembles that of non-NF pseudarthrosis or fibrous dysplasia.

Anterolateral bowing of the tibias is common in NF1 (Fig. 23.21) and may suggest the diagnosis in young children. Fracture is common before age 3 years, and this may be followed by pseudarthrosis of the lower tibia (see Fig. 23.21). Although pseudarthrosis of the tibia can develop in the general population, it is especially common in NF1, occurring in up to 11 % of patients with this diagnosis (conversely, approximately 50 % of patients with tibial pseudarthrosis have NF1). (See Chap. 13 for further discussion of tibial pseudarthrosis.) A similar pathologic process may occur in the fibula, radius, ulna, humerus, clavicle, and other sites. Bowing of the

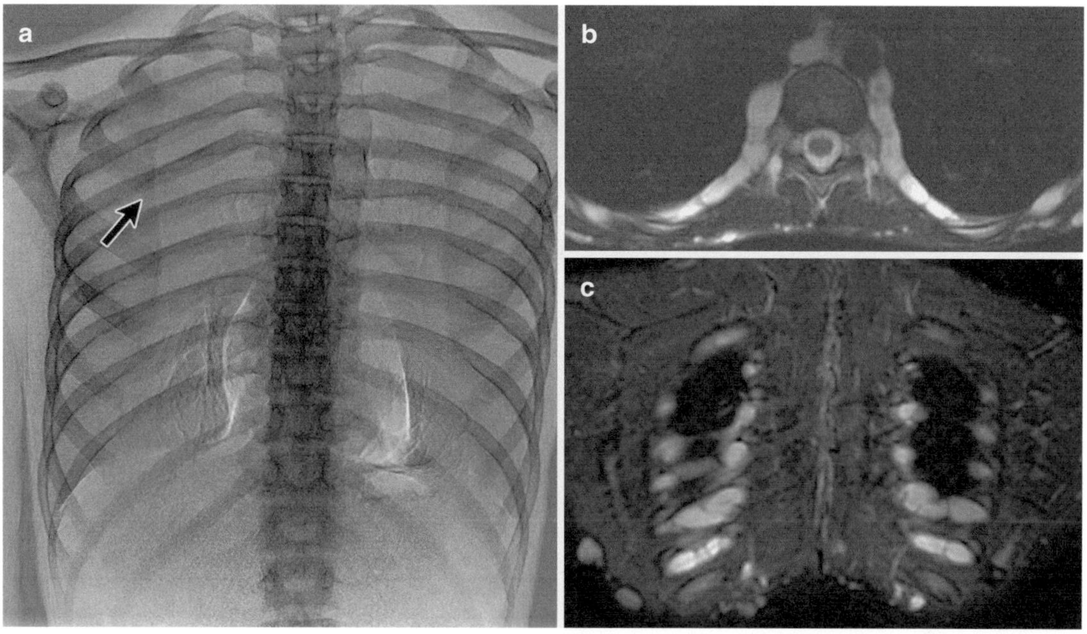

Fig. 23.20 Intercostal neurofibromas in a 16-year-old boy with NF1 (same patient as Fig. 23.15). (**a**) Dual-energy chest radiograph with bone algorithm shows rib notching at multiple levels, most evident at the posterior fifth right rib (*arrow*). Axial (**a**) and coronal (**b**) T2-W MRI shows multiple hyperintense neurofibromas along the lower edges of the ribs (Courtesy of Sandra L Wootton-Gorges)

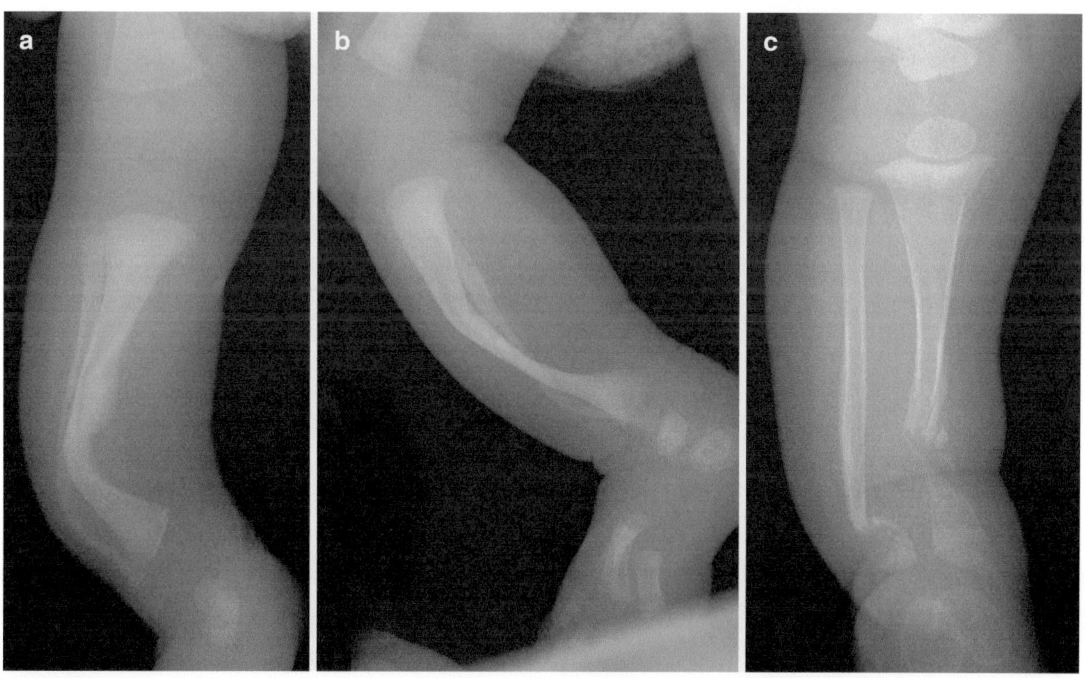

Fig. 23.21 Anterolateral bowing and subsequent pseudarthrosis in a boy with NF1. (**a**, **b**) During infancy, there is anterolateral tibial and fibular bowing. (**c**) Tibial and fibular pseudarthroses develop by about age 2 years (Courtesy of Sandra L. Wootton-Gorges)

radius with radial head dislocation can be associated with ulnar pseudarthrosis.

Other focal intrinsic and extrinsic osseous abnormalities also occur. Intrinsic fibrous cortical defects and nonossifying fibromas are more common in NF1 than in the general population, and indeed multiple bilaterally symmetric nonossifying fibromas about the knee suggest the presence of NF1 [41]. Multiple nonossifying fibromas accompanied with café-au-lait spots characterize Jaffe-Campanacci syndrome; this may be a manifestation of NF1 (see Chap. 21). Mesodermal dysplasia and intraosseous neurofibromas may be responsible for some cystic lesions (Fig. 23.22). Extrinsic cortical erosions, in contrast, result from pressure caused by adjacent expanding plexiform neurofibromas or localized periosteal thickening. The periosteum in patients with NF1 is abnormally loose, and this can allow extensive subperiosteal hemorrhage.

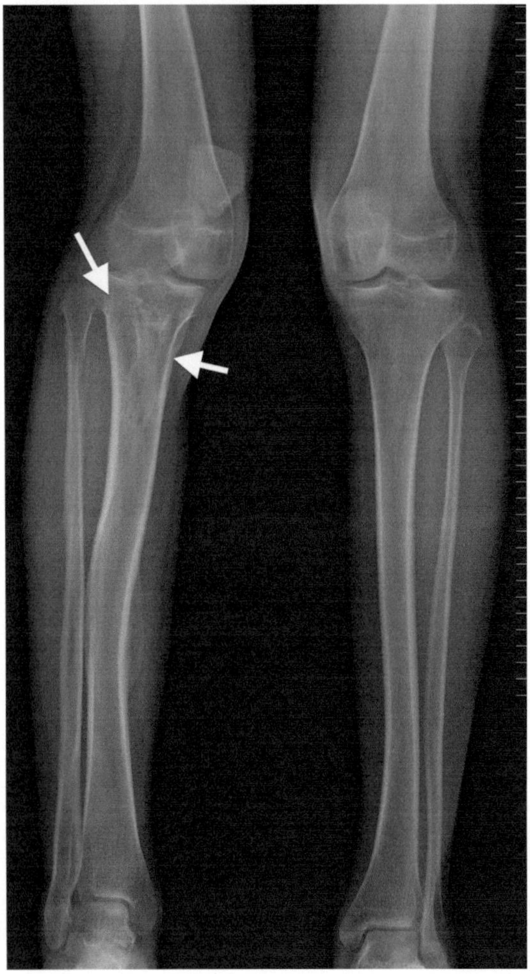

Fig. 23.22 Lucent lesions resembling nonossifying fibromas in the proximal tibia in a patient with NF1. *Arrows* identify lesions. Dysmorphic growth has resulted in genu valgum (Courtesy of Rebecca Stein-Wexler)

Dysplasia of individual bones may take the form of irregular cortical contour, angular deformity, and irregular cortical sclerosis and lucency. If extreme, sclerosis may resemble melorheostosis. The iliac wing of the pelvis may be enlarged, with a narrow sclerotic base and enlarged obturator foramen. The femoral necks often demonstrate valgus alignment.

Neurofibromatosis can also cause hypertrophy and deformity in limbs. The soft tissues, muscles, and bones are all involved, with an increase in both length and width; plexiform neurofibromas are often present. The resulting massive limb enlargement has been termed "elephantiasis neuromatosa." This must be differentiated from hemangioma, vascular/lymphatic malformation, and Proteus syndrome.

3 Arthrogryposis

Arthrogryposis constitutes a clinical description ("hooked joint") rather than a single discrete pathologic entity and is defined as two or more joint contractures in multiple body areas [47]. Approximately 1 in 4,300 live births is affected [47]. Individuals often have reduced or absent skinfolds at involved joints, skin dimples at large joints, adducted shoulder joints, and reduced muscle mass. The condition results from decreased fetal movement, which may be secondary to underlying neurologic or muscle disease, connective tissue or skeletal abnormality, or intrauterine constraint. The clinical features range from nonspecific combinations of joint contractures to well-known, complex syndromes. More than 300 specific disorders exhibit arthrogrypotic features, and a definite diagnosis other than arthrogryposis can be made in approximately 50 % of patients with congenital contractures. As our knowledge of disease genotypes improves, fewer and fewer patients are diagnosed with arthrogryposis.

Arthrogrypotic conditions are generally classified as arthrogryposis multiplex congenita or as classic arthrogryposis (amyoplasia congenital) [48, 49]. Arthrogryposis multiplex congenita is defined as having multiple congenital contractures of all four limbs but can be limited to the upper or lower extremities and can also involve the jaw and trunk. Amyoplasia is more specific: the limbs are affected symmetrically, with the elbows extended, the wrist flexed, camptodactyly, severe equinovarus, knee flexion or extension, and dislocated hips, with no truncal involvement. Cases of arthrogryposis can also be divided into three categories that facilitate diagnosis: group I, only limbs involved; group II, limb and other malformations; group III, limb malformations along with lethality or central nervous system involvement [50]. Patients in groups II and III can often be diagnosed with a specific disorder [48].

In patients with arthrogryposis, fetal development is initially normal, but joint movement becomes constrained, leading to collagen proliferation, fibrotic replacement of muscle, and marked thickening of joint capsules (the collagenic response). The most extreme form of arthrogryposis is fetal akinesia deformation sequence (Pena-Shokeir syndrome), characterized by—in addition to joint contractures—facial and jaw abnormalities, lung hypoplasia, short umbilical cord, growth retardation, and polyhydramnios.

Arthrogryposis is often found incidentally during routine second trimester ultrasound (US), before the usual maternal perception of fetal movement. However, it may also be identified by third trimester US if the mother reports decrease in fetal movement. Immobilization lasting longer than 3 weeks likely produces pathologic joint contracture, the severity of which is determined by the age at onset and duration of immobility [51]. In the classic picture of arthrogryposis, the newborn is delivered with internally rotated shoulders, extended elbows, pronated forearms, and flexed wrists in ulnar deviation (Fig. 23.23). The scapulae may be non-descended. The hips are usually also flexed, whereas the knees are either flexed or extended. Joint abnormalities are usually bilateral and fairly symmetric, although the degree of contracture is not necessarily equal on both sides (e.g., valgus deformity on one side and varus on the other is rare). The contractures

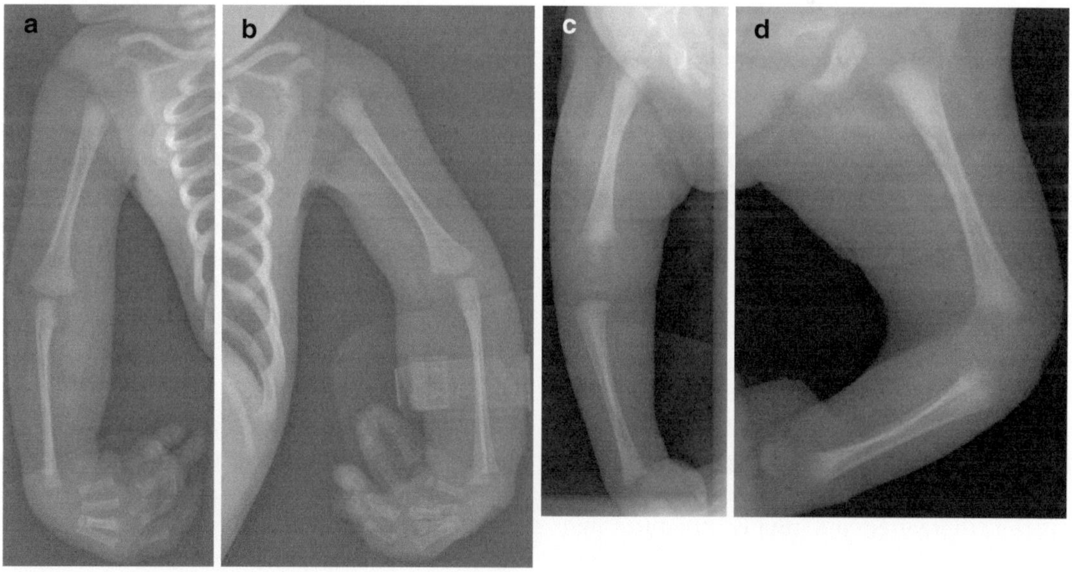

Fig. 23.23 Arthrogryposis in a newborn. (**a**, **b**) Bilateral extended elbows and flexed wrists in ulnar deviation. (**c**, **d**) The right knee is hyperextended, and there is a flexion contracture at the left knee. Bilateral hindfoot equinus is incompletely imaged. All four extremities show fusiform and featureless tissues (Courtesy of Rebecca Stein-Wexler)

associated with arthrogryposis are severe at birth, and although the underlying abnormalities do not change, untreated deformities worsen as the child grows [52].

The extremities are tubular; joints have fusiform swelling and lack normal skin creases. The skin is smooth, and subcutaneous fat tissues appear diminished. Articular changes are more severe distally than proximally. These findings are usually symmetric and involve all four limbs more often than only two. Diagnosis is difficult if abnormalities are unilateral. In that case, infants are labeled arthrogrypotic only after other diagnoses are excluded.

Nonskeletal abnormalities associated with arthrogryposis include cryptorchidism and other genitourinary anomalies, gastroschisis, biliary atresia, congenital heart disease, and congenital hernias.

The disease is lethal in 27 % of live births, usually within the first month [48]. Dysphagia, dyspnea, dysphonia, and other laryngeal problems can lead to aspiration or respiratory failure. However, the patient with arthrogryposis who survives infancy may live a long time, with normal sensation and intelligence. Intense treatment, aimed to prevent further contractures and allow functional positioning of the extremities, increases the likelihood of a satisfactory life in those who survive. Since deformities often progress without treatment and recur after treatment, multiple operations are often necessary. However, three fourths of patients who are surgically treated will eventually ambulate to a degree.

Imaging (Box 23.4)

No radiographic findings are specific for arthrogryposis, with the possible exception of altered carpal bone orientation. Joint contractures and deformities may also occur with other syndromes or as isolated findings. The bones are thin and prone to fracture at birth or any time thereafter, and joint contractures may cause the long bones to appear bent. Contractures may induce radiographically apparent soft tissue webbing. Muscles are small, and both subcutaneous and intramuscular fat are increased (Fig. 23.24).

Box 23.4: Radiographic Features of Classic Arthrogryposis (Amyoplasia)

Fusiform soft tissues of extremities without discernible joint demarcation

Usually symmetric, 4 limbs >2 limbs, lower > upper limbs

Thin bones, fractures not uncommon

Elbows: flexion or extension contractures, dislocated radial head

Carpal synostoses common, increased carpal angle

Hips: may be dislocated, often bilateral

Knee: fixed contractures, flexion > extension; small/absent patella

Foot: equinus or equinovarus > congenital vertical talus

Scoliosis common; hip contractures may induce lordosis

In most patients, all four limbs are affected, while some have leg-only and a few have arm-only involvement [51]. The humeri may be internally rotated but are usually otherwise normal. The elbows exhibit flexion or extension contractures, and the radial heads may be or become dislocated (Fig. 23.25). As with other joints, an initially normal articular relationship deforms with progressive capsular and ligamentous contracture.

Some degree of carpal fusion is seen in 40 % of patients. Carpal coalitions begin in the proximal row of the wrist and eventually involve the distal. The carpal bones eventually fuse into one conglomerate mass. In two thirds of patients the orientation of the carpal bones also changes. The carpal angle is increased in two thirds of older patients with arthrogryposis. (The normal carpal angle, defined by lines tangent to the navicular, lunate, and triquetrum, is between 124 and 138°.) Syndactyly may be present.

The lower extremities are affected in most children with arthrogryposis. The hips area

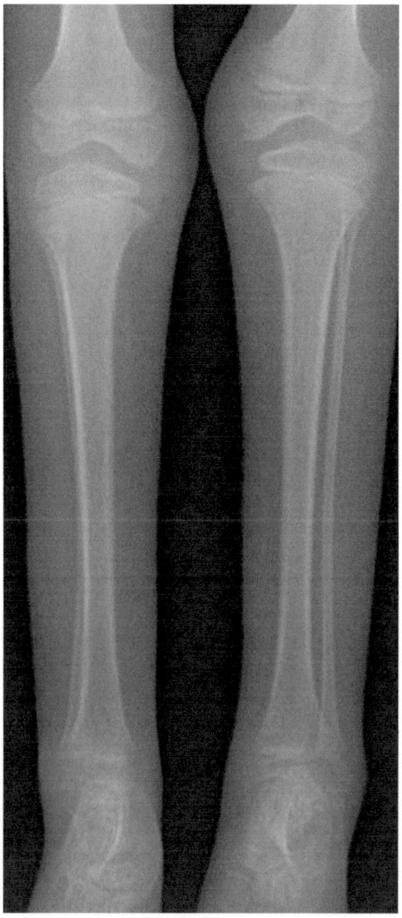

Fig. 23.24 Arthrogryposis in a 9-year-old girl. Gracile bones, osteopenia, diminished muscle bulk, increased adipose tissue, and featureless soft tissue contours

dislocated in one third of patients, and two thirds of these dislocations are bilateral (Fig. 23.26). These are teratologic intrauterine dislocations, and the hips are stiff and difficult to reduce. Pseudoacetabula may be present at birth, and abnormal muscle pull can lead to coxa vara deformity.

Fixed flexion contractures are common in the knee. Extension contractures with anterior subluxation of the tibia may also be present, and bilateral involvement is characteristic. Patellae may be small or absent.

Equinovarus foot deformity is seen in three fourths of patients, and more than 90 % are bilateral. Vertical talus is the second most common abnormality; calcaneovalgus and rocker-bottom deformity, as well as syndactyly and polydactyly, have also been reported. In contrast to the carpal area, tarsal fusions are uncommon.

Between 15 and 40 % of patients with arthrogryposis have scoliosis, occasionally present at birth but more often developing within the first few years of life [53]. As in other neuromuscular disorders, a long, C-shaped thoracolumbar scoliosis is common. These curves are rigid and progressive in more than half of cases and are infrequently associated with such anomalies as hemivertebrae, bars, and fusion. Abnormal lordosis may be induced by flexion contractures of the hips (Fig. 23.27). Pelvic obliquity is common.

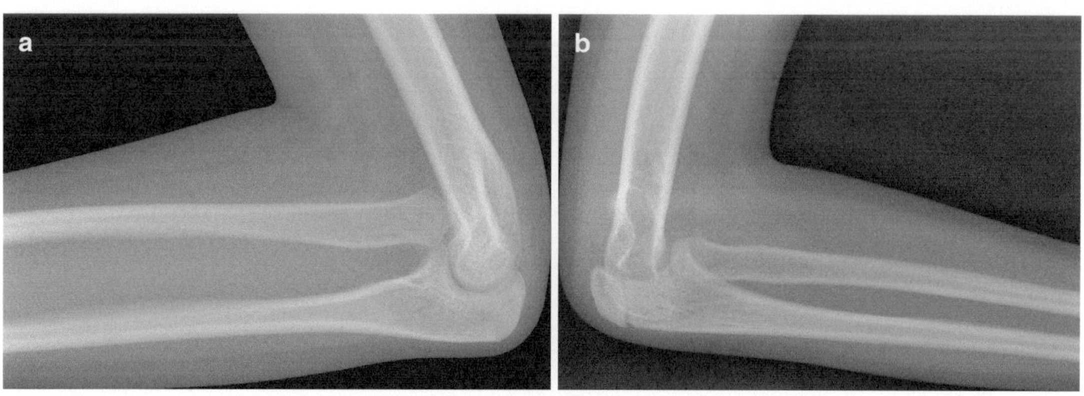

Fig. 23.25 Bilateral elbow dislocations in a child with arthrogryposis (**a**, **b**)

Differential Diagnosis

The differential diagnosis of classic arthrogryposis (amyoplasia) includes other diseases with articular dislocations or contractures. There are over 300 syndromes associated with multiple contractures [48].

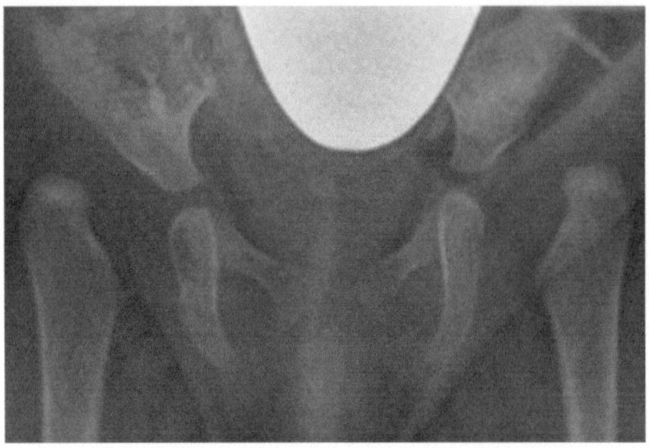

Fig. 23.26 Bilateral hip dislocation with acetabular dysplasia in a 7-month-old girl with arthrogryposis

4 Down Syndrome (Trisomy 21)

This disorder results from the presence of all or part of an extra chromosome 21. Its incidence is estimated at 1 in 600–2,000 live births [1]. Both the specific manifestations of the syndrome and their severity vary considerably among affected individuals. The gene-dosage hypothesis of its pathogenesis states that specific gene dosages are linked to specific phenotypic abnormalities [54].

Down syndrome is characterized by mental impairment and multiple malformations, including hypotonia, small brachycephalic head, epicanthic folds, flat nasal bridge, upward slanting palpebral fissures, small mouth, small

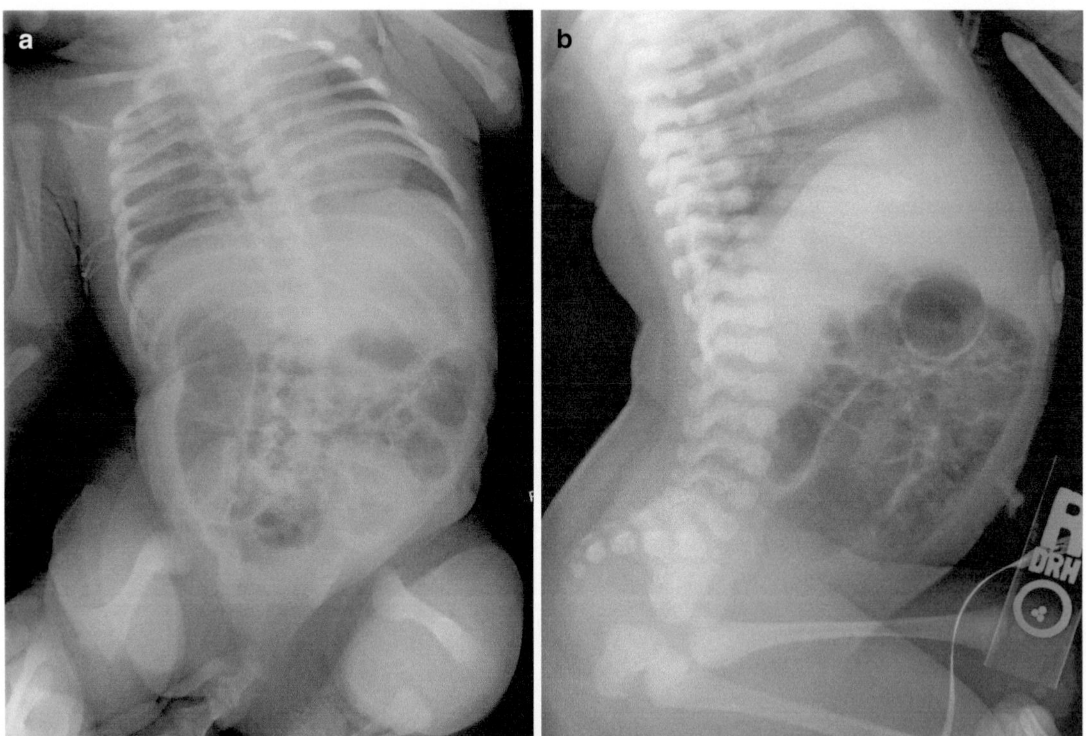

Fig. 23.27 Scoliosis and lordosis in a newborn with arthrogryposis. (**a**, **b**) Flexion contractures at the hips lead to excessive lordosis. Note the right humeral fracture

ears, excessive skin at the nape of the neck, single transverse palmar crease, and short fifth finger with clinodactyly. A wide space, often with a deep fissure between the first and second toes, is also common [55]. However, the expression of the syndrome varies enormously. The following features are encountered in at least 50 % of patients: congenital heart defects, hearing loss, otitis media, eye disease (including cataracts and severe refractive errors), and obstructive sleep apnea. Thyroid disease is encountered in 15 %, gastrointestinal atresias in 12 %, hip dislocation in 6 %, and Hirschsprung disease or leukemia in less than 1 % [55].

Neurological complications include cognitive deficits, seizures, early-onset dementia that resembles Alzheimer disease, and neurological complications of systemic disorders. The degree of mental impairment usually varies from mild to moderate and is only occasionally severe. The level of social function varies greatly and can be improved with early intervention. Children with Down syndrome tend to function better in social situations than is expected based on their IQ.

Interventions in Down syndrome increase longevity, with estimated life expectancy in countries with advanced medical care now averaging 60 years (increased from an average of 12 years in the 1940s). However, children with Down syndrome have increased risk of anesthetic complications and prolonged postoperative recovery due to atlantoaxial subluxation, gastroesophageal reflux and subsequent aspiration, and generalized hypotonia. Treatment of scoliosis, hip instability, slipped capital femoral epiphysis, patellar instability, and foot deformities can be challenging for the orthopedic surgeon [56].

Imaging (Box 23.5)

Orthopedic manifestations are common in the lower extremities and in the spine, mostly related to hypotonia, joint hypermobility, and ligamentous laxity [56]. There is also rhizomelic shortening, with relatively short femurs and humeri.

Box 23.5: Radiographic Features of Down Syndrome (Trisomy 21)

Spine	Instability at C1–2 in 20 %
	Occipitocervical laxity in up to 60 %
	Thoracic kyphosis; occasional scoliosis
Hip	Horizontal acetabular roof in infancy, with increased acetabular anteversion
	Dysplasia/dislocation, AVN, or SCFE in 8 %
Patella	Hypermobile, subluxate/dislocate
Foot	Hindfoot/hallux valgus, occasional clubfoot

The transverse ligament that holds the odontoid to the axis may be lax and the cervical vertebrae dysmorphic, resulting in atlanto-occipital, atlantoaxial, and lower cervical instability. About 20 % of patients develop subluxation at C1–2. Whether and how to screen for instability—especially before participating in sports—is controversial, but lateral flexion/extension radiographs are commonly employed (Fig. 23.28). MRI may be useful to assess spinal cord impingement in symptomatic patients. Thoracic kyphosis may develop, resembling idiopathic juvenile kyphosis, with decreased intervertebral disc space height and end-plate irregularities. The height of lumbar vertebral bodies is increased, whereas their anteroposterior diameter is diminished. Scoliosis develops in a minority of patients, usually without underlying segmentation abnormalities.

The iliac wings have a characteristic flared configuration, resulting in the "Mickey Mouse" pelvis. The acetabulum in patients with trisomy 21 is more horizontal than usual, and there is increased acetabular anteversion (Fig. 23.29). Approximately 8 % of patients eventually develop hip dysplasia or dislocation (Fig. 23.30), avascular necrosis, or slipped capital femoral epiphysis [57]. The patella may be unusually mobile, predisposing these patients to subluxation or dislocation. Foot deformities include hindfoot and hallux valgus, and clubfoot is occasionally seen.

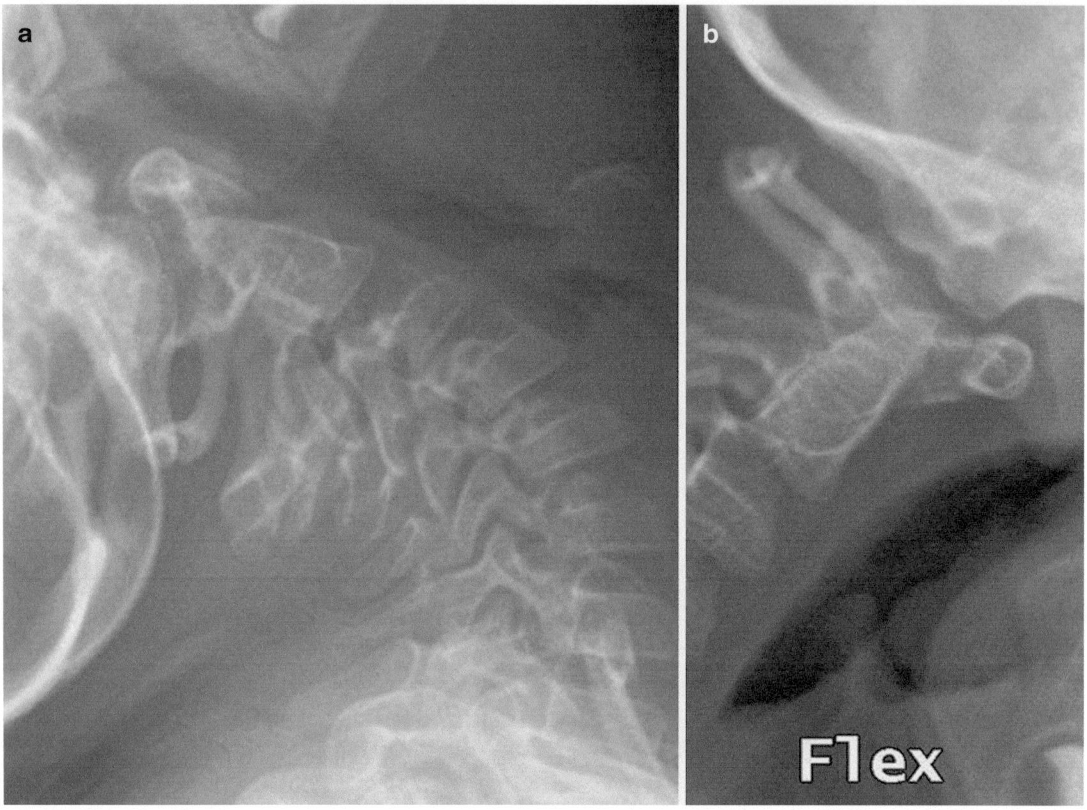

Fig. 23.28 Atlanto-occipital and atlantoaxial instability in a 4-year-old girl with Down syndrome. Extension (**a**) and flexion (**b**) views show the atlantoaxial interval increases with flexion, and the occiput moves anteriorly

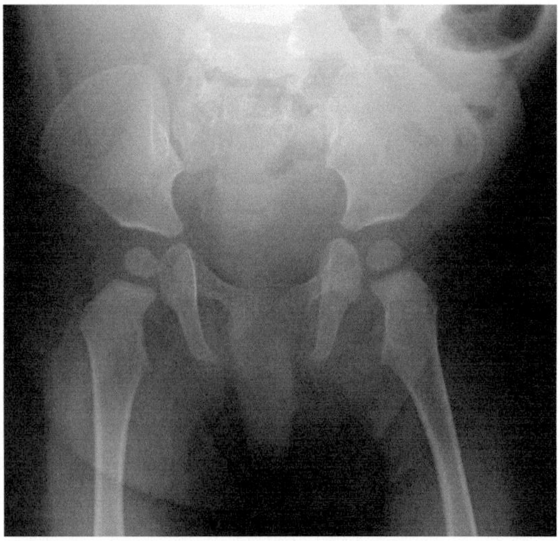

Fig. 23.29 Classic findings in the pelvis in a 6-month-old girl with Down syndrome. Iliac wings are flared (Mickey Mouse pelvis), and acetabular roofs are flat (Courtesy of Sandra L. Wootton-Gorges)

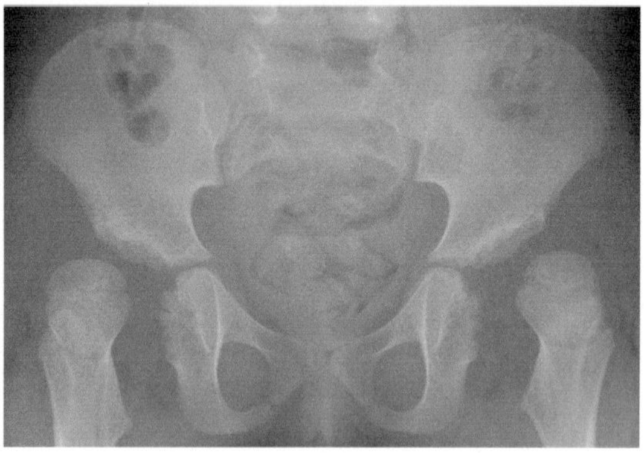

Fig. 23.30 Bilateral hip subluxation with acetabular dysplasia and apparent coxa valga in a 4-year-old with Down syndrome

5 Sickle Cell Disease

Sickle cell disease (SCD) is an autosomal recessive disorder that can seriously impair many organ systems. Hemoglobin polymerization, leading to erythrocyte rigidity and vaso-occlusion, is central to the pathophysiology, although chronic anemia, hemolysis, and vasculopathy are also important [58]. "Sickle cell disease" refers to the various genotypes that cause the syndrome, whereas "sickle cell anemia," the most common manifestation, refers specifically to homozygous βS alleles. Around 80 % of affected children live in sub-Saharan Africa. The yearly estimate of affected births is 2,600 in North America and 1,300 in Europe [59].

Diagnosis is based on hemoglobin analysis. Protein electrophoresis and chromatography are inexpensive and widely available. Hemoglobin mass spectrometry and DNA analysis are increasingly employed and enable high-throughput testing. Antenatal screening helps identify at-risk couples and can diagnose sickle cell disease in utero [58].

The clinical course of SCD varies greatly. Pain, varying in severity and frequency, is the main symptom. About 50 % of children between the ages of 6 months and 2 years present with sickle cell dactylitis, manifested by tender and swollen hands and feet, reduced movement, and fever (dactylitis occurs because persistent red marrow predisposes the small tubular bones to infarction). Splenic sequestration is also common, seen in 30 % of patients under 6. Acute chest syndrome is a life-threatening complication most common in early childhood, characterized by pulmonary opacities and at least two of the following: fever, cough, wheezing, tachypnea, and chest pain. Stroke occurs in 11 % of children, but screening transcranial Doppler can decrease this to 1 %, as those with elevated cerebral velocity should receive transfusion therapy. Urinary concentrating defects and glomerular hyperfiltration are common. Proliferative sickle retinopathy peaks between age 15 and 24. Extramedullary hematopoiesis leads to hepatosplenomegaly as well as intrathoracic, adrenal, and cutaneous masses.

Therapy includes antibacterial prophylaxis, hydroxyurea, and chronic monthly blood transfusions. Genetic-based studies aim for curative therapy to prevent disease-related sequelae. However, clinical management is relatively limited and, although blood transfusion and hydroxycarbamide can be beneficial in some circumstances, no drugs specifically target the pathophysiology of SCD.

Imaging (Box 23.6)

Box 23.6: Imaging Features of Sickle Cell Disease

Red marrow persists in wrists, ankles, diaphyses
- Wide medullar space, coarse trabeculae, osteopenia
- MRI: persistent red marrow signal

Infarcts: shoulders, hips, diaphyses, vertebral bodies
- Osteolysis, patchy intramedullary lucency/sclerosis
- Infarcts femoral head and humerus: like infarcts elsewhere, but bilateral
- H-shaped vertebrae: infarct affects central growth plate
  - Dactylitis (infarcts in small tubular bones of hand) in 50 % of 6–24 months old
- MRI of infarcts: serpiginous double line on T2
  - Hyperintense marrow on T1-W unenhanced FS sequences

Osteomyelitis, especially of long bones

Infants with sickle cell disease have red marrow throughout all their bones. Marrow gradually recedes from the small bones of the hands and feet but persists in the wrists, ankles, and diaphyses of the long bones [60]. Increased red cell production results in wide medullary spaces and thin cortical bone, which predisposes patients to pathologic fractures. Radiographs demonstrate coarsened trabeculae and osteopenia in both long and flat bones.

Infarcts develop in many bones, and these have a characteristic appearance in the hands, shoulders, hips, diaphyses of long bones, and vertebral bodies. Infants and young children develop infarcts in the diaphyses of the small tubular bones of the hands and feet, termed "sickle cell dactylitis" or "hand-foot" syndrome. Radiographs demonstrate patchy lucencies and periosteal reaction. Bone destruction, premature

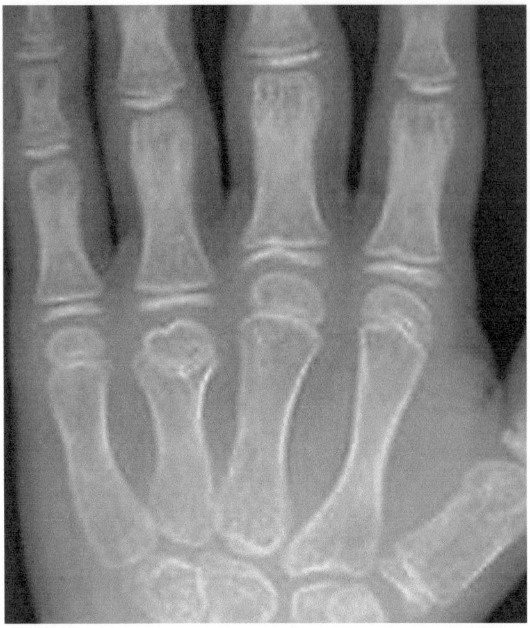

Fig. 23.31 Short fourth metacarpal in a 5-year-old girl with sickle cell anemia. Premature fusion of the growth plate is due to a previous bone infarct

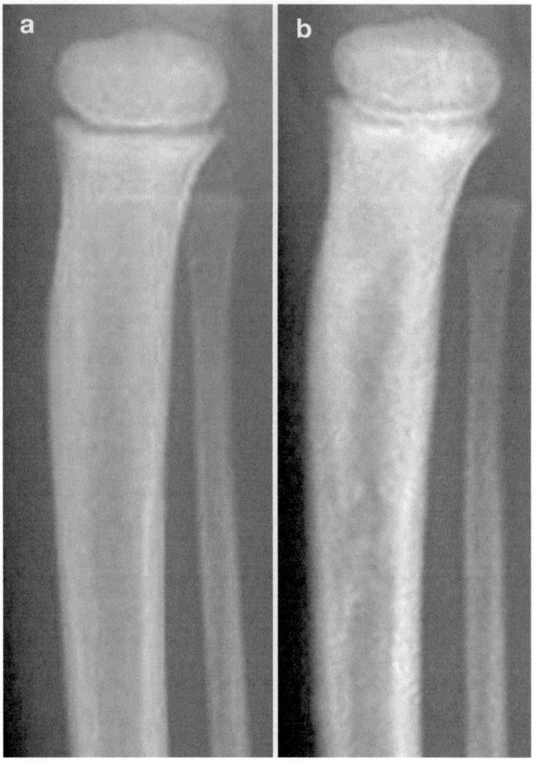

Fig. 23.32 Bone infarct in a 4-year-old with sickle cell anemia. (**a**) Initial radiograph is normal. (**b**) Six weeks later, the medullary cavity appears heterogeneous, and the cortex is thickened due to endosteal new bone formation

physeal closure, and resultant deformity and growth disturbance characterize severe cases (Fig. 23.31). Medullary infarcts in the ribs, pelvis, and spine may demonstrate striking sclerosis due to dystrophic calcification.

Long bone infarcts are common in both children and adults. Radiographs are initially normal but are useful to exclude other pathology. Osteolysis develops, followed by patchy intramedullary lucencies and sclerosis. Cortical infarcts may lead to subperiosteal or endosteal new bone (Fig. 23.32).

The appearance on bone scan evolves. In the first few days after the acute episode, radiotracer uptake is decreased or normal, and uptake increases during revascularization and remodeling [60]. If there is adequate revascularization, bone may return to normal after a few months; otherwise, focal photopenia may persist. MRI readily demonstrates early evidence of bone infarcts. Sequestration of red blood cells in the marrow results in hyperintensity on unenhanced T1-W fat saturated images. T2-weighted (T2-W) images show a serpiginous double line consisting of a hyperintense inner border and hypointense periphery (Fig. 23.33).

Epiphyseal infarction is common, occurring in about half of patients with sickle cell disease by the fourth decade. Most common in the femoral (Fig. 23.34) and humeral heads, the appearance resembles avascular necrosis encountered in other diseases—except it is more often bilateral (see Chap. 12 for further discussion of radiographic and MRI findings) [60].

Bone infarcts can lead to premature physeal closure and subsequent growth disturbance, such as malalignment and limb shortening. H-shaped vertebrae (Fig. 23.35) result from end-plate depression caused by infarcts affecting the central growth plate.

Osteomyelitis is relatively common (between 15 and 20 %) and often affects the long bones, although vertebrae and other bones may be involved. Salmonella species are the most

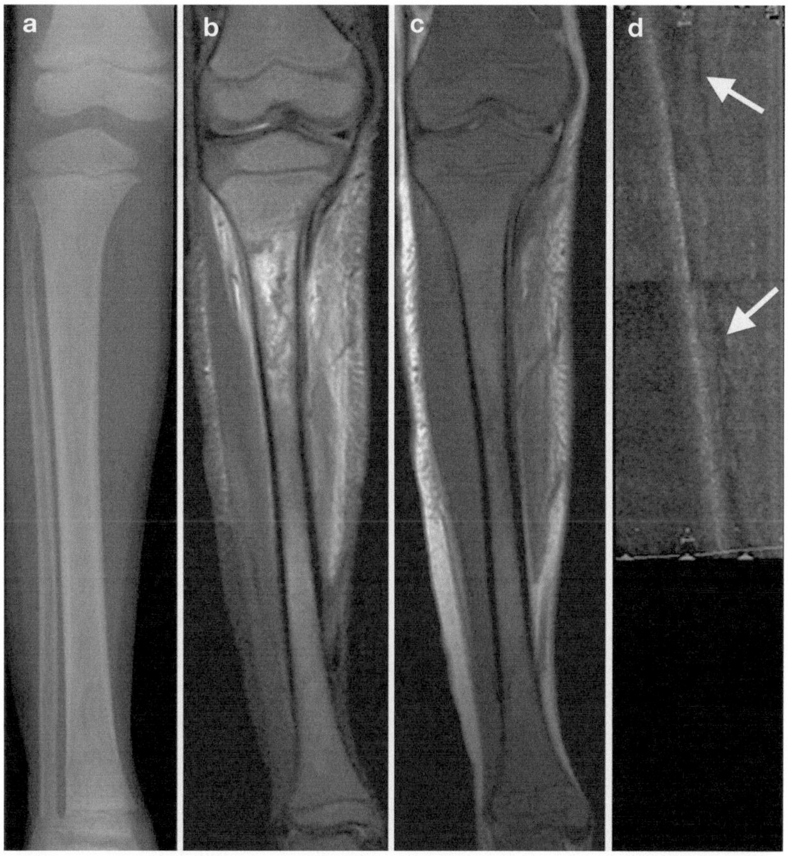

Fig. 23.33 Acute bone marrow infarct at the proximal tibia in a 4-year-old girl with sickle cell anemia. (**a**) Initial radiograph is normal. (**b**) Coronal T2-W short tau inversion recovery (STIR) image shows heterogeneous foci of increased signal in the marrow, muscle, and subcutaneous tissues. (**c**) Coronal T1-W image shows patchy irregular and decreased signal intensity. (**d**) Ultrasound (US) shows irregular hypoechoic lines (*arrows*) paralleling the periosteum and in the more superficial tissues, consistent with edema. Bone biopsy was negative for infection

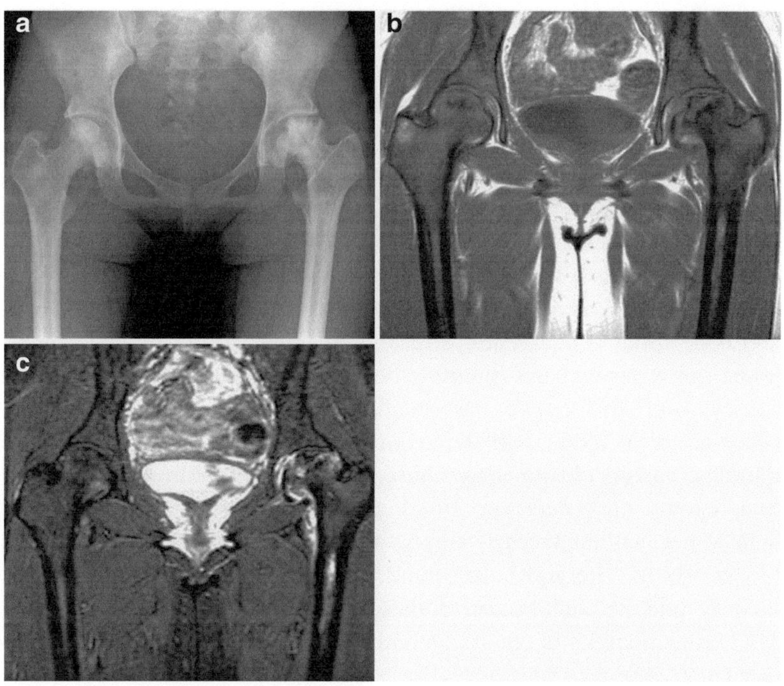

Fig. 23.34 Bilateral femoral head epiphyseal infarction in a 21-year-old female with sickle cell anemia. (**a**) Femoral head contour is irregular, and there is patchy sclerosis; findings are more severe on the left. (**b**) Coronal T1-W image shows fibrous and calcified tissue in the femoral heads with hypointense red marrow throughout the femurs. (**c**) Coronal STIR image shows marrow edema and an effusion on the left, with markedly hypointense fibrous and calcified tissue in both femoral heads. Hyperintensity in the diaphyses results from marrow infarcts (Courtesy of Sandra L. Wootton-Gorges)

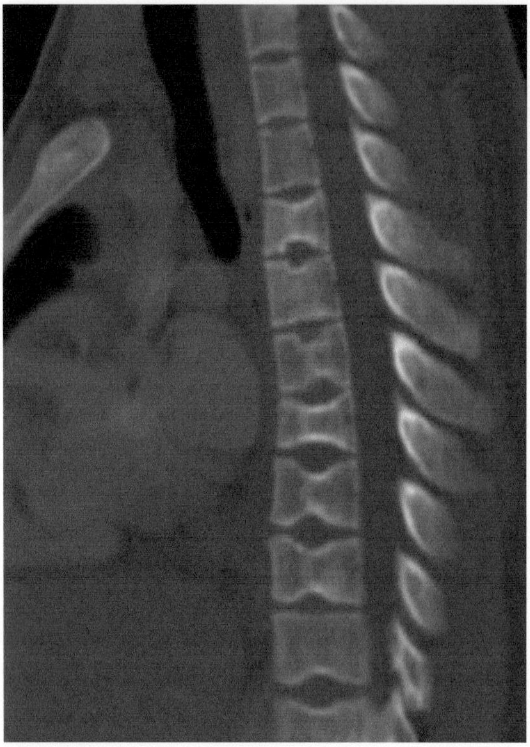

Fig. 23.35 H-type vertebrae in a patient with sickle cell disease (sagittal reformatted CT) (Courtesy of Sandra L. Wootton-Gorges)

common bacterial pathogens, followed by *Staphylococcus aureus* [60]. Gram-negative organisms are occasionally implicated. Clinical features resemble those of painful bone crisis, and infarct and infection can be difficult to differentiate by radiographs. Nuclear imaging can be helpful, and MRI may demonstrate fluid collections and sequestra (see Chap. 19).

Septic arthritis is less common than osteomyelitis and may accompany vaso-occlusive crises and bone infarction. Aseptic effusions at large joints may accompany painful bone crises. Muscle and soft tissue vaso-occlusion may occur alone or along with bone infarction. In muscles, vaso-occlusion may cause inflammation, edema, and necrosis. Fluid collections, hematomas, and fat necrosis may be seen in soft tissues [60]. Although ultrasound (US) can identify and help characterize these findings, MRI is the modality of choice for complex cases (see Chap. 22).

6 Mucopolysaccharidosis

The mucopolysaccharidoses (MPS), or lysosomal storage disorders, are a group of inheritable, metabolic diseases with an estimated prevalence of 4–6 per 100,000 births [61]. There are many clinical types and even more additional subtypes; each is caused by a specific deficient lysosomal enzyme required for glycosaminoglycan degradation [62]. Accumulation of partially degraded lysosomal glycosaminoglycans results in progressive cellular damage, affecting multiple organ systems and leading to organ failure, cognitive impairment, and premature death. Growth plate architecture is disrupted.

The MPSs have been categorized as types I through IX (with no V or VIII) but are also often referred to by their common names (Table 23.3). Type I (and its subtypes) are known as Hurler and Scheie syndromes; II, Hunter syndrome; III, Sanfilippo syndrome; IV, Morquio syndrome; VI, Maroteaux-Lamy syndrome; VII, Sly syndrome; and IX, Natowicz syndrome. The following discussion will refer to these disorders by their designated roman numeral. All except for MPS II are inherited in an autosomal recessive pattern and affect males and females equally. MPS II is X-linked recessive and almost exclusively affects males.

All are heterogeneous, progressive disorders with highly variable clinical manifestations that vary in severity both between and within different types. Patients usually appear normal at birth, with clinical onset during early childhood. Skeletal, respiratory, cardiac, and neurological systems are affected, and both hearing and vision are impaired. Other findings include coarse facial features; decreased pulmonary function and obstructive sleep apnea, frequent and recurrent respiratory infections, cardiac valvular disease, hepatosplenomegaly, umbilical and inguinal hernias, chronic diarrhea, and neurologic problems (carpal tunnel syndrome, communicating hydrocephalus, and spinal cord compression). MPS II patients may also have a distinctive appearance to the skin (pebbling), described as ivory-white papules from 2 to 10 mm in diameter that often coalesce in ridges.

Patients with severe forms of MPS I, II, VII, as well as all subtypes of III may be severely mentally

Table 23.3 Clinical and radiographic features of mucopolysaccharidoses subtypes

Name (Eponym)	Defective enzyme	Clinical features	Dysostosis multiplex
MPS IH (Hurler)	α-L-iduronidase	Coarse face, mental retardation, corneal clouding, visceromegaly	Severe
MPS IH/S (Hurler-Scheie)		Phenotype between IH and IH/S	Moderate
MPS IS (Scheie)		Corneal clouding, stiff joints, normal IQ	Mild
MPS IIA (Hunter A)	Iduronate sulfatase	Similar to IH but clear corneas	Severe
MPS IIB (Hunter B)		Mild somatic changes, normal intelligence, clear corneas	Moderate
MPS IIIA (Sanfilippo A)	Sulfatase	Profound mental retardation, behavioral changes, mild somatic manifestation	Mild
MPS IIIB (Sanfilippo B)	α-N-Ac-glucosaminidase	Profound mental retardation, behavioral changes, mild somatic manifestation	
MPS IIIC (Sanfilippo C)	Ac-CoA: α-gluc-acetyltransferase	Profound mental retardation, behavioral changes, mild somatic manifestation	
MPS IIID (Sanfilippo D)	N-Ac-gluc-6-sulfatase	Profound mental retardation, behavioral changes, mild somatic manifestation	
MPS IVA (Morquio A)	Galactose-6-sulfatase	Dwarfism, fine corneal opacities, normal IQ	Distinct
MPS IVB (Morquio B)	β-galactosidase	Milder somatic changes, adult height usually >125 cm	
MPS VIA (Maroteaux-Lamy A)	N-Ac-gal-4-sulfatase	Hurler-phenotype with corneal clouding, normal IQ	Severe
MPS VIB (Maroteaux-Lamy B)		Small stature, stiff joints, corneal clouding, normal IQ	Mild
MPS VII (Sly)	β-glucuronidase	Wide phenotype spectrum	Moderate

Adapted from [3]

disabled [62]. Development is globally delayed and eventually plateaus; progressive and inexorable regression follows. Life expectancy is short in untreated and severe forms of MPS I, II, and VII. Patients with severe forms of MPS I rarely reach age 10, whereas those with severe MPS II rarely survive beyond their teens [62]. However, patients with mild disease have little or no cognitive impairment and often live into adulthood, although they may die prematurely due to progressive airway or cardiac disease. MPS III is primarily a central nervous system disease. All patients with MPS should be considered to have high anesthesia risk [63].

The extent of skeletal abnormalities varies. The term dysostosis multiplex encompasses a set of radiological features characteristic of MPS, involving malformation of the skull, thorax, spine, pelvis, long bones, and hands, with mild or profoundly decreased range of joint motion, delayed or arrested growth, and short stature. Moderate to severe dysostosis multiplex is seen in types I, II, IV, VI, and VII (see Table 23.3). Restricted joint motion is typical, although patients with MPS IV generally have hypermobility. Even patients with severe MPS III have only mild skeletal manifestations. Patients with mucolipidosis and other storage diseases may have similar skeletal findings as those with MPS. However, MPS is more likely if many features of dysostosis multiplex are present.

Diagnosis is often delayed, particularly in those presenting with mild signs and symptoms.

For example, patients with attenuated disease may present with decreased range of joint motion, and although they often also have mild multisystemic disease, this can easily be missed. The configuration of the hands is distinctive in patients with dysostosis multiplex, and this may precipitate diagnosis (Fig. 23.36). Decreased range of wrist motion, stiff interphalangeal joints, and curved fingers result in a clawlike appearance and can impair function [62]. Positive urinary glycosaminoglycan levels suggest MPS, but false negatives occur. Enzyme activity essays based on cultured fibroblasts are required to secure a definite diagnosis and establish MPS type, and a skeletal survey showing characteristic features of dysostosis multiplex is useful to support the diagnosis.

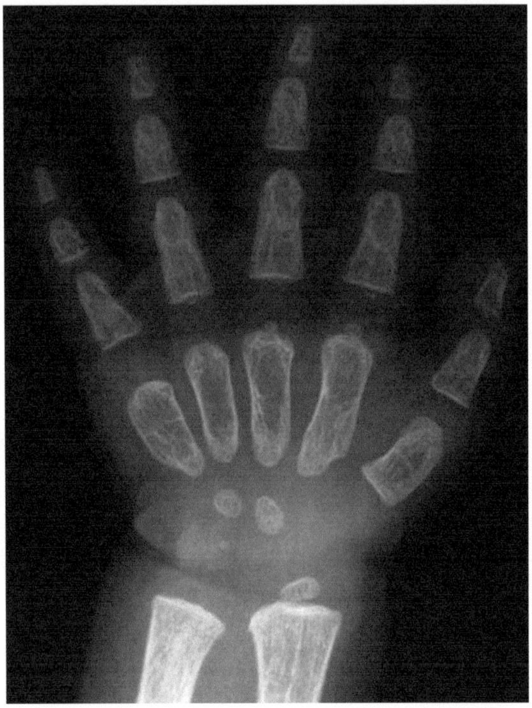

Fig. 23.36 Typical findings in the hand of a 2-year-old with MPS, who presented with swollen wrist and suspected juvenile idiopathic arthritis. The phalanges and metacarpals are broad, whereas the proximal ends of the second to fifth metacarpals are clustered together and pointed. The carpal angle is mildly decreased

Treatment is directed at the underlying pathophysiology: hematopoietic stem cell transplantation is useful for selected patients, and recombinant enzyme replacement therapy is available for MPS I, II, and VI. Early diagnosis and treatment can ameliorate many clinical manifestations of MPS but does not appear to significantly change the natural course of musculoskeletal abnormalities [64].

Surgical intervention is often required for some of the skeletal manifestations of MPS. For example, thoracolumbar kyphosis greater than 40° generally progresses despite stem cell transplantation and may require surgical stabilization to halt progression. Bracing has limited success in treatment of spinal deformity but may limit progression in young children who are not surgical candidates [63]. Craniocervical instability is common in MPS IV patients and can lead to catastrophic cord compression; these patients are often treated prophylactically with decompression and spinal fusion.

Hip dysplasia has been treated with abduction bracing in young children, but this is not necessarily effective [63]. It does not seem to respond to stem cell transplant or enzyme replacement therapy either, and corrective hip surgery is eventually required in many patients with MPS I (Fig. 23.37).

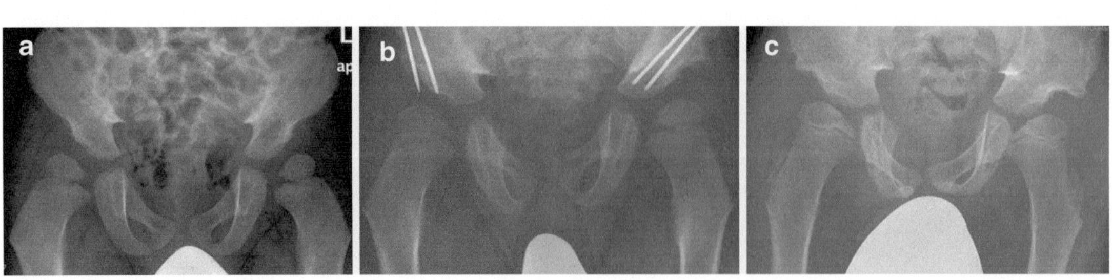

Fig. 23.37 Hip dysplasia in a boy with MPS type I, treated with periacetabular osteotomy. (**a**) At age 2 years, the acetabula are shallow, and the femoral heads are subluxated. There is underdevelopment of the medial portion of the capital femoral epiphyses along with coxa valga. (**b**) A periacetabular osteotomy was performed at age 3 years. (**c**) At age 7 years, the femoral heads are well centered

The role of surgery in treating hip dysplasia in other MPS types is debatable, as postoperative avascular necrosis is common [59]. Osteotomies do heal well.

Growth in MPS can be difficult to predict, and therefore criteria dictating intervention cannot be based upon growth parameters of normal children [63].

Imaging (Box 23.7)

Box 23.7: Radiographic Features of Dysostosis Multiplex

Decreased joint range of motion (type IV: hypermobile joints)

Delayed/arrested growth

Distinctive hands: pointed, clustered second–fifth MC base; short, broad small bones

Delayed ossification of odontoid, ligamentous instability (maybe only on CT)

Vertebrae: flat, irregular, oval, with posterior scalloping (especially L1–2)

- Central tongue, severe platyspondyly: type IV
- Inferior beaking: types I and II
- Kyphosis at TL junction (anterior wedging, retrolisthesis)

Oar-shaped ribs; short/thick clavicles

Acetabular dysplasia and femoral head (dysplasia, fragmentation)

Long bones: thick, short diaphyses; hypoplastic epiphyses

Proximal humeral notches

There is considerable overlap in the radiologic appearance of the different types of MPS, and diagnosis does not rest on imaging findings alone [65].

Skull radiographs may demonstrate a J-shaped sella turcica (Fig. 23.38) and thickening of the diploic space—the former probably due to pressure from glycosaminoglycan accumulation in the brain [65], and the latter due to accumulation in the diploic space. Platybasia may be seen as well. However, the skull is usually normal in patients with MPS IV.

Abnormalities at the craniocervical junction include delayed ossification of the odontoid process and ligamentous instability (Fig. 23.39). Resultant atlantoaxial instability is common, but often not apparent on flexion-extension radiographs. Deposition of glycosaminoglycans contributes to spinal stenosis, but this cannot be appreciated on radiographs.

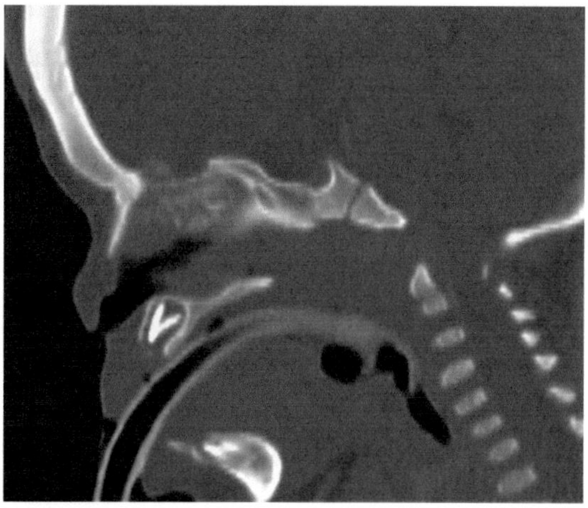

Fig. 23.38 J-shaped sella in a patient with MPS I. Also note cervical platyspondyly and unusually wide diploic space at frontal bone (Courtesy of Sandra L. Wootton-Gorges)

Vertebral bodies are typically flat, irregular, and oval shaped, with central tongues or inferior beaking as well as posterior scalloping (Fig. 23.40); these findings are most pronounced at the L1–2 levels. In MPS IVA, platyspondyly is usually severe, and beaks typically protrude anteriorly from the middle of the vertebral body (Fig. 23.41). Impaired bone growth at the superoanterior upper lumbar vertebrae causes anterior wedging and retrolisthesis at the thoracolumbar (TL) junction. This may lead to kyphosis (or gibbus deformity), found in nearly all children with severe MPS I and common in other MPS's as well (Fig. 23.42). Scoliosis may be seen in patients with MPS I, II, and III.

Ribs are paddle (or oar) shaped, wide anteriorly, and tapered posteriorly (Fig. 23.43). Clavicles are short and thick (Fig. 23.44).

The pelvis is narrow, the iliac wings rounded, and the inferior iliac bones tapered (Fig. 23.45). Ossification of the lateral acetabular corner is delayed, contributing to a shallow acetabulum. The medial portion of the capital femoral

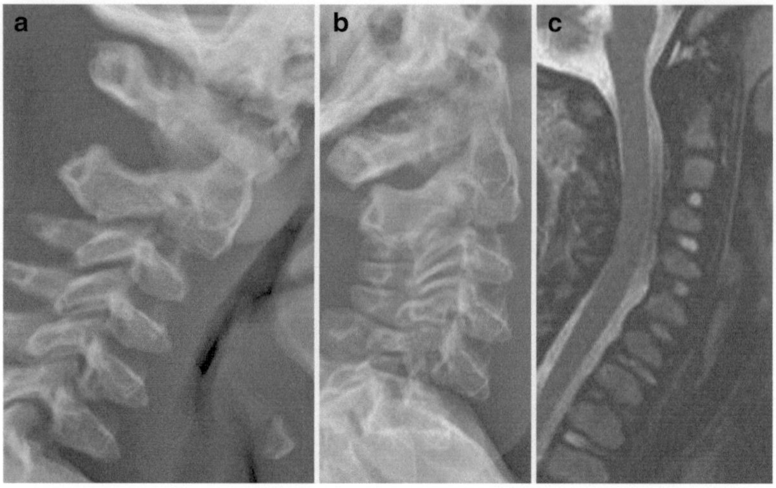

Fig. 23.39 Cervical spine in a 7-year-old with MPS. Flexion (**a**) and extension (**b**) views show a relatively small odontoid process but no instability. Vertebrae are ovoid and pointed anteriorly. (**c**) Sagittal T2-W image shows a periodontoid soft tissue mass without spinal cord compression

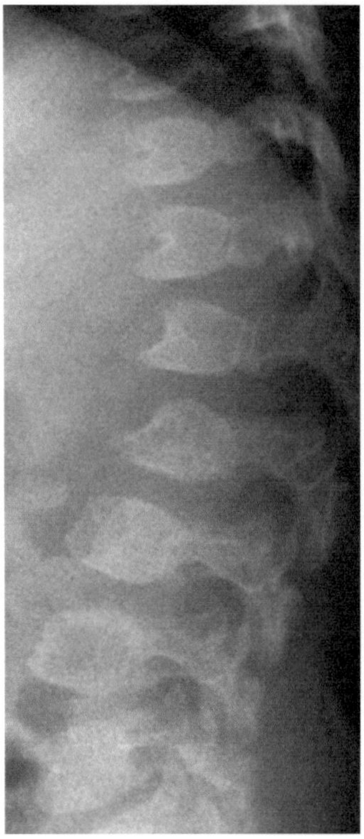

Fig. 23.40 Thoracolumbar kyphosis in a 2-year-old with mucopolysaccharidosis (MPS). The superior and inferior end plates are convex, and there is inferior beaking of L1 and L2. L2 is hypoplastic

epiphysis is underdeveloped, and there is coxa valga. Acetabular dysplasia and proximal femoral deformities result in progressive hip instability and eventual dislocation, limiting function by adolescence or early adulthood in many patients with MPS. The femoral head may become fragmented as a result of progressive resorption.

The diaphyses of all the long bones may be thick and short. The epiphyses of the long bones may be slightly hypoplastic, and indeed the femoral heads may appear fragmented. The femoral necks may be long and narrow, with both medial and lateral erosions. Genu valgum is common, especially in patients with MPS I and IV. If the tibial-femoral angle exceeds 15°, surgery may be required. There are notches at the proximal humeri. The distal ulnae may be hypoplastic, with resultant Madelung-type deformity.

The appearance of the hands is distinctive. The bases of the second through fifth metacarpals (MC) appear pointed, and the medial ends of these bones are clustered together. Metacarpals and phalanges and short and broad but cortices thin, and the carpal angles are decreased (see Fig. 23.36). Carpal tunnel syndrome may develop, as a result of glycosaminoglycan deposition along the flexor retinaculum and tenosynovium.

Although radiographs may not demonstrate instability, flexion-extension CT may assess cervical spine instability in those with significant skeletal changes or equivocal diagnoses (see Fig. 23.39).

MRI provides important information about spinal cord and nerve root compression due to ligamentous laxity, osseous deformity, and

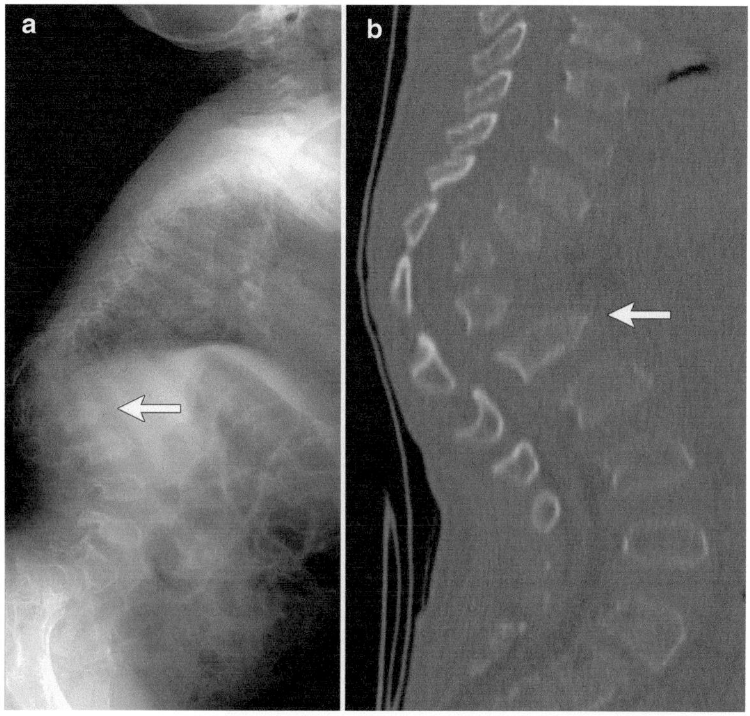

Fig. 23.41 Kyphosis in a 9-year-old boy with MPS IV. (**a**) There is platyspondyly, middle vertebral beaking (*arrow*) and thoracolumbar kyphosis due anterior hypoplasia at T11–L1 vertebrae. (**b**) Sagittally reformatted CT delineates the middle vertebral beaking (*arrows*) and truncated vertebral bodies (Courtesy of Sandra L. Wootton-Gorges)

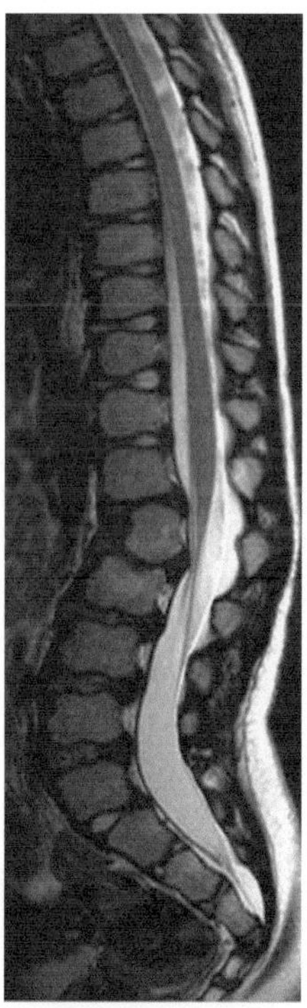

Fig. 23.42 Thoracolumbar kyphosis in a 7-year-old with MPS type I. Sagittal T2-W image shows L2 is hypoplastic and slightly retropulsed. Note hypointensity in adjacent bulging discs. Additional vertebrae demonstrate biconvex contour as well

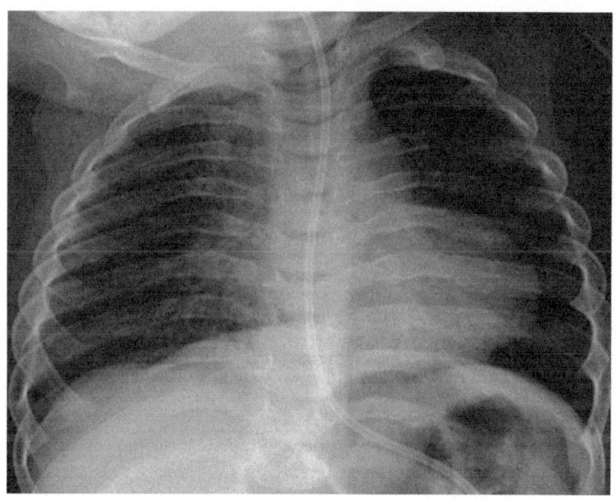

Fig. 23.43 Broad ribs with posterior constrictions in a 2-year-old with MPS

deposition of glycosaminoglycans (see Fig. 23.39) in the tissues around the spinal cord. Spinal cord compression may occur at any level but is most common at the cervicocranial junction (see Fig. 23.39) or thoracolumbar region. Atlantoaxial instability, myelopathy, and spastic quadriparesis can lead to premature death, usually in patients with MPS IV and MPS VI.

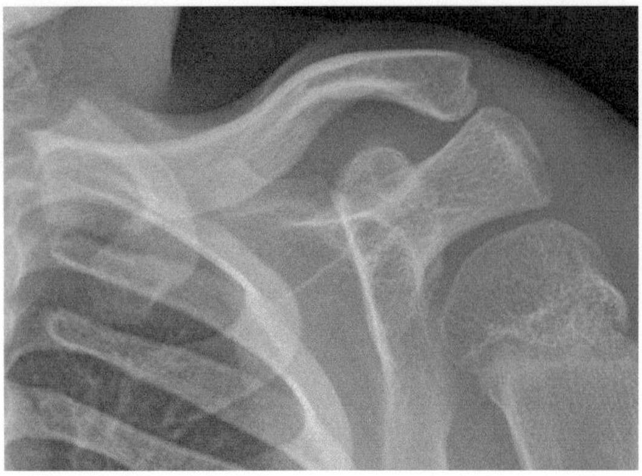

Fig. 23.44 Broad clavicle with coarse trabeculae in a 7-year-old with MPS type I

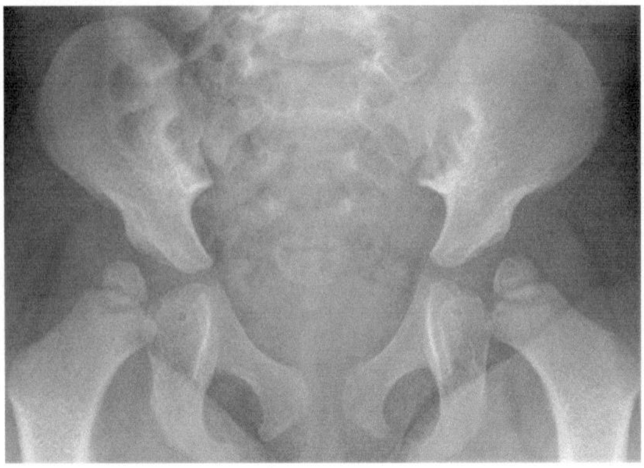

Fig. 23.45 Narrow pelvis, with rounded iliac wings, constricted inferior iliac bones, and acetabular dysplasia in a 2-year-old with MPS type I

MRI also demonstrates typical abnormalities in the brain, including white matter disease, hydrocephalus, and atrophy.

7 Gaucher Disease

Gaucher disease is the most common lysosomal storage disorder, with a prevalence of about 1.1 per 100,000 births [61], and it is more common in people of Eastern European (Ashkenazi) Jewish descent. Inherited as an autosomal recessive trait, Gaucher disease is characterized by the accumulation of glucocerebroside in the lysosomes due to a glucocerebrosidase enzyme deficiency (lysosomal acid β-glucosidase). The glucocerebrosidase gene (GBA) is mapped to chromosome 1, band q21. Over 200 mutations can lead to Gaucher disease.

This heterogeneous and progressive disorder exhibits highly variable clinical manifestations and severity. It affects several organ systems, particularly the bone marrow, spleen, liver, lungs, and central nervous system. There are three major clinical phenotypes, differentiated by primary central nervous system involvement and disease severity [66, 67].

Type 1, the non-neuronopathic form, is the most prevalent, accounting for 90–95 % of cases. It is characterized by adult onset and no involvement of the central nervous system. However, some individuals with severe mutations present early in childhood [68]. Type 2 is characterized by severe neurological involvement, onset during infancy, and death within the first 2 years of life. Type 3 exhibits neurological abnormalities in the late first decade of life, and its severity falls between types 1 and 2.

Gaucher cells derive from the monocyte-macrophage system and are present throughout the body, but they are most concentrated in the spleen, liver, bone marrow, and lymph nodes, where they cause enlargement and lead to dysfunction. As with the mucopolysaccharidoses, patients are typically normal at birth, and clinical features become apparent as substrate accumulates. Hepatosplenomegaly, anemia, and bleeding due to thrombocytopenia are common early features. Bone involvement is seen in 80 % of patients with type 1 Gaucher disease and may be asymptomatic or mildly to extremely painful. Pathophysiology of bone disease is incompletely understood but probably includes altered bone formation and resorption, focal deposition, and increased intraosseous pressure [67]. Growth is delayed in moderate to severe forms of Gaucher disease. The neurological symptoms encountered in types 2 and 3 include oculomotor apraxia, opisthotonus, bulbar signs (problems with breathing, swallowing, and talking), and seizures. Death may result from infection or from complications of neurological impairment.

Gaucher disease is diagnosed by determining the glucocerebrosidase activity of peripheral leukocytes or cultured skin fibroblasts. DNA analysis can diagnose the disease and determine prognosis [69]. Imaging assesses the severity of disease, identifies complications, and monitors response to treatment [67].

Current therapy involves enzyme replacement, substrate reduction, and stem cell transplantation. Enzyme replacement can decrease the likelihood of skeletal complications, including bone pain, bone crisis, infarction, and fracture. Stem cell transplantation is risky but can confer long-term benefits, such as regression of skeletal and neurological changes.

Imaging (Box 23.8)

Box 23.8: Imaging Features of Gaucher Disease

Bone involvement in 80 % with type 1

Erlenmeyer flask deformity (diaphyseal construction; metaphyseal/metadiaphyseal flaring)

Increased red marrow

Avascular necrosis of femoral and humeral heads; vertebral bodies

MRI for bone infarcts, infection, fracture

Skeletal disease affects more than 80 % of Gaucher type 1 patients and is more debilitating than the hematological or visceral manifestations. Bone manifestations include generalized osteopenia, deformity, infarcts, avascular necrosis, lytic lesions, osteosclerosis, pathological fractures, and rarely acute osteomyelitis. The vertebrae, femurs, humeri, and tibias are affected most often (Figs. 23.46 and 23.47).

With the exception of detecting fractures, radiography plays a limited role in Gaucher disease, as it detects abnormal morphology in only 30–40 % of cases [67]. However, the presence of classic radiological findings may suggest the diagnosis. For example, the Erlenmeyer flask deformity, which results from diaphyseal constriction, metaphyseal and metadiaphyseal flaring, and cortical thinning, may be seen in patients with Gaucher disease (Fig. 23.48), although it occurs with other disorders as well. Sequelae of ischemia may be seen in the femoral heads, proximal humeri, and vertebral bodies (see Figs. 23.46 and 23.47). During an acute

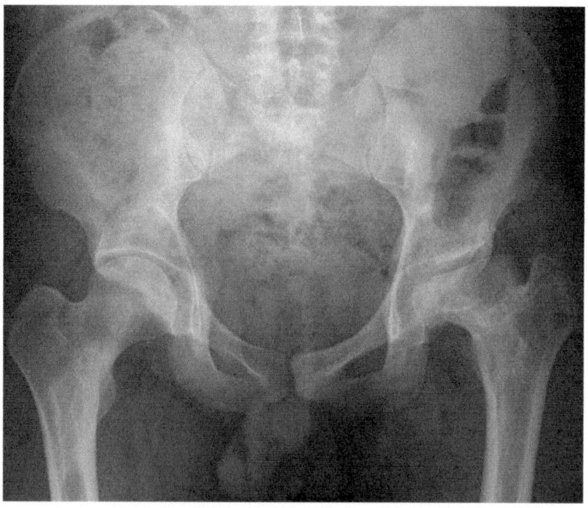

Fig. 23.46 Gaucher disease in a 30-year-old. Avascular necrosis (AVN) of the left femoral head and associated acetabular remodeling, with sclerotic proximal femoral metadiaphyses due to medullary infarcts (Same patient as Fig. 23.47)

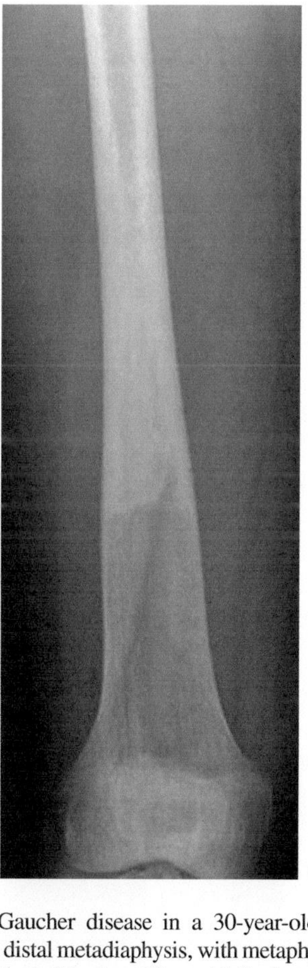

Fig. 23.47 Gaucher disease in a 30-year-old. Increased lucency at the distal metadiaphysis, with metaphyseal expansion and cortical thinning. The mid-diaphyseal sclerosis results from medullary infarcts (Same patient as Fig. 23.46)

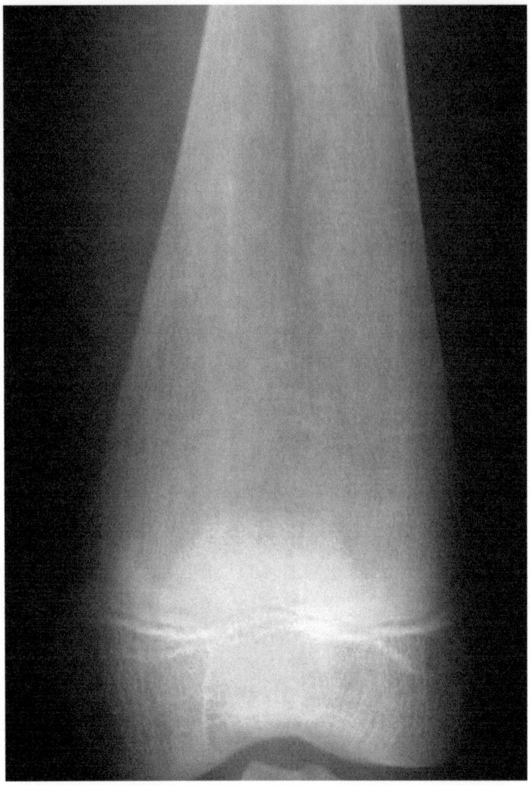

Fig. 23.48 Erlenmeyer flask deformity in a patient with Gaucher disease. There is metaphyseal and metadiaphyseal flaring along with cortical thinning and osteopenia (Courtesy of Rebecca Stein-Wexler)

"bone crisis," which is characterized by severe bone pain, fever, leukocytosis, and elevated erythrocyte sedimentation rate, radiographs may demonstrate periosteal reaction without osteolysis [70].

Bone densitometry is helpful for assessing osteopenia in patients with Gaucher disease. Bone marrow scintigraphy (such as 99m-sestamibi) can be employed to assess the extent of Gaucher cell infiltration, but MRI provides similar information with better spatial resolution and no radiation exposure. When performed within 3 days of onset of pain, Tc-99m MDP scintigraphy can help differentiate aseptic infarction ("bone crisis") from acute osteomyelitis.

MRI is highly sensitive to Gaucher cells in bone marrow and to complications such as bone infarction, infection, and fracture. Evaluating the lumbar spine and femurs determines the extent and severity of bone marrow involvement and detects musculoskeletal complications secondary to Gaucher infiltration [67] (Fig. 23.49) (see Chap. 25). T2 hyperintensity is seen with recent bone infarcts, osteomyelitis, and bone crisis (which precedes frank osteonecrosis) [67].

Several MRI techniques and scoring systems have been devised to quantify bone marrow

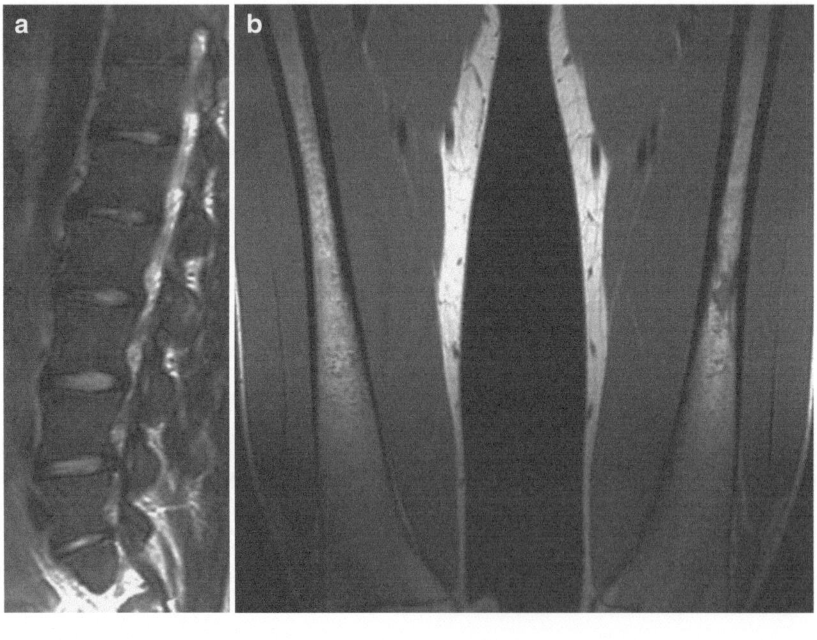

Fig. 23.49 Diffuse marrow replacement in an 18-year-old with Gaucher disease. (**a**) Sagittal T1-W spine MRI shows decreased signal in all vertebrae due to increased cellularity secondary to marrow infiltration. (**b**) Coronal T1-W image of the femurs shows mild diffuse hypointensity in the diaphyses and distal metaphyses (Courtesy of Rikin Hargunani)

involvement. These assess the extent to which Gaucher cells displace normal bone marrow adipocytes and thus reduce marrow fat. However, bone marrow change in children must be interpreted with caution due to the normal presence of red marrow in the vertebrae and long bones. Quantitative chemical shift imaging (QCSI), which measures fat in bone marrow, is the most accurate MRI assessment technique. However, the technology is not widely available and is fairly cumbersome. For this reason, a number of semiquantitative scoring systems based on standard MRI sequences have been devised. These are based on the fact that bone marrow infiltration follows a specific sequential pattern, starting in the axial skeleton and progressing to the proximal and then distal appendicular skeleton. In the long bones, infiltration starts in the metaphyses, progresses to the diaphyses, and finally involves the epiphyses and apophyses [67]. Scores are based on altered signal intensity at various anatomic locations and may be helpful in monitoring disease (see Chap. 26).

8 VACTERL (VATER) Association

This condition is defined by the presence of at least three of the following congenital malformations from which the acronym is derived: vertebral defects, anal atresia, cardiac defects, tracheoesophageal fistula (TEF), renal anomalies, and limb anomalies [1, 71]. However, there are no strict diagnostic criteria, and the designation VACTERL is purely descriptive and does not imply a uniform pathogenesis. In addition to these defining elements, patients may have other congenital anomalies, including vascular abnormalities, auricular defects, and rib anomalies [1], but neurocognitive function is usually normal. Although diagnostic criteria vary, the prevalence is estimated at approximately 1 in 10,000–40,000 live births [71]. The etiology is believed to be multifactorial and has been identified in only a small fraction of patients. Thorough clinical and laboratory analysis is essential, as the differential diagnosis is broad. Prenatal US can demonstrate most of the elements of the VACTERL complex.

Of the core components, vertebral anomalies have been reported in approximately 60–80 % of patients, imperforate anus/anal atresia in 55–90 %, genitourinary anomalies in up to 25 %, cardiac malformations in 40–80 %, tracheoesophageal fistula in 50–80 %, and limb malformations in 40–50 % [71].

Management of VACTERL association in the immediate postnatal period is directed at surgical correction of specific congenital anomalies (typically anal atresia, certain types of cardiac malformations, and tracheoesophageal fistula). Long-term medical management is often necessary, and although some patients have relatively minor clinical sequelae, the malformations can be quite debilitating.

Imaging

Characteristic vertebral anomalies include segmentation defects, such as hemivertebrae, butterfly vertebrae, wedge vertebrae, vertebral fusion, and supernumerary or absent vertebrae, sometimes accompanied with anomalous ribs (see Chap. 3) (Figs. 23.50 and 23.51). These abnormalities often result in scoliosis, and assessment of scoliosis may prompt diagnosis of occult VACTERL association. Limb malformations have been defined as radial anomalies, including thumb aplasia/hypoplasia (Fig. 23.52) (see Chaps. 7 and 9); however, many other limb anomalies have been ascribed (perhaps erroneously) to VACTERL association, including polydactyly and lower limb anomalies [1, 71].

The differential diagnosis is broad. A few diagnoses to consider are: Baller-Gerold syndrome, CHARGE syndrome, Currarino syndrome, deletion 22q11.2 syndrome, Fanconi anemia, Feingold syndrome, Fryns syndrome, oculo-auriculo-vertebral syndrome, Opitz G/BBB syndrome, Pallister-Hall syndrome, and Townes-Brocks syndrome, and VACTERL with hydrocephalus [71].

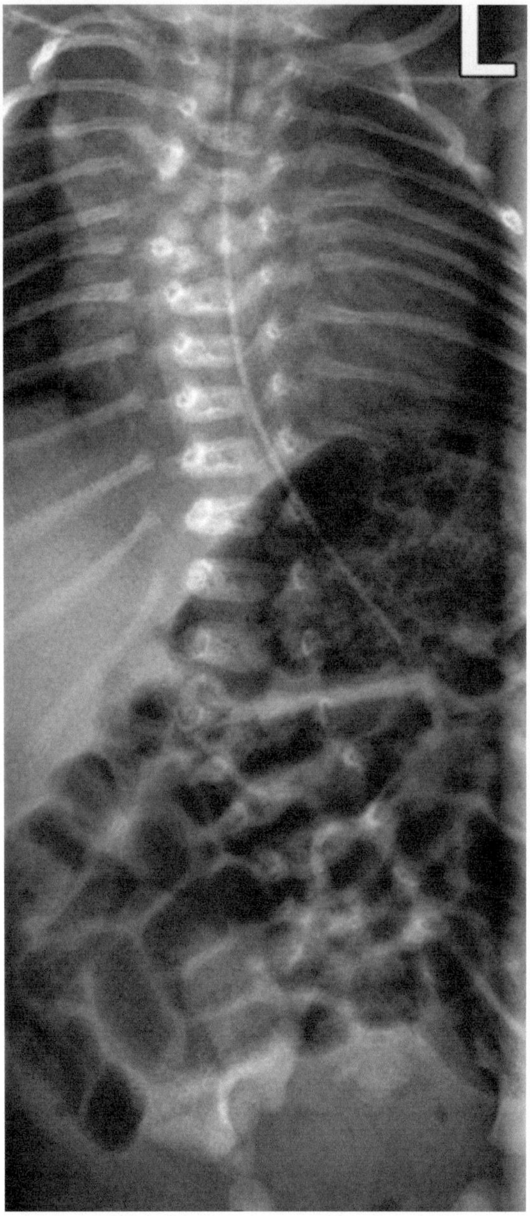

Fig. 23.50 Vertebral and rib anomalies, along with scoliosis in a newborn girl with VACTERL association

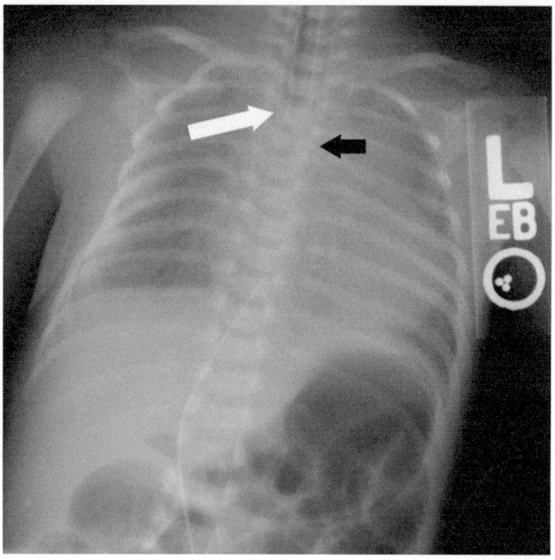

Fig. 23.51 Newborn with esophageal atresia/tracheoesophageal fistula (note esophageal catheter terminating at the thoracic inlet (*white arrow*)) and T3 butterfly vertebral segmentation anomaly (*black arrow*) (Courtesy of Sandra L. Wootton-Gorges)

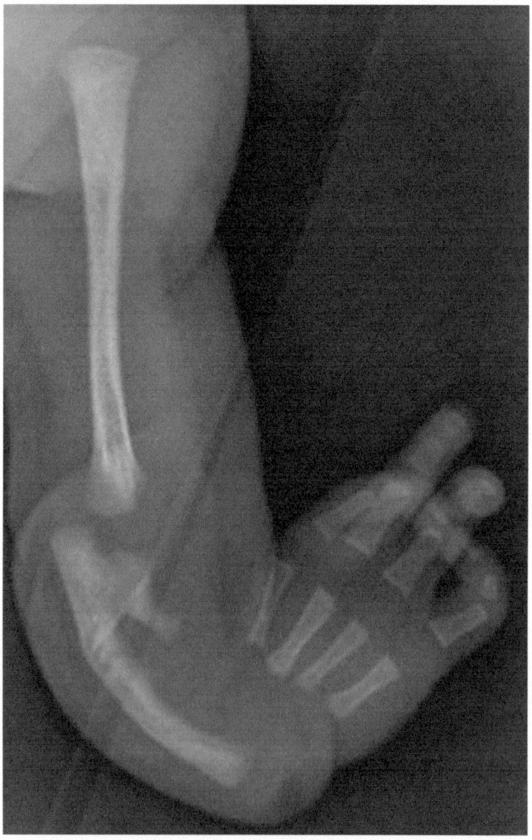

Fig. 23.52 Radial longitudinal deficiency in newborn with VACTERL, along with absent thumb and radial clubhand

9 Limb-Body Wall Defects

Limb-body wall defects include a variety of malformations involving the ventral body wall, limbs, viscera, face, and cranium. The disorder has also been termed amniotic band disruption complex, amnion rupture sequence, limb-body wall complex, and simply body wall complex [72]. The reported incidence is 0.33 per 1,000 live births. The association of malformations can originate as early as the embryonic disc stage, with some of the associated anomalies resulting from the primary disturbance in embryogenesis.

The limb anomalies in this spectrum of disorders vary, as does their etiology. They range from mild deformities to major positional anomalies, hypoplasia of all or part(s) of one or more limbs, intercalary and terminal deficiencies, amelia, syndactylies (sometimes associated with amniotic bands), amputation-like anomalies (see Chap. 9), pseudosyndactyly associated with constrictions, and/or bands that may or may not connect to the amnion.

10 Achondroplasia

Achondroplasia is the most common form of short-limbed dwarfism, with a reported birth prevalence of 1 in 10,000–30,000. Although it is autosomal dominant, the mutation rate is high and therefore 80 % of children with achondroplasia have parents of average stature [73]. Over 95 % of cases are caused by one of two recurrent mutations in the gene encoding fibroblast growth factor receptor type 3 (FGFR3), both resulting in the same amino acid substitution (G380R).

Prenatal US by 25 weeks can show short femurs (often below the 3rd percentile) [74] along with a head size of greater than the 50th percentile, bowed femurs, frontal bossing, small chest, and polyhydramnios. Diagnosis at birth is based upon the clinical findings of predominantly rhizomelic limb shortening, dysmorphic features, a prominent forehead, and depressed nasal bridge. Respiratory distress may develop, caused by short ribs and a narrow thorax. If the diagnosis is in question, chromosomal analysis can detect G380R/FGFR3 mutations.

Most children with achondroplasia develop thoracolumbar kyphosis in the first few months of life, but this usually corrects spontaneously as truncal muscle tone and strength improve. When the child starts to walk, kyphosis occasionally progresses but is usually replaced by painful lumbar lordosis. Bracing is used to treat those with progressive kyphosis, but occasionally surgical stabilization of the spine may be required [73]. A small number of children also have odontoid hypoplasia and cervical spine instability.

As the child matures, narrowed interpediculate distances and short pedicles may lead to spinal stenosis and cord compression. As a result, approximately 20 % of individuals with achondroplasia develop lower extremity weakness, numbness, and other neurological findings by age 20.

Neurological problems involving the brain and cervicomedullary junction are also common. Restricted movement of cerebrospinal fluid due to a narrow foramen magnum increases the likelihood of hydrocephalus (Fig. 23.53). However,

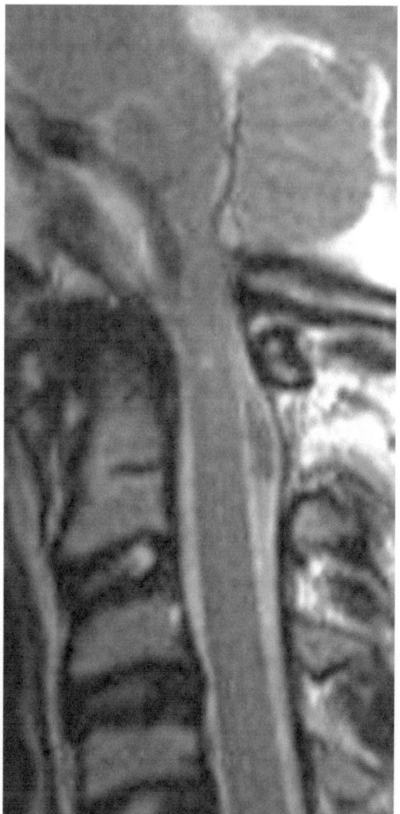

Fig. 23.53 Narrow foramen magnum in an 11-year-old boy with achondroplasia. Sagittal T2-W MRI shows resultant cervical cord compression

non-pathological megalencephaly is also common, as normal patients with achondroplasia often have increased intraventricular and extra-axial fluid. The small foramen magnum may cause cervicomedullary compression and lead to cervical myelopathy and central apnea. This rare but severe complication must be monitored closely. Additionally, there is commonly a degree of megalencephaly with increased ventricular volume and extra-axial fluid volumes. To avoid overdiagnosis of hydrocephalus and unnecessary intervention, it is essential that neuroimaging is interpreted based on achondroplasia-specific standards and not those of the average stature child [70]. The American Academy of Pediatrics recommends baseline neuroimaging for all infants with achondroplasia.

Significant and progressive tibial bowing is seen in about 10 % of children by age 5 and up to 40 % of older children. Fibular overgrowth may contribute to both tibial bowing and genu varum [75]. Corrective surgery to realign the lower limb may be performed in the setting of recurrent knee or ankle pain, gait disturbance, frequent falls, or a "lateral thrust" of the knee (uncontrolled lateral movement on weight bearing). Most joints are hypermobile (except the elbows and hips, where flexion contractures are common).

Limb lengthening by distraction osteotomy has been successful in a number of children with achondroplasia. A significant increase in limb length (over 10 cm) can be achieved. However, the process is painful and involves several operations followed by long periods in external fixation. Many centers therefore insist on extensive psychological assessment prior to surgery, that children are at least 10 years of age, and that they they are both able and allowed to participate in the decision to undergo surgery.

A multidisciplinary approach to children with achondroplasia should include a clinical geneticist, pediatrician, and an occupational therapist with expertise in achondroplasia. In addition, specialists in pediatric radiology, orthopedics, neurology, and pulmonology should be involved. Despite its potential neurological complications, achondroplasia has the best long-term prognosis of all short-limb dwarfisms.

Imaging (Box 23.9)

Box 23.9: Radiographic Features of Achondroplasia

Long bones	Newborn: Short, tubular, with sloping metaphyses
	Progressive: Apparent increased thickness of long bones (disproportional)
	Short femoral necks
	Prominent metaphyseal irregularities (knees)
Skull	Large, with small base
Vertebrae	Short, flat, bullet shaped
	Decreasing interpediculate distance level L1 to 5, short pedicles
Pelvis	Squared iliac wings, small sacrosciatic notches
	Trident acetabula (horizontal, with lateral and medial spurs)
Hands	Trident shaped with short fingers, bullet-shaped phalanges

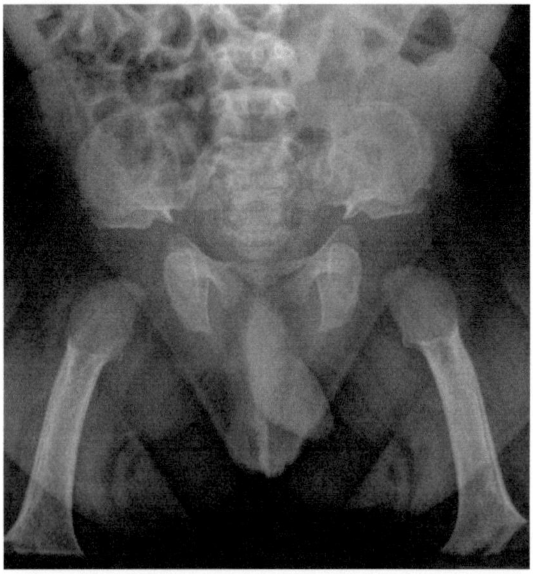

Fig. 23.54 Achondroplasia in a newborn. Short, broad femurs with sloping metaphyses and characteristic oval lucency of the proximal femurs due to decreased anteroposterior diameter. Note the characteristic configuration of the pelvis, with broad iliac bones, small sacrosciatic notches, and horizontal acetabula

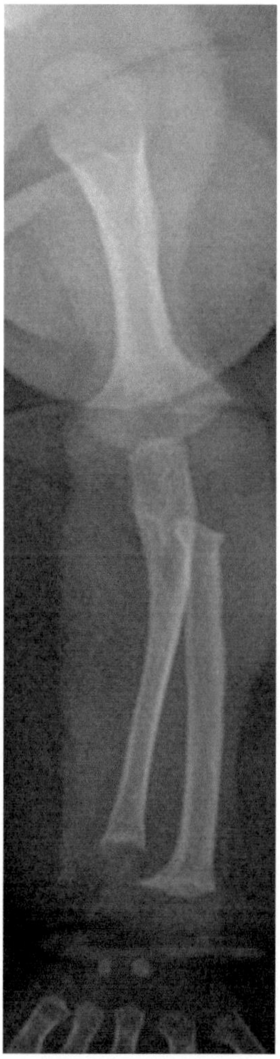

Fig. 23.55 Achondroplasia. The tubular bones are short, especially the humerus (rhizomelic limb shortening). Note characteristic lucency of proximal humeri

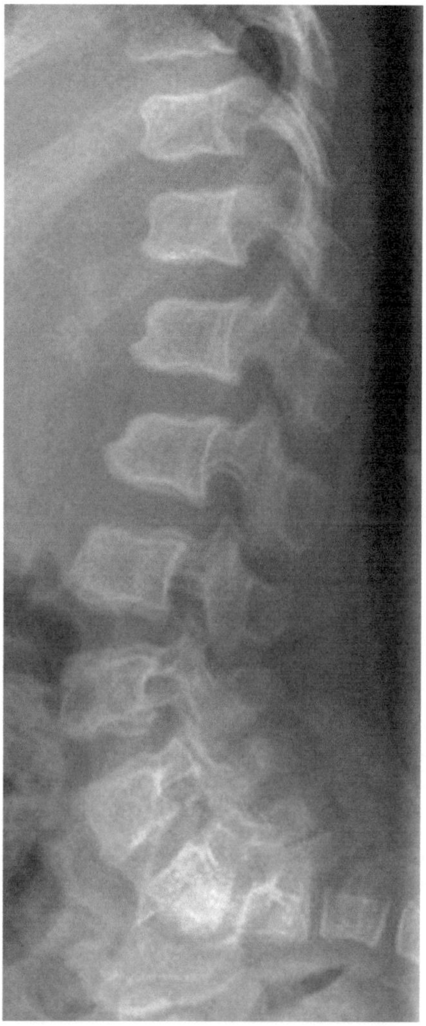

Fig. 23.56 Achondroplasia in a newborn. Short, slightly flat vertebral bodies, with short pedicles. L3 is bullet shaped

In infancy, bones are short and tubular with sloping metaphysis; the upper femurs and humeri are oval and relatively lucent due to decreased anteroposterior diameter (Figs. 23.54 and 23.55). The skull is large, with a relatively small base. The vertebral bodies are short, flat, and often bullet shaped (Figs. 23.56 and 23.57), with short pedicles on the lateral view. There is progressive narrowing of the interpediculate distance in the lower spine (Fig. 23.58). The configuration of the pelvis is characteristic, with squared iliac wings and small sacrosciatic notches, as well as horizontal acetabula with lateral and medial spurs (trident acetabula) (see Fig. 23.54). The hands are trident shaped with short fingers, bullet-shaped phalanges with broad metaphyses, and distal tapering (Fig. 23.59).

The tubular bones are short even in the neonate, but their thickness appears to increase as the patient matures due to more pronounced disproportion between normal width and short length. Short femoral necks become progressively more impressive, and metaphyseal irregularities develop, most striking at the knee and at other areas with prominent muscle attachments [3] (Fig. 23.60). As the patient matures, decreased

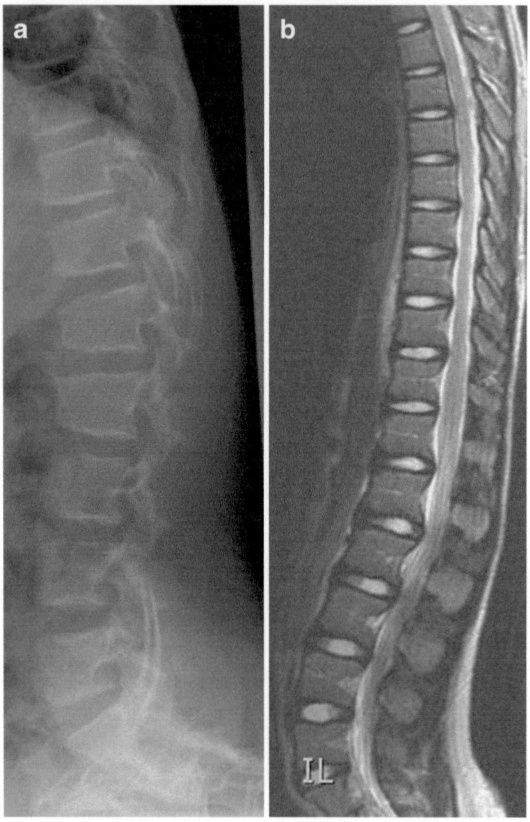

Fig. 23.57 Spinal stenosis and cord compression in a boy with achondroplasia. (**a**) The pedicles are extremely short. (**b**) T2-W MRI shows very narrow anteroposterior diameter

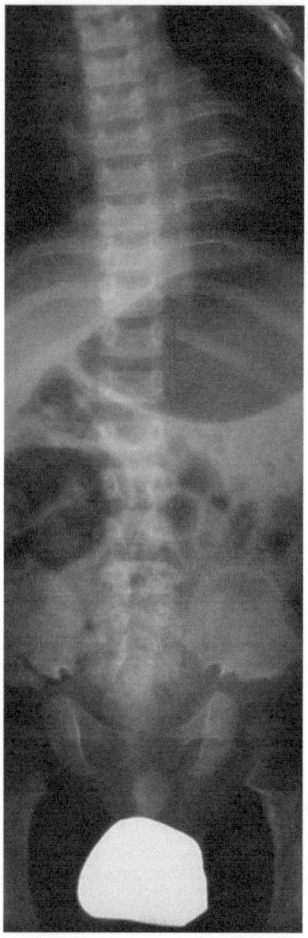

Fig. 23.58 Achondroplasia in a 6-month-old boy. There is narrowing of the interpediculate distance in the lower lumbar spine (Courtesy of Sandra L. Wootton-Gorges)

interpediculate distances at the lumbar spine become evident.

Differential Diagnosis

The major differential is hypochondroplasia, which has similar but milder skeletal changes (Fig. 23.61). In thanatophoric dysplasia, the abnormalities are more severe, with markedly underossified, band-like vertebrae; these infants often die in early infancy. Homozygous achondroplasia—usually diagnosed by parental history—is lethal in early infancy. In pseudoachondroplasia, the skull is normal but ossification of the epiphyses is severely disturbed. Other dysplasias are often incorrectly diagnosed as achondroplasia.

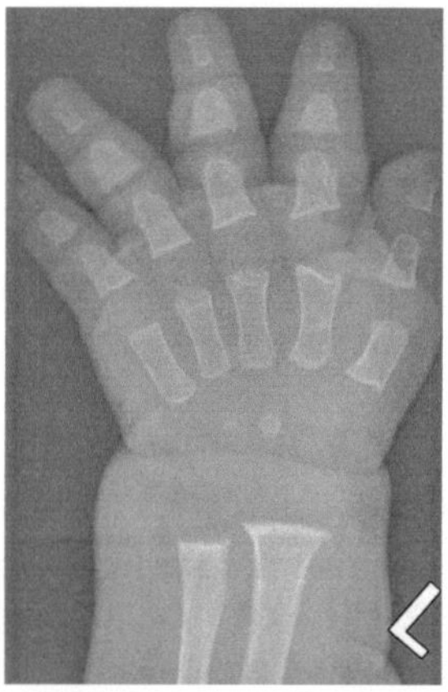

Fig. 23.59 Achondroplasia in a 3-month-old. The hand is trident shaped with short fingers and bullet-shaped phalanges that have broad metaphyses. The digits taper distally

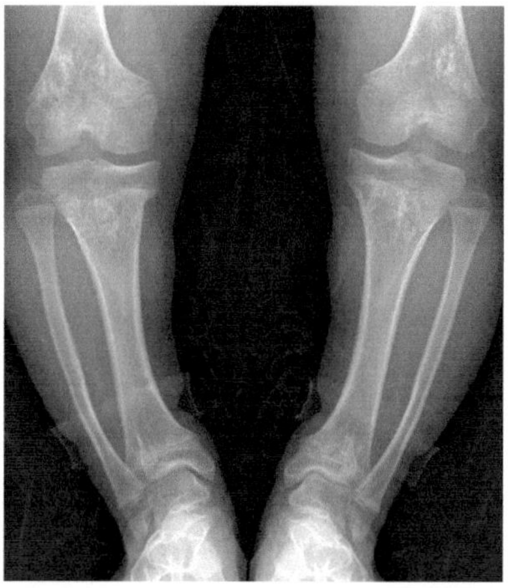

Fig. 23.60 Massive-appearing long bones in a 15-year-old boy with achondroplasia. Although the tubular bones are short at all ages, they appear more massive as patients age. Typical metaphyseal irregularities

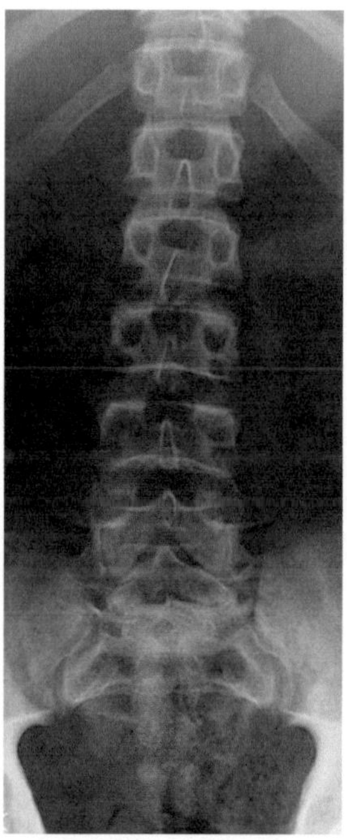

Fig. 23.61 Hypochondroplasia in a 13-year-old boy. The interpediculate distances in the lumbar spine decrease distally

11 Multiple Epiphyseal Dysplasia (MED) and Pseudoachondroplasia

MED and pseudoachondroplasia are also common skeletal dysplasias, characterized by short-limbed dwarfism, joint pain, and stiffness (Table 23.4). The two conditions are part of the same spectrum of disease. Although pseudoachondroplasia is transmitted only by autosomal dominant inheritance, MED can be either autosomal dominant (AD-MED) or autosomal recessive (AR-MED). Most cases of AD-MED and pseudoachondroplasia result from mutations in cartilage oligomeric matrix protein (COMP). However, AD-MED is genetically heterogeneous and can also result from mutations in matrilin-3 (MATN3) and type IX collagen (COL9A1, COL9A2, and COL9A3) [76]. The phenotype of familial hip dysplasia (Beukes type), mapped to chromosome 4q35, overlaps with MED and is grouped with AD-MED [2]. AR-MED appears to result exclusively from mutations in sulfate transporter solute carrier family 26 (SLC26A2). The reported birth prevalence of MED is 9 per 100,000 [1].

MED is a clinically variable disease that manifests in early to mid-childhood with joint pain and stiffness, particularly involving the hips and knees; mild to moderate short stature; and early-onset osteoarthritis [76]. Body proportions are normal, but fingers may be short. Accentuated thoracic kyphosis and back pain can be present. MED can be extremely difficult to diagnose due to relatively subtle abnormalities and wide clinical variability, both between and within families. Various complications, such as osteochondritis dissecans and mild myopathy, mimic other diseases, creating further confusion.

Pseudoachondroplasia typically manifests in the second year of life and is characterized by moderate to severe disproportionate short stature (long trunk with accentuated lumbar lordosis), ligamentous laxity, and degenerative joint disease.

Table 23.4 Features of multiple epiphyseal dysplasia and pseudoachondroplasia

Disorder	Multiple epiphyseal dysplasia	Pseudoachondroplasia
Inheritance	AR, AD	AD
Age of onset	Early to mid-childhood	1–2 y/o
Stature	Mild/moderately short	Moderate/severely short
Joints	Pain/stiffness Hip/knee	Laxity Many joints
Epiphyses	Hip, knee: irregular, fragmented Others: near normal, normal, or slightly small	All are small, irregular
Metaphyses	Normal	Flared, irregular
Spine	Increased thoracic kyphosis End-plate irregularities Platyspondyly	Increased lumbar lordosis Long trunk Mild platyspondyly Biconvex vertebrae Improves with age
Mutations and associated deformities		
COMP	Shallow, irregular acetabula, marginal spikes Fragmented, cracked distal femoral epiphyses Delayed bone age Irregular carpal contour, small MC epiphyses Mild spine abnormalities	
MATN3	Vertical striations: epiphyses at knee Mild spine abnormalities	
DTDST	Double-layered patella	

y/o years old

There may be an associated mild to moderate scoliosis and/or kyphosis as well as genu varus or valgus. In general, the skeletal findings are more severe than for MED, with characteristic spinal involvement as well as marked epiphyseal and metaphyseal abnormalities [3].

Diagnosing pseudoachondroplasia and MED can be difficult and often requires genetic analysis. Distinctive radiological features are associated with specific mutations and may help guide genetic testing. For example, patients with COMP mutations are likely to have shallow, irregular acetabula with marginal spikes, along with fragmented or cracked distal femoral epiphyses. Their hands and wrists typically demonstrate delayed bone age, irregular carpal contours, small, round metacarpal epiphyses, and brachydactyly. Vertical striations in the distal femoral and/or proximal tibial metaphyses with distinct epiphyseal changes increase the probability of MATN3 mutation. A double-layered patella is associated with, but not diagnostic of, a DTDST mutation (Fig. 23.62) [76]. The spine may be mildly abnormal in both COMP and MATN3 mutations.

Imaging

In MED, epiphyses at the hips and knees are often irregular, flat, fragmented, and sclerotic; the ankles, wrists, and hands may also be affected but can be normal (Fig. 23.63). Sometimes epiphyses are small but otherwise normal, and it may be necessary to correlate imaging with age-matched controls in order to suggest or confirm the diagnosis (Fig. 23.64). Irregularities of the articular surfaces can develop later. The metaphyses are often normal (Fig. 23.65). The spine may demonstrate various degrees of vertebral end-plate irregularity and decreased vertebral body height, particularly at the thoracolumbar junction (see Fig. 23.63).

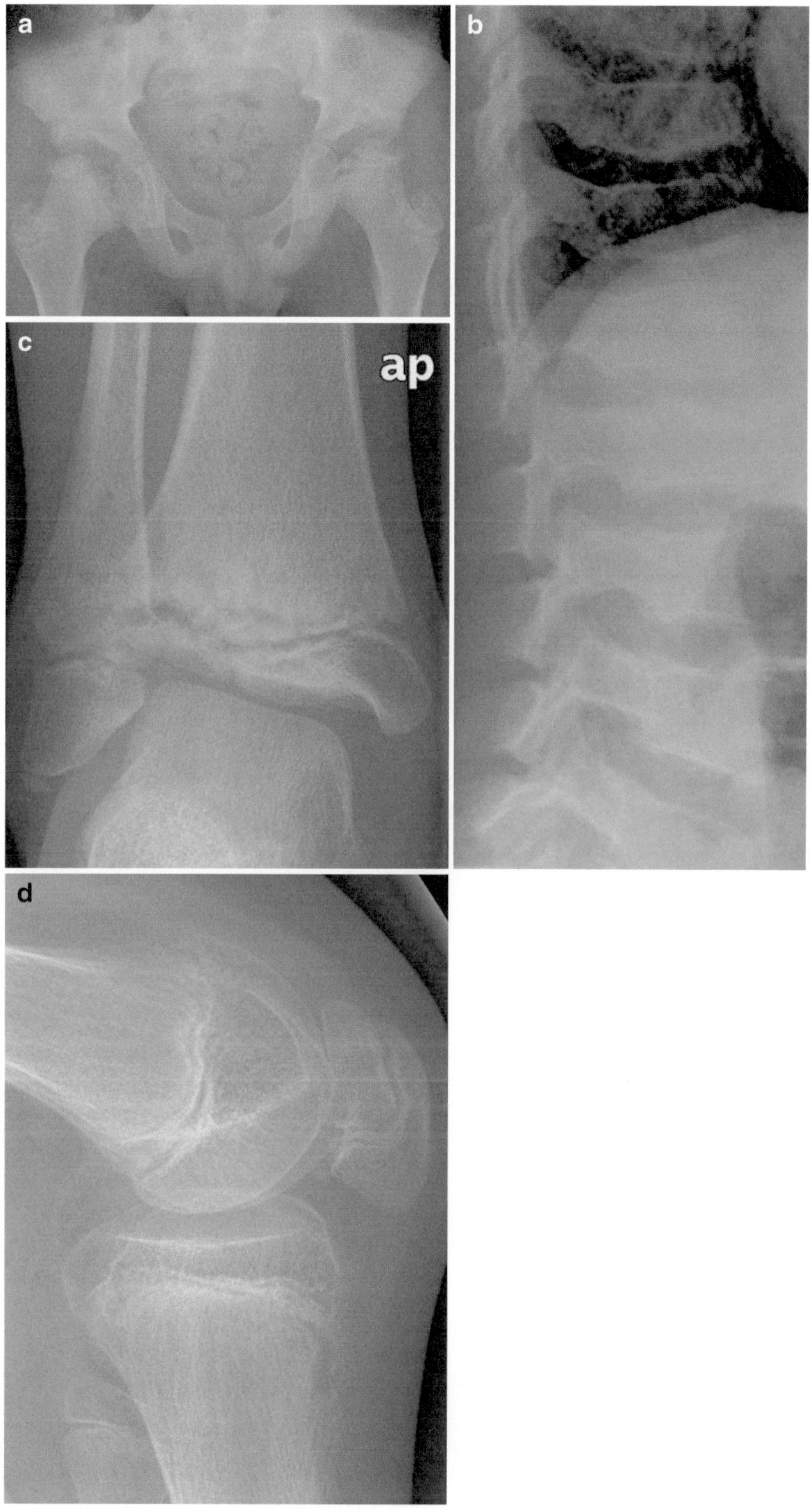

Fig. 23.62 Multiple epiphyseal dysplasia (MED) in a 9-year-old boy. (**a**) Bilateral irregular, flattened femoral heads, with irregular acetabula. (**b**) Mild platyspondyly, with irregular end plates. (**c**) Small, slightly fragmented distal tibial epiphysis, with mild metaphyseal irregularity and striation. (**d**) Double-layered patella, associated with DTDST mutation

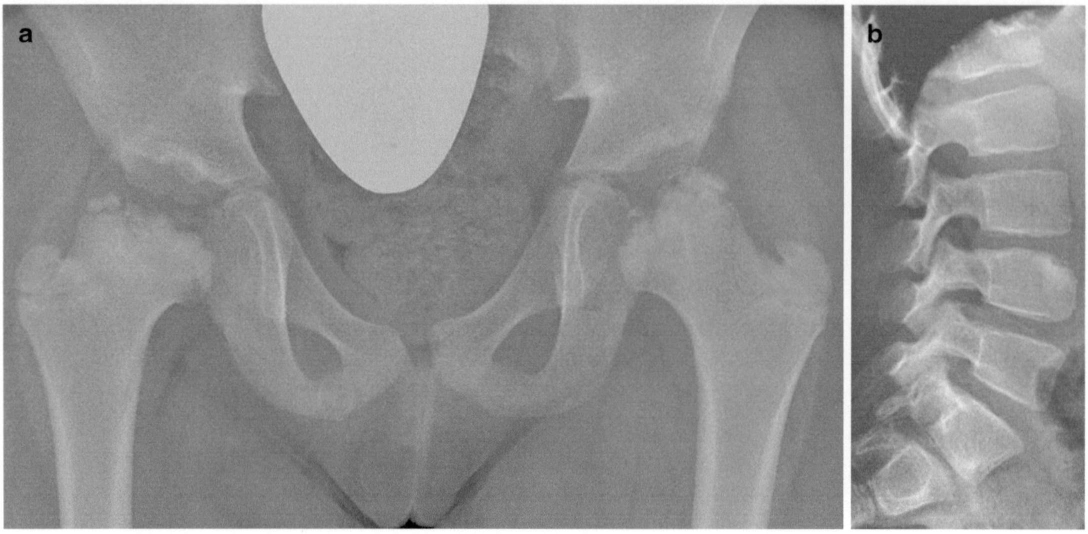

Fig. 23.63 MED in a 7-year-old asymptomatic girl, imaged because of a positive family history. (**a**) Epiphyses are small and fragmented. (**b**) The superior end plates at L1 and L4 are irregular

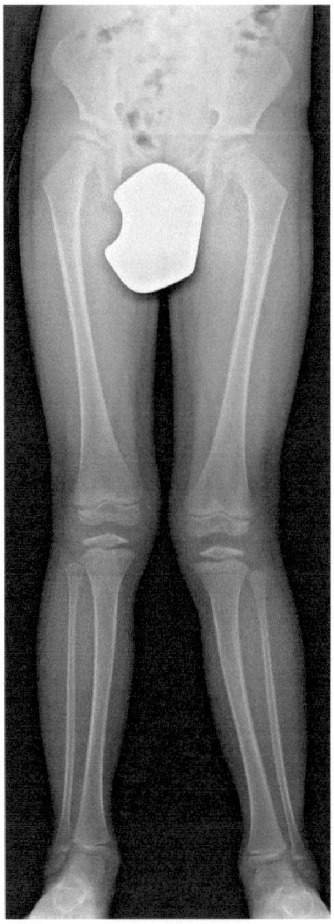

Fig. 23.64 MED in a 6-year-old. Most epiphyses appear small for age but otherwise almost normal (Courtesy of Rebecca Stein-Wexler)

In pseudoachondroplasia, the metaphyses are involved, as well as the epiphyses and spine (Fig. 23.66). The metaphyses may appear flared and irregular, and the epiphyses may appear small and irregular. The subchondral margins of the acetabula may be irregular, and the triradiate cartilage in the pelvis may be unusually wide. Mild platyspondyly with biconvex vertebral bodies and irregular end plates is common, but the appearance of the spine tends to improve with age.

Differential Diagnosis

Achondroplasia is differentiated from pseudoachondroplasia because it manifests at a younger age and is characterized by more severe abnormalities, an abnormal head, and relatively normal epiphyses. MED can be mistaken for bilateral Legg-Perthes or Meyer disease; careful clinical examination and radiographic evaluation of knees and ankles as well as the spine facilitates diagnosis.

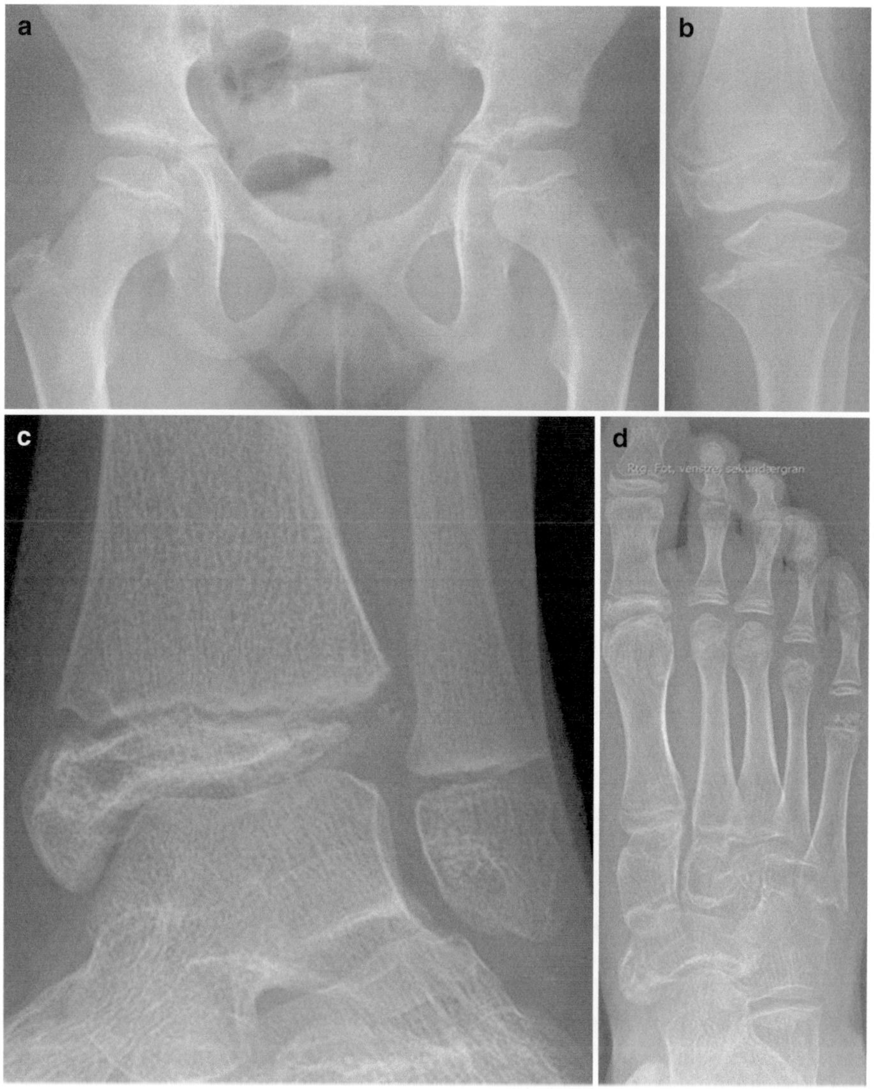

Fig. 23.65 MED in an 8-year-old girl who presented 5 years earlier with painful hips. Although the hip involvement is mild (**a**), with only slight flattening of the femoral heads, the epiphyses at the knee (**b**), ankle (**c**), and foot (**d**) are quite small and irregular. (**e**) The spine is almost normal

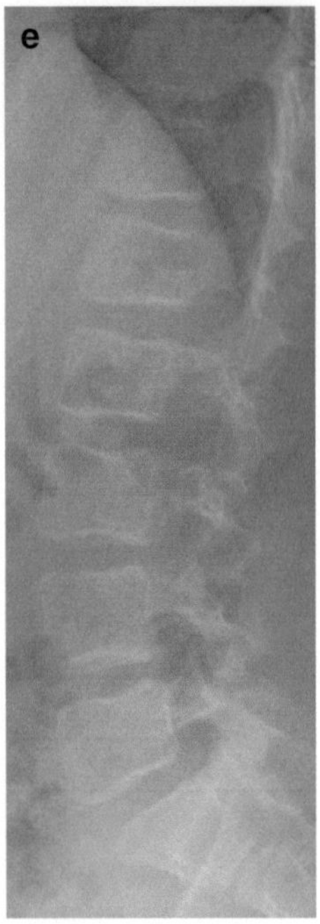

Fig. 23.65 (continued)

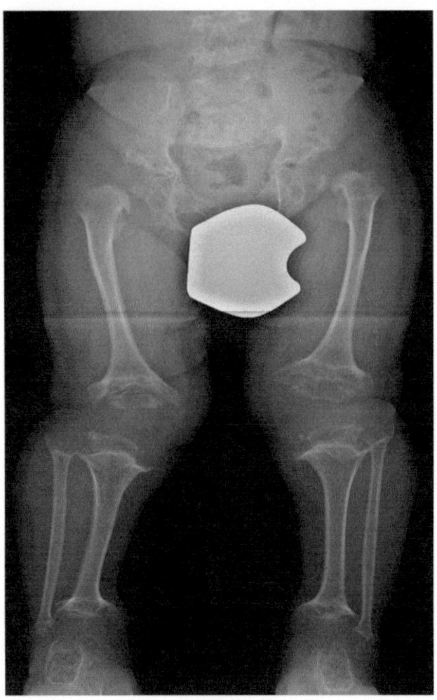

Fig. 23.66 Pseudoachondroplasia. All epiphyses are small and irregular. The tubular bones are shortened with wide, irregular metaphyses (a ball-in-socket appearance is seen at the ends of the femora and tibiae). The fibulae are disproportionately long. Acetabula are irregular, and vertebrae are short (Courtesy of Rebecca Stein-Wexler)

12 Brachyolmia

Also referred to as spondylodysplasia, this skeletal dysplasia is characterized by a short trunk and abnormal vertebrae. Inheritance is either autosomal dominant or autosomal recessive, and the disorder is believed to be a mild form of spondylo/spondylometaphyseal dysplasia (SMD) [77]. TRPV4 mutations have been found in patients diagnosed with the autosomal dominant form of brachyolmia, spondylometaphyseal dysplasia Kozlowski type, and metatropic dysplasia.

Different forms of brachyolmia are distinguished by their modes of inheritance and comorbidities. In all types, trunk length is normal at birth, but the spine fails to grow normally, and a short trunk manifests during childhood. Type I (Hobaek and Toledo, autosomal recessive) is characterized by short stature (late childhood) limited to the trunk, with associated spinal stenosis (in the Toledo subtype, there are also punctate corneal calcifications). Type 2 (Maroteaux, also autosomal recessive) shows similar childhood onset but has hypoplastic nails. Type 3 (autosomal dominant) demonstrates mild short stature and often presents with scoliosis [77].

Imaging

Platyspondyly is usually present, but it may be mild in type 3. Type 3 brachyolmia demonstrates "over-faced" pedicles (lateral extension of the lateral margins of the vertebral bodies and more medial appearance of the pedicles). In addition, there are end-plate irregularities and anterior vertebral body rounding (Fig. 23.67). Type 2 shows similar changes, along with narrowing of intervertebral disks. Type 1 is characterized by platyspondyly and end-plate interdentations, along with spinal stenosis, but the pedicles do not appear over faced. All types can exhibit mild metaphyseal abnormalities at the hips [77] (see Fig. 23.67).

Differential Diagnosis

Mild forms of spondylometaphyseal dysplasia are differentiated by more generalized metaphyseal

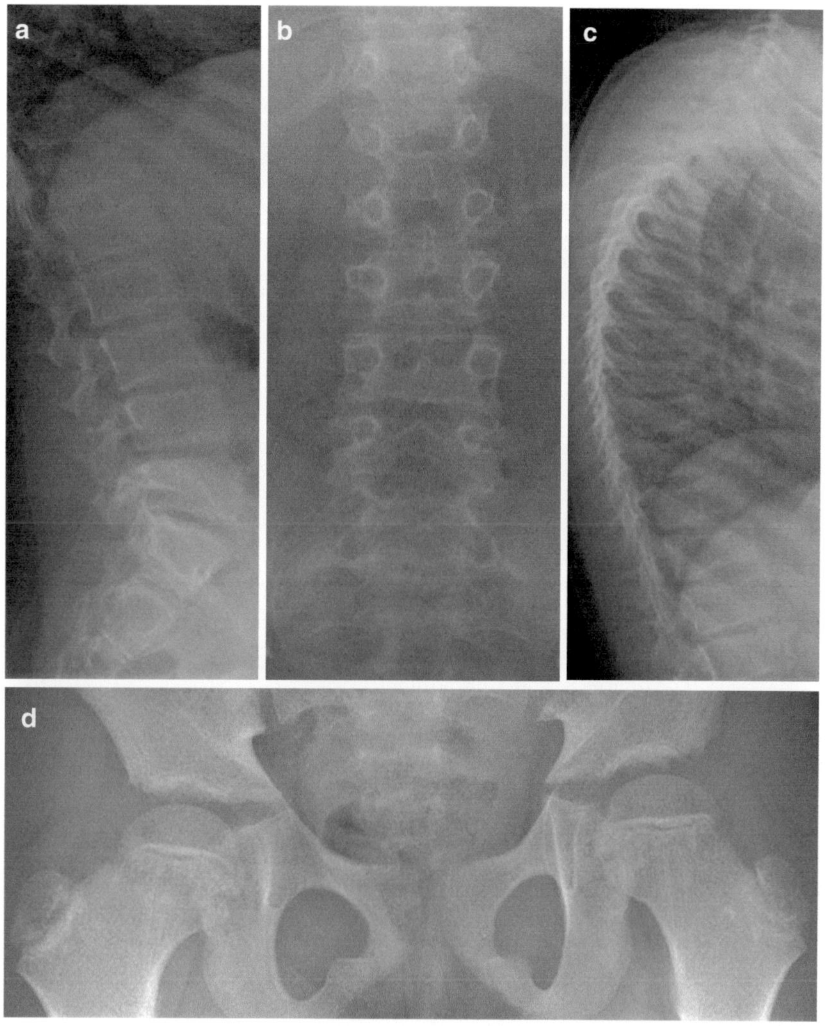

Fig. 23.67 Brachyolmia in a 12-year-old boy who presented at age 4 with back pain, stiffness, and short stature. (**a**–**c**) Moderate diffuse platyspondyly, end-plate irregularity, and decreased disc space. The pedicles appear over faced. (**d**) Irregular proximal femoral metaphyses, with mixed sclerosis and lucency, but relatively normal epiphyses

change. Scheuermann disease can resemble the autosomal dominant form of brachyolmia.

References

1. Lachman RS. Taybi and Lachman's radiology of syndromes, metabolic disorders and skeletal dysplasias. 5th ed. Philadelphia: Mosby Elsevier; 2007.
2. Warman ML, Cormier-Daire V, Hall C, Krakow D, Lachman R, LeMerrer M, et al. Nosology and classification of genetic skeletal disorders: 2010 revision. Am J Med Genet A. 2011;155A(5):943–68.
3. Spranger JW, Brill PW, Superti-Furga A, Unger S, Nishimura G. Bone dysplasias: an atlas of genetic disorders of skeletal development. 3rd ed. New York: Oxford University Press; 2012.
4. Schumacher R, Seaver L, Spranger J. Fetal radiology. A diagnostic atlas. Berlin: Springer; 2004.
5. Hall CM, Offiah AC, Forzano F. Fetal and perinatal skeletal dysplasias. An atlas of multimodality imaging. London: Radcliffe Publishing Ltd; 2012.
6. Steiner RD, Pepin MG, Byers PH. Osteogenesis imperfecta. In: Pagon RA, Bird TD, Dolan CR, Stephens K, editors. Gene reviews. Seattle: University of Washington; 1993. Available at: http://www.ncbi.nlm.gov/books/NBK1116/. Accessed April 11, 2014.
7. Rauch F, Glorieux FH. Osteogenesis imperfecta. Lancet. 2004;363(9418):1377–85.
8. van Dijk FS, Cobben JM, Kariminejad A, Maugeri A, Nikkels PG, van Rijn RR, et al. Osteogenesis imperfecta: a review with clinical examples. Mol Syndromol. 2011;2(1):1–20.
9. Jepsen KJ, Schaffler MB, Kuhn JL, Goulet RW, Bonadio J, Goldstein SA. Type I collagen mutation alters the strength and fatigue behavior of Mov13 cortical tissue. J Biomech. 1997;30(11–12):1141–7.
10. Jepsen KJ, Goldstein SA, Kuhn JL, Schaffler MB, Bonadio J. Type-I collagen mutation compromises the

post-yield behavior of Mov13 long bone. J Orthop Res. 1996;14(3):493–9.
11. Kleinman PK. Differentiation of child abuse and osteogenesis imperfecta: medical and legal implications. AJR Am J Roentgenol. 1990;154(5):1047–8.
12. Carty H. Differentiation of child abuse from osteogenesis imperfecta. AJR Am J Roentgenol. 1991;156(3):635–6.
13. Malmgren B, Norgren S. Dental aberrations in children and adolescents with osteogenesis imperfecta. Acta Odontol Scand. 2002;60(2):65–71.
14. Baljet B. Aspects of the history of osteogenesis imperfecta (Vrolik's syndrome). Ann Anat. 2002;184(1):1–7.
15. Sillence DO, Senn A, Danks DM. Genetic heterogeneity in osteogenesis imperfecta. J Med Genet. 1979; 16(2):101–16.
16. Sillence DO, Rimoin DL. Classification of osteogenesis imperfect. Lancet. 1978;1(8072):1041–2.
17. van Dijk FS, Pals G, van Rijn RR, Nikkels PG, Cobben JM. Classification of osteogenesis imperfecta revisited. Eur J Med Genet. 2010;53(1):1–5.
18. Byers PH, Wallis GA, Willing MC. Osteogenesis imperfecta: translation of mutation to phenotype. J Med Genet. 1991;28(7):433–42.
19. Marini JC, Forlino A, Cabral WA, Barnes AM, San Antonio JD, Milgrom S, et al. Consortium for osteogenesis imperfecta mutations in the helical domain of type I collagen: regions rich in lethal mutations align with collagen binding sites for integrins and proteoglycans. Hum Mutat. 2007;28(3):209–21.
20. Wallis GA, Sykes B, Byers PH, Mathew CG, Viljoen D, Beighton P. Osteogenesis imperfecta type III: mutations in the type I collagen structural genes, COL1A1 and COL1A2, are not necessarily responsible. J Med Genet. 1993;30(6):492–6.
21. Cabral WA, Chang W, Barnes AM, Weis M, Scott MA, Leikin S, et al. Prolyl 3-hydroxylase 1 deficiency causes a recessive metabolic bone disorder resembling lethal/severe osteogenesis imperfecta. Nat Genet. 2007; 39(3):359–65.
22. Bellary SS, Steinberg A, Mirzayan N, Shirak M, Tubbs RS, Cohen Gadol AA, et al. Wormian bones: a review. Clin Anat. 2013;26:922–7.
23. Dent JA, Paterson CR. Fractures in early childhood: osteogenesis imperfecta or child abuse? J Pediatr Orthop. 1991;11(2):184–6.
24. Carty H, Brunelle F, Stringer DA, Kao SCS, editors. Imaging children. 2nd ed. Edinburgh: Elsevier Churchill Livingstone; 2005.
25. Goldman AB, Davidson D, Pavlov H, Bullough PG. "Popcorn" calcifications: a prognostic sign in osteogenesis imperfecta. Radiology. 1980;136(2):351–8.
26. Glorieux FH, Rauch F, Plotkin H, Ward L, Travers R, Roughley P, et al. Type V osteogenesis imperfecta: a new form of brittle bone disease. J Bone Miner Res. 2000;15(9):1650–8.
27. Banta JV, Schreiber RR, Kulik WJ. Hyperplastic callus formation in osteogenesis imperfecta simulating osteosarcoma. J Bone Joint Surg Am. 1971;53(1):115–22.
28. Whyte MP, Obrecht SE, Finnegan PM, Jones JL, Podgornik MN, McAlister WH, et al. Osteoprotegerin deficiency and juvenile Paget's disease. N Engl J Med. 2002;347(3):175–84.
29. Kemp AM, Dunstan F, Harrison S, Morris S, Mann M, Rolfe K, et al. Patterns of skeletal fractures in child abuse: systematic review. BMJ. 2008;337:a1518.
30. Binkovitz LA, Sparke P, Henwood MJ. Pediatric DXA: clinical applications. Pediatr Radiol. 2007;37(7):625–35.
31. Uhlmann E, Plotkin S. Neurofibromatosis. In: Ahmad SI, editor. Neurodegenerative diseases. New York: Landes Bioscience and Springer Science+Business Media; 2012.
32. Huson SM, Compston DA, Clark P, Harper PS. A genetic study of von Recklinghausen neurofibromatosis in south east Wales. I. Prevalence, fitness, mutation rate, and effect of parental transmission on severity. J Med Genet. 1989;26(11):704–11.
33. Lammert M, Friedman JM, Kluwe L, Mautner VF. Prevalence of neurofibromatosis 1 in German children at elementary school enrollment. Arch Dermatol. 2005;141(1):71–4.
34. Bollag G, McCormick F, Clark R. Characterization of full-length neurofibromin: tubulin inhibits Ras GAP activity. EMBO J. 1993;12(5):1923–7.
35. Legius E, Marchuk DA, Collins FS, Glover TW. Somatic deletion of the neurofibromatosis type 1 gene in a neurofibrosarcoma supports a tumour suppressor gene hypothesis. Nat Genet. 1993;3(2):122–6.
36. Jouhilahti EM, Peltonen S, Heape AM, Peltonen J. The pathoetiology of neurofibromatosis 1. Am J Pathol. 2011;178(5):1932–9.
37. Melean G, Sestini R, Ammannati F, Papi L. Genetic insights into familial tumors of the nervous system. Am J Med Genet C Semin Med Genet. 2004;129C(1): 74–84.
38. Evans DG, Baser ME, McGaughran J, Sharif S, Howard E, Moran A. Malignant peripheral nerve sheath tumours in neurofibromatosis 1. J Med Genet. 2002;39(5):311–4.
39. Evans DG. Neurofibromatosis 2 [Bilateral acoustic neurofibromatosis, central neurofibromatosis, NF2, neurofibromatosis type II]. Genet Med. 2009;11(9): 599–610.
40. Baser ME, Friedman JM, Aeschliman D, Joe H, Wallace AJ, Ramsden RT, et al. Predictors of the risk of mortality in neurofibromatosis 2. Am J Hum Genet. 2002;71(4):715–23.
41. Patel NB, Stacy GS. Musculoskeletal manifestations of neurofibromatosis type 1. AJR Am J Roentgenol. 2012;199(1):W99–106.
42. Winter RB, Moe JH, Bradford DS, Lonstein JE, Pedras CV, Weber AH. Spine deformity in neurofibromatosis. A review of one hundred and two patients. J Bone Joint Surg Am. 1979;61(5):677–94.
43. Scott JC. Scoliosis and neurofibromatosis. J Bone Joint Surg Br. 1965;47:240–6.
44. Calvert PT, Edgar MA, Webb PJ. Scoliosis in neurofibromatosis. The natural history with and without operation. J Bone Joint Surg Br. 1989;71(2):246–51.
45. Ramachandran M, Tsirikos AI, Lee J, Saifuddin A. Whole-spine magnetic resonance imaging in

patients with neurofibromatosis type 1 and spinal deformity. J Spinal Disord Tech. 2004;17(6):483–91.
46. Ton J, Stein-Wexler R, Yen P, Gupta M. Rib head protrusion into the central canal in type 1 neurofibromatosis. Pediatr Radiol. 2010;40(12):1902–9.
47. Hall JG. Arthrogryphosis. In: Management of genetic syndromes. 2nd ed. Hoboken: Wiley; 2005. p. 63–75.
48. Lowry RB, Sibbald B, Bedard T, Hall JG. Prevalence of multiple congenital contractures including arthrogryposis multiplex congenita in Alberta, Canada, and a strategy for classification and coding. Birth Defects Res A Clin Mol Teratol. 2010;88(12):1057–61.
49. Sarwark JF, MacEwen GD, Scott Jr CI. Amyoplasia (a common form of arthrogryposis). J Bone Joint Surg Am. 1990;72(3):465–9.
50. Hall JG. Arthrogryposes (multiple congenital contractures). In: Principles and practice of medical genetics, vol. 3. 5th ed. Philadelphia: Churchill Livingstone–Elsevier; 2007. p. 3785–856.
51. Bevan WP, Hall JG, Bamshad M, Staheli LT, Jaffe KM, Song K. Arthrogryposis multiplex congenita (amyoplasia): an orthopaedic perspective. J Pediatr Orthop. 2007;27(5):594–600.
52. Wynne-Davies R, Williams PF, O'Connor JC. The 1960s epidemic of arthrogryposis multiplex congenita: a survey from the United Kingdom, Australia and the United States of America. J Bone Joint Surg Br. 1981;63-B(1):76–82.
53. Daher YH, Lonstein JE, Winter RB, Moe JH. Spinal deformities in patients with arthrogryposis. A review of 16 patients. Spine (Phila Pa 1976). 1985;10(7):609–13.
54. Megarbane A, Ravel A, Mircher C, Sturtz F, Grattau Y, Rethore MO, et al. The 50th anniversary of the discovery of trisomy 21: the past, present, and future of research and treatment of Down syndrome. Genet Med. 2009;11(9):611–6.
55. American Academy of Pediatrics Committee on Genetics. American Academy of Pediatrics: health supervision for children with Down syndrome. Pediatrics. 2001;107(2):442–9.
56. Caird MS, Wills BP, Dormans JP. Down syndrome in children: the role of the orthopaedic surgeon. J Am Acad Orthop Surg. 2006;14(11):610–9.
57. Shaw ED, Beals RK. The hip joint in Down's syndrome. A study of its structure and associated disease. Clin Orthop Relat Res. 1992;278:101–7.
58. Rees DC, Williams TN, Gladwin MT. Sickle-cell disease. Lancet. 2010;376(9757):2018–31.
59. Modell B, Darlison M. Global epidemiology of haemoglobin disorders and derived service indicators. Bull World Health Organ. 2008;86(6):480–7.
60. Ejindu VC, Hine AL, Mashayekhi M, Shorvon PJ, Misra RR. Musculoskeletal manifestations of sickle cell disease. Radiographics. 2007;27(4):1005–21.
61. Poupetova H, Ledvinova J, Berna L, Dvorakova L, Kozich V, Elleder M. The birth prevalence of lysosomal storage disorders in the Czech Republic: comparison with data in different populations. J Inherit Metab Dis. 2010;33(4):387–96.
62. Muenzer J. Overview of the mucopolysaccharidoses. Rheumatology (Oxford). 2011;50 Suppl 5:v4–12.
63. White KK. Orthopaedic aspects of mucopolysaccharidoses. Rheumatology (Oxford). 2011;50 Suppl 5:v26–33.
64. Weisstein JS, Delgado E, Steinbach LS, Hart K, Packman S. Musculoskeletal manifestations of Hurler syndrome: long-term follow-up after bone marrow transplantation. J Pediatr Orthop. 2004;24(1):97–101.
65. Lachman R, Martin KW, Castro S, Basto MA, Adams A, Teles EL. Radiologic and neuroradiologic findings in the mucopolysaccharidoses. J Pediatr Rehabil Med. 2010;3(2):109–18.
66. Brady RO. Gaucher's disease: past, present and future. Baillieres Clin Haematol. 1997;10(4):621–34.
67. Katz R, Booth T, Hargunani R, Wylie P, Holloway B. Radiological aspects of Gaucher disease. Skeletal Radiol. 2011;40(12):1505–13.
68. Somaraju UR, Tadepalli K. Hematopoietic stem cell transplantation for Gaucher disease. Cochrane Database Syst Rev. 2012;7:CD006974.
69. Beutler E. Gaucher disease: multiple lessons from a single gene disorder. Acta Paediatr Suppl. 2006; 95(451):103–9.
70. McHugh K, Olsen EOE, Vellodi A. Gaucher disease in children: radiology of non-central nervous system manifestations. Clin Radiol. 2004;59(2):117–23.
71. Solomon BD. VACTERL/VATER association. Orphanet J Rare Dis. 2011;6:56.
72. Hunter AG, Seaver LH, Stevenson RE. Limb-body wall defect. Is there a defensible hypothesis and can it explain all the associated anomalies? Am J Med Genet A. 2011;155A(9):2045–59.
73. Wright MJ, Irving MD. Clinical management of achondroplasia. Arch Dis Child. 2012;97(2):129–34.
74. Chitty LS, Griffin DR, Meaney C, Barrett A, Khalil A, Pajkrt E, et al. New aids for the non-invasive prenatal diagnosis of achondroplasia: dysmorphic features, charts of fetal size and molecular confirmation using cell-free fetal DNA in maternal plasma. Ultrasound Obstet Gynecol. 2011;37(3):283–9.
75. Lee ST, Song HR, Mahajan R, Makwana V, Suh SW, Lee SH. Development of genu varum in achondroplasia: relation to fibular overgrowth. J Bone Joint Surg Br. 2007;89(1):57–61.
76. Jackson GC, Mittaz-Crettol L, Taylor JA, Mortier GR, Spranger J, Zabel B, et al. Pseudoachondroplasia and multiple epiphyseal dysplasia: a 7-year comprehensive analysis of the known disease genes identify novel and recurrent mutations and provides an accurate assessment of their relative contribution. Hum Mutat. 2012;33(1):144–57.
77. Nemec SF, Cohn DH, Krakow D, Funari VA, Rimoin DL, Lachman RS. The importance of conventional radiography in the mutational analysis of skeletal dysplasias (the TRPV4 mutational family). Pediatr Radiol. 2012;42(1):15–23.

Neuromuscular Diseases

24

Elka Miller and Nagwa Wilson

Contents

E. Miller, MD (✉)
Department of Diagnostic Imaging,
Children's Hospital of Eastern Ontario,
Room 2148A, 401 Smyth Road,
Ottawa, ON K1H 8L1, Canada
e-mail: emiller@cheo.on.ca

N. Wilson, MS, MD, PhD
Department of Medical Imaging,
Montreal Children's Hospital, McGill University,
2300 Tupper Street, Montreal, QC H3H 1P3, Canada
e-mail: nagwa.wilson@muhc.mcgill.ca

Abstract

This chapter addresses neuromuscular disorders of the brain/upper motor neuron (cerebral palsy) and spinal cord/lower motor neuron (myelomeningocele, spinal muscular atrophy, spinal cord injury, and poliomyelitis). It then addresses Charcot-Marie-Tooth disease, an example of a disorder affecting the peripheral nerves. Muscular diseases are then discussed, such as Duchenne muscular dystrophy, myotonic disorders, and dermatomyositis. The chapter concludes with Friedrich ataxia and complex regional pain syndrome type 1. Imaging modalities and issues for each condition are considered by anatomic region, with focus on the manifestations and sequelae of common pathophysiologic processes.

Neuromuscular diseases encompass a large group of conditions affecting muscles and the nerves that control them; they can occur in utero or develop at any time from infancy through adulthood. Localizing the lesion to the brain/upper motor nerve, spinal cord/motor nerve, peripheral nerve, and muscle is essential to narrow the differential diagnosis. The type of weakness and the presence of increased muscle tone or bulk, Babinski sign, hypotonia, and delayed motor skills help determine whether the disorder is peripheral or centrally mediated. In either case, respiratory and cardiac complications, along with

R. Stein-Wexler et al. (eds.), *Pediatric Orthopedic Imaging*,
DOI 10.1007/978-3-642-45381-6_24, © Springer-Verlag Berlin Heidelberg 2015

joint contractures and other musculoskeletal abnormalities, may manifest at any time.

Genetic testing should be considered, as many pediatric neuromuscular disorders have a genetic basis. The World Muscle Society classification divides these diseases into genetic and acquired disorders in a regularly updated and extensive online genotype-phenotype table (http://194.167.35.195:3000/).

1 Brain/Upper Motor Neuron

1.1 Cerebral Palsy (Box 24.1)

Box 24.1: Musculoskeletal Imaging Abnormalities in Cerebral Palsy

Cerebral palsy

Location	Common musculoskeletal imaging abnormalities	Comment
Spine	Long C-shaped thoracolumbar scoliosis with pelvic obliquity, elongated vertebral bodies, increased thoracic kyphosis, lumbar lordosis	Early detection and treatment may prevent severe deformities
Upper extremity	Radial head dislocation, contractures, negative ulnar variance	Uncommon or often overlooked
Hip	Windblown deformity, increased femoral anteversion, coxa valga, subluxation, deformed femoral head	Early acetabular index measurements may predict future dislocation
Knee	Flexion contracture deformity (crouch knee), patella alta, patellar fragmentation, chondromalacia of patella	
Foot	Equinovalgus malalignment, hallux valgus	Associated ankle valgus

Cerebral palsy (CP) affects the brain and neurons above the anterior horn cells of the spinal cord; it results in spasticity and difficulty in controlling muscles. The most common cause of physical disability in childhood, it has an incidence of 2.0–2.5 per 1,000 live births [1]. A heterogeneous group of neurodevelopmental disorders, CP causes persistently impaired movement and posture. In 2004, the International Working Group on the Definition and Classification of Cerebral Palsy [2] defined CP as "a group of permanent disorders of the development of movement and posture, causing activity limitation, that are attributed to non-progressive disturbances that occurred in the developing fetal or infant brain. The motor disorders of CP are often accompanied by disturbances of sensation, perception, cognition, communication, and behavior; by epilepsy; and by secondary musculoskeletal problems."

Four major components determine the classification of CP: (1) type and severity of motor abnormalities, (2) anatomical and neuroimaging distribution, (3) associated non-motor impairments, and (4) timing of the presumed causal event (prenatal, perinatal, or postnatal) [3]. A widely used classification system differentiates motor abnormalities according to neuromuscular tone (hypotonia or hypertonia) by spastic (most common, 70 %), ataxic (5–20 %), dyskinetic (dystonia or choreoathetosis, 10–20 %), and mixed forms. The trunk and each of the limbs are assessed separately to define distribution (monoplegia, hemiplegia, diplegia, triplegia, and total body involvement). Although this system is clinically significant, it lacks inter-user reliability [4]. Palisano and colleagues [5] developed the gross motor function classification system (GMFCS), a five-level classification based on the child's motor abilities, functional limitations, and need for wheel mobility or assistive devices. This has become a simple, intuitive, complementary, and reliable tool to classify gross motor function in children with CP and has been implemented worldwide.

The underlying causes of CP are poorly understood. Several risk factors have been identified, but less is known about their interactions and how they relate to different pathophysiological pathways. A wide range of prenatal, perinatal, and postnatal

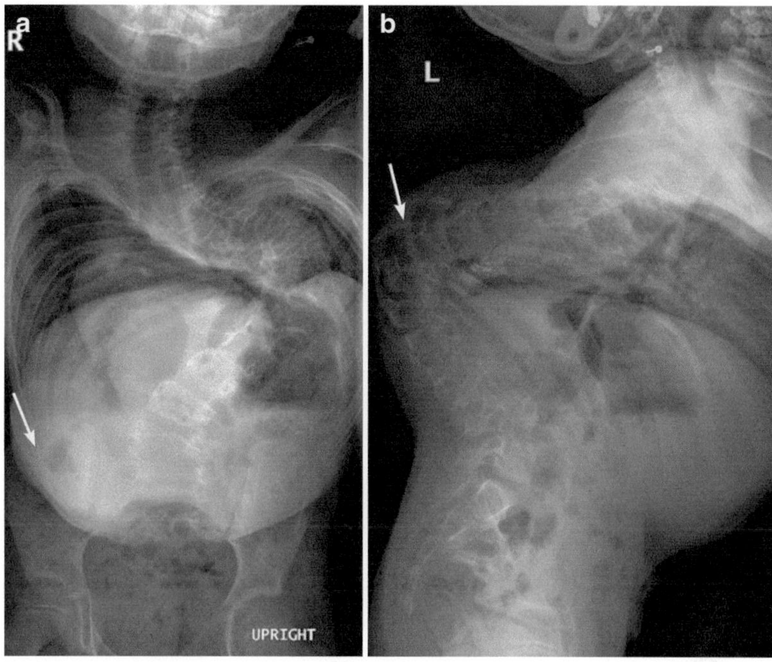

Fig. 24.1 Kyphoscoliosis in an 8-year-old with spastic diplegia. (**a**) Severe C-shaped levoconvex thoracolumbar scoliosis. The right ribs override the iliac crest (*arrow*). (**b**) Marked kyphosis centered at the lower thoracic spine (*arrow*)

factors can occur alone or in combination. Common risk factors include prematurity, low birth weight, birth asphyxia, fetal intrauterine exposure to maternal infection and inflammation, maternal fever during labor, multiple gestations, coagulation disorders, pre- or perinatal stroke, maternal thyroid disease, and placental pathology [6]. Recent evidence that CP may be caused by multiple genetic factors will likely influence future therapy [7]. Hypoxic ischemic encephalopathy is the major perinatal cause of neurological morbidity in both premature and full term newborns. Resulting from asphyxia in the preterm brain, mild to moderate injury results in damage to white matter, manifesting as periventricular leukomalacia or parenchymal hemorrhage; gray matter damage occurs in premature infants with profound hypoxic ischemic encephalopathy or in full-term infants [8].

Spasticity, which typically develops between 6 and 18 months of age, alters previously normal skeletal anatomy [9]. The paraspinal muscles, hip flexors, hip adductors, hamstrings, gastrocnemius, and soleus muscles are most commonly affected. Scoliosis, hip dislocation, and fixed contractures develop during periods of rapid growth and represent the most common progressive manifestations of CP.

In addition, children with CP are at increased risk of fractures due to disuse osteoporosis. Bisphosphonates may be used to increase bone density, reducing fracture risk from 30.6 to 13 % [10]. However, after bisphosphonate therapy fractures may occur at locations where there are large differences in bone density [11]; the transition in density may produce a so-called stress concentration or stress riser, which predisposes to fracture.

Spine

The prevalence of scoliosis in patients with spastic CP ranges from 15 to 61 % [12, 13]. Scoliosis in CP is more common in males and may be painful, whereas idiopathic scoliosis has an eight to one female predominance and is rarely painful. The risk of developing scoliosis increases with GMFCS level and age. Children in GMFCS level IV or V have a 50 % risk of developing moderate or severe scoliosis by 18 years of age, whereas children in GMFCS level I or II have almost no risk [12].

Patients with CP, especially those with spastic diplegia, often suffer from low back pain, which restricts their ability to walk and impairs their quality of life [14]. This may be due to increased thoracic kyphosis (Fig. 24.1) along with lumbar lordosis that results in compression and shearing

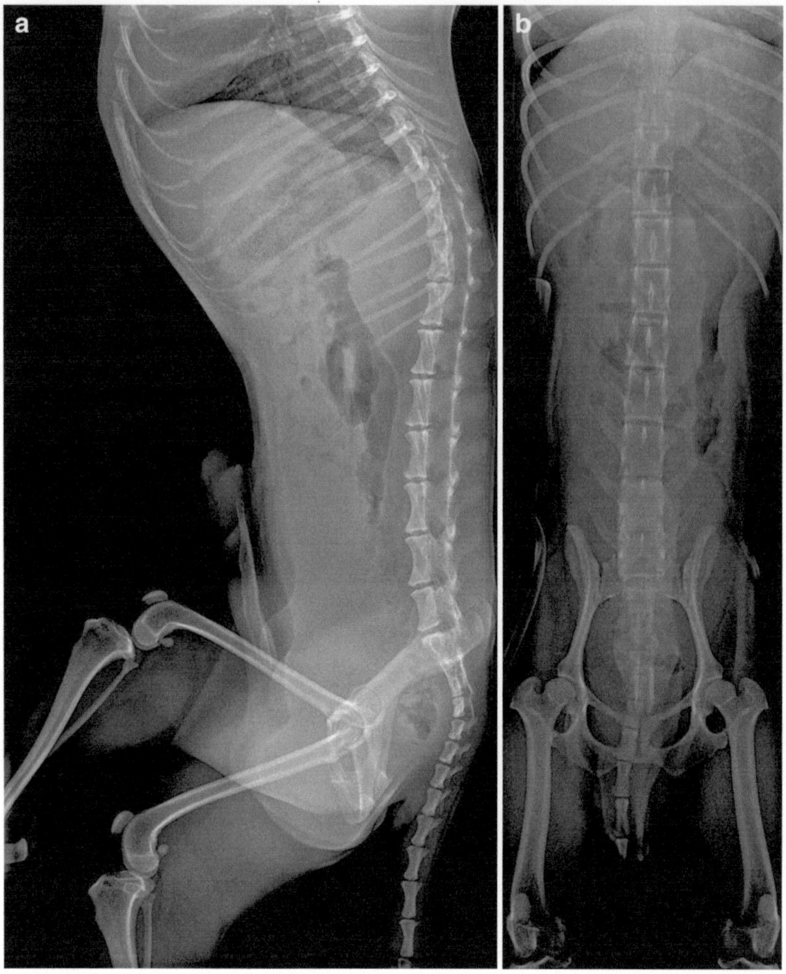

Fig. 24.2 (**a**, **b**) Canine vertebrae in a 2-year-old Maltese Terrier. The vertebral bodies are elongated and narrow, similar to those in patients with severe CP who have never born weight (Courtesy of Lynda Zucca)

forces, leading to spondylolysis and spondylolisthesis. Spondylolysis of the fifth lumbar vertebra is found in 21 % of children with CP, four times more often than in normal subjects [14].

In severely disabled patients, developmental abnormalities of the spine become evident in early childhood, presumably the result of decreased activity, lack of erect weight bearing, abnormal posture, and muscle imbalance. The vertebral bodies are elongated, with increased vertical height and decreased anteroposterior dimensions, resembling those of a dog (Fig. 24.2)—hence the term caninization. The end plates are often convex and the disk spaces small (Fig. 24.3).

In both mild and severe cases, a long C-shaped thoracolumbar curve is most common, followed by a lumbar curve (Fig. 24.4). Most curves evolve from postural to fixed deformities. Progression is greatest during rapid growth in middle adolescence and may continue after skeletal maturity (Fig. 24.5), especially when associated with pelvic obliquity [15]. In patients whose curve is less than 50° at skeletal maturity, researchers have reported an annual progression of 0.8°, whereas the annual progression is 1.4° in those whose curve exceeds 50° at maturity [16].

Two thirds of patients with scoliosis have fixed pelvic obliquity, and almost as many have hip subluxation. A characteristic "windblown" configuration with both femurs deviated toward the concave side of the curve may be seen, and in severe cases the ribs may override the iliac

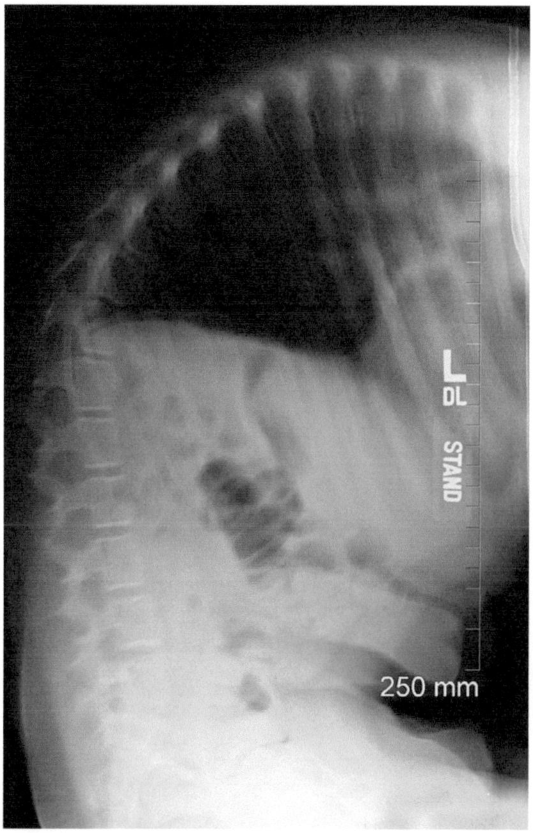

Fig. 24.3 Caninization of vertebrae in CP. The vertebral bodies are relatively tall, and the intervertebral spaces are narrow and aligned in severe kyphosis, likely due to muscle weakness (Courtesy of Rebecca Stein-Wexler)

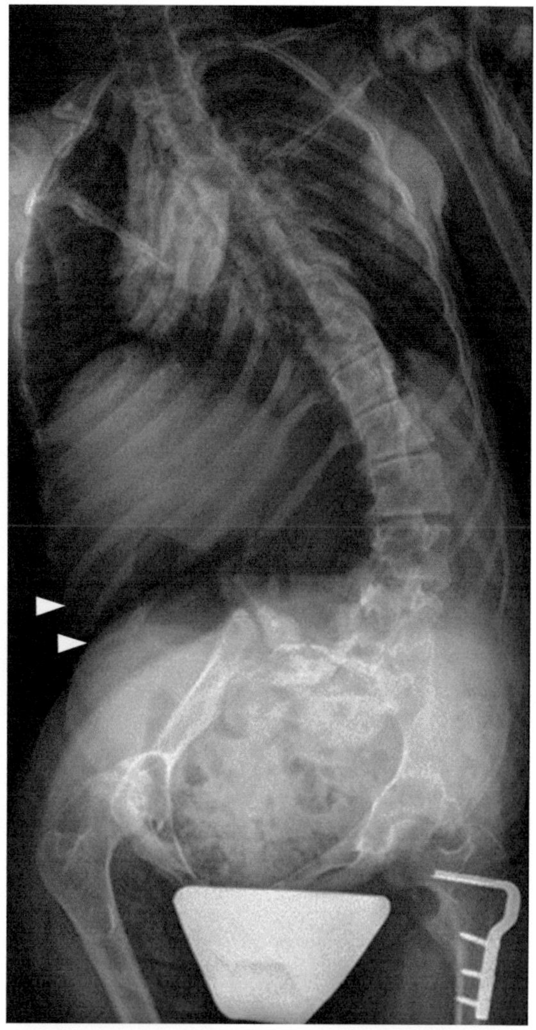

Fig. 24.4 Long C-shaped scoliosis in a 15-year-old girl with CP. The ribs are almost overriding the right iliac bone (*arrowheads*). Note the "windblown" configuration of the pelvis. Femoral hardware is from the right varus osteotomy

crest or even lie within the pelvic brim (see Fig. 24.4).

Treatment

The primary goal of treatment is to improve sitting balance and prevent curve progression. External bracing is poorly tolerated and rarely successful, and therefore, surgical procedures such as anterior release or fusion combined with posterior fusion may be necessary. Correction of increased kyphosis, pelvic obliquity, hip flexion deformity, and hip dislocation is also helpful [17] and contributes to improved quality of life [18].

Upper Extremity

Radial head dislocation is rarely reported, and the incidence of the condition is unknown. Posterior dislocation is most common and is probably caused by combined effects of muscle imbalance, spasticity, and contracture. Elbow, wrist, and finger contractures also occur. Negative ulnar variance can be seen in children with more severe muscle imbalance and tone [19] (Fig. 24.6). If radial head dislocation is painful, excision may be more successful than reconstruction [20].

Lower Extremity

Hip

The prevalence of hip subluxation and dislocation in CP ranges between 3 and 75 % [21]. Progressive

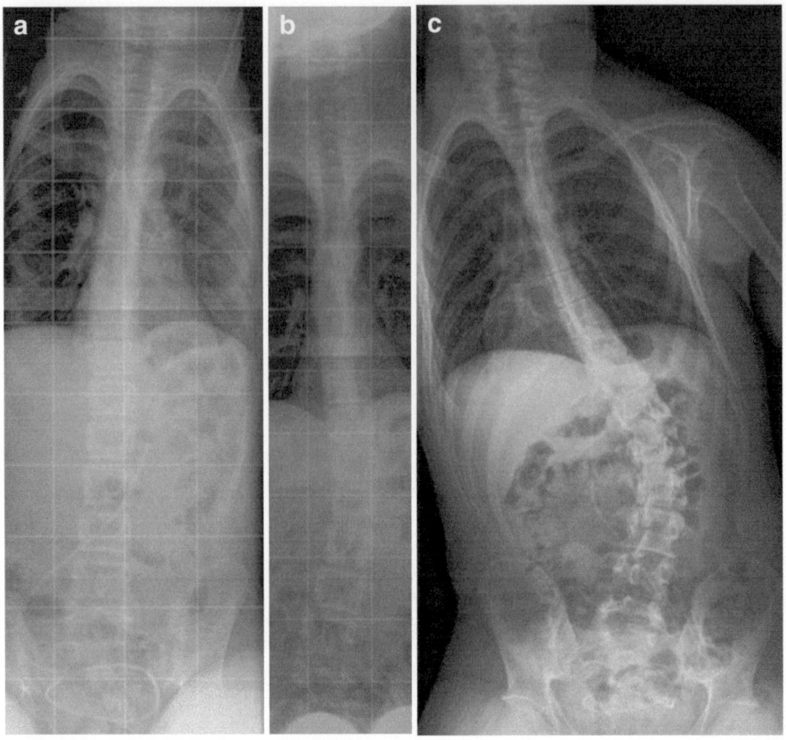

Fig. 24.5 Progressive thoracolumbar scoliosis in CP. Sequential radiographs demonstrate (**a**) normal alignment at age 13, (**b**) 19° of scoliosis at age 15, and (**c**) further progression at age 17

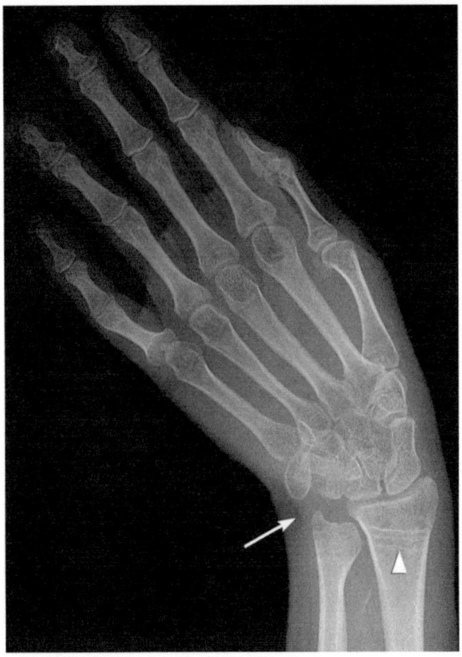

Fig. 24.6 Varus deviation of the hand in a 16-year-old with CP and developmental delay. There is minimal negative ulnar variance (*arrow*). Note diffuse osteopenia with multiple growth arrest lines in the proximal radial metaphysis (*arrowhead*)

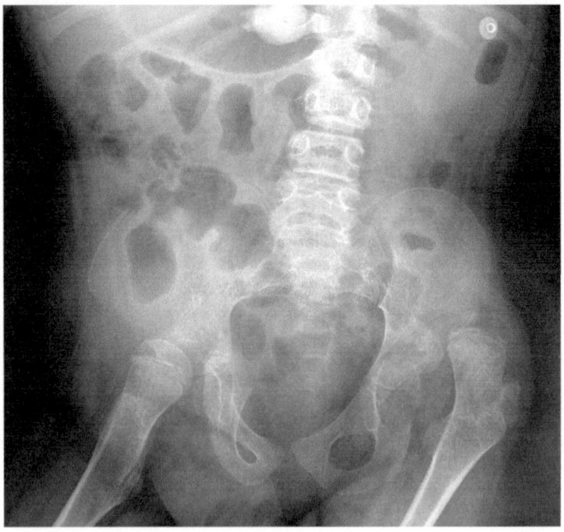

Fig. 24.7 Windblown pelvis in a 10-year-old boy. The right hip is abducted, and the left adducted and also dislocated. Shallow left acetabulum (Courtesy of Tal Laor, Cincinnati Children's Hospital)

hip flexion and adduction lead to windblown deformity (Fig. 24.7), increased femoral anteversion, coxa valga (real or apparent), subluxation, and deformity of the femoral head (Fig. 24.8).

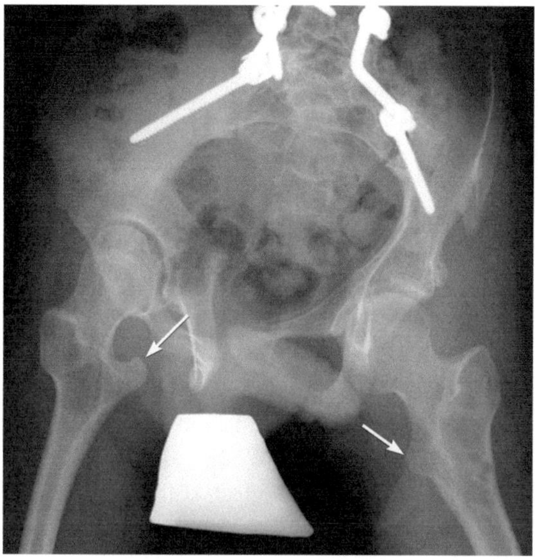

Fig. 24.8 Pelvic deformity in a 16-year-old boy with CP. There is bilateral external rotation and abduction. The pelvis is oblique, with apparent right acetabular protrusion. Prominent lesser trochanters (*arrows*)

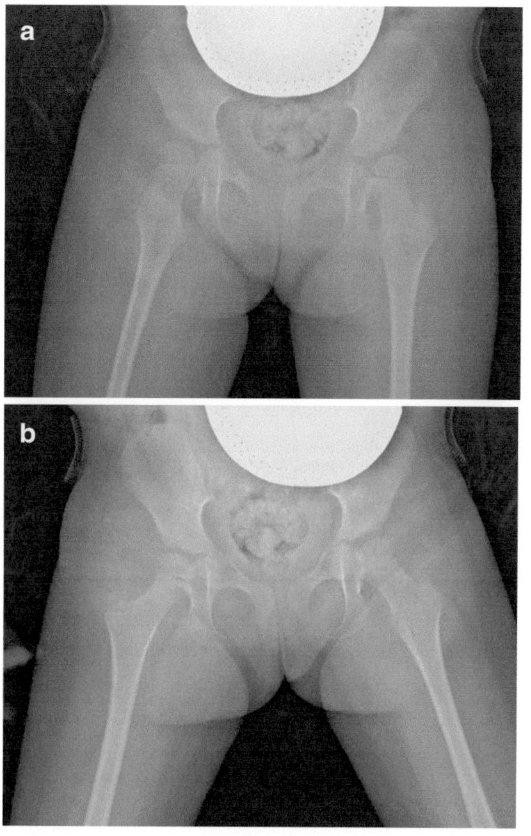

Fig. 24.9 Apparent coxa valga in a 4-year-old girl with CP (GMFCS V). (**a**) Supine frontal view with hips in external rotation shows apparent coxa valga on the *right*, with a neck-shaft angle of 180°. (**b**) Frontal view on the same date with hips internally rotated (and abducted). The femoral neck-shaft angle now appears normal at 160° (Courtesy of Jon R. Davids)

Complete hip dislocation is uncommon in patients with CP. Typically, the spastic adductor and iliopsoas muscles induce a twisting or internal rotation of the femur along its longitudinal axis. Thirty to fifty degrees in normal infants, this anteversion should diminish during childhood and measure 8–15° by skeletal maturity.

Patients with spastic CP have normal anteversion at birth, but abnormal muscle forces prevent the decrease in torsion that typically occurs after age 2 or 3, causing increased femoral neck anteversion to persist. The anteversion angle averages 55° in children with CP and is even larger in nonambulatory patients [15, 22].

The extent of anteversion is usually assessed clinically, but it can also be calculated from limited magnetic resonance imaging (MRI) [23] or computer tomography (CT) [24, 25], with cuts through the hips and knees. The angle is determined by measuring the angle that the femoral neck makes to a transverse plane through the femoral condyles when the femur is viewed on end [15]. (See Chap. 13 for detailed presentation of measurement technique.)

The femoral neck-shaft angle, measured on a true frontal radiograph, is the angle between the mid-axis of the femoral shaft and a line along the mid-axis of the femoral head and neck. This can be measured on a true frontal radiograph. However, both increased femoral anteversion and improper positioning of the femur can result in projectional foreshortening of the femoral neck, generating the false impression of an increased neck-shaft angle [15]. This should be described as "apparent coxa valga" (Fig. 24.9). In cases of severe CP, valgus may truly be present.

A radiograph with hips internally rotated accurately depicts the neck-shaft angle. Optimal alignment of the proximal femur for radiographic analysis can be assessed by the appearance of the greater and lesser trochanters. The lesser trochanter should not be visualized, whereas the greater trochanteric apophysis should be seen in its entirety. If the lesser trochanter is visualized and the apophysis of the greater trochanter is obscured, then the femur is externally rotated and not properly positioned for accurate assessment of the neck-shaft angle; this positioning results in apparent coxa valga. External rotation of the upper femur causes the lesser trochanter to appear prominent (Fig. 24.10).

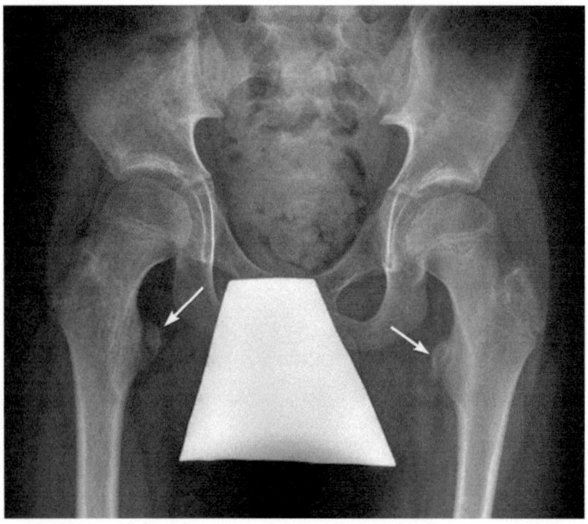

Fig. 24.10 External rotation with increased femoral anteversion in a patient with CP causing valgus appearance of the femoral necks as well as lesser trochanter prominence (*arrows*)

Femoral head position is initially normal or only slightly subluxated, but severe subluxation is common by age 7 (Fig. 24.11) [26]. Incomplete lateral coverage of the femoral head is not necessarily due to subluxation, but can result from pelvic obliquity, adductor contracture, increased femoral neck anteversion/valgus, or disparity in size between the femoral head and the acetabulum. Furthermore, acetabular dysplasia and secondary degenerative joint disease result from chronic subluxation, and mobility may be impaired [27]. Medial flattening and a triangular or V shape of the femoral head may develop as subluxation progresses (Fig. 24.12) [27]. Abnormal forces may result in irregular ossification of the femoral heads (Fig. 24.13).

The aim of treatment is to prevent adduction and flexion deformity and progression to subluxation or dislocation [26]. Nonsurgical management entails stretching the spastic agonist muscles, strengthening the weaker antagonist muscles, and splinting in abduction. Surgical procedures include tenotomy. Correction of actual coxa valga and femoral anteversion can be achieved by varus derotation osteotomy.

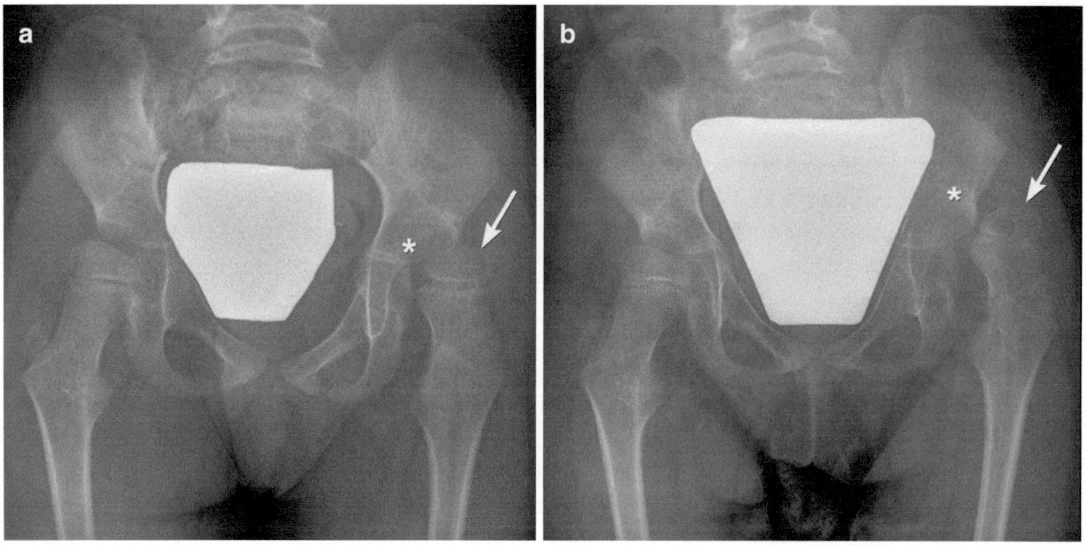

Fig. 24.11 Progressive superolateral migration of the left femoral head in a patient with severe dyskinetic CP. (**a**) At 3 years old, there is mild superolateral migration of the left femoral head (*arrow*) and acetabular dysplasia (*). (**b**) Three years later, the hip is dislocated (*arrow*), and a pseudoacetabulum has formed (*). Bilateral apparent coxa valga

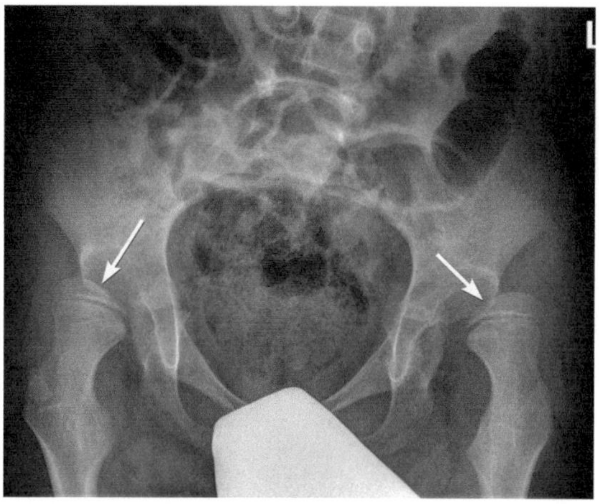

Fig. 24.12 Bilateral superolateral dislocation of the hips in a 9-year-old boy with CP. Note symmetric flattening of the medial aspects of both femoral heads (*arrows*)

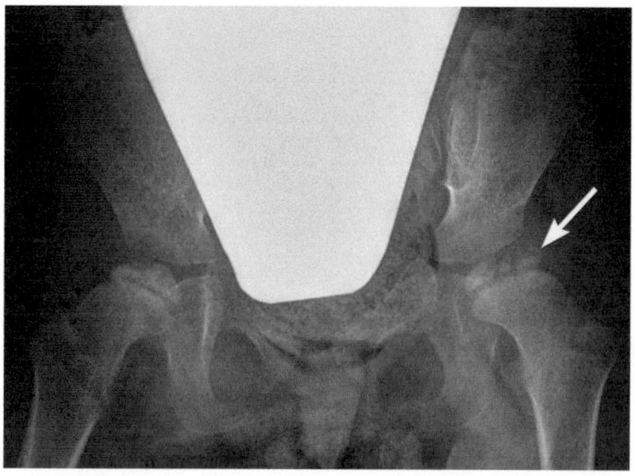

Fig. 24.13 Disturbed ossification of the femoral heads in a 5-year-old patient with spastic quadriplegic CP. Abnormal forces result in irregular ossification of the femoral heads, more pronounced on the left (*arrow*). However, the overlying cartilage is probably intact

Knee

Flexion contracture deformity (crouch knee) is the most common knee abnormality in spastic CP. Crouch knee is associated with hip and ankle flexion contractures. Increased force on the quadriceps muscles as well as overstretch of the infrapatellar tendon lead to patella alta, patellar fragmentation, chondromalacia, joint instability, muscle weakness, and pain [28]. Projectional overriding of the femoral condyles and tibial plateau due to fixed flexion contracture may make it difficult to obtain a satisfactory frontal radiograph (See Chap. 11 for discussion of techniques for measuring patella alta.)

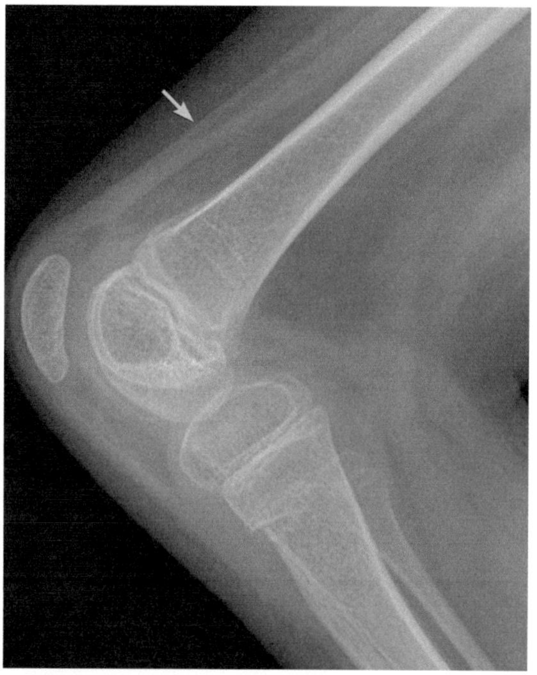

Fig. 24.14 Knee in a 9-year-old boy with paraplegic CP. The patella is elongated and crescent shaped. Bones are osteopenic, and muscles atrophic due to disuse (*arrow*)

Other patellar abnormalities include an elongated or crescent-shaped patella (Fig. 24.14), fragmentation of the lower pole of the patella, chondromalacia, and Osgood-Schlatter-like changes in the tibial tubercle. Hyperextension of the knee (genu recurvatum) is common in spastic CP due to progressive rectus femoris contracture together with abnormally long hamstrings and equinus foot deformity [29].

Ankle and Foot

The most common complaint related to foot deformity in children with CP is pain with ambulation or use of orthoses. Abnormal shoe wear patterns are often evident. Foot deformities usually result from imbalance between the extrinsic muscles of the lower leg that control foot and ankle alignment [30]. This may be secondary to spasticity, disrupted motor control, and/or impaired balance. Typically, the ankle plantar flexors (gastrocnemius and soleus) are overactive, and the ankle dorsiflexors are ineffective.

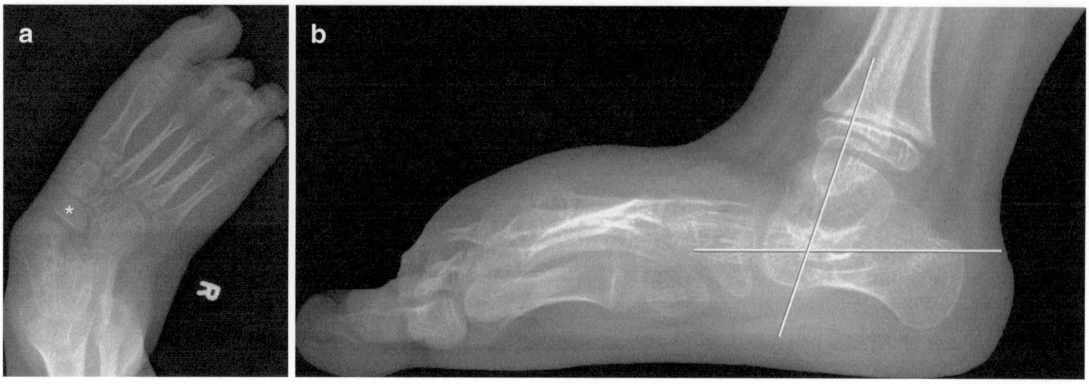

Fig. 24.15 Foot deformity in a patient with spastic CP. (**a**) There is hindfoot and forefoot valgus with the talus directed medial to the base of the first metatarsal. The navicular (*) is laterally displaced relative to the talus. (**b**) The talus is almost vertical, with its long axis almost parallel to that of the tibia. The talocalcaneal angle is increased

In children with CP, there are three common coupled foot and ankle segmental malalignment patterns: equinus, equinoplanovalgus, and equinocavovarus. In addition, there are two common secondary malalignments, ankle valgus and hallux valgus, which may be associated with any of the three segmental malalignment patterns. (See Chap. 15 for more detailed discussion of these abnormalities, as well as specific information on measurement techniques.) Standardized radiographic analysis of foot deformity in these children should include three views: frontal and lateral views of the foot, along with a frontal view of the ankle. Although it is difficult to obtain weight-bearing projections in severely disabled children, they are necessary for standardization and later comparison.

Equinus at the Ankle

Equinus results from fixed spastic contracture of the gastrocnemius and soleus, causing the characteristic tiptoe or toe-heel gait. Equinus is commonly associated with knee flexion and valgus or varus deformity of the hindfoot and forefoot.

Equinovalgus Malalignment

This is characterized by equinus deformity of the hindfoot, coupled with pronation deformity of the midfoot and forefoot. As the contracture worsens, the calcaneus becomes displaced posterolaterally and everts, allowing the talus to drop into a vertical position (Fig. 24.15), with eventual rocker-bottom deformity (increased talocalcaneal angle) (Fig. 24.16). Ankle valgus and hallux valgus deformities are frequently associated with equinovalgus foot. Equinovarus is less common but can be present in up to 20 % in patients with spastic CP.

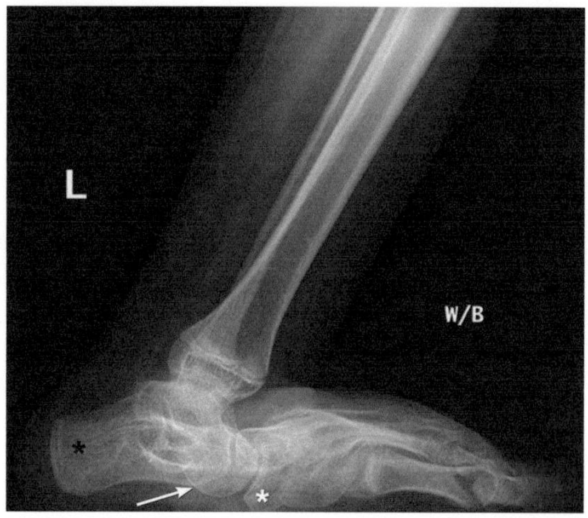

Fig. 24.16 Rocker-bottom deformity in a 13-year-old boy with spastic CP. Lateral weight-bearing view shows posterior displacement of the calcaneus (*black asterisk*) and vertical talus (*arrow*) resulting in rocker-bottom deformity. The navicular (*) is displaced downward by the vertical talus. The tibia and fibula are inclined anteriorly with respect to the long axis of the foot. Note fatty infiltration of the muscles

Ankle Valgus

This is determined by the tibiotalar angle, assessed on a frontal weight-bearing ankle radiograph (Fig. 24.17). Ankle valgus is often corrected when it contributes to hindfoot valgus deformity. The goal of treatment of ankle and

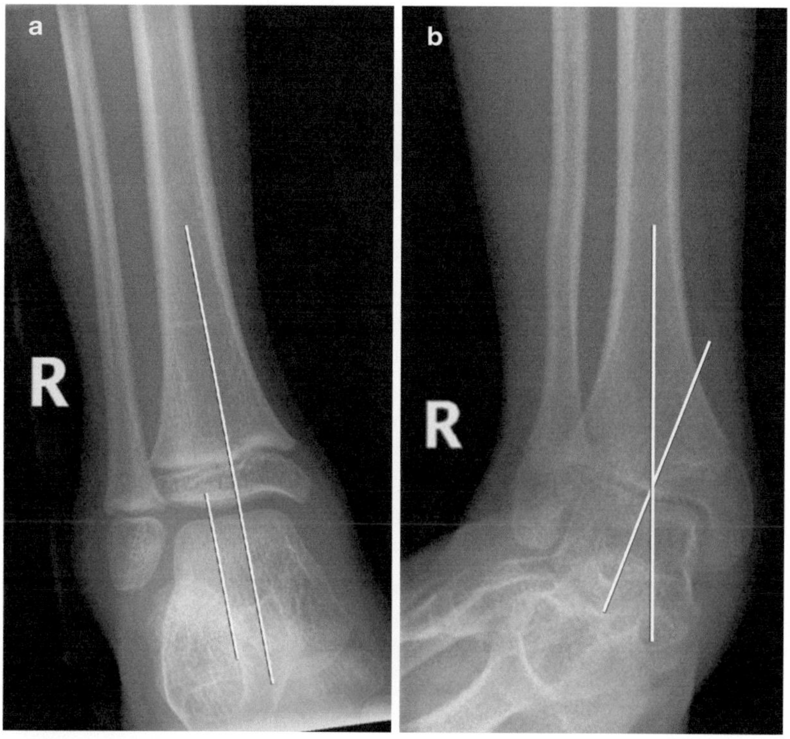

Fig. 24.17 Ankle valgus deformity in a 13-year-old boy with spastic diplegia. (**a**) Normal ankle for comparison, with the long axis of the talus parallel to that of the tibia. (**b**) There is lateral tilt of the talus with respect to the long axis of the tibia

foot deformities is to increase function by preventing and correcting deformities.

Treatment
Early management of spasticity with pharmacologic injections (e.g., *Botulinum* toxin), neurosurgery (selective dorsal rhizotomy, intrathecal baclofen), and application of orthotics helps prevent the development of fixed deformities of the muscle-tendon unit. Musculoskeletal surgeries include tendon transfer to address dynamic muscle imbalance and osteotomies/arthrodeses to fix malalignment that cannot be corrected simply by manipulation [15, 30].

2 Spinal Cord/Motor Unit Lesions

Spinal cord/motor unit lesions constitute a group of disorders that affect nerve fibers traveling from the spinal cord to the muscles. They include developmental disorders of the spinal cord (neural tube defects), spinal cord trauma, and hereditary and infectious disorders of the anterior horn cells (spinal muscular atrophy, poliomyelitis).

Flaccid paralysis, which is accompanied by muscle atrophy, helps identify lower motor neuron defects. Neural tube defects, such as myelomeningocele, are among the most common disorders requiring imaging prior to orthopedic management. Although myelomeningocele is often characterized as a typical lower motor neuron lesion, it is frequently accompanied with upper motor neuron signs, including spinal cord reflex activity and spasticity. Loss of proprioception and sensation challenges bony stabilization procedures in patients with myelomeningocele.

2.1 Developmental: Neural Tube Defects (Dysraphism)

Spinal dysraphism encompasses a group of congenital anomalies caused by defective neural tube closure and anomalous differentiation of the caudal cell mass. Neural tube defects refer to a wide range of abnormalities that result from the maldevelopment of the neuropore and the adjacent mesodermal and ectodermal structures during embryogenesis (see Chap. 3 for further discussion of spine development). The defects are classified as open or closed according to the presence or absence of exposed neural tissue. Open spina bifida ("spina bifida aperta") is caused by the failure of primary neurulation, resulting in exposed neural tissue or meninges with or without cerebrospinal fluid leakage. It includes two main types: myelomeningocele and meningocele. Myelomeningocele is a severe form in which the neural tissue and the meninges protrude through an opening in the spine, whereas with meningocele only the meninges protrude. Incidence in males and females is equal.

Spina bifida occulta is caused by defects in secondary neurulation and includes diastematomyelia, diplomyelia, dorsal dermal sinus, spinal lipoma, and isolated bone defects. In these forms, skin covers the neural elements, but there may be overlying cutaneous lesions such as nevi or depigmentation, hairy patches, hemangiomas, dimples, and subcutaneous lipomas. Occult lesions are more common in boys than in girls [31].

Neural tube defects result from multifactorial genetic, environmental, and combined factors. Chromosome malformations are present in a small minority of individuals, most frequently trisomy 13 or 18. Maternal diabetes, folic acid deficiency, and anticonvulsant drugs are a few common environmental risk factors that may cause neural tube defects; with widespread use of antenatal screening and folic acid dietary supplementation, the incidence has fallen [32].

Prenatal diagnosis of open spina bifida is common in countries with advanced medical care and is based on ultrasound (US) evidence of associated cerebral signs, including ventriculomegaly, scalloping of the frontal bones, and abnormal curvature of the cerebellar hemispheres. Evaluation of the spine may show absence of the dorsal arches or interrupted skin contour with or without meningocele and splaying of the laminae (Fig. 24.18). The antenatal diagnosis of closed spina bifida is difficult since cranial signs are absent and diagnosis relies only on direct evidence of the lesion, hydrosyringomyelia, or a low-lying cord—all difficult to identify by prenatal US although they are readily apparent at MRI (Fig. 24.19).

Myelomeningocele (Box 24.2) accounts for more than 98 % of open spinal dysraphisms [33]. Up to 85 % of myelomeningocele patients

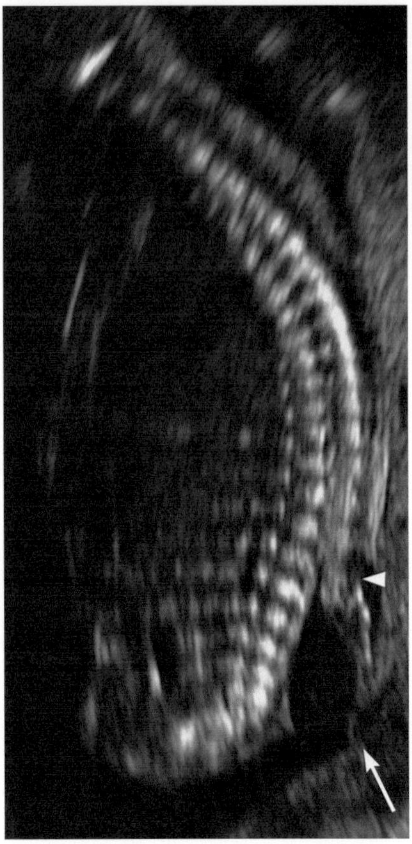

Fig. 24.18 Prenatal sagittal US at 17 weeks gestational age shows a meningocele sac (*arrow*) and a defect in the posterior elements of the spine (*arrowhead*) (Courtesy of Felipe Moretti)

Box 24.2: Common Musculoskeletal Imaging Abnormalities in Myelomeningocele

Myelomeningocele

Location	Common musculoskeletal imaging abnormalities
Spine	Scoliosis: congenital or acquired
	Kyphosis: congenital or acquired
	Developmental lordosis
Hip	Subluxation and dislocation
	Coxa valga
	Contractures
Knee	Extension and flexion contractures deformities
Foot	Equinus deformity
	Calcaneus foot
	Valgus deformity
	Clubfoot
	Vertical talus

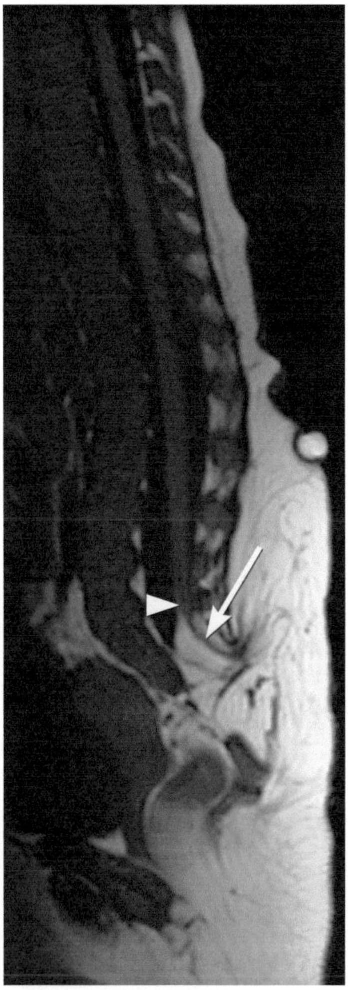

Fig. 24.19 Newborn with lipomyeloschisis, a type of skin-covered spina bifida. Sagittal T1-W MRI shows a low lying cord (*arrowhead*) reaching the sacral level and connecting with deep extension of a subcutaneous lipoma through spinal dysraphism (*arrow*)

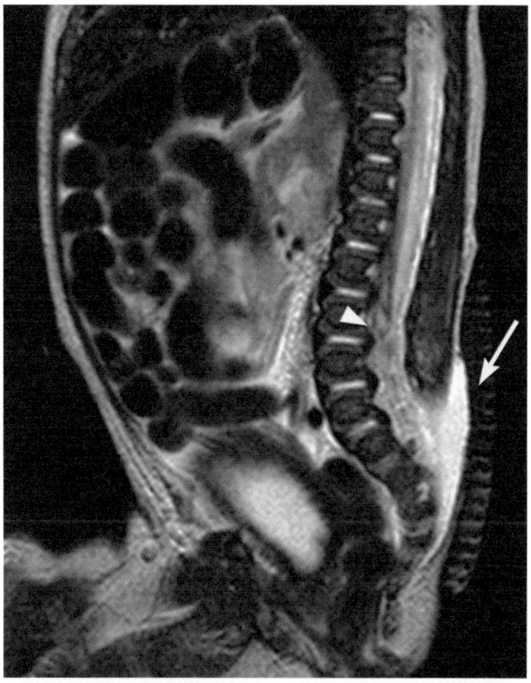

Fig. 24.20 Newborn with a lumbosacral myelomeningocele. A sagittal T2-W MRI shows complete absence of the midline posterior cartilage, muscle, and skin layers at the level of the open spinal dysraphism (*arrow*). The distal spinal cord is low lying (*arrowhead*). There was also a Chiari II malformation of the brain (not shown)

have coexisting hydrocephalus, and nearly all have an associated Chiari II malformation [34] (Fig. 24.20).

The child with myelomeningocele needs intensive support from a multidisciplinary team that includes radiologists, neurosurgeons, orthopedic surgeons, urologists, neurologists, and rehabilitation therapists. Bone abnormalities associated with myelomeningocele may be congenital or acquired, specific to myelomeningocele or similar to deformities seen in other conditions. Most of these deformities occur in childhood. Acquired abnormalities are caused by paralysis, muscle imbalance, bone malformation, or a combination of factors. The level of dysraphism may cause weakness or paralysis of agonist muscle groups and spasticity of antagonist groups, leading to dynamic muscle imbalance, disrupted musculoskeletal growth, and functional impairment.

All children with myelomeningocele have some degree of tethered cord, and this typically persists or recurs after surgical release due to scarring or adhesions. This tethering of the neural elements may not cause problems, but pain, decreased function in the lower extremities, and progressive scoliosis may be clinical signs of a significant tethering lesion. Tethered cord should be suspected as a cause of scoliosis in children younger than 6 years old with a high lumbar lesion.

Imaging

Prenatal imaging often begins with US. Fetal MRI is complementary, providing superior anatomic resolution regardless of maternal body

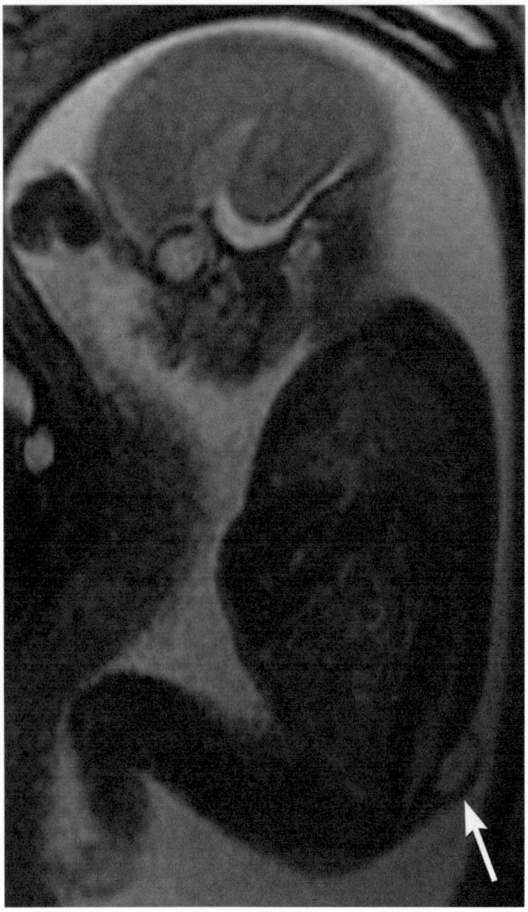

Fig. 24.21 Meningocele in a 23-week-old fetus. Sagittal FIESTA (fast imaging employing steady-state acquisition) MRI shows a lumbosacral defect and meningocele (*arrow*)

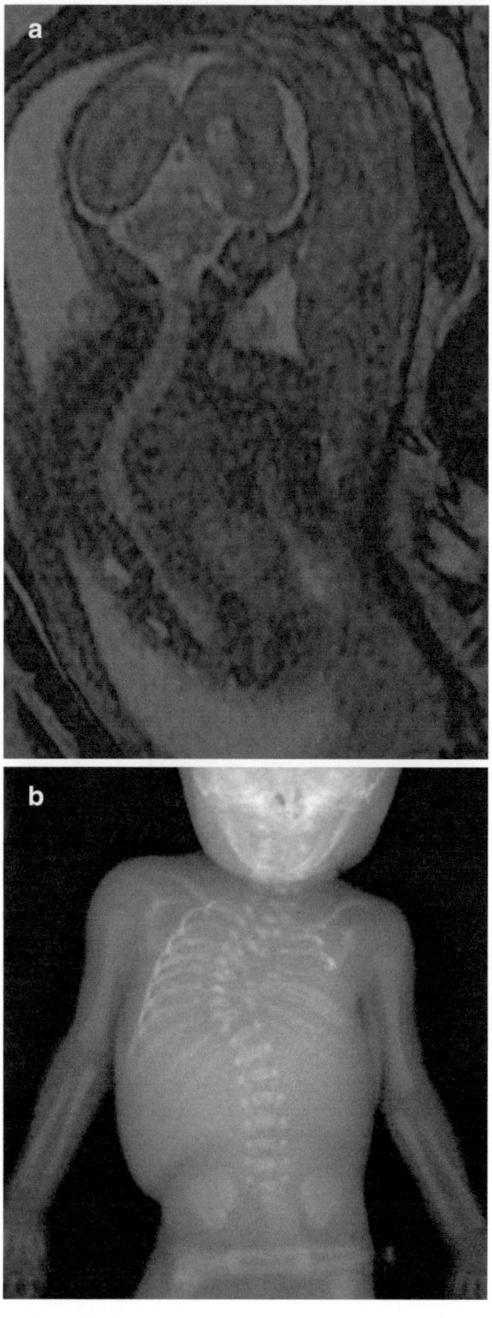

Fig. 24.22 Thoracic scoliosis in a 22-week-old fetus. (**a**) Coronal FIESTA MRI shows dextroscoliosis. (**b**) Postmortem radiograph shows fixed scoliosis with multiple vertebral segmentation anomalies and chest deformity (Courtesy of Julie Hurteau-Miller)

habitus or fetus position. Fetal MRI facilitates recognition of the craniocervical abnormalities of Chiari II malformation and delineation of less common types of dysraphism (Fig. 24.21), such as terminal myelocystocele [35] or lipomeningocele [36]. It also provides the opportunity to evaluate congenital scoliosis (Fig. 24.22).

Postnatal imaging should include cranial and renal ultrasound, which can be performed after surgical correction of dysraphism. Severe kyphosis may displace the psoas muscles anteriorly, which pushes the kidneys together so they may abut each other at the midline, putting them at risk during surgery. In addition, cross-sectional imaging may show that the aorta is unusually short, and it may have an abnormal branching pattern. Brain MRI is especially important in the neonate with brainstem-related symptoms, as it allows

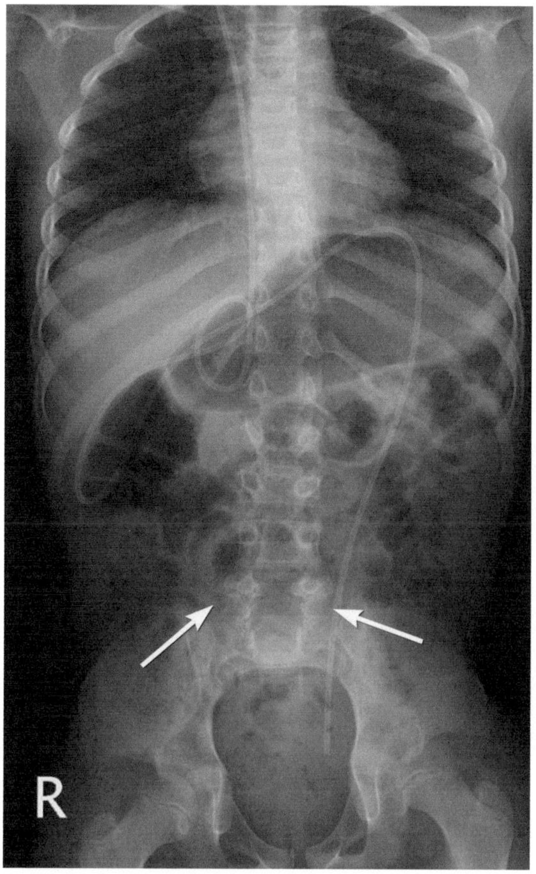

Fig. 24.23 Spinal dysraphism, L5 and sacrum (*arrows*). Note absent spinous processes from L5 to S5. Ventriculoperitoneal shunt

assessment of the brainstem and craniocervical junction. Presurgical spine radiographs are helpful, and spine MRI may be needed if the clinical features are atypical or to help with surgical decision-making.

Radiographs are helpful later in life to assess scoliosis, hip position, and other associated bone abnormalities. If there is spinal deformity, spine radiographs should be performed annually, but rapidly progressive curves or curves associated with neurological manifestations should be imaged with MRI of the brain and spine [37]. Supine frontal and lateral spine radiographs allow assessment of structural dysraphism and hip position, but as the child matures, upright views are essential to demonstrate the effect of gravity.

The frontal projection demonstrates fusiform increase in interpediculate distance, with the widest separation at the midsegment; this point also corresponds to the apex of the kyphosis (if present). Disk spaces are narrowed and vertebral bodies appear to be widened, although measurement may not confirm this. The spinous processes are absent and laminae cannot be identified, as they are forced outward by the expanding meningocele and therefore project anteriorly and laterally (Fig. 24.23). The transverse processes project forward and the pedicles laterally. The facets may be fused into a continuous mass that is initially cartilaginous and later osseous (Fig. 24.24). In infants, the normal anterior vertebral body notch is often absent at the defect level.

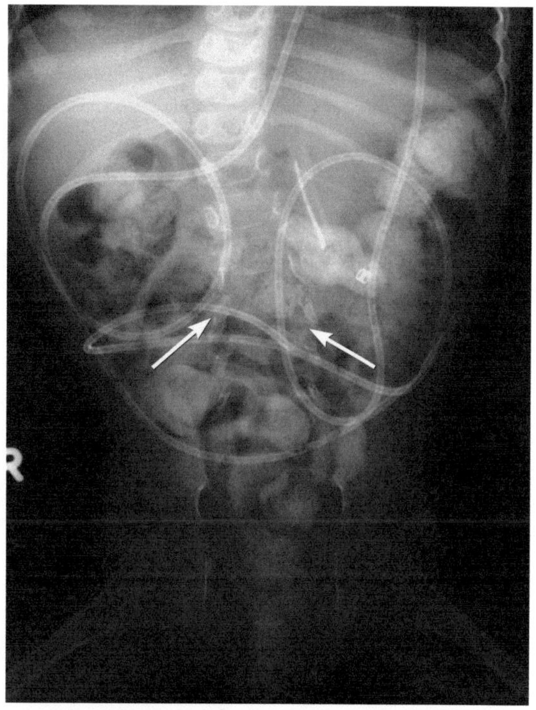

Fig. 24.24 Lumbosacral dysraphism. The vertebrae are wide, and the interpediculate distance is increased. There are no identifiable lumbar laminae or spinous processes, and the pedicles project laterally (*arrows*). Note fecal retention, gastrostomy tube, and ventriculoperitoneal shunt tubing, all associated findings in patients with meningomyelocele

Scoliosis

Spinal curvature is common, including scoliosis, kyphosis, and lordosis. These deformities

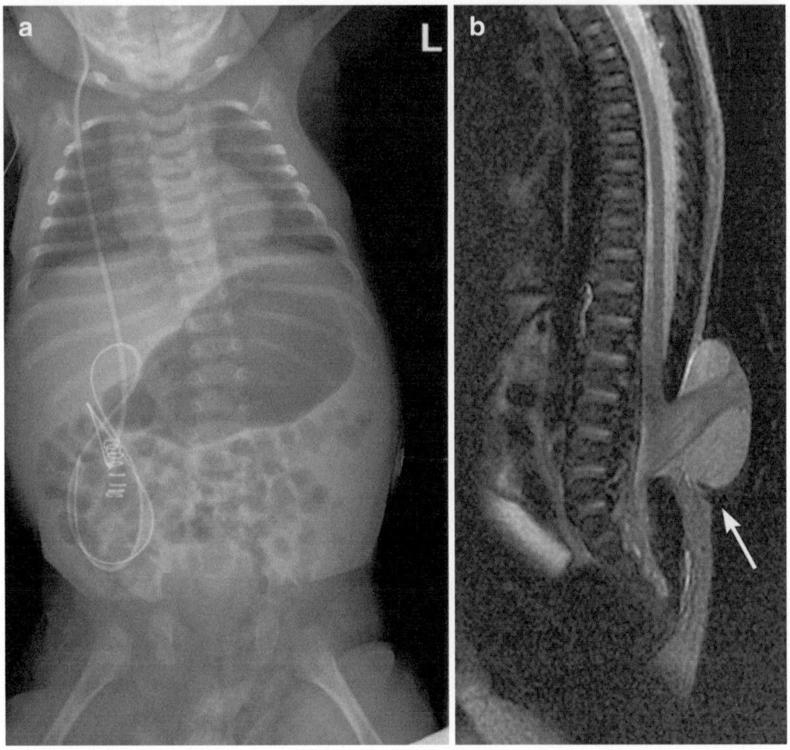

Fig. 24.25 Newborn with myelomeningocele and congenital scoliosis. (**a**) There is mild thoracolumbar C-shaped levoscoliosis. (**b**) Sagittal T2-W MRI shows low-lying cord, lumbar dysraphism, and herniation of the meninges and neural tissue (*arrow*), fusing with neural placode

can be congenital or acquired. Congenital curves are less common, present in only about 15 % of children, and associated with hemivertebrae or bony bars. They are unlikely to progress. Most curves are acquired, caused by mechanical instability; these tend to increase during childhood, as paresis progresses [38, 39]. The progressive nature of these deformities may cause severe disability and interfere with both rehabilitation and ambulation. A review of the predictors of scoliosis in patients with myelomeningocele found that most curves develop early in life (Fig. 24.25) [40], about 40 % of curves begin to form after age 9, and a few develop later, up to about 15 years of age.

Clinically significant scoliosis in patients with myelomeningocele is defined as a curve with a Cobb angle measuring more than 20°, because smaller curves often fluctuate, resolve, or even reverse direction [40]. Children with a thoracic neurological injury level have a 90 % incidence of scoliosis [41], with curves often greater than 45°. The lower the dysraphic defect, the less the incidence of scoliosis. Only 10 % of those with dysraphism at or below L4 will develop scoliosis.

Scoliosis in children with myelomeningocele can be attributed to muscle weakness due to high paraplegia, asymmetric paralysis, or spastic hemiplegia due to hydrocephalus. This usually causes a C-shaped scoliosis with associated kyphosis (Fig. 24.26). S-shaped scoliosis can occur in children with hydromyelia or hydrosyringomyelia with hydrocephalus [42]; shunting may halt the progression of neurological deficits, but usually does not result in recovery of function, and scoliosis may still progress. Scoliosis may be accompanied by pelvic obliquity, which may compromise seating balance and lead to ischial pressure sores.

Increasing scoliosis should prompt assessment for hydrocephalus, shunt-related complications, syrinx, and recurrent tethering of the cord (Fig. 24.27). Recurrent tethering at the site of the initial neural canal closure is quite common [43]. MRI of the brain and spine depicts most of these entities, but re-tethering of the cord can be difficult to assess and requires

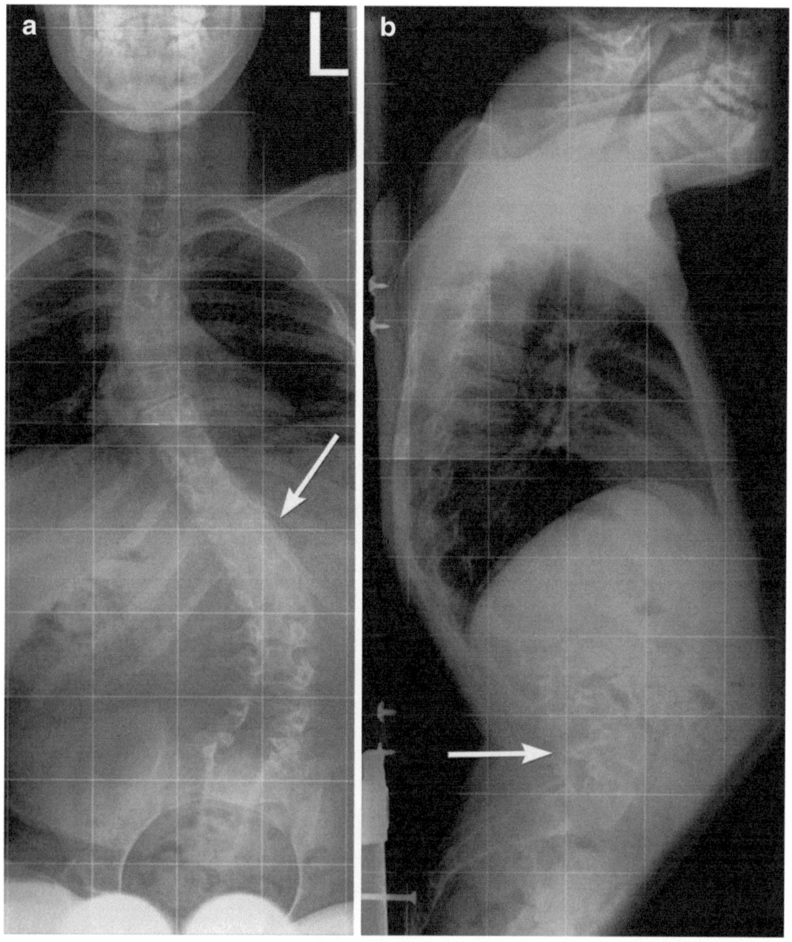

Fig. 24.26 Kyphoscoliosis in a 14-year-old boy with myelomeningocele. (**a**) The neural arch defect begins at about T10 (*arrow*). (**b**) Thoracic kyphosis is centered at this level, and there is also exaggerated lumbar lordosis (*arrow*)

clinical correlation. CT or limited MRI can be used to follow hydrocephalus.

Large curves may cause pain, make sitting in a chair difficult, and restrict pulmonary function (Fig. 24.28). If scoliosis continues to progress (Fig. 24.29) after neurological problems have been corrected, orthopedic treatment should be considered, as symptoms may improve following spinal realignment with fusion [44]. Conservative orthotic treatment is relatively ineffective for curve correction. Spinal fusion with correction of scoliotic deformity can improve pulmonary function and sitting balance as well as prevent further progression of the curve. Careful planning for spinal surgery is required as children with myelomeningocele are at increased risk of wound infections, pseudarthrosis, and progression of deformity.

Kyphosis

Kyphosis usually occurs in the lower thoracic and upper lumbar spine, with an incidence of 10–46 %. Lumbar kyphosis at birth can make closing the skin and meningeal defects difficult. Later, progression of the kyphosis can lead to breathing difficulties because crowded abdominal structures press upward on the diaphragm. Children also have difficulty feeding, since they often lean forward and must therefore use their hands to support themselves; this may lead to failure to thrive [45]. Treatment is not easy but should be initiated early to increase abdominal space, avoid pressure on the diaphragm and lungs, and improve truncal balance.

Congenital kyphosis is characterized by a severe angular deformity with a prominent gibbus at the apex of the curve. Paralytic kyphosis is more

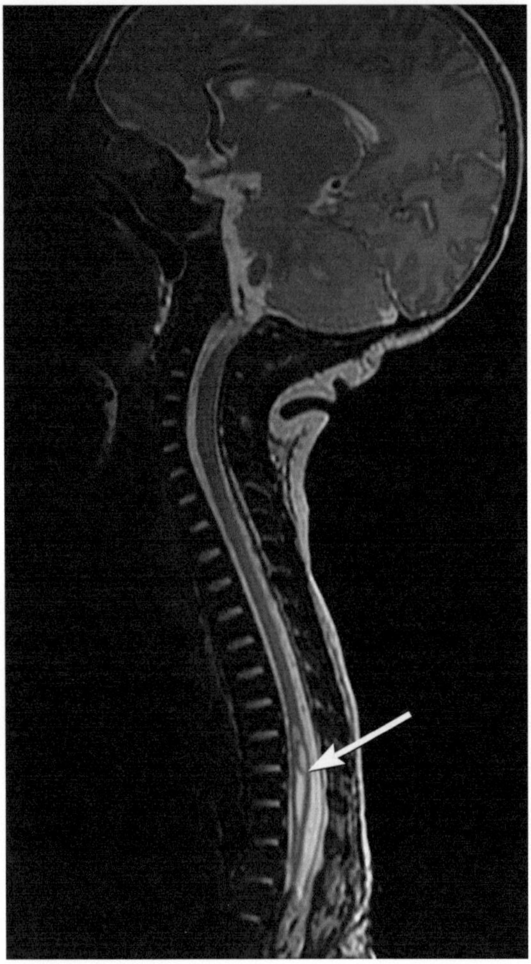

Fig. 24.27 Newly developed syrinx in a child with repaired myelomeningocele and increasing scoliosis. Sagittal T2-W MRI shows a cavity (*arrow*) in the spinal cord

common than the congenital form and is classified as collapsing kyphosis or rigid-sharp angle kyphosis. Collapsing kyphosis is often C shaped and initially flexible. The apex may occur anywhere in the lower thoracic or lumbar spine (see Fig. 24.26). Rigid sharp-angle kyphosis is more common in older children and is usually S shaped with an accompanying upper thoracic lordosis. All kyphotic curves tend to progress [42, 46, 47]. Vertebrae are wedged or bullet shaped in lateral projection.

Developmental lordosis with or without scoliosis is usually compensatory, counteracting instability caused by pelvic obliquity or a dislocated hip. In the past, this deformity was associated with lumboperitoneal shunting, but this method of shunting is rarely used today [48].

Hip and Lower Extremity

Hip Subluxation

Deformity and instability of the hip in myelomeningocele is common, ranging from joint contracture to subluxation and dislocation. The presence of hip deformity and dislocation is related to the neurological level of the disorder and resultant muscle imbalance. Nerves for the hip flexors and adductors originate at L1–L3, whereas innervation of the hip abductors and extensors originates at L5–S2. The myelo-hip can be divided into three groups, based upon the level of the neurological injury. The first is thoracic/high lumbar level, in which none of the muscles about the hip are significantly innervated, and dislocation develops slowly over time due to flaccid paralysis. The second is low lumbar level, in which the hip flexors, hip adductors, and knee extensors are functionally innervated, whereas the hip extensors, hip abductors, and knee extensors are flail. Hip subluxation and dislocation occur rapidly due to muscle imbalance. The final group is injured at the sacral level. In this group, all muscles about the hip are functionally innervated, and subluxation/dislocation is unusual.

Subluxation and dislocation are very common in children with myelomeningocele, occurring in up to 50 %. In most cases, hips are normal at birth and become dislocated or dysplastic after the first year of life. However, infants who were in the breech position or those who are placed on their side after surgical closure of dysraphism frequently develop early dislocation. Hip US allows early diagnosis in these cases, but because most patients with myelomeningocele develop dysplasia or dislocation more than 1 year after birth, radiographs are in general most useful [38] (Fig. 24.30). The same measurements apply in myelomeningocele as in developmental dysplasia of the hip (Chap. 11).

Pavlik harness and closed reduction are used to treat hip dysplasia or instability in preambulatory patients with a sacral level of neurological impairment. However, due to the underlying muscle imbalance, reduction is usually

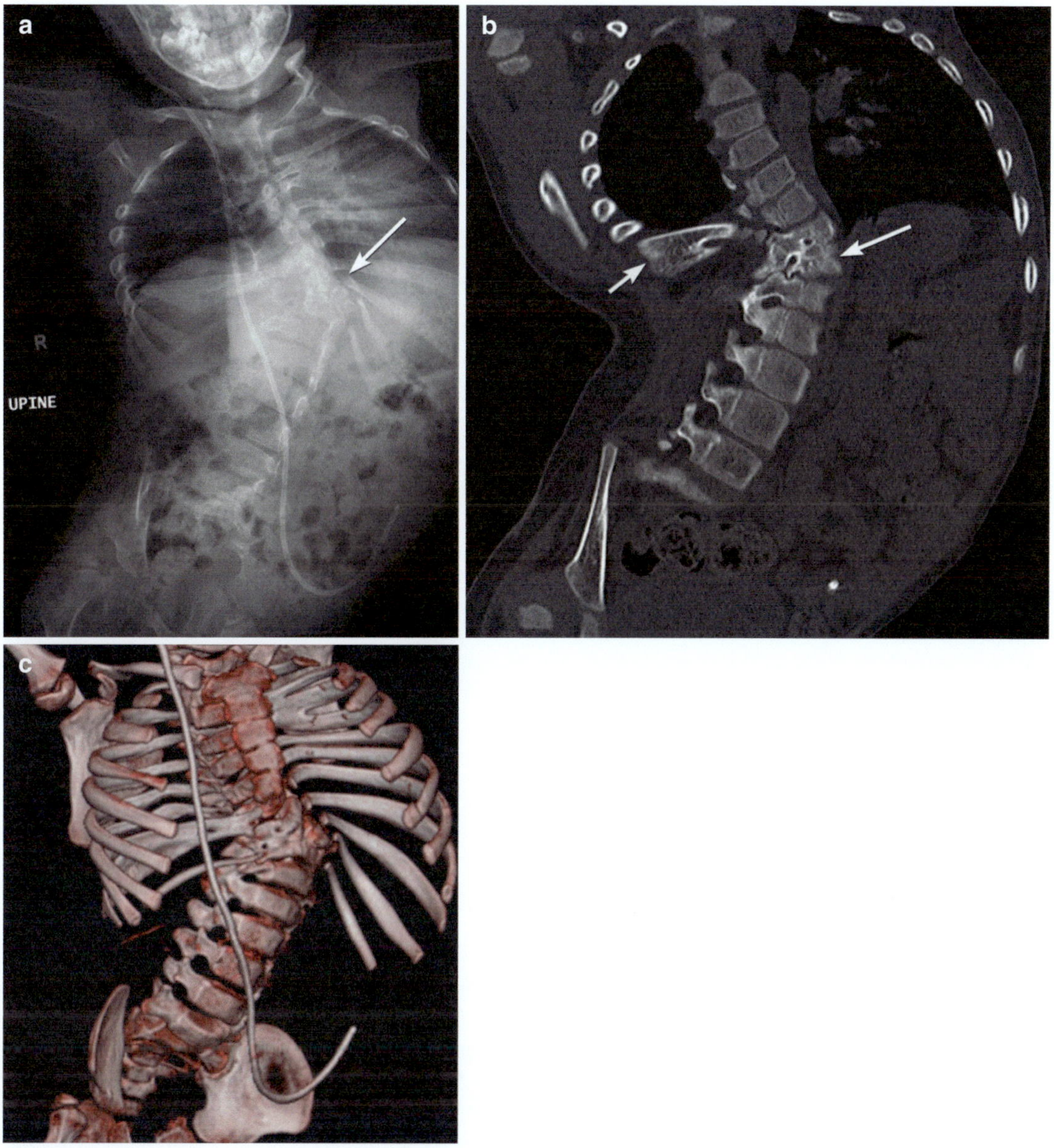

Fig. 24.28 Spina bifida and multiple segmentation abnormalities resulting in small lung volumes in a 5-year-old boy. Radiograph (**a**), coronal CT reconstruction (**b**), and 3-D CT reformatted image (**c**) demonstrate dysraphism extending from the mid-thoracic spine distally, with fused vertebrae on the right as well as multiple hemivertebrae on the left at the apex of the scoliosis (*arrow*, (**a**); *long arrow*, (**b**)). Ribs are fused (*short arrow*, (**b**)) Additional fused ribs at the upper left chest. Note dislocated right hip

followed by recurrent dislocation. Treatment of hip deformity in older children depends on the neurological level, the specific deformity, and the potential for ambulation. Reduction of a dislocated hip may involve both femoral and acetabular surgery.

Hip Flexion

Hip flexion deformity may be seen in patients with thoracic or lumbar defects and is frequently associated with abduction contracture, which results from unusually tight tensor fascia lata. When unilateral, there is also pelvic obliquity

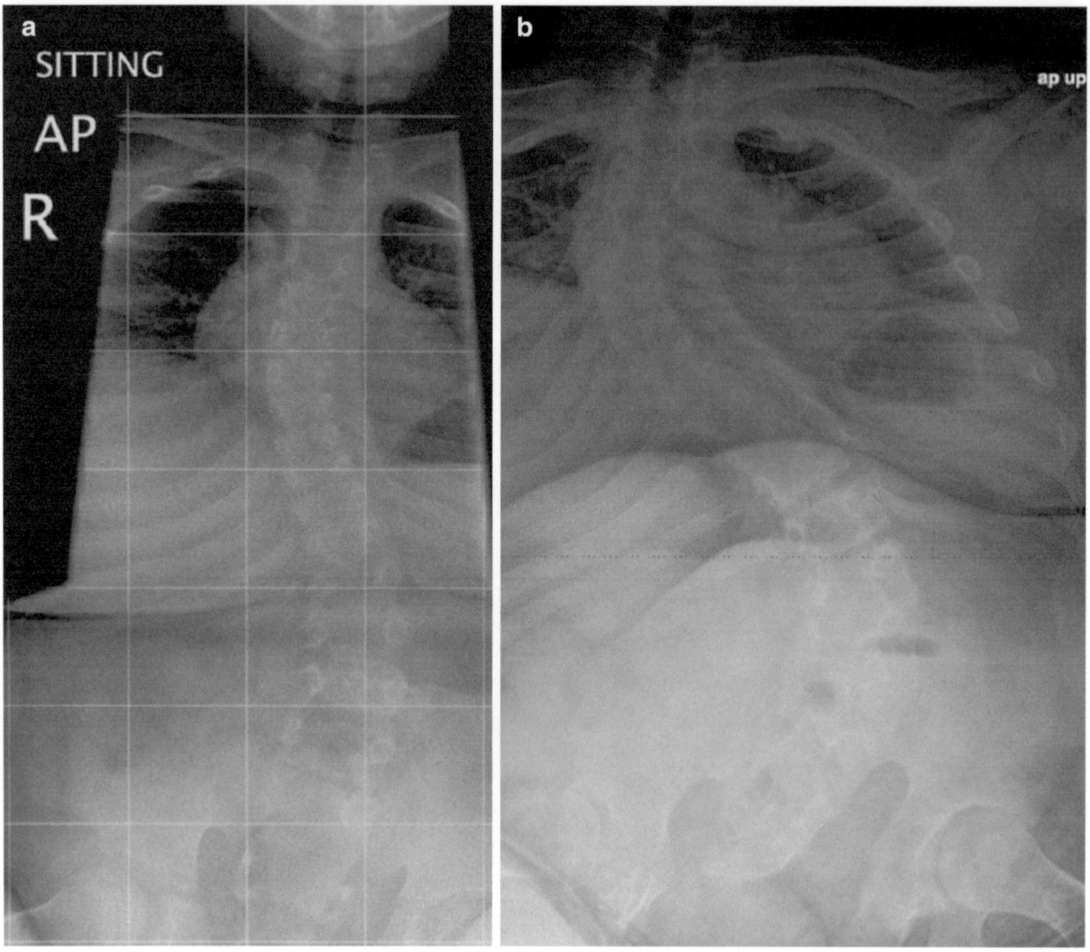

Fig. 24.29 Progressive S-shaped scoliosis in a boy ((**a**), 9 years old; (**b**), 15 years old) with spina bifida, sacral agenesis, tethered cord, and cloacal exstrophy

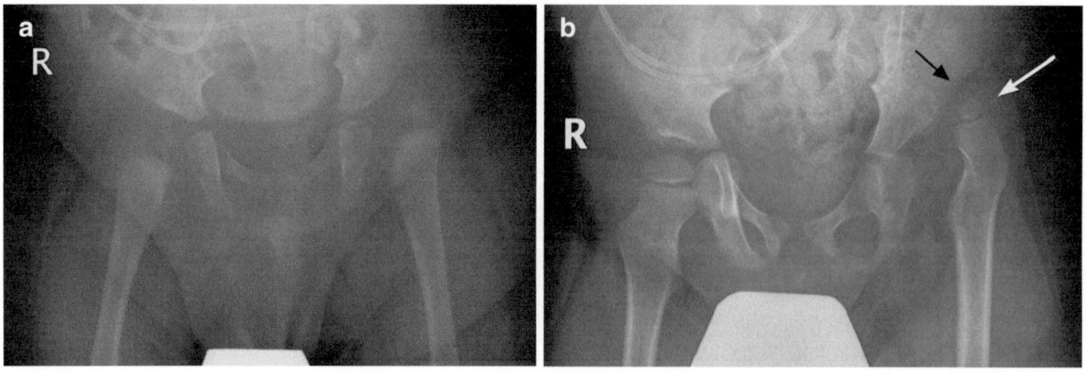

Fig. 24.30 Progressive hip dislocation in patient with myelomeningocele. (**a**) At 1 year of age, the left hip is dislocated and the acetabulum dysplastic. Note sacral defect. (**b**) Two years later, the degree of dislocation has increased (*white arrow*), and a pseudoacetabulum is present (*black arrow*). The femoral head is smaller than on the normal side. Bilateral coxa valga

and scoliosis. Surgery is directed at release of hip muscles.

Femoral Torsion

In children with myelomeningocele who have abnormal gait and activity levels, femoral torsion fails to decrease normally as the child grows. This results in inward rotation at the knees and in-toeing of the legs and feet, as in patients with CP [38] (see Chap. 13 for discussion of measurement techniques). Both flexion and extension contractures may develop at the knee, interfering with ambulation, upright position, and orthotic fitting. Flexion contractures are probably the most common knee deformity, and contractures greater than 30° often impair the ability to walk. Extension contractures are infrequent and most often encountered in children who were in breech presentation, as intrauterine compression can lead to hyperflexed hips, hyperextended knees, and clubfoot. Extension contractures may also result from extensive immobilization.

Rotational Deformities

Rotational deformities of the lower extremities are common in both ambulatory and nonambulatory children with myelomeningocele. An in-toeing gait is usually dynamic if secondary to medial hamstring dominance or fixed if secondary to internal tibial torsion. A short fibula and a weak soleus muscle can lead to excessive lateral twisting of the tibia, resulting in external tibial torsion and an out-toeing gait. Selective fibular shortening is common in children with myelomeningocele. Normally, by age 4 the distal fibular growth plate should be at the level of the talar dome, and it should be even lower in older children. In many patients with myelomeningocele, the distal fibular physis is at or above the level of the distal tibial physis (Fig. 24.31). A short distal fibula causes ankle valgus deformity. This

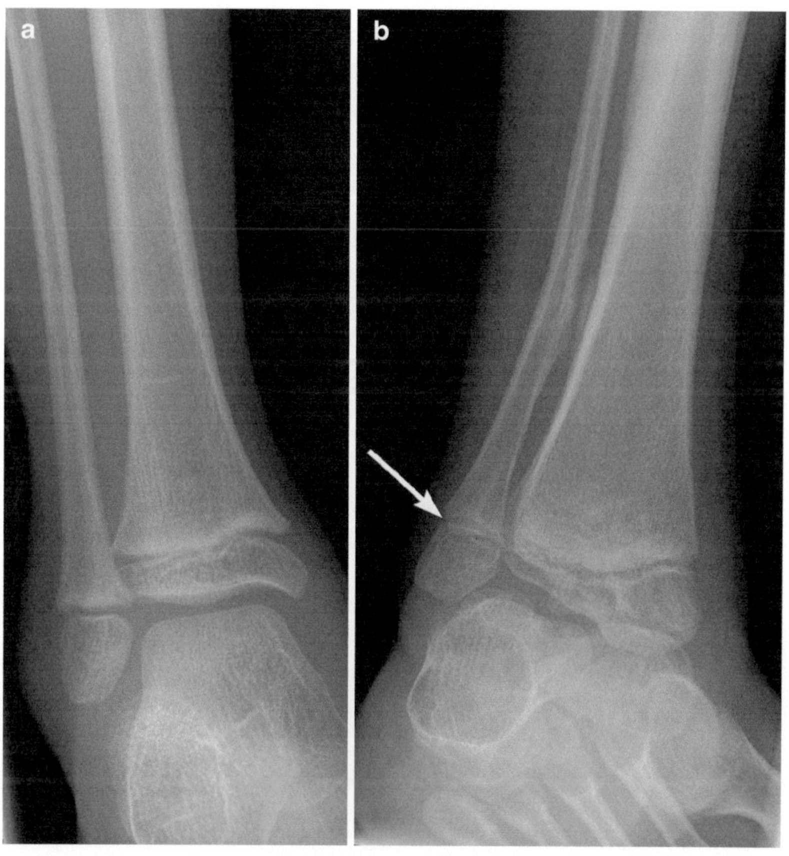

Fig. 24.31 Selective fibular underdevelopment in a 13-year-old with spina bifida. (**a**) In a normal 10-year-old (supplied for comparison), the fibular growth plate is at the level of the talar dome. (**b**) In the patient with dysraphism, the fibular growth plate (*arrow*) is at the same level as the tibial growth plate. The tibial epiphysis is deformed

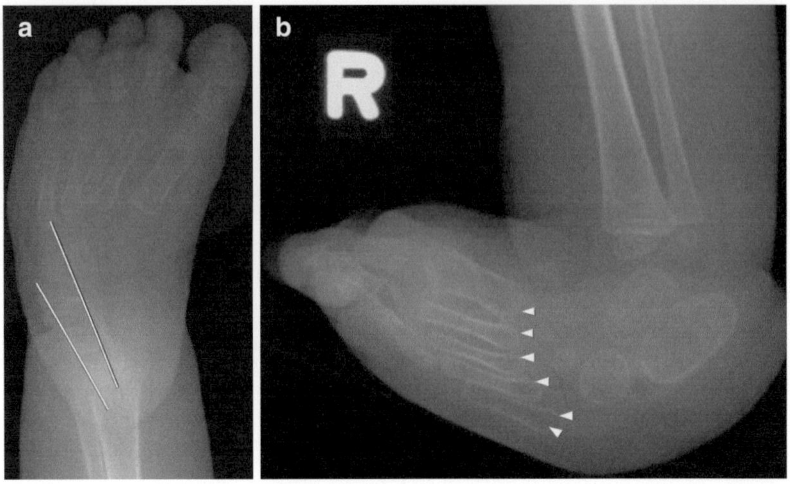

Fig. 24.32 Severe equinovarus clubfoot in a 2-year-old girl with myelomeningocele. (**a**) There is hindfoot varus with abnormal parallelism of the talus and calcaneus. The talus points lateral to the first metatarsal. (**b**) Abnormal talocalcaneal angle. The ladderlike arrangement of the metatarsals (*arrowheads*) indicates severe forefoot inversion

combined with external tibial torsion results in abnormal loading of the ankle, leading to a wedge-shaped distal tibial epiphysis, which is narrower laterally. This deformity contributes to planovalgus foot malalignment, which can compromise standing and use of orthoses.

Foot

Both congenital and acquired foot deformities are common in children with myelomeningocele, occurring in 64–90 %. Equinus is most common, but calcaneus, cavus, valgus, clubfoot, and vertical talus deformity also occur [49]. Several factors besides external tibial torsion are associated with ankle and foot deformity, including intrauterine pressure and malposition, positional deformity, abnormal posture, and weight bearing. Foot deformities are addressed briefly below (see Chap. 15 for more thorough discussion).

Clubfoot (equinovarus) deformity is common, present at birth, rigid, and quite severe. However, it does respond reasonably well to serial casting [50]. It has several components that are demonstrated on a lateral weight-bearing view. Hindfoot equinus denotes plantar flexion of the calcaneus, whereas hindfoot varus denotes a decreased talocalcaneal angle. Forefoot varus appears as a ladderlike arrangement of the metatarsals. On the frontal projection the talocalcaneal angle is decreased, and the talus points lateral to the first metatarsal [38] (Fig. 24.32).

Calcaneus foot consists of abnormal dorsiflexion and is commonly associated with ankle valgus. The talocalcaneal angle on the lateral view is decreased (Fig. 24.33). Often resulting from a tibialis anterior muscle that is spastic or overbalances a weak or paralyzed gastrocnemius, this deformity is usually encountered in children with L5–S1 paralysis. Calcaneus deformity usually progresses until the calcaneus becomes vertical under the talus. This is an extremely disabling malformation because the weight-bearing surface of the foot is very short. In addition, pressure on the calcaneus leads to ulceration with increased risk for osteomyelitis.

Congenital vertical talus (rocker-bottom deformity) accounts for about 10 % of the abnormal feet in patients with myelomeningocele. It is often associated with calcaneovalgus deformity, with the midfoot and forefoot dorsiflexed on a rigid plantar-flexed talus. The talus assumes a vertical position and may become parallel to the long axis of the tibia (Fig. 24.34). It is best to image the talus in extreme plantar flexion.

Fractures

Paralysis and immobilization cause the femur, tibia, and fibula to become thin and osteopenic. The combination of sensory deficit, osteopenia, muscular-ligamentous atrophy and laxity, absence of deep tendon reflexes, and abnormal

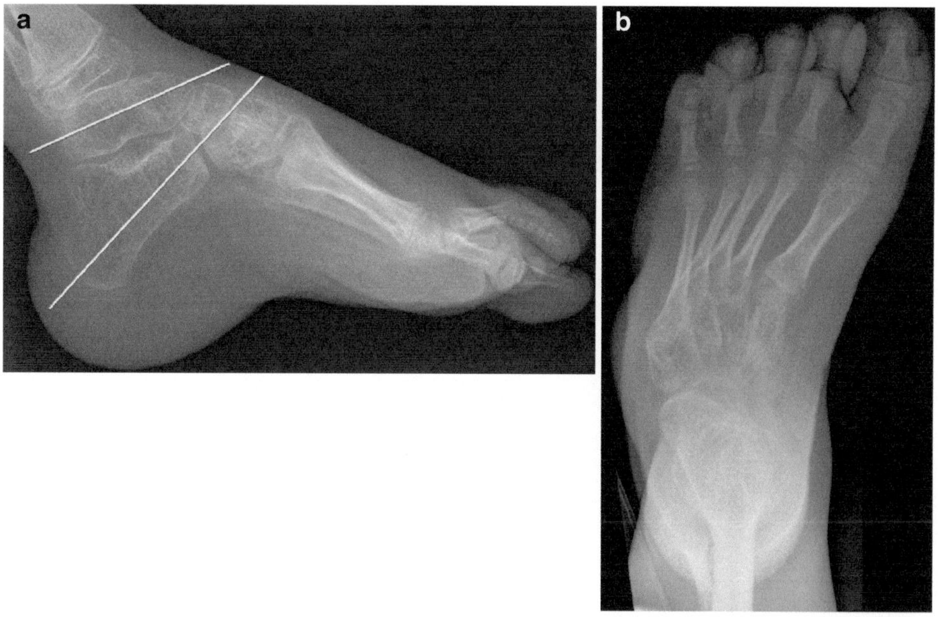

Fig. 24.33 Calcaneus foot in a 10-year-old boy with spina bifida. On lateral (**a**), the anterior calcaneus is dorsiflexed, and the metatarsals are plantar flexed, increasing the depth of the plantar arch. The talocalcaneal angle is diminished at 28°. Slight ankle obliquity gives the false impression of talar dome flattening. Note fibular shortening. The frontal view (**b**) shows mild metatarsus adductus along with calcaneal varus deformity. Diffuse osteopenia

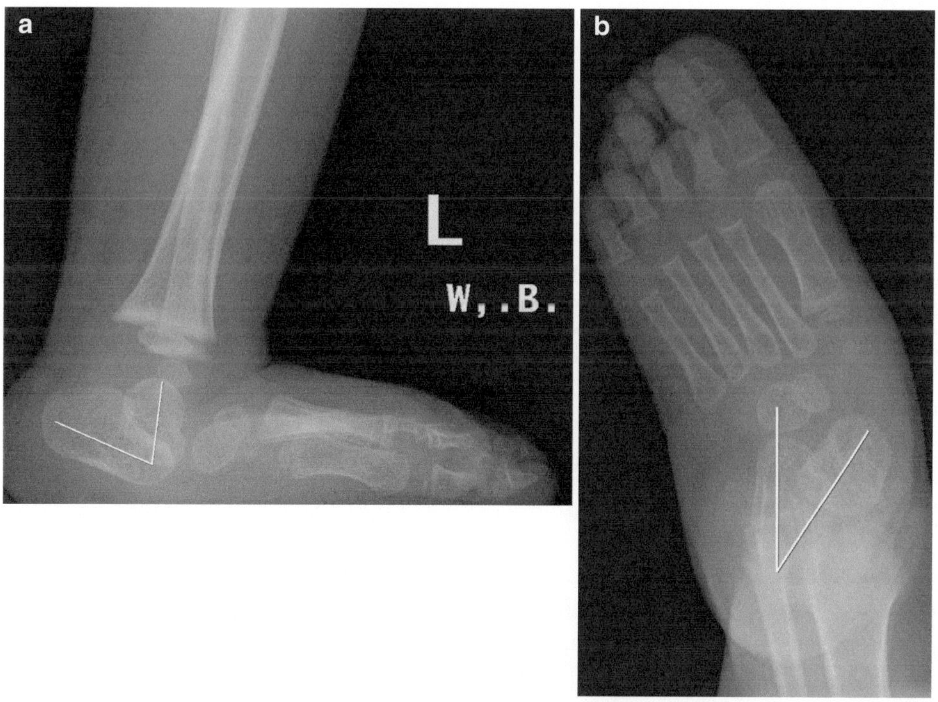

Fig. 24.34 Congenital vertical talus in a 2-year-old girl with myelomeningocele. (**a**) On the lateral, the talus is almost vertical, parallel to the long axis of the tibia. The calcaneus is plantar flexed with an increased talocalcaneal angle of 60°, resulting in rocker-bottom deformity. (**b**) There is hindfoot valgus with increased talocalcaneal angle measuring 46°. The talus is directed medial to the first metatarsal, and the navicular assumes a more lateral relationship to the talus

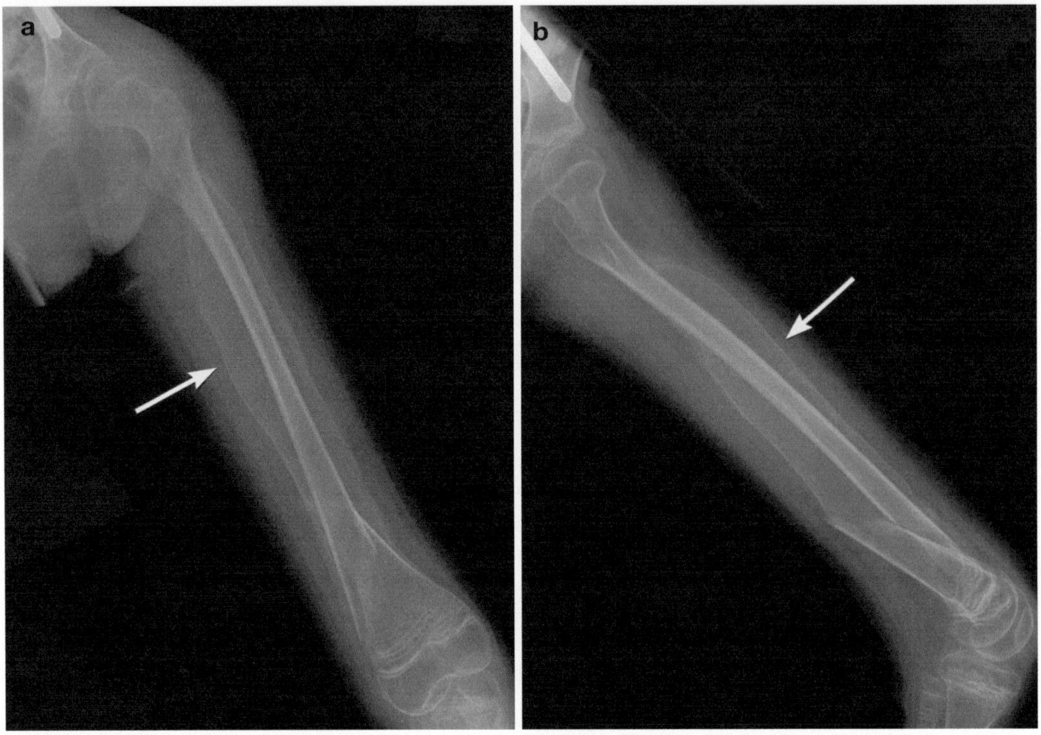

Fig. 24.35 (**a**, **b**) Fractured femur in a patient with myelomeningocele. There is diffuse osteopenia, an oblique overriding distal femoral fracture, and large enveloping callus (*arrow*) caused by motion and late recognition in this insensate limb

joint relationships results in increased risk of fracture. Pathological fractures may occur in 20 % of children with myelomeningocele [51]. Nonambulatory children with high thoracic lesions are at highest risk for fractures. Neonates with thoracic and upper lumbar lesions also have increased risk [52]. Fractures occur after minor trauma, not infrequently during mild physical activity. Fractures can also occur in postoperative patients immobilized in casts.

The clinical manifestations of these pathological fractures resemble infection, with a swollen, red limb, possibly accompanied by fever. Injuries may not be noticed due to lack of sensation (Fig. 24.35). Fractures are often located in the supracondylar region of the femur. Exuberant callus is common, since fracture recognition may be delayed. Callus may be so prolific that the lesion resembles osteomyelitis or osteosarcoma, necessitating biopsy [53, 54]. Fracture healing can be complicated by pseudarthrosis, malunion, and delayed union. Soft tissue ulceration may lead to osteomyelitis.

Physeal Fractures

Fractures involving the physes carry a poor prognosis. These fractures are less common and tend to occur with no known antecedent trauma in children with low lumbar neurologic involvement who are ambulatory [38, 54]. Radiographs initially demonstrate growth plate widening with an irregular, broad metaphysis (Fig. 24.36). The appearance results from recurrent fracture, hematoma formation, and callus deposition. With healing, the growth plate narrows and may fuse either partially or in its entirety, causing angular deformity or complete growth arrest.

Charcot Arthropathy

Charcot or neurotrophic arthropathy is progressive degeneration of a joint caused by lack of protective sensation. This occurs most commonly in children with a motor level at or below L4 and a sensory level slightly higher and can affect the hips, knees, and ankles [55]. Radiographs demonstrate severe bone fragmentation, joint destruction, and sclerosis.

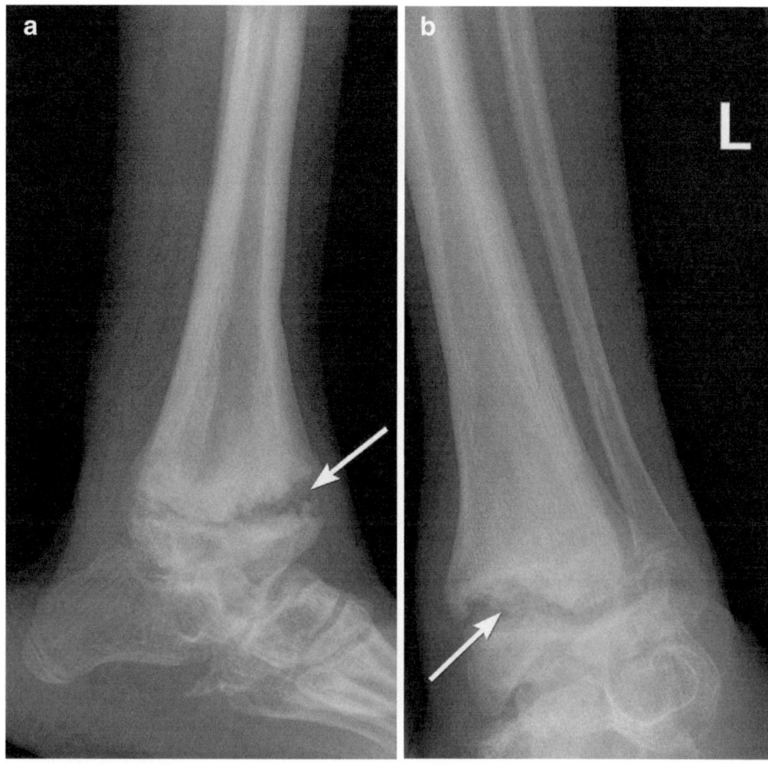

Fig. 24.36 (**a**, **b**) Recurrent physeal fracture, hematoma, and callus deposition in a patient with myelomeningocele. There is fragmentation and sclerosis at the adjacent metaphysis, with irregularity and widening of the tibial physis (*arrows*). The talus has collapsed

2.2 Hereditary: Spinal Muscular Atrophy

Spinal muscular atrophy (SMA) is an incurable autosomal recessive disease caused by a genetic defect in the SMN1 gene which codes SMN (survival motor neuron), a protein necessary for the survival of motor neurons. The result is death of neuronal cells in the anterior horn of the spinal cord and subsequent system-wide muscle atrophy. Different forms of SMA vary in severity but share general muscle wasting and impaired mobility. SMA is the second most common fatal autosomal recessive disorder after cystic fibrosis, with an estimated incidence of 1 in 6,000–10,000 live births and a carrier frequency of 1 in 40–60 [56].

The disease spectrum is divided into four types, according to the age at onset of symptoms and the highest attained milestone of motor development.

SMA Type I (Werdnig-Hoffmann Disease)

This is the most common and most severe type, accounting for about 50 % of patients diagnosed with SMA. Classically, infants with SMA type I have onset of clinical signs before 6 months of age, never acquire the ability to sit unsupported, and without intervention generally do not survive beyond age 2. These patients have profound hypotonia, symmetrical flaccid paralysis, and no control of head movement. Respiratory failure develops by age 2, and pneumonia is the most frequent cause of death. In the most severe forms, reduced intrauterine movements suggest prenatal onset; patients present at birth with severe weakness and joint contractures. These children may have congenital fractures and extremely thin ribs.

SMA Type II (Intermediate Form)

These children never stand or walk, but they can maintain a sitting position. The onset of weakness is usually noticed between 6 and 18 months of age. Disease course varies greatly: some patients gradually weaken, while those who receive careful maintenance do not progress. Muscles are weak, and the respiratory system is a major concern. Life expectancy is reduced, but most SMA II patients live well into adulthood. Deep tendon reflexes are absent, and fine tremors of upper extremities are common. Joint contractures and kyphoscoliosis are very common.

SMA Type III (Kugelberg-Welander Disease)

This juvenile form manifests after 18 months of age and describes patients who are at some point able to walk without support, although many later lose this ability. They develop little to no respiratory muscle weakness, and life expectancy is near normal. Patients who lose ambulation often develop scoliosis and other medical problems related to poor mobility, such as obesity and osteoporosis [56].

SMA Type IV

Late-onset SMA describes patients with adult onset (>18 years) and a mild disease course. These patients are able to walk and have no respiratory or nutritional problems.

Imaging

The radiographic findings parallel both clinical severity and course of disease. In severe cases, the thoracic diameter is decreased, and ribs are thin with an oblique course due to weak intercostal muscles (Figs. 24.37 and 24.38). Frequent complications include atelectasis and pneumonia. Bones are gracile, and fractures are common. Thoracolumbar or lumbar scoliosis is common [57] and correlates with age at presentation, especially in those who cannot walk. Scoliosis is almost universal in the infantile form. In types II and III, scoliosis almost always begins in the first decade of life due to severe truncal weakness (Fig. 24.39). Progression correlates with the degree of muscle weakness. Spinal deformity may become very severe by mid childhood, and although initially flexible it becomes rigid as

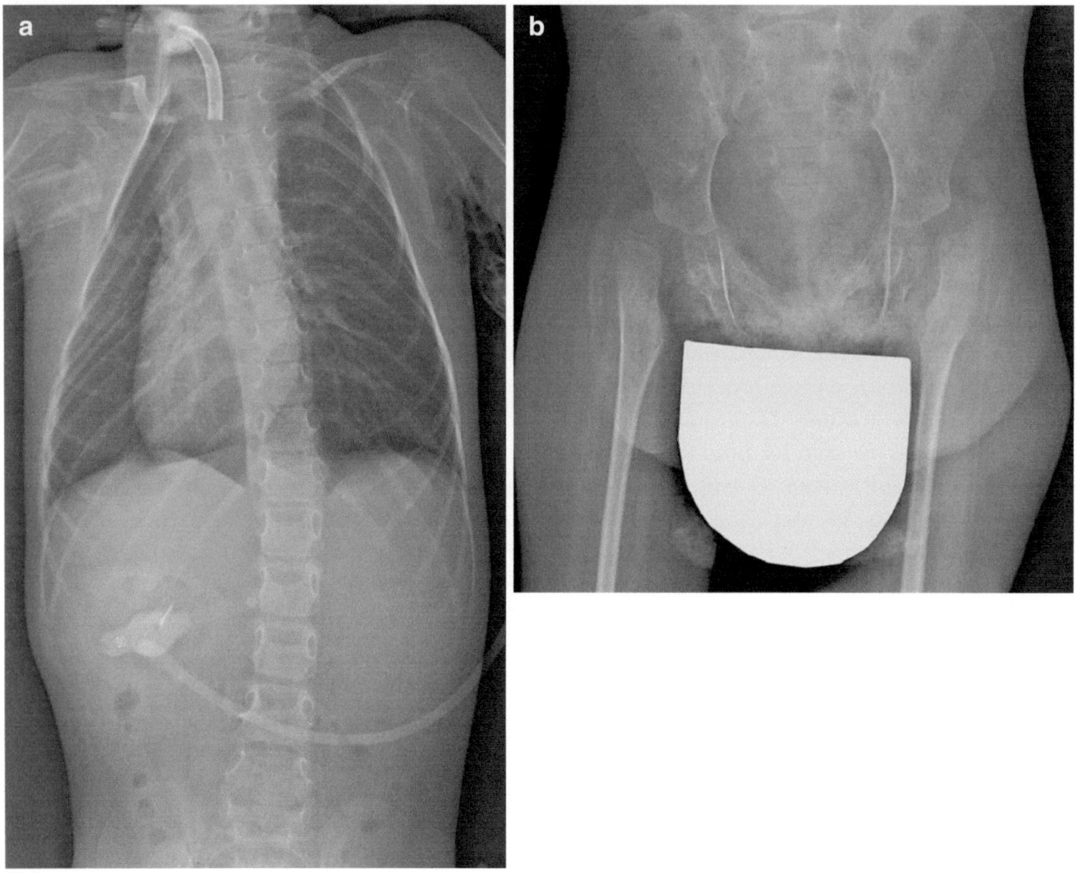

Fig. 24.37 Spinal muscular atrophy type I in a 3-year-old ventilator-dependent boy. (**a**) There is mild scoliosis. Vertebrae are elongated, bones extremely gracile, and ribs thin and oblique. Muscle mass is profoundly diminished. (**b**) Both hips are dislocated, and there is coxa valga

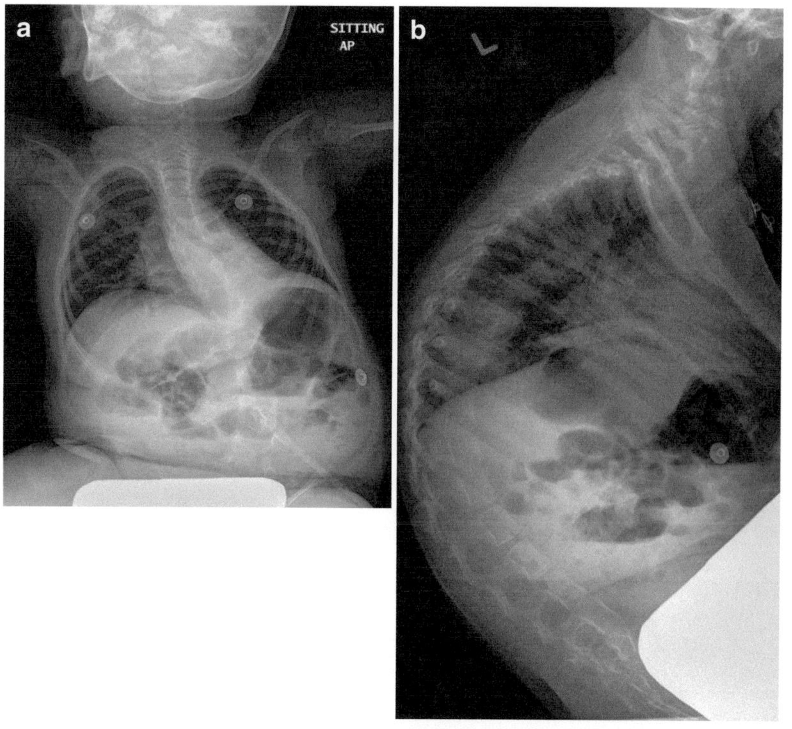

Fig. 24.38 (**a**, **b**) Spinal muscular atrophy type II in a 4-year-old girl with severe C-shaped thoracolumbar scoliosis and kyphosis, as well as caninization of vertebrae. The thorax is small, the ribs have an oblique course, and the humeri are extremely thin. There is atelectasis at the left base

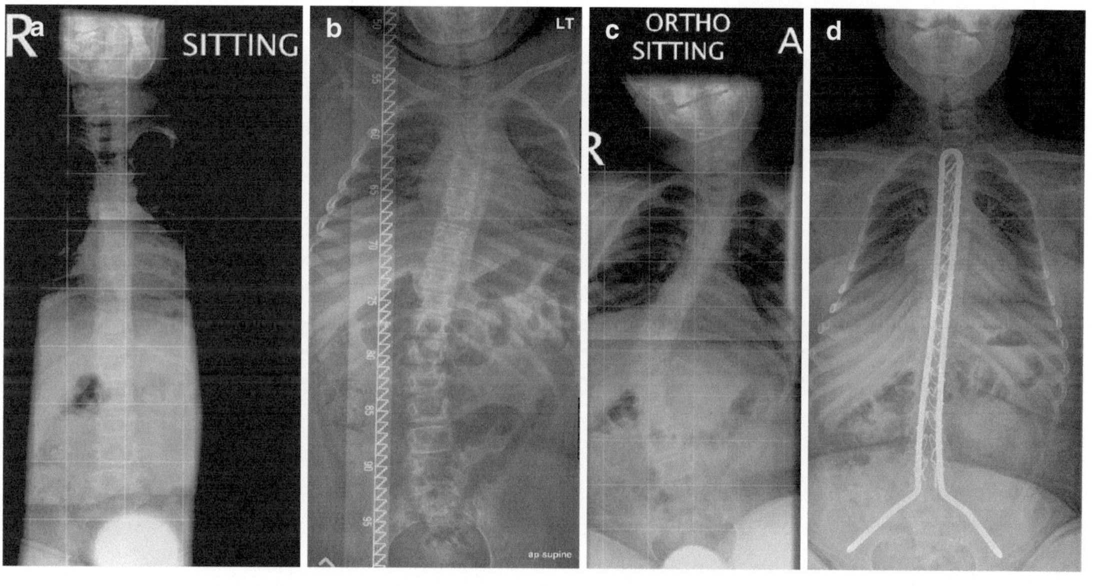

Fig. 24.39 Progressive C-shaped thoracolumbar scoliosis in a patient with spinal muscular atrophy type II, showing characteristic progression of curve. The patient is normal at age 8 (**a**), but scoliosis has developed by age 10 (**b**), becomes more severe with typical narrow thorax and oblique, thin ribs at age 12 (**c**), and finally requires fusion at age 14 (**d**)

structural deformities develop in the vertebrae. Pelvic obliquity with the iliac crest elevated toward the concave side of the spinal curve is common, sometimes associated with unilateral hip dislocation. Valgus deformity of the proximal femur and acetabular dysplasia with subluxation

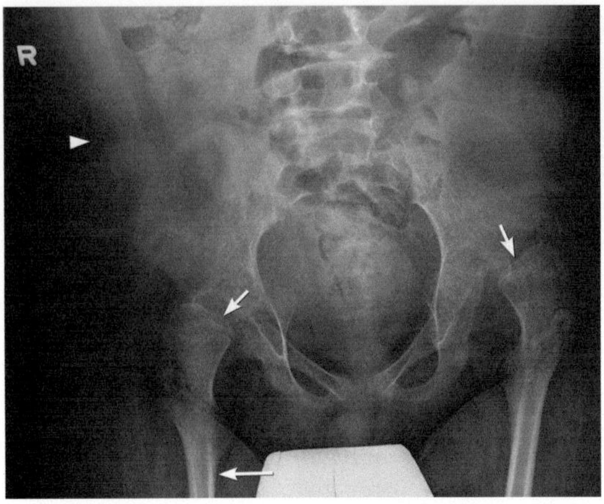

Fig. 24.40 Dislocated left and subluxated right hips in a 10-year-old with spinal muscular atrophy type II. Note valgus deformity of the proximal femurs, acetabular dysplasia, gracile femoral diaphyses (*long arrow*), flat medial aspects of both femoral heads (*short arrows*), and muscle atrophy (*arrowhead*)

and dislocation of the hip occur early and often in the severe forms of the disease (Fig. 24.40) but are less frequent and milder with late-onset disease.

Ultrasound and MRI of the extremities both demonstrate severe muscle atrophy (Fig. 24.41), the extent varying with disease severity. Infantile type I SMA shows severe atrophy of all the muscle bundles of the thigh and the calf [58, 59]. The intermediate type demonstrates ragged atrophy of muscle bundles of the thigh and calf, and there may be selective preservation of the adductor longus muscle. Mild SMA (type III) has fatty infiltration of muscle bundles and increased intramuscular fat planes.

Differential Diagnosis

The infant presenting with hypotonia and/or weakness may have a congenital myopathy, congenital myotonic dystrophy, congenital myasthenic syndrome, metabolic myopathy, or congenital disorder of the motor neuron and the peripheral nerve (congenital hypomyelinating neuropathy). Non-neuromuscular pathology including neonatal sepsis, hypoxic ischemic encephalopathy, metabolic conditions, and genetic syndromes such as Prader-Willi should also be considered.

2.3 Trauma: Spinal Cord Injury

Traumatic spinal cord injury (SCI) is relatively unusual in the pediatric population, accounting for less than 4 % of all SCI [60]. The mechanism of injury in pediatric patients differs from that in adults, as the pediatric spine has unique anatomic properties. The immature spine is hypermobile due to ligamentous laxity, shallow facet joints, underdeveloped spinous processes, and physiologic wedging of the vertebral bodies. These findings are most notable in the cervical spine, where hypermobility combined with a large head-to-body ratio and poorly developed cervical musculature predisposes younger children to high torque forces. The fulcrum of the cervical axis changes as children grow. In children younger than 8 years, maximal mobility occurs at C1–C3. As the ossification centers form and the C2 body fuses with the odontoid process (3–6 years), the fulcrum moves to the C3–C5 level. At 12 years of age, the fulcrum settles at C5–C6, where it remains throughout adulthood. Younger children are therefore at higher risk of upper cervical injury [61].

Spinal cord injury follows direct cord laceration or transection, pressure necrosis from expanding hematoma, or ischemic infarction due to disruption of vessels. Vertebral fractures are initially diagnosed in the emergency situation with radiographs and CT (Fig. 24.42a). MRI is helpful in the acute situation to evaluate hematoma and ligamentous injury and later to define cord disruption, cyst formation, and atrophy (Fig. 24.42b). Spinal cord injury without radiologic abnormality (SCIWORA) is defined as a cord injury without abnormality depicted on conventional radiographs or CT [62]. These lesions are usually related to transient ligamentous injury or transient vertebral displacement of the cervical spine secondary to hyperextension, flexion, or distracting injury and are diagnosed only by MRI.

SCI lesions can be classified as complete or incomplete based on sacral sparing. Sacral sparing denotes the presence of sensory or motor function in the most caudal sacral segments (i.e., preservation of light touch or pinprick sensation

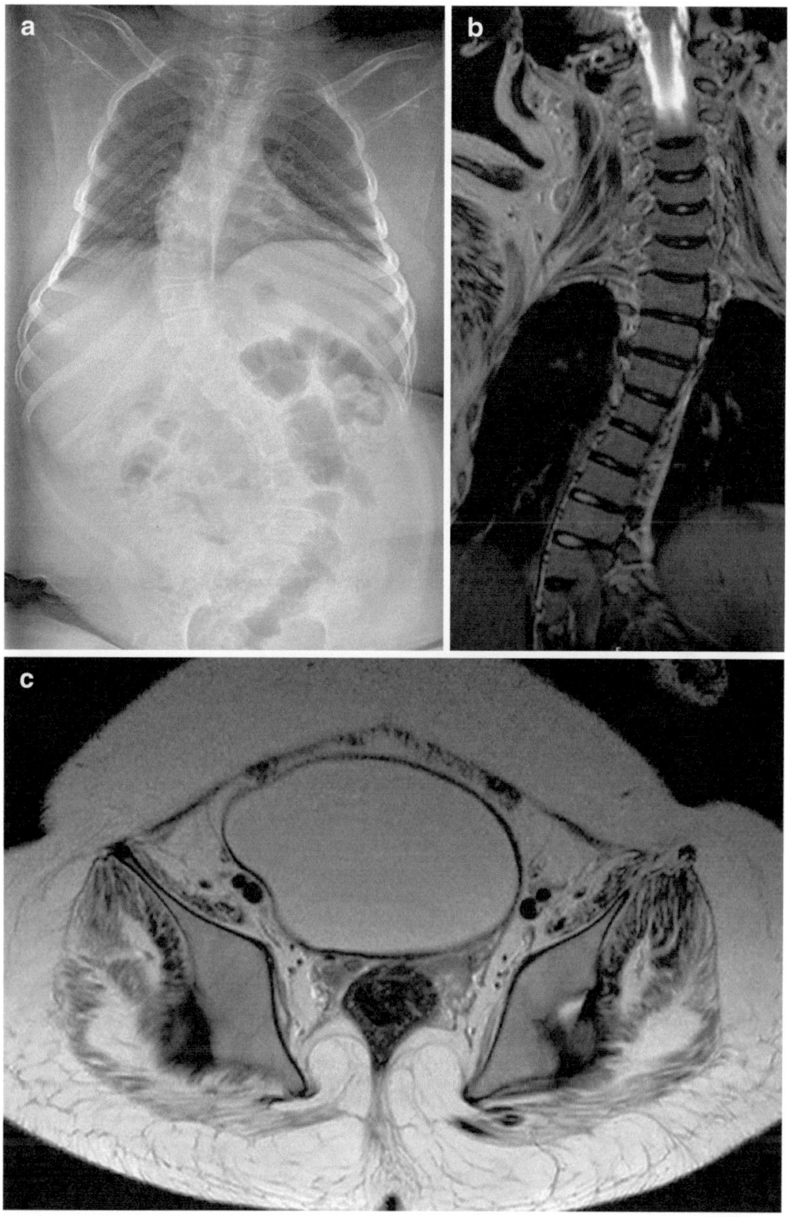

Fig. 24.41 Spinal muscular atrophy in a 13-year-old boy. (**a**) Scoliosis and downsloping ribs with characteristic extensively lucent soft tissues, delineating severely atrophic musculature (best seen over the right scapula and axilla). Coronal (**b**) and axial (**c**) T2-W images show increased adipose tissue and severe fatty degeneration of musculature (Courtesy of Tal Laor, Cincinnati Children's Hospital)

at the S4–S5 dermatome, deep anal pressure, and voluntary anal sphincter contraction). A complete injury is defined by the absence of sacral sparing (i.e., no sensory or motor function in the lowest sacral segments), whereas an incomplete injury is defined by the presence of at least some sacral sparing (i.e. partial preservation of sensory and/or motor function) (Table 24.1) [63]. Incomplete injuries have been described as central, posterior, and anterior cord as well as Brown-Séquard hemisection syndromes.

Quadriplegia refers to impairment or loss of motor and possibly sensory control and transmission in the cervical cord, resulting in impaired function in all four extremities, the trunk, and the pelvic organs. In paraplegia, patients with lesions below T2 retain use of the upper extremities, with various degrees of motor and sensory impairment

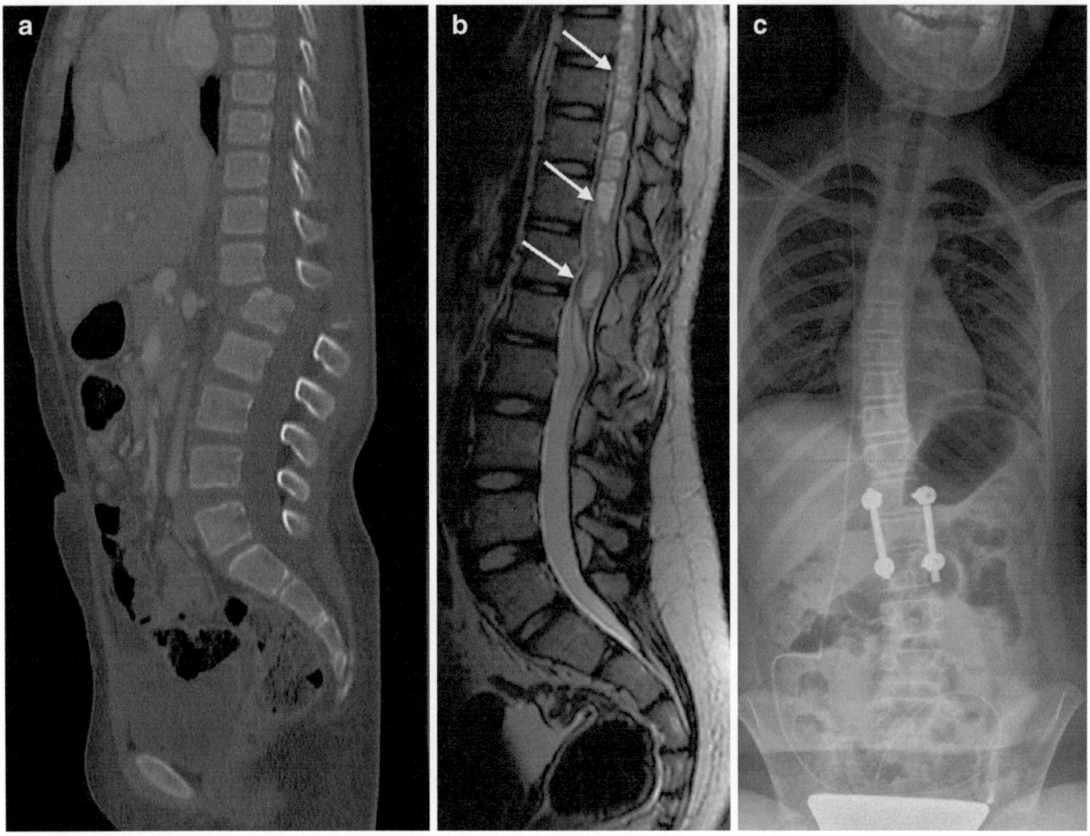

Fig. 24.42 Spinal cord injury in a 9-year-old girl. (**a**) Sagittal reformatted CT at the time of injury shows an L1 vertebral body fracture and T12 spinous process fracture. There is dorsal displacement of L1, with resultant spinal cord injury. (**b**) Sagittal T2-W MRI 3 years later shows multiple posttraumatic syrinx cavities (*arrows*), with artifact from the spine hardware. (**c**) Three years after surgery, dextroconvex scoliosis has developed above the surgical level

Table 24.1 American Spinal Injury Association (ASIA) Impairment Scale [1]

A = Complete: no motor or sensory function is preserved in the sacral segments S4–S5
B = Incomplete: sensory but not motor function is preserved below the neurological level and includes the sacral segments S4–S5
C = Incomplete: motor function is preserved below the neurological level, and more than half of the key muscles below the neurological level have a muscle grade less than 3
D = Incomplete: motor function is preserved below the neurological level, and at least half of the key muscles below the neurological level have a muscle grade of 3 or more
E = Normal: motor and sensory functions are normal

Adapted from the American Spinal Injury Association [108]
Adapted with permission from Kirshblum et al. [63]
For an individual to receive a grade of C or D, he or she must be incomplete, that is, has sensory or motor function in the sacral segments S4–S5. In addition, the individual must have either (a) voluntary anal sphincter contraction or (b) sparing of motor function more than three levels below the motor level

below this. Ambulation in orthoses is possible with T7–T12 lesions but is usually impractical owing to severe energy requirement. Bowel and bladder dysfunction can occur with spinal cord injury at all levels.

Kyphoscoliosis is common, but the age of the child at the time of injury has enormous impact on orthopedic course. Essentially all children injured before the adolescent growth spurt will develop progressive scoliosis due to neurologic

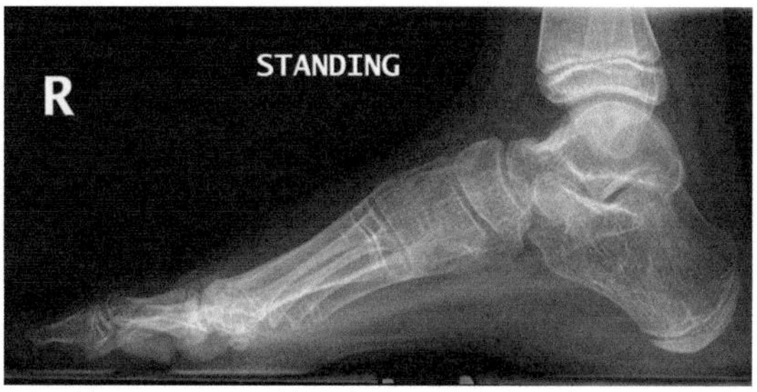

Fig. 24.43 Pes cavus and osteopenia 2 years after spine injury, with fatty infiltration of the plantar musculature (the other foot was similarly affected)

paresis or imbalance and structural alteration in vertebral architecture; two thirds require surgical correction (Fig. 24.42c). Older children tend to have nonprogressive acute angulation or kyphosis at the level of the vertebral injury [64]. Of those injured after skeletal maturity, only 20 % develop scoliosis and 5 % require surgery [65, 66]. Kyphosis in young children is characterized by a rounded thoracolumbar curve with gradual loss of normal lumbar lordosis. Emergency surgical laminectomy without surgical fusion increases the likelihood that kyphosis will develop and progress.

Children who sustain SCI before puberty are also at increased risk of hip dislocation or subluxation [67]. Hip instability has been reported in all children injured before 5 years of age and in 60–83 % of those injured before age 10. Pelvic obliquity results from unbalanced trunk and hip musculature and often becomes fixed as contracture supervenes. With severe pelvic obliquity, the rib cage overrides the pelvis or protrudes into it. The hip on the high side of the obliquity is often dislocated. Pes cavus deformity may develop as well (Fig. 24.43).

Disuse can rapidly lead to cartilage atrophy, along with impaired joint morphology and function. This is seen in adults as early as 6 months after SCI, with cartilage volume at the knee decreased by 10 % 12 months post injury [68]. The joint space at the hip may narrow more than 50 % [69]. Cartilage atrophy probably results from decreased synovial fluid production leading to decreased nutrition of the cartilage, since immobilization prevents the normal pumping action that induces fluid production and hydrates cartilage.

Osteoporosis is common in individuals with SCI. Bone loss begins immediately after injury and reaches as much as 22 % in the first 3 months. SCI may also alter bone structure and microstructure, affecting trabecular more than cortical bone. The pathogenesis of osteoporosis after SCI is incompletely understood, but disuse and neural factors appear to play an important role.

In general, demineralization occurs below the level of injury and results in an increased incidence of lower extremity fractures. Lack of sensation causes these fractures to be asymptomatic and therefore diagnosed late, increasing the need for lengthy immobilization and the likelihood of heterotopic ossification and pressure sores.

Dual x-ray absorptiometry (DXA) can be used to evaluate bone density and fracture risk (see Chap. 26). SCI can also affect the parathyroid hormone (PTH)-vitamin D axis, leading to impaired calcium and phosphate metabolism. Pharmacologic intervention with calcium, phosphate, vitamin D, calcitonin, bisphosphonate, and functional stimulation exercises may help prevent bone loss [70, 71].

Myositis ossificans (see Chap. 22) develops in approximately 10 % of children with spinal cord injury, generally 6–18 months post trauma. In this population, bone forms in the soft tissues around paralyzed joints. Pathogenesis may be related to circulatory stasis, edema, and tissue hypoxia. The most common site of involvement is the hip, followed by the shoulder and elbow. The knee is usually spared. Most children complain of pain or decreased range of motion. The incidence of myositis ossificans is lower in children with SCI than in adults, and it occurs later and with fewer associated signs and symptoms. Unlike in adults, pediatric myositis ossificans may eventually reabsorb [72]. However, myositis ossificans can lead to restricted joint motion and ankylosis with subsequent loss of independence. MRI findings of myositis ossificans can mimic infection, and it is especially important to avoid confusing these diagnoses in paralyzed children, as many have accompanying decubitus ulcers and florid soft tissue infections.

Decubitus or pressure ulcers over bony prominences are common in the pediatric patient population with any sensory-motor impairment but especially in SCI. Dystrophic calcification and heterotopic bone formation may then develop. Extrinsic pressure on soft tissue that exceeds capillary perfusion pressure is the principal cause of skin breakdown. The location provides information about the cause. Ischial ulcers are typically due to prolonged sitting. Trochanteric ulcers commonly result from excessive side-lying. Sacral ulcers, if high, may be due to supine lying, whereas lower intergluteal ulcers may result from sitting at an angle.

The presence of decubitus ulcers can raise concern for osteomyelitis. Osseous cortical erosions frequently result from local erythema and do not demonstrate histologic evidence of osteomyelitis. However, periostitis, permeative osteolysis, reactive sclerosis, and sequestrum formation indicate osseous infection. MRI helps determine the depth and extent of soft tissue involvement adjacent to decubitus ulcers, including the presence of fluid collections and/or abscesses as well as heterotopic ossification. It also identifies findings suspicious for osteomyelitis (see Chap. 19).

2.4 Infectious: Poliomyelitis

Poliomyelitis is an acute viral infection that largely affects children under 2 years of age. Polio peaked in the United States in 1952, with more than 21,000 paralytic cases. However, following the introduction of effective vaccines, incidence rapidly declined. The last case of wild-virus polio acquired in the United States was in 1979. While the virus is still endemic in isolated parts of Asia and Africa, global polio eradication may be imminent.

Poliomyelitis is caused by infection with *poliovirus—enterovirus* subgroup, family *Picornaviridae*. These RNA viruses colonize the gastrointestinal tract and usually incubate from 6 to 20 days. The virus only infects humans and is spread via the fecal-oral route. Three serotypes have been identified. All are extremely virulent and produce the same disease symptoms, but polio virus 1 (PV1) is most common and most closely associated with paralysis. The polio virus targets anterior horn cells (motor neurons) of the spinal cord and brainstem. Acute anterior poliomyelitis leads to varying degrees of asymmetric paralysis and is sometimes associated with respiratory and bulbar involvement.

Up to 95 % of all polio infections are asymptomatic. Approximately 4–8 % present as minor, nonspecific illness without clinical or laboratory evidence of nervous system invasion. Less than 1 % develop flaccid paralysis. MRI can help establish the initial diagnosis of poliomyelitis. T2-weighted images demonstrate hyperintense signal in the bilateral substantia nigra and anterior horns of the spinal cord.

After acute infection, there is a slow and progressive recovery phase. Denervated by the initial acute polio infection, motor function improves through reinnervation of muscle fibers. Some of the brainstem and spinal cord motor neurons that were not destroyed develop new branches, or axonal sprouts, generating enlarged motor neurons. This recovery process does not affect all denervated fibers, and thus, motor sequelae are common. Residual muscular atrophy varies according to the individual subject and topography.

Although new cases are limited to parts of Asia and Africa, orthopedic sequelae can be encountered in patients who have moved from endemic countries.

Children with polio can develop scoliosis, usually in the lumbar region, and this affects walking and sitting. Standing spine radiographs provide important information about leg length discrepancy and pelvic obliquity. Before puberty, scoliosis secondary to polio is generally more flexible (assessed with traction or bending views) than idiopathic scoliosis. After puberty, polio-related scoliosis becomes rigid. Therefore, progression of a curve before puberty can often be followed clinically until it becomes stiff.

In the pelvis, contracture of the tensor fascia lata and gluteus medius tendon inhibits hip extension. This makes walking and standing difficult and accentuates lateral pelvic obliquity, which in turn makes the higher hip more likely to subluxate. Secondary scoliosis may result. Knee contractures can accentuate those in the hip [73].

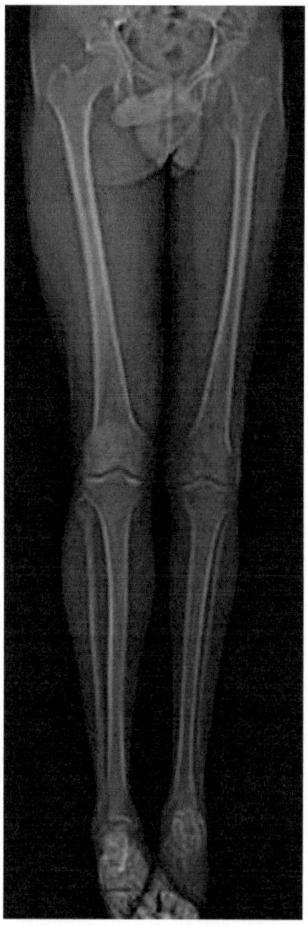

Fig. 24.44 Leg length discrepancy, gracile long bones, and reduced muscle bulk in a patient with polio (Courtesy of Marcos Sampaio)

Polio causes profound asymmetric muscle weakness and wasting. Radiographs and cross-sectional imaging demonstrate fatty replacement, as with other neuromuscular disorders. When the disease affects a very young child, lack of normal weight bearing causes bones to model improperly, resulting in a gracile appearance. Leg length discrepancy is normally associated with soft tissue atrophy and small, fat-replaced muscles (Fig. 24.44). The hips may be dysplastic.

Foot deformities such as equinus, equinovarus, drop foot, and valgus may require early treatment to promote stable and confident walking. Calcaneocavus (hindfoot cavus) results from weak gastrocnemius function, and claw toes develop due to imbalance and overactivity of the long toe flexors and extensors (compensating for weak ankle plantarflexor and dorsiflexor muscles).

In the upper extremities, flail shoulder is common. Other abnormalities include contractures of the elbow, wrist, and both the metacarpal-phalangeal and the interphalangeal joints.

Differential Diagnosis

The muscle wasting of polio resembles a muscular dystrophy, but the clinical presentation is very different. Spinal cord tumors and Guillain-Barre syndrome can also affect the anterior horn cells, but cerebrospinal fluid (CSF) examination and MRI help differentiate between these disorders. Whereas in Guillain-Barre the CSF exhibits increased protein levels and a relatively normal cell count, in polio CSF shows relatively normal protein levels and up to 300 nucleated cells. MRI excludes spinal cord tumor as well as the enlarged anterior nerve roots of Guillain-Barre.

3 Peripheral Nerve

3.1 Charcot-Marie-Tooth Disease

Charcot-Marie-Tooth (CMT) disease, also termed hereditary motor and sensory neuropathy, includes several forms of chronic, peripheral sensory and/or motor neuropathies with variable genetic causes, patterns of inheritance, and penetrance. CMT disease is the most common hereditary neuropathy, with a prevalence of 10–82/100,000. It is slightly more common in females [74]. There are several different subtypes, but CMT type 1A accounts for 70 % of cases. Initial complaints are nonspecific, including clumsiness, frequent ankle sprains, and difficulty buttoning clothing and climbing stairs. Physical examination can disclose distal weakness and wasting beginning at the lower legs, variable amounts of distal sensory loss, depressed or absent deep tendon reflexes, foot and ankle deformities including foot drop and claw toes, spinal deformity, and hip dysplasia [75].

Imaging

Scoliosis, kyphoscoliosis, and thoracic kyphosis are common in adults with CMT. However, spinal deformities are unusual in most children with

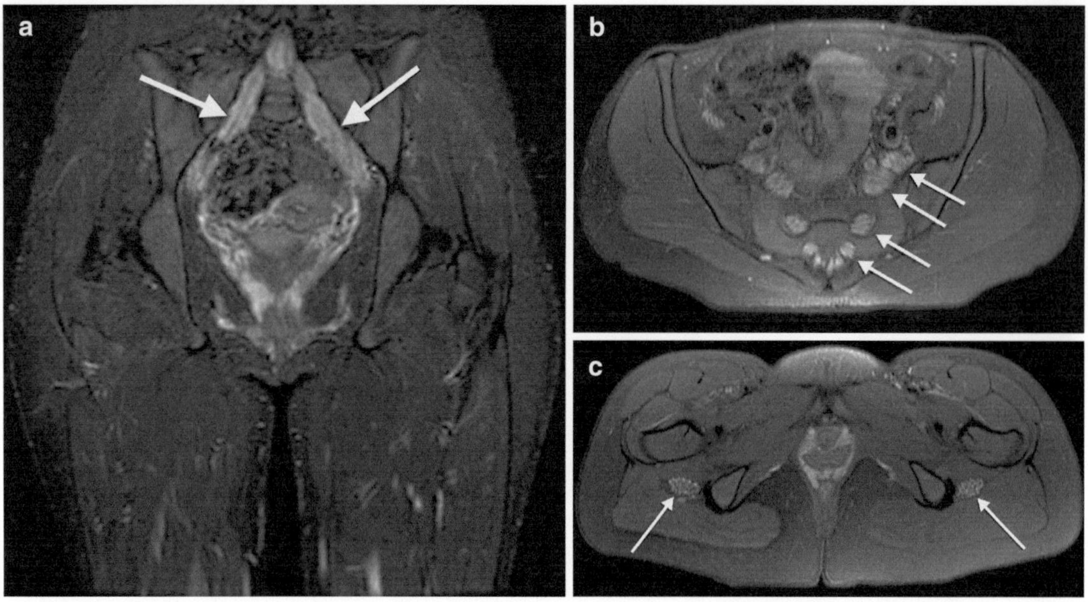

Fig. 24.45 Sciatic nerve involvement in Charcot-Marie-Tooth disease. (**a**) Coronal short-tau inversion recovery (STIR) image of the pelvis and hips shows marked thickening and increased signal of the sciatic nerves (*arrows*). Axial T2-W fat-suppressed images demonstrate (**b**) thickening and increased signal of multiple sacral nerve roots (*arrows* indicate those on the left) as well as (**c**) thickening and separation of individual fascicles of the sciatic nerve (*arrows*) (Courtesy of Rebecca Stein-Wexler)

this disease, unless they have specific mutations. For example, all children with a mutation of the myelin protein zero (MPZ) gene develop scoliosis by age 10 [76]. Scoliosis is usually biphasic, with thc dominant curve in the thoracic region.

In CMT type 1A, MRI evaluation of the pelvis and thighs may show symmetrical moderate to marked enlargement of the nerves (Fig. 24.45). There is interfascicular fatty infiltration as well as demyelinization and atrophy of the fascicles, and nerves may enhance [77].

A review of 74 radiographs of 100 children with CMT found hip dysplasia in six children and minor hip abnormalities in 21 [78]. Hip anomalies are more commonly associated with CMT1 than CMT2 and should be suspected in children developing hip disease or abnormal gait after age 8 [79]. Shallow acetabula and coxa valga are the most common abnormalities.

The typical deformities of the foot result from progressive and selective muscle weakness and include cavus (most common) and hindfoot varus, along with characteristic muscle wasting [80]. Surgical management of foot and ankle deformities is indicated if symptoms—such as ankle sprain, difficulty with shoe wear, stress fractures, or pain—progress.

4 Muscle

4.1 General Considerations

Muscle diseases are categorized as muscular dystrophies (pseudohypertrophic [Duchenne], limb girdle, facioscapulohumeral), myotonic disorders, and inflammatory myopathies (dermatomyositis).

The US appearance of muscle can help differentiate between neuromuscular disorders. For example, Duchenne muscular dystrophy results in severe, homogeneous increased echogenicity with normal muscle thickness, whereas spinal muscular atrophy shows heterogeneously

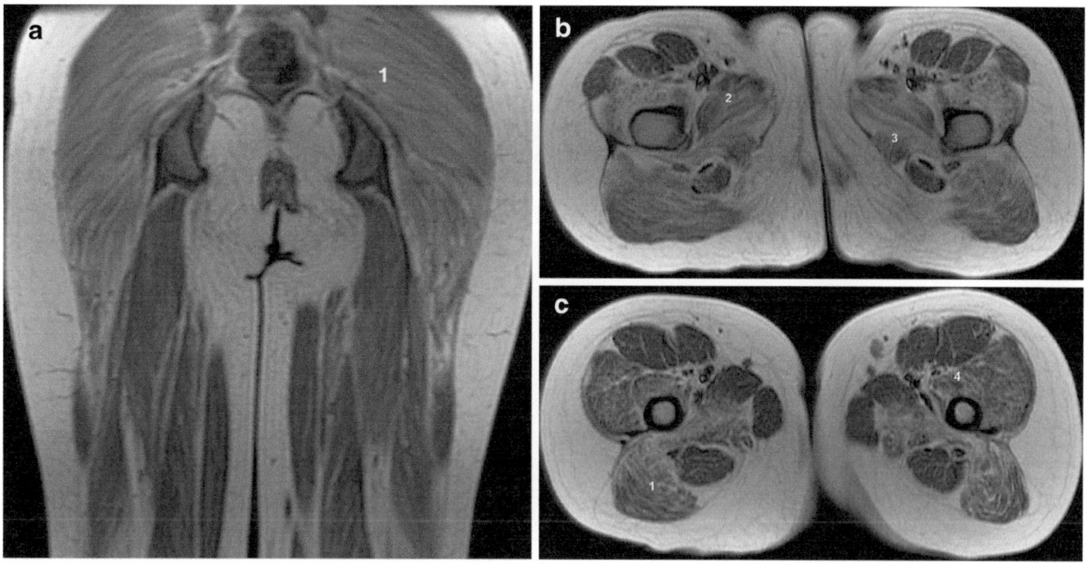

Fig. 24.46 Muscle abnormalities in limb girdle dystrophy (Erb muscular dystrophy) in a 10-year-old boy. Coronal (**a**) and axial (**b**, **c**) T1-W images show hyperintense fatty infiltration of select musculature (*1* gluteus maximus, *2* obturator externus, *3* obturator internus, and *4* vastus intermedius)

increased echogenicity with severe atrophy. A major advantage of muscle US is that it allows dynamic imaging of muscle contraction and fasciculation [81]. High-frequency transducers should be used.

MRI is employed more frequently in the diagnosis of neuromuscular disorders. It can detect the degree of muscular involvement, assessing muscle shape, volume, and tissue architecture. The main goal is delineating altered fat-water composition. T1-weighted imaging is essential for depicting high-signal-intensity fat and low-signal-intensity water (Fig. 24.46). Short-tau inversion recovery (STIR) sequences are sensitive to edematous processes, as they suppress fat signal. Alternative T2 chemical shift sequences offer a relatively short scanning time. Fast T2 spin echo sequences should be avoided because they provide insufficient fat signal suppression. Gadolinium-enhanced T1-weighted imaging may differentiate inflammatory or neoplastic lesions from edematous fluid and also target appropriate sites for biopsy. Coronal images provide an overview of the longitudinal extent of disease and identify palpable bony landmarks that may prove useful at biopsy, whereas axial images best delineate muscle groups and characterize tissue. MRI also helps assess therapeutic success [58, 82, 83].

Computed tomography can detect fatty infiltration caused by neuromuscular disorders and is better than MRI at depicting calcifications caused by inflammatory myopathies. However, its use is limited as it has poor soft tissue contrast, cannot depict the mild edema of early disease, and requires exposure to ionizing radiation.

4.2 Duchenne Muscular Dystrophy

This is the most common and severe muscular dystrophy, causing muscle degeneration and eventual death. A recessive X-linked disorder, Duchenne muscular dystrophy is caused by a mutation in the dystrophin gene (*DMD*; locus

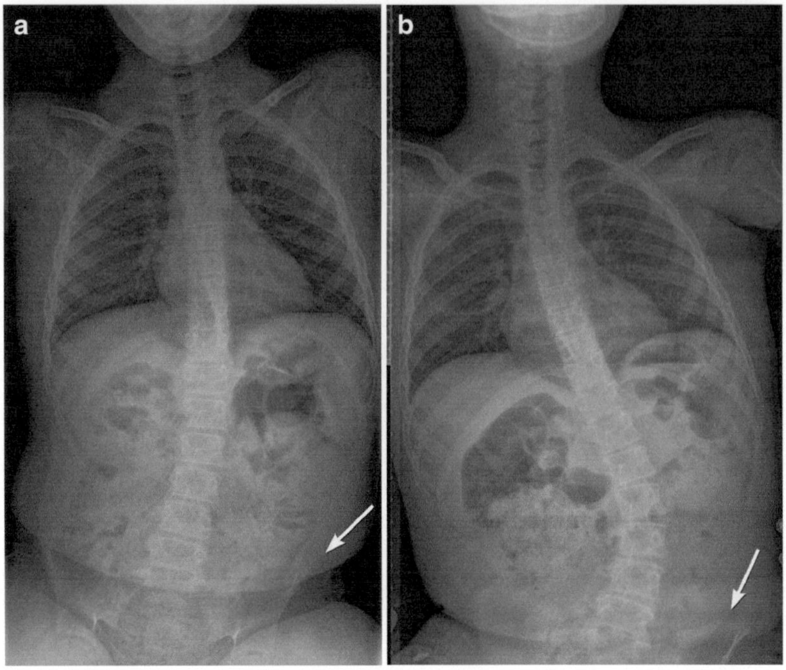

Fig. 24.47 Progressive thoracolumbar scoliosis in a boy with Duchenne muscular dystrophy. (**a**) At age 10, there is mild levoscoliosis and minimal pelvic tilt (*arrow*). (**b**) By age 12, both the curve and the pelvic tilt (*arrow*) have progressed

Xp21.2), which codes for a protein that provides structural stability to muscle cell membranes. Although both sexes can carry the mutation, females rarely exhibit signs of the disease.

Symptoms usually appear in boys before age 5 and may be evident in early infancy. The muscles of the pelvis and upper legs gradually weaken, and there is loss of muscle mass. Weakness eventually spreads to the arms, neck, and other areas. Patients experience difficulty standing unaided and become unable to climb stairs. The calf, deltoid, and triceps muscles are gradually also replaced with fat, resulting in characteristic pseudohypertrophic enlargement in 90 %. However, similar changes occasionally occur in other dystrophies. As the condition progresses, fat and fibrous tissue eventually replace wasted muscle. Most patients are wheelchair dependent by age 12. Respiratory, orthopedic, and cardiac complications develop, and without intervention the mean age at death is approximately 19 years. There may be nonprogressive cognitive dysfunction [84].

Scoliosis is a common complication (68–90 %) and progresses rapidly during puberty in nonambulatory children (Fig. 24.47). It causes discomfort and leads to compromised respiratory function. Attempts to prevent or delay scoliosis with spinal support systems are rarely effective. Corticosteroids are the standard of care for treatment of DMD. Corticosteroids prolong ambulation, improve cardiac and pulmonary function, reduce the incidence of scoliosis, and improve survival. Side effects reported with the use of corticosteroids include weight gain, decreased height, and cataract formation [85]. Progressive curvature, despite bracing, usually mandates surgical fusion. Spinal surgery improves sitting comfort, appearance, and quality of life. However, the timing of spine surgery and its effect on respiratory function and long-term survival are controversial [86].

Thoracic deformity is evident in older patients, with thin, downward sloping ribs and narrow upper thoracic diameter (Fig. 24.48). Cardiac disease and chronic respiratory insufficiency due to restrictive lung disease are terminal findings. Dilated cardiomyopathy affects one third of patients by age 14 and is present in all patients over 18 years of age; fibrosis leads to conduction abnormalities and disturbed rhythm.

Osteoporosis is present in most children with Duchenne (Fig. 24.49). Bone density begins to decrease while boys are still ambulatory and worsens with age [87]. Long bones are thin, osteopenic (Fig. 24.50), and prone to fracture in

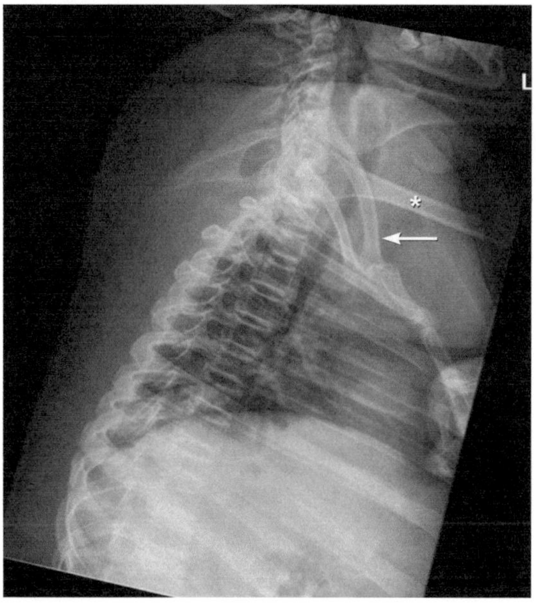

Fig. 24.48 Duchenne muscle dystrophy in a 19-year-old. The upper thorax is small. Ribs and clavicles (*arrow*) are oblique. Note the thin humerus (*) and diffuse osteopenia

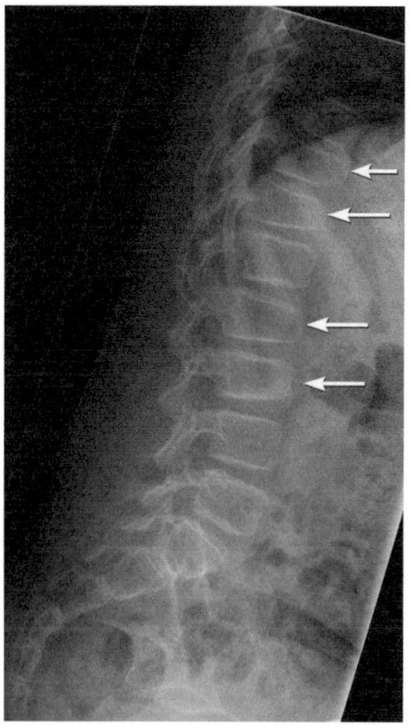

Fig. 24.49 Diffuse osteopenia and multiple compression fractures (*arrows*) in a 10-year-old boy with Duchenne muscle dystrophy

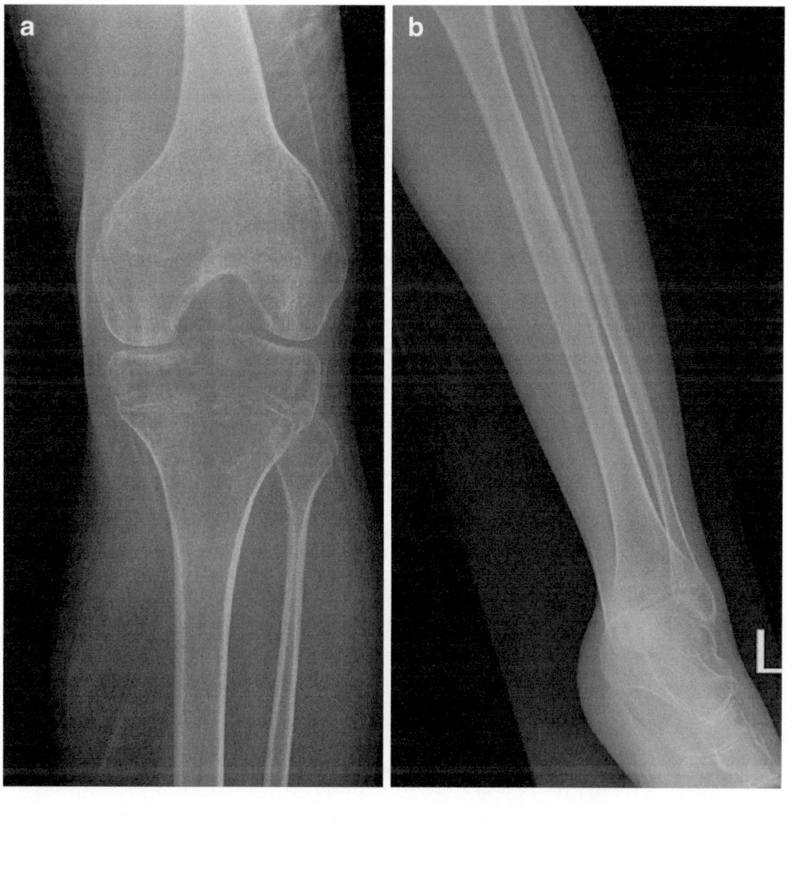

Fig. 24.50 (**a**, **b**) Duchenne muscle dystrophy in an 18-year-old. There is striking osteopenia with thin cortices and a paucity of trabecular markings. Gracile fibula. Muscles planes are extremely faint, due to atrophy and fatty infiltration

21–44 % of cases, usually due to falls. Fractures in ambulatory boys cause many to lose the ability to walk [88]. Knee flexion contracture usually follows wheelchair confinement. The calf muscles are large but appear abnormally lucent. Ankle equinus is often severe.

Ultrasound and MRI reveal the presence, magnitude, and progression of muscle involvement and reflect the clinical stage. Muscle US may be normal in asymptomatic patients, but by the time clinical signs develop, muscle appears abnormal in almost everyone, demonstrating homogeneously increased muscle echogenicity with normal thickness [89]. T1-weighted MRI reveals hyperintense fatty infiltration of diseased muscles.

The other muscular dystrophies are less common and are differentiated from Duchenne by specific clinical patterns. Becker dystrophy is a slowly progressive primary degeneration of skeletal muscle, with onset at approximately 11 years of age and survival to the fourth decade. The disease is inherited as an X-linked recessive disorder, predominantly in boys. Duchenne and Becker muscular dystrophies involve the same muscles, but Becker is less severe. The lower limbs are affected 5–10 years before the upper limbs. Increased serum creatine kinase activity in Becker muscular dystrophy is high, as with Duchenne. Some dystrophies such as facioscapulohumeral type progress slowly and are much less disabling. Limb-girdle dystrophy also progresses slowly but eventually causes severe disability.

Various degrees of scoliosis, femoral neck valgus, hip subluxation, and equinovarus foot occur in all these syndromes.

4.3 Myotonic Disorders

These are a group of diseases that demonstrate involuntary muscle contraction and delayed muscle relaxation. They are hereditary conditions classified into myotonic dystrophies (type 1 and 2) and nondystrophic myotonias, depending on the symptoms.

Myotonic dystrophy type 1 is a multisystem disorder that affects skeletal and smooth muscle as well as the eye, heart, endocrine system, and central nervous system. Myotonic dystrophy type 2 is characterized by myotonia in 90 % of affected individuals and muscle dysfunction (weakness, pain, and stiffness) in 82 %. Cardiac conduction defects, iridescent posterior subcapsular cataracts, insulin-insensitive type 2 diabetes mellitus, and testicular failure are less common. MRI demonstrates nonuniform fatty degeneration of musculature and loss of muscle bulk [90] (Fig. 24.51).

The nondystrophic myotonias are the channelopathies, characterized by impaired transmembrane conductance of either chloride or sodium ions that results in myotonia [91]. These pure skeletal muscle diseases do not involve the heart, brain, eye, or other tissues [92]. Thomsen myotonia congenita, Becker myotonia congenita, myotonia levior, and fluctuating myotonia congenital are all chloride channelopathy-based nondystrophic myotonias. They are caused by mutations that result in loss of function of the chloride channel ClC-1, which is expressed exclusively in skeletal muscle membrane.

In Thomsen myotonia congenita, physical examination may reveal muscle hypertrophy in the extremities and in the facial muscles, handgrip myotonia, and eyelid myotonia. Patients may have trouble sitting up quickly after lying supine for several minutes, as a result of myotonia in the paraspinal muscles and in the proximal muscles of the extremities [93]. Becker myotonia is an autosomal recessive chloride channel myotonia that, like Thomsen myotonia, is characterized by generalized myotonia and muscle hypertrophy. However, Becker myotonia has an insidious onset in later childhood, initially manifests in the lower extremities (hence the synonym "ascending myotonia congenital"), and may present with slowly progressive weakness and with transient episodes of proximal muscle weakness that last seconds or minutes [94, 95].

Sodium channelopathy myotonias are characterized by sensitivity to cold exposure, potassium ingestion, and paradoxical worsening after exercise [96]. Muscle MRI of nondystrophic myotonias demonstrates evidence of fatty infiltration and/or edema [97].

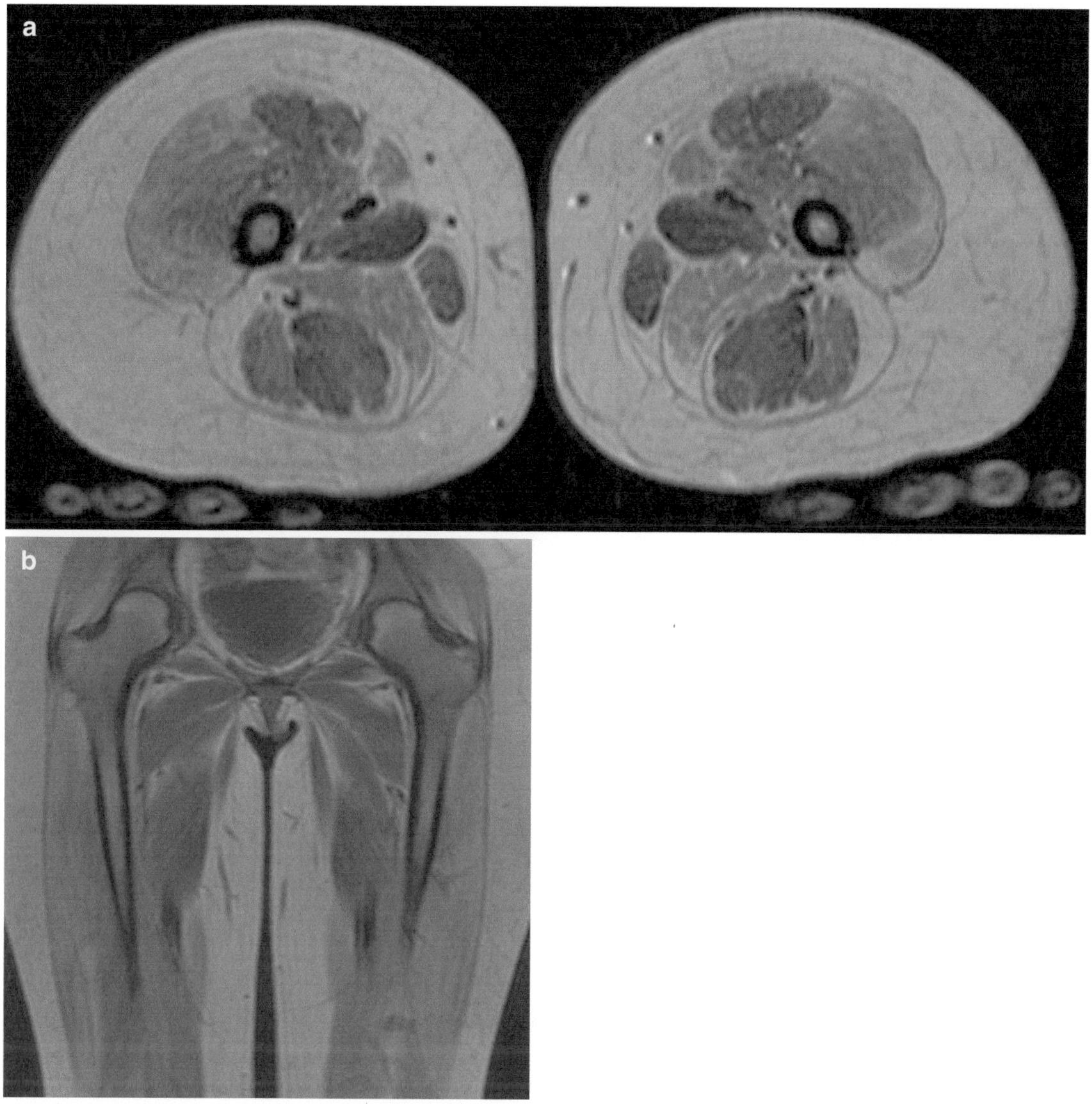

Fig. 24.51 Muscular dystrophy in a 17-year-old girl. Axial (**a**) and coronal (**b**) T1-W MRI images show fatty degeneration of musculature and overall loss of bulk, along with diffuse increase in fatty tissue. The adductor magnus, vastus lateralis, and sartorius muscles are most severely affected (Courtesy of Tal Laor, Cincinnati Children's Hospital)

4.4 Dermatomyositis

Juvenile dermatomyositis is a rare autoimmune disease and the most common inflammatory myopathy of childhood. This systemic vasculopathy is characterized by proximal muscle weakness, elevated levels of muscle enzymes, and characteristic skin rashes, including Gottron papules over the extensor surfaces of the extremities and discoloration of the upper lids and cheeks.

MRI is useful for managing dermatomyositis, as it helps diagnose the condition, monitor treatment, and identify sites for muscle biopsy. The diagnostic sensitivity of MRI has been reported at 76 %, compared with 64 % for creatine kinase [98]. MRI reveals increased water content that is generally symmetric within edematous muscles, particularly in the deep musculature. The anterior muscles of the thigh are most frequently involved. T2-weighted and

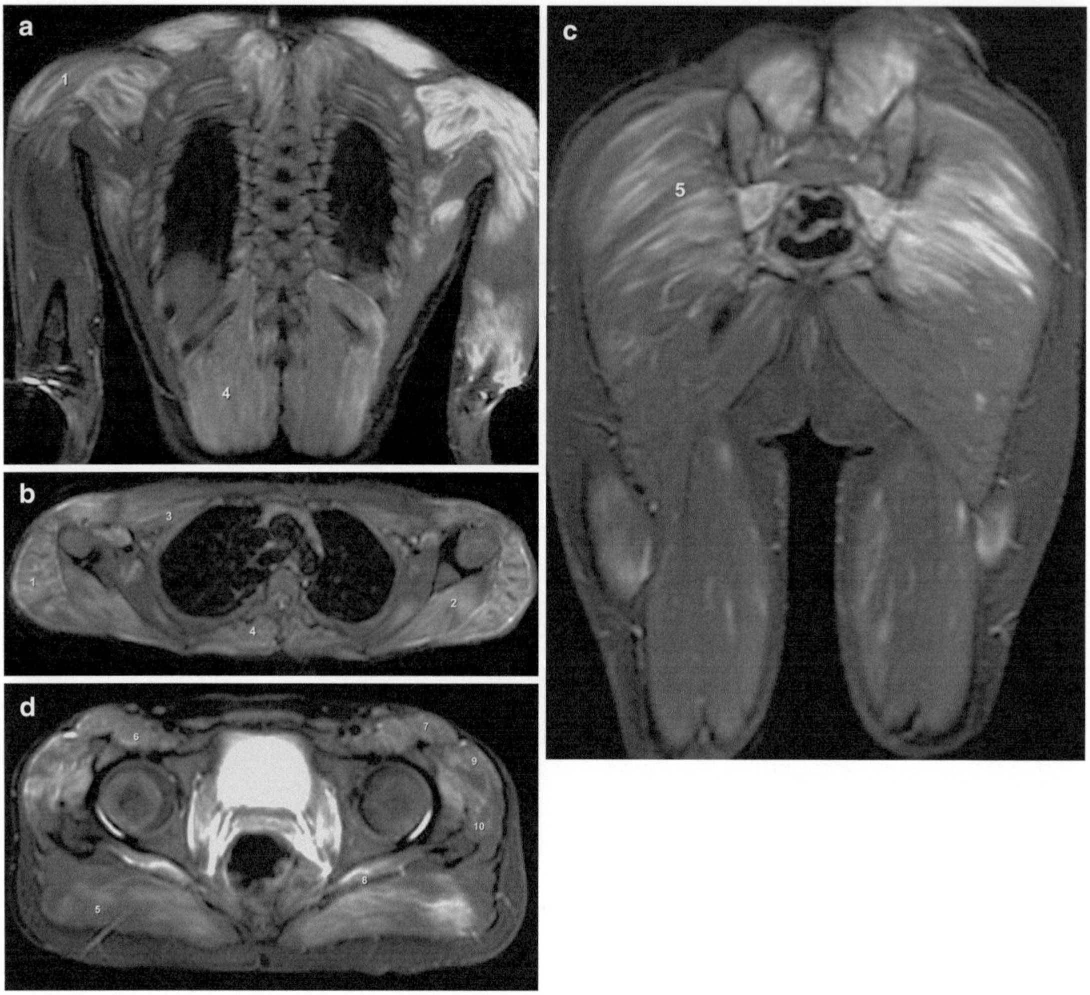

Fig. 24.52 Dermatomyositis in a 14-year-old boy. Coronal and axial short-tau inversion recovery (STIR) images of the chest and shoulders (**a**, **b**) and of the pelvis and thighs (**c**, **d**) show roughly symmetric increased signal in essentially all visualized muscles. Deltoid (*1*), rotator cuff (*2*), pectoralis major (*3*), erector spinae and latissimus dorsi (*4*), gluteus maximus (*5*), iliopsoas (*6*), sartorius (*7*), quadratus femoris (*8*), rectus femoris (*9*), and tensor fascia lata (*10*)

short-tau inversion recovery (STIR) MRI sequences are important to depict muscle edema, perimuscular edema, and fascial abnormalities (Fig. 24.52). T1-weighted images demonstrate muscle atrophy and fatty infiltration in the presence of chronic muscle damage. Children with dermatomyositis may also have extensive subcutaneous and intermuscular fluid collections, whose margins may demonstrate mild enhancement after administration of gadolinium (if abscesses, their peripheral enhancement will be more intense) [58, 99].

5 Multifocal Neuromuscular Disease

5.1 Friedreich Ataxia

Friedreich ataxia is the most common autosomal recessive hereditary ataxia. It is caused by mutations in the FRDA (Friedreich ataxia) gene [100], which produces frataxin, a protein involved in iron-sulfur cluster synthesis. The lack of frataxin results in early loss of large sensory neurons in the dorsal root ganglia, with subsequent deterio-

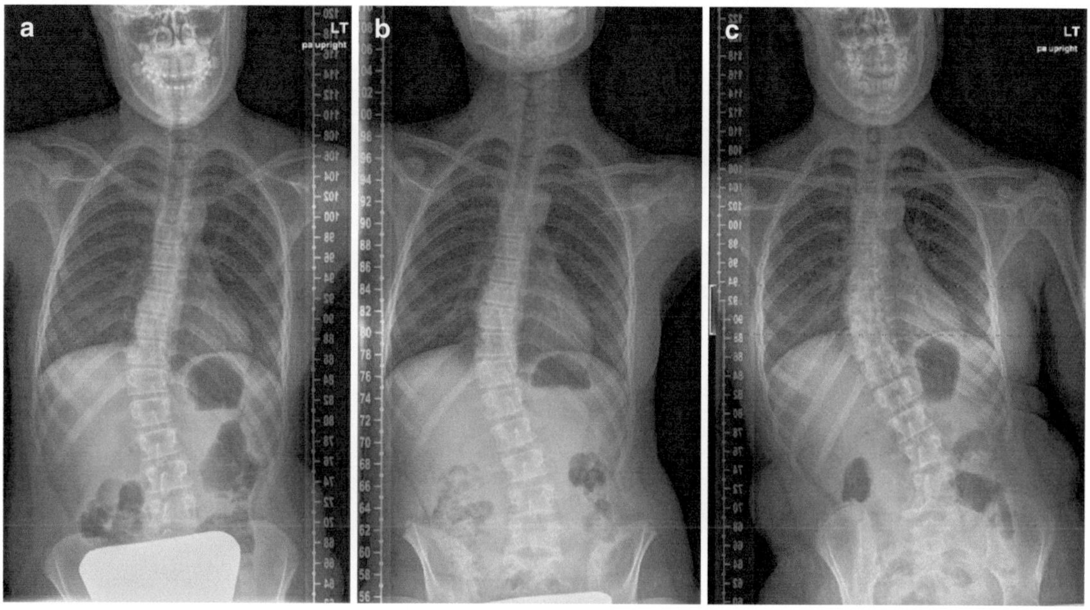

Fig. 24.53 (**a**–**c**) Gradual progression of biphasic thoracolumbar scoliosis in a boy with Friedreich ataxia. The non-compensated scoliosis with upper body lean (**c**) is typical of muscle weakness

ration of the spinocerebellar tract, pyramidal tract, and dorsal columns.

Friedreich ataxia typically presents before age 25, with the average onset of symptoms in the early teen to mid-teen period. This slowly progressive disorder is characterized by ataxia of limbs and gait, absence of knee and ankle reflexes, and dysarthria. Brain MRI is often normal but may show atrophy of the superior vermis, inferior cerebellar hemispheres, spinal cord, and occasionally brainstem. Cardiomyopathy occurs in 70 % of patients and diabetes in 10 % [101].

Scoliosis develops in 75 % of patients. Like idiopathic scoliosis, it is not necessarily progressive, and the curvature is unrelated to muscle weakness or duration of disease (Fig. 24.53). Also like idiopathic scoliosis, biphasic thoracolumbar curvature—with the thoracic curve convex to the right and the lumbar curve convex to the left—is common. Onset before puberty increases the likelihood of progression. Increased thoracic kyphosis is encountered in about 75 % of patients. Coxa valga may develop as well, with subsequent hip subluxation. Pes cavus is common, occurring in 55–75 %.

6 Sensory/Autonomic

6.1 Complex Regional Pain Syndrome: Type 1 (CRPS-1)

Previously known as reflex sympathetic dystrophy and reflex neurovascular dystrophy, this rare clinical syndrome affects one or more extremities. CRPS-1 is an incompletely understood response to an external stimulus that results in pain that is usually nonanatomic and disproportionate to the inciting event or expected healing response (CRPS-2 has underlying causality). Patients with CRPS-1 present with pain, hyperesthesia, and vasomotor disturbances, and there must be at least one sign of autonomic dysfunction in the affected limb(s) [102]. Later, more permanent or serious symptoms may develop, including muscle atrophy, bone demineralization, and contractures of soft tissue around affected joints—however, complete resolution of symptoms is more likely in children than in adults. Major disability and profound psychological dysfunction may follow, but sympathetic denervation can relieve symptoms.

CRPS-1 is well known in adults but is a relatively new and frequently unrecognized diagnosis in children; clinical features may vary widely between children and adults. Most children present in late childhood or early adolescence, with mean onset at age 12–13 and a higher incidence in girls (four to one) [103]. Symptoms have often been present for 6 months. The most common complaint is pain that exceeds the severity of injury, and in children the lower extremities are involved most often. The affected extremity demonstrates altered color and temperature (mostly cooler) and impaired active range of motion [104].

There is no uniform cause of CRPS-1. The precipitating event in children may be quite minor, or CRPS-1 may follow fracture, sprain, illness, infection, surgical procedure, psychological distress, or a combination thereof. Psychological factors appear to play a larger role in children, but children tend to have milder neurological or sympathetic symptoms. Early mobilization, pain control, physical therapy, and psychotherapy decrease pain and improve function. In children and adolescents, physiotherapy is more effective than other more invasive treatments (such as sympathetic blocks), and most recover fully.

Imaging

Diagnosis is usually based on history and physical, as laboratory tests are not helpful.

Radiographs eventually demonstrate demineralization and soft tissue swelling, but these late findings are nonspecific (Fig. 24.54). Most importantly, radiographs exclude other conditions such as stress fracture, infection, and neoplasm. Findings on three-phase bone scan vary. There may be increased blood flow to the affected limb as well as increased uptake on delayed images, especially around the joints. However, radiotracer uptake in children may be decreased [105]. Bone scan has a higher negative predictive value and is also more sensitive to CRPS-1 than MRI or radiographs [106]. There has been little work on MRI of CRPS-1 in children, but in adults MRI findings are nonspecific, with soft tissue thickening that shows variable enhancement [107]. Bone marrow findings vary and are nonspecific.

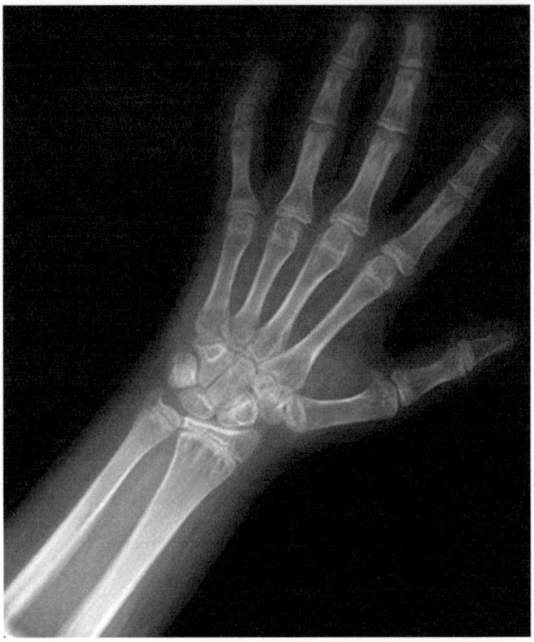

Fig. 24.54 Complex regional pain syndrome type 1 in a 13-year-old boy with neurological impairment several months after meningitis. There is periarticular osteopenia at the interphalangeal and metacarpophalangeal joints as well as osteopenia at the distal radius and ulna. Soft tissue swelling at the digits. These findings would be present in atrophy due to disuse as well and must be correlated with the clinical findings of complex regional pain syndrome type 1

Acknowledgments We would like to thank Dr. Hugh McMillan, Dr. Kristin Udjus, and Dr. Rita Putnins (Children's Hospital of Eastern Ontario, University of Ottawa) for their contribution of cases.

References

1. Standley F, Blair E, Alberman E. Cerebral palsies: epidemiology and causal pathways. Clinics in developmental medicine. London: Mac-Keith Press; 2000. p. 151.
2. Rosenbaum P, Paneth N, Leviton A, Goldstein M, Bax M, Damiano D, et al. A report: the definition and classification of cerebral palsy April 2006. Dev Med Child Neurol Suppl. 2007;109:8–14. PubMed PMID: 17370477. Epub 2007/03/21. eng.
3. Bax M, Goldstein M, Rosenbaum P, Leviton A, Paneth N, Dan B, et al. Proposed definition and classification of cerebral palsy, April 2005. Dev Med Child Neurol. 2005;47(8):571–6. PubMed PMID: 16108461. Epub 2005/08/20. eng.
4. Howard J, Soo B, Graham HK, Boyd RN, Reid S, Lanigan A, et al. Cerebral palsy in Victoria: motor types, topography and gross motor function. J Paediatr Child Health. 2005;41(9–10):479–83. PubMed PMID: 16150063. Epub 2005/09/10. eng.

5. Palisano R, Rosenbaum P, Walter S, Russell D, Wood E, Galuppi B. Development and reliability of a system to classify gross motor function in children with cerebral palsy. Dev Med Child Neurol. 1997;39(4):214–23. PubMed PMID: 9183258. Epub 1997/04/01. eng.
6. Nelson KB. Causative factors in cerebral palsy. Clin Obstet Gynecol. 2008;51(4):749–62. PubMed PMID: 18981800. Epub 2008/11/05. eng.
7. Moreno-De-Luca A, Ledbetter DH, Martin CL. Genetic [corrected] insights into the causes and classification of [corrected] cerebral palsies. Lancet Neurol. 2012;11(3):283–92. PubMed PMID: 22261432. Pubmed Central PMCID: 3296129. Epub 2012/01/21. eng.
8. Chao CP, Zaleski CG, Patton AC. Neonatal hypoxic-ischemic encephalopathy: multimodality imaging findings. Radiographics. 2006;26 Suppl 1:S159–72. PubMed PMID: 17050513. Epub 2006/10/20. eng.
9. Beals RK. Developmental changes in the femur and acetabulum in spastic paraplegia and diplegia. Dev Med Child Neurol. 1969;11(3):303–13. PubMed PMID: 5794162. Epub 1969/06/01. eng.
10. Bachrach SJ, Kecskemethy HH, Harcke HT, Hossain J. Decreased fracture incidence after 1 year of pamidronate treatment in children with spastic quadriplegic cerebral palsy. Dev Med Child Neurol. 2010;52(9):837–42. PubMed PMID: 20573180.
11. Harcke HT, Stevenson KL, Kecskemethy HH, Bachrach SJ, Grissom LE. Fracture after bisphosphonate treatment in children with cerebral palsy: the role of stress risers. Pediatr Radiol. 2012;42(1):76–81. PubMed PMID: 21877116.
12. Persson-Bunke M, Hagglund G, Lauge-Pedersen H, Ma PW, Westbom L. Scoliosis in a total population of children with cerebral palsy. Spine (Phila Pa 1976). 2012;37(12):E708–13. PubMed PMID: 22218299. Epub 2012/01/06. eng.
13. Robson P. The prevalence of scoliosis in adolescents and young adults with cerebral palsy. Dev Med Child Neurol. 1968;10(4):447–52. PubMed PMID: 5681556. Epub 1968/08/01. eng.
14. Harada T, Ebara S, Anwar MM, Kajiura I, Oshita S, Hiroshima K, et al. The lumbar spine in spastic diplegia. A radiographic study. J Bone Joint Surg Br. 1993;75(4):534–7. PubMed PMID: 8331105. Epub 1993/07/01. eng.
15. Morrell DS, Pearson JM, Sauser DD. Progressive bone and joint abnormalities of the spine and lower extremities in cerebral palsy. Radiographics. 2002;22(2):257–68. PubMed PMID: 11896216. Epub 2002/03/16. eng.
16. Thometz JG, Simon SR. Progression of scoliosis after skeletal maturity in institutionalized adults who have cerebral palsy. J Bone Joint Surg Am. 1988;70(9):1290–6. PubMed PMID: 3182881. Epub 1988/10/01. eng.
17. Ferguson RL, Allen Jr BL. Considerations in the treatment of cerebral palsy patients with spinal deformities. Orthop Clin North Am. 1988;19(2):419–25. PubMed PMID: 3357689. Epub 1988/04/01. eng.
18. Bohtz C, Meyer-Heim A, Min K. Changes in health-related quality of life after spinal fusion and scoliosis correction in patients with cerebral palsy. J Pediatr Orthop. 2011;31(6):668–73. PubMed PMID: 21841443. Epub 2011/08/16. eng.
19. Nishioka E, Yoshida K, Yamanaka K, Inoue A. Radiographic studies of the wrist and elbow in cerebral palsy. J Orthop Sci. 2000;5(3):268–74. PubMed PMID: 10982668. Epub 2000/09/12. eng.
20. Abu-Sneineh AK, Gabos PG, Miller F. Radial head dislocation in children with cerebral palsy. J Pediatr Orthop. 2003;23(2):155–8. PubMed PMID: 12604942. Epub 2003/02/27. eng.
21. Persiani P, Molayem I, Calistri A, Rosi S, Bove M, Villani C. Hip subluxation and dislocation in cerebral palsy: outcome of bone surgery in 21 hips. Acta Orthop Belg. 2008;74(5):609–14. PubMed PMID: 19058693. Epub 2008/12/09. eng.
22. Sauser DD, Hewes RC, Root L. Hip changes in spastic cerebral palsy. AJR Am J Roentgenol. 1986;146(6):1219–22. PubMed PMID: 3486566. Epub 1986/06/01. eng.
23. Tomczak RJ, Guenther KP, Rieber A, Mergo P, Ros PR, Brambs HJ. MR imaging measurement of the femoral antetorsional angle as a new technique: comparison with CT in children and adults. AJR Am J Roentgenol. 1997;168(3):791–4. PubMed PMID: 9057536.
24. Davids JR, Marshall AD, Blocker ER, Frick SL, Blackhurst DW, Skewes E. Femoral anteversion in children with cerebral palsy. Assessment with two and three-dimensional computed tomography scans. J Bone Joint Surg Am. 2003;85-A(3):481–8. PubMed PMID: 12637435.
25. Jarrett DY, Oliveira AM, Zou KH, Snyder BD, Kleinman PK. Axial oblique CT to assess femoral anteversion. AJR Am J Roentgenol. 2010;194(5):1230–3. PubMed PMID: 20410408.
26. Samilson RL, Tsou P, Aamoth G, Green WM. Dislocation and subluxation of the hip in cerebral palsy. Pathogenesis, natural history and management. J Bone Joint Surg Am. 1972;54(4):863–73.
27. Bleck EE. The hip in cerebral palsy. Orthop Clin North Am. 1980;11(1):79–104. PubMed PMID: 7360505. Epub 1980/01/01. eng.
28. Sutherland DH, Davids JR. Common gait abnormalities of the knee in cerebral palsy. Clin Orthop Relat Res. 1993;288:139–47. PubMed PMID: 8458127. Epub 1993/03/01. eng.
29. Svehlik M, Zwick EB, Steinwender G, Saraph V, Linhart WE. Genu recurvatum in cerebral palsy–part A: influence of dynamic and fixed equinus deformity on the timing of knee recurvatum in children with cerebral palsy. J Pediatr Orthop B. 2010;19(4):366–72. PubMed PMID: 20442674. Epub 2010/05/06. eng.
30. Davids JR. The foot and ankle in cerebral palsy. Orthop Clin North Am. 2010;41(4):579–93. PubMed PMID: 20868886. Epub 2010/09/28. eng.

31. Eubanks JD, Cheruvu VK. Prevalence of sacral spina bifida occulta and its relationship to age, sex, race, and the sacral table angle: an anatomic, osteologic study of three thousand one hundred specimens. Spine (Phila Pa 1976). 2009;34(15):1539–43. PubMed PMID: 19564762. Epub 2009/07/01. eng.
32. Prevention of neural tube defects: results of the Medical Research Council Vitamin Study. MRC Vitamin Study Research Group. Lancet. 1991;338(8760):131–7. PubMed PMID: 1677062. Epub 1991/07/20. eng.
33. Tortori-Donati P, Rossi A, Cama A. Spinal dysraphism: a review of neuroradiological features with embryological correlations and proposal for a new classification. Neuroradiology. 2000;42(7):471–91. PubMed PMID: 10952179. Epub 2000/08/22. eng.
34. Miller E, Widjaja E, Blaser S, Dennis M, Raybaud C. The old and the new: supratentorial MR findings in Chiari II malformation. Childs Nerv Syst. 2008;24(5):563–75. PubMed PMID: 18026960. Epub 2007/11/21. eng.
35. Midrio P, Silberstein HJ, Bilaniuk LT, Adzick NS, Sutton LN. Prenatal diagnosis of terminal myelocystocele in the fetal surgery era: case report. Neurosurgery. 2002;50(5):1152–4. PubMed PMID: 11950422. discussion 4–5; Epub 2002/04/13. eng.
36. Leung EC, Sgouros S, Williams S, Johnson K. Spinal lipoma misinterpreted as a meningomyelocele on antenatal MRI scan in a baby girl. Childs Nerv Syst. 2002;18(6–7):361–3. PubMed PMID: 12172948. Epub 2002/08/13. eng.
37. Breningstall GN, Marker SM, Tubman DE. Hydrosyringomyelia and diastematomyelia detected by MRI in myelomeningocele. Pediatr Neurol. 1992;8(4):267–71. PubMed PMID: 1388414. Epub 1992/07/01. eng.
38. Westcott MA, Dynes MC, Remer EM, Donaldson JS, Dias LS. Congenital and acquired orthopedic abnormalities in patients with myelomeningocele. Radiographics. 1992;12(6):1155–73. PubMed PMID: 1439018. Epub 1992/11/01. eng.
39. Muller EB, Nordwall A, Oden A. Progression of scoliosis in children with myelomeningocele. Spine (Phila Pa 1976). 1994;19(2):147–50. PubMed PMID: 8153821. Epub 1994/01/15. eng.
40. Trivedi J, Thomson JD, Slakey JB, Banta JV, Jones PW. Clinical and radiographic predictors of scoliosis in patients with myelomeningocele. J Bone Joint Surg Am. 2002;84-A(8):1389–94. PubMed PMID: 12177269. Epub 2002/08/15. eng.
41. Samuelsson L, Bergstrom K, Thuomas KA, Hemmingson A, Wallensten R. Scoliosis in myelomeningocele. Significance of syringohydromyelia and Chiari malformations studied with magnetic resonance imaging. Rev Chir Orthop Reparatrice Appar Mot. 1988;74 Suppl 2:310–1. PubMed PMID: 3231810. Epub 1988/01/01. eng.
42. Ozek MM, Erol B, Tamai J. Management of vertebral problems and deformities. In: Ozek MM, Cinalli G, Maixner WJ, editors. Spina bifida management and outcome. New York: Springer; 2008. p. 305–17.
43. Mehta VA, Bettegowda C, Ahmadi SA, Berenberg P, Thomale UW, Haberl EJ, et al. Spinal cord tethering following myelomeningocele repair. J Neurosurg Pediatr. 2010;6(5):498–505. PubMed PMID: 21039176.
44. Muller EB, Nordwall A. Brace treatment of scoliosis in children with myelomeningocele. Spine (Phila Pa 1976). 1994;19(2):151–5. PubMed PMID: 8153822. Epub 1994/01/15. eng.
45. Leatherman KD, Dickson RA. Congenital kyphosis in myelomeningocele. Vertebral body resection and posterior spine fusion. Spine (Phila Pa 1976). 1978;3(3):222–6. PubMed PMID: 715551. Epub 1978/09/01. eng.
46. Carstens C, Koch H, Brocai DR, Niethard FU. Development of pathological lumbar kyphosis in myelomeningocele. J Bone Joint Surg Br. 1996;78(6):945–50. PubMed PMID: 8951012. Epub 1996/11/01. eng.
47. Hoppenfeld S. Congenital kyphosis in myelomeningocele. J Bone Joint Surg Br. 1967;49(2):276–80. PubMed PMID: 5338247. Epub 1967/05/01. eng.
48. Steel HH, Adams DJ. Hyperlordosis caused by the lumboperitoneal shunt procedure for hydrocephalus. J Bone Joint Surg Am. 1972;54(7):1537–42. PubMed PMID: 4653637. Epub 1972/10/01. eng.
49. Broughton NS, Graham G, Menelaus MB. The high incidence of foot deformity in patients with high-level spina bifida. J Bone Joint Surg Br. 1994;76(4):548–50. PubMed PMID: 8027137. Epub 1994/07/01. eng.
50. Gerlach DJ, Gurnett CA, Limpaphayom N, Alaee F, Zhang Z, Porter K, et al. Early results of the Ponseti method for the treatment of clubfoot associated with myelomeningocele. J Bone Joint Surg Am. 2009;91(6):1350–9. PubMed PMID: 19487512. Epub 2009/06/03. eng.
51. Barnett J, Menelaus MB. Pressure sores and pathological fractures. In: Broughton N, Menelaus MB, editors. Menelaus' orthopaedic management of spina bifida cystica. Philadelphia: WB Saunders; 1998. p. 51–65.
52. Boytim MJ, Davidson RS, Charney E, Melchionni JB. Neonatal fractures in myelomeningocele patients. J Pediatr Orthop. 1991;11(1):28–30. PubMed PMID: 1988474. Epub 1991/01/01. eng.
53. Kumar SJ, Cowell HR, Townsend P. Physeal, metaphyseal, and diaphyseal injuries of the lower extremities in children with myelomeningocele. J Pediatr Orthop. 1984;4(1):25–7. PubMed PMID: 6693564. Epub 1984/01/01. eng.
54. Lock TR, Aronson DD. Fractures in patients who have myelomeningocele. J Bone Joint Surg Am. 1989;71(8):1153–7. PubMed PMID: 2777841. Epub 1989/09/01. eng.
55. Nagarkatti DG, Banta JV, Thomson JD. Charcot arthropathy in spina bifida. J Pediatr Orthop. 2000;20(1):82–7. PubMed PMID: 10641695. Epub 2000/01/21. eng.
56. D'Amico A, Mercuri E, Tiziano FD, Bertini E. Spinal muscular atrophy. Orphanet J Rare Dis.

2011;6:71. PubMed PMID: 22047105. Pubmed Central PMCID: 3231874. Epub 2011/11/04. eng.
57. Mesfin A, Sponseller PD, Leet AI. Spinal muscular atrophy: manifestations and management. J Am Acad Orthop Surg. 2012;20(6):393–401. PubMed PMID: 22661569. Epub 2012/06/05. eng.
58. Chan WP, Liu GC. MR imaging of primary skeletal muscle diseases in children. AJR Am J Roentgenol. 2002;179(4):989–97. PubMed PMID: 12239053. Epub 2002/09/20. eng.
59. Pillen S, Arts IM, Zwarts MJ. Muscle ultrasound in neuromuscular disorders. Muscle Nerve. 2008;37(6):679–93. PubMed PMID: 18506712. Epub 2008/05/29. eng.
60. Center NSCIS. The 2004 Annual Statistical Report for the Model Spinal Cord Injury Care Systems. Birmingham: University of Alabama; 2004.
61. Bilston LE, Brown J. Pediatric spinal injury type and severity are age and mechanism dependent. Spine (Phila Pa 1976). 2007;32(21):2339–47. PubMed PMID: 17906576. Epub 2007/10/02. eng.
62. Pang D, Wilberger Jr JE. Spinal cord injury without radiographic abnormalities in children. J Neurosurg. 1982;57(1):114–29. PubMed PMID: 7086488. Epub 1982/07/01. eng.
63. Kirshblum SC, Burns SP, Biering-Sorensen F, Donovan W, Graves DE, Jha A, et al. International standards for neurological classification of spinal cord injury (revised 2011). J Spinal Cord Med. 2011;34(6):535–46. PubMed PMID: 22330108. Pubmed Central PMCID: 3232636. Epub 2012/02/15. eng.
64. Parent S, Mac-Thiong JM, Roy-Beaudry M, Sosa JF, Labelle H. Spinal cord injury in the pediatric population: a systematic review of the literature. J Neurotrauma. 2011;28(8):1515–24. PubMed PMID: 21501096. Pubmed Central PMCID: 3143390. Epub 2011/04/20. eng.
65. Apple Jr DF, Anson CA, Hunter JD, Bell RB. Spinal cord injury in youth. Clin Pediatr (Phila). 1995;34(2):90–5. PubMed PMID: 7729113. Epub 1995/02/01. eng.
66. Dearolf 3rd WW, Betz RR, Vogel LC, Levin J, Clancy M, Steel HH. Scoliosis in pediatric spinal cord-injured patients. J Pediatr Orthop. 1990;10(2):214–8. PubMed PMID: 2312704. Epub 1990/03/01. eng.
67. Rink P, Miller F. Hip instability in spinal cord injury patients. J Pediatr Orthop. 1990;10(5):583–7. PubMed PMID: 2394810. Epub 1990/09/01. eng.
68. Vanwanseele B, Eckstein F, Knecht H, Spaepen A, Stussi E. Longitudinal analysis of cartilage atrophy in the knees of patients with spinal cord injury. Arthritis Rheum. 2003;48(12):3377–81. PubMed PMID: 14673989. Epub 2003/12/16. eng.
69. Pool Jr WH. Cartilage atrophy. Radiology. 1974;112(1):47–50. PubMed PMID: 4832511. Epub 1974/07/01. eng.
70. Jiang SD, Dai LY, Jiang LS. Osteoporosis after spinal cord injury. Osteoporos Int. 2006;17(2):180–92. PubMed PMID: 16217589. Epub 2005/10/12. eng.
71. Maimoun L, Fattal C, Sultan C. Bone remodeling and calcium homeostasis in patients with spinal cord injury: a review. Metabolism. 2011;60(12):1655–63. PubMed PMID: 21632079. Epub 2011/06/03. eng.
72. Garland DE, Shimoyama ST, Lugo C, Barras D, Gilgoff I. Spinal cord insults and heterotopic ossification in the pediatric population. Clin Orthop Relat Res. 1989;245:303–10. PubMed PMID: 2502349. Epub 1989/08/01. eng.
73. Hugh GW. Orthopedic techniques in the management of the residua of paralytic poliomyelitis. Techniques in orthopaedics. Philadelphia: Lippincott Williams & Wilkins, Inc; 2005. p. 179–89.
74. Braathen GJ, Sand JC, Lobato A, Hoyer H, Russell MB. Genetic epidemiology of Charcot-Marie-Tooth in the general population. Eur J Neurol. 2011;18(1):39–48. PubMed PMID: 20482598. Epub 2010/05/21. eng.
75. Yagerman SE, Cross MB, Green DW, Scher DM. Pediatric orthopedic conditions in Charcot-Marie-Tooth disease: a literature review. Curr Opin Pediatr. 2012;24(1):50–6. PubMed PMID: 22189393. Epub 2011/12/23. eng.
76. Horacek O, Mazanec R, Morris CE, Kobesova A. Spinal deformities in hereditary motor and sensory neuropathy: a retrospective qualitative, quantitative, genotypical, and familial analysis of 175 patients. Spine (Phila Pa 1976). 2007;32(22):2502–8. PubMed PMID: 18090092. Epub 2007/12/20. eng.
77. Wadhwa V, Thakkar RS, Maragakis N, Hoke A, Sumner CJ, Lloyd TE, et al. Sciatic nerve tumor and tumor-like lesions—uncommon pathologies. Skeletal Radiol. 2012;41(7):763–74. PubMed PMID: 22410805. Epub 2012/03/14. eng.
78. Walker JL, Nelson KR, Heavilon JA, Stevens DB, Lubicky JP, Ogden JA, et al. Hip abnormalities in children with Charcot-Marie-Tooth disease. J Pediatr Orthop. 1994;14(1):54–9. PubMed PMID: 8113373. Epub 1994/01/01. eng.
79. Bamford NS, White KK, Robinett SA, Otto RK, Gospe Jr SM. Neuromuscular hip dysplasia in Charcot-Marie-Tooth disease type 1A. Dev Med Child Neurol. 2009;51(5):408–11. PubMed PMID: 19388151. Epub 2009/04/24. eng.
80. Guyton GP, Mann RA. The pathogenesis and surgical management of foot deformity in Charcot-Marie-Tooth disease. Foot Ankle Clin. 2000;5(2):317–26. PubMed PMID: 11232233. Epub 2001/03/10. eng.
81. Pillen S, van Alfen N, Zwarts MJ. Muscle ultrasound: a grown-up technique for children with neuromuscular disorders. Muscle Nerve. 2008;38(3):1213–4. PubMed PMID: 18642384. Epub 2008/07/22. eng.
82. Mercuri E, Pichiecchio A, Allsop J, Messina S, Pane M, Muntoni F. Muscle MRI in inherited neuromuscular disorders: past, present, and future. J Magn Reson Imaging. 2007;25(2):433–40. PubMed PMID: 17260395. Epub 2007/01/30. eng.
83. Wattjes MP, Kley RA, Fischer D. Neuromuscular imaging in inherited muscle diseases. Eur Radiol. 2010;20(10):2447–60. PubMed PMID: 20422195. Pubmed Central PMCID: 2940021. Epub 2010/04/28. eng.

84. Poysky J. Behavior patterns in Duchenne muscular dystrophy: report on the Parent Project Muscular Dystrophy behavior workshop 8–9 of December 2006, Philadelphia, USA. Neuromuscul Disord. 2007;17(11–12):986–94. PubMed PMID: 17720499. Epub 2007/08/28. eng.
85. McAdam LC, Mayo AL, Alman BA, Biggar WD. The Canadian experience with long-term deflazacort treatment in Duchenne muscular dystrophy. Acta Myol. 2012;31(1):16–20. PubMed PMID: 22655512. Pubmed Central PMCID: 3440807. Epub 2012/06/05. eng.
86. Kinali M, Main M, Eliahoo J, Messina S, Knight RK, Lehovsky J, et al. Predictive factors for the development of scoliosis in Duchenne muscular dystrophy. Eur J Paediatr Neurol. 2007;11(3):160–6. PubMed PMID: 17257866. Epub 2007/01/30. eng.
87. Aparicio LF, Jurkovic M, DeLullo J. Decreased bone density in ambulatory patients with Duchenne muscular dystrophy. J Pediatr Orthop. 2002;22(2):179–81. PubMed PMID: 11856925. Epub 2002/02/22. eng.
88. McDonald DG, Kinali M, Gallagher AC, Mercuri E, Muntoni F, Roper H, et al. Fracture prevalence in Duchenne muscular dystrophy. Dev Med Child Neurol. 2002;44(10):695–8. PubMed PMID: 12418795. Epub 2002/11/07. eng.
89. Heckmatt JZ, Pier N, Dubowitz V. Assessment of quadriceps femoris muscle atrophy and hypertrophy in neuromuscular disease in children. J Clin Ultrasound. 1988;16(3):177–81. PubMed PMID: 3150399. Epub 1988/03/01. eng.
90. Damian MS, Bachmann G, Herrmann D, Dorndorf W. Magnetic resonance imaging of muscle and brain in myotonic dystrophy. J Neurol. 1993;240(1):8–12. PubMed PMID: 8423464.
91. Morales Montero F, Cuenca Berger P. [Molecular and genetic aspects of the myotonic conditions]. Rev Neurol. 2004;38(7):668–74. PubMed PMID: 15098190. Epub 2004/04/21. Aspectos geneticos y moleculares de las enfermedades miotonicas. spa.
92. Mankodi A. Myotonic disorders. Neurol India. 2008;56(3):298–304. PubMed PMID: 18974556. Epub 2008/11/01. eng.
93. Pusch M. Myotonia caused by mutations in the muscle chloride channel gene CLCN1. Hum Mutat. 2002;19(4):423–34. PubMed PMID: 11933197. Epub 2002/04/05. eng.
94. Heatwole CR, Moxley 3rd RT. The nondystrophic myotonias. Neurotherapeutics. 2007;4(2):238–51. PubMed PMID: 17395134. Epub 2007/03/31. eng.
95. Ryan AM, Matthews E, Hanna MG. Skeletal-muscle channelopathies: periodic paralysis and nondystrophic myotonias. Curr Opin Neurol. 2007;20(5):558–63. PubMed PMID: 17885445. Epub 2007/09/22. eng.
96. Cannon SC. Pathomechanisms in channelopathies of skeletal muscle and brain. Annu Rev Neurosci. 2006;29:387–415. PubMed PMID: 16776591. Epub 2006/06/17. eng.
97. Morrow JM, Matthews E, Raja Rayan DL, Fischmann A, Sinclair CD, Reilly MM, et al. Muscle MRI reveals distinct abnormalities in genetically proven non-dystrophic myotonias. Neuromuscul Disord. 2013;23(8):637–46. PubMed PMID: 23810313. Epub 2013/07/03. Eng.
98. McCann LJ, Juggins AD, Maillard SM, Wedderburn LR, Davidson JE, Murray KJ, et al. The Juvenile Dermatomyositis National Registry and Repository (UK and Ireland)–clinical characteristics of children recruited within the first 5 yr. Rheumatology (Oxford). 2006;45(10):1255–60. PubMed PMID: 16567354. Epub 2006/03/29. eng.
99. Davis WR, Halls JE, Offiah AC, Pilkington C, Owens CM, Rosendahl K. Assessment of active inflammation in juvenile dermatomyositis: a novel magnetic resonance imaging-based scoring system. Rheumatology (Oxford). 2011;50(12):2237–44. PubMed PMID: 21972421. Epub 2011/10/06. eng.
100. Delatycki MB, Williamson R, Forrest SM. Friedreich ataxia: an overview. J Med Genet. 2000;37(1):1–8. PubMed PMID: 10633128. Pubmed Central PMCID: 1734457. Epub 2000/01/14. eng.
101. Delatycki MB, Corben LA. Clinical features of Friedreich ataxia. J Child Neurol. 2012;27(9):1133–7. PubMed PMID: 22752493. Epub 2012/07/04. Eng.
102. Richards S, Chalkiadis G, Lakshman R, Buttery JP, Crawford NW. Complex regional pain syndrome following immunisation. Arch Dis Child. 2012;97(10):913–5. PubMed PMID: 22858647.
103. Wilder RT, Berde CB, Wolohan M, Vieyra MA, Masek BJ, Micheli LJ. Reflex sympathetic dystrophy in children. Clinical characteristics and follow-up of seventy patients. J Bone Joint Surg Am. 1992;74(6):910–9. PubMed PMID: 1634582. Epub 1992/07/01. eng.
104. Tan EC, Zijlstra B, Essink ML, Goris RJ, Severijnen RS. Complex regional pain syndrome type I in children. Acta Paediatr. 2008;97(7):875–9. PubMed PMID: 18410465. Epub 2008/04/16. eng.
105. Goldsmith DP, Vivino FB, Eichenfield AH, Athreya BH, Heyman S. Nuclear imaging and clinical features of childhood reflex neurovascular dystrophy: comparison with adults. Arthritis Rheum. 1989;32(4):480–5. PubMed PMID: 2706031. Epub 1989/04/01. eng.
106. Cappello ZJ, Kasdan ML, Louis DS. Meta-analysis of imaging techniques for the diagnosis of complex regional pain syndrome type I. J Hand Surg. 2012;37(2):288–96. PubMed PMID: 22177715.
107. Schweitzer ME, Mandel S, Schwartzman RJ, Knobler RL, Tahmoush AJ. Reflex sympathetic dystrophy revisited: MR imaging findings before and after infusion of contrast material. Radiology. 1995;195(1):211–4. PubMed PMID: 7892471. Epub 1995/04/01. eng.
108. American Spinal Injury Association. International standards for neurological classification of spinal cord injury. Chicago: ASIA; 2002.

Bone Marrow

25

Paul Babyn and Jennifer Stimec

Contents

Abstract

It is important to recognize the magnetic resonance imaging (MRI) appearance of normal and abnormal bone marrow. With its high tissue contrast, MRI is an excellent technique to evaluate bone marrow well before osseous destruction becomes apparent on radiographs or computed tomography. This chapter discusses the role of various MRI techniques for assessing bone marrow. It also describes normal marrow maturation and reconversion of fatty to hematopoietic marrow. It concludes with a review of neoplastic marrow disorders, emphasizing metastases and hematologic malignancies, and a brief discussion of other infiltrative and reactive marrow disorders.

One of the largest and most dynamic tissues in the body, bone marrow is the main site of hematopoiesis, producing and regulating the supply of erythrocytes, platelets, and leukocytes [1]. The cellular constituents of bone marrow include stem cells, erythrocytes, mast cells, myeloid cells, megakaryocytes, and fat cells, all supported within a framework of cancellous bone trabeculae. At least some bone marrow is visible in essentially every magnetic resonance imaging (MRI) study, underscoring the importance of recognizing the MRI appearance of normal and abnormal bone marrow. With its high tissue contrast, MRI is an excellent technique to evaluate bone marrow, allowing earlier assessment of bone marrow infiltration by

P. Babyn, MDCM (✉)
Department of Medical Imaging, University of Saskatchewan and Saskatoon Health Region, 103 Hospital Drive, Room 1566.1, Royal University Hospital, Saskatoon, SK S7N 0W8, Canada
e-mail: paul.babyn@saskatoonhealthregion.ca

J. Stimec, MD, FRCPC
Department of Diagnostic Imaging, The Hospital for Sick Children, 555 University Avenue, Toronto, ON M5G 1X8, Canada
e-mail: jennifer.stimec@sickkids.ca

R. Stein-Wexler et al. (eds.), *Pediatric Orthopedic Imaging*,
DOI 10.1007/978-3-642-45381-6_25, © Springer-Verlag Berlin Heidelberg 2015

tumor or other marrow disorders, well before osseous destruction becomes apparent on radiographs or computed tomography (CT) [2]. MRI may be used to assess focal or diffuse bone lesions found on other imaging tests or for evaluation of localized signs or symptoms. In comparison with the more limited sampling by marrow aspirate or biopsy, MRI has the ability to provide an overview of the entire marrow cavity [2].

1 Normal Bone Marrow

1.1 Physiology

Development of marrow depends on the formation of the marrow cavity. During the fetal period and throughout early childhood, there is significant bone formation, accompanied by enlargement of the marrow space [3]. In the fetus, hematopoiesis starts in the yolk sac and then, by the second trimester, extends to the liver and, to a lesser degree, the spleen [1, 4]. By the fourth fetal month, hematopoiesis begins within the marrow space as bone cavities develop. Bone marrow soon becomes the exclusive site of granulocyte and megakaryocyte proliferation; however, it is not until the end of the third trimester that the marrow environment supports erythroblasts. At birth, bone marrow is the major site of red cell production [1, 4].

On visual examination, bone marrow appears red (hematopoietic marrow) or yellow (fatty marrow), depending on its predominant components. Hematopoietic marrow is red because of the presence of hemoglobin within erythrocytes and their precursor cells and is actively involved in hematopoiesis (Fig. 25.1). Fatty marrow is yellow due to its high lipid content. Fat is a major component of yellow and to a lesser extent red marrow. The amount of fatty marrow responds to the need for hematopoietic marrow and can increase or decrease accordingly. When the need for hematopoietic marrow volume increases, for example, in response to severe blood loss, fatty adventitial cells lose fat and increase the space available for hematopoiesis [5]. During periods of decreased hematopoiesis, fat cells increase in size and number.

Fat cells may be actively involved in hematopoiesis, supplying metabolic or nutritional support, possibly along with growth factors [5]. The cellular composition of adult red marrow is 60 % hematopoietic cells and 40 % adipocytes, while its chemical composition is 40–60 % lipid, 30–40 % water, and 10–20 % proteins [6]. In contrast, yellow marrow is almost entirely composed of adipocytes (95 %), with its chemical composition being 80 % lipid, 15 % water, and 5 % protein [6–8]. In neonates and young infants, little or no marrow fat is present. Red marrow is significantly more cellular than yellow, with 100 % cellularity at birth; this decreases to 80–90 % in infancy and 60–80 % in young children [8]. Cancellous bone, composed of primary and secondary bridging trabeculae, provides the underlying structural framework for the cellular elements of marrow and also serves as a mineral depot [9].

The MRI signal of marrow reflects its cellular composition. Hematopoietic marrow is usually similar to or slightly more hyperintense than muscle on T1-weighted (T1-W) and T2-weighted (T2-W) sequences, although in neonates it can be slightly darker than muscle on T1-W images as a result of its relatively high cellularity [10, 11]. On T1-W sequences, yellow marrow is isointense to subcutaneous fat, whereas on T2-W images it appears similar to or slightly more hypointense than subcutaneous fat and slightly more hyperintense than muscle. This is discussed in greater detail below, in the section on MRI technique and the appearance of bone marrow.

Bone Marrow Conversion

The cellular composition of normal marrow changes significantly with age (Box 25.1). This is termed marrow conversion. Thorough understanding of the rate and anatomic pattern of marrow conversion has allowed for MRI mapping of the expected age-related distribution of marrow throughout the skeleton [8, 11–15]. At birth, hematopoietic marrow is present throughout the entire skeleton. Various regions of hematopoietic marrow then rapidly undergo conversion to fatty marrow. This begins in the periphery of the skeleton—first in the distal phalanges of the fingers and toes (Fig. 25.2) and then extending in a symmetric, centripetal manner into the more proximal skeleton [6, 16]. During the first decade, but especially during the first 5 years of life, the long bones undergo marrow conversion [17].

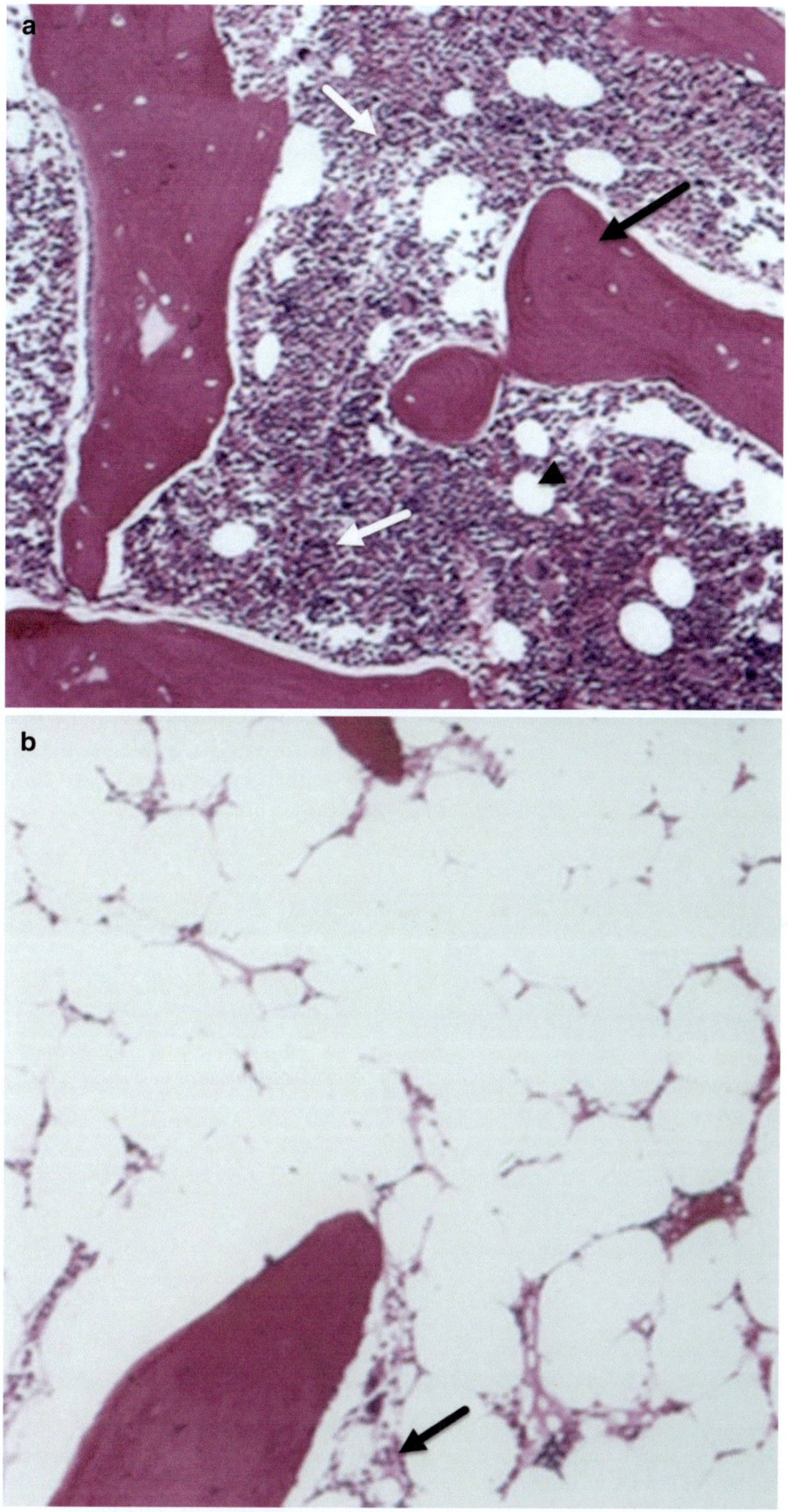

Fig. 25.1 Histology of normal hematopoietic and fatty marrow. (**a**) Hematopoietic marrow is very cellular (*white arrows*) and has little fat (*arrowhead*). Supporting trabeculae (*black arrow*). (**b**) Fatty marrow has low cellularity (*black arrow*) and extensive fat

Box 25.1: Conversion of Hematopoietic to Fatty Marrow

Neonate	Hematopoietic marrow everywhere
Conversion	Progression: distal to proximal (distal phalanges to proximal long bones)
	Epiphysis: rapid conversion to fatty marrow (within several months of ossification)
	Residual red marrow common in humeral head
	Diaphysis to distal metaphysis to proximal metaphysis
	Spine: on T1-W imaging

<1 year old	Vertebral body darker than intervertebral disk
1–3 to 5 years old	Vertebral body similar to intervertebral disk
>3 to 5 years old	Vertebral body brighter than intervertebral disk

The epiphyses are the first areas to develop fatty marrow, as discussed below and in Chap. 2. Marrow conversion then occurs in the diaphysis and progresses to the distal and finally proximal metaphyses [6, 16] (Fig. 25.3). Slight early fatty conversion can result in subtle increased signal in the diaphysis as soon as age 3 months, and by 1 year of age, some degree of heterogeneity is routinely evident. By age 5 years, the femoral diaphysis is homogeneously hyperintense due to fatty conversion [17]. Persistence of significant hematopoietic marrow in the diaphysis after about age 10 is abnormal.

Cartilaginous epiphyses and apophyses lack marrow until they ossify. Once ossified, these centers initially contain hematopoietic marrow that is hypointense on T1-W and hyperintense on T2-W images. This is rapidly converted to fatty marrow within months of ossification (with resultant hyperintense signal on both T1- and T2-W images) (Fig. 25.4). In the mid- to late third decade of life, bone marrow distribution achieves its adult state [16], confined to the axial skeleton and proximal humeri and femurs.

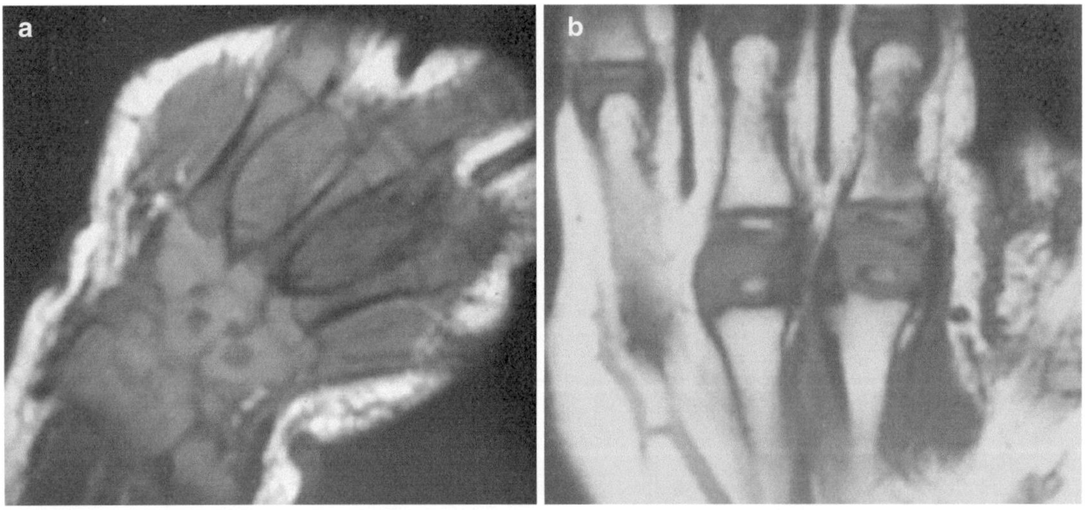

Fig. 25.2 Normal rapid conversion from hematopoietic to fatty marrow in the peripheral appendicular skeleton. (**a**) Coronal T1-weighted (T1-W) hand in a *neonate* shows T1-hypointense hematopoietic marrow in the metacarpals. The epiphyses and carpal bones are cartilaginous and mildly hyperintense. (**b**) Coronal T1-W hand in a *1-year-old* shows fatty conversion of the metacarpals and phalanges, which are now hyperintense, brighter than the cartilaginous portions of the epiphyses

Even though red marrow persists in the axial skeleton, it too undergoes conversion—though later and more gradually than in the appendicular skeleton (Fig. 25.5). For example, the amount of hematopoietic marrow in the vertebral bodies diminishes, with corresponding slight increase in fatty marrow. Before age 1 year, the vertebral body appears hypointense on T1-W images compared with the intervertebral disks. It then becomes isointense to the disks. After age 3–5 the vertebral body is mildly hyperintense compared with the disks, and this hyperintensity gradually increases [18, 19] (Box 25.1).

Box 25.2: Characteristics of Metaphyseal Residual Red Marrow

Symmetric, with base near physis (flame shape)
Margins: vertical, feathery, ill defined
Center: ± fat
T1-W: brighter than muscle
No trabecular distortion or mass effect

These are only general guidelines on marrow maturation, and variation and incomplete conversion are very common. For example, prominent

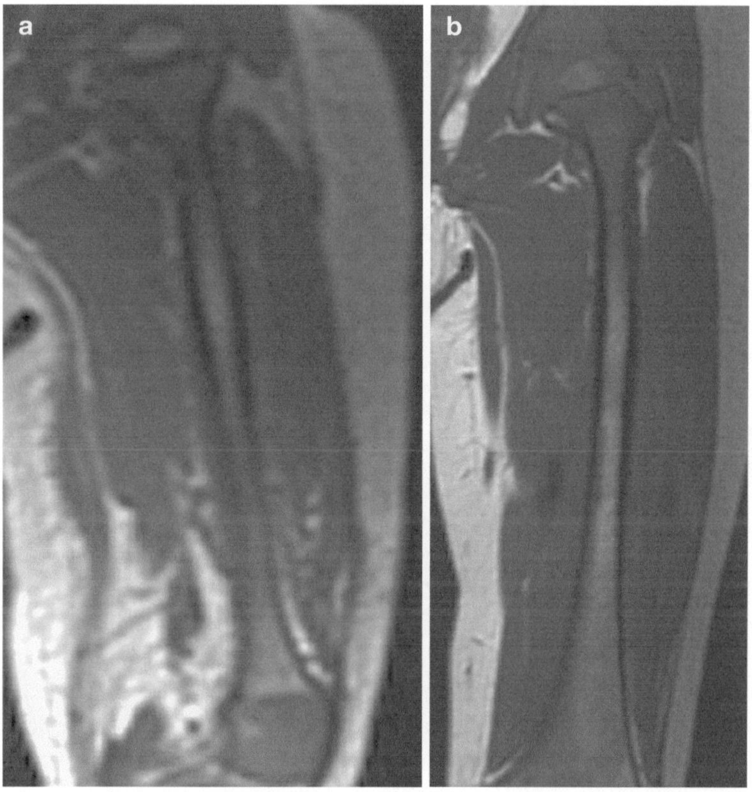

Fig. 25.3 Normal marrow conversion in the femur on coronal T1-W images. (**a**) *1-year-old* boy: the diaphysis has subtle hyperintensity, but the metadiaphysis is predominantly hypointense. The ossification center at the proximal femur is hyperintense due to fatty marrow (the distal femoral ossification center is almost entirely out of plane). (**b**) *4-year-old* girl: heterogeneous hyperintensity is evident in the diaphysis and distal metaphysis. (**c**) *6-year-old* boy: hyperintensity at the distal femur has increased. (**d**) *7-year-old* girl: the distal femoral metaphysis is almost uniformly hyperintense, and the proximal metaphysis is becoming brighter. (**e**) *9-year-old* boy: there is now heterogeneous hyperintensity at the proximal femoral metaphysis (Courtesy of Rebecca Stein-Wexler)

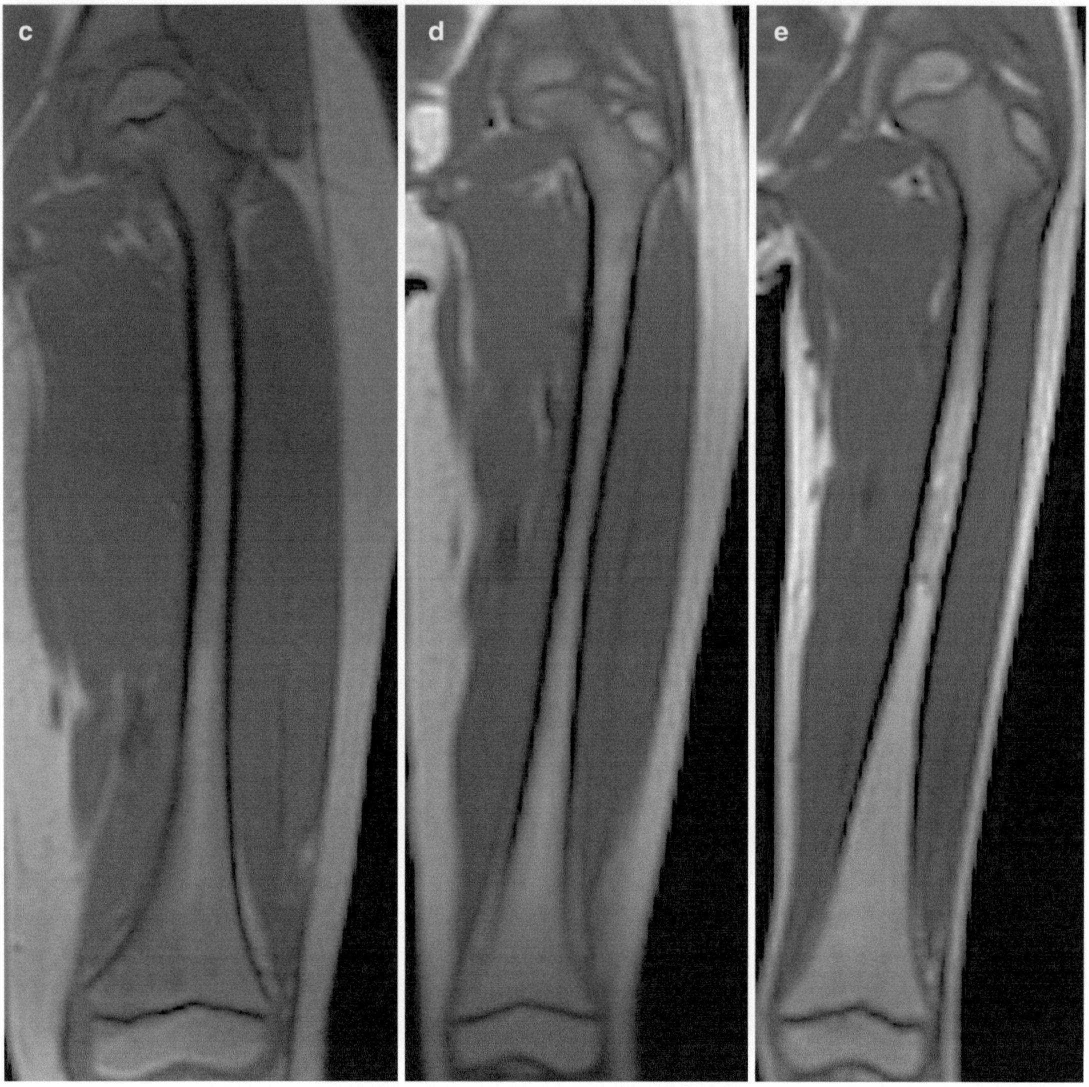

Fig. 25.3 (continued)

hematopoietic marrow in the metaphyses is normal until the end of the second decade. In fact, the lack of red marrow in the proximal femoral metaphyses in the young child is abnormal and raises concern for myeloid depletion.

Heterogeneous, sharply demarcated linear areas or focal islands of red marrow are common normal variants (Fig. 25.6). Although they can be confused with marrow lesions, several features help to differentiate. Residual red marrow typically has a symmetric distribution and abuts or almost abuts the physis. It is flame shaped and often has vertical or feathery margins, with a central focus of fatty marrow (target sign). It does not disturb the trabeculae. Finally, residual marrow should be brighter than muscle on T1-W imaging and similar to marrow on short-tau inversion recovery (STIR) (Box 25.2).

Small foci of high-signal T2 changes of the bone marrow are common within the foot and ankle, wrist, and cervical spine in children up to the age of 15 years (Fig. 25.7). These may

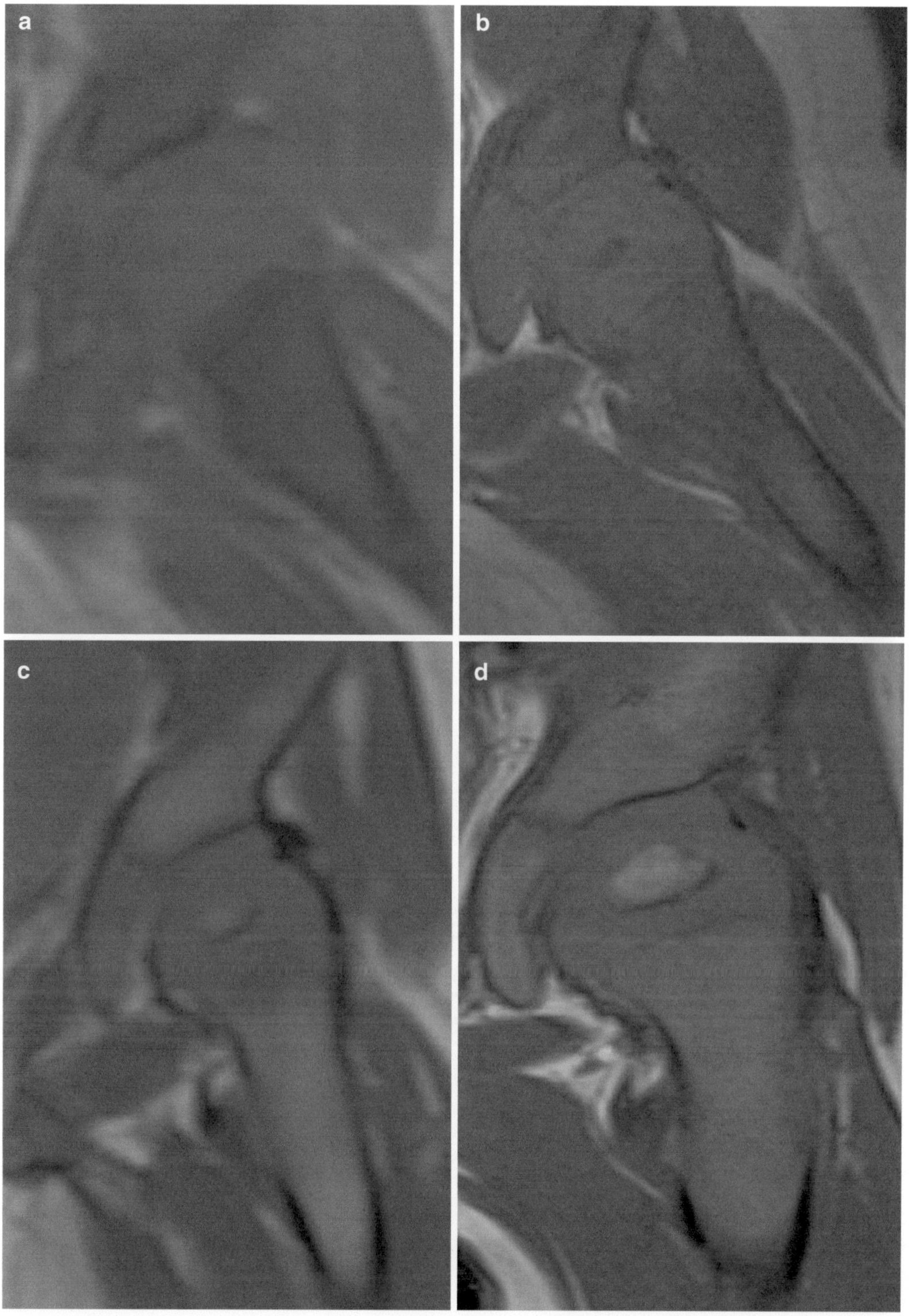

Fig. 25.4 Changes in the appearance of the proximal femur on coronal T1-W images during early childhood. (**a**) The femoral head of this *3-month-old* girl is uniformly isointense to muscle; there is no ossification center. (**b**) The femoral head of another *3-month-old* girl is hypointense, with early ossification and formation of hypointense red marrow. In both a and b, the proximal femur is hypointense due to red marrow. (**c**) The femoral head in a *6-month-old* girl is converting to fatty marrow, slightly hyperintense to muscle. (**d**) The femoral head in this *8-month-old* boy is larger and demonstrates hyperintense fatty marrow (Courtesy of Tal Laor, Cincinnati Children's Hospital)

reflect residual regions of red marrow or possibly asymptomatic changes from subclinical trauma. Out-of-phase imaging may help differentiate hematopoietic marrow from metastasis.

Prominent hematopoietic marrow can occasionally be normal in the subchondral regions of some epiphyses, most often in the distal femur, proximal tibia, and proximal humerus (Fig. 25.8). Although this is often interpreted as evidence of

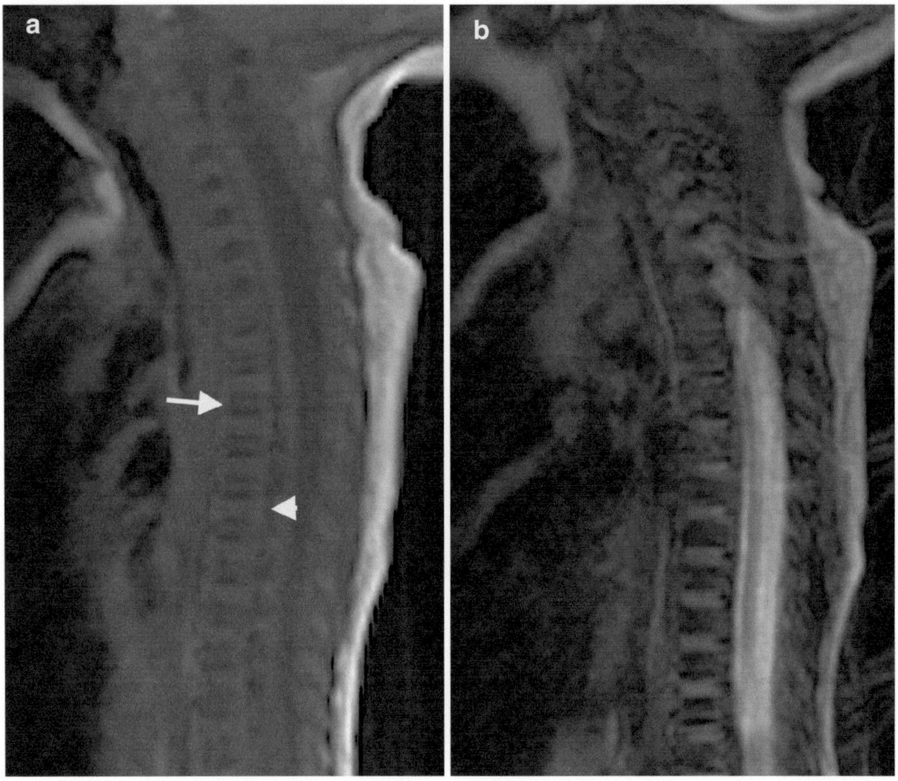

Fig. 25.5 T1 and T2 signal alterations in the vertebral bodies during early childhood in a girl followed for Chiari I malformation and syrinx (*sagittal views*). At *1 week*, T1-W image (**a**) shows marrow (*arrow*) that is hypointense compared with the hyperintense intervertebral disk (*arrowhead*) and adjacent vertebral body cartilage; T2-W image (**b**) shows the vertebral bodies are hypointense compared to hyperintense intervertebral disks. At *6 months*, T1-W image (**c**) shows that the vertebral body (*arrow*) is heterogeneous but predominantly isointense to the intervertebral disk (*arrowhead*); T2-W image (**d**) shows uniform marrow and cartilage hypointensity compared to the disk. At *14 months*, T1-W image (**e**) shows that the marrow (*arrow*) is slightly more hyperintense than the disk (*arrowhead*); T2-W image (**f**) shows little change. At *2 years*, T1-W image (**g**) shows marrow (*arrow*) is brighter than disk (*arrowhead*); T2-W image (**h**) shows decreasing marrow signal intensity (compared to disk) due to progressive increase in fatty marrow. At *3.5 years*, T1-W image (**i**) shows that hyperintense marrow fills the marrow space more completely and is hyperintense to disk; T2-W image (**j**) shows no significant change (Courtesy of Rebecca Stein-Wexler)

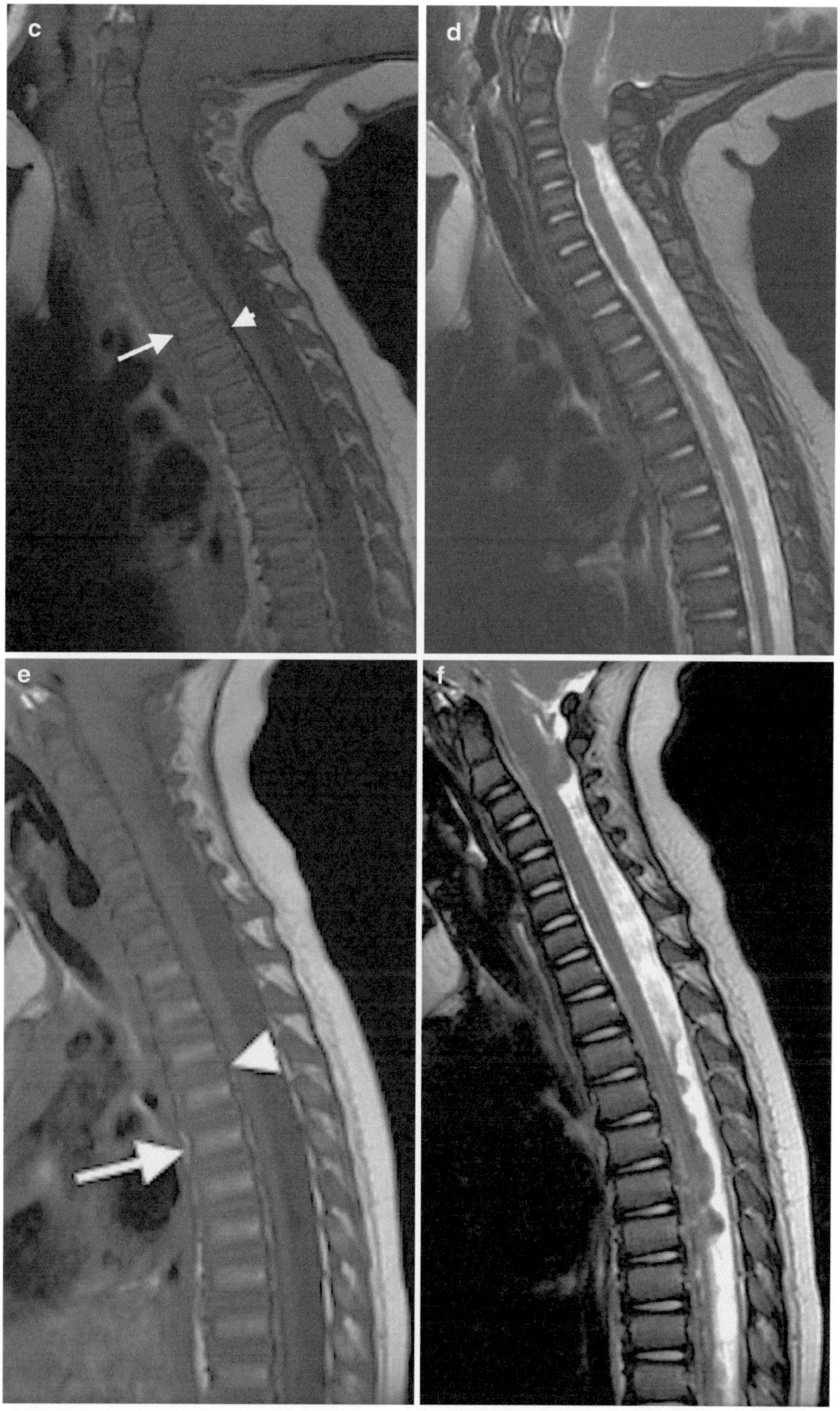

Fig. 25.5 (continued)

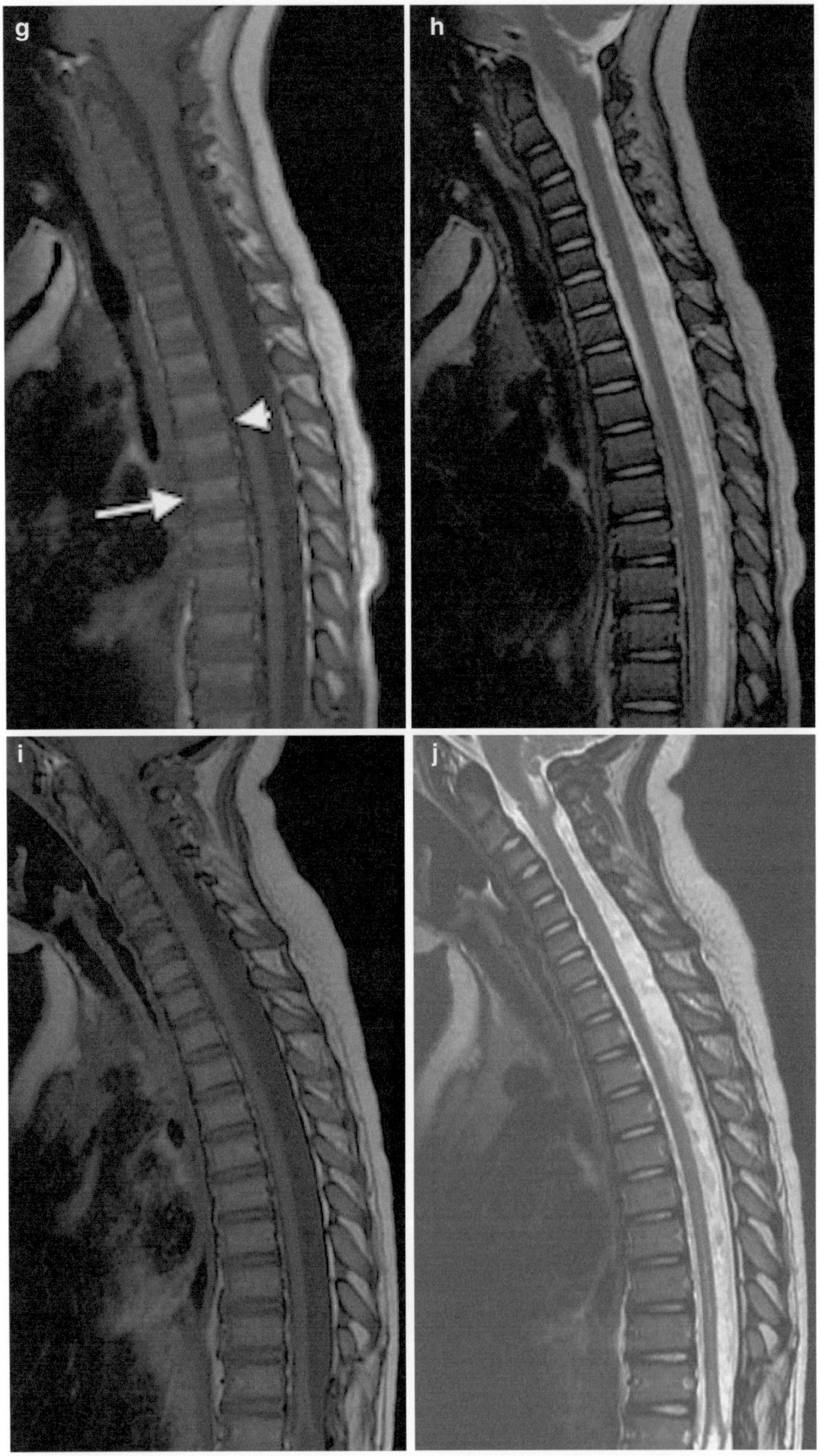

Fig. 25.5 (continued)

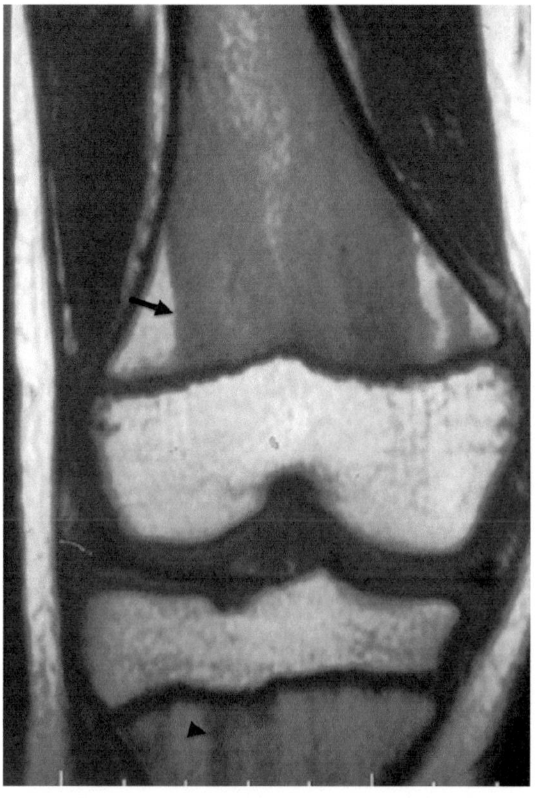

Fig. 25.6 Prominent persistent hematopoietic marrow. Coronal T1-W image shows hypointense hematopoietic marrow that has the typical straight margins (*arrow*) and is brighter than muscle. At the proximal tibial metaphysis, residual hematopoietic marrow appears feathery and flame shaped (*arrowhead*)

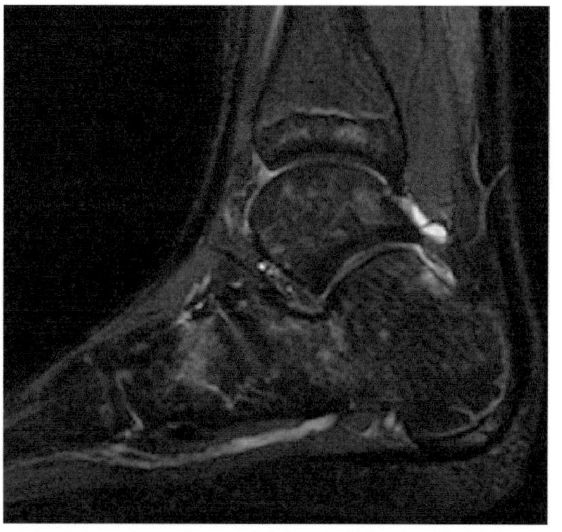

Fig. 25.7 Normal hyperintense foci in tarsal bones of a 9-year-old. Sagittal inversion recovery (IR) image (Courtesy of Rebecca Stein-Wexler)

marrow reconversion, it likely represents residual hematopoietic marrow [20].

Bone Marrow Reconversion

In the event of increased functional demand for hematopoiesis, yellow marrow may reconvert to red marrow. Conditions triggering reconversion include chronic hemolytic anemias (such as sickle-cell disease and thalassemia) (Fig. 25.9), physiologic stress, endurance running, obesity, extensive marrow replacement from marrow proliferative or replacement disorders, and chemotherapy with marrow-stimulating agents such as granulocyte colony-stimulating factor [12, 16] (Fig. 25.10). The extent of reconversion depends on the severity and duration of the stimulus. This reconversion process typically reverses the order of initial conversion, first in the central and then the peripheral skeleton, and in the long bones from the metaphyses to the diaphyses [6].

2 MRI Technique and Appearance of Bone Marrow

MRI is the mainstay of clinical marrow evaluation. The MRI characteristics of bone marrow are influenced by a number of factors, including the choice of imaging sequence, use of contrast agents, marrow cellularity (especially its hematopoietic, lipid, and iron content), and surrounding trabecular bone [3].

On *T1-weighted (T1-W) and T2-weighted (T2-W) fast spin-echo (FSE) sequences*, differences in T1 and T2 relaxation times generally allow the differentiation of normal red and yellow marrow from pathologic marrow. The trabecular bone itself has little direct signal but contributes to T2 shortening, producing local magnetic field gradients [7, 21].

Since fatty marrow is composed primarily of low-cellular lipids, its signal characteristics are

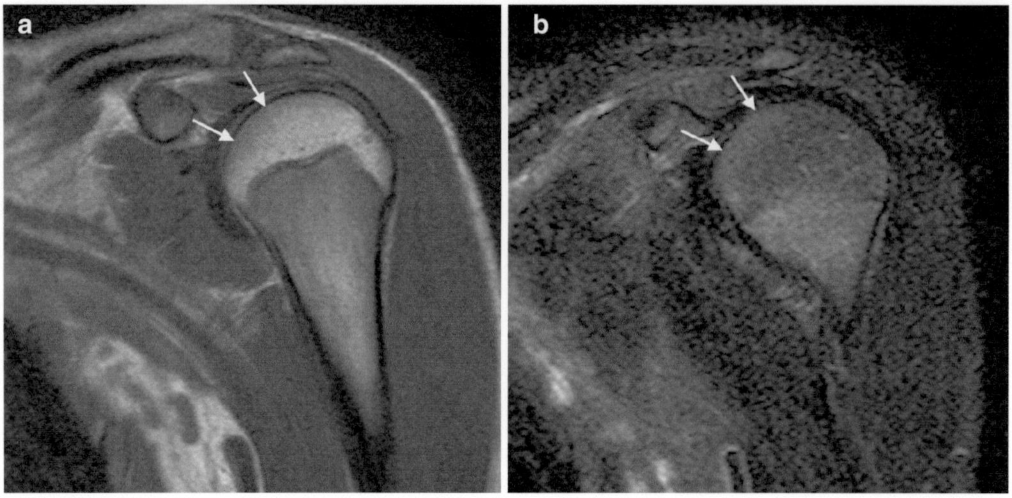

Fig. 25.8 Subchondral epiphyseal hematopoietic marrow, a normal variant. (**a**) Coronal T1-W image shows subchondral hypointensity (*arrows*). (**b**) Coronal T2-W FS image shows increased signal in the corresponding area (*arrows*). Vascularity in the subchondral region is slightly increased, and hematopoietic marrow may persist within the epiphysis

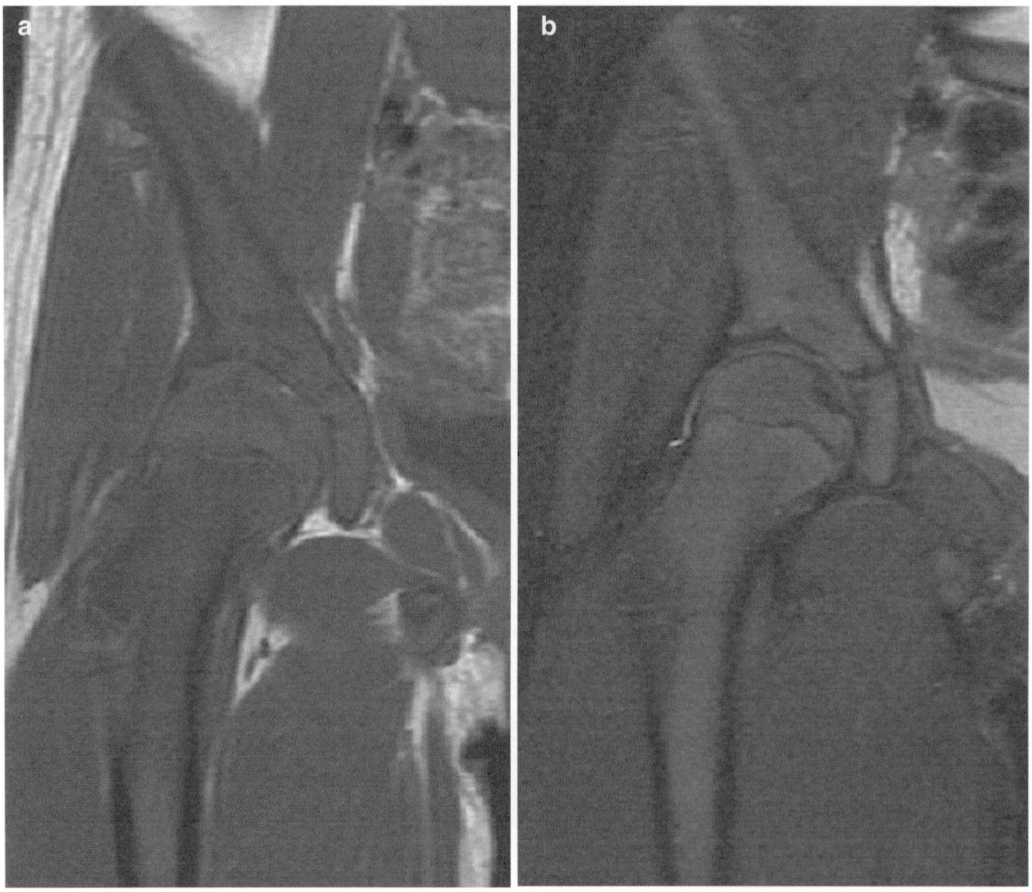

Fig. 25.9 Marrow reconversion in a young adolescent girl with sickle-cell disease. (**a**) T1-W coronal image shows diffuse hypointensity throughout the marrow due to replacement of all expected fatty marrow with hematopoietic marrow. This is especially striking at the femoral head, which should be hyperintense. (**b**) T2-W FS image shows diffuse intermediate signal due to marrow reconversion

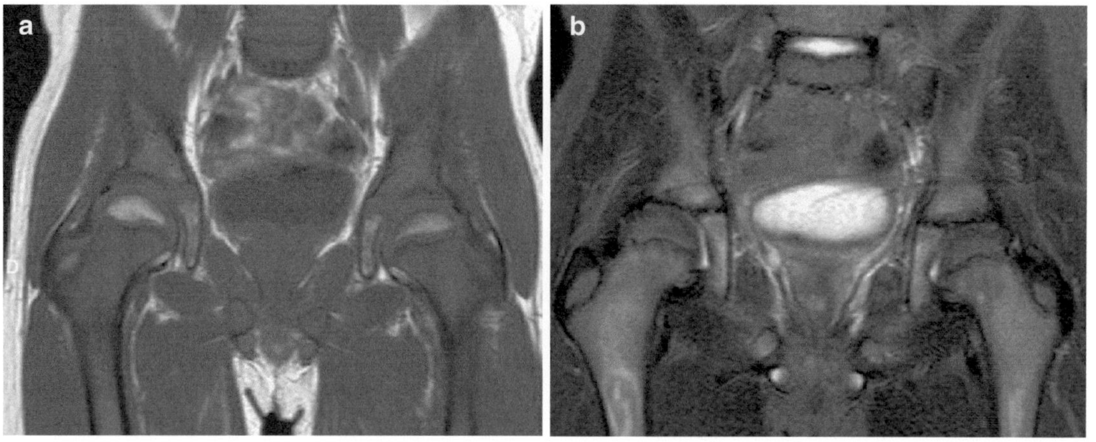

Fig. 25.10 Marrow reconversion after therapy with granulocyte colony-stimulating factor in a child with osseous metastases in the proximal femurs due to rhabdomyosarcoma. (**a**) On T1-W coronal image, diffuse hypointensity in the femoral metaphysis results from combination of hematopoietic marrow and metastases. (**b**) On T2-W FS image, heterogeneous signal better delineates these two processes

similar to those of subcutaneous fat on both T1-W and T2-W spin-echo (SE) sequences. Red marrow is more cellular but still contains significant lipid, and therefore, the signal characteristics of fat are averaged with the longer T1 and T2 relaxation times of water and protein [7, 12]. On T1-W images, the signal intensity of red marrow is less than that of fatty marrow but typically higher than that of adjacent muscle or intervertebral disks (except in the very young child, in whom the fat content of hematopoietic marrow can be quite low). The exact marrow signal intensity will depend on the specific water and lipid content [7, 12]. On T2-W images, the signal intensity of red marrow is similar to that of adjacent muscle and approximates the signal intensity of fatty marrow. Hence, the contrast between red and fatty marrow is more evident on T1-W sequences. SE imaging underestimates the proportion of hematopoietic marrow because the short T1 relaxation time of fat overwhelms the longer T1 relaxation time of red marrow.

Fast spin-echo (FSE) T2-W sequences have largely replaced conventional T2-W SE imaging because of the marked reduction in acquisition times as well as improved signal-to-noise ratio for similar acquisition times [3]. Fat is much brighter on T2-W FSE images compared with conventional T2-W images, and selective fat suppression is therefore generally applied to FSE T2-W images to improve other tissue contrast [12]. With fat suppression, T2-W FSE images have been shown to be highly effective in the evaluation of marrow abnormalities, improving lesion conspicuity [22] (Fig. 25.11). As most marrow lesions are rich in free water, they are brighter than both red and yellow marrow on T2-W images and thus easily detected [12].

Short-tau inversion recovery (STIR) or FSE inversion recovery (FSE IR) demonstrates lesions well. STIR is widely used for bone marrow imaging because it offers excellent delineation of marrow abnormalities and, depending on technical parameters, may yield improved lesion visibility compared with T2-W SE imaging. STIR images have additive T1 and T2 characteristics, so lesions with long T1 and T2 relaxation times are bright on STIR. Normal fatty marrow is low in signal intensity, while red marrow demonstrates intermediate signal intensity, similar to muscle [3]. The chemical shift/selective fat suppression techniques used in FS T2-W FSE images may cause field heterogeneity, particularly with large fields of view. STIR imaging is less susceptible to magnetic field inhomogeneity, and therefore, a large volume of bone marrow can be assessed with large field of view STIR imaging [12]. Fast

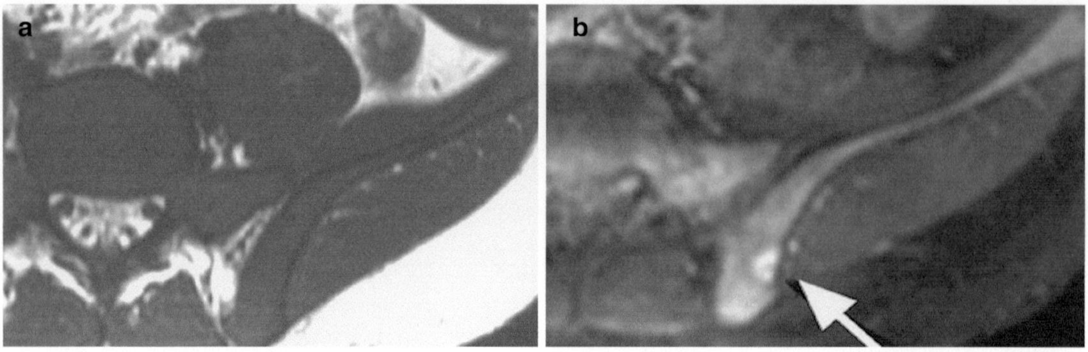

Fig. 25.11 Hypercellular marrow with focus of metastatic Wilms tumor evident only on T2-W FS imaging in a 2-year-old. (**a**) On T1-W axial image, marrow signal is uniformly hypointense. (**b**) T2-W FS image shows intermediate signal in most of the marrow and a focal hyperintense lesion (*arrow*) that was obscured by adjacent hematopoietic marrow on T1

STIR sequences can demonstrate marrow lesions as well as conventional STIR sequences, with considerable savings in imaging time.

Intermediate proton density (*PD*) images lack sufficient contrast resolution between normal marrow and pathologic processes to be primarily useful for marrow evaluation.

Gradient-echo (*GRE*) sequences are sometimes helpful in musculoskeletal imaging, especially for delineation of hemosiderin. Many factors influence the appearance of normal marrow on GRE, including tissue characteristics and acquisition technique. Unlike SE techniques, local magnetic field inhomogeneities are not rephased on GRE, making it more sensitive to susceptibility differences and signal loss, especially with 3-Tesla (T) imaging. This includes the effects induced by trabecular bone and marrow heterogeneity [3]. On GRE imaging, this leads to a loss of marrow signal intensity that is greatest in the regions with the most trabecular bone (e.g., epiphyses, metaphyses, and vertebrae) and is even greater when there is iron, such as in hematopoietic marrow. Hence, there is more signal loss for epiphyseal marrow than for metaphyseal marrow and more for metaphyseal marrow than for trabeculae-poor diaphyseal marrow [23].

Fat suppression offers important information. In GRE sequences, if fat and water protons are in phase (typically an echo time [TE] of 4.2 ms at 1.5 T), their signals are added; if they are opposed phase (a TE of 2.1 ms at 1.5-Tesla (1.5 T)), the image obtained represents the difference between the lipid and water signals. This can be used to help identify the presence or absence of marrow fat. Since both hematopoietic and fatty marrow contain fat, normal marrow signal is suppressed and appears dark on opposed-phase imaging (see Fig. 25.8). However, if normal marrow is replaced by a lesion (with loss of marrow fat), no subtraction will be apparent on opposed-phase imaging, and the lesion will remain bright [24]. This is useful for differentiating neoplasia from normal marrow as well as in evaluation of nonneoplastic processes, such as ischemia and injury, where marrow fat persists [20].

Gadolinium-enhanced images are particularly useful for the detection of diffusely abnormal marrow that may not be recognized on unenhanced MRI [25, 26]. However, normal hematopoietic marrow of some infants and young children may also enhance, as it can be quite vascular. The degree of enhancement depends on the type of marrow present and is generally much more evident with hematopoietic than with fatty marrow. Normal marrow enhancement decreases with advancing age, paralleling an increasing proportion of marrow fat and accompanying decreasing vascularity [3]. In addition, delay in scanning after gadolinium injection reduces the degree of enhancement [25].

Dynamic gadolinium-enhanced imaging can be useful for tumor evaluation, as it assesses capillary blood flow, permeability, and the relative volume of the extravascular extracellular space. It may allow differentiation of tumor from the many other processes that also cause abnormal marrow enhancement, such as inflammation and infection. Angiogenesis, which is common with neoplastic involvement of the marrow, leads to increased initial flow [20]. Peak normal marrow enhancement is evident within the first minute after injection (between 45 and 60 s). Dynamic contrast-enhanced MRI allows quantitative estimates of tumor necrosis, which correlate well with pathologic determination of percent necrosis. The dynamic MRI's ability to distinguish between tumors that are less or more than 90 % necrotic is especially important clinically, as this noninvasive assessment of treatment response during neoadjuvant therapy can suggest which patients would benefit from a change in therapy [27].

Studies in adults suggest that *diffusion-weighted* MRI allows excellent distinction between neoplastic and benign causes of collapsed vertebral bodies [20], and there may be similar applications in children. Diffusion-weighted imaging is based on the principle of Brownian motion of water molecules. The apparent diffusion coefficient (ADC) of tissues quantifies this microscopic motion in tissues and reflects local water mobility. The free motion of water molecules in normal tissues results in relatively high ADC values. Both densely packed cells within a tumor and cytotoxic edema restrict the motion of free water molecules, thus decreasing the ADC and resulting in low signal on an ADC map. High-resolution diffusion-weighted MRI with STIR-echo planar imaging sequence and free-breathing scanning can be used to create three-dimensional displays of the marrow [28].

In the neonate and young child, assessment of the marrow is often more challenging. For example, in the developing spine, striking marrow enhancement results from hypervascularity, increased marrow cellularity, and extensive extravascular space where contrast can pool. From the neonatal period through early childhood, increased cellularity due to especially active hematopoiesis results in unusually hyperintense T2 signal (brighter than muscle), no loss of signal on out-of-phase imaging, and regions of restricted diffusion that may mimic lesions.

Whole-body MRI (*WB-MRI*) allows noninvasive and relatively rapid survey of the entire body and bone marrow (usually with STIR technique). This supplements standard multimodality imaging both for initial tumor staging and to screen for tumor recurrence [2] and may help detect distant metastatic disease. Pediatric patients may benefit especially from WB-MRI, as marrow metastases in the peripheral skeleton are more common in children than in adults [29]. The use of WB-MRI has also been reported in Langerhans cell histiocytosis, chronic osteomyelitis, and systemic muscle diseases [30–33]. WB-MRI facilitates accurate biopsy by identifying the exact location of marrow involvement in cases of focal disease.

Fluorodeoxyglucose positron emission tomography (FDG PET) may be more sensitive for detecting bone metastasis than WB-MRI in children, but it may have more false-positives [34]. Furthermore, FDG PET requires complementary CT or MRI to localize areas of increased glucose metabolism. In addition, FDG PET may not display or demonstrate skull metastases because the high glucose metabolism of normal brain may obscure lesions [35]. Positron emission tomography-magnetic resonance imaging (PET-MRI) may improve both sensitivity and specificity for detecting marrow metastases. MRI techniques employing injection of ultrasmall super-paramagnetic iron oxide particles have the potential to improve the contrast between tumor and normal marrow (the reticuloendothelial system of normal marrow phagocytizes the particles, resulting in signal loss) [36, 37].

3 Abnormal Bone Marrow

A variety of disorders may lead to abnormal marrow. These include disorders of marrow hyperplasia and reconversion, disorders with diffuse marrow infiltration (including neoplasia and nontumoral infiltration), and disorders of marrow depletion and failure. MRI has proven to be a sensitive method for detecting focal, multifocal, and diffuse bone marrow lesions, including those of neoplastic, infectious, and ischemic origin (see Table 25.1). Careful consideration of the morphologic signal characteristics of any marrow lesion, its distribution, and its location facilitates diagnosis.

The appropriate choice of MRI sequences depends not only on the suspected underlying condition but also on the signal characteristics of the surrounding normal marrow so that lesion conspicuity may be maximized. Since most marrow lesions (benign or malignant) contain more free water than either hematopoietic or fatty marrow, they appear brighter than marrow on T2-W sequences [7] (recall that normal red marrow in children older than 2 or 3 years is brighter than muscle or non-degenerated intervertebral disks [44]). Marrow lesions have a longer T1 relaxation time and therefore appear isointense or hypointense compared to muscle on T1-W imaging and conspicuously hypointense against a background of the hyperintense yellow marrow in adults, adolescents, and older children [16]. However, especially in younger children, marrow lesions may appear similar to normal red marrow on T1-W images [6, 7, 10], and other techniques such as in-phase and out-of-phase imaging may be necessary.

With diffuse marrow abnormalities, there is extensive or complete replacement of normal bone marrow. The differential diagnosis of diffuse marrow disorders is broad (see Table 25.1) and includes neoplastic disorders such as leukemias, lymphomas, and metastatic disease (especially neuroblastoma and rhabdomyosarcoma). Other nonneoplastic conditions include aplastic anemia, myelodysplastic syndromes, myelofibrosis, hemosiderosis, Gaucher disease, and osteopetrosis. Diffuse hematopoietic marrow may be difficult to distinguish from diffuse marrow disease in young children [45], particularly in the setting of acute leukemias.

Quantitative serial assessment of the fat fraction of bone marrow may further help distinguish normal from abnormal marrow. It may also be useful for monitoring patients' response to therapy for leukemia, aplastic anemia, and Gaucher disease [46].

Table 25.1 Marrow disorders by anatomic distribution

Diffuse marrow disorders
Normal variant
Gaucher disease
Iron overload
Langerhans cell histiocytosis
Lymphoma
Marked red cell hyperplasia
Marrow reconversion
Metastases from certain solid tumors including neuroblastoma and rhabdomyosarcoma
Myelodysplastic disorder
Myelofibrosis
Myeloproliferative disorders including
Acute myelogenous leukemia
Acute lymphoblastic leukemia
Chronic myelogenous leukemia
Essential thrombocythemia
Idiopathic hypereosinophilic syndrome
Idiopathic myelofibrosis
Juvenile myelomonocytic leukemia
Mastocytosis
Polycythemia vera
Transient myeloproliferative disorder of Down syndrome
Multifocal marrow disorders
Langerhans cell histiocytosis
Lymphoma
Metastasis
Osteonecrosis
Focal marrow disorders
Benign or malignant tumors—primary or secondary
Infection
Inflammatory arthritis
Osteonecrosis
Radiation
Trauma including fracture, contusion, and stress reaction

Adapted from [7, 8, 11, 13–15, 38, 39–43]

3.1 Neoplasia

Tumors affecting the bone marrow can be classified according to the site of origin: they arise from myeloid elements of marrow (leukemia, lymphoma), mesenchymal elements of marrow (primary sarcomas of bone), or hematogenous spread to the marrow cavity. MRI is more sensitive than radiography, CT, or scintigraphy for the detection of bone metastases in children and young adults, even if the trabecular bone is not destroyed [34, 47]. It also assists with diagnosis, staging, and follow-up of hematologic malignancies [47].

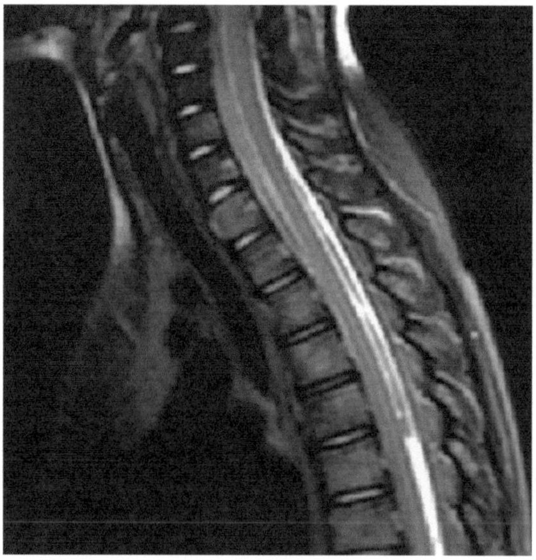

Fig. 25.12 Metastatic neuroblastoma. T2-W sagittal image shows heterogeneous increased signal intensity in multiple vertebral bodies

Metastases to Bone Marrow

Bone marrow metastases are most often seen with neuroblastoma and the primary bone and soft tissue sarcomas, including Ewing sarcoma and rhabdomyosarcoma. Focal or multifocal, they occur anywhere in the marrow space but are most common in red marrow (Fig. 25.12). The MRI appearance of metastases varies depending on the tumor and the host response; metastases can be osteolytic, osteoblastic, or mixed. Some tumors grow between trabeculae within marrow, without causing gross trabecular or cortical destruction. MRI is superior to radiography and bone scan in detecting such intertrabecular tumor deposits [27]. Neuroblastoma and rhabdomyosarcomas may diffusely infiltrate marrow, resembling leukemia.

On T1-W sequences, tumor is typically identified by replacement of fatty marrow, resulting in hypointensity. T1-W imaging alone provides excellent delineation of tumor extent in areas where fatty marrow predominates, although it is less reliable where the normal marrow is hematopoietic. Lesions that are hyperintense on T1-W imaging are typically benign, with the exception of metastatic melanoma, whose hemorrhage or melanin content may cause T1 hyperintensity [38]. Increased water in tumor cells causes most neoplasms to appear hyperintense on fat-suppressed sequences, such as STIR. However, the appearance of osteoblastic metastases on STIR sequences varies from hypointense for densely sclerotic lesions to hyperintense if more cellular components are present [2]. Table 25.2 presents marrow lesions with low signal on both T1-W and T2-W images.

Table 25.2 Causes of low signal intensity marrow on both T1-W and T2-W imaging

Focal
Benign bone islands
Sclerotic metastases
Diffuse
Gaucher disease
Iron overload
Myelofibrosis
Osteopetrosis

In adults, MRI has been shown to be more sensitive than bone scan for demonstrating marrow metastases [48–50]. However, the normal hypointensity of highly cellular hematopoietic marrow in children may result in misdiagnosis of marrow lesions [12, 34]. In addition, as discussed in the section above on marrow maturation, foci of residual marrow may be mistaken for marrow lesions (see Box 25.2). Metastatic disease has more rounded and sharply defined contours, is usually asymmetric, and appears less bright than muscle on T1-W imaging [16].

As described in detail in the section above on MRI technique, in-phase and out-of-phase imaging employ the inherent differences in the resonance frequencies of water and lipid protons to differentiate metastatic disease (or other marrow lesions) from normal red or yellow marrow. Whereas the fat content of normal marrow leads to hypointense signal on out-of-phase imaging, the vast majority of tumor deposits remain bright due to their high fluid content and lack of fat [16, 51, 52].

See Chap. 21 for discussion of primary bone malignancies.

Hematologic Malignancy

MRI provides valuable information that can aid in diagnosis, staging, and follow-up of

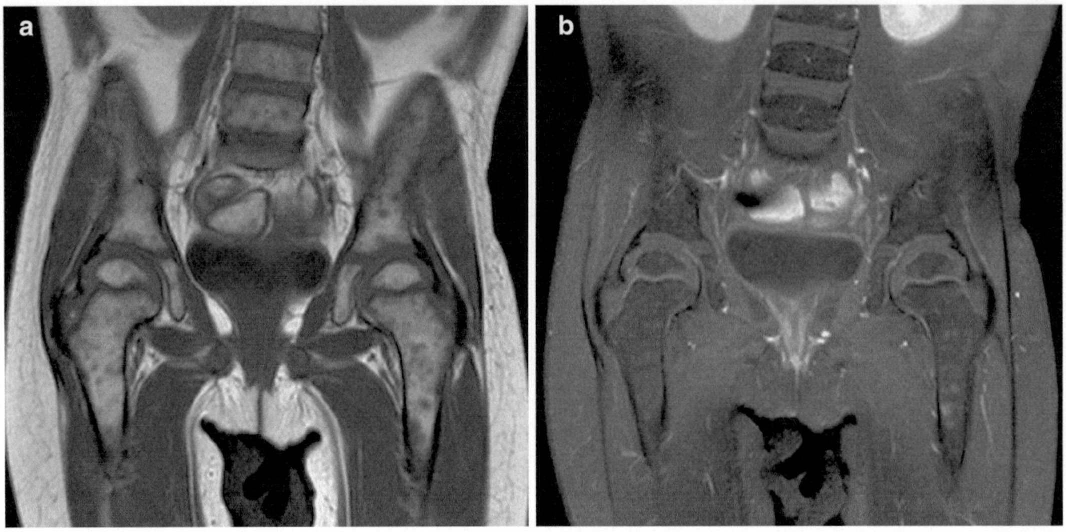

Fig. 25.13 Diffuse nodular pattern of acute lymphocytic leukemia in a 3-year-old. (**a**) Coronal T1-W image shows multiple hypointense foci within the marrow due to leukemic deposits. (**b**) Coronal T1-W FS gadolinium-enhanced image shows corresponding abnormal enhancement

hematologic malignancies [47]. It readily demonstrates replacement of normal marrow with leukemic cells in cases of acute leukemia [53] and may occasionally depict early marrow changes of *subleukemic leukemia*, prior to the development of extensive blood leukocytosis. However, the marrow may appear normal if the tumor load is low. Three patterns of leukemic marrow infiltration have been described: diffuse uniform, diffuse patchy, and focal [20] (Fig. 25.13). The diffuse patterns are most common but are not specific for the disease (Figs. 25.14 and 25.15). MRI cannot differentiate between the various leukemias, such as acute myelocytic leukemia (AML) and acute lymphoid leukemia (ALL).

MRI can demonstrate posttreatment residual disease in patients with ALL, and sequential quantitative assessment appears to have value in predicting treatment response in this group of patients [54]. Due to inherent differences between lymphoid and myeloid cells, it is less helpful in patients with AML [12]. In this group, responders and nonresponders show no significant difference in posttreatment T1 measurements during and after the first induction course of treatment [55].

Avascular necrosis (AVN) results in cellular demise following interruption of blood supply to the bone and commonly complicates malignancy. The classic MRI appearance is a geographic region with serpiginous margins that are hypointense on T1-W imaging. The "double-line" sign results from an inner band of high signal representing granulation tissue, with outer low signal intensity representing sclerotic bone. Marrow necrosis is infrequently associated with malignancy, most commonly ALL. Found in less than 0.5 % of marrow biopsies, marrow necrosis is characterized by loss of myeloid tissue and marrow fat. Unlike with AVN, trabeculae are not destroyed. The appearance on MRI otherwise resembles AVN, but marrow necrosis tends to be more diffuse and involve the axial skeleton without vertebral collapse [27].

Marrow infiltration occurs in 5–15 % of patients with Hodgkin disease and in 25–45 % of patients with non-Hodgkin lymphoma [12, 27, 29]; it indicates stage IV disease, with significant therapeutic and prognostic implications [29]. On MRI, lymphomatous involvement of marrow is seen as diffuse heterogeneous replacement and less frequently as focal marrow lesions [27]. Demonstration of focal involvement has important consequences, affecting patient prognosis and therapy selection [27].

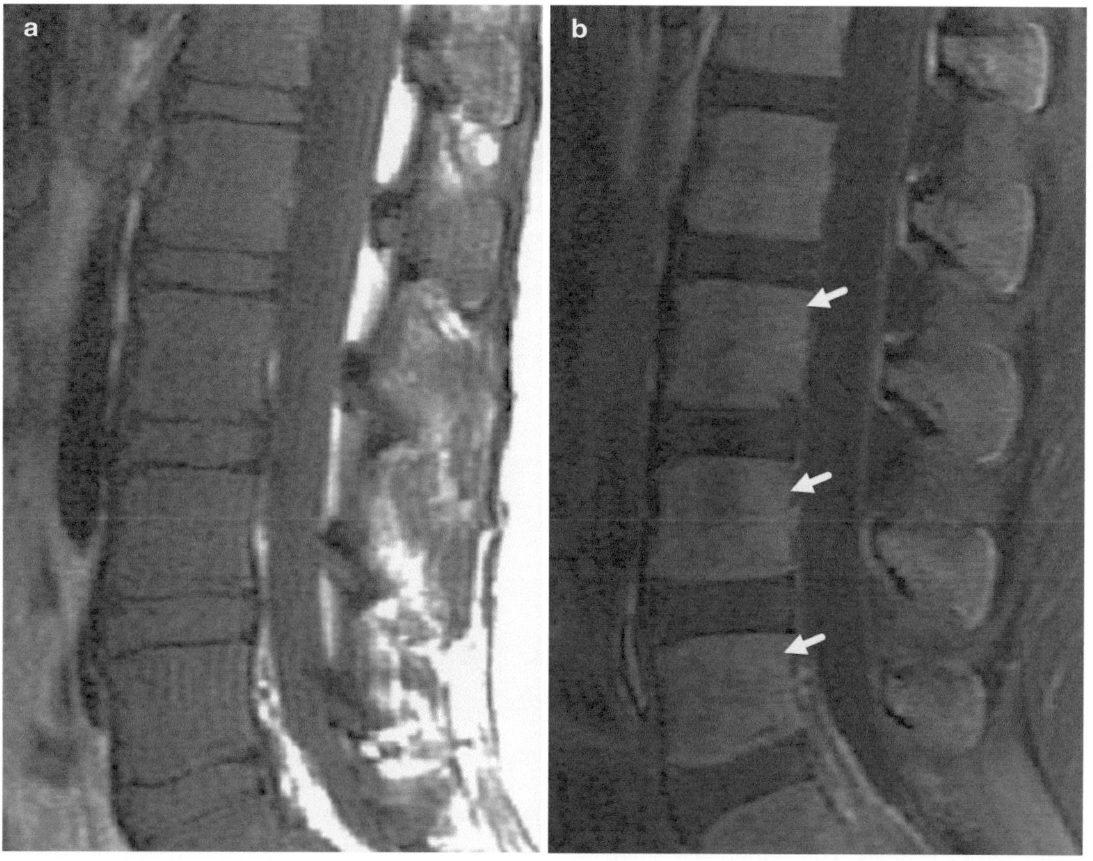

Fig. 25.14 Diffuse but subtle leukemic infiltration of vertebral bodies. (**a**) On T1-W sagittal image, the vertebral bodies are uniformly too dark, darker than the intervertebral disks. (**b**) Fat-suppressed (FS) T1-W gadolinium-enhanced (GE) image shows subtle abnormal enhancement resulting in a blotchy appearance (*arrows*)

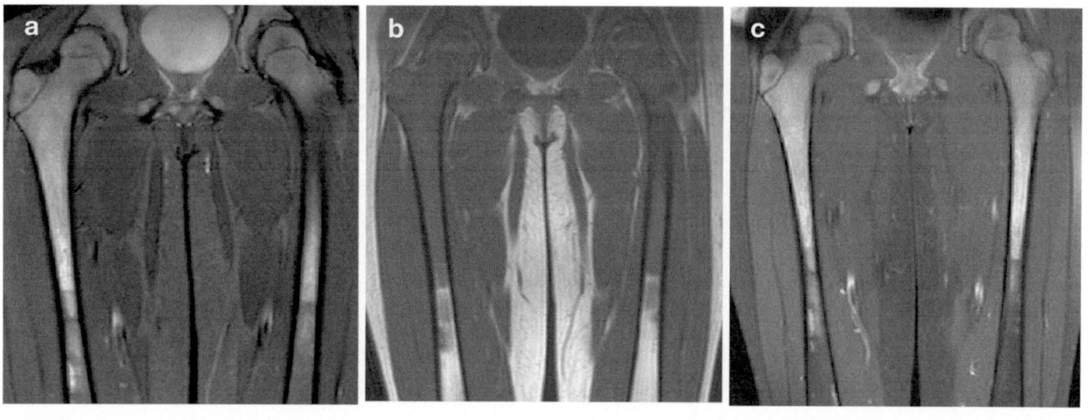

Fig. 25.15 Extensive leukemic marrow infiltration. (**a**) Short-tau inversion recovery (STIR) coronal image shows diffuse hyperintensity in the mid and proximal femurs. (**b**) T1-W image shows corresponding hypointensity. (**c**) Gadolinium-enhanced FS T1-W image shows marked enhancement

Extraosseous tumor extension in patients with lymphoma may have a characteristic (although not pathognomonic) appearance, allowing the radiologist to suggest the possibility of lymphoma: due to the permeative nature of the tumor, there may be an extraosseous mass with no obvious destruction of cortical bone [12].

In patients with lymphoma, MRI has been shown to be superior to scintigraphy in the evaluation of bone marrow. However, it does not appear to be sufficiently sensitive to exclude marrow involvement [29]. Furthermore, it cannot differentiate between the different histologic subtypes of lymphoma. The diagnosis of marrow involvement is therefore established with marrow biopsies, which are usually obtained from the bilateral posterior superior iliac crests. Because only a small volume of bone is examined, sampling errors exist [29]. The diagnostic yield of bone marrow biopsy may be increased if the biopsy site is selected with the aid of MRI [12, 29]. MRI may also direct harvest procedures for autologous bone marrow transplantation to sites of relatively uninvolved marrow [12, 56].

MRI has been applied to the posttreatment follow-up of patients with lymphoma. Dynamic contrast-enhanced MRI may help assess treatment response, as a decrease in the degree of contrast enhancement has been shown to correlate with a good response or remission [27]. Patients who respond to treatment may show a decrease in T1 relaxation time on quantitative T1-W serial MRI [12, 57].

Posttreatment Changes

MRI is useful for evaluating post-chemotherapy and postradiation tumor response. It can also demonstrate systemic response to chemotherapy.

Patients undergoing chemotherapy generally develop fatty transformation of bone marrow, readily apparent on MRI as increased hyperintensity on T1-W images (Fig. 25.16). The administration of hematopoietic growth factors may delay this process or may cause reconversion of fatty to hematopoietic marrow, which can simulate persistent disease or relapse [27, 58] (Fig. 25.17). Additionally, several drugs used in oncology patients (such as granulocyte colony-stimulating factor [G-CSF]) can cause side effects in the immature skeleton, some of which may be misdiagnosed as neoplastic involvement on MRI [27]. For example, osteopenia, fractures, osteonecrosis (Fig. 25.18), and AVN are well-known complications of prolonged administration of steroids in patients of all ages, and their MRI appearance can resemble neoplasia. In children, methotrexate can cause bone pain and metaphyseal insufficiency fractures (termed *methotrexate osteopathy*) [27].

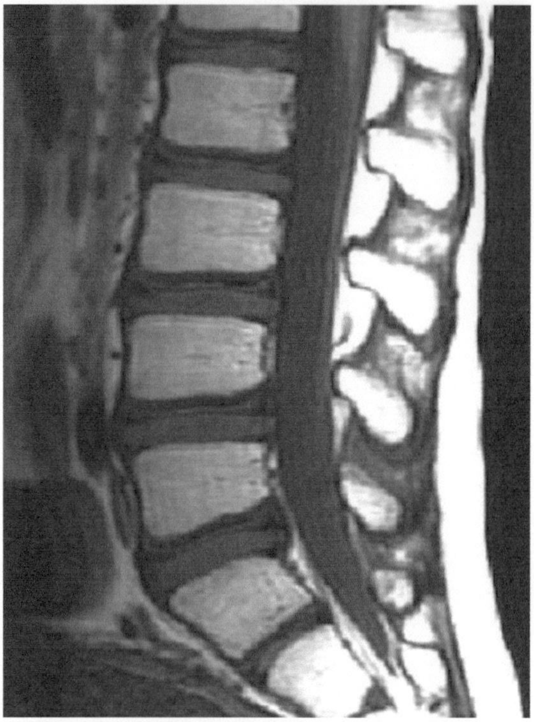

Fig. 25.16 Diffuse fatty marrow due to chemotherapy. Sagittal T1-W image shows hyperintensity throughout vertebral bodies

Radiation therapy kills the hematopoietic cells and destroys the vascular sinusoids, and like chemotherapy this causes conversion of hematopoietic to fatty marrow [2]. The initial marrow response to irradiation consists of a short period of cellular depletion, vascular congestion, edema, and hemorrhage [27]; STIR magnetic resonance (MR) images may demonstrate hyperintensity in the distribution of the radiation portal within a few days of initiation of treatment [20]. The chronic phase follows, characterized by fatty

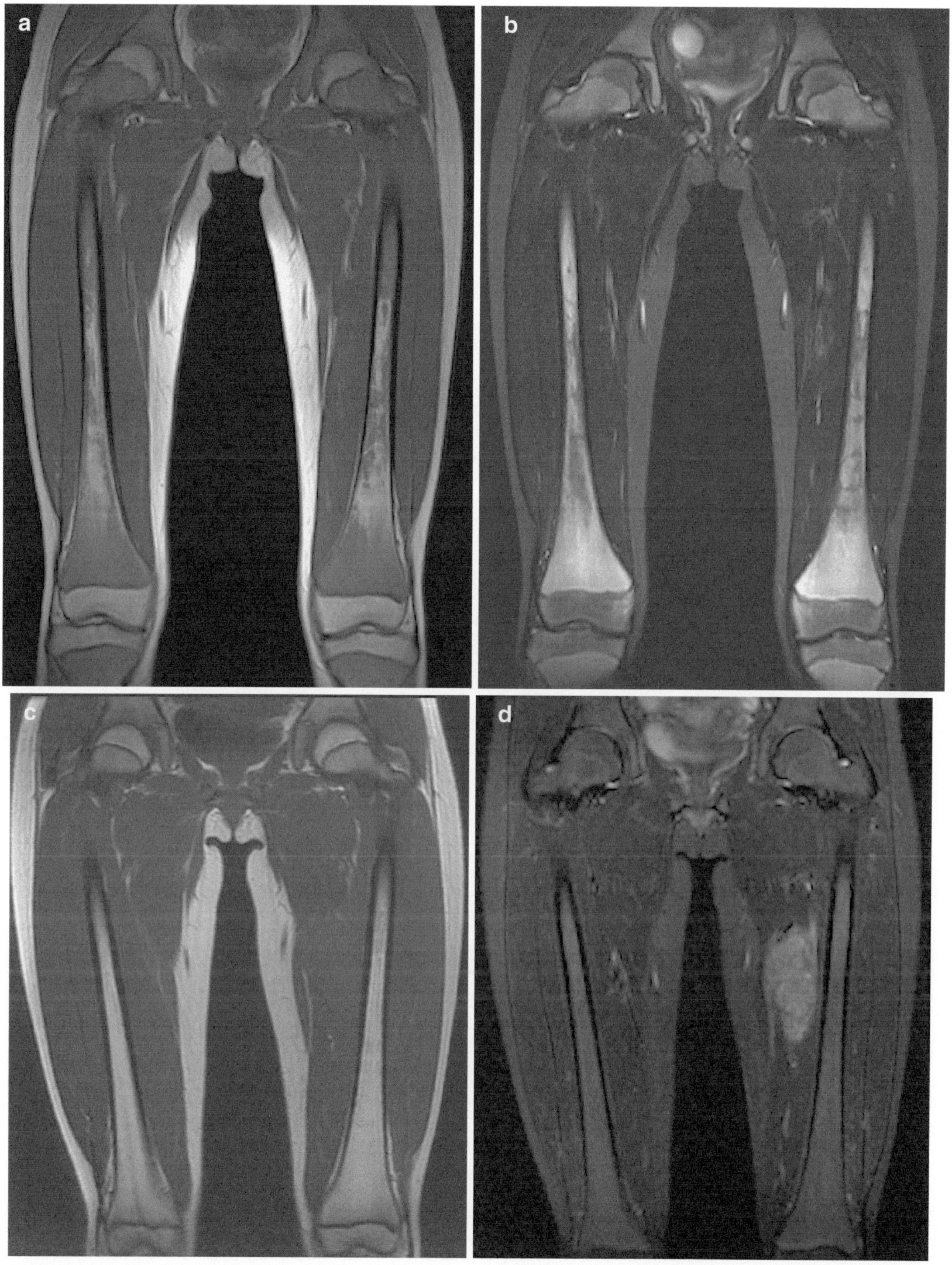

Fig. 25.17 Marrow reconversion in a 12-year-old after chemotherapy for soft tissue Ewing sarcoma. (**a**) Coronal T1-W image (**a**) shows metadiaphyseal hypointensity, with corresponding hyperintensity on coronal STIR image (**b**). 3 months earlier, prior to chemotherapy, coronal T1-W (**c**) and STIR (**d**) images show normal fatty marrow in the metadiaphyses. Note soft tissue mass

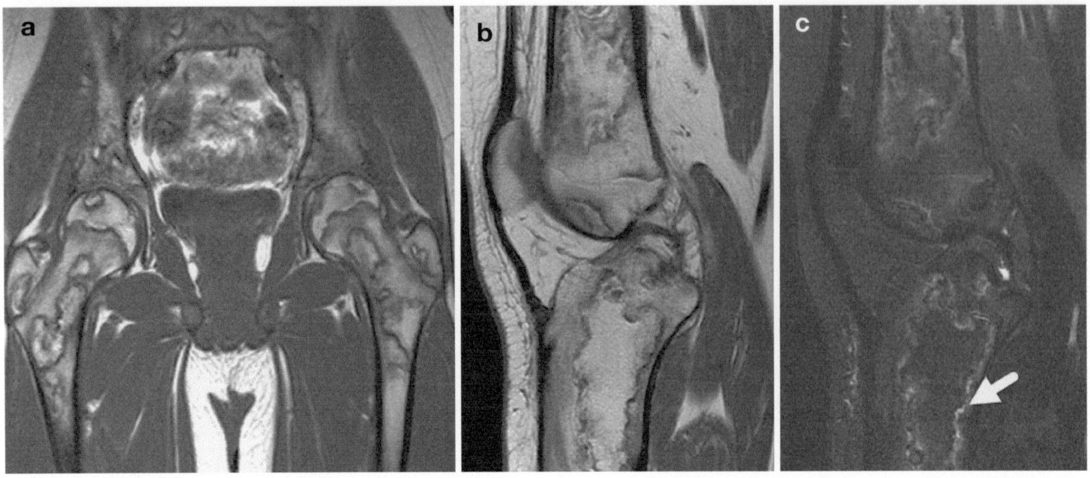

Fig. 25.18 Extensive bilateral osteonecrosis after corticosteroid treatment of leukemia. (**a**) Coronal T1-W image shows multiple mildly hyperintense foci with irregular hypointense margins in the femurs and to a lesser extent the iliac bones. (**b**) Sagittal T1-W image shows similar appearance at the knee. (**c**) Corresponding T2-W FS image shows the "double-line" sign (*arrow*) with inner hyperintense margins representing granulation tissue, paralleling the low signal intensity serpiginous borders

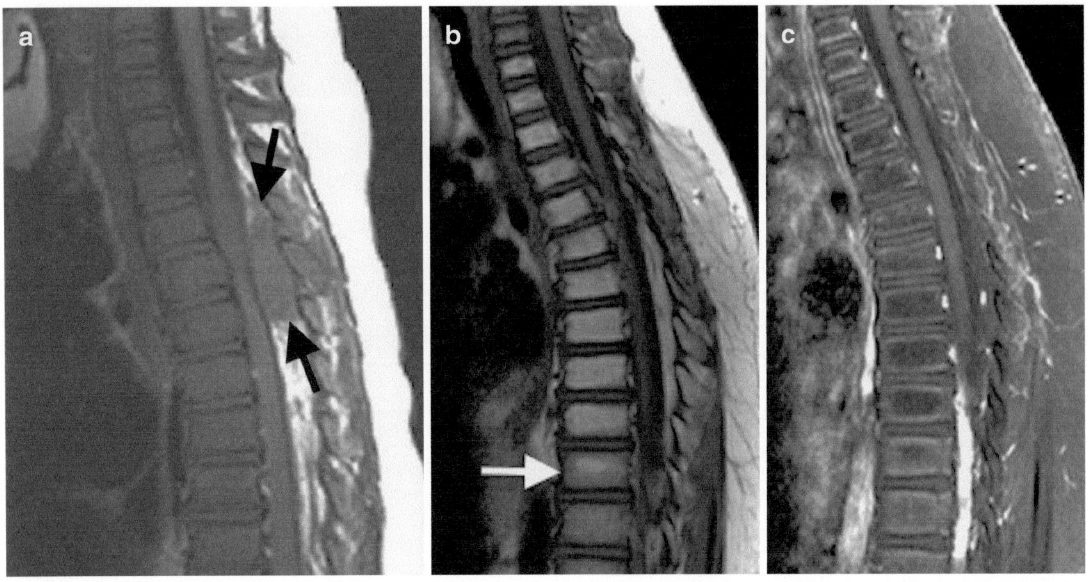

Fig. 25.19 Diffuse neuroblastoma metastases before and after radiation therapy. (**a**) T1-W sagittal image shows diffuse hypointense marrow and parathecal mass (*arrows*). (**b**) T1-W image after treatment shows diffuse hyperintense signal in lower cervical and upper thoracic vertebrae, due to fatty marrow replacement. *Arrow* delineates the distal-most extent of the radiation portal. (**c**) FS T1-W gadolinium-enhanced image after treatment shows limited enhancement

marrow transformation that is more sharply limited to the radiation portals (Fig. 25.19). This progresses rapidly during the first 6 weeks of therapy and then continues at a much slower rate [20]. With time, however, marrow may regenerate. Marrow recovery is better in younger patients, and in patients younger than 18 years of age, marrow regeneration may be complete [27].

After radiation therapy, MRI is especially helpful because new lesions are easily distinguishable from irradiated marrow, which appears hyperintense on T1-W images due to fatty conversion [2]. MRI also delineates other radiation-induced complications, such as osteonecrosis, fractures, and radiation-induced neoplasm.

Differentiation between regenerating hematopoietic marrow, disease relapse, peri-tumoral reactive change, and posttreatment marrow fibrosis can be challenging, as all these entities demonstrate contrast enhancement at MRI. Out-of-phase imaging may supply additional information by demonstrating the presence of fat within marrow foci. Dynamic enhanced MRI may be helpful, as viable tumor may demonstrate early enhancement and early washout of contrast, whereas the other entities show delayed and more prolonged enhancement [12, 59].

3.2 Non-tumoral Infiltrative Disorders

Hemochromatosis and Hemosiderosis

Increased marrow iron stores can result from iron deposition, as in hemosiderosis and hemochromatosis. Increased marrow iron is also seen when marrow reconversion results in markedly hypercellular marrow, such as with sickle-cell disease. By MRI criteria, iron overload may be present if bone marrow signal intensity is less than that of muscles on both T1- and T2-W images [3] and is also lower than non-degenerated intervertebral disks [44]. However, normal signal intensity on T1-W images does not exclude iron overload. T2* images are more sensitive to iron overload and may be abnormal even if T1-W images are normal [60]. Knowledge of the patient's transfusion history is very important for correct interpretation of the MRI findings of bone marrow. Table 25.2 lists entities that cause low signal on both T1 and T2.

Sickle-Cell Disease

Patients with sickle-cell disease may demonstrate persistence, hyperplasia, or reconversion of hematopoietic marrow. Intramedullary marrow hyperplasia is characterized by increased width of the medullary and diploic spaces as well as cortical thinning, with signal characteristics of hematopoietic marrow. With severe disease, extramedullary hematopoiesis may also be present. In addition, infarcts and osteomyelitis occur with increased frequency in patients with sickle-cell disease and manifest as marrow edema and corresponding high T2 signal (see Chap. 23 for further discussion).

Gaucher Disease

Gaucher disease, the most common of the inherited lysosomal storage disorders, is characterized by accumulation of glucocerebroside in lysosomes in the reticuloendothelial system. Potential clinical manifestations include hepatomegaly, splenomegaly, anemia, thrombocytopenia, and marrow infiltration by lipid-engorged Gaucher cells [61]. Marrow involvement generally follows the distribution of red marrow and progresses from a proximal to distal direction in the appendicular skeleton. With more advanced disease, epiphyseal involvement and secondary osteonecrosis may develop. Replacement of bone marrow by Gaucher cells produces low signal intensity lesions on both T1- and T2-W images (Fig. 25.20). Both homogeneous and inhomo-

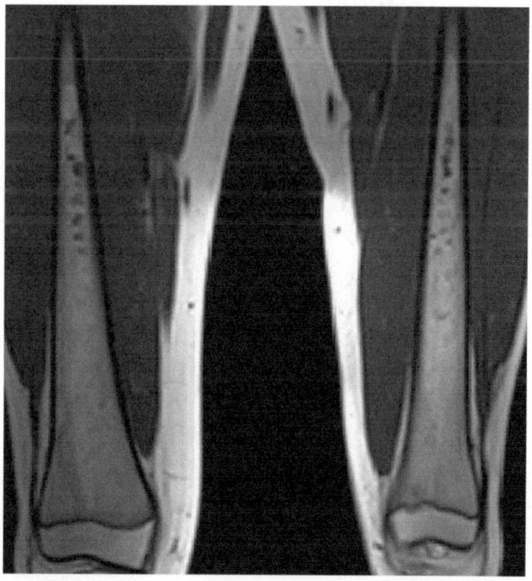

Fig. 25.20 Gaucher disease. T1-W coronal image shows heterogeneous metadiaphyseal hypointensity due to accumulation of glucocerebroside. Erlenmeyer flask deformity

geneous patterns of altered signal intensity have been described. In addition, infection or osteonecrosis may result in high signal intensity on fluid-sensitive sequences.

Quantitative assessment of marrow involvement in Gaucher disease helps determine treatment efficacy. Various scoring systems have been developed, including Dixon quantitative chemical shift imaging and bone marrow burden scores [20]. The bone marrow burden scoring method is preferred, as it assesses both the lumbar spine and the femur, key anatomical sites for Gaucher cell infiltration. Furthermore, it has been validated against other methods and researched in multiple studies [61].

Osteopetrosis

Patients with the infantile form of osteopetrosis have the most severe marrow involvement, characterized by reduced marrow space that demonstrates low signal intensity on both T1- and T2-W images. This results in a "black bones" appearance [20] (Fig. 25.21).

3.3 Marrow Aplasia and Myelodysplastic Disorders

Aplastic anemia may be idiopathic or result from exposure to drugs, toxic substances, ionizing radiation, or viral infections. MRI demonstrates fatty replacement of the bone marrow [53] due to the absence of cellular elements. On T1-W images, the marrow may be entirely fatty or predominantly fatty with small hypointense nodules [47]. The presence of either focal or diffuse hypointense nodules may suggest an underlying myelodysplastic disorder [12]. Increase in the extent of marrow involvement and signal intensity on STIR images indicates disease progression. As with other infiltrative marrow disorders, MRI can guide marrow sampling procedures to sites of hypercellular marrow.

Myelofibrosis

The bone marrow in myelofibrosis may be either hypercellular or fibrotic (depleted of hematopoietic elements). Fibrotic marrow usually manifests as multiple foci of markedly low signal intensity on all MRI sequences. Alternatively, the appearance may resemble the metaphyses in Gaucher disease, with additional T1 and T2 hypointensity in the epiphyses and apophyses [20].

3.4 Ischemia

Marrow blood supply is derived from two major sources: the major nutrient artery, which supplies most of the marrow, and smaller periosteal arteries, which directly penetrate the bone [1, 4].

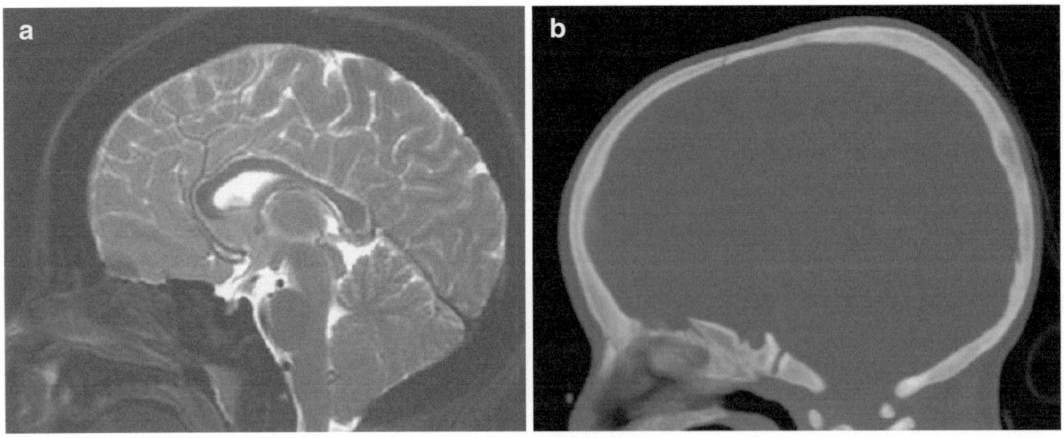

Fig. 25.21 Osteopetrosis. (**a**) T2-W FS sagittal image shows marked thickening and hypointensity of the cortices. (**b**) Corresponding sagittal CT reformat shows thickening and diffuse sclerosis of the calvarium

Blood then flows from these transosteal vessels into a highly branched network of medullary venous sinuses. These sinuses form an extensive anastomosis of thin-walled, relatively large vascular channels that drain into a large central sinus before joining the systemic venous circulation [5]. The vascular supply of red marrow is typically rich and arborized, whereas that of yellow marrow is much sparser [5, 7]. Osteonecrosis therefore predominates in the fatty marrow [20]. In addition, there is relatively little collateral circulation in the metaphyses, and therefore, the majority of non-epiphyseal infarcts in the long tubular bones occur in this region.

The initial ischemic insult is followed by cell loss. Hematopoietic cells die within the first 6–12 h of anoxia. Osteocytes, osteoblasts, and osteoclasts begin to show evidence of cellular death after 48 h. The adipocytes are most resistant and survive for 2–5 days. MRI is a very sensitive method for detecting osteonecrosis. In its earliest stage, osteonecrosis produces a nonspecific pattern of poorly defined T2 hyperintensity, identical to the appearance of bone marrow edema. Typical low signal intensity margins of reactive bone then become evident, sometimes demonstrating the double-line sign that is considered characteristic of osteonecrosis (see Fig. 25.18).

After allogeneic hematopoietic stem cell transplantations, bone infarcts appear as a geographical area of decreased signal on T1-W imaging and increased signal on STIR. Involvement is often multifocal, most often affecting both knees. MRI is also used to evaluate bone infarcts in patients with sickle-cell anemia, characterizing foci of osteonecrosis as acute or remote. Unlike patients with normal hemoglobin, whose bone infarcts occur predominantly in fatty marrow, patients with sickle-cell anemia develop infarcts in both hematopoietic and fatty marrow [20].

3.5 Trauma

In the setting of fracture, contusion, osteochondral injury, and stress reaction, edema and/or hemorrhage may be observed. Fractures may be radiographically occult but appear on MRI as a linear band that is hypointense on both T1- and T2-W sequences. However, if the edema is extensive, fracture lines may be obscured, particularly on T1-W sequences [20]. Prominent marrow edema may be the only MRI finding in cases of stress-related response. This is most often encountered in the tibial diaphysis (see Chap. 14).

3.6 Arthritis

MRI demonstrates both the articular soft tissue and the osseous inflammatory and destructive features of arthritis. It is more sensitive than radiographic examination for the detection of inflammatory soft tissue and bone changes, including bone marrow edema and inflammatory infiltrates. In patients with spondyloarthropathy, MRI can diagnose sacroiliitis and other focal or multifocal bone marrow pathologies when radiographs are still normal [62] (see Chap. 20).

3.7 Scurvy

Prolonged vitamin C deficiency may cause scurvy and defective collagen fiber formation, leading to bony demineralization, microfractures, and poor healing. Conventional radiographs may demonstrate prominent zones of provisional calcification (the white lines of Frankel), subjacent lines of demineralization (scurvy lines), and lateral spurs off the epiphyses (Pelkan spurs). However, radiographs are often normal. In these cases, MRI may demonstrate multifocal patchy abnormal marrow signal in the femoral diaphyses and/or subperiosteal fluid collections (consistent with hematomas). Bilateral, symmetric, broad, band-like metadiaphyseal marrow that is hypointense on T1-W imaging and hyperintense on T2 may be evident, simulating malignancy. This results from gelatinous transformation of bone marrow and should raise suspicion of scurvy [63, 64].

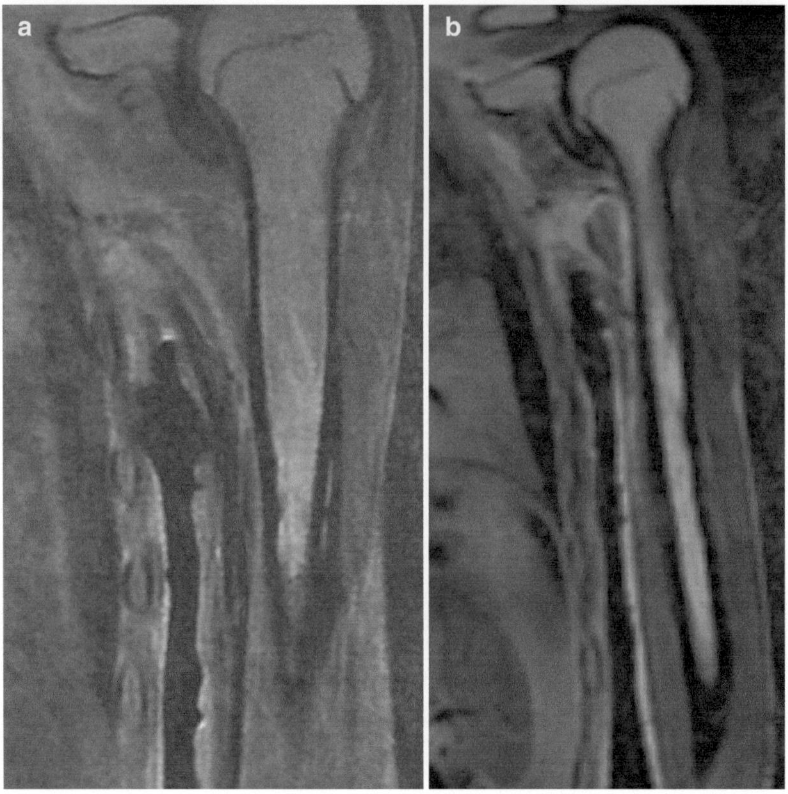

Fig. 25.22 Gelatinous transformation of bone marrow in a 17-year-old girl with anorexia nervosa and hepatitis. (**a**) Coronal T1-W image of the arm shows abnormally hypointense bone marrow. (**b**) Fast spin-echo inversion recovery (FSEIR) image shows abnormal marrow hyperintensity. There is minimal adipose tissue in the arm and chest wall (Courtesy of Tal Laor, Cincinnati Children's Hospital)

3.8 Anorexia Nervosa

Severe malnutrition may lead to diffuse gelatinous transformation of bone marrow. Increase in extracellular gelatinous material (mucopolysaccharides) accompanies decrease in the size and number of hematopoietic and fat cells, leading to bone fragility and increased likelihood of insufficiency fractures. The condition begins in the periphery. It may be reversible if the underlying cause is treated. Gelatinous transformation may also be seen with cancer and infection.

On T1-W imaging performed without fat suppression, the signal intensity appears reversed from normal: marrow appears diffusely hypointense (Fig. 25.22). On STIR or T2-W fat-suppressed (FS) imaging, marrow appears too hyperintense. It is important to note that there is no evidence of other underlying pathology, and erosions and marrow lesions are absent. The overall appearance may suggest failed fat suppression (but fat suppression was not applied). There is minimal subcutaneous and intermuscular fat, and deep fat may appear hyperintense on T2-W FS imaging. In the setting of gelatinous transformation, stress fractures may be difficult to see (personal communication (Robert Boutin and Tal Laor)).

References

1. Abboud C, Lichtman M. Structure of the bone marrow. In: Beutler E, Lichtman M, Coller B, et al., editors. Williams hematology, vol. 1. 5th ed. New York: McGraw-Hill; 1995. p. 25–38.
2. Schmidt GP, Reiser MF, Baur-Melnyk A. Whole-body imaging of the musculoskeletal system: the value of MR imaging. Skeletal Radiol. 2007;36(12):1109–19. PubMed PMID: 17554538. Pubmed Central PMCID: 2042033.
3. Babyn PS, Ranson M, McCarville ME. Normal bone marrow: signal characteristics and fatty conversion. Magn Reson Imaging Clin N Am. 1998;6(3):473–95. PubMed PMID: 9654581.
4. Weiss L. Bone marrow. In: Weiss L, editor. Cell and tissue biology: a textbook of histology. Baltimore: Urban and Schwarzenberg; 1988.

5. Trubowitz S, Davis S. The bone marrow matrix. In: Trubowitz S, Davis S, editors. The human bone marrow: anatomy, physiology, and pathophysiology. Boca Raton: CRC Press; 1982. p. 43–75.
6. Steiner RM, Mitchell DG, Rao VM, Schweitzer ME. Magnetic resonance imaging of diffuse bone marrow disease. Radiol Clin North Am. 1993;31(2):383–409. PubMed PMID: 8446756.
7. Vogler 3rd JB, Murphy WA. Bone marrow imaging. Radiology. 1988;168(3):679–93. PubMed PMID: 3043546.
8. Bracken J, Nandurkar D, Radhakrishnan K, Ditchfield M. Normal paediatric bone marrow: magnetic resonance imaging appearances from birth to 5 years. J Med Imaging Radiat Oncol. 2013;57(3):283–91. PubMed PMID: 23721136.
9. Moore S. Pediatric musculoskeletal magnetic resonance. In: International Pediatric Radiology, editor. Pediatric imaging: update 91. Stockholm: Institute for Diagnostik Radiologi; 1991. p. 217–23.
10. Siegel MJ, Luker GG. Bone marrow imaging in children. Magn Reson Imaging Clin N Am. 1996;4(4):771–96. PubMed PMID: 8832854.
11. Siegel MJ. MRI of bone marrow [PDF download]. Available from: www.arrs.org/shoparrs/products/pdf.cfm?thefile=s06p_sample.pdf. Accessed on 7 Apr 2014.
12. Moulopoulos LA, Dimopoulos MA. Magnetic resonance imaging of the bone marrow in hematologic malignancies. Blood. 1997;90(6):2127–47. PubMed PMID: 9310464.
13. Guillerman RP. Marrow: red, yellow and bad. Pediatr Radiol. 2013;43 Suppl 1:S181–92. PubMed PMID: 23478934.
14. Shah LM, Hanrahan CJ. MRI of spinal bone marrow: part 1, techniques and normal age-related appearances. Am J Roentgenol. 2011;197(6):1298–308.
15. Muller L-SO, editor. MRI of bone marrow. The European society of paediatric radiology 50th annual meeting. Budapest. 2013.
16. Hwang S, Panicek DM. Magnetic resonance imaging of bone marrow in oncology, part 1. Skeletal Radiol. 2007;36(10):913–20. PubMed PMID: 17492443.
17. Waitches G, Zawin JK, Poznanski AK. Sequence and rate of bone marrow conversion in the femora of children as seen on MR imaging: are accepted standards accurate? AJR Am J Roentgenol. 1994;162(6):1399–406. PubMed PMID: 8192007.
18. Sebag GH, Dubois J, Tabet M, Bonato A, Lallemand D. Pediatric spinal bone marrow: assessment of normal age-related changes in the MRI appearance. Pediatr Radiol. 1993;23(7):515–8. PubMed PMID: 8309751.
19. Laor T, Jaramillo D. MR imaging insights into skeletal maturation: what is normal? Radiology. 2009;250(1):28–38. PubMed PMID: 19092089.
20. Resnick D, Sik Kang H, Pretterklieber M. Bone and bone marrow: anatomy and pathophysiology, Internal derangements of joints, vol. 1. 2nd ed. Philadelphia: Saunders Elsevier; 2007. p. 231–57.
21. Caldemeyer KS, Smith RR, Harris A, Williams T, Huang Y, Eckert GJ, et al. Hematopoietic bone marrow hyperplasia: correlation of spinal MR findings, hematologic parameters, and bone mineral density in endurance athletes. Radiology. 1996;198(2):503–8. PubMed PMID: 8596857.
22. Pui MH, Chang SK. Comparison of inversion recovery fast spin-echo (FSE) with T2-weighted fat-saturated FSE and T1-weighted MR imaging in bone marrow lesion detection. Skeletal Radiol. 1996;25(2):149–52. PubMed PMID: 8848745.
23. Sebag GH, Moore SG. Effect of trabecular bone on the appearance of marrow in gradient-echo imaging of the appendicular skeleton. Radiology. 1990;174(3 Pt 1):855–9. PubMed PMID: 2305069.
24. Vanel D, Dromain C, Tardivon A. MRI of bone marrow disorders. Eur Radiol. 2000;10(2):224–9. PubMed PMID: 10663751.
25. Baur A, Stabler A, Bartl R, Lamerz R, Scheidler J, Reiser M. MRI gadolinium enhancement of bone marrow: age-related changes in normals and in diffuse neoplastic infiltration. Skeletal Radiol. 1997;26(7):414–8. PubMed PMID: 9259099.
26. Moulopoulos LA, Varma DG, Dimopoulos MA, Leeds NE, Kim EE, Johnston DA, et al. Multiple myeloma: spinal MR imaging in patients with untreated newly diagnosed disease. Radiology. 1992;185(3):833–40. PubMed PMID: 1438772.
27. Hwang S, Panicek DM. Magnetic resonance imaging of bone marrow in oncology, Part 2. Skeletal Radiol. 2007;36(11):1017–27. PubMed PMID: 17492444.
28. Takahara T, Imai Y, Yamashita T, Yasuda S, Nasu S, Van Cauteren M. Diffusion weighted whole body imaging with background body signal suppression (DWIBS): technical improvement using free breathing, STIR and high resolution 3D display. Radiat Med. 2004;22(4):275–82. PubMed PMID: 15468951.
29. Kwee TC, Kwee RM, Verdonck LF, Bierings MB, Nievelstein RA. Magnetic resonance imaging for the detection of bone marrow involvement in malignant lymphoma. Br J Haematol. 2008;141(1):60–8. PubMed PMID: 18324967.
30. Ghanem N, Lohrmann C, Engelhardt M, Pache G, Uhl M, Saueressig U, et al. Whole-body MRI in the detection of bone marrow infiltration in patients with plasma cell neoplasms in comparison to the radiological skeletal survey. Eur Radiol. 2006;16(5):1005–14. PubMed PMID: 16463030.
31. Buhmann S, Schoenberg S, Becker C, Lang N, Reiser M, Baur-Melnyk A. Whole-body imaging approach of patients with multiple myeloma: comparing MR imaging with MD-CT. Eur Radiol. 2006;16 Suppl 1:13–003.
32. O'Connell MJ, Powell T, Brennan D, Lynch T, McCarthy CJ, Eustace SJ. Whole-body MR imaging in the diagnosis of polymyositis. AJR Am J Roentgenol. 2002;179(4):967–71. PubMed PMID: 12239048.
33. Lenk S, Fischer S, Kotter I, Claussen CD, Schlemmer HP. Possibilities of whole-body MRI for investigating

musculoskeletal diseases. Radiologe. 2004;44(9):844–53. PubMed PMID: 15349730. Moglichkeiten der Ganzkorper-MRT zur Diagnostik muskuloskelettaler Erkrankungen.
34. Daldrup-Link HE, Franzius C, Link TM, Laukamp D, Sciuk J, Jurgens H, et al. Whole-body MR imaging for detection of bone metastases in children and young adults: comparison with skeletal scintigraphy and FDG PET. AJR Am J Roentgenol. 2001;177(1):229–36. PubMed PMID: 11418435.
35. Hoh CK, Glaspy J, Rosen P, Dahlbom M, Lee SJ, Kunkel L, et al. Whole-body FDG-PET imaging for staging of Hodgkin's disease and lymphoma. J Nucl Med. 1997;38(3):343–8. PubMed PMID: 9074514.
36. Seneterre E, Weissleder R, Jaramillo D, Reimer P, Lee AS, Brady TJ, et al. Bone marrow: ultrasmall superparamagnetic iron oxide for MR imaging. Radiology. 1991;179(2):529–33. PubMed PMID: 2014305.
37. Daldrup-Link HE, Mohanty A, Cuenod C, Pichler B, Link T. New perspectives on bone marrow contrast agents and molecular imaging. Semin Musculoskelet Radiol. 2009;13(2):145–56. PubMed PMID: 19455477.
38. McMenamin DS, Stuckey SL, Potgieter GJ. T1 hyperintense vertebral column melanoma metastases. AJNR Am J Neuroradiol. 2007;28(9):1817–8. PubMed PMID: 17885232.
39. Howe BM, Johnson GB, Wenger DE. Current concepts in MRI of focal and diffuse malignancy of bone marrow. Semin Musculoskelet Radiol. 2013;17(2):137–44. PubMed PMID: 23673545.
40. Khung S, Budzik JF, Amzallag-Bellenger E, Lambilliote A, Soto Ares G, Cotten A, et al. Skeletal involvement in Langerhans cell histiocytosis. Insights Imaging. 2013;4(5):569–79. PubMed PMID: 23907805. Pubmed Central PMCID: 3781243.
41. Kung JW, Yablon CM, Eisenberg RL. Bone marrow signal alteration in the extremities. AJR Am J Roentgenol. 2011;196(5):W492–510. PubMed PMID: 21512037.
42. Long SS, Yablon CM, Eisenberg RL. Bone marrow signal alteration in the spine and sacrum. AJR Am J Roentgenol. 2010;195(3):W178–200. PubMed PMID: 20729415.
43. Hanrahan CJ, Shah LM. MRI of spinal bone marrow: part 2, T1-weighted imaging-based differential diagnosis. AJR Am J Roentgenol. 2011;197(6):1309–21. PubMed PMID: 22109284.
44. Carroll KW, Feller JF, Tirman PF. Useful internal standards for distinguishing infiltrative marrow pathology from hematopoietic marrow at MRI. J Magn Reson Imaging. 1997;7(2):394–8. PubMed PMID: 9090597.
45. Vande Berg BC, Lecouvet FE, Galant C, Maldague BE, Malghem J. Normal variants and frequent marrow alterations that simulate bone marrow lesions at MR imaging. Radiol Clin North Am. 2005;43(4):761–70. ix. PubMed PMID: 15893536.
46. Rosen BR, Fleming DM, Kushner DC, Zaner KS, Buxton RB, Bennet WP, et al. Hematologic bone marrow disorders: quantitative chemical shift MR imaging. Radiology. 1988;169(3):799–804. PubMed PMID: 3187003.
47. Imamura F, Kuriyama K, Seto T, Hasegawa Y, Nakayama T, Nakamura S, et al. Detection of bone marrow metastases of small cell lung cancer with magnetic resonance imaging: early diagnosis before destruction of osseous structure and implications for staging. Lung Cancer. 2000;27(3):189–97. PubMed PMID: 10699692.
48. Flickinger FW, Sanal SM. Bone marrow MRI: techniques and accuracy for detecting breast cancer metastases. Magn Reson Imaging. 1994;12(6):829–35. PubMed PMID: 7968282.
49. Frank JA, Ling A, Patronas NJ, Carrasquillo JA, Horvath K, Hickey AM, et al. Detection of malignant bone tumors: MR imaging vs scintigraphy. AJR Am J Roentgenol. 1990;155(5):1043–8. PubMed PMID: 2120933.
50. Eustace S, Tello R, DeCarvalho V, Carey J, Wroblicka JT, Melhem ER, et al. A comparison of whole-body turboSTIR MR imaging and planar 99mTc-methylene diphosphonate scintigraphy in the examination of patients with suspected skeletal metastases. AJR Am J Roentgenol. 1997;169(6):1655–61. PubMed PMID: 9393186.
51. Disler DG, McCauley TR, Ratner LM, Kesack CD, Cooper JA. In-phase and out-of-phase MR imaging of bone marrow: prediction of neoplasia based on the detection of coexistent fat and water. AJR Am J Roentgenol. 1997;169(5):1439–47. PubMed PMID: 9353477.
52. Zajick Jr DC, Morrison WB, Schweitzer ME, Parellada JA, Carrino JA. Benign and malignant processes: normal values and differentiation with chemical shift MR imaging in vertebral marrow. Radiology. 2005;237(2):590–6. PubMed PMID: 16244268.
53. Cohen MD, Klatte EC, Baehner R, Smith JA, Martin-Simmerman P, Carr BE, et al. Magnetic resonance imaging of bone marrow disease in children. Radiology. 1984;151(3):715–8. PubMed PMID: 6585859.
54. Vande Berg BC, Michaux L, Scheiff JM, Malghem J, Lecouvet FE, Bourgois MP, et al. Sequential quantitative MR analysis of bone marrow: differences during treatment of lymphoid versus myeloid leukemia. Radiology. 1996;201(2):519–23. PubMed PMID: 8888252.
55. Vande Berg BC, Schmitz PJ, Scheiff JM, Filleul BJ, Michaux JL, Ferrant A, et al. Acute myeloid leukemia: lack of predictive value of sequential quantitative MR imaging during treatment. Radiology. 1995;197(1):301–5. PubMed PMID: 7568842.
56. Smith MR, Schilder R, Padavic-Shaller K, Shaer A, Al-Saleem T, Negendank W. Lymphoma staging with bone marrow MRI. Proc Am Soc Clin Oncol. 1995;14:390.
57. Smith SR, Williams CE, Edwards RH, Davies JM. Quantitative magnetic resonance studies of lumbar vertebral marrow in patients with refractory or relapsed Hodgkin's disease. Ann Oncol. 1991;2 Suppl 2:39–42. PubMed PMID: 2049319.

58. Fletcher BD, Wall JE, Hanna SL. Effect of hematopoietic growth factors on MR images of bone marrow in children undergoing chemotherapy. Radiology. 1993;189(3):745–51. PubMed PMID: 7694312.
59. van der Woude HJ, Bloem JL, Verstraete KL, Taminiau AH, Nooy MA, Hogendoorn PC. Osteosarcoma and Ewing's sarcoma after neoadjuvant chemotherapy: value of dynamic MR imaging in detecting viable tumor before surgery. AJR Am J Roentgenol. 1995;165(3):593–8. PubMed PMID: 7645476.
60. Ishijima H, Ishizaka H, Aoki J, Inoue T, Endo K. T2 relaxation time of bone marrow water and lipid: correlation with serum ferritin in normal individuals. J Comput Assist Tomogr. 1997;21(3):506–8. PubMed PMID: 9135666.
61. Maas M, Hangartner T, Mariani G, McHugh K, Moore S, Grabowski GA, et al. Recommendations for the assessment and monitoring of skeletal manifestations in children with Gaucher disease. Skeletal Radiol. 2008;37(3):185–8. PubMed PMID: 18094966. Pubmed Central PMCID: 2226077.
62. Babyn P, Doria AS. Radiologic investigation of rheumatic diseases. Rheum Dis Clin North Am. 2007;33(3):403–40. PubMed PMID: 17936172.
63. Weinstein M, Babyn P, Zlotkin S. An orange a day keeps the doctor away: scurvy in the year 2000. Pediatrics. 2001;108(3):E55. PubMed PMID: 11533373.
64. Brennan CM, Atkins KA, Druzgal CH, Gaskin CM. Magnetic resonance imaging appearance of scurvy with gelatinous bone marrow transformation. Skeletal Radiol. 2012;41(3):357–60. PubMed PMID: 22223127.

26 Bone Density

Tishya A.L. Wren and Vicente Gilsanz

Contents

Abstract

This chapter presents several noninvasive imaging techniques for measuring bone properties in children and adolescents. Dual-energy x-ray absorptiometry (DXA) is the most widely used but has several major limitations because it depends on two-dimensional projections. Quantitative computed tomography (QCT) allows for three-dimensional imaging, but it is more costly and delivers more radiation. Peripheral QCT (pQCT) delivers less radiation but has lower resolution and applies only to peripheral sites. High-resolution pQCT and magnetic resonance imaging (HR-MRI) help estimate bone microarchitectural parameters but require further development before clinical use. Quantitative ultrasound (QUS) is simple and inexpensive but can only measure bone quality at a single peripheral site. Clinical interpretation of bone measurements is challenging.

T.A.L. Wren, PhD
Children's Orthopaedic Center,
Children's Hospital Los Angeles,
4650 Sunset Blvd., MS #69,
Los Angeles, CA 90027, USA
e-mail: twren@chla.usc.edu

V. Gilsanz, MD, PhD (✉)
Department of Radiology,
Children's Hospital Los Angeles,
4650 Sunset Blvd., MS #81,
Los Angeles, CA 90027, USA
e-mail: vgilsanz@chla.usc.edu

Bone is assessed to evaluate fracture risk (Fig. 26.1). Numerous studies in elderly adults have linked osteoporosis, low bone mass, and low bone density to increased fracture risk [1]. Studies in children and adolescents have also related low bone mass or small bone size to fractures [2–4]. Weak bones may play a role in certain types of pediatric fractures, such as

R. Stein-Wexler et al. (eds.), *Pediatric Orthopedic Imaging*,
DOI 10.1007/978-3-642-45381-6_26, © Springer-Verlag Berlin Heidelberg 2015

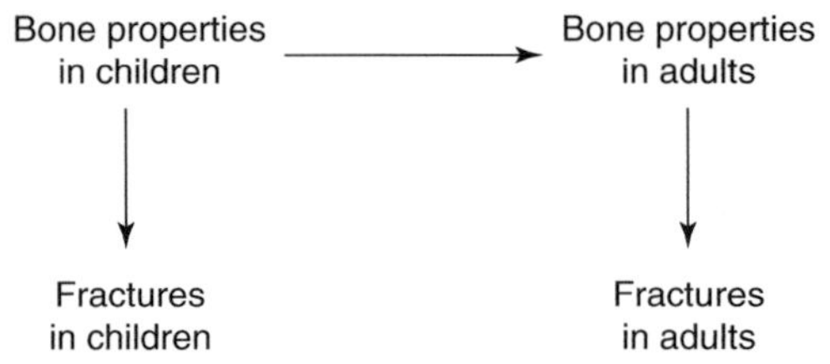

Fig. 26.1 Rationale for measuring bone in children. Bone properties in children may predict childhood fractures as well as osteoporosis and fractures during adulthood

repeat fractures [5] or low impact forearm fractures [2, 3]. In addition, many childhood disorders, or their treatment, may lead to osteopenia and fragility fractures. Imaging helps monitor these patients and determine appropriate intervention.

Assessing bone deficiency in children is fundamentally different from assessing osteoporosis in elderly adults. Since children are growing, low bone mass reflects deficient bone accrual, rather than excessive bone loss. The bone accumulated during childhood determines the peak bone mass reached in early adulthood. Peak bone mass is one of the most important determinants of the risk of osteoporosis.

Genetic susceptibility to osteoporosis and fractures manifests in early childhood. Even before puberty, girls and their mothers share similar bone traits [6]. In addition, genes associated with normal variations in bone mass in the elderly may be related to variations in bone density in children [7]. Finally, measures of bone appear to "track" during growth, with bone mass at a younger age predicting bone mass at older ages. Dual-energy x-ray absorptiometry (DXA) measures of bone mineral content and bone mineral density track over at least a 3-year period, with correlations of 0.76–0.88 between baseline Z-scores (number of standard deviations above or below the mean of normal) and Z-scores in the same individual 3 years later [8]. Perhaps more importantly, bone measures also track through puberty, the critical period for bone acquisition. Bone density and volume in the axial and appendicular skeleton track from the beginning of puberty (Tanner stage 2) through sexual maturity (Tanner 5) [9]. Early identification of individuals at risk for future development of osteoporosis allows for counseling and lifestyle modifications.

1 Bone Properties

Whether a bone fractures depends on the balance between the load applied to the bone and the bone's mechanical properties, or strength. If the load exceeds the bone's strength, the bone breaks. If the load approaches the bone's failure strength, the bone may be damaged, making it more susceptible to future fracture or to overuse injuries with repetitive loading. On the other hand, loading that does not damage the bone may stimulate bone remodeling, resulting in a stronger structure that can resist typical loading patterns.

In terms of engineering mechanics, the geometry and material properties of a structure determine its characteristics. *Geometric properties* commonly used to describe bones include cross-sectional area, bone area, and bone volume. *Material properties* refer to the mechanical behavior of bone tissue. These include elastic modulus (resistance to deformation), strength, and density. Bone density can be described in terms of either tissue density (mass per volume of actual bone material, such as the trabeculae in cancellous bone) or apparent density (mass per volume of bulk material, such as a volume of cancellous bone including both trabeculae and pores). Cortical and cancellous bones have similar tissue density but very different apparent density. *Structural properties* combine the effects of geometry and material. Structural properties include stiffness, mass, and properties derived from the spatial distribution of bone, which are related to torsional (twisting) strength and bending strength. Bones can be compromised in terms of geometry, material, or both (Fig. 26.2).

Imaging is used to assess bone microarchitecture. High-resolution imaging can show cortical porosity, trabecular number, trabecular thickness, trabecular separation, and bone volume fraction. These architectural or morphometric properties are analogous to

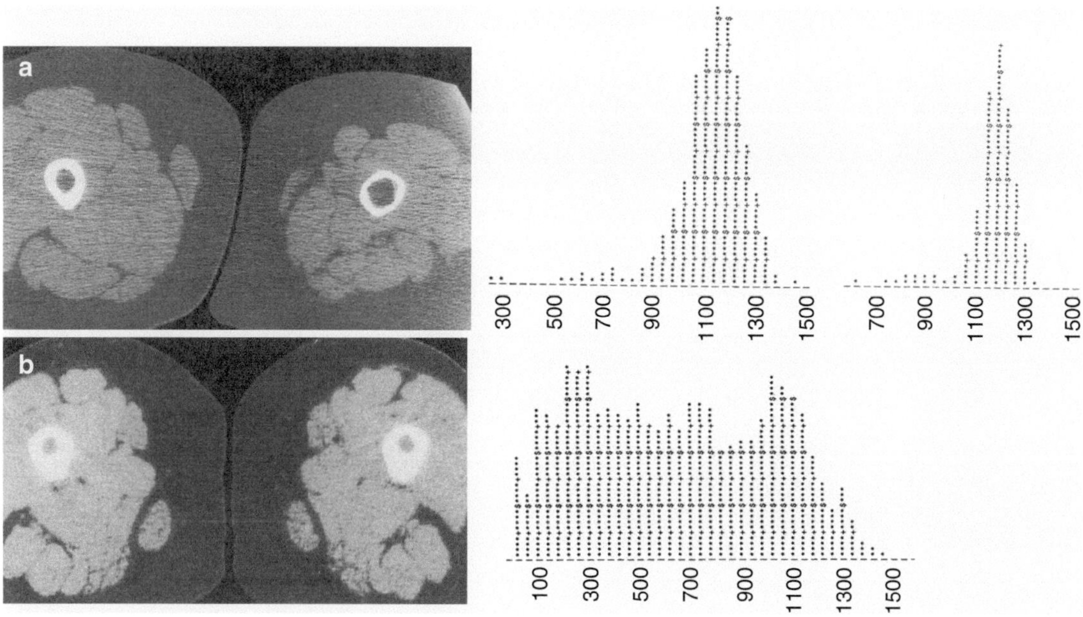

Fig. 26.2 Two examples of abnormal bone demonstrated by CT. (**a**) Compromised bone geometry at the mid shaft of the femur in a 14-year-old boy 2 months after completion of casting for an injury. The left (injured) leg has a thinned cortex but normal bone density (1,135 ± 115 mg/cm^3 K2HPO4) compared with the contralateral leg (1,100 ± 141 mg/cm^3 K2HPO4), as indicated by the density histograms on the right of the figure. (**b**) Compromised material properties at the mid shaft of a 3-year-old boy with familial hypophosphatemic rickets. Bone density (619 ± 366 mg/cm^3 K2HPO4) is lower than normal and broadly distributed, while bone geometry is enhanced by increased cortical thickness (Images reprinted from Kovanlikaya et al. [48])

traditional histomorphometric measures. A number of noninvasive imaging techniques can assess and quantify bone properties. The most commonly used techniques include dual-energy x-ray absorptiometry (DXA), quantitative computed tomography (QCT), peripheral quantitative computed tomography (pQCT), magnetic resonance imaging (MRI), and quantitative ultrasound (QUS). The following sections describe these techniques.

2 Dual-Energy X-ray Absorptiometry (DXA)

This technique is most commonly used to assess bone in children and adults, particularly in clinical settings. Advantages of DXA include low cost, widespread availability, ease of use, short scan times, and very low radiation exposure (<4 μSv per scan). Standardized scanning and analysis protocols exist for commonly assessed sites such as the whole body, spine, hip, and forearm. Normative data specific to children are available [10]. However, DXA has several major limitations particularly problematic to measuring bone in growing children and adolescents. These limitations include size dependence of the density measurements due to the two-dimensional (2-D) nature of DXA (Fig. 26.3), inaccuracies associated with nonhomogeneous soft tissue, inclusion of posterior elements in anterior-posterior imaging of the spine, and discrepancies that occur when using different densitometers.

DXA measurements of bone rely on the difference in attenuation between high- and low-energy x-ray beams as they pass through soft tissue and bone. The low-energy beam is attenuated more than the high-energy beam in both soft

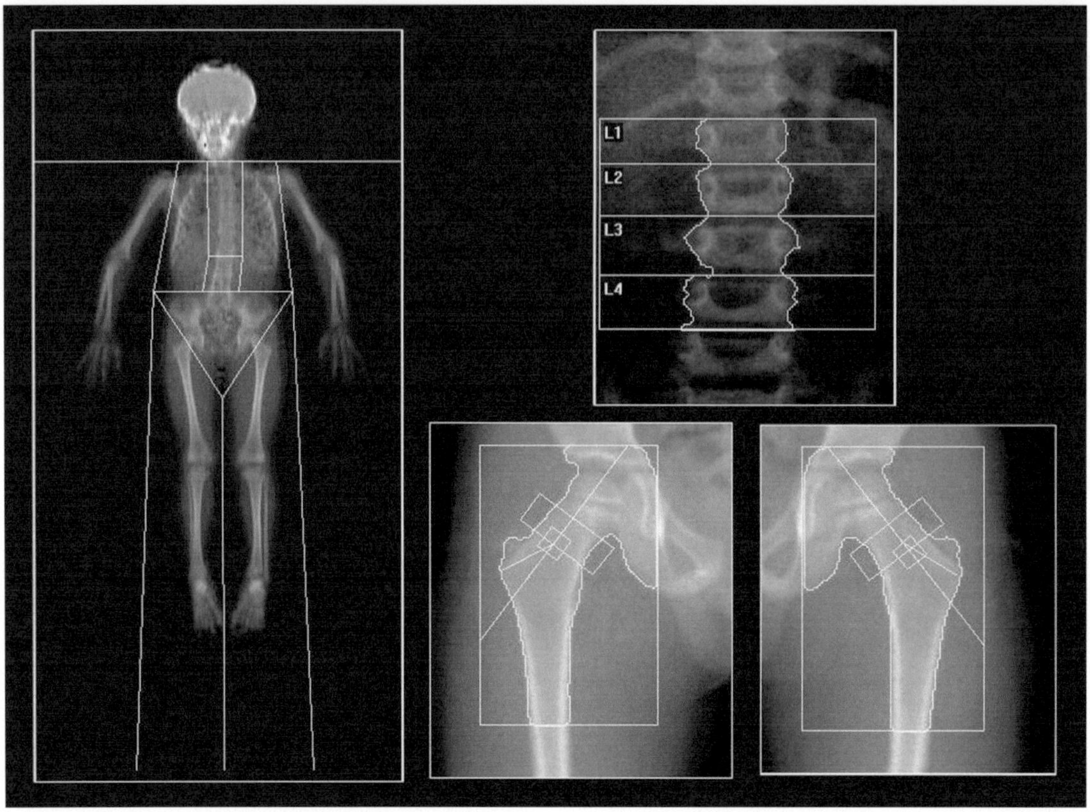

Fig. 26.3 DXA projection images of the whole body, spine, and hips from a healthy 6-year-old boy

tissue and bone, but the differential is much greater in bone. Subtracting soft tissue attenuation from regions not containing bone yields bone attenuation. Attenuation can then be converted to mass and density by internal phantom calibration.

The resulting measurements provide estimates of bone mineral content (BMC, measured in grams), bone mineral density (BMD, measured in g/cm^2), and bone area (BA, measured in cm^2). Bone area is the projected area of the bone in a plane perpendicular to the x-ray beams. Bone mineral density is calculated as BMD = BMC/BA. Since BMD is determined using an area rather than a volume, it is referred to as areal BMD (aBMD) to emphasize that it is not a true volumetric density. DXA aBMD can explain approximately 70 % of the variance in bone strength and is a significant predictor of fracture risk in adults [1]. DXA measures may also predict fractures in children and adolescents [11, 12]. Clinical interpretation of DXA results is complex because the World Health Organization (WHO) definition of osteoporosis based on T-scores does not apply to children. Rather, the International Society for Clinical Densitometry (ISCD) recommends the use of Z-scores, with Z-scores of less than −2 considered low for chronological age. In addition, height adjustment is recommended for children with linear growth disturbances or delay in maturation; however, there is no consensus on the method of adjustment.

For populations that commonly present with skeletal deformities, joint contractures, or indwelling hardware, DXA scanning of the lateral distal femur (LDF) is useful. This approach was first developed for use in children with cerebral palsy; the existing protocols were inappropriate for these patients due to their inability to be properly positioned and/or the presence of metal implants at the spine and hips [13]. The method is now used in other pediatric patient populations including children with spina bifida, muscular dystrophy, osteogenesis imperfecta, juvenile arthritis, and other diagnoses [14]. Generally, LDF scanning is feasible in patients for whom standard scans cannot be obtained. In a review of pediatric DXA examinations performed on orthopedic patients, only LDF scans could be obtained in 21 % of children. Hip, spine, and whole body assessments could not be performed in these patients due to contractures or metal instrumentation [15]. Pediatric normative data are available for the LDF scan [16], facilitating estimation of Z-scores and interpretation of the results.

Despite its widespread use, DXA has several major limitations that particularly affect bone measurements in children and adolescents. First, because it is a two-dimensional projection technique, DXA cannot account for the dimensions of the bone in the direction of the x-ray beams. Consequently, larger bones produce higher aBMD measurements even if they do not have higher volumetric density. Various corrections have been proposed to account for this size bias. Unfortunately, these corrections do not work as well in children as in adults, probably because of the osseous changes that occur during growth [17]. To account for the size dependence of DXA, the ISCD recommends that, in addition to chronological age, a measure of growth, such as height or height-age (the age at which a child's height is the median height-for-age), be taken into account when comparing an individual child to reference data. However, this usually does not completely remove age or height bias [18]. Height-for-age percentiles or Z-scores may provide the best adjustment [18].

The second major limitation of DXA is that it assumes that soft tissue adjacent to bone and soft tissue overlying bone has the same attenuation. Because fat has significantly lower attenuation than other soft tissues, which are considered "lean," the assumption of homogeneous soft tissue attenuation breaks down when the soft tissue overlying and adjacent to bone contain different proportions of fat. The resulting errors in aBMD can be up to 15 % in adults [19] and 18 % in adolescents, with an average error of 7 % in a large cohort of adolescents and young adults ages 16–25 years [20]. Errors due to soft tissue artifacts may be particularly problematic in overweight or obese individuals and in those who undergo large changes in weight and body composition [21].

A third major limitation of DXA is inclusion of the posterior elements in anterior-posterior imaging of the lumbar spine. Since DXA is a projection technique, the bone measured by DXA includes all bone along the beam path. This includes the cortical and cancellous compartments of the vertebral body, as well as the posterior elements. Although the posterior elements contribute little to vertebral fracture resistance, they add a significant volume of cortical bone, greatly increasing the BMC and aBMD measured by DXA. In fact, the posterior elements contribute approximately half of the total vertebral BMC in children [22]. The percentage of BMC contributed by the posterior elements increases during development but stabilizes after sexual maturity [22]. Therefore, the posterior elements should be considered when measuring DXA aBMD of the lumbar spine in growing children. They are of less concern in older adolescents and young adults.

Finally, DXA measurements are repeatable when acquired on the same machine using the same software but may differ when with different densitometers or software. Discrepancy occurs when manufacturers implement the basic DXA concepts differently. To account for these differences, "universal" measures have been proposed [23]. Unfortunately, these methods have not been widely adopted and are seldom practiced. However, despite its lack of accuracy, DXA is reasonably precise. The short-term in vivo precision of DXA measurements is 0.8–2.5 % in children and 1.5–2.5 % in infants [24, 25]. For longitudinal evaluations, patients should be measured on the same densitometer using the same software. However, care should be exercised in interpreting results since measurements may be influenced by bone morphology or growth.

3 Quantitative Computed Tomography (QCT)

QCT is a three-dimensional imaging technique that allows for segmentation of cortical and trabecular bone regions and separate assessments of bone density, size, and geometry. Unlike DXA, QCT measurements are largely unaffected by soft tissue artifacts. However, QCT is expensive and uses ionizing radiation. QCT assessments of bone mass are mostly used in research but are sometimes performed clinically.

QCT bone measurements are obtained with a standard clinical computed tomography (CT) scanner. X-rays pass through the body in different directions, usually in a spiral or helical pattern, and attenuation is measured for each x-ray transmission. Since each voxel in the region of interest is traversed by multiple x-ray beams traveling in different directions, the data set can be resolved to determine an attenuation value (CT number) for each voxel. The attenuation values are expressed in terms of Hounsfield units (HU), calibrated so water has a value of 0. Cancellous and cortical bones range from 400 to 3,000 HU; fat and air have negative values. In QCT imaging, a bone mineral reference phantom is placed under the patient during scanning (Fig. 26.4). The phantom enables conversion of HU to a hydroxyapatite equivalent density measured in mg/cm^3.

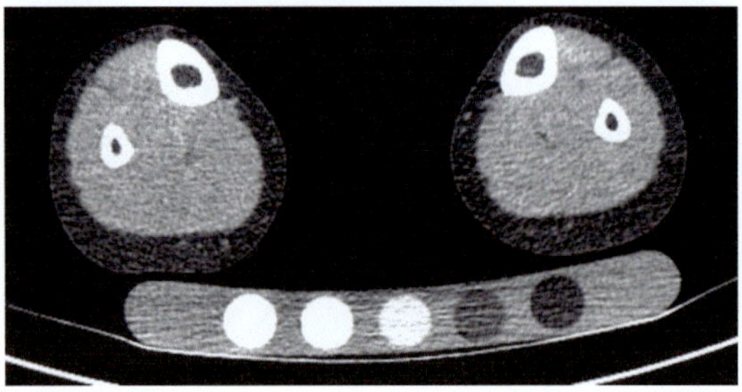

Fig. 26.4 QCT image of a healthy 11-year-old boy at the mid-tibia level showing bone mineral reference phantom. The phantom allows for quantification of hydroxyapatite equivalent volumetric bone mineral density

QCT measurements of cortical bone density represent the bone's material density as long as the cortex is sufficiently thick to avoid volume averaging errors (>2.0–2.5 mm) [26]. The CT value of cortical bone depends primarily on the calcified bone volume fraction because bone mineral has a very high attenuation coefficient.

In cancellous bone, the trabeculae are small relative to the size of the voxel. QCT values therefore reflect not only the amount of mineralized bone and osteoid but also the amount of marrow in each voxel [27]. On average, the CT values of cortical bone are eight times higher than those of cancellous bone. This reflects the porous nature of cancellous bone, not a difference in bone material.

In addition to measures of cortical and cancellous bone density, QCT can be used to obtain measures of three-dimensional bone geometry.

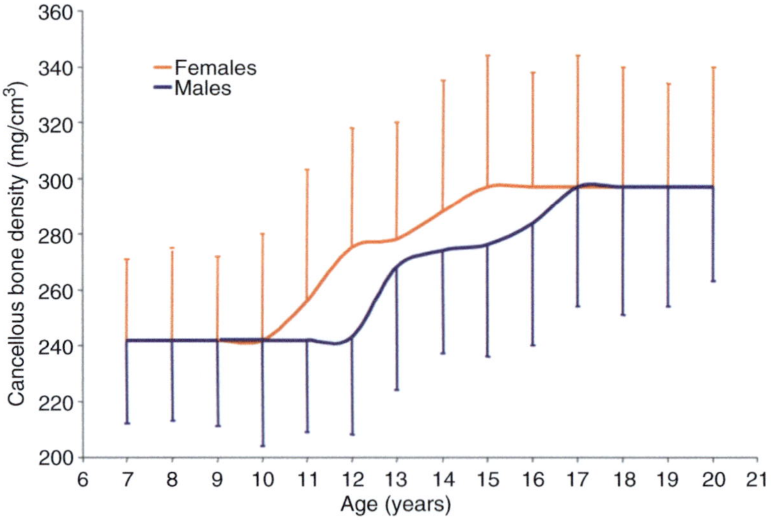

Fig. 26.5 Changes in vertebral cancellous bone density during growth. Density does not begin increasing until approximately age 10 years in females and age 12 years in males. Density reaches its peak by age 15 years in females and age 17 years in males (Reprinted with permission from Gilsanz et al. [49])

Cross-sectional area and volume are often measured, along with cortical bone area for diaphyseal sites. The cross-sectional images can also determine structural parameters that reflect bone stiffness and strength such as moments of inertia, section modulus, and stress-strain index. The coefficients of variation for QCT measurements of bone density and geometry are between 1 and 2 %.

QCT measures of volumetric cancellous bone density in the lumbar vertebrae increase primarily during puberty and peak by late adolescence (Fig. 26.5) indicating that puberty is the critical period for building cancellous bone mass. In contrast, long bones increase in diameter throughout life due to the ongoing processes of periosteal apposition and endosteal resorption. This difference in growth patterns may contribute to the increasing susceptibility of cancellous sites such as the hip and spine to fracture with aging.

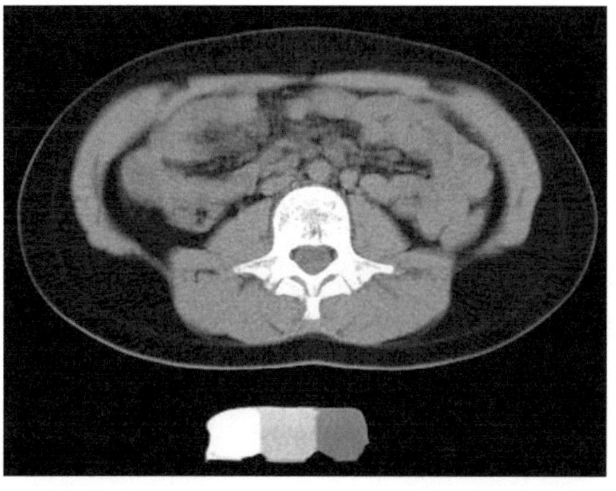

Fig. 26.6 QCT image of the L3 vertebra in an ambulatory 10-year-old girl with diplegic cerebral palsy

Most clinical assessments of bone using QCT evaluate a localized region such as a slice through the middle of the vertebral body or femur (Fig. 26.6). Volumetric QCT can be performed but is not widely used due to radiation concerns. Clinical studies in adults have used volumetric QCT to examine the hip and spine [28], but this has not been done in children. However, volumetric QCT has been used in children at peripheral sites such as the tibia and radius (Fig. 26.7) where relatively low radiation exposure is possible.

The main advantage of volumetric QCT is that it allows for assessment of entire structures. Examining a single slice may miss the weakest and most vulnerable section of the bone. In addition, certain regions such as the metaphyses of long bones are not uniform, making measurement at a single site problematic. In the proximal tibial metaphysis, for example, cancellous bone

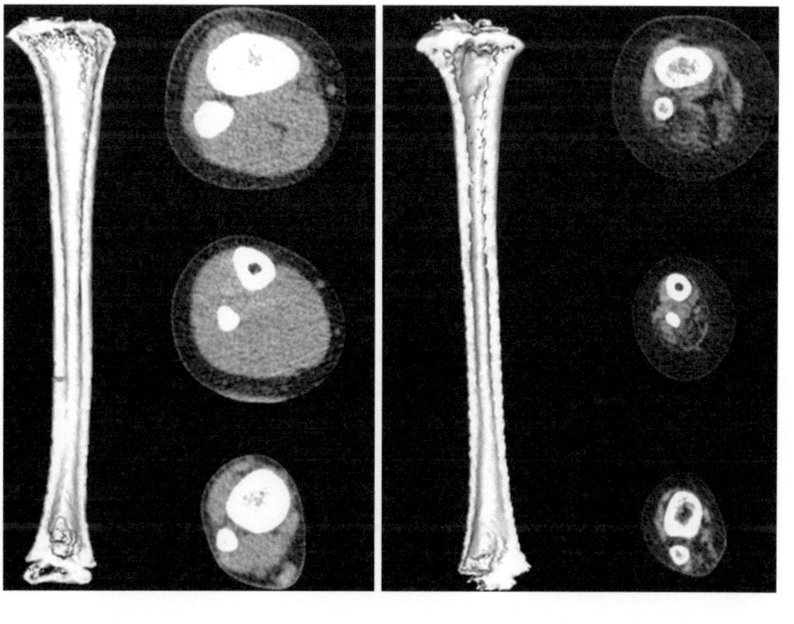

Fig. 26.7 Volumetric QCT images of the tibia in a healthy 6-year-old boy (*left*) and a 6-year-old boy with lumbar level myelomeningocele (*right*). The child with myelomeningocele has a smaller bone with thinner cortices. Muscle volume and density are also greatly reduced in the child with myelomeningocele

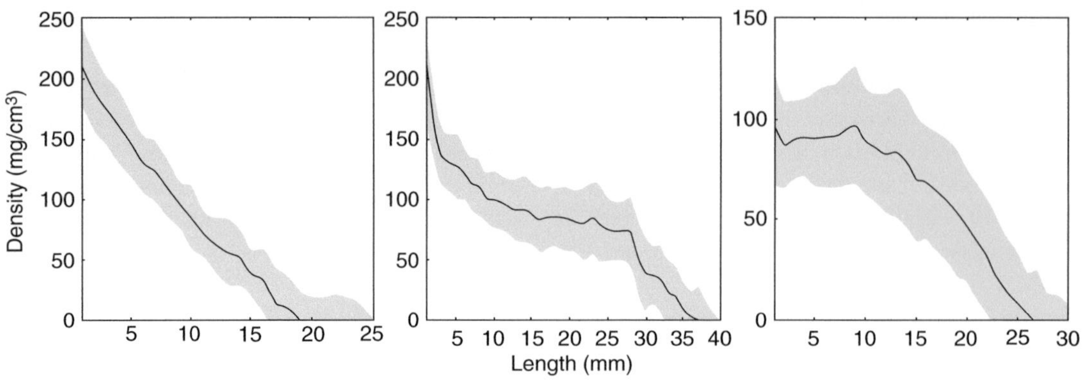

Fig. 26.8 Change in cancellous bone density along the length of the metaphysis in three ambulatory children with cerebral palsy (Reprinted with permission from Lee et al. [29])

density changes by an average of 7 mg/cm^3 or 17 % for each millimeter along the length of the metaphysis [29] (Fig. 26.8). A small change in slice location therefore results in a large change in measured density. In longitudinal studies, even if the site of measurement can be replicated exactly, changes in morphology due to growth make it difficult to compare measurements.

Radiation exposure is QCT's main drawback. For QCT measurements of bone, the radiation exposure can be as low as 1.5 mSv localized to the region of interest, with a total body equivalent dose of approximately 40–90 μSv including the localizer images [30, 31]. This is similar to the amount of radiation exposure that occurs during a round-trip flight across North America [30, 31] and much lower than the radiation associated with other CT imaging procedures.

4 Peripheral Quantitative Computed Tomography (pQCT)

PQCT is similar to QCT except that it uses scanners specifically designed to deliver doses of radiation that are generally less than 5 mSv. This is comparable to DXA and much lower than conventional CT [32]. In addition to lower radiation exposure, pQCT scanners are smaller, more portable, and less expensive. The main limitation of pQCT is that it is only used for peripheral sites. PQCT is most commonly used to measure the distal radius and tibia (Fig. 26.9), although some scanners can image the pediatric femur and humerus. The primary measurements obtained are the same as for QCT, i.e., the density and cross-sectional properties of trabecular and cortical bone.

The innovation of high-resolution scanners (high-resolution peripheral quantitative computed tomography, or HR-pQCT) has allowed for volumetric pQCT imaging. The improved resolution allows for estimation of common bone architectural parameters such as trabecular connectivity, anisotropy, structure model index (characterizing rod- or platelike trabecular shape), and cortical porosity [32]. Reproducibility of HR-pQCT measures is quite high with coefficients of variation of less than 1 % for densities and 4–5 % for architectural parameters [28]. However, positioning the scan region must be done carefully, particularly in growing children and adolescents whose anatomy and growth plate location change [33]. Currently, scans can cover only a 9 mm section and require a scan time of approximately 3 min, during which movement must be minimized since HR-pQCT is susceptible to motion artifacts. In addition, HR-pQCT is limited to distal peripheral sites; even diaphyseal sites of the radius and tibia cannot be imaged [32]. While pQCT and HR-pQCT are promising clinical tools, they are currently used primarily for research.

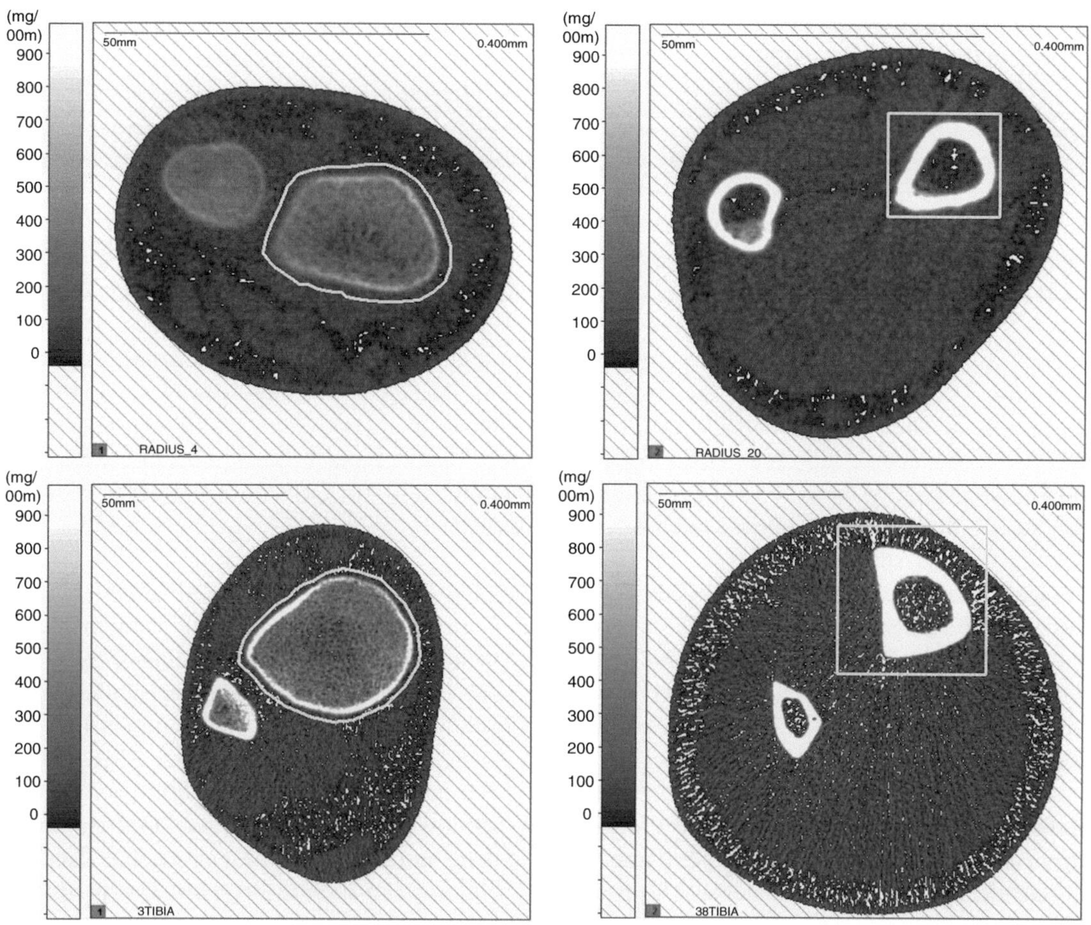

Fig. 26.9 pQCT images of the radius (*top*) and tibia (*bottom*) metaphysis (*left*) and diaphysis (*right*) (Courtesy of Dr. Babette Zemel)

5 Magnetic Resonance Imaging (MRI)

Like pQCT, MRI allows volumetric assessment of bone. The main advantage of MRI is lack of ionizing radiation. Disadvantages include lower spatial resolution than pQCT and the inability to quantify bone mass or density. Spatial resolution is on the order of trabecular dimensions (150–300 μm in-plane with a section thickness of 0.3–1 mm), resulting in significant partial volume effects [28]. As with HR-pQCT, high-resolution MRI (HR-MRI) has primarily been used to analyze trabecular bone architecture at peripheral locations, such as the distal radius, distal tibia, phalanges, and calcaneus [34, 35]. Initial studies suggest that measurements using specialized coils, optimized pulse sequences, and high-strength magnets may also be feasible at more proximal sites such as the proximal femur [35].

Using MRI to obtain quantitative measures of bone is still in the development phase. It is costly, technically difficult, and requires long scan times and sophisticated post-processing. It is susceptible to technical artifacts such as overestimation of trabecular thickness and bone volume fraction [36, 37]. Although HR-MRI measures are reasonably reproducible with coefficients of variation of 2–10 % [35, 38], there are large discrepancies between HR-MRI measures of trabecular architecture and morphometric parameters derived from HR-pQCT [36]. Further improvements are needed before HR-MRI is useful in a clinical setting.

6 Quantitative Ultrasound (QUS)

QUS offers low cost, portability, ease of use, and lack of ionizing radiation. It is widely used in Europe but has not been readily adopted in the United States. The calcaneus is the most common measurement site, although QUS has also been used for the patella, tibia, and phalanges.

QUS measures the transmission properties of sound waves. QUS machines are generally designed with fixed transducers for a specific measurement site. Consequently, they do not readily accommodate different sized patients. Since commercial systems are usually configured for adults, they must be adapted with smaller transducers and special footpads or calipers to study children. A coupling medium, such as rubber pads or sonographic gel, is needed between the ultrasound transducers and the patient's body. The temperature of the coupling medium must be kept constant to avoid temperature-associated errors in the ultrasound measurements.

QUS does not directly measure bone mass. Rather, it measures bone "quality," which depends on bone density, bone size, and trabecular architecture [39]. In the calcaneus, for example, QUS measurements primarily reflect the number, thickness, mineral content, and spatial arrangement of the trabeculae. QUS values may vary by as much as 50 % depending on the size of the bone [40] and the principal orientation of the trabeculae [27]. In addition to being influenced by bone properties, QUS measurements are also influenced by the composition of the cancellous bone and the surrounding soft tissues [27].

QUS measures speed of sound (SOS, measured in m/s) and broadband ultrasound attenuation (BUA, measured in dB/MHz). SOS is the distance between transducers divided by the wave transit time. SOS decreases with lower-density bone. BUA is the slope of attenuation versus the frequency curve in the 200–600 kHz range, where the curve is linear. BUA increases in lower-density bone. BUA and SOS are sometimes combined into a single parameter referred to as "stiffness" or Quantitative Ultrasound Index (QUI) [41].

In children, SOS and BUA values generally correlate with age and pubertal stage but exhibit considerable variability [39, 42–44]. Different measurement sites give very different values [40]. During puberty, values increase at different rates in boys and girls [44]; SOS is higher in girls between the ages of 9 and 15 years [39].

Reported SOS intra-observer variations for children range from 0.5 to 1.2 % [42, 43] and from 2 to 5 % for BUA [43, 44]. Unfortunately, numerous studies in adults and children have found that QUS and measurements using other methods do not correlate [27, 43, 44]. Therefore, QUS cannot replace other modalities, and the interpretation of QUS measurements remains unclear.

Conclusion

Currently, the ability to obtain bone measurements exceeds our understanding of the clinical implications of these measurements in children. In adults, a clear relationship has been established between DXA BMD values and fracture risk through multiple large, prospective, controlled studies [45]. However, there is relatively little comparable data for children and adolescents. Furthermore, different measurement techniques yield conflicting information about pediatric bone. For example, children are classified as having low bone mass more often when assessed by DXA than when evaluated with QCT [46].

Case-controlled studies examining the relationship between bone density and fracture incidence in children have yielded conflicting results [2, 3, 47]. A recent meta-analysis concluded that there is probably an association between bone density and fractures in children [4]. However, studies have found that other factors, such as bone cross-sectional area or body weight, are more important in identifying children at risk for fractures [2, 3]. Prospective studies have found a significant relationship between DXA bone measures and fractures in children [11, 12], although Caucasian boys paradoxically exhibit higher fracture risk with higher DXA scores [11].

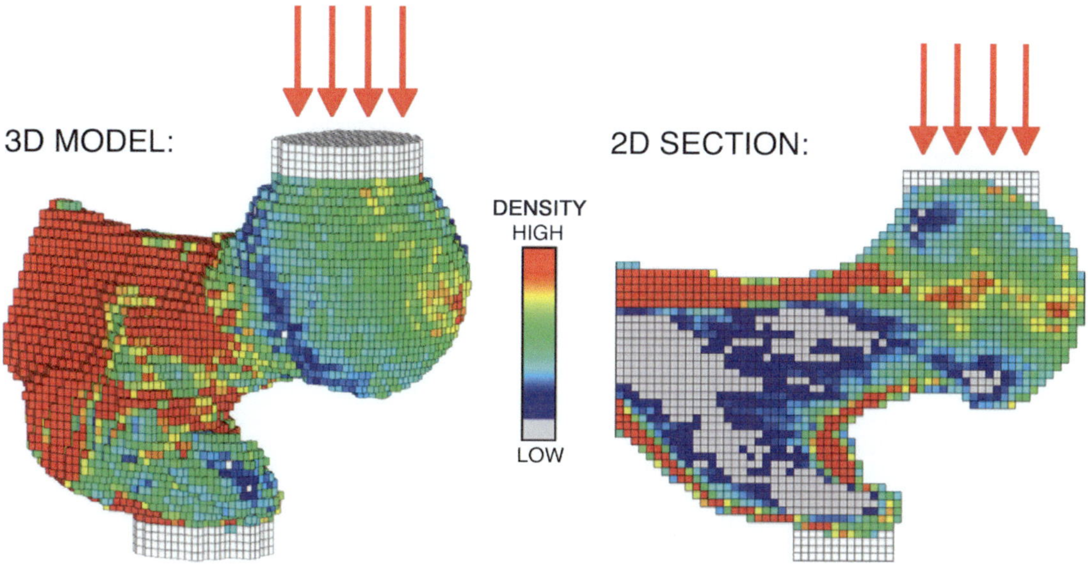

Fig. 26.10 Finite element model of the proximal femur with applied loading simulating a sideways fall. The geometry and material properties of the model were derived from clinical CT scans. The color coding indicates the material strength of each element determined based on the calibrated QCT density (Reprinted from Keaveny et al. [50])

Studies correlating childhood bone density with eventual osteoporosis and fracture risk are not yet available. However, longitudinal QCT measurements of bone density and cross-sectional area of the vertebrae and femurs have shown that measures in early puberty predict values at sexual maturity [9]. Children in the lowest quartile at the start of puberty generally remain in the lowest quartile post puberty, suggesting that they will have low peak values and be at increased risk for osteoporosis as they age. DXA values also track during childhood and adolescence [8]. Since bone measures appear to track during peak bone mass development, it is likely that they will track throughout the entire life span.

Improvements in technology and methodology will facilitate faster imaging, better image resolution, and more accurate estimation of bone measures including mass, quality, and strength. Computer modeling techniques, such as finite element analysis, may better model the mechanical response of bones to loading (Fig. 26.10), enabling prediction of whether a bone will fail under specific loading conditions.

References

1. NIH Consensus Development Panel on Osteoporosis Prevention. Osteoporosis prevention, diagnosis, and therapy. JAMA. 2001;285(6):785–95. PubMed PMID: 11176917, Epub 2001/02/15. eng.
2. Goulding A, Jones IE, Taylor RW, Williams SM, Manning PJ. Bone mineral density and body composition in boys with distal forearm fractures: a dual-energy x-ray absorptiometry study. J Pediatr. 2001;139(4):509–15. PubMed PMID: 11598596, Epub 2001/10/13. eng.
3. Skaggs DL, Loro ML, Pitukcheewanont P, Tolo V, Gilsanz V. Increased body weight and decreased radial cross-sectional dimensions in girls with forearm fractures. J Bone Miner Res. 2001;16(7):1337–42. PubMed PMID: 11450710.
4. Clark EM, Tobias JH, Ness AR. Association between bone density and fractures in children: a systematic review and meta-analysis. Pediatrics. 2006;117(2): e291–7. PubMed PMID: 16452336, Pubmed Central PMCID: 2742730, Epub 2006/02/03. eng.
5. Goulding A, Grant AM, Williams SM. Bone and body composition of children and adolescents with repeated forearm fractures. J Bone Miner Res. 2005;20(12): 2090–6. PubMed PMID: 16294262, Epub 2005/11/19. eng.
6. Ferrari S, Rizzoli R, Slosman D, Bonjour JP. Familial resemblance for bone mineral mass is expressed before puberty. J Clin Endocrinol Metab. 1998;83: 358–61.

7. Ferrari S, Rizzoli R, Chevalley T, Slosman D, Eisman JA, Bonjour JP. Vitamin-D-receptor-gene polymorphisms and change in lumbar-spine bone mineral density. Lancet. 1995;345:423–4.
8. Kalkwarf HJ, Gilsanz V, Lappe JM, Oberfield S, Shepherd JA, Hangartner TN, et al. Tracking of bone mass and density during childhood and adolescence. J Clin Endocrinol Metab. 2010;95(4):1690–8. PubMed PMID: 20194709, Epub 2010/03/03. eng.
9. Loro ML, Sayre J, Roe TF, Goran MI, Kaufman FR, Gilsanz V. Early identification of children predisposed to low peak bone mass and osteoporosis later in life. J Clin Endocrinol Metab. 2000;85(10):3908–18. PubMed PMID: 11061556.
10. Zemel BS, Kalkwarf HJ, Gilsanz V, Lappe JM, Oberfield S, Shepherd JA, et al. Revised reference curves for bone mineral content and areal bone mineral density according to age and sex for black and non-black children: results of the bone mineral density in childhood study. J Clin Endocrinol Metab. 2011;96(10):3160–9. PubMed PMID: 21917867, Epub 2011/09/16. eng.
11. Wren TA, Shepherd JA, Kalkwarf HJ, Zemel BS, Lappe JM, Oberfield S, et al. Racial disparity in fracture risk between white and nonwhite children in the United States. J Pediatr. 2012;161(6):1035–40 e2. PubMed PMID: 22974572. Pubmed Central PMCID: 3504618. Epub 2012/09/15. eng.
12. Clark EM, Ness AR, Bishop NJ, Tobias JH. Association between bone mass and fractures in children: a prospective cohort study. J Bone Miner Res. 2006;21(9):1489–95. PubMed PMID: 16939408, Pubmed Central PMCID: 2742714, Epub 2006/08/31. eng.
13. Harcke HT, Taylor A, Bachrach S, Miller F, Henderson RC. Lateral femoral scan: an alternative method for assessing bone mineral density in children with cerebral palsy. Pediatr Radiol. 1998;28(4):241–6. PubMed PMID: 9545479, Epub 1998/06/20. eng.
14. Henderson RC, Berglund LM, May R, Zemel BS, Grossberg RI, Johnson J, et al. The relationship between fractures and DXA measures of BMD in the distal femur of children and adolescents with cerebral palsy or muscular dystrophy. J Bone Miner Res. 2010;25(3):520–6. PubMed PMID: 19821773, Pubmed Central PMCID: 3153393, Epub 2009/10/14. eng.
15. Szalay EA, Harriman D. Adapting pediatric DXA scanning to clinical orthopaedics. J Pediatr Orthop. 2006;26(5):686–90. PubMed PMID: 16932112. Epub 2006/08/26. eng.
16. Zemel BS, Stallings VA, Leonard MB, Paulhamus DR, Kecskemethy HH, Harcke HT, et al. Revised pediatric reference data for the lateral distal femur measured by Hologic discovery/Delphi dual-energy X-ray absorptiometry. J Clin Densitom. 2009;12(2):207–18. PubMed PMID: 19321369. Epub 2009/03/27. eng.
17. Wren TA, Liu X, Pitukcheewanont P, Gilsanz V. Bone acquisition in healthy children and adolescents: comparisons of dual-energy x-ray absorptiometry and computed tomography measures. J Clin Endocrinol Metab. 2005;90(4):1925–8. PubMed PMID: 1563 4720.
18. Zemel BS, Leonard MB, Kelly A, Lappe JM, Gilsanz V, Oberfield S, et al. Height adjustment in assessing dual energy x-ray absorptiometry measurements of bone mass and density in children. J Clin Endocrinol Metab. 2010;95(3):1265–73. PubMed PMID: 20103654, Pubmed Central PMCID: 2841534, Epub 2010/01/28. eng.
19. Tothill P, Pye DW. Errors due to non-uniform distribution of fat in dual X-ray absorptiometry of the lumbar spine. Br J Radiol. 1992;65(777):807–13. PubMed PMID: 1393420.
20. Lee DC. Optimizations in the assessment of pediatric bone [Dissertation]. Los Angeles: University of Southern California; 2009 [updated May 2009; cited Doctor of Philosophy].
21. Tothill P, Hannan WJ, Cowen S, Freeman CP. Anomalies in the measurement of changes in total-body bone mineral by dual-energy X-ray absorptiometry during weight change. J Bone Miner Res. 1997;12(11):1908–21. PubMed PMID: 9383696, Epub 1998/02/07. eng.
22. Lee DC, Campbell PP, Gilsanz V, Wren TA. Contribution of the vertebral posterior elements in anterior-posterior DXA spine scans in young subjects. J Bone Miner Res. 2009;24(8):1398–403. PubMed PMID: 19257831, Epub 2009/03/05. eng.
23. Hui SL, Gao S, Zhou XH, Johnston Jr CC, Lu Y, Gluer CC, et al. Universal standardization of bone density measurements: a method with optimal properties for calibration among several instruments. J Bone Miner Res. 1997;12(9):1463–70. PubMed PMID: 9286763.
24. Zanchetta JR, Plotkin H, Alvarez Filgueira ML. Bone mass in children: normative values for the 2–20-year-old population. Bone. 1995;16(4 Suppl):393S–9. PubMed PMID: 7626329.
25. Koo WW, Massom LR, Walters J. Validation of accuracy and precision of dual energy X-ray absorptiometry for infants. J Bone Miner Res. 1995;10(7):1111–5. PubMed PMID: 7484287.
26. Hangartner TN, Gilsanz V. Evaluation of cortical bone by computed tomography. J Bone Miner Res. 1996;11(10):1518–25. PubMed PMID: 8889852.
27. Genant HK, Engelke K, Fuerst T, Gluer CC, Grampp S, Harris ST, et al. Noninvasive assessment of bone mineral and structure: state of the art. J Bone Miner Res. 1996;11(6):707–30. PubMed PMID: 8725168.
28. Link TM. Osteoporosis imaging: state of the art and advanced imaging. Radiology. 2012;263(1):3–17. PubMed PMID: 22438439, Pubmed Central PMCID: 3309802, Epub 2012/03/23. eng.
29. Lee DC, Gilsanz V, Wren TA. Limitations of peripheral quantitative computed tomography metaphyseal bone density measurements. J Clin Endocrinol Metab. 2007;92(11):4248–53. PubMed PMID: 17684050, Epub 2007/08/09. eng.

30. Kalender WA. Effective dose values in bone mineral measurements by photon absorptiometry and computed tomography. Osteoporos Int. 1992;2(2):82–7. PubMed PMID: 1536984.
31. Cann CE. Why, when and how to measure bone mass: a guide for the beginning user. In: Frey GD, Yester MV, editors. Expanding the role of medical physics in nuclear medicine. Washington DC: American Physics Institute; 1991. p. 250–79.
32. Krug R, Burghardt AJ, Majumdar S, Link TM. High-resolution imaging techniques for the assessment of osteoporosis. Radiol Clin North Am. 2010;48(3):601–21. PubMed PMID: 20609895, Pubmed Central PMCID: 2901255, Epub 2010/07/09. eng.
33. Burrows M, Liu D, McKay H. High-resolution peripheral QCT imaging of bone micro-structure in adolescents. Osteoporos Int. 2010;21(3):515–20. PubMed PMID: 19322507, Epub 2009/03/27. eng.
34. Link TM, Majumdar S, Grampp S, Guglielmi G, van Kuijk C, Imhof H, et al. Imaging of trabecular bone structure in osteoporosis. Eur Radiol. 1999;9(9):1781–8. PubMed PMID: 10602950.
35. Krug R, Banerjee S, Han ET, Newitt DC, Link TM, Majumdar S. Feasibility of in vivo structural analysis of high-resolution magnetic resonance images of the proximal femur. Osteoporos Int. 2005;16(11):1307–14. PubMed PMID: 15999292.
36. Kazakia GJ, Hyun B, Burghardt AJ, Krug R, Newitt DC, de Papp AE, et al. In vivo determination of bone structure in postmenopausal women: a comparison of HR-pQCT and high-field MR imaging. J Bone Miner Res. 2008;23(4):463–74. PubMed PMID: 18052756. Epub 2007/12/07. eng.
37. Phan CM, Matsuura M, Bauer JS, Dunn TC, Newitt D, Lochmueller EM, et al. Trabecular bone structure of the calcaneus: comparison of MR imaging at 3.0 and 1.5 T with micro-CT as the standard of reference. Radiology. 2006;239(2):488–96.
38. Gomberg BR, Wehrli FW, Vasilic B, Weening RH, Saha PK, Song HK, et al. Reproducibility and error sources of micro MRI-based trabecular bone structural parameters of the distal radius and tibia. Bone. 2004;35(1):266–76. PubMed PMID: 15207767.
39. Baroncelli GI, Federico G, Bertelloni S, de Terlizzi F, Cadossi R, Saggese G. Bone quality assessment by quantitative ultrasound of proximal phalanxes of the hand in healthy subjects aged 3–21 years. Pediatr Res. 2001;49(5):713–8. PubMed PMID: 11328957.
40. Fricke O, Tutlewski B, Schwahn B, Schoenau E. Speed of sound: relation to geometric characteristics of bone in children, adolescents, and adults. J Pediatr. 2005;146(6):764–8. PubMed PMID: 1597 3315.
41. Fogelman I, Blake GM. Different approaches to bone densitometry. J Nucl Med. 2000;41(12):2015–25. PubMed PMID: 11138687.
42. Schonau E, Radermacher A, Wentzlik U, Klein K, Michalk D. The determination of ultrasound velocity in the os calcis, thumb and patella during childhood. Eur J Pediatr. 1994;153(4):252–6. PubMed PMID: 8194557.
43. Jaworski M, Lebiedowski M, Lorenc RS, Trempe J. Ultrasound bone measurement in pediatric subjects. Calcif Tissue Int. 1995;56(5):368–71. PubMed PMID: 7621343.
44. Mughal MZ, Langton CM, Utretch G, Morrison J, Specker BL. Comparison between broad-band ultrasound attenuation of the calcaneum and total body bone mineral density in children. Acta Paediatr. 1996;85(6):663–5. PubMed PMID: 8816199.
45. Johnell O, Kanis JA, Oden A, Johansson H, De Laet C, Delmas P, et al. Predictive value of BMD for hip and other fractures. J Bone Miner Res. 2005;20(7):1185–94. PubMed PMID: 15940371.
46. Wren TA, Liu X, Pitukcheewanont P, Gilsanz V. Bone densitometry in pediatric populations: discrepancies in the diagnosis of osteoporosis by DXA and CT. J Pediatr. 2005;146:776–9.
47. Ma DQ, Jones G. Clinical risk factors but not bone density are associated with prevalent fractures in prepubertal children. J Paediatr Child Health. 2002;38(5):497–500. PubMed PMID: 12354268.
48. Kovanlikaya A, Loro ML, Hangartner TN, et al. Osteopenia in children: CT assessment. Radiology. 1996;198:781–4.
49. Gilsanz V, Perez FJ, Campbell PP, Dorey FJ, Lee DC, Wren TA. Quantitative CT reference values for vertebral trabecular bone density in children and young adults. Radiology. 2009;250(1):222–7.
50. Keaveny TM, McClung MR, Wan X, Kopperdahl DL, Mitlak BH, Krohn K. Femoral strength in osteoporotic women treated with teriparatide or alendronate. Bone. 2012;50(1):165–70.

Orthopedic Procedures

27

Brian M. Haus and Debra Templeton Popejoy

Contents

B.M. Haus, MD (✉) • D.T. Popejoy, MD
Department of Orthopaedic Surgery,
UC Davis Children's Hospital and Shriners Hospital for Children Northern California,
2425 Stockton Blvd, Sacramento, CA 95817, USA
e-mail: brihaus@gmail.com; dpopejoy@shrinenet.org

Abstract

A wide variety of surgical procedures may be employed to treat pediatric orthopedic problems. This chapter presents some of the more common procedures, focusing on those involving the spine, lower extremities, and foot. The procedures address issues of

R. Stein-Wexler et al. (eds.), *Pediatric Orthopedic Imaging*,
DOI 10.1007/978-3-642-45381-6_27, © Springer-Verlag Berlin Heidelberg 2015

alignment (e.g., scoliosis, extremity angulation or asymmetry, and foot deformities), correct sequelae of hip disorders by redirecting the femoral head or by increasing acetabular coverage, or compensate for—or take advantage of—the potential for continued skeletal growth.

Radiologists must be familiar with the radiographic appearance of orthopedic procedures and must also be able to recognize their many possible complications. However, several factors combine to challenge mastery of this information. First, there are numerous different orthopedic procedures, and new ones are constantly being developed. In addition, there are innumerable innovations and alterations of these basic procedures. Finally, the nomenclature describing these procedures is confusing, in part due to widespread use of eponyms (naming a procedure or piece of hardware after a person) instead of more descriptive, generic terms.

Many surgical procedures have been devised to ameliorate problems specific to, and adversely affected by, growth in children. The following descriptions, grouped anatomically, are limited to those procedures that are generally performed only in children, are in common use, and present observable radiographic alterations. Soft tissue procedures often accompany osseous procedures, but these are not commonly visible on radiographs (and hardware may limit satisfactory use of computed tomography (CT) and magnetic resonance imaging (MRI)).

Both local customs and evolution of surgical practice have led to modifications of many basic techniques, with the changes often indicated by a new or altered eponym. The procedures described in this chapter reflect the practices of the surgical staff at Shriners Hospital for Children, Northern California, and the University of California, Davis. Salient points have been chosen to highlight alterations that should be observed postoperatively. Pertinent complications related to specific surgical procedures are also discussed.

1 Spine

1.1 General Considerations

Surgical fusion is a definitive procedure designed to prevent progressive deformity in developmental conditions such as scoliosis and/or kyphosis or to stabilize the spinal column in the setting of instability caused by trauma or tumors.

In most cases, spinal fusion is performed from a posterior approach, and instrumentation is employed (posterior spinal fusion with instrumentation (PSFI)) to facilitate deformity correction and to stabilize the spine. Anterior fusion is used less frequently, sometimes to augment PSFI in cases of posterior element dysplasia or in patients with severe, rigid deformities. Anterior fusion alone may also be used in certain patterns of isolated idiopathic lumbar curves.

Although spinal fusion is an effective surgery in older children and adolescents, it cannot be performed in younger patients with spinal deformity because it halts linear growth of the spinal column and can lead to thoracic insufficiency. For this reason, temporizing techniques are employed, which stabilize the spine and which also expand during growth. Growing rods and vertical expandable prosthetic titanium rib (VEPTR) devices are utilized in young children with significant spinal deformity and large growth potential until they can have spinal fusion near or upon reaching skeletal maturity. At skeletal maturity, these patients may also require thoracoplasty to remove posterior rib elements and facilitate correction of thoracic wall deformity.

Spinal instrumentation alone is not enough to stabilize the spine, and the long-term success of surgery depends upon the ultimate bony fusion of the spinal column into a corrected position. To achieve fusion, laminae are decorticated and cartilage is resected from the facets; bone graft is then interpositioned to facilitate fusion along the spinal column.

If the spine fails to fuse postoperatively, spinal curvature may recur and/or hardware may fail. Late breakage or loosening of spine implants suggests the presence of a pseudarthrosis. Bone graft and fusion mass are usually visible along the concavity of the curve on posteroanterior images, but they are often better visualized on lateral and oblique views. CT may be helpful as well.

Complications include hardware failure (see Fig. 3.69), pseudarthrosis, malposition of hardware, superior mesenteric artery (SMA) syndrome (attributed to postoperative lengthening and stretching of the mesentery and/or weight loss) (see Fig. 3.68), infection, and neurological compromise.

1.2 Posterior Spinal Fusion with Instrumentation (PSFI) [1] (Figs. 27.1–27.4) (See Also Figs. 3.54, 3.65, and 3.69)

Clinical Application

Idiopathic scoliosis, neuromuscular scoliosis.

Specific Indications

This procedure is used to halt progression of scoliosis, to restore coronal and sagittal balance, and to improve the appearance of chest wall deformity.

Surgical Technique

Hooks are placed around the pedicles or laminae, or pedicle screws are inserted through the pedicles into the vertebral body (Fig. 27.1). Vertical rods are then inserted through this hardware. The posterior spinal elements are decorticated, the facet joints removed, and bone graft applied. For patients with neuromuscular scoliosis, the distal extent of hardware may be embedded in the iliac bones, in order to improve spine stability (Fig. 27.2).

Postoperative Evaluation

Hooks, screws, and rods are visible on the right and left sides of the spine. Bone graft is usually visible primarily on the concave side of the curve.

Complications

Hooks may erode the spine and subsequently pull out (Fig. 27.3). Pullout of pedicle screws is extremely rare. Pedicle screws may be malpositioned, potentially damaging the spinal cord, nerve roots, or soft tissues adjacent to the spine. If pedicle screws are

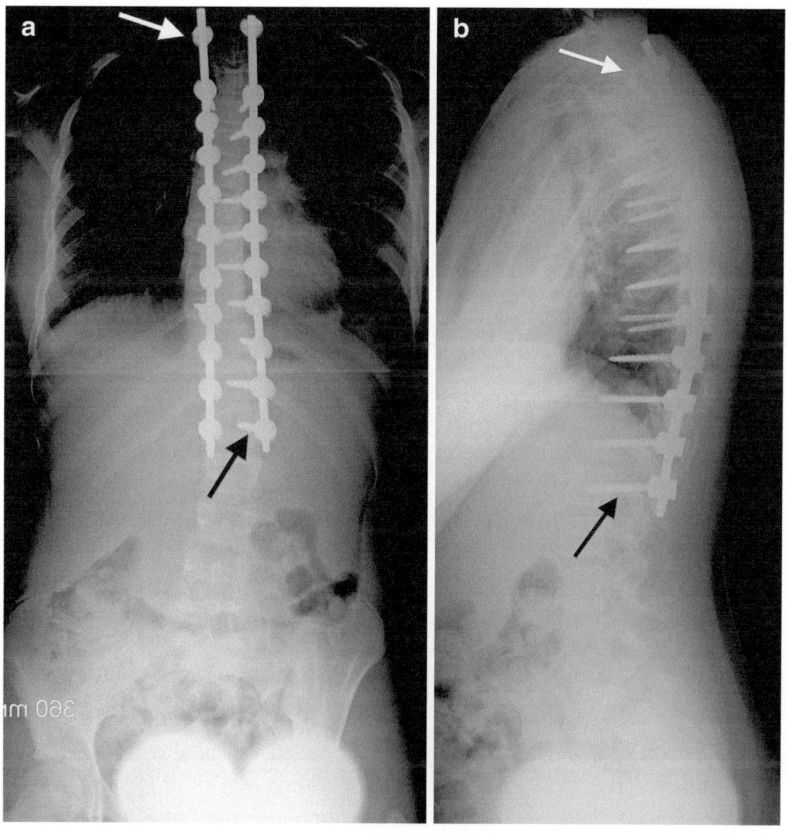

Fig. 27.1 Posterior spinal fusion (PSFI) with instrumentation. (**a**, **b**) There are hooks (*white arrows*) above the laminae of T2, and screws (*black arrows*) have been inserted through the pedicles and then into the vertebral bodies at multiple levels. Vertical rods connect the instrumentation

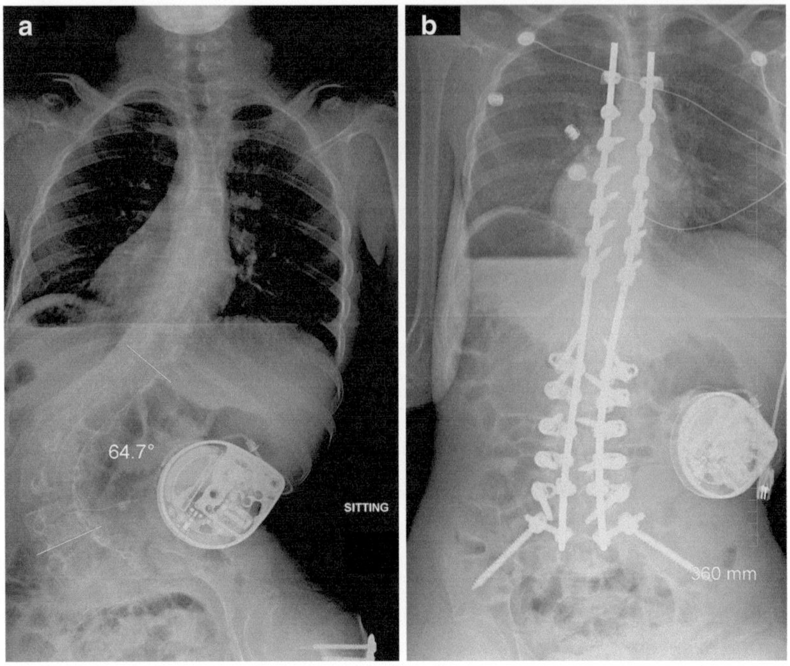

Fig. 27.2 PSFI anchored in iliac bones in patient with cerebral palsy (CP). (**a**) Preoperative image shows a neuromuscular-appearing curve, along with a baclofen pump and hardware from prior femoral varus derotational osteotomy. (**b**) This flexible curve almost straightens with posterior fusion. Hardware is anchored in the iliac bones (Courtesy of Rebecca Stein-Wexler)

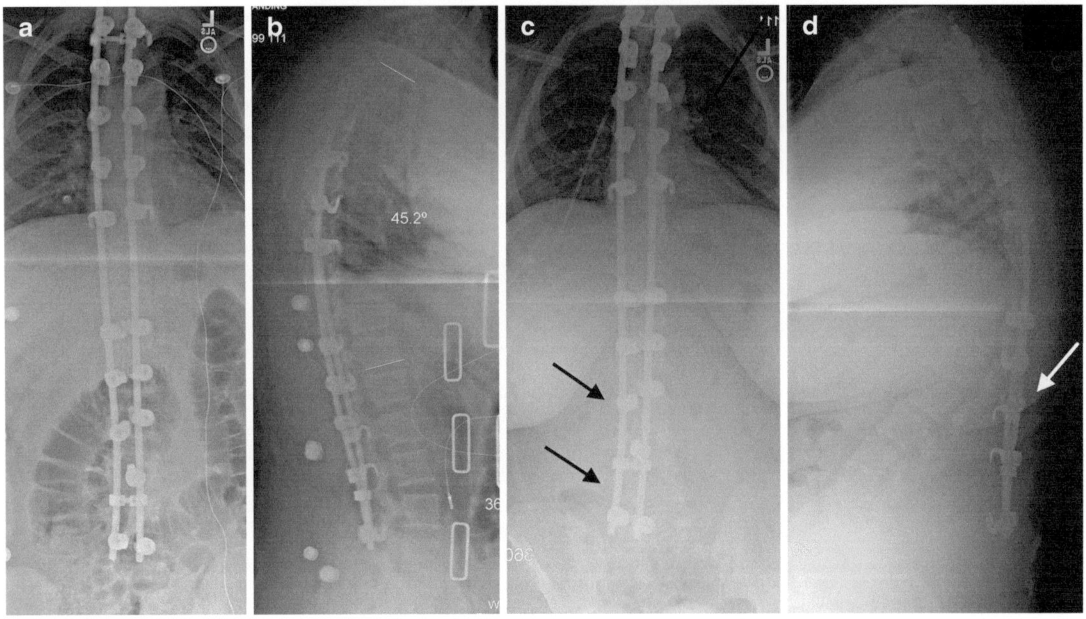

Fig. 27.3 PSFI failure due to pullout of the hooks. (**a**, **b**) Perioperative images demonstrate hooks at multiple levels, with mild wedging of multiple lower thoracic vertebral bodies due to underlying Scheuermann disease. (**c**, **d**) The three distal pairs of hooks have detached from the laminae, and the rods now arc to the right of (*black arrows*) and posterior to (*white arrow*) the lumbar spine (Courtesy of Rebecca Stein-Wexler)

positioned too far to the left, the aorta may be endangered (this is generally seen on the concave side, near the apex). A major increase in scoliosis implies failed fusion. Rod breakage (Fig. 27.4; see also Fig. 3.69) indicates motion, which may signify incomplete fusion or pseudarthrosis.

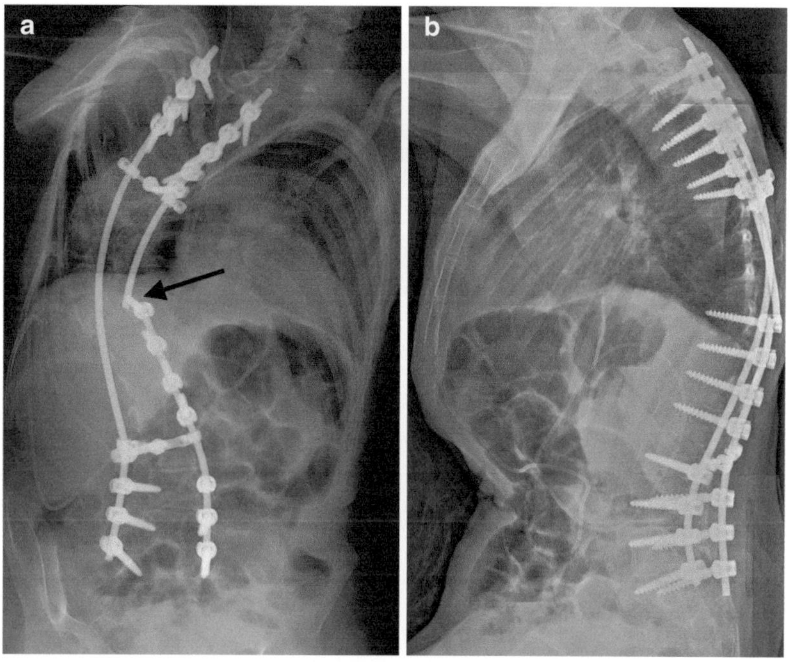

Fig. 27.4 PSFI with rod fracture. (**a**, **b**) The rod on the left has fractured (*black arrow*) just above a pedicle screw (Courtesy of Leslie E. Grissom)

1.3 Growing Rod Technique [2] (Figs. 27.5–27.9)

Clinical Application
Progressive early-onset scoliosis.

Specific Indications
This procedure is employed in young children with progressive deformity that (in general) exceeds 50°, who have failed nonoperative measures. The goal is to postpone definitive spinal fusion in order to allow the child to achieve maximal spinal growth, overall growth of the entire thoracic cavity, and optimal lung maturation.

Surgical Technique
Distal and proximal foundation sites are prepared by exposing the subperiosteal bone. Hooks or screws may be used at either site. Each foundation is composed of four anchors (hooks and/or screws), which are attached to vertical rods (Fig. 27.5). These rods are placed by a solely subcutaneous or subfascial approach. This is important, since premature spine fusion is avoided by not disturbing the remainder of the spine. Rods are connected transversely by a subcutaneous transverse connector. The vertical rods are lengthened at the tandem connector about every 6 months to accommodate growth.

Postoperative Evaluation
Hooks and/or screws are attached to the spine at each foundation site. Elongation of the rods is best appreciated by evaluating the length of the rod distraction gap.

Complications
If the foundation sites are not stable enough to accept corrective loads, hooks and/or screws may dislodge (Fig. 27.6). Pedicle screws and hooks may also pull out during growth. Rod breakage may occur. Screws may loosen and fracture (Figs. 27.7 and 27.8). With this and other procedures, improper alignment of pasted images may give the false impression that rods are fractured (Fig. 27.9). Although infection is a risk with any surgical procedure, the manipulation involved with lengthening increases the likelihood of infection with this procedure.

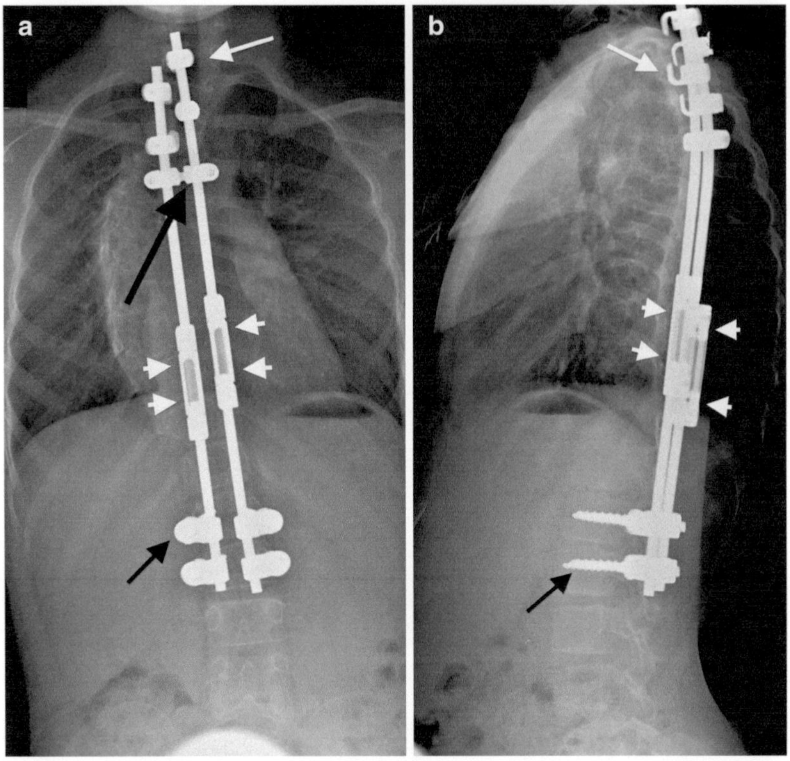

Fig. 27.5 Growing rod technique. (**a**, **b**) There are hooks (*short white arrows*) and pedicle screws (*short black arrows*) at the foundation sites. The two expandable growing rods are connected by a transverse connector (*long black arrow*). The expandable growing rod is extended through the tandem connector (*arrowheads*)

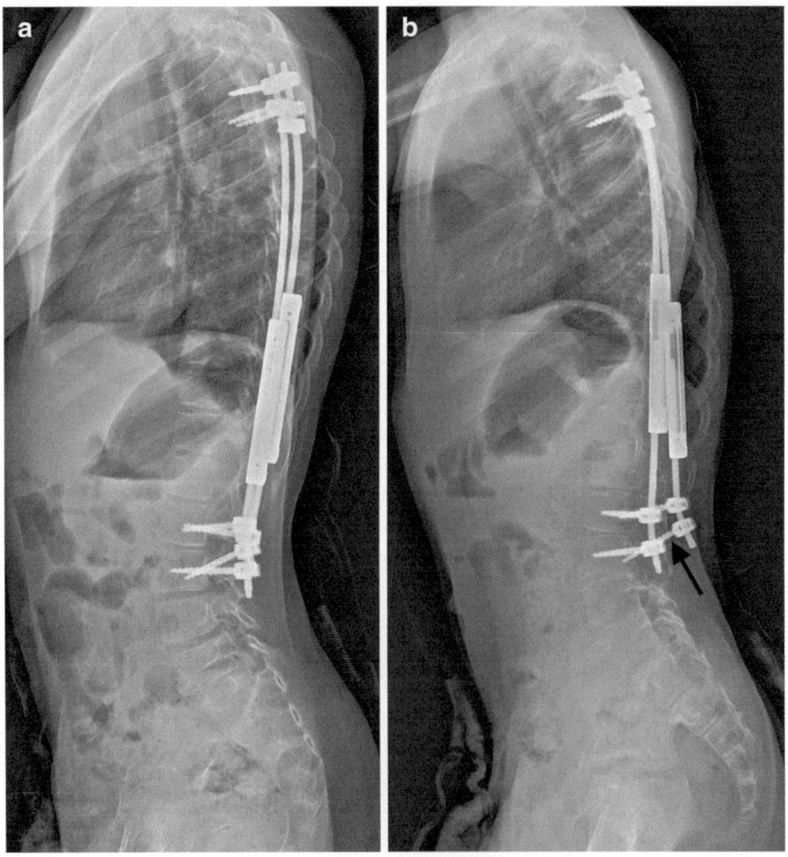

Fig. 27.6 Screw retraction from growing rods. (**a**) After surgery, one of the four distal foundation pedicle screws is angled and may not adequately engage with the pedicle. (**b**) Later, both the angled screw (*arrow*) and the screw above are dorsally displaced, no longer engaged with the pedicle. The associated rod arcs posteriorly (Courtesy of Leslie E. Grissom)

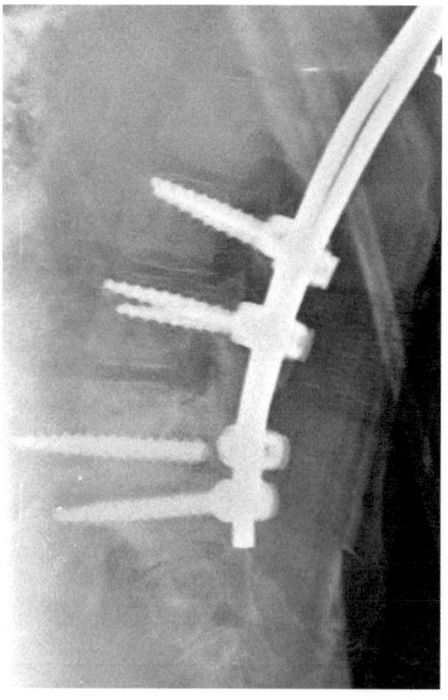

Fig. 27.7 Growing rods with screw fracture. There is an obvious break in one of the two most distal foundation screws. Furthermore, ill-defined lucency surrounds both distal screws, suggesting loosening (Courtesy of Leslie E. Grissom)

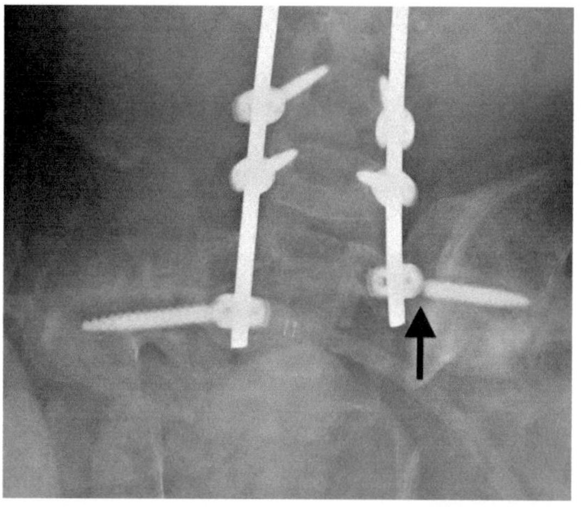

Fig. 27.8 Growing rods with screw fracture and loosening. One of the distal anchoring screws at the iliac bone has fractured (*black arrow*) near its base. Ill-defined lucency surrounds that screw as well as its counterpart on the right, indicating loosening (Courtesy of Leslie E. Grissom)

1.4 Vertical Expandable Prosthetic Titanium Rib (VEPTR) [3, 4] (Fig. 27.10; See Also Fig. 3.66)

Clinical Application

Patients with thoracic insufficiency syndrome due to a primary spine or rib deformity.

Specific Indications

This procedure is used to treat thoracic insufficiency syndrome in children who have fused ribs and severe scoliosis, flail chest, or a hypoplastic thorax.

Surgical Technique

The proximal portion of the VEPTR device is attached to the ribs via a cradle. The distal portion is attached to the ribs, lumbar spine, or ilium (the ilium is usually used if the patient has neuromuscular impairment). No spinal fusion is performed. The device is expanded twice per year to accommodate patient growth.

Postoperative Evaluation

The VEPTR should be securely attached both proximally and distally. Expansion is apparent at the tandem connector (see Fig. 3.66).

Complications

Cradle detachment and VEPTR displacement are not uncommon. The device is bulky and may induce soft tissue complications such as skin breakdown. Manipulation of the rods increases risk of infection.

1.5 Anterior Spinal Fusion [5–9] (Fig. 27.11; See Also Fig. 3.67)

Clinical Application

Thoracolumbar or lumbar curves in patients with idiopathic scoliosis, kyphosis, and dysplastic spinal instability.

Specific Indications

Anterior spinal fusion with instrumentation is used to treat certain curve patterns in adolescent

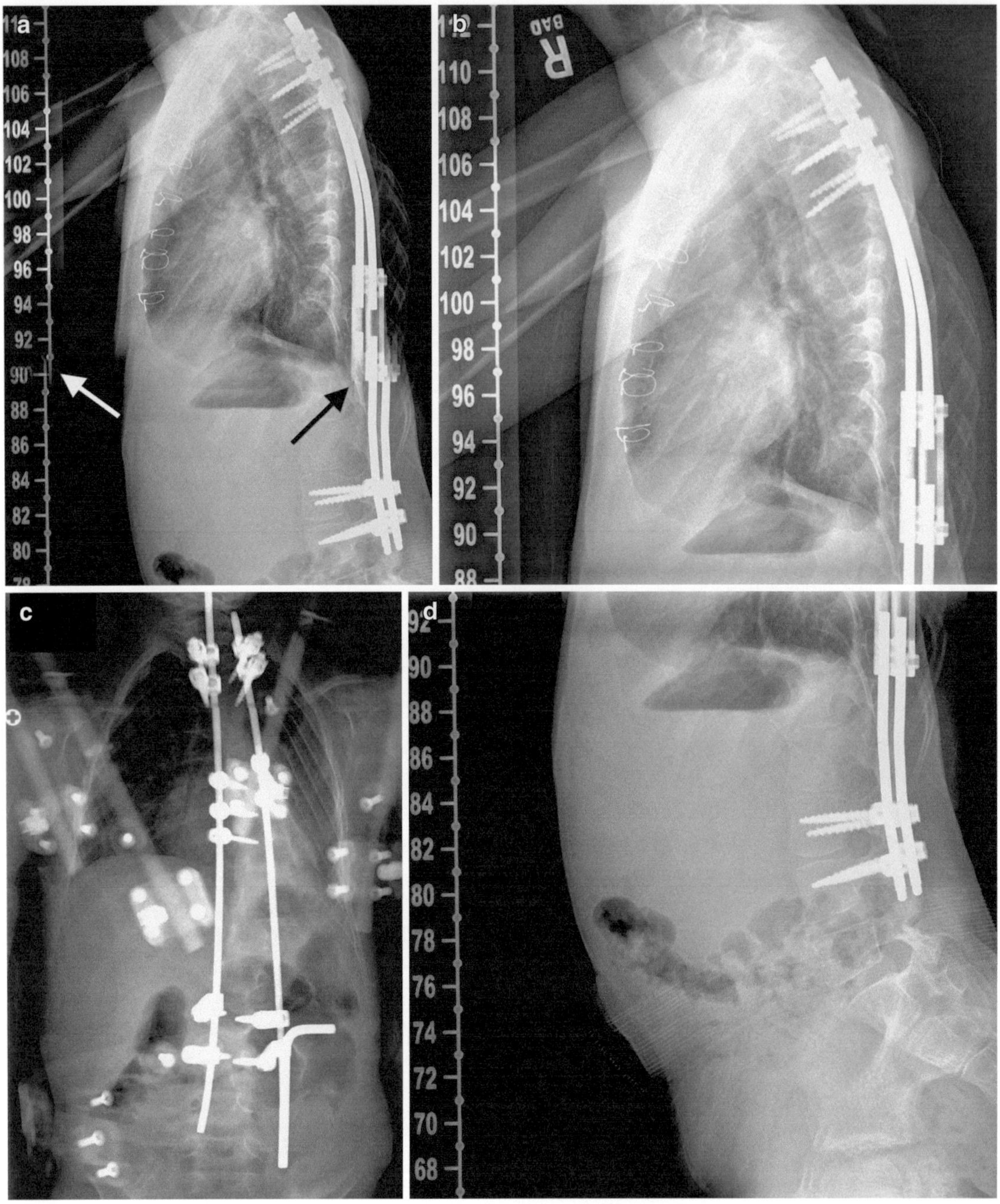

Fig. 27.9 PSFI with rod breakage simulated by stitching artifact. (**a**) On the lateral view, the more anterior rod appears fractured (*black arrow*). However, duplication of the measurement numbers (*white arrow*) indicates that this break results from stitching artifact. (**b**, **d**) Review of the source images shows no evidence of rod fracture. (**c**) On the frontal projection, the rods appear intact (Courtesy of Leslie E. Grissom)

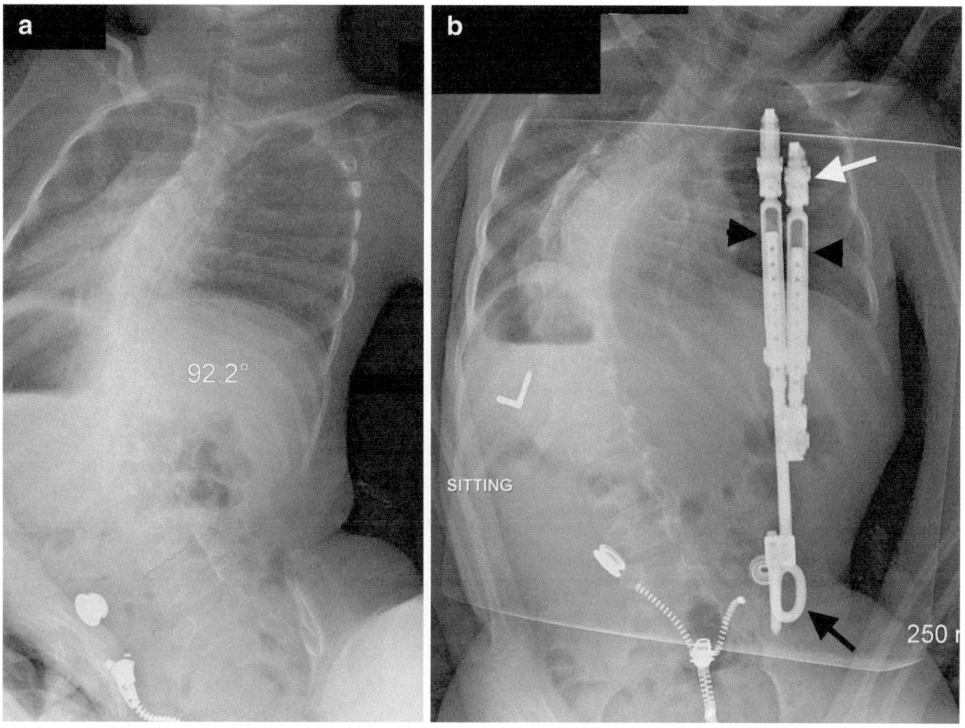

Fig. 27.10 Vertical expandable prosthetic titanium rib (VEPTR) technique. (**a**) Preoperative image demonstrates severe neuromuscular scoliosis and a small thoracic cage. (**b**) The VEPTR device is attached proximally to the ribs via a cradle (*white arrow*). The distal portion of the device is attached to the iliac bone (*black arrow*). The device is expanded through the tandem connector (*arrowheads*)

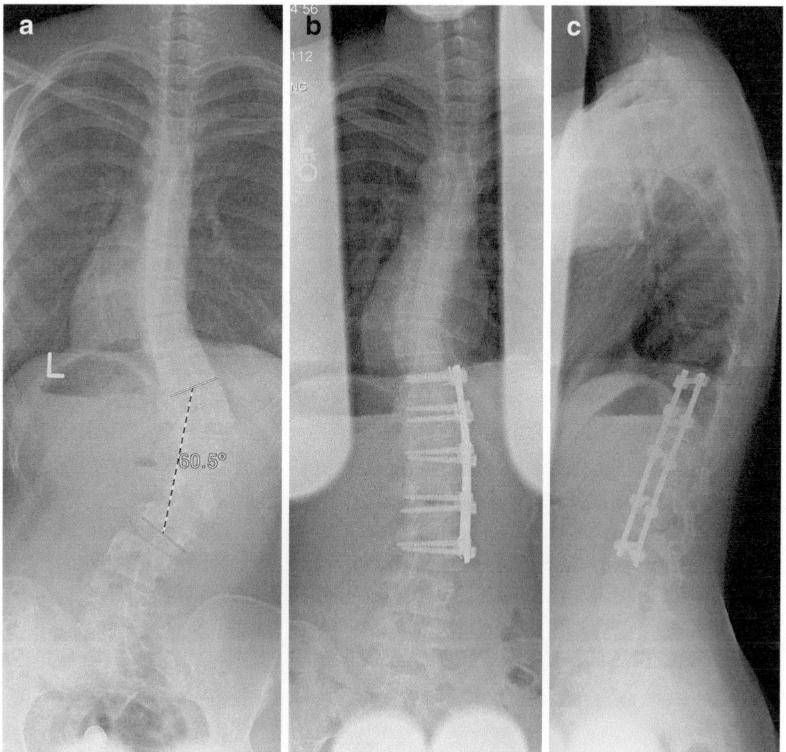

Fig. 27.11 Anterior spinal fusion. (**a**) Preoperative image shows focal lower thoracic/upper lumbar dextroscoliosis. (**b**, **c**) Screws traverse each vertebral body and are linked together by vertical rods. Grafting material fills the disk spaces

idiopathic scoliosis, usually in the thoracolumbar spine. Applying anterior as well as posterior fusion may make it possible to decrease the extent of distal fusion, preserving more spine mobility. Anterior spinal fusion is also usually combined with posterior fusion in cases with deficient posterior structures, such as myelodysplasia, or dystrophic healing, as in neurofibromatosis. In addition, by restricting anterior growth in young children who also undergo PSFI, anterior spinal fusion may prevent the "crankshaft" phenomenon, which occurs when abnormal spinal curvature develops due to continued anterior growth after posterior fusion.

Surgical Technique

Disks are removed from an anterior approach, which in some cases adequately corrects the abnormal curvature. In cases that also require instrumentation, screws are placed across the vertebral body and then linked together by rods. Bone graft and/or a structural cage is placed in the disk space to facilitate fusion and maintain lordosis.

Postoperative Evaluation

Hardware is clearly visualized. Eventually the disk spaces are obliterated by mature bone, although if a structural cage has been placed, it will remain evident.

Complications

Screw loosening, hardware failure, and pseudarthrosis may occur.

2 Pelvic Acetabuloplasty

2.1 General Considerations

Pelvic acetabuloplasty procedures reorient or change the depth or version of the acetabulum to improve hip joint congruence and to achieve a more normal weight-bearing surface. These surgeries are performed in patients with developmental dysplasia of the hip (DDH), Legg-Perthes disease, cerebral palsy, and other disorders that contribute to the development of a dysplastic acetabulum.

There are three general types of acetabuloplasty procedures: rotational acetabuloplasty, reduction acetabuloplasty, and augmentation acetabuloplasty. Each is performed by cutting the pelvis to reorient the articular surface over the femoral head. The indications for each depend on the degree and direction of acetabular deficiency, as well as the age and skeletal maturity of the patient.

Rotational acetabuloplasties, such as the Salter, Steel triple osteotomy, and periacetabular osteotomy, rotate the dysplastic acetabulum around a concentric femoral head after performance of a series of pelvic osteotomies. These procedures are generally used for patients with more significant deformity or for those whose hip dysplasia is not recognized until late childhood (or later).

Reduction acetabuloplasties, such as the Pemberton and Dega, redirect the acetabulum around a concentric femoral head, decreasing acetabular volume. These osteotomies are performed on the youngest patients, whose hips are best able to respond to decreased volume by continuing to grow and develop after the osteotomy.

Augmentation acetabuloplasties, such as the Chiari and shelf procedures, are generally utilized as salvage procedures, when additional acetabular coverage is needed but a concentric reconstruction cannot be achieved with other acetabuloplasties. These approaches are often employed in children with aspherical femoral heads or premature arthritis.

2.2 Rotational Acetabuloplasty with Innominate Osteotomy (Salter) [10, 11] (Figs. 27.12 and 27.13)

Clinical Applications

DDH and Legg-Perthes disease.

Specific indications: This procedure provides increased anterior and lateral coverage of the femoral head. It is performed in younger children whose pubic symphysis is still flexible. Congruent hip reduction and a spherical femoral head are prerequisites.

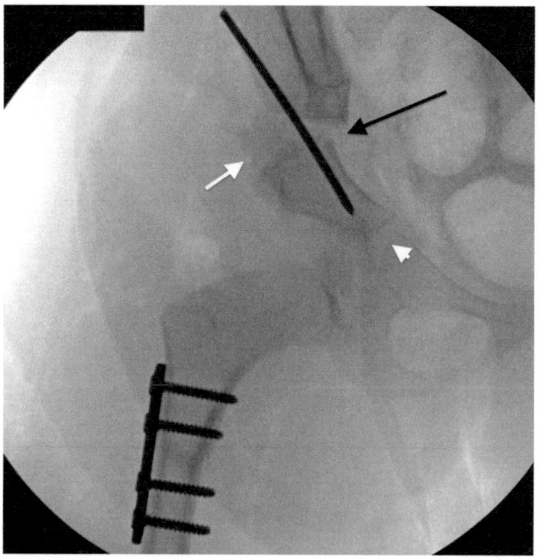

Fig. 27.12 Rotational acetabuloplasty with innominate osteotomy (Salter). There is a horizontal osteotomy of the ilium just above the acetabulum (*long black arrow*). A triangular-shaped bone graft (*short white arrow*), taken from the iliac crest, is held in the osteotomy site by a pin. The osteotomy is hinged medially without offset of the lower segment (*white arrowhead*). A varus femoral osteotomy has also been performed in this patient with developmental dysplasia of the hip (DDH)

Surgical Technique

A horizontal osteotomy of the ilium is performed just above the acetabulum. The osteotomy is opened anteriorly and laterally by hinging and rotating the acetabular segment, using the pubic symphysis as the axis of rotation. A triangular-shaped bone graft is taken from the iliac crest and is held in the osteotomy site by transfixing pins.

Postoperative Evaluation

The osteotomy is hinged medially without offset of the lower segment. The lower ilia and obturator foramina should be asymmetrical on the two sides due to the rotation of the segment (bilateral symmetry is later regained through remodeling). Pins should not penetrate into the hip joint or pelvic basin. The bone graft donor site is usually identifiable.

Complications

Loss of angulation and rotation may occur in the immediate postoperative period. Pin extrusion, graft dislodgement, medial migration of the lower segment, and disruption of the ipsilateral sacroiliac joint are also possible. Avascular necrosis (AVN) may develop (Fig. 27.13).

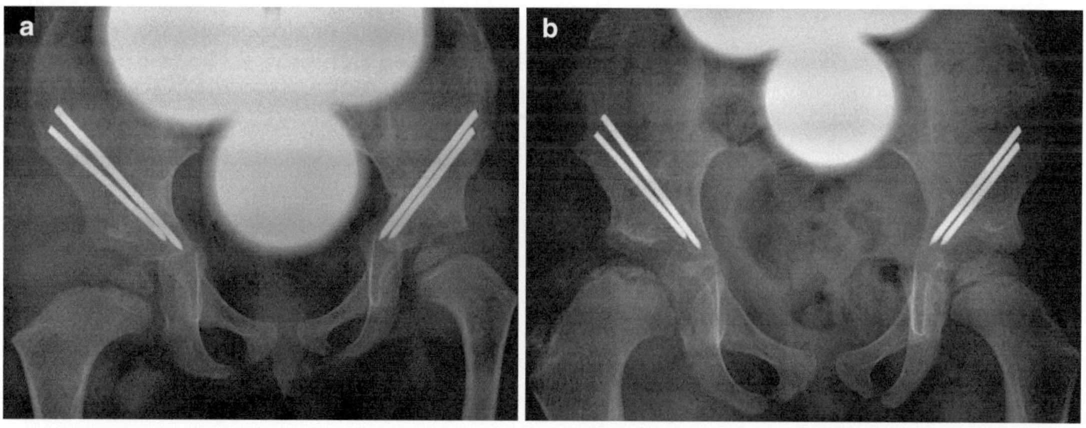

Fig. 27.13 Avascular necrosis (AVN) after rotational acetabuloplasties with innominate osteotomies. (**a**) Bilateral osteotomies have healed in this 2-year-old girl with history of bilateral DDH, and hardware is intact. Femoral heads are reduced. (**b**) 1.5 years later, the right femoral head is small and sclerotic; the metaphysis is broad and demonstrates subphyseal cysts. The left hip is developing normally (Courtesy of Rebecca Stein-Wexler; images copyright Shriners Hospital for Children, Los Angeles)

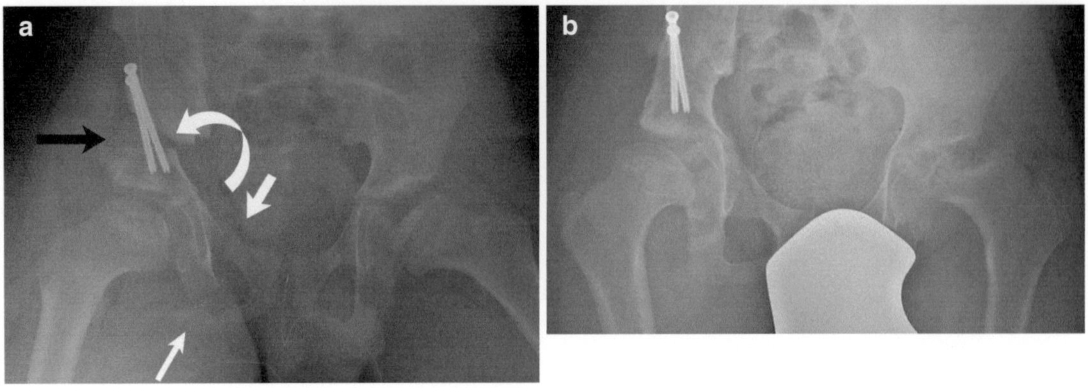

Fig. 27.14 Triple innominate osteotomy (Steel). (**a**) A perioperative image in a patient with bilateral AVN shows a supra-acetabular horizontal iliac osteotomy with bone graft (*black arrow*), a vertical osteotomy of the pubis (*thick white arrow*), and excision of a small segment of the ischium (*thin white arrow*). The acetabular fragment is rotated (*curved arrow*) to cover the femoral head. Transfixing screws hold the osteotomy in place. (**b**) Two years later, bone graft material is smoothly incorporated into a fully healed osteotomy

2.3 Triple Innominate Osteotomy (Steel) [12, 13] (Fig. 27.14)

Clinical Applications

DDH, neuromuscular hip dislocation, AVN.

Specific Indications

As with the Salter procedure, a congruent hip joint is a prerequisite for this procedure. The triple innominate osteotomy is utilized to improve acetabular coverage in the older child whose pubic symphysis is no longer flexible.

Surgical Technique

A horizontal osteotomy of the ilium is performed just above the acetabulum. A vertical osteotomy of the pubis is also performed. A small segment of the ischium is excised. The acetabular fragment is completely free and is rotated where coverage is needed. Bone graft is placed into the gapped iliac osteotomy, and transfixing screws are used to hold the osteotomy in place.

Postoperative Evaluation

Femoral head coverage is improved, and there should be no pins or screws penetrating the pelvic basin or hip joint.

Complications

Pin or screw penetration, graft extrusion, and loss of correction may occur.

2.4 Pericapsular Iliac Osteotomy of Pemberton (Reduction Acetabuloplasty) [14–17] (Fig. 27.15)

Clinical Applications

DDH with acetabular dysplasia.

Specific Indications

Acetabular dysplasia with a capacious acetabulum relative to the size of the femoral head. The acetabular index angle is larger than normal (>20° at age 2 or older). The triradiate cartilage must be open and mobile. The Dega procedure achieves the same goals as the Pemberton and appears radiographically similar.

Surgical Technique

The ilium is cut circumferentially around the acetabulum down to the triradiate cartilage. The acetabular rim is displaced downward and held with a bone graft. Unlike the Salter or Steel osteotomies, the bone graft is inherently stable and fixation is typically not needed.

Postoperative Evaluation

The femoral head is reduced and the acetabular index improved.

Complications

Intra-articular extension of the osteotomy, graft extrusion, and hip subluxation may occur.

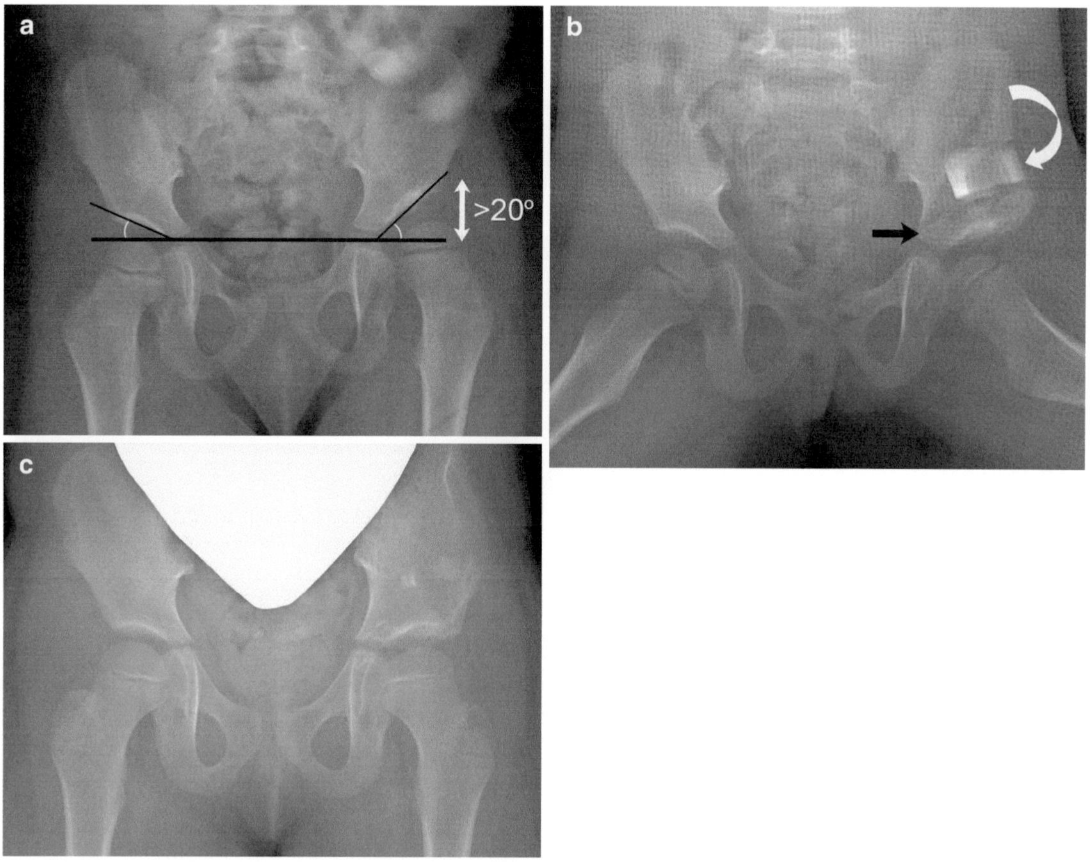

Fig. 27.15 Pericapsular iliac osteotomy of Pemberton (reduction acetabuloplasty). (**a**) Preoperative image shows a shallow left acetabulum with an acetabular angle of greater than 20° (*double arrow*) and left hip subluxation. (**b**) The ilium has been cut around the acetabulum, down to the triradiate cartilage (*black arrow*). The acetabular rim has been displaced downward and is held in place with a bone graft (*curved arrow*). The acetabular index is improved and the femoral head reduced. (**c**) Two years later, the osteotomy has healed, and the left iliac bone remains mildly distorted

2.5 Augmentation Acetabuloplasty: Medial Displacement Osteotomy (Chiari) [18–21] (Fig. 27.16)

Clinical Applications

DDH, AVN

Specific Indications

This procedure is performed for symptomatic, nonconcentric hips that cannot be treated with concentric acetabuloplasty procedures. Since the bone and not the cartilage is placed over the femoral head, this is considered to be a salvage procedure.

Surgical Technique

A supra-acetabular osteotomy is performed, extending from the anterior ilium into the sciatic notch. The leg is then abducted, and axial pressure is applied to cause the acetabular fragment to displace medially underneath the ilium. Pins or screws are used to hold the pelvis in its corrected position.

Postoperative Evaluation

The supra-acetabular portion below the osteotomy is displaced medially, with offset at the inner margin of the pelvis. The femoral head is shifted medially and covered by the enlarged acetabulum. The procedure may be performed in conjunction with femoral procedures, such as

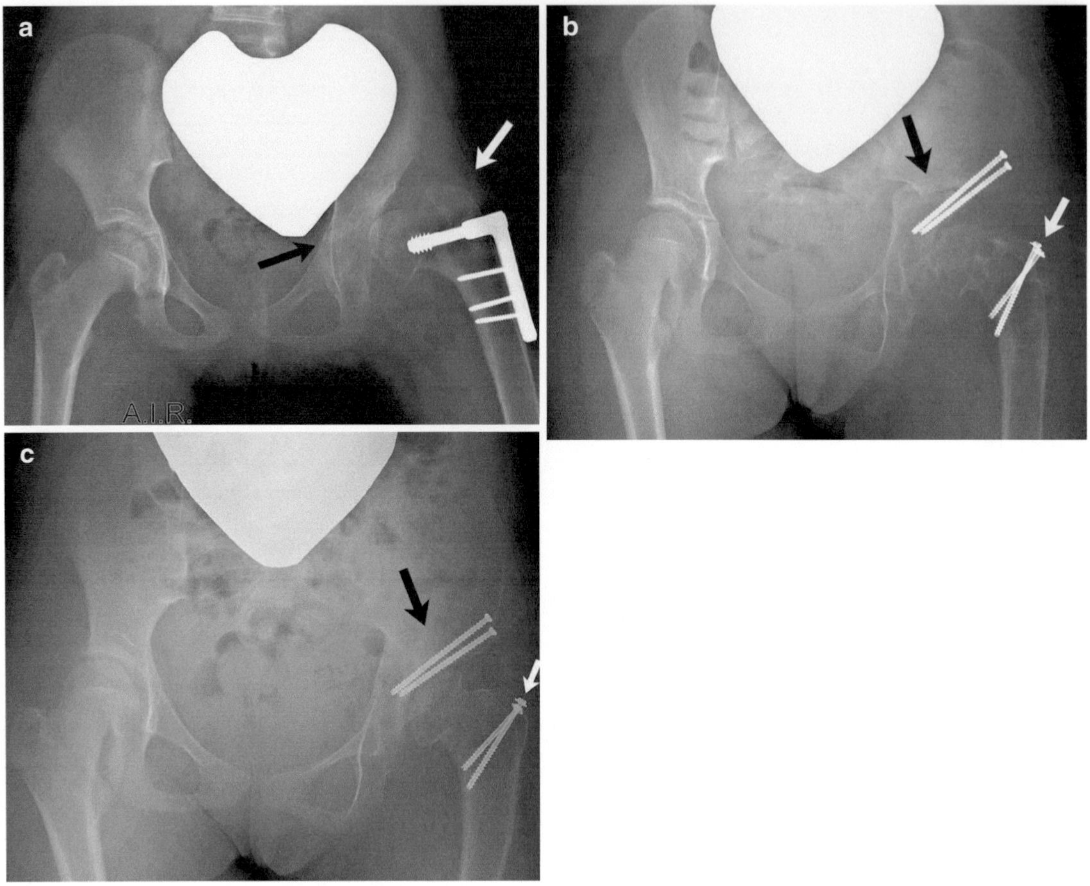

Fig. 27.16 Augmentation acetabuloplasty-medial displacement osteotomy (Chiari) with greater trochanter transfer. (**a**) Preoperative image obtained in abduction and internal rotation (AIR) shows a nonconcentric hip (*black arrow*) and a shallow acetabulum. The patient had already been treated with an unsuccessful varus derotational proximal femoral osteotomy, and the greater trochanter is higher than the femoral articulation (*white arrow*). (**b**) After surgery, the cut bony margin of the ileum forms a large neo-acetabulum that covers the medially shifted femoral head. Note offset (*black arrow*) at inner margin of the pelvis. Trochanteric advancement (*white arrow*) has also been performed, so that the greater trochanter is now distal to the level of the femoral articulation. (**c**) 1.5 years later, osteotomies have healed, and the pelvic offset has remodeled, with residual narrowing of the pelvic outlet. The contour of the femoral head is smoother

trochanteric advancement or intertrochanteric osteotomy.

Complications

Loss of medial displacement, insufficient medial movement of the lower segment, over-displacement with loss of bony contact, and pin or screw migration may occur. Later, there may be narrowing of the pelvic outlet or degenerative arthritis of the hip, as the femoral head rests on interposed capsule.

2.6 Staheli Shelf Procedure [22–24] (Fig. 27.17)

Clinical Indications

DDH

Specific Indications

To increase the load-bearing area of the femoral head. This procedure is only performed if the acetabulum cannot be redirected to provide better coverage. Like the Chiari, this is a salvage proce-

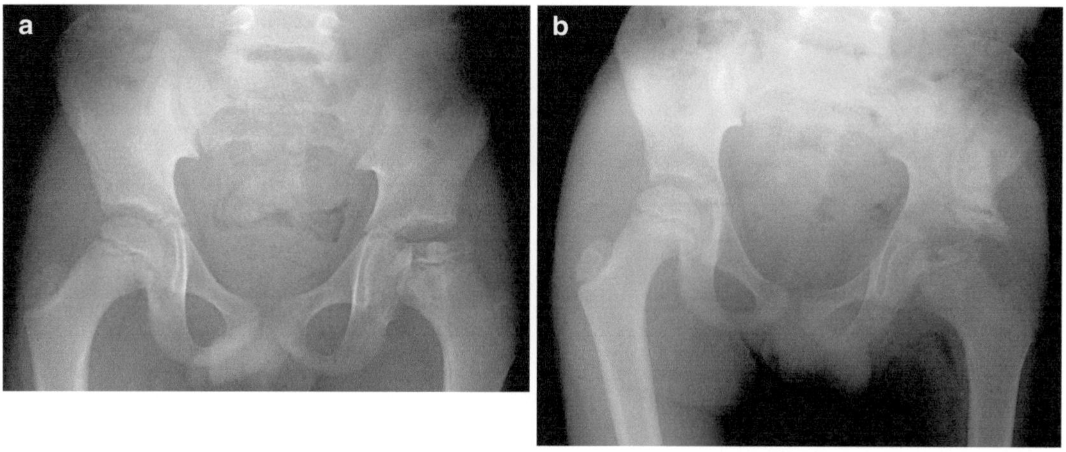

Fig. 27.17 Staheli shelf procedure. (**a**) Preoperative image shows the left femoral head is flat, broad, sclerotic, partially uncovered, and non-congruent after Legg-Perthes disease. (**b**) After surgery, a block of bone extends the acetabulum laterally, improving coverage of the femoral head. The inferior surface of the bone buttress is at the level of the lateral acetabular rim (Courtesy of Leslie E. Grissom)

dure because the bone and not the cartilage is being placed over the femoral head.

Surgical Technique

A bone block is placed in a slot at the edge of the acetabulum and may be fixed with a pin or screw.

Postoperative Evaluation

The femoral head is reduced and laterally covered by bone buttress. The inferior surface of the bone block should be at the level of the lateral acetabular rim.

Complications

Displacement or pressure resorption of the bone block due to continued lateral subluxation of the femoral head may occur. Degenerative arthritis may develop.

3 Hip and Proximal Femur

3.1 General Considerations

Most operative procedures performed on the proximal femur correct abnormally increased rotation and angulation of the femoral neck by means of a varus or valgus derotational intertrochanteric ostetomy. In other cases screws may be placed across an acute or subacute slip of the proximal femoral epiphysis, intended to stabilize the epiphysis and prevent further displacement; proximal femoral osteotomies may be performed later on, in order to correct the position of the femoral head. Trochanteric transfer may be performed to shift the insertion of the abductor force distally in patients in whom shortening of the femoral neck has reduced the normal articular-trochanteric distance. Hip joint fusion is a temporizing measure, decreasing the symptoms of a degenerative joint in a child who is considered too young for joint replacement.

3.2 Varus Derotational Femoral Osteotomy [25] (Fig. 27.18)

Clinical Applications

Cerebral palsy, Legg-Perthes disease, hip dysplasia, and increased femoral anteversion.

Specific Indications

This procedure is used to correct abnormally increased femoral anteversion and/or valgus deformity. It is also used to increase varus and

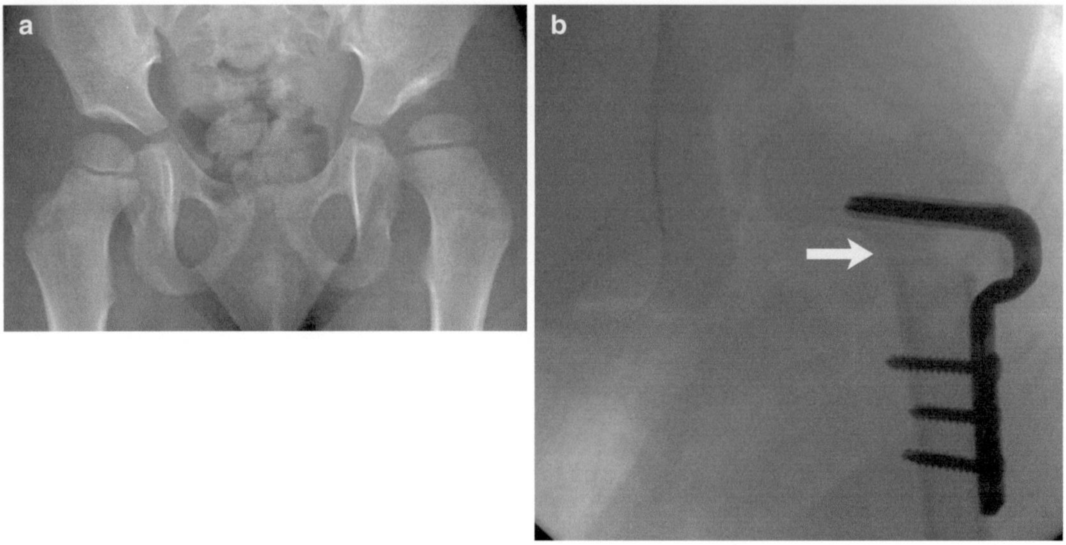

Fig. 27.18 Varus derotational femoral osteotomy. (**a**) There is bilateral coxa valga in this patient with CP. The left acetabulum is shallow, and the hip is subluxated. (**b**) Transverse femoral osteotomy at the level of the lesser trochanter (*arrow*) results in improved femoral head coverage. A blade plate holds the osteotomy fragments together

contain the femoral head in some cases of AVN or Legg-Perthes disease.

Surgical Technique

A transverse femoral osteotomy is performed at the level of the lesser trochanter. A wedge of bone may be removed to achieve varus, but this is not always necessary. The desired amount of varus and anteversion is achieved and either a blade plate or a hip screw placed to hold the osteotomy together. Ideally, the distal shaft is positioned more medially in order to maintain normal weight-bearing forces.

Postoperative Evaluation

The blade is in the femoral neck and does not breach the bone (the "calcar," the vertically oriented posteromedial bone above the lesser trochanter, is especially prone to penetration). The lesser trochanter may be displaced from its usual position.

Complications

Complications include inadequate blade penetration, which may result in loss of fixation, blade breakage, and delayed union due to rigid fixation and lack of compression across the osteotomy site. In addition, the femoral neck may fracture due to blade penetration (especially at the calcar), and the proximal femur may fracture after plate removal.

3.3 Pinning of Slipped Capital Femoral Epiphysis (SCFE) [26] (Figs. 27.19 and 27.20)

Clinical Application

Stable or unstable SCFE.

Specific Indications

This procedure is used to stabilize the epiphysis, prevent further slippage, and promote closure of the proximal femoral growth plate.

Surgical Technique

Pinning is performed using fluoroscopy. A central screw is placed from the femoral neck

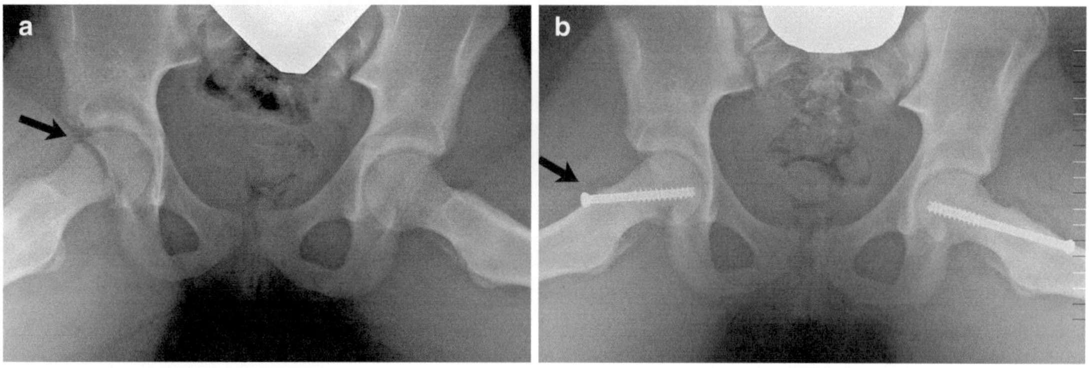

Fig. 27.19 Pinning of slipped capital femoral epiphysis (SCFE). (**a**) Preoperative image shows a moderate SCFE (*arrow*) on the right. (**b**) Central screws have been placed on the right (*arrow*) as well as on the left, from the femoral neck through the growth plate, ending in the femoral head. The screws are perpendicular to the physis, and there are five threads beyond the physis

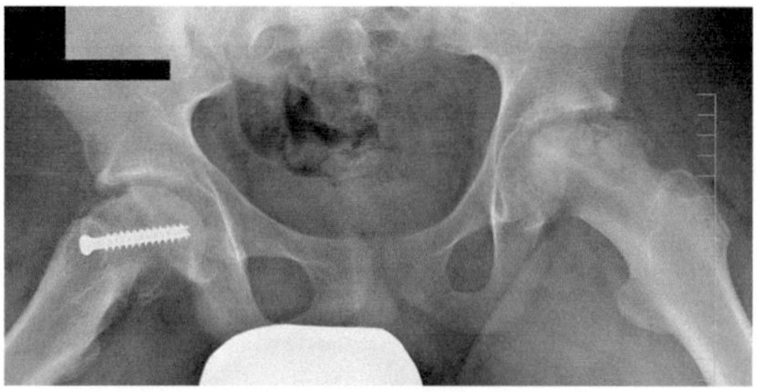

Fig. 27.20 AVN after prophylactic pinning for contralateral SCFE. There is sclerosis, collapse, and fragmentation of the left femoral head, status post removal of a pin that had been placed prophylactically for SCFE. The patient had frank SCFE on the right, also treated with pin placement

through the growth plate, ending in the femoral head. It should be placed perpendicular to the physis, with five threads crossing the growth plate. If the slip is unstable, two screws may be employed. The contralateral hip may be treated as well (see Chap. 12).

Postoperative Evaluation

The screw should not penetrate into the hip joint. However, since the femoral head is spherical, penetration may be difficult to assess. In a stable slip, no reduction is attempted, and the epiphyseal position is therefore similar to the preoperative position. Unstable SCFEs typically reduce in the course of positioning the patient for surgery, so the epiphysis is often in a better position than it was preoperatively.

Complications

Screw extrusion, screw cutout with resultant further progression of the slip, and screw penetration into the joint may occur. Chondrolysis, AVN (Fig. 27.20), and screw head impingement on the acetabular rim may also be seen.

3.4 Biplane Proximal Femoral Osteotomy [27] (Fig. 27.21)

Clinical Application

Old healed or severe chronic SCFE.

Specific Indications

An osteotomy is usually performed after growth plate fusion to correct symptomatic deformity from prior SCFE. The proximal femoral neck deformity may cause impingement with hip flexion, and the biplane osteotomy is used to direct the deformity away from the acetabulum, thus limiting impingement. The procedure may infrequently be performed before growth plate closure to prevent additional slippage.

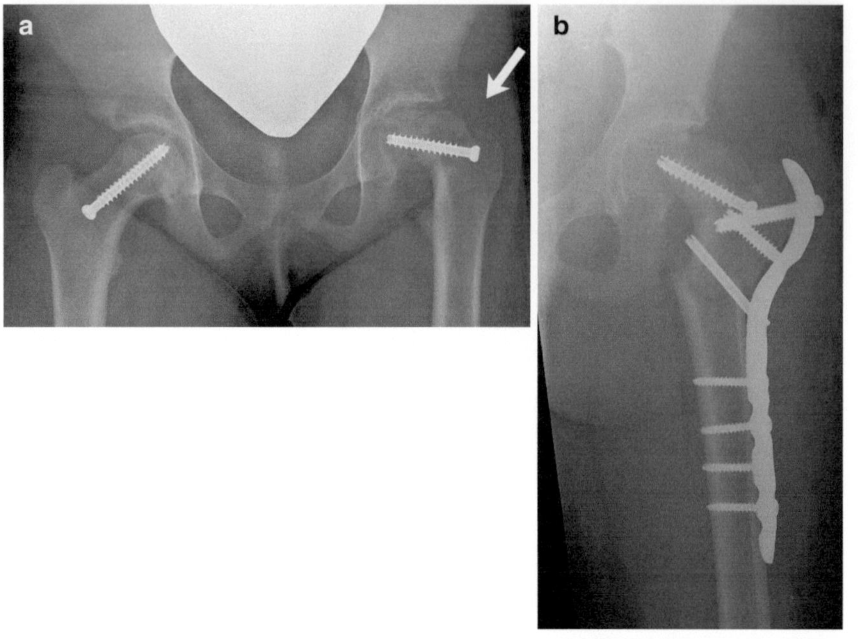

Fig. 27.21 Biplane proximal femoral osteotomy. (**a**) Preoperative image shows screws from prior pinning of SCFE. On the left, there is deformity at the femoral head-neck junction (*arrow*), which causes impingement with hip flexion. (**b**) After biplane osteotomy of the proximal femur, valgus has increased, and the proximal femoral deformity is directed away from the acetabulum. A plate and screws fixate the osteotomy fragments

Surgical Technique

A biplane osteotomy of the proximal femur is performed to redirect the proximal femoral deformity away from the hip articulation. The osteotomy is usually designed to eliminate impingement by increasing valgus and/or flexing or derotating the femoral neck, depending on the deformity. The osteotomy fragments are held together with a plate and screws.

Postoperative Evaluation

The osteotomy site should be evaluated for bony union.

Complications

Nonunion or delayed union may occur. Hardware failure, chondrolysis, and AVN may occur.

3.5 Greater Trochanter Transfer [28] (See Fig. 27.16)

Clinical Application

Legg-Perthes disease or healed AVN of the femoral head (typically from treatment of DDH), in which associated growth plate dysfunction causes decreased femoral neck growth and relative overgrowth of the greater trochanter.

Specific Indications

Femoral neck shortening and overgrowth of the greater trochanter resulting from Legg-Perthes or AVN cause decreased range of motion, a gluteus medius limp, and femoroacetabular impingement. This procedure treats femoral neck shortening by moving the greater trochanter distally, which then increases the articular-trochanteric distance, decreasing limp and hip impingement. Epiphyseodesis of the greater trochanter before age 8 years may avoid the need for a transfer.

Surgical Technique

The greater trochanter is resected at its base, leaving the gluteus medius attachment intact. The trochanter is then displaced distally and attached to the lateral femoral shaft by screws or wires. This procedure is often done in conjunction with other hip procedures.

Postoperative Evaluation

The greater trochanter should be located distal to the original site and inferior to the level of the femoral articulation. Screws should be intact.

Complications

Wire or screw failure, displacement of the trochanter resulting in loss of correction, and trochanteric resorption may complicate this procedure.

3.6 Hip Joint Fusion [29, 30] (Fig. 27.22)

Clinical Application

Septic, avascular, or traumatic femoral head collapse with joint incongruity and degenerative joint disease.

Specific Indications

Fusion is performed to relieve pain or instability secondary to degenerative joint disease. It may be converted to joint replacement when indicated.

Surgical Technique

Joint surfaces are denuded of cartilage. Bone graft is placed into the joint interval and sometimes along the surface of the adjacent pelvis and proximal femur. The femur is held in the appropriate position by screws or plates. A subtrochanteric osteotomy is performed to achieve the desired position of the femur relative to the pelvis.

Postoperative Evaluation

The femur should be in 30–40° of flexion and adduction relative to the pelvis. The joint space is obliterated, and external bone graft may be visible.

Complications

Failure of fixation, loss of correction, nonunion, and femoral shaft fracture below the fusion level may occur.

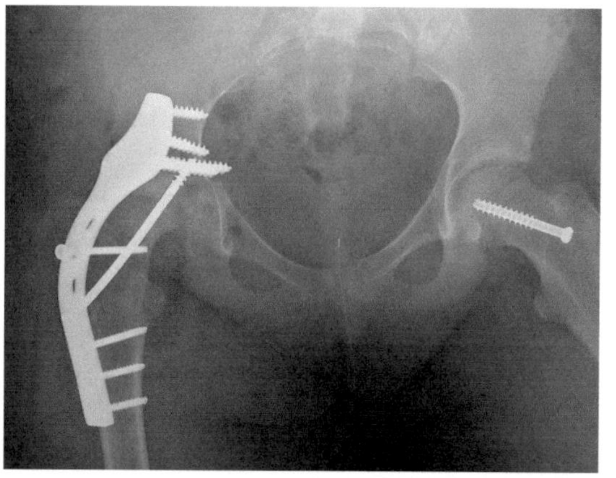

Fig. 27.22 Hip joint fusion. The joint space has been denuded and grafted with bone, and the femur is held in adduction and flexion by a plate and screws (the patient had bilateral SCFE, and severe deformity and osteoarthritis developed on the right despite treatment)

3.7 Core Decompression [31, 32] (Fig. 27.23)

Clinical Application

AVN of the femoral head.

Surgical Indications

Core decompression may be performed in the early stages of AVN, before there is evidence of collapse of the femoral head. The procedure is contraindicated if there is evidence of collapse.

Surgical Technique

One large or multiple small bone tunnels are drilled through the femoral neck into the head beneath the zone of AVN. This relieves the pressure within the bone and creates channels for angiogenesis to nourish the area of AVN, promoting healing. Bone graft or bone graft substitute is often introduced into the bone tunnel(s) beneath the lesion to further augment healing.

Postoperative Evaluation

The bony tunnel(s) and zone of AVN should be evaluated for healing, although complete bony

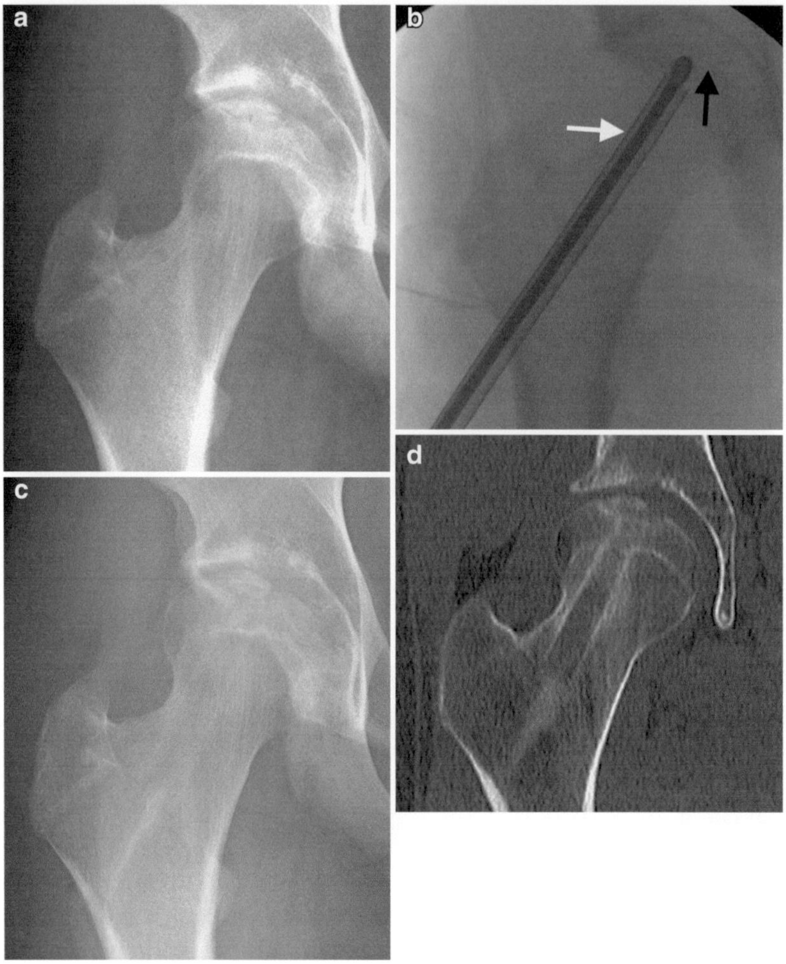

Fig. 27.23 Core decompression. (**a**) Preoperative image demonstrates early AVN of the femoral head in a 16-year-old boy, with subchondral lucency but no evidence of collapse. (**b**) Intraoperative image shows hardware drilling a bone tunnel through the femoral neck (*white arrow*) into the head beneath the zone of AVN (*black arrow*). (**c**) One month after surgery, the proximal portion of the tract is lucent, whereas the distal portion is dense due to bone graft substitute. (**d**) Coronally reformatted CT, performed 4 months after surgery to assess for bony integration, shows bone substitute separates the zone of healing AVN from the remainder of the femoral head

integration may take quite a while. The femoral head should be assessed for healing or progressive collapse. CT may be helpful to evaluate bony integration.

Complications

Intra-articular spillage of bone graft substitute may occur if the drill is driven into the joint.

4 Extremities

4.1 General Considerations

Surgical procedures performed on the extremities are typically intended to correct abnormal rotation, abnormal alignment, or leg length discrepancy. With the exception of extensible intramedullary rodding designed to adjust growth, most stabilization procedures and devices utilized in children are similar in design to those used in adults.

Length inequality is typically only clinically significant in the lower extremities (see Chap. 13). All methods of correction depend on accurate assessment and prediction of ultimate discrepancy at skeletal maturity. The ideal time for surgical intervention is determined by bone age assessment (see Chap. 2) and estimation of residual growth.

Leg length inequality may be corrected by shortening the longer leg, interrupting growth of the longer leg, or lengthening the shorter leg. In general, shortening the longer leg is performed

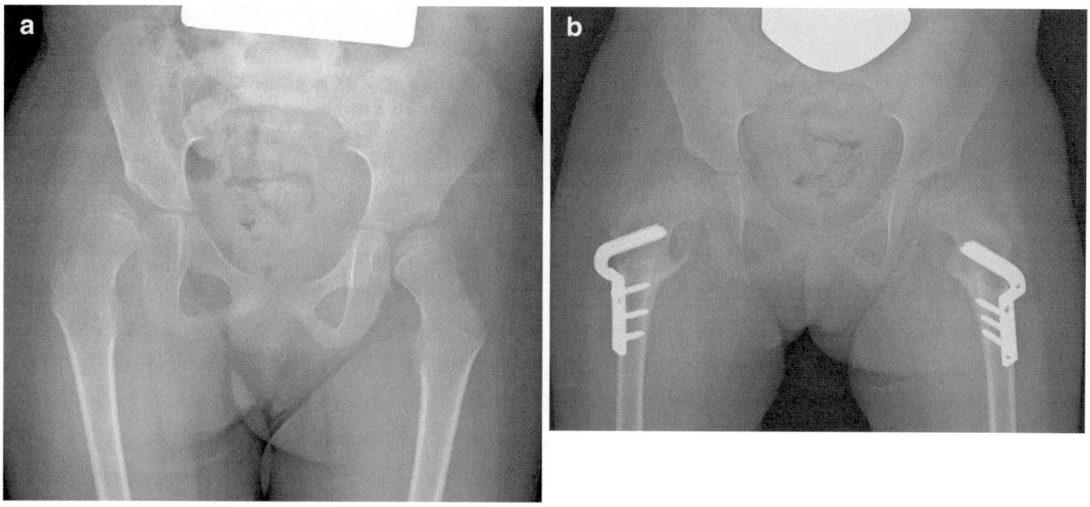

Fig. 27.24 Angulation derotational osteotomy. (**a**) Preoperative image shows bilateral femoral anteversion and apparent coxa valga. (**b**) After bilateral opening wedge osteotomies, bone graft was inserted into the osteotomy sites. Femoral head positioning is improved. The fragments are held together with a blade plate and screws

only if the disparity is great and the child is tall and relatively mature. When the difference is small and/or the child is still growing, growth inhibition of the longer leg is preferable. The inhibition may be permanent (epiphyseodesis) or temporary (stapling). Leg lengthening is utilized if discrepancy will be more than 6 cm at maturity.

Leg lengthening techniques are based on gradual distraction at a rate that allows bone to form and nerves and vessels to grow. Bone formation occurs by one of two mechanisms: either by filling in the distraction gap with bone formed from the periosteum and marrow elements or by stretching of callus formed between the bone ends before distraction is initiated.

4.2 Angulation Derotational Osteotomy [30] (Fig. 27.24)

Clinical Applications

Cerebral palsy, abnormal femoral rotation, tibial torsion, and angular deformities in children whose growth is complete or nearly complete.

Specific Indications

This procedure is used to correct abnormal femoral anteversion or retroversion as well as excessive varus or valgus.

Surgical Technique

Parallel guide pins placed above and below the site of the osteotomy are used to ascertain the degree of rotation. The primary surgical site is transected. If derotation only is being performed, the fragments are rotated in relation to each other. If angular correction is desired, the bone is either wedged open or a wedge is removed to achieve the desired angular correction. The fragments are held together with a plate and screws or with crossed pins. When osteotomies are performed on the tibia, a segment of the fibula is often removed as well in order to aid in correction.

Postoperative Evaluation

Small holes above and below the surgical line may indicate guide pin defects. Slight offset of the upper and lower cortical margins may be deliberate or secondary to unequal bone diameter after rotation.

Complications

Pins may bend or migrate. Hardware may fail. Fractures may occur at the ends of the plate due to a stress riser effect. There may be nonunion as well as loss of correction.

4.3 Epiphyseodesis (Percutaneous or Phemister-Green Technique) [33, 34] (Fig. 27.25)

Clinical Application

Leg length discrepancy in a skeletally immature child.

Specific Indications

Epiphyseodesis is used to inhibit growth of the longer leg by permanent growth plate closure.

Surgical Technique

The cartilage cells at the periphery of both sides of the growth plate are curetted and removed by an open or percutaneous medial and lateral approach. Most surgeons now favor the percutaneous approach, as it is equally efficacious and has a more benign postoperative course. When

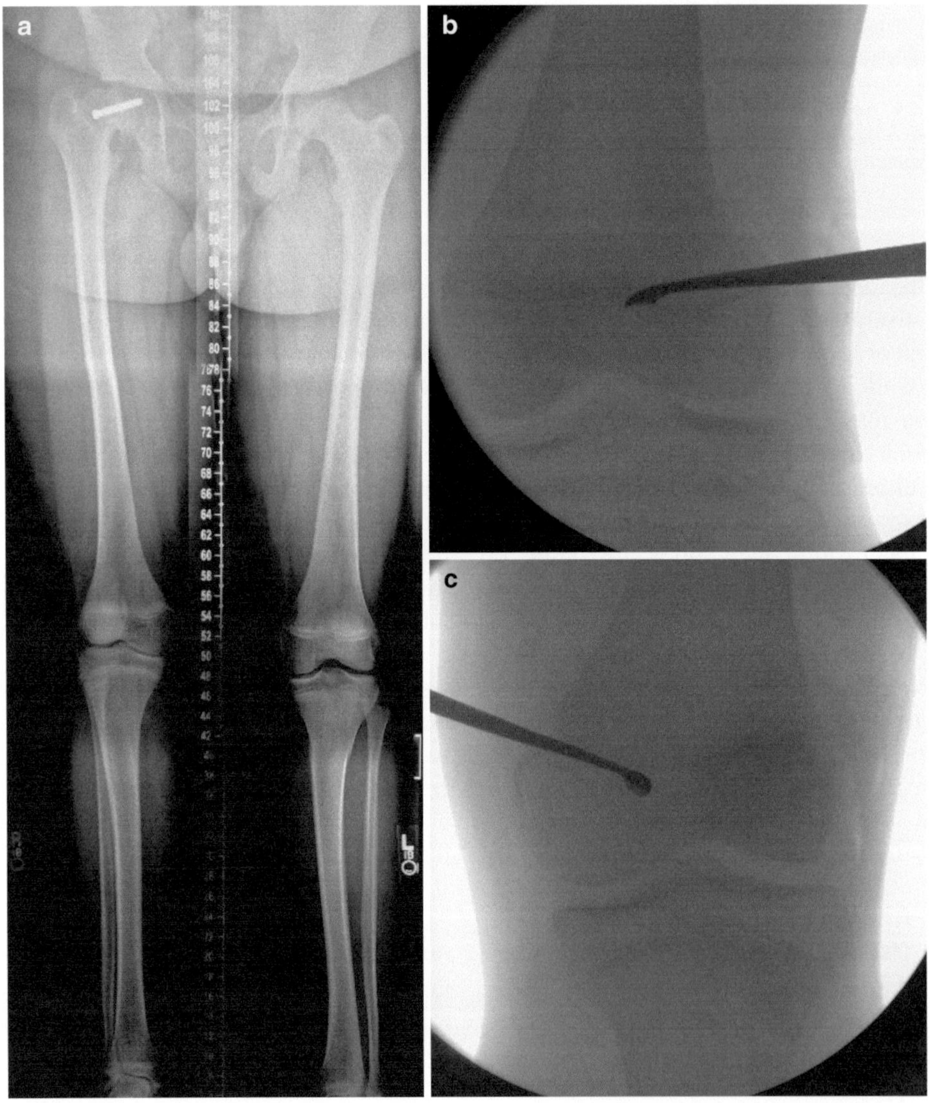

Fig. 27.25 Epiphyseodesis employing percutaneous technique (Phemister-Green). (**a**) Preoperative image with the right foot elevated on a block shows the right lower extremity is shorter than the left, secondary to sequelae of SCFE. (**b**, **c**) The cartilage cells at the periphery of both sides of the left distal femoral growth plate are curetted and removed by a percutaneous lateral (**b**) and medial (**c**) approach

an open technique is utilized, a small portion of the adjacent metaphysis and growth plate is removed, inverted, and replaced to provide a further tethering effect (Phemister-Green technique).

Postoperative Evaluation
Bony fragments may be seen in the adjacent soft tissues with the percutaneous technique. The growth plate may be narrowed or widened initially; narrowing and fusion should follow.

Complications
Growth may continue if curettage was incomplete. If growth plate removal was asymmetrical, unilateral tethering may cause angulation with further growth.

4.4 Limb Deformity Correction by Hemiepiphyseodesis [35] (Fig. 27.26)

Clinical Applications
Asymmetrical growth causing angular deformity.

Specific Indications
This procedure is used for temporary manipulation of growth. Growth is planned to resume after the tension band plates, "eight plates," or staples are removed, but cannot be guaranteed.

Surgical Technique
Fluoroscopic guidance is utilized to position the two-holed eight plate across the physis. Screws

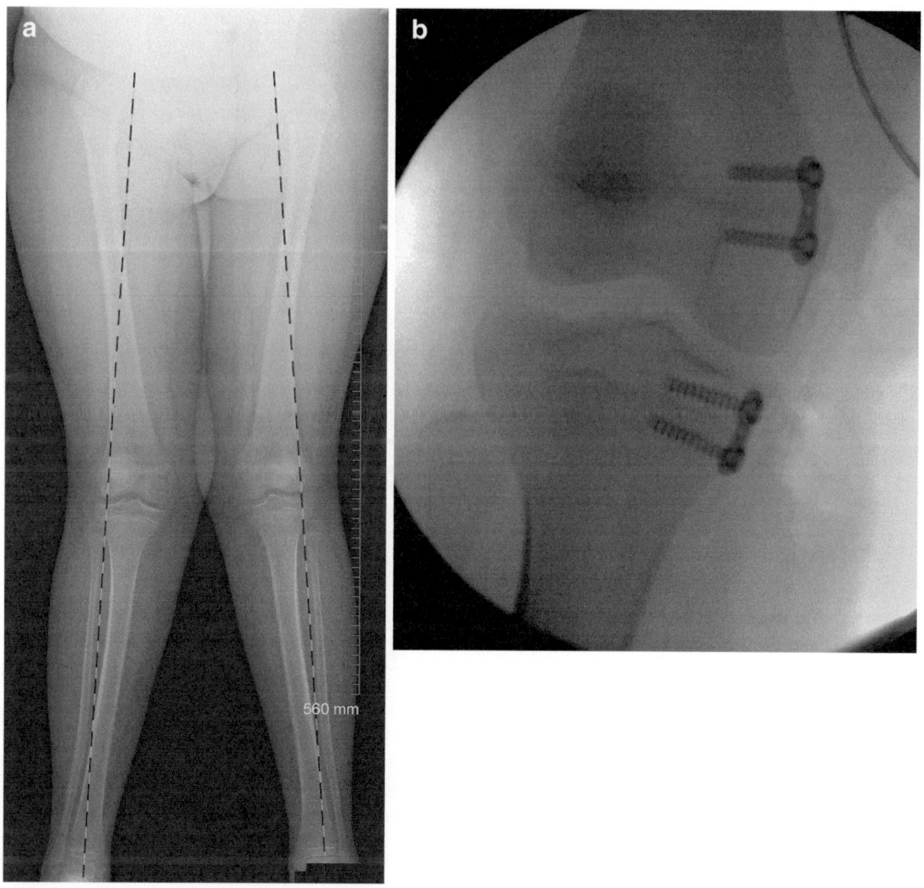

Fig. 27.26 Limb deformity correction by hemiepiphyseodesis. (**a**) Preoperative image shows bilateral genu valgum, right worse than left. (**b**) Eight plates have been placed at the right medial distal femur and proximal tibia, bridging the physis to tether medial growth

are then inserted proximal and distal to the physis in order to create a tethering effect. Once desired inhibition has been achieved, the plates are typically removed. This procedure can also be performed with staples.

Postoperative Evaluation

The plate is closely applied to the bone, and screws extend transversely into the epiphysis and metaphysis. With time, continued growth on the side that has not been manipulated should gradually correct angular deformity.

Complications

The tension band plate may fracture or lose purchase over time. When the device is removed, growth may fail to resume or rebound overgrowth may occur.

4.5 Limb Lengthening by Diaphyseal Distraction and Callotasis (Ilizarov) [36, 37] (Figs. 27.27 and 27.28)

Clinical Applications

Leg length inequality.

Specific Indications

Patients with significant leg length discrepancy not amenable to contralateral epiphyseodesis. Simultaneous correction of torsional and angular deformities may also be performed.

Surgical Technique

Wires under tension and/or half pins are inserted through the bone shaft above and below the planned level of the osteotomy (Fig. 27.27). Transverse osteotomy is performed, leaving as much periosteum as possible intact. The wires and pins are connected to a framework of rings and telescoping threaded rods that allow control of angulation, rotation, and displacement. Distraction is initiated after 7–10 days, once early callus is allowed to form. Controlled distraction then progresses, stretching out callus in the bone gap. This procedure is sometimes performed over an intramedullary nail (Fig. 27.28). Once there is adequate distraction and the leg is lengthened, the Ilizarov device is removed to allow better mobilization. Callus formation around the intramedullary nail confers increased stability.

Postoperative Evaluation

Callus initially appears as calcific strings aligned in the axis of distraction. This then ossifies, becomes denser, and remodels. Later on, corticomedullary differentiation occurs.

Complications

Unplanned angulation or rotation may develop. If detected early, this may be corrected by adjusting the distraction apparatus. Osteomyelitis may be suggested by ill-defined lucency surrounding the pins. Fracture of the regenerate bone and pseudarthrosis may occur. Joint subluxation may develop above or below the operative site.

Fig. 27.27 Limb lengthening by diaphyseal distraction and callotasis (Ilizarov). (**a**) Preoperative image shows the short right tibia and fibula resulting in marked leg length discrepancy. (**b**) A proximal wire under tension (*black arrow*) and a distal half pin (*white arrow*) traverse the tibia above and below the transverse osteotomy (*arrowhead*). The wire and pin are connected to an external framework of rings and telescoping threaded rods (*double white arrow*). (**c**) With distraction, callus stretches, filling the bone gap. Note expansion (*double white arrow*) of the framework. (**d**) The ossifying callus (*black arrow*) resembles giant strings, aligned in the axis of distraction. There has also been further distraction

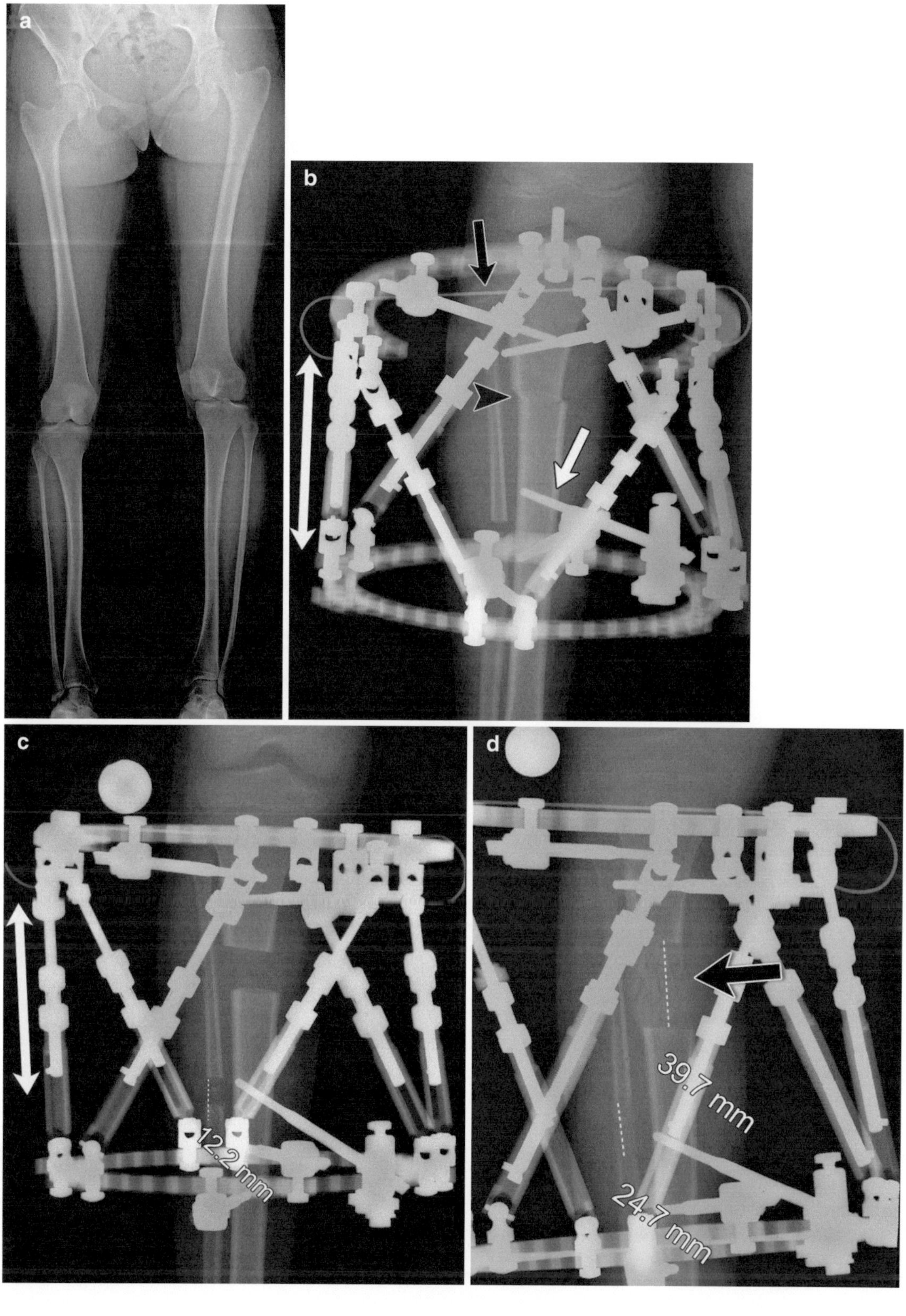
a
b
c
12.2 mm
d
39.7 mm
24.7 mm

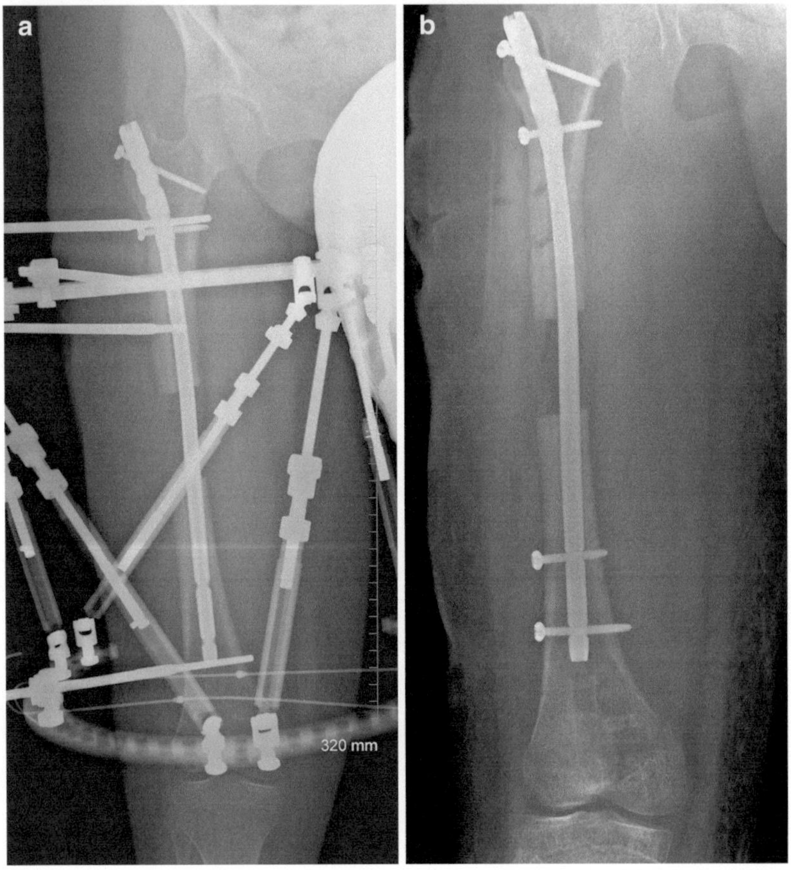

Fig. 27.28 Limb lengthening by diaphyseal distraction and callotasis, performed over an intramedullary nail. (**a**) Half pins anchor the framework of rings and telescoping threaded wires, and there are also two distal wires under tension. An intramedullary nail traverses the osteotomy, placed via the greater trochanter. There is a large gap at the osteotomy site, with faint callus aligned with the axis of distraction. (**b**) The framework, half pins, and wires have been removed. Callus bridging the osteotomy site is denser

4.6 Intramedullary Rodding (Fassier-Duval Rod) [38, 39] (Fig. 27.29)

Clinical Application

Osteogenesis imperfecta.

Specific Indications

The Fassier-Duval rod is a specialized rod that is usually implanted after multiple osteotomies to straighten a deformed long bone shaft. The extensible feature, in which one end telescopes into the other, allows for continued stabilization and alignment during growth.

Surgical Technique

Multiple transverse osteotomies are performed. The diaphysis is realigned on the intramedullary rod. Both ends of the extensible rod pass through the growth plate and are anchored in the epiphysis so that extension of the rod occurs during growth.

Postoperative Evaluation

Shaft deformity is realigned. The rod is anchored in the epiphysis. Gradual lengthening of the rod occurs during growth.

Complications

Rods may bend or fracture. The telescoping mechanism may fail. There may be delayed or nonunion of the osteotomy sites.

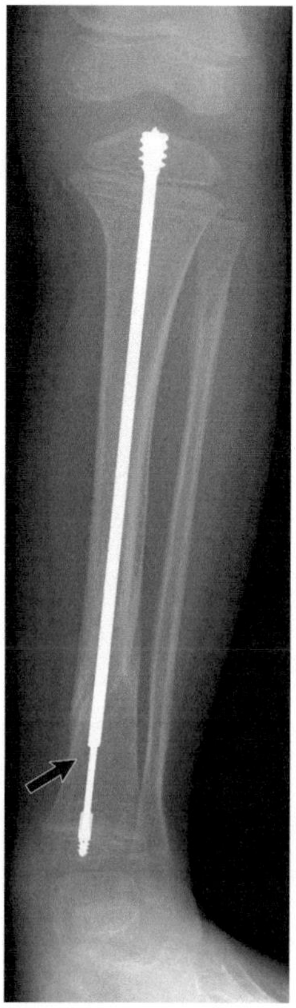

Fig. 27.29 Intramedullary rodding. An extensible (*black arrow*) telescoping rod was placed after segmental osteotomy. The rod passes through the diaphysis, terminating in both epiphyses to allow for extension with growth. Callus is forming along the diaphysis

5 Foot

5.1 General Considerations

Surgical treatment of the foot is performed to correct deformity. Arthrodesis is a corrective procedure that simplifies joint mechanics, produces stability, and relieves pain. Since fusion in a young child inhibits further growth and may lead to disparity in foot size, this operation is carefully timed to allow as much growth as possible.

Joint stabilization includes both bony fusion and reorientation of abnormal joint mechanics resulting from fixed deformity of angulated articular planes. In addition to osseous surgery, tendon transfers may be necessary to eliminate deforming forces that may defeat the bony realignment and fusion.

5.2 Posteromedial Release (PMR) [40–43] (Fig. 27.30)

Clinical Application
Clubfoot.

Specific Indications
This procedure is used to correct hindfoot varus and equinus in children who have failed casting.

Surgical Technique
The posterior and medial capsules and ligaments are released. The foot is realigned and held in position by pins and/or a cast. The Achilles and posterior tibial tendons are typically lengthened.

Postoperative Evaluation
Pins may be present. Talocalcaneal relationships are realigned to more normal angles. The calcaneus may be more horizontal than normal on the lateral film.

Complications
There may be pin extrusion or penetration, loss of correction, skin slough, AVN of the talus, and a convex arch secondary to excessive anterior foot dorsiflexion in an attempt to correct equinus.

5.3 Hindfoot Tarsal Arthrodesis (Triple Arthrodesis) [44] (Fig. 27.31)

Clinical Applications
Residual foot deformity and unstable paretic foot.

Specific Indications
Triple arthrodesis is utilized as a salvage procedure to provide a flat platform with lateral stability in an unstable or painful, deformed foot. This

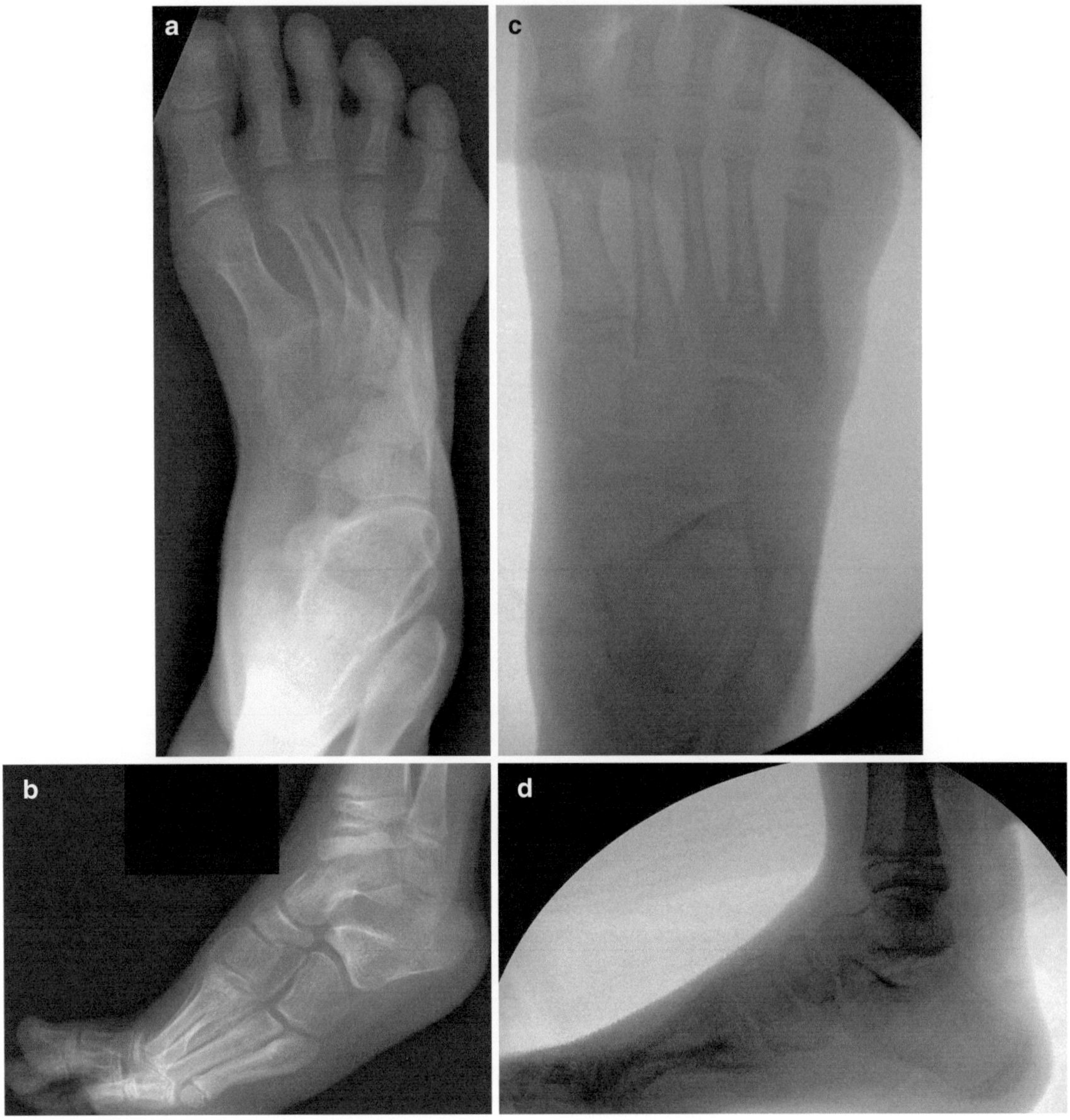

Fig. 27.30 Posteromedial release. (**a**, **b**) Preoperative imaging shows hindfoot varus and equinus as well as metatarsus adductus. (**c**, **d**) Intraoperative imaging shows improved alignment after posterior and medial capsular along with ligamentous soft tissue release. Although in this case the calcaneal angle has been corrected, it is often more horizontal than normal after the procedure

operation is best performed near skeletal maturity to prevent an unacceptably short foot.

Surgical Technique

The hindfoot (talus and calcaneus) is fused to the proximal tarsus (navicular and cuboid). In a triple arthrodesis, the talocalcaneal, talonavicular, and calcaneocuboid joints are fused. Wedges of bone are removed based on the specific deformity being addressed as well as the patient age. When the wedges are removed, the foot is placed in the corrected position and held together with staples, screws, or a plate/screw device.

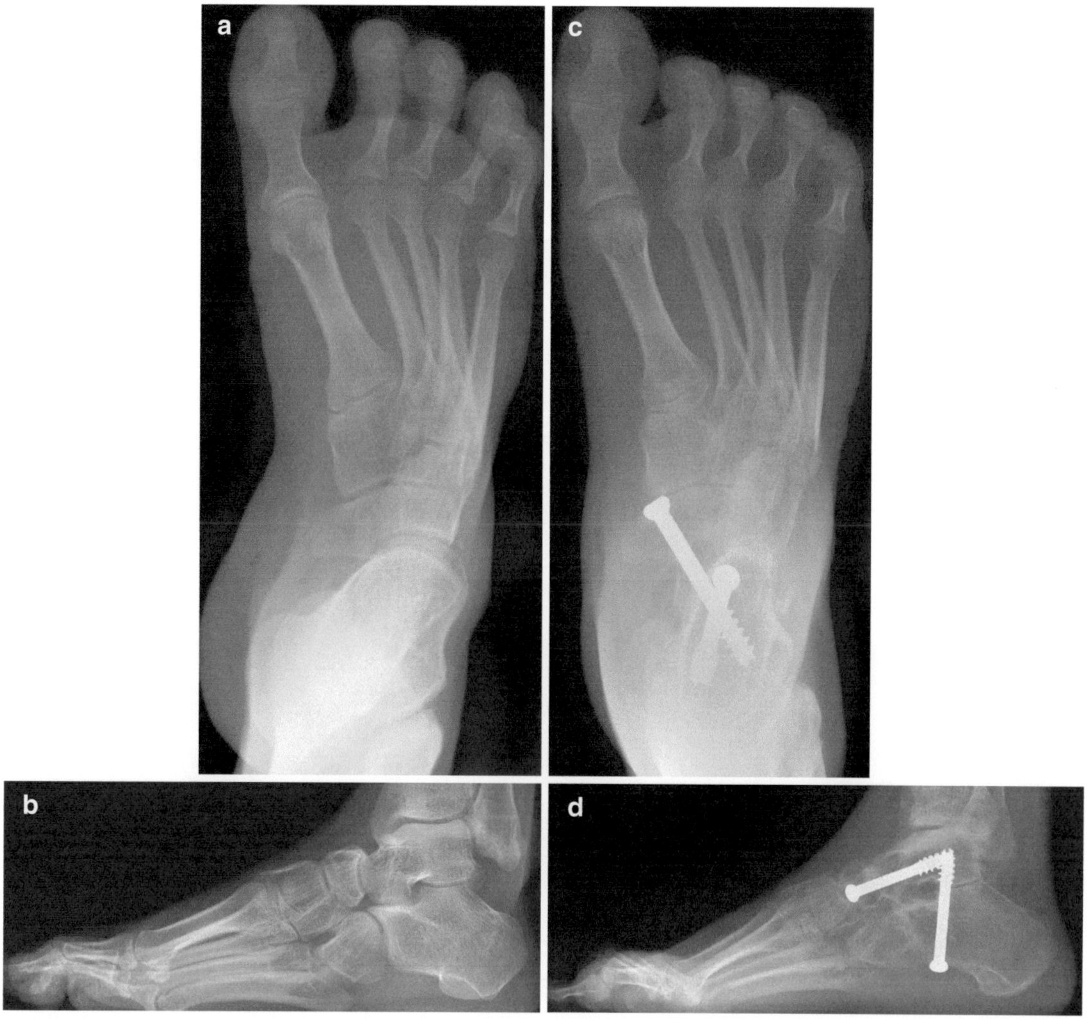

Fig. 27.31 Triple arthrodesis. (**a**, **b**) Severe hindfoot varus and metatarsus adductus in a patient whose deformity did not correct with casting. (**c**, **d**) A screw fixates the navicular to the talus, and a second screw fixates the calcaneus to the talus. Both gaps are filled with remodeled bone graft material. Calcaneocuboid fusion is evident as well

Postoperative Evaluation

The hindfoot should be normally aligned. Joint surfaces are resected with loss of cartilage intervals. Over time, mature osseous fusion should be seen across former joint planes.

Complications

Complications may include loss of correction, failure of fixation, AVN of the talus or navicular, nonunion of arthrodesed joints, and degenerative arthritis at joints proximal and distal to the fusion.

5.4 Lateral Column Lengthening [45] (Figs. 27.32, 27.33, and 27.34)

Clinical Applications

Hindfoot valgus deformity.

Specific Indications

Lateral column lengthening is utilized to treat conditions that cause hindfoot valgus, including rigid flatfoot; severe, symptomatic flatfoot; and cerebral palsy.

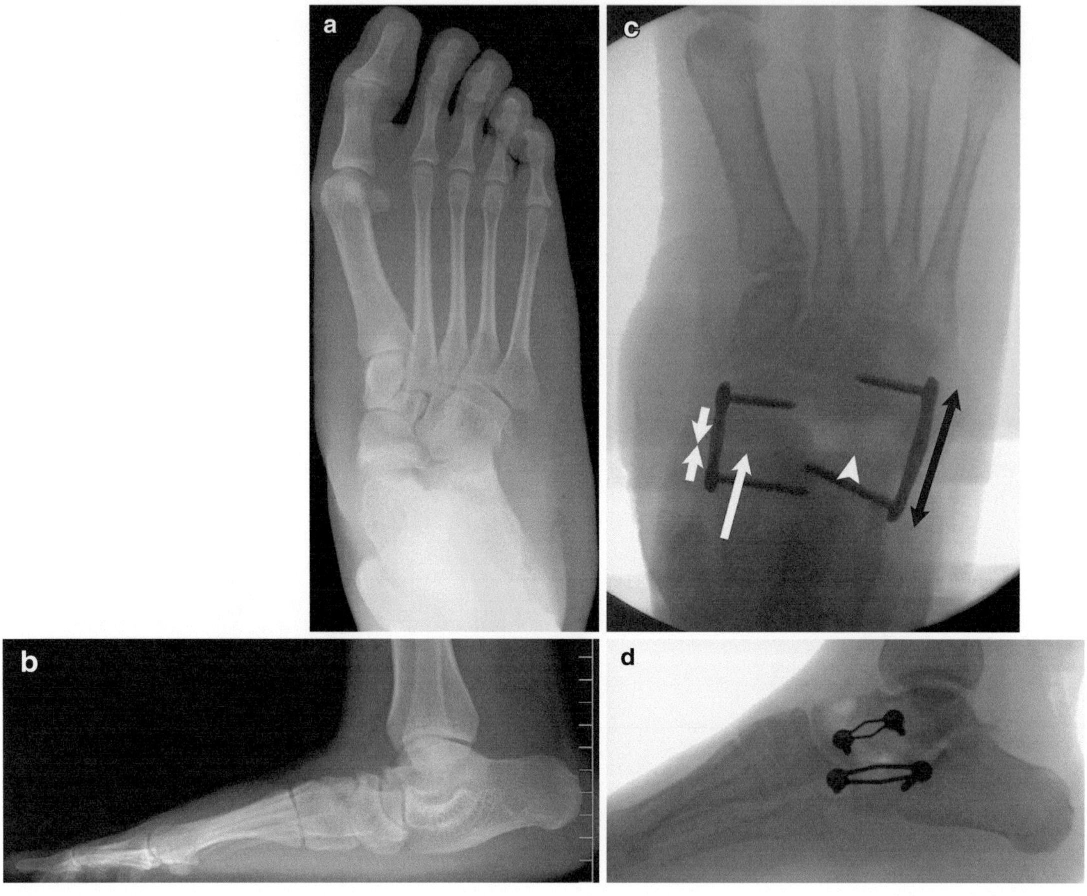

Fig. 27.32 Lateral column lengthening. (**a**, **b**) Preoperative imaging shows severe hindfoot valgus and pes planus (as well as hallux valgus) in a patient with CP. (**c**, **d**) There has been a calcaneal osteotomy with distraction proximal to the calcaneocuboid joint, and structural bone graft (*white arrowhead*) has been placed in the gap, lengthening the lateral column. This osteotomy is fixated with a plate and screws (*double black arrow*). Medial column shortening was also performed by resecting the distal talus and proximal navicular and juxtaposing the cut fragments (*white arrow*), which are held in place with plate and screws (*double white arrow*). Alignment is much improved

Surgical Technique

The distal calcaneus is exposed and an osteotomy made proximal to the calcaneocuboid joint (Fig. 27.32). The osteotomy is distracted to lengthen the lateral column, and a structural bone graft is placed. The osteotomy is fixed with either pins or a plate with screws. Alternatively, in an older child, the lengthening may be performed at the calcaneocuboid joint (Figs. 27.33 and 27.34). For additional correction, medial column shortening may also be performed by making a closing wedge osteotomy in the medial cuneiform or by cutting and juxtaposing the distal talus and the proximal navicular (Fig. 27.32).

Postoperative Evaluation

The navicular should be reduced on the head of the talus after lengthening. Alignment of the talus should also be improved on the lateral projection (decreased "talar sag").

Complications

The distal fragment of the calcaneus may subluxate dorsally. Collapse may occur around the

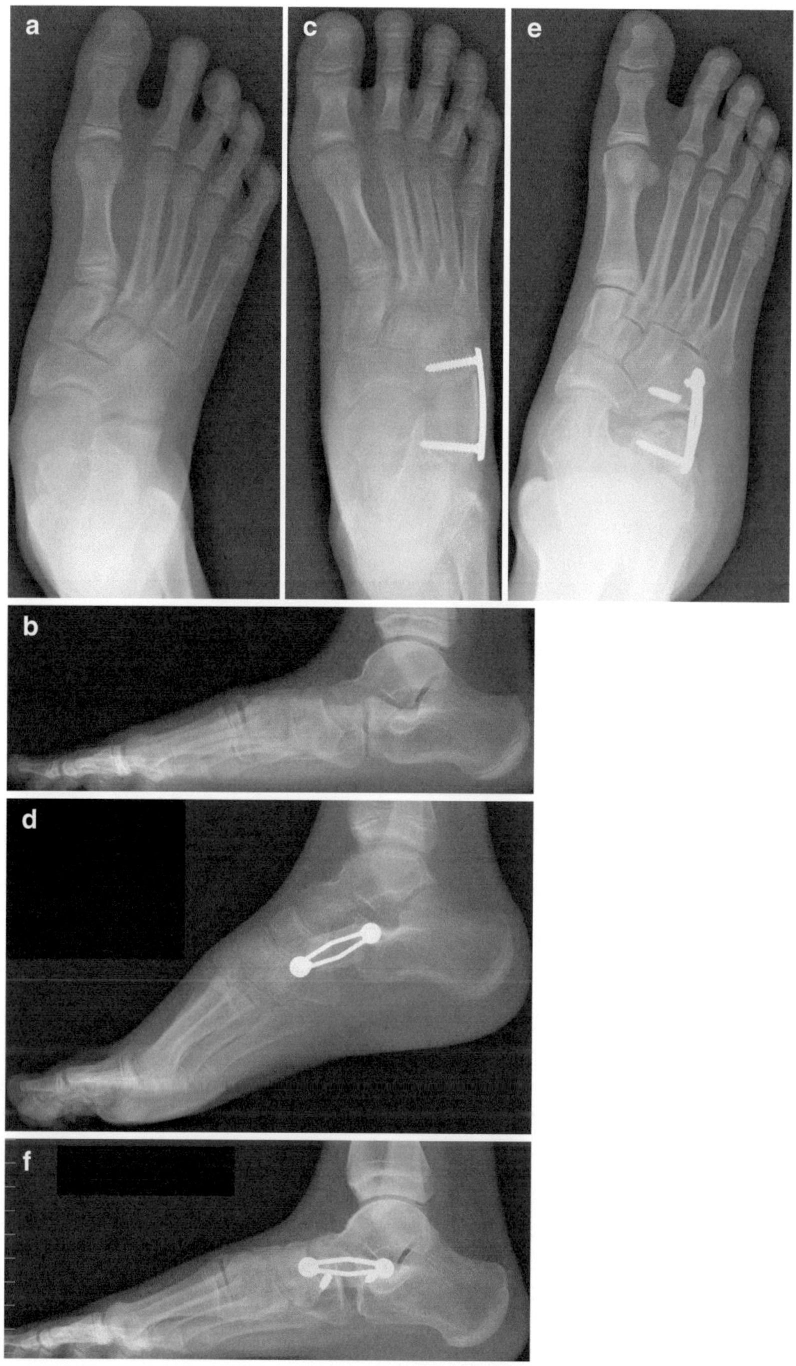

Fig. 27.33 Lateral column lengthening with failed bone graft and fractured screw. (**a**, **b**) Preoperative standing images show hindfoot valgus and pes planus. (**c**, **d**) After calcaneal and cuboid osteotomies and placement of structural bone graft in the gap, a plate and screws have been applied. (**e**, **f**) One year after surgery, bone graft has been absorbed without bridging bone formation, and there is a resultant lucent gap between the irregular, cut surfaces of the calcaneus and cuboid. The more distal screw has fractured. Hindfoot valgus has recurred, though it is not as severe as before surgery (Courtesy of Sandra L. Wootton-Gorges)

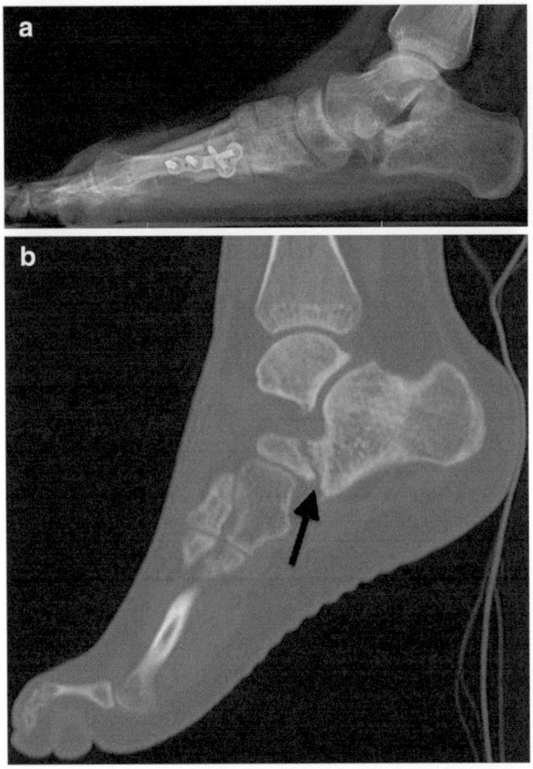

Fig. 27.34 Lateral column lengthening with nonunion of calcaneal osteotomy in a 15-year-old girl. (**a**) Two months after distal calcaneal osteotomy with graft placement, a standing view shows a lucent gap at the calcaneal osteotomy site, with angulation of the distal fragment. (**b**) Sagittally reformatted CT confirms complete absence of bridging bone formation (*arrow*) (Courtesy of J. Herman Kan)

structural graft, resulting in loss of correction. Hardware may fracture and bone graft fail (Fig. 27.33), and cut bone surfaces may fail to fuse (Fig. 27.34).

5.5 Boyd Amputation (Calcaneotibial Fusion) [46] (Fig. 27.35)

Clinical Application

Postaxial limb bud deficiency, congenital longitudinal deficiencies of the tibia and fibula, proximal focal femoral deficiency (PFFD), congenital pseudarthrosis of the tibia, resistant clubfoot, and acquired deformities secondary to trauma and chronic osteomyelitis.

Specific Indications

Boyd amputation is used in various conditions in the pediatric population for late salvage of a foot resistant to other means of establishing a weight-bearing limb. It is an ankle-level amputation, which retains the calcaneus and heel pad by fusing the calcaneus to the distal tibia. The advantages of this procedure are that it provides heel pad stabilization, improves prosthetic suspension, and allows for complete weight bearing through the end of the residual limb. The Boyd procedure provides a sta-

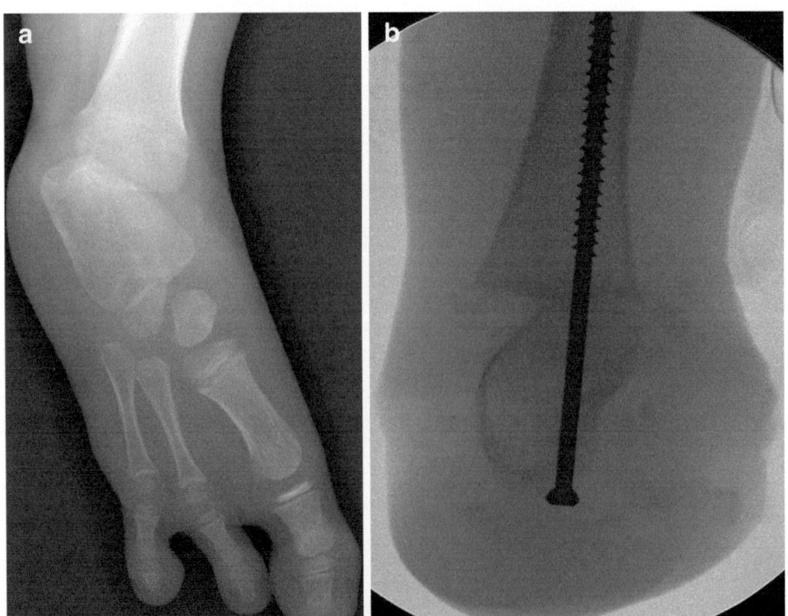

Fig. 27.35 Boyd amputation. (**a**) Preoperative image shows longitudinal deficiency of the fibula, failure of formation of the lateral rays, and tarsal deformity and deficiency. (**b**) The talus has been removed and the calcaneus rotated and fused with the distal tibia

ble heel pad with an excellent end-bearing residual limb which allows for improved proprioception and control of the foot of the prosthesis. By removal of the talus, distal tibia, and superior surface of calcaneus, the limb is shortened to allow for adequate space for foot and ankle prosthetic components.

Surgical Technique

The calcaneus is preserved with a large plantar soft tissue flap, and the talus and all distal bones are removed. Approximately 1/3 of the superior surface of the calcaneus is removed with a saw-cut that is parallel to the plantar aspect of the heel pad. The distal tibial physis and epiphysis are removed by a transverse saw-cut at the level of the metaphysis just proximal to the physis. The calcaneus and the heel pad are then positioned so that the heel pad is perpendicular to the long axis of the tibia and posteriorly translated so that the anterior edge of the tibia is in line with the anterior edge of the calcaneus. Steinmann pins or screws are placed to maintain alignment. The procedure is commonly performed with concomitant procedures, such as correction of an anterior tibial bow, proximal tibial epiphyseodesis, and knee fusion.

Postoperative Evaluation

The calcaneus is everted and pseudo-articulates with the distal tibia. A small remnant of the talus may be left behind. The calcaneotibial fusion is assessed for bony union, malunion, or nonunion, as well as for hardware failure.

Complications

A residual talar remnant may increase in size. Arthritis and hindfoot ankle collapse may occur as late complications.

6 Bone Cyst Opacification and Corticosteroid Injection [47] (Fig. 27.36)

Clinical Application

Simple bone cyst.

Specific Indications

Corticosteroid injection is postulated to reduce fluid secretion and promote internal cyst ossification. Injection of calcium phosphate may also promote internal ossification. It is possible, however, that the healing effect results from bleeding that is engendered by the puncture and not by the actual substance injected. When steroids are used, a series of three injections at 6-week intervals are performed. Therapeutic injection of simple bone cysts is usually performed after injecting contrast into the cyst to outline the extent of the cavity.

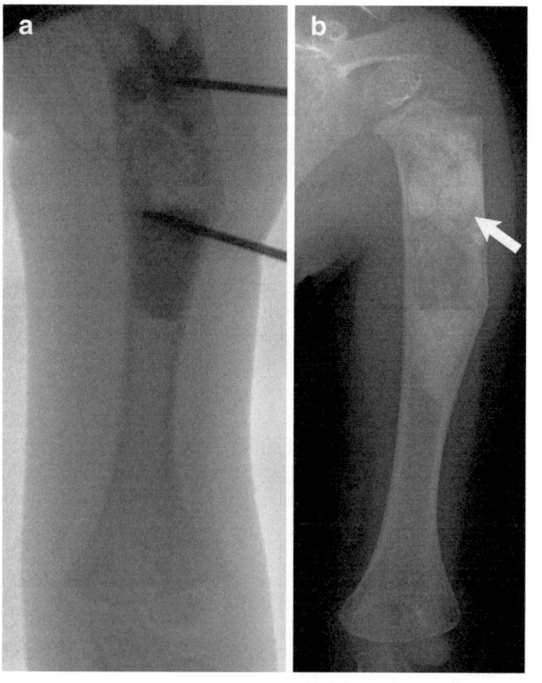

Fig. 27.36 Bone cyst opacification and corticosteroid injection. (**a**) Intraoperative image shows two bone marrow biopsy needles inserted into the cyst cavity. Contrast medium outlines the cyst. (**b**) Two months later, dense bone graft (*arrow*) fills the contours of the cyst, stimulating new bone formation

Surgical Technique

Two bone marrow biopsy needles are inserted into the cyst cavity under fluoroscopic control. Contrast medium is injected to outline the cyst. Saline is vigorously irrigated through the cyst cavity to help separate the cyst lining from the bone. Corticosteroid or bone substitute is then injected.

Postoperative Evaluation

There may be gradual loss of lucency as the cyst calcifies internally.

Complications
Pathologic fracture may occur, and isolated loculations of the lesion may remain cystic.

References

1. Sucato DJ, Duchene C. The position of the aorta relative to the spine: a comparison of patients with and without idiopathic scoliosis. J Bone Joint Surg Am Vol. 2003;85-A(8):1461–9. PubMed PMID: 12925625. Epub 2003/08/20. eng.
2. Akbarnia BA, Marks DS, Boachie-Adjei O, Thompson AG, Asher MA. Dual growing rod technique for the treatment of progressive early-onset scoliosis: a multicenter study. Spine. 2005;30(17 Suppl):S46–57. PubMed PMID: 16138066. Epub 2005/09/03. eng.
3. Campbell Jr RM, Smith MD, Mayes TC, Mangos JA, Willey-Courand DB, Kose N, et al. The characteristics of thoracic insufficiency syndrome associated with fused ribs and congenital scoliosis. J Bone Joint Surg Am Vol. 2003;85-A(3):399–408. PubMed PMID: 12637423. Epub 2003/03/15. eng.
4. Campbell Jr RM, Smith MD. Thoracic insufficiency syndrome and exotic scoliosis. J Bone Joint Surg Am Vol. 2007;89 Suppl 1:108–22. PubMed PMID: 17272428. Epub 2007/02/03. eng.
5. Lenke LG, Betz RR, Harms J, Bridwell KH, Clements DH, Lowe TG, et al. Adolescent idiopathic scoliosis: a new classification to determine extent of spinal arthrodesis. J Bone Joint Surg Am Vol. 2001;83-A(8):1169–81. PubMed PMID: 11507125. Epub 2001/08/17. eng.
6. Betz RR, Harms J, Clements 3rd DH, Lenke LG, Lowe TG, Shufflebarger HL, et al. Comparison of anterior and posterior instrumentation for correction of adolescent thoracic idiopathic scoliosis. Spine. 1999;24(3):225–39. PubMed PMID: 10025017. Epub 1999/02/20. eng.
7. Foley MJ, Calenoff L, Hendrix RW, Schafer MF. Thoracic and lumbar spine fusion: postoperative radiologic evaluation. AJR Am J Roentgenol. 1983;141(2):373–80. PubMed PMID: 6603137. Epub 1983/08/01. eng.
8. Lauerman WC, Bradford DS, Transfeldt EE, Ogilvie JW. Management of pseudarthrosis after arthrodesis of the spine for idiopathic scoliosis. J Bone Joint Surg Am Vol. 1991;73(2):222–36. PubMed PMID: 1993718. Epub 1991/02/01. eng.
9. McMaster MJ. Anterior and posterior instrumentation and fusion of thoracolumbar scoliosis due to myelomeningocele. J Bone Joint Surg Br Vol. 1987;69(1):20–5. PubMed PMID: 3818727. Epub 1987/01/01. eng.
10. Saran N, Varghese R, Mulpuri K. Do femoral or salter innominate osteotomies improve femoral head sphericity in Legg-Calve-Perthes disease? A meta-analysis. Clin Orthop Relat Res. 2012;470(9):2383–93. PubMed PMID: 22467420. Epub 2012/04/03. eng.
11. Salter RB. Role of innominate osteotomy in the treatment of congenital dislocation and subluxation of the hip in the older child. J Bone Joint Surg Am Vol. 1966;48(7):1413–39. PubMed PMID: 5921797. Epub 1966/10/01. eng.
12. Steel HH. Triple osteotomy of the innominate bone. J Bone Joint Surg Am Vol. 1973;55(2):343–50. PubMed PMID: 4572223. Epub 1973/03/01. eng.
13. Steel HH. Triple osteotomy of the innominate bone. A procedure to accomplish coverage of the dislocated or subluxated femoral head in the older patient. Clin Orthop Relat Res. 1977;122:116–27. PubMed PMID: 837597. Epub 1977/01/01. eng.
14. Pemberton PA. Pericapsular osteotomy of the ilium for treatment of congenital subluxation and dislocation of the hip. J Bone Joint Surg Am Vol. 1965;47:65–86. PubMed PMID: 14256975. Epub 1965/01/01. eng.
15. Pemberton PA. Pericapsular osteotomy of the ilium for the treatment of congenitally dislocated hips. Clin Orthop Relat Res. 1974;98:41–54. PubMed PMID: 4817244. Epub 1974/01/01. eng.
16. Faciszewski T, Kiefer GN, Coleman SS. Pemberton osteotomy for residual acetabular dysplasia in children who have congenital dislocation of the hip. J Bone Joint Surg Am Vol. 1993;75(5):643–9. PubMed PMID: 8501078. Epub 1993/05/01. eng.
17. Berkeley ME, Dickson JH, Cain TE, Donovan MM. Surgical therapy for congenital dislocation of the hip in patients who are twelve to thirty-six months old. J Bone Joint Surg Am Vol. 1984;66(3):412–20. PubMed PMID: 6699058. Epub 1984/03/01. eng.
18. Klaue K, Sherman M, Perren SM, Wallin A, Looser C, Ganz R. Extra-articular augmentation for residual hip dysplasia. Radiological assessment after Chiari osteotomies and shelf procedures. J Bone Joint Surg Br Vol. 1993;75(5):750–4. PubMed PMID: 8376432. Epub 1993/09/01. eng.
19. Kotz R, Chiari C, Hofstaetter JG, Lunzer A, Peloschek P. Long-term experience with Chiari's osteotomy. Clin Orthop Relat Res. 2009;467(9):2215–20. PubMed PMID: 19521741. Pubmed Central PMCID: 2866931. Epub 2009/06/13. eng.
20. Chiari K. Medial displacement osteotomy of the pelvis. Clin Orthop Relat Res. 1974;98:55–71. PubMed PMID: 4817245. Epub 1974/01/01. eng.
21. Ito H, Tanino H, Yamanaka Y, Nakamura T, Minami A, Matsuno T. The Chiari pelvic osteotomy for patients with dysplastic hips and poor joint congruency: long-term follow-up. J Bone Joint Surg Br Vol. 2011;93(6):726–31. PubMed PMID: 21586768. Epub 2011/05/19. eng.
22. Bickel WH, Breivis JS. Shelf operation for congenital subluxation and dislocation of the hip. Clin Orthop Relat Res. 1975;106:27–34. PubMed PMID: 1126084. Epub 1975/01/01. eng.
23. Hamanishi C, Tanaka S, Yamamuro T. The Spitzy shelf operation for the dysplastic hip. Retrospective 10 (5–25) year study of 124 cases. Acta Orthop Scand. 1992;63(3):273–7.
24. Nishimatsu H, Iida H, Kawanabe K, Tamura J, Nakamura T. The modified Spitzy shelf operation for

patients with dysplasia of the hip. A 24-year follow-up study. J Bone Joint Surg Br Vol. 2002;84(5):647–52. PubMed PMID: 12188478. Epub 2002/08/22. eng.
25. Coates CJ, Paterson JM, Woods KR, Catterall A, Fixsen JA. Femoral osteotomy in Perthes' disease. Results at maturity. J Bone Joint Surg Br Vol. 1990;72(4):581–5. PubMed PMID: 2380208. Epub 1990/07/01. eng.
26. Larson AN, Sierra RJ, Yu EM, Trousdale RT, Stans AA. Outcomes of slipped capital femoral epiphysis treated with in situ pinning. J Pediatr Orthop. 2012;32(2):125–30. PubMed PMID: 22327445. Epub 2012/02/14. eng.
27. Kartenbender K, Cordier W, Katthagen BD. Long-term follow-up study after corrective Imhauser osteotomy for severe slipped capital femoral epiphysis. J Pediatr Orthop. 2000;20(6):749–56. PubMed PMID: 11097248. Epub 2000/11/30. eng.
28. Rab GT. The geometry of slipped capital femoral epiphysis: implications for movement, impingement, and corrective osteotomy. J Pediatr Orthop. 1999;19(4):419–24. PubMed PMID: 10412987. Epub 1999/07/21. eng.
29. Sponseller PD, McBeath AA, Perpich M. Hip arthrodesis in young patients. A long-term follow-up study. J Bone Joint Surg Am Vol. 1984;66(6):853–9. PubMed PMID: 6234319. Epub 1984/07/01. eng.
30. Schafroth MU, Blokzijl RJ, Haverkamp D, Maas M, Marti RK. The long-term fate of the hip arthrodesis: does it remain a valid procedure for selected cases in the 21st century? Int Orthop. 2010;34(6):805–10. PubMed PMID: 19697025. Pubmed Central PMCID: 2989023. Epub 2009/08/22. eng.
31. Tooke SM, Nugent PJ, Bassett LW, Nottingham P, Mirra J, Jinnah R. Results of core decompression for femoral head osteonecrosis. Clin Orthop Relat Res. 1988;228:99–104. PubMed PMID: 3342594.
32. Rajagopal M, Balch Samora J, Ellis TJ. Efficacy of core decompression as treatment for osteonecrosis of the hip: a systematic review. Hip Int. 2012;22(5):489–93. PubMed PMID: 23100153.
33. Inan M, Chan G, Littleton AG, Kubiak P, Bowen JR. Efficacy and safety of percutaneous epiphysiodesis. J Pediatr Orthop. 2008;28(6):648–51. PubMed PMID: 18724201.
34. Bowen JR, Johnson WJ. Percutaneous epiphysiodesis. Clin Orthop Relat Res. 1984;190:170–3. PubMed PMID: 6488627.
35. Stevens PM. Guided growth for angular correction: a preliminary series using a tension band plate. J Pediatr Orthop. 2007;27(3):253–9. PubMed PMID: 17414005.
36. Birch JG, Samchukov ML. Use of the Ilizarov method to correct lower limb deformities in children and adolescents. J Am Acad Orthop Surg. 2004;12(3):144–54. PubMed PMID: 15161167.
37. Paley D, Fink B, Herzenberg JE. Pseudarthrosis following slipped capital femoral epiphysis: treatment with reduction with use of gradual distraction. A case report. J Bone Joint Surg Am Vol. 1997;79(10):1552–5. PubMed PMID: 9378742.
38. Ruck J, Dahan-Oliel N, Montpetit K, Rauch F, Fassier F. Fassier-Duval femoral rodding in children with osteogenesis imperfecta receiving bisphosphonates: functional outcomes at one year. J Child Orthop. 2011;5(3):217–24. PubMed PMID: 22654983. Pubmed Central PMCID: 3100465.
39. Birke O, Davies N, Latimer M, Little DG, Bellemore M. Experience with the Fassier-Duval telescopic rod: first 24 consecutive cases with a minimum of 1-year follow-up. J Pediatr Orthop. 2011;31(4):458–64. PubMed PMID: 21572286.
40. Halanski MA, Davison JE, Huang JC, Walker CG, Walsh SJ, Crawford HA. Ponseti method compared with surgical treatment of clubfoot: a prospective comparison. J Bone Joint Surg Am Vol. 2010;92(2):270–8. PubMed PMID: 20124052.
41. Levin MN, Kuo KN, Harris GF, Matesi DV. Posteromedial release for idiopathic talipes equinovarus. A long-term follow-up study. Clin Orthop Relat Res. 1989;242:265–8. PubMed PMID: 2706856.
42. DePuy J, Drennan JC. Correction of idiopathic clubfoot: a comparison of results of early versus delayed posteromedial release. J Pediatr Orthop. 1989;9(1):44–8. PubMed PMID: 2915038.
43. van Gelder JH, van Ruiten AG, Visser JD, Maathuis PG. Long-term results of the posteromedial release in the treatment of idiopathic clubfoot. J Pediatr Orthop. 2010;30(7):700–4. PubMed PMID: 20864856.
44. Child BJ, Hix J, Catanzariti AR, Mendicino RW, Saltrick K. The effect of hindfoot realignment in triple arthrodesis. J Foot Ankle Surg. 2009;48(3):285–93. PubMed PMID: 19423028.
45. Westberry DE, Davids JR, Anderson JP, Pugh LI, Davis RB, Hardin JW. The operative correction of symptomatic flat foot deformities in children: the relationship between static alignment and dynamic loading. Bone Joint J. 2013;95-B(5):706–13. PubMed PMID: 23632686.
46. Westberry DE, Davids JR, Pugh LI. The Boyd amputation in children: indications and outcomes. J Pediatr Orthop. 2014;34(1):86–91. PubMed PMID: 23872807.
47. Canavese F, Wright JG, Cole WG, Hopyan S. Unicameral bone cysts: comparison of percutaneous curettage, steroid, and autologous bone marrow injections. J Pediatr Orthop. 2011;31(1):50–5. PubMed PMID: 21150732.

Index

R. Stein-Wexler et al. (eds.), *Pediatric Orthopedic Imaging*,
DOI 10.1007/978-3-642-45381-6, © Springer-Verlag Berlin Heidelberg 2015

B

P

Q

R